SURGICAL ANATOMY

By

C. LATIMER CALLANDER, A.B., M.D., F.A.C.S.

Late Associate Clinical Professor of Surgery and Topographic Anatomy, University
of California Medical School; Member of Founders' Group of the
American Board of Surgery; Member of American Association
for Traumatic Surgery; Associate Visiting Surgeon
to the San Francisco Hospital

With a Foreword by
DEAN LEWIS, M.D., Sc.D., LL.D., F.A.C.S.

WITH 819 ILLUSTRATIONS

SECOND EDITION, REVISED REPRINT

PHILADELPHIA AND LONDON

W. B. SAUNDERS COMPANY

1948

MADE IN U. S. A.

PRESS OF
W. B. SAUNDERS COMPANY
PHILADELPHIA

FOREWORD

Anatomical studies of the human body initiated the Renaissance of medicine. A good understanding of anatomy adds to the keenness of the diagnostician and to the efficiency and comfort of the surgeon. During the past few years many changes have occurred in the teaching of anatomy. As anatomy has come to be regarded more and more as an abstract science, gross anatomy and its direct application to medicine and surgery have been neglected. There are definite reasons for this. Discoveries are no longer to be made in gross anatomy, and it has become, as far as research is concerned, a more or less sterile field. The importance of gross anatomy to the clinic has not changed.

In order to obtain the best results, as far as the clinic is concerned, regional and topographical anatomy must be emphasized. The systems should not be regarded as entities. When the breast is studied anatomically, all the structures entering into its formation should be visualized in their proper relationship. Acini and ducts, for example, should be considered in their relation to the lymphatics; both the normal and accessory lymphatic channels in relation to their central connections and to the lymph nodes. Muscles and bones should be considered together, so that the student may determine while the subject is fresh in his mind the relation of muscles to the displacement of fragments in fractures. The strengthening bands in the capsules of joints may be advantageously studied in their relation to the reduction of dislocations, and bursae in their relation to different types of inflammation. To give the name "monkey hand" to the deformity caused by combined division of the ulnar and median nerve no longer satisfies, for the student should know the muscles affected, the action of each, and the relation of the antagonistic groups causing the deformity. Such an approach stimulates thinking and vitalizes a subject which to many may seem dead. Visualization rather than memory alone should be cultivated. In medical schools the surgical department should hold itself responsible for the proper approach to gross anatomy, and as early as the second year should attempt to develop an interest in anatomy which has a direct application in the clinic.

In this book the anatomy of the organ or region is first considered, and then its surgical application fully discussed. The principles and anatomy of the commoner operations are discussed, and the steps in sequence fully illustrated. The book is planned with the definite idea of indicating the paths of surgical approach to the pathologic process which is to be removed or corrected.

We have long been in need of a book in which anatomy and its surgical application are considered together or in close sequence. In this book systems and organs are studied in relation to each other, and knowledge which can be used in the ward and operating room is imparted. The book's appearance should be eminently satisfying.

Dean Lewis.

PREFACE TO THE SECOND EDITION

In this, the first revision of our textbook on Surgical Anatomy, I have rearranged, and in many instances rewritten, much of the text. These changes were necessary to accommodate the required additions and to allow deletions of unessential text and illustrations.

I have endeavored to carry correct anatomic detail, which was stressed in the first edition, not only into the paths of surgical approach, but also into the depiction of the steps of most of the standardized commoner operations. To this end, many large pen-and-ink illustrations have been added, showing these operations in some detail. Under each illustration has been given a descriptive legend in order further to clarify the operative maneuver illustrated.

The more recent advances in the surgical anatomy of many topographic regions have been recorded. Lumbar sympathetic ganglionectomy and resection of the sacral plexus have been illustrated. New fields in nerve surgery in connection with the scalenus anticus and cervical rib syndromes and the surgery of the intervertebral disks and of the ligamenta flava have been introduced. Spondylolisthesis has been covered adequately. One hundred new figures, most of them original, will be found.

The volume has been made smaller by the deletion of obsolete text and out-of-date illustrations. A great many of the illustrations have been spaced more economically.

We are obligated to many doctors, to the editors of surgical journals, and to many of the medical-book publishers for cooperation in this revision. Many surgeons have given generously of their text and illustrations; constructive criticism from the profession at large has been of great value. If any courtesy acknowledgment to doctor or publisher has been overlooked, it is hoped it may be excused as unintentional.

Ralph Sweet, our artist, has again put his best work into our new illustrations, many of them multifigured drawings of operative procedures. Miss Kay Gehlken has made many useful diagrams and sketches. Mrs. C. L. Callander has been most helpful in working out the structure of the text. I am deeply grateful to my friend, Thomas F. Ryan, III, for a gift which made possible many of the new drawings in the present edition of this work. The officers of W. B. Saunders Company, as before, have cooperated wholeheartedly.

C. Latimer Callander.

450 Sutter Street,
San Francisco, California.

PREFACE

As this book comes to print, I feel a profound regret that my father is not living and sharing with me the high feeling that arises from completion of the work we planned together. Twelve years ago we felt and discussed the need for a text which would meet the anatomic demands of the student and of the practitioner confronting everyday surgical problems. Recognizing accurate anatomic knowledge as the basis of surgical technic, we planned to present anatomic facts in terms of their clinical importance. With this in view, we have described topographically the anatomic surgical approaches, the paths of extension of pathologic processes, and the common operations. We worked together assembling and organizing material until three years ago when I was left to finish alone.

This text is not a systematic treatise; it is intended to be explanatory and utilitarian rather than encyclopedic. To avoid repetition of material, cross referencing is used throughout. Most of the illustrations are original drawings of dissected material. If any of them are derived from sources not credited, the oversight is unintentional.

I wish to acknowledge my appreciation for assistance with many sections of manuscript, especially to Dr. O. W. Jones and Dr. Howard A. Brown for neurosurgical suggestions; Dr. Warren D. Horner and Dr. Joseph William Crawford for aid in preparation of the text on the visual apparatus; Dr. John C. W. Taylor and Dr. Arthur C. Gibson for ear, nose, and throat guidance; Dr. Alson R. Kilgore and Dr. R. J. Millzner for information concerning the neck and breast; Dr. William B. Faulkner, Jr., for thoracic surgery considerations; Dr. Roscoe C. Webb for notes on the gastro-intestinal tract; Dr. Miley B. Wesson for urological facts; Dr. R. Glenn Craig for gynecological criticism; Dr. Horace C. Pitkin for aid in the section devoted to the extremities and spine; Dr. John Saunders for proof reading the manuscript and furnishing many valuable anatomic and surgical criticisms.

I am indebted to Miss J. N. Forsythe and Miss Ellen Green for assistance in preparation of the manuscript; to Mrs. Josephine Quayle for proof reading the entire manuscript and assisting in construction; and to Dr. Mary Olney who has labored with me for three years and has rendered invaluable assistance in arranging material and clarifying construction throughout.

I am sincerely grateful to Kay Hyde and Ralph Sweet, the artists, whose skill, untiring energy, patience, and intelligent aid are responsible for the illustrations of this text.

An enumeration of those contributing to the completion of this work would be incomplete without mention of my wife who has worked untiringly and painstakingly in the preparation and construction of the manuscript.

I wish to acknowledge my indebtedness to the Staff of the San Francisco Hospital, a unit of the San Francisco Department of Health, for the cooperation shown me in the surgical wards. In these wards most of the surgical and many of the anatomic applications of this book have been worked out.

I wish to thank W. B. Saunders Company for their splendid cooperation, patience, and unfailing generosity in meeting my many demands.

C. LATIMER CALLANDER.

450 SUTTER STREET,
SAN FRANCISCO, CALIFORNIA.

CONTENTS

HEAD

THE PELVIS

MALE PERINEUM AND EXTERNAL GENITALIA

SURGICAL ANATOMY

HEAD

I. SCALP, CRANIUM, MENINGES, AND BRAIN

A. EXTRACRANIAL SOFT PARTS

THE scalp is of particular surgical interest not only as a covering for the skull, but also as a frequent site of many skin lesions. Scalp injuries and infections may lead to osteomyelitis of the skull with septic thrombosis of the dural sinuses, and to involvement of the cranial meninges and brain. Various superficial cysts have a decided predilection for the scalp, and vascular tumors may communicate with the intracranial sinuses.

The soft parts over the skull consist of five layers: the skin, subcutaneous tissue, epicranius (occipitofrontalis) muscle and its galeal aponeurosis, a lax layer of subaponeurotic connective tissue, and the pericranium or outer periosteum of the skull. From the surgical standpoint, the first three strata are considered as forming a single layer, the scalp proper, since they are connected intimately and are not separated easily.

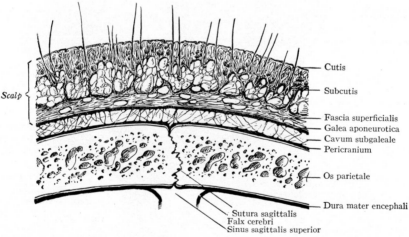

FIG. 1.—FRONTAL SECTION THROUGH THE EXTRACRANIAL SOFT PARTS AND THE PARIETAL BONES.

1. **Skin.**—The skin of the scalp is very thick, particularly in the occipital region, and is attached by tough fibrous septa to the underlying galea (epicranial aponeurosis), from which it is detached with difficulty. It has an abundant arterial and lymphatic supply; the arteries are derived from the vessels in the subcutaneous tissue. Within the skin are numerous sweat and sebaceous glands. Cysts occasionally develop in connection with the sebaceous glands as a result of occlusion of their ducts. These cysts (wens) are contained within the true skin, do not invade the subcutaneous tissue, and move with the scalp.

2. **Subcutaneous Tissue.**—The subcutaneous tissue is remarkable for its density and toughness, characteristics which may be attributed to its short fibrous septa, which enclose small fat lobules and form an inelastic layer carrying the blood vessels. Several decided peculiarities of the scalp result from this arrangement. The blood vessels, embedded in this unyielding tissue, do not contract fully, but bleed freely when divided. Because

2

of the abundant anastomoses of the scalp vessels, scalp flaps with only a small pedicle survive and large flaps heal with very little tissue-loss from sloughing. Superficial infections are prone to remain localized in the subcutaneous tissue because of the fibrous septa; these infections are exceedingly painful because the nerves are compressed. There is a comparative lack of swelling of the subcutaneous tissue in skin inflammations such as erysipelas, and a negligible difference in the amount of subcutaneous fat in obesity and emaciation. Fatty tumors and fluid collections are encountered rarely, but *caput succedaneum*, an edema of the elements of the scalp, follows prolonged pressure in difficult labor.

3. **Epicranius (Occipitofrontalis) Muscle and Its Galeal (Epicranial) Aponeurosis.**— The paired, double-bellied epicranius muscles and their intervening aponeuroses are attached posteriorly to the external occipital protuberance and to the superior nuchal

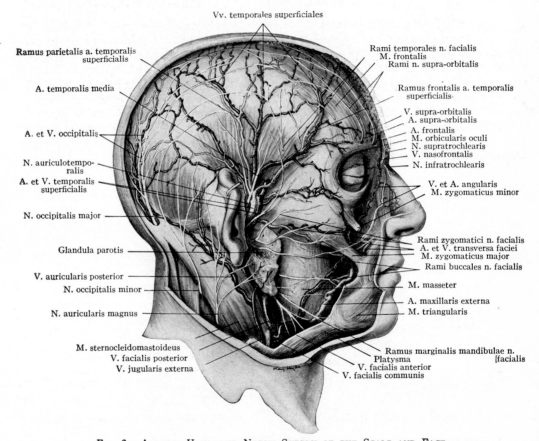

Vv. temporales superficiales

Ramus parietalis a. temporalis superficialis

A. temporalis media

A. et V. occipitalis

N. auriculotemporalis

A. et V. temporalis superficialis

N. occipitalis major

Glandula parotis

V. auricularis posterior

N. occipitalis minor

N. auricularis magnus

M. sternocleidomastoideus
V. facialis posterior
V. jugularis externa

Rami temporales n. facialis
M. frontalis
Rami n. supra-orbitalis

Ramus frontalis a. temporalis superficialis

V. supra-orbitalis
A. supra-orbitalis

A. frontalis
M. orbicularis oculi
N. supratrochlearis
V. nasofrontalis
N. infratrochlearis

V. et A. angularis
M. zygomaticus minor

Rami zygomatici n. facialis
A. et V. transversa faciei
M. zygomaticus major
Rami buccales n. facialis

M. masseter

A. maxillaris externa
M. triangularis

Ramus marginalis mandibulae n.
Platysma   [facialis
V. facialis anterior
V. facialis communis

FIG. 2.—ARTERY, VEIN, AND NERVE SUPPLY OF THE SCALP AND FACE.

(curved) line of the occipital bone. The muscles have no well-defined lateral margins where they are prolonged over the temporal fascia. Anteriorly, they are attached through the frontal bellies mainly to the superciliary ridges and subcutaneous tissue over the eyebrows and nose and to the orbicularis oculi muscles.

4. **Subepicranial Connective Tissue Space.**—The subepicranial space lies between the epicranius muscle and the pericranium. This potential space is traversed by small arteries and by the important emissary veins connecting the intracranial venous sinuses with the superficial veins of the scalp. Subepicranial abscess is likely to occur when infection following a galeal laceration cannot find easy exit. Pus within the space can spread in all directions and elevate the scalp, which, on palpation, feels as though it were lying upon a water-bed. Incisions for the evacuation of the abscess are made near the lateral

attachments of the scalp, parallel to the larger vessels. The pus may destroy the pericranium and cause necrosis of the bones of the skull. It also may cause thrombosis of the emissary veins and allow emboli to spread to the dural sinuses. Because of the possibility of this intracranial spread, the subepicranial space is called the "danger zone" of the scalp

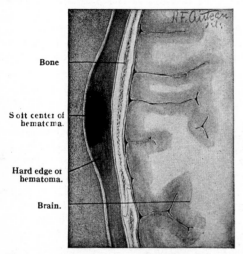

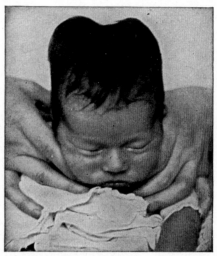

FIG. 3.—HEMATOMA OF THE SCALP WITH SOFT CENTER AND FIRM EDGES. This condition simulates fracture closely. (Scudder, "The Treatment of Fractures.")

FIG. 4.—BIPARIETAL CEPHALHEMATOMA. (A. B. Davis.)

5. Pericranium.—The pericranium is the outer periosteum of the skull. In the fetal skull, the membranous spaces or fontanels lying between the undeveloped cranial bones

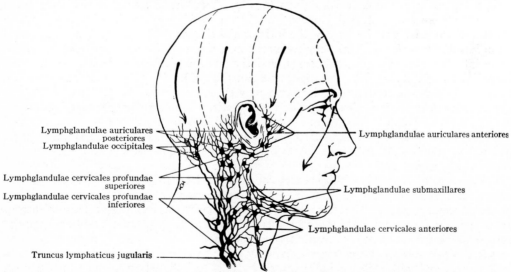

Lymphglandulae auriculares posteriores
Lymphglandulae occipitales
Lymphglandulae cervicales profundae superiores
Lymphglandulae cervicales profundae inferiores
Truncus lymphaticus jugularis
Lymphglandulae auriculares anteriores
Lymphglandulae submaxillares
Lymphglandulae cervicales anteriores

FIG. 5.—REGIONAL LYMPH DRAINAGE FROM THE SCALP AND FACE.

are bridged by the pericranium externally and the dura mater internally. When these fontanels are obliterated, the sutural membrane of connective tissue connects the pericranium with the dura mater across the suture line. This explains the ease of stripping the pericranium off the bones except at the suture lines. Where the bones have fused, the sutures are obliterated and the pericranium stretches from one bone to the other with no strong sutural attachment. *Cephalhematoma* is an extravasation of blood between the pericranium and skull. It is caused by pressure upon the head at birth at the point of presentation and may be limited to one or both parietal bones.

Subpericranial abscesses are comparatively rare and usually arise from secondary infection of a hematoma deep to the pericranium, or from carious bone. Pus, like hemorrhage, often is limited to the confines of a single bone because of the intimate attachment of the pericranial membrane to the suture lines.

The pericranium differs in certain respects from periosteum elsewhere; it nourishes the underlying bone to only a very limited degree and its bone-forming power is slight. Extensive strips of pericranium can be detached without any subsequent bone necrosis; when part of the skull is removed at operation, the pericranium makes little attempt to re-form bone. The blood vessels, which traverse the pericranium and the small channels in the outer table of the skull, afford paths along which infection may reach the diploë and set up an osteomyelitis.

6. **Vessels and Nerves.**—Aside from the small frontal and supra-orbital branches of the ophthalmic artery (p. 71), the *arterial supply* is derived from the superficial temporal, posterior auricular, and occipital branches of the external carotid artery. These branches run in the subcutaneous layer from the periphery toward the vertex and anastomose freely across the median line. In flap preparation, the pedicle should include one of these trunks. A peculiar form of vascular growth, called *cirsoid aneurysm* (racemose angioma), occasionally is observed in connection with the superficial temporal artery and, less frequently, with the occipital artery. It is composed of a number of large, tortuous, and pulsating vessels which form an irregularly circumscribed bluish-red swelling beneath the skin, to which enlarged pulsating arteries and veins are tributary.

The frontal, parietal, and occipital *veins* follow the arteries roughly as anterior, lateral, and posterior venous stems and empty into the external jugular vein. The frontal and supra-orbital veins unite at the median angle of the eye and communicate there with the angular vein which is the beginning of the facial vein. The supra-orbital vein has an anterior diploic branch and a branch which engages through the orbit with the ophthalmic vein, a tributary to the cavernous sinus (p. 32). The lateral and posterior scalp veins drain mainly into the external jugular, but some pass by way of the diploic veins into the internal jugular vein by way of the intracranial sinuses. The parietal emissary veins drain into the superior sagittal (longitudinal) sinus, the mastoid and condyloid emissaries drain into the transverse (lateral) sinus, and the supra-orbital veins drain into the ophthalmic vein and thence into the cavernous sinus (p. 32). By these main channels and by many others less conspicuous, infection may spread from the scalp to the interior of the skull and lead to sinus thrombosis and meningitis. Without these emissary communications, scalp and skull infections and injuries would lose much of their significance.

The *lymph vessels* of the scalp drain downward from the occipital region to the occipital glands; from the parietal and temporal regions to the pre-auricular and postauricular glands; and from the frontal and frontoparietal regions to the submaxillary glands.

The *nerves* of the scalp, with the exception of the facial supply to the epicranius muscle, are sensory. The supratrochlear, supra-orbital, and auriculotemporal nerves are branches of the trigeminal nerve. The great auricular, lesser occipital, and major occipital nerves are of spinal origin. Any of these sensory nerves are affected by neuralgia, but the occipital and supra-orbital nerves are involved most frequently.

7. **Scalp Wounds.**—Lacerations commonly extend through the epicranius muscle and aponeurosis, and, although generally caused by falls or inflicted with blunt instruments, their edges usually are clean-cut because of the division of the tissues against the unyielding surface of the subjacent skull. When these wounds are directed anteroposteriorly, their edges show little tendency to separate and are easy to approximate. When they cross the plane of action of the muscle, and particularly when the muscle elements are involved, they are prone to gape and curl inward at the edges.

The extraordinary vitality of the scalp, resulting from its vascularity, explains why

wounds involving it heal so rapidly.   Large areas may be stripped off by injury or under-
mined by suppuration to the point of detachment and, if replaced, often heal with little
loss from sloughing.   The bleeding in these wounds is free and difficult to arrest and depends more on vessel retraction into the dense subcutaneous tissue than upon the number
of vessels severed.   Hemorrhage can be arrested by pressure against the underlying bone.
Digital pressure applied on each side of an incision materially reduces hemorrhage in the
wound.

B. CRANIUM IN GENERAL

1. **Landmarks.**—The cranial vault, superciliary arches, orbital margins, and angular
processes of the cranium are palpable.   The zygomatic arch, supramastoid crest, suprameatal spine, and the mastoid process are superficial and easy to locate.   The *external
occipital protuberance* (*inion*) is one of the most important landmarks in cranio-encephalic
topography.   At the junction of the coronal and sagittal sutures is the *bregma*, found on a
line drawn vertically upward from a point just anterior to the external auditory meatus
At the point of union of the sagittal and lambdoid sutures is the *lambda*, lying about 6 cm.

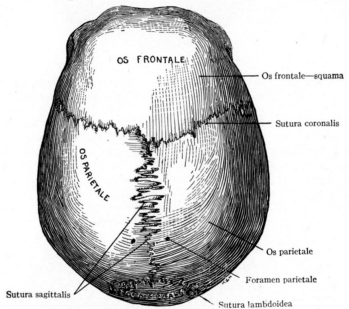

FIG. 6.—VAULT OF THE ADULT SKULL.

superior to the external occipital protuberance.   Treves locates the *lambdoid suture* as the
upper two thirds of a line drawn from the lambda to the apex of the mastoid process.
Along a line from the bregma to a point midway on the zygomatic arch lies the *coronal
suture*.   The middle of the nasofrontal suture marks the *nasion*, while the bulge midway
between the two superciliary ridges marks the *glabella*.

2. **Development of the Cranium.**—It is necessary to review the development of the
skull to explain the fontanels, which are so important in obstetric diagnosis and in congenital cranial malformations.   Ossification in the vault bones takes place in membrane.
However, complete transformation of membrane into bone is not completed at birth, so
that areas of membrane are present about the periphery of these bones.   The larger,
diamond-shaped, *anterior fontanel* is formed by the confluence of the frontal, interparietal
(sagittal) and coronal sutures; the triangular *posterior* (*occipital*) *fontanel*, by the junction
of the sagittal and lambdoid sutures.   The apex of the posterior fontanel extends forward
between the two parietal bones and the sides pass laterally into the lambdoid suture.
These membranous areas are in the midline of the cranium, and are of great value in
determining the position of the fetal head during labor.   When the posterior fontanel

presents, the occiput is anterior, by far the most common position of the head at birth
When the examining finger encounters the anterior fontanel and can be carried posteriorly
along the sagittal suture, the occiput is posterior.   To make delivery easy, the head must
rotate to an occiput anterior position.

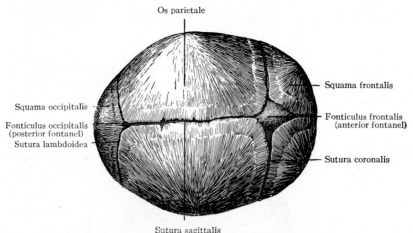

FIG. 7.—SUPERIOR VIEW OF INFANT SKULL TO SHOW THE SUTURES AND FONTANELS.
The radial development of the individual bones is emphasized.

Normally, all traces of the membranous fontanels disappear during the first year after
birth.   In *hydrocephalus* the fontanels and sutures are open widely; in that condition the
ventricles can be tapped through the anterior fontanel or at some point along the coronal
suture.   The needle must be introduced lateral to the median line to avoid injury to the
superior longitudinal sinus.

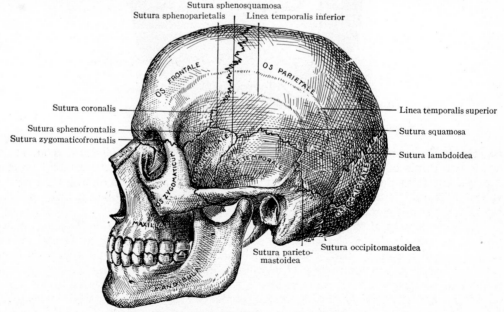

FIG. 8.—LATERAL VIEW OF THE ADULT SKULL.

3. **Exterior and Interior of the Skull.**—The *exterior* of the cranial vault is readily palpable and surgically accessible.   It is set apart artificially from the less accessible base
of the skull by a line passing a little above the zygomatic arch and connecting the super-

ciliary arches and the external occipital protuberance. Over the lateral aspect, the cranium is somewhat flattened to form a very important surgical region, the temporal fossa.

The extracranial surface of the base is difficult to palpate or to approach surgically. It is divided into two portions, one articulating with the bones of the face, and the other made up of the temporal and occipital bones, the basal portion proper.

The *interior* of the skull, like the exterior, is divided into vault and base. The base contains three fossae, an anterior ethmoidofrontal, a middle sphenotemporal, and a posterior occipitotemporal.

4. Structure.—The bones of the skull are adapted to undergo great change in shape during birth, as they are laid down in primitive membrane and are pliable. As the bony centers grow in the membrane, an outer periosteum, or pericranial layer, and an inner

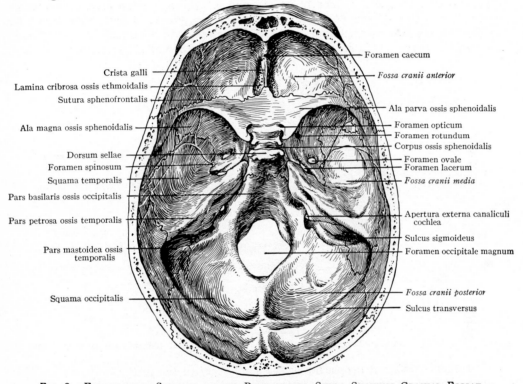

FIG. 9.—ENDOCRANIAL SURFACE OF THE BASE OF THE SKULL SHOWING CRANIAL FOSSAE.

periosteum, or dural layer, develop. Both layers early play a part in bone formation, but later lose, to a great extent, the bone-forming function. With the laying down of bony deposits, inner and outer dense deposits form about an intervening spongy diploic layer. Varying amounts of diploic bone explain the difference in thickness of different skull areas. Over the base, bone may be composed of a single layer of compact tissue; for example, the paper-thin cribriform plate of the ethmoid. The bony channels of the diploic veins can be seen in x-rays of the skull and easily may be mistaken for fractures. Circulation is not active in the cranial bones and losses of substance are slow to repair, gaps being replaced by fibrous tissue. Exuberant callus may so irritate the subjacent cortical tissue as to cause jacksonian epilepsy.

SURGICAL CONSIDERATIONS

1. Skull in Rickets.—In *rickets* there are pronounced alterations in the cranial bones because of impaired nutrition, the essential condition being deficiency of mineral matter in the bone cells. "Craniotabes" is the term applied to the yielding parchment-like membrane in the squamous portions of the parietal and occipital bones.

2. Infectious Processes.—*Pyogenic osteomyelitis* rarely is primary in the cranium, but may occur from infection secondary to pericranial laceration in scalp wounds. Collections of blood under the pericranium may become infected, producing subpericranial abscesses which cause secondary changes in the underlying bone. The resulting bony necrosis may be so extensive that portions of the outer table or of the entire thickness of the vault are sequestrated. The complications of osteomyelitis are serious when the infection spreads into the subcranial areas where sinusitis, meningitis, or brain abscess may develop. When this occurs, prompt and efficient drainage down to, and sometimes through, the dura must be instituted. The osteomyelitic process may become chronic and sequestration be retarded so that granulation and discharge persist for years.

The usual manifestation of *syphilis of the cranium* is a gummatous inflammation of the pericranium, and, less frequently, of the diploë. This, if progressive, may produce remarkably widespread bone changes. Reactionary overgrowth of hard bone causes the irregularly-shaped, worm-eaten appearance so characteristic of the disease in its late stage Scalp infection may be transmitted through the honeycombed bone to the dura

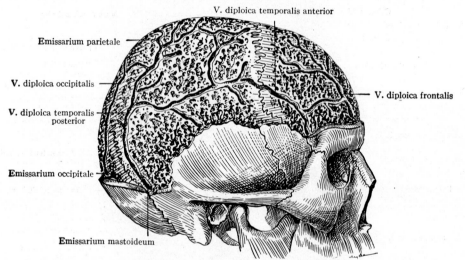

FIG. 10.—VASCULAR CHANNELS IN THE DIPLOË.
The outer table of compact bone has been removed from the frontal, parietal, and occipital bones.

3. Tumors.—Isolated neoplasms of the skull occur in the form of *osteomata*. These exostoses of compact bone arise either from the pericranial or dural surfaces of the skull and increase slowly in size. The larger the tumor, the more irregular is the shape. An osteoma projecting into the cranial cavity may grow to a considerable size without causing symptoms. Skull *sarcoma* differs in no essential detail from that in long bones. It may arise as a diploic growth or originate in the pericranial or dural coverings where it is accompanied by abundant new bone formation. Trauma apparently plays an important rôle in the growth and may be the cause of skull sarcoma. Progress of the tumor is by true bone invasion rather than by bone destruction through pressure and absorption. Sarcoma occurs less frequently in the base than in the vault of the cranium.

4. Acromegaly and Paget's Disease.—*Acromegaly* is characterized by a general skeletal hypertrophy, usually with symmetrical enlargement of the bones and soft parts of the extremities and face. The undershot lower jaw, unduly prominent cheeks, nasal bones, and supra-orbital ridges, together with the thick lips, large nose, and spadelike hands present a remarkable picture and identify the disease at a glance. Hypersecretion or perverted secretion of the anterior lobe of the hypophysis is considered responsible.

Paget's disease is rare, and of unknown etiology; it affects the bones of the lower extremities, spine, and skull. The skull enlargement is limited to the cranial vault. The hypertrophy is eccentric and rarely encroaches on the intracranial space and the bony overgrowth is smooth. As the bones in the frontal, temporal, and occipital regions thicken and project, the head acquires a characteristic heavy appearance.

5. **Fractures of the Cranial Bones.**—The cranium, a hollow, somewhat elastic shell, differs from other bones in the mechanics of its fracture. Considering the skull as an elastic globe, it may be seen that a blow lessens the diameter along the line of trauma. The point of impact is brought somewhat nearer to the point of the globe directly opposite. As the impact forces the poles of this diameter toward each other, the equatorial diameter increases correspondingly, and the sides of the sphere bulge or burst. In a lesser degree, all the other circumferences perpendicular to the line of impact will be increased. If the distortion is inconsiderable, the cranium, because of its elasticity, will resume its former shape unimpaired. If, on the other hand, the distortion is serious enough, cohesion will be disrupted and a break will result, either at the pole of impact or

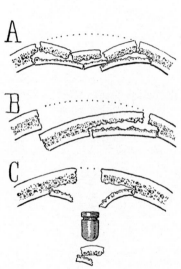

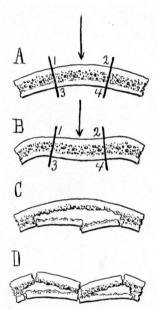

FIG. 11.—DIAGRAMS OF FRAGMENT DISPLACEMENT IN COMMINUTED FRACTURE OF THE VAULT.

A, is a fracture with central depression; B, fracture with peripheral depression; C, fracture with loss of bony substance. (Cushing.)

FIG. 12.—DIAGRAMS ILLUSTRATING THE MECHANICAL PRINCIPLES OF BENDING FRACTURES.

In A and B, the arrow indicates the direction of impact; points 3 and 4 are dragged apart until the tensile strength is overcome; C, shows the possible effect on the inner table alone; D, shows the possible effect on both tables. (Teevan.)

where the cranial circumference has been increased to the point of overcoming the tensile strength of the bony particles.

The variety of fracture is influenced by the structural peculiarity of cranial bone. The dense inner and outer tables of the cranial bones are separated by spongy diploë. Any blow which leads to a bending fracture or fracture at the pole of impact will cause the inner table to give way and splinter before the outer table is affected. In consequence, fractures may be limited to the inner table, as is illustrated in the breaking of a green stick. The cranial impact leads to a local indentation which tends to pull apart or burst the particles comprising the inner table and to drive together those of the outer. If the force of the blow has been expended when the inner table is broken, it alone suffers fracture. If the force is continued, the outer table as well gives way and the inner table splinters over a wider area.

A blow to the cranium by a flat surface is likely to produce injury at a distance from the point of impact, while that from a small body tends to cause local changes. It is, however, common enough for the forms of impact which cause local changes to cause a bursting of the skull, which takes place if there is not adequate rebound and if enough force is exerted for a sufficient length of time.

Meridional fractures are found radiating from the point of impact of a local bending fracture. Most fissured fractures are the expression of the bursting effect of a blow and occur readily in the base of the cranium which is more fragile than the vault. As they may have no connection with lesions at the point of impact, they are spoken of as the indirect result of violence. Clinical observations demonstrate that there need be no displacement of bone in bursting fractures, but that linear cracks may extend into the nearest weak portion of the cranial base. Such fissures terminate in the middle cranial fossa rather than in the anterior or posterior fossa, and often involve the sella turcica,

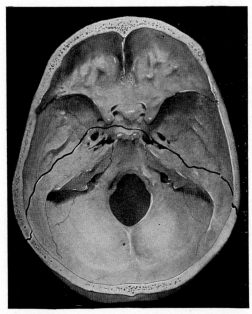

FIG. 13.—BASE OF SKULL SHOWING TYPICAL BURST-
ING FRACTURE PASSING THROUGH THE MIDDLE
FOSSAE AND THE SELLA TURCICA. (Cushing.)

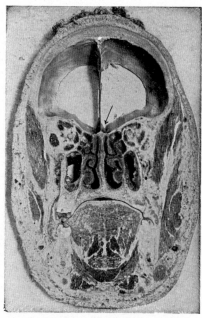

FIG. 14.—FRONTAL FROZEN SECTION SHOWING THE
CLOSE PROXIMITY OF THE DURA AND THE
ETHMOID CELLS.

The thin plate of bone (arrow), perforated by olfactory nerves, is a common seat of basal fracture; here cerebrospinal fluid often escapes into the nose. (Cushing.)

presumably one of the weakest points in the base of the skull. Here, more than elsewhere, the distinction must be made between the importance of the management of the fracture and that of its complications, chief among which are brain damage and hemorrhage. Life is lost in acute head injuries, not necessarily because of skull fracture, but because of excessive intracranial pressure. This increased pressure is due to hemorrhage, brain edema, or both.

In basal fracture, there usually are external bleeding and escape of cerebrospinal fluid, valuable signs in diagnosing the existence of fracture and its location. Should fracture involve the anterior cranial fossa, the frontal, ethmoidal, or sphenoidal cells may be injured, and bleeding may occur from the nose and mouth. If cerebrospinal fluid escapes from the nose, there is, in addition to fracture of the nasal roof, a laceration of the mucous membrane along the sheaths of the olfactory nerves. When the fracture is in the frontal region through the roof of the orbit, hemorrhage works its way forward, presents under the bulbar conjunctiva, and advances to the edge of the cornea.   Hemorrhage into the lids and loose cellular tissue about the eye usually results from rupture of subcutaneous vessels by external violence, and is not necessarily the result of basal fracture.

When fracture involves the middle cranial fossa, the fracture line may pass through the sphenoid bone or the base of the occipital bone and cause bleeding into the mouth.   The line of fracture may pass through the petrous portion of the temporal bone and involve the internal as well as the external auditory meatus.   Bleeding from the ear through a ruptured tympanic membrane, however, may be caused by intracranial extravasation or torn vessels in the membrane.   Hemorrhage into the middle ear may pass down the auditory tube and escape from the mouth or nose, or be swallowed and vomited at a later time.   If cerebrospinal fluid escapes from the external ear, the fracture has involved the internal auditory meatus or has torn its dural prolongation.   There also is traumatic communication between the internal and middle ear cavities, and rupture of the tympanic membrane.

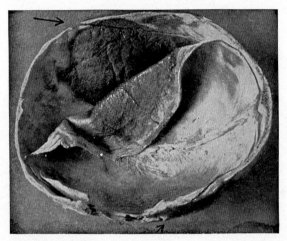

Fig. 15.—Inner Surface of the Calvarium with the Dura Reflected Showing Extradural Hematoma.
The clot is grooved by the meningeal artery which has been torn in a linear fissure from a meridional fracture.   (Cushing.)

In vault fractures, detached bony fragments or a penetrating instrument may injure the superior longitudinal and lateral sinuses.   Extradural hemorrhage follows injury to the middle meningeal artery, occurring, of necessity, in fractures passing through the squamous portion of the temporal bone, since here for 2 to 3 cm. the course of the artery is often in a bony canal.   Since branches of the middle meningeal artery nourish the bone as well as the dura, hemorrhage occurs when the dura is loosened from the overlying bone. In children, the dural attachment is so firm that separation involves great risk of injury to the artery and its branches.   Extradural middle meningeal hemorrhage may arise from any skull injury which detaches the dura; fracture is not necessary.   In operations in the temporal region which involve separation of the dura, bleeding may be free.

C. MENINGES (CRANIAL ENVELOPES AND EPENDYMA)

A thorough knowledge of the cerebral membranes, their contained fluids, and the parts they play in cranial and intracranial disease is of great importance.   The cranial mass is separated from its bony covering by three superimposed envelopes, the dura mater, arachnoid, and pia.   These membranes form at least three intracranial spaces.   Between the skull and the dura is the potential extradural space.   Between the dura and arachnoid is the subdural or extra-arachnoid space, and deep to the arachnoid, between it and the pia mater, is the subarachnoid space which contains the cerebrospinal fluid.

(I) Dura Mater, Its Venous Sinuses, and the Middle Meningeal Artery

1. Dura Mater.—The dura is a thick resistant membrane possessing little elasticity and carrying on its outer surface ramifications of the middle meningeal arteries. Duplications of the dura enclose the great intracranial venous sinuses.

There is a somewhat firm adhesion between the outer surface of the dura and the skull; the outer layer assists in bone formation in the young. The strength of *dural attachment* to the vault is variable, and decreases with advancing years. Attachment is particularly strong at the base, which explains laceration of the basal dura in head trauma. In linear basal fractures, the membrane usually is torn. The dural prolongation along the cerebral nerves contributes to the firm adhesion, making basal extradural hemorrhage unusual. In the newborn, attachment is so compact at the margins of the bones that

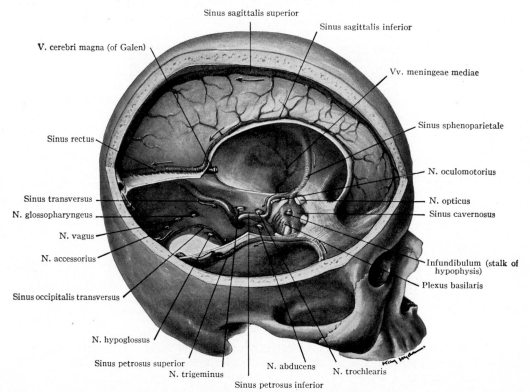

Fig. 16.—Right Lateral Half of the Cranial Vault Removed to Show the Topography of the Dural Sinuses.

A segment is removed from the cerebellar tentorium to show the foramen magnum and the transverse sinus; arrows indicate the direction of venous flow.

extradural hemorrhage is likely to be limited to the inner surface of one bone. The loose attachment in the occipital and temporal regions is the rationale for the choice of these regions as paths of access to the brain.

Because of its toughness and smooth inner surface, the dura furnishes excellent enveloping protection to the brain. A dural defect is replaced by scar tissue which adheres to the cortical meninges only when the subjacent pia-arachnoid is damaged. A well-sutured dural wound with edges approximated accurately should not cause adhesions, as the apposed edges unite quickly.

The dura may be dissected into two layers, an outer applied directly over the cranial wall, serving as its periosteum, and an inner, constituting the dura proper. The semilunar (gasserian) ganglion and venous sinuses lie within duplications of the dura. The intracranial dural layers split and descend separately into the vertebral canal at the occipital foramen.   The outer periosteal layer lines the bony canal and the inner layer becomes the spinal dura.   The space between the two layers, the intradural, more commonly known as the epidural space, while continuous over the whole of the spinal canal, does not exist within the cranium.   Therefore, an epidural spinal infection cannot spread into the cranial cavity.

From the mesial surface of the dura, folds or prolongations are interposed as partitions between the different segments of the brain, separating and maintaining them in their respective locations, and permitting free intercommunication.   These folds are the falx of the cerebrum, the tentorium of the cerebellum, and the diaphragm of the sella.   The *falx of the cerebrum* is a sagittal, sickle-shaped, membranous partition descending into the great longitudinal fissure and separating the cerebral hemispheres.   The *tentorium of the cerebellum* is the transverse crescentic septum which separates the cerebrum from the

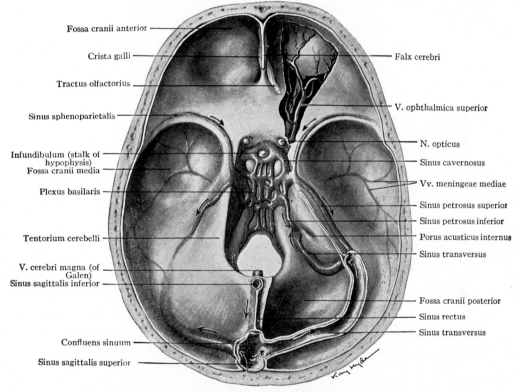

Fossa cranii anterior

Crista galli

Tractus olfactorius

Sinus sphenoparietalis

Infundibulum (stalk of hypophysis)
Fossa cranii media

Plexus basilaris

Tentorium cerebelli

V. cerebri magna (of Galen)
Sinus sagittalis inferior

Confluens sinuum

Sinus sagittalis superior

Falx cerebri

V. ophthalmica superior

N. opticus

Sinus cavernosus

Vv. meningeae mediae

Sinus petrosus superior

Sinus petrosus inferior

Porus acusticus internus

Sinus transversus

Fossa cranii posterior

Sinus rectus

Sinus transversus

FIG. 17.—SINUSES IN THE DURA VIEWED FROM ABOVE.
The cerebellar tentorium has been removed on the right.

cerebellum.   It is well adapted to support pressure from above and protects the important structures resting upon it.   The *diaphragm of the sella* is a small circular fold of dura forming a roof over the pituitary (hypophyseal) fossa and transmitting the infundibulum, or stalk of the hypophysis, through an opening in its center.

2. **Dural Venous Sinuses.**—The dura, in addition to carrying the important middle meningeal arteries on its outer surface, encloses in its duplications the great venous sinuses which collect the blood after it has nourished the brain and carry it to the internal jugular veins.   Of these, the superior sagittal, transverse (lateral), and cavernous sinuses are of particular surgical importance.

The *superior sagittal sinus* lies a little to the right of the median line and, because of the large vessels opening into it, increases in size from its origin in the anterior cranial fossa to its termination at the *confluence of sinuses* (torcular Herophili).   In the anterior cranial fossa, the superior sagittal sinus communicates through the foramen cecum with the veins of the nasal cavities and the upper veins of the face. It receives the veins of the mesial surface and those of a portion of the lateral surfaces of the cerebral hemispheres. The emissary veins which traverse the cranial wall from the scalp enter it and furnish direct communication with the scalp (p. 20). The parietal veins which cover the motor areas of the lower extremities also drain into it. The superior sagittal sinus usually is continued into the right transverse (lateral) sinus, sidetracking the unimportant, small, vertically placed occipital sinus.

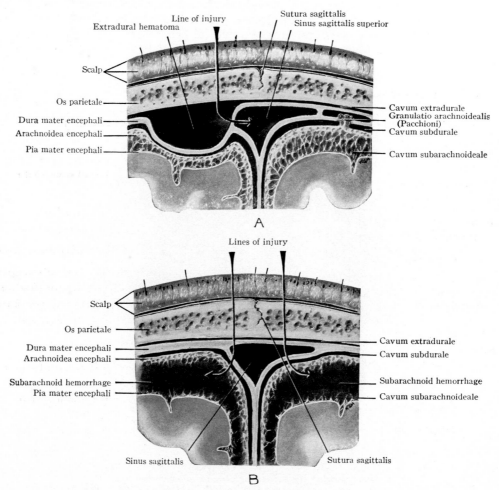

FIG. 18.—DIAGRAMMATIC FRONTAL SECTIONS THROUGH THE SUPERIOR SAGITTAL SINUS TO ILLUSTRATE THE MECHANISM OF EXTRADURAL AND SUBARACHNOID HEMORRHAGE.

A, Laceration of the superior sagittal sinus producing an extradural hematoma. B, Laceration of the superior sagittal sinus producing an extravasation of blood into the subarachnoid space.

Most of the veins, notably the more important of the superior cerebral veins, do not empty into the superior sagittal sinus directly, but into lateral lacunae, a series of spaces which extend laterally a variable distance between the dural layers. The most important of these lacunae overlie the anterior and posterior central convolutions. Into these venous lacunae project tuftlike derivatives of the subjacent arachnoid (p. 35), the brain envelope immediately underneath the dura. The granulations almost completely fill the lacunae and by pressure-atrophy even cause depressions on the under surface of the cranium. Skull injury and operative intervention here may be attended by serious hemorrhage because it is difficult to remove the bone from the dura without tearing the thinned-out dural coverings of the granulations.   Neither can the dura be lifted from the brain without injuring the cerebral veins which, with the granulations, fix it to the cortex.

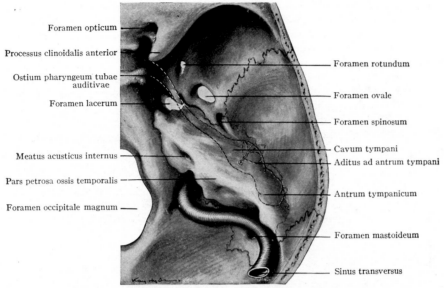

FIG. 19.—TRANSVERSE SINUS AND ITS RELATIONS; MIDDLE CRANIAL FOSSA.
The auditory apparatus is projected to the surface of the petrous portion of the temporal bone.

The *transverse (lateral) sinuses* are right and left bifurcations of the superior sagittal sinus at the confluence of sinuses.   They are the largest of the cranial sinuses and the right is usually larger than the left.   Each runs to the corresponding jugular foramen where

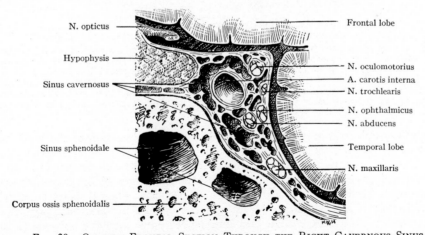

FIG. 20.—OBLIQUE FRONTAL SECTION THROUGH THE RIGHT CAVERNOUS SINUS.
Note the relation of the sinus to the hypophysis, sphenoid sinus, and brain; attention is called to the possibility of basal skull fracture producing arteriovenous fistula between the internal carotid artery and cavernous sinus, and the many possibilities for production of nerve pressure.

it terminates at the internal jugular vein.   The continuity of sinus and vein explains the propagation of transverse sinus thrombosis to the internal jugular vein, and supports the rationale of ligation of the internal jugular vein to prevent the carrying of septic emboli to the heart.

Each transverse sinus lies in the triangular space at the attachment of the cerebellar tentorium to a groove in the occipital bone. It turns downward to the medial surface of the mastoid portion of the temporal bone which it grooves or canalizes. Destruction of the occipital bone may injure the sinus and produce grave hemorrhage with rapid brain compression. The greatest danger of injury to the sinus, however, occurs in mastoid operations. At the posterior portion of the mastoid process is an emissary vein which unites the veins of the scalp with the transverse sinus. Injury to this communicating vein in bone removal, especially when there is venous stasis, may lead to serious hemorrhage; this accident is equivalent to an injury of the sinus itself. At the occipital protuberance, there are communicating vessels between the scalp and the confluence of sinuses, necessitating special care in the removal of bone. Along the main body of the transverse sinus there are no important vascular communications and the overlying bone may be removed by rongeur with little risk of bleeding.

At the sides of the body of the sphenoid bone lie the *cavernous sinuses* with their anterior and posterior intercavernous connections. At the orbital fissure, each sinus

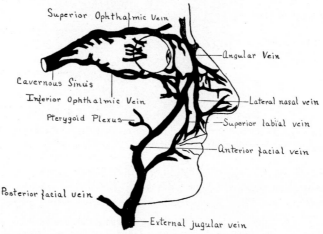

FIG. 21.—DRAWING SHOWING THE ANASTOMOSES OF THE SUPERFICIAL VEINS OF THE NOSE AND LIPS WITH THE OPHTHALMIC VEINS, CAVERNOUS SINUS, AND EXTERNAL JUGULAR VEIN.

The angular vein leads directly into the superior ophthalmic vein which runs backward in the upper portion of the orbit through the superior orbital fissure and terminates in the anterior part of the cavernous sinus. The lateral nasal vein communicates with the superior ophthalmic vein and with the anterior facial vein. The majority of the veins of the nasal fossae, both from the septum and lateral walls, unite and form the sphenopalatine vein which terminates in the pterygoid plexus; this plexus of veins also communicates directly with the cavernous sinus and with the anterior facial vein. (Ingersoll in Jackson and Coates, "Nose, Throat, and Ear and Their Diseases.")

receives tributary ophthalmic veins which readily propagate infection to the sinus (p. 32). At the apex of the petrous portion of the temporal bone, these sinuses terminate by emptying into the superior and inferior petrosal sinuses which drain into the internal jugular vein The cavity of each cavernous sinus is divided by fibrous strands so that it has the appearance of cavernous tissue. In its walls are embedded the internal carotid artery, the oculomotor, trochlear, and abducens nerves and the ophthalmic and maxillary divisions of the trigeminal nerve. The medial and inferior relations with the sphenoidal sinuses furnish the possibility of cavernous sinus thrombosis resulting from sphenoid sinusitis. Relations with the internal carotid artery are so intimate that arteriovenous fistula sometimes complicates basal skull fracture at this point. The sinus may be injured in operations upon the gasserian ganglion which rests in close proximity to it.

3. **Middle Meningeal Artery.**—The middle meningeal artery, a large branch of the internal maxillary artery, is the chief arterial supply of the dura and is remarkable for its long course and surgical importance. After passing into the cranium through the foramen spinosum, it runs horizontally outward for a distance of 3 to 4 cm. where

it divides into anterior and posterior terminal branches. The larger *anterior branch* passes upward along the great wing of the sphenoid where it may be enclosed in a distinct bony canal. The artery clings intimately to the dura, so that separation of the dura from the bone is difficult and often is impossible without troublesome hemorrhage. A linear fracture crossing the temporal region and the region of the sutures around the great wing of the sphenoid bone is likely to injure the vessel. The *posterior branch* passes posteriorly from the great wing of the sphenoid to the squamous part of the temporal bone, which it crosses on the way to the middle of the inner surface of the parietal bone. Injury to this branch may result in an extradural temporoparietal hematoma.

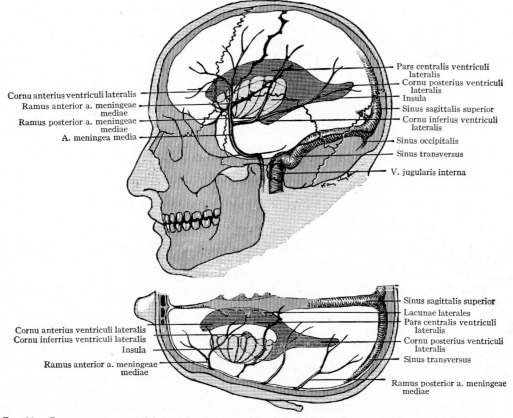

FIG. 22.—RELATIONS OF THE MIDDLE MENINGEAL ARTERY WITH THE CRANIUN, INSULA, AND THE LATERAL VENTRICLES. (After Cushing.)

4. **Subdural Space.**—The dura mater and the arachnoid are applied closely to each other and the subdural space is the interval which separates them. Like the pleural cavity, it is a potential space which becomes real only when an effusion, serous, purulent, or hemorrhagic, collects between the membranes. The small amount of fluid it contains has no communication with the subarachnoid spaces which hold the cerebrospinal fluid.

SURGICAL CONSIDERATIONS

1. **Pachymeningitis,** or inflammation of the dura mater, may occur on its outer or inner surface, constituting respectively pachymeningitis externus or internus. The dense dural membrane with its paucity of vessels is quite resistant to infection, and acts as a barrier to further extension. Large extradural collections of pus may exist for a considerable time without brain involvement.

Pachymeningitis externus frequently accompanies pyogenic and syphilitic osteomyelitis of the vault. Lateral dural involvement with local abscess formation usually is secondary to chronic suppuration of the middle ear, and prompt evacuation of the abscess may limit further extension. The dural sinuses may become involved early in dural disease, and result in sinus thrombosis and bacteremia. This occurs most commonly about the ear whence infection may involve the transverse sinus.

*Pachymeningitis internus (haemorrhagica)*is a chronic hematoma of the inner surface of the dura, covering the surface of one or both hemispheres. It is generally a chroni affair with the formation of an easily-detached hemorrhagic membrane, and occurs in poorly nourished children, patients suffering from anemia, and in the insane; most frequently it occurs late after skull trauma. Whatever the cause of formation of the membrane, repeated extravasations of blood occur. The cerebral veins which pass directly from the brain to the tributaries of the superior sagittal sinus are acknowledged to be the source of hemorrhage in most of these cases. They are short trunks which pass at right angles from brain to dura. With the cranial end of the veins fixed in rigid dura and the cerebral end attached to a movable hemisphere, it is easy to understand how venous injury occurs in movements of the hemispheres which result in anteroposterior displacement.

2. **Extradural Hemorrhage.**—Hemorrhage from the dura caused by injury in skull fracture has been discussed (p. 27). Extradural hemorrhage may occur from skull trauma without fracture, as a result of detachment of the membrane from the bone. Operations involving separation of the dura from the skull may be accompanied by free bleeding from the vessels which pass from the dura to the overlying bone. Birth injuries cause subdural hemorrhage at the wedge of the superior sagittal sinus. When the dura is torn by bony fragments, generally the top of the wedge is injured and, unless the tear involves the sides of the sinus, the bleeding is extradural (Fig. 18, A).

3. **Sinus Thrombosis.**—Suppurations in the paranasal sinuses are in close relationship to the dural venous channels, an anatomic proximity overlooked too often and regarded too indifferently. Any infection in an area tributary to the dural sinuses may cause death even though the original infection may not appear serious.

Chronic suppuration in the middle ear is the commonest focus for *transverse sinus infection*. When the mastoid antrum and air cells are involved, and particularly when there is obstruction to free discharge of purulent material, the bone between these cavities and the dura is destroyed and intracranial complications may ensue. The size, location, and structure of the mastoid air cells, the persistence of cranial sutures, and the presence of bone defects determine largely the extent of infection. A mastoid abscess may extend into the transverse sinus directly by continuity, or may involve it by infection from the small veins emptying into the sinus over the jugular bulb. In some such manner, the wall of the sinus is involved, a local thrombosis occurs, and the condition advances until the vessel is occluded. This infection may spread into the superior sagittal sinus or, by way of the jugular vein, into the general circulation.

Thrombosis in the cavernous sinus results commonly from infection about the brow, orbt, inose, or upper lip; more rarely, by direct extension from an infected sphenoid sinus. Cavernous sinus thrombosis is unapproachable surgically and, therefore, is infinitely more serious than transverse sinus thrombosis. Lesions of the nerves in and about the sinus, with a marked degree of exophthalmus caused by stasis in the ophthalmic veins, generally result.

Thrombosis in the superior sagittal sinus is rare and usually is the result of cranial osteomyelitis, infected wounds of the scalp, or erysipelas of the scalp. Early evacuation of the infected clot in the sinus may prevent death.

(II) ARACHNOID, PIA MATER, SUBARACHNOID SPACE, AND CEREBROSPINAL FLUID

1. **Arachnoid and Pia Mater.**—These membranes are applied more closely to the surface of the brain than is the dura. Over the convolutions they are in contact, but over the sulci they are separated more or less widely. The pia mater fits the convolutions

closely like a glove, while the arachnoid stretches over most of the fissures, save the longitudinal and lateral, and may be likened to a mitten drawn over the pial glove.

The *arachnoid* extends as a distinct sheet over the convolutions, sulci, and minor depressions. Over special areas, such as the venous sinuses, particularly the superior sagittal, it develops villi (pacchionian bodies). These tuftlike processes contain cerebrospinal fluid which is separated from the venous blood by the arachnoid covering of the tufts and the thin endothelial walls of the lateral lacunae. Through these bodies, cerebrospinal fluid can pass into the sinuses to relieve the fluid pressure within the cerebrospinal system.

The *pia mater* intimately invests the brain, following all its irregularities. While the larger blood vessels of the brain lie in the subarachnoid space, the smaller vessels ramify in the pia before proceeding into the substance of the brain. It is about these vessels that most of the lesions of tuberculous and syphilitic meningitis occur.

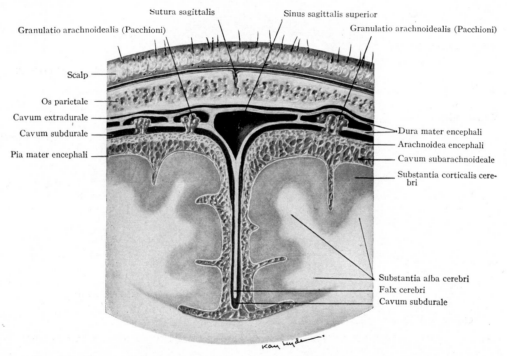

FIG. 23.—FRONTAL SECTION THROUGH THE SCALP, CRANIUM, MENINGES, AND BRAIN.
Attention is called to the invasion of the lateral lacunae of the superior sagittal sinus by the arachnoid villi; the trabeculated subarachnoid space lies between the arachnoid and pial membranes.

2. **Subarachnoid Space.**—A cushion for the brain is furnished by the cerebrospinal fluid in the subarachnoid space, enclosed between the arachnoid and pia. Familiarity with this space is becoming progressively more important. When the brain is congested and swollen, it does not impinge against nonyielding bone, but rests upon an adjustable bed of cerebrospinal fluid, part of which it can displace into the subarachnoid space of the spine. The communicating spinal subarachnoid space may be tapped by lumbar puncture and fluid be drained from the cranial subarachnoid space to lessen intracranial pressure. One danger in this procedure lies in the possibility of forcing the brain stem into the foramen magnum because of decompression of the spinal subarachnoid space.

The subarachnoid space over the vault is divided into intercommunicating channels by delicate connective tissue trabeculae. Over certain portions of the brain, however, the arachnoid is separated from the pia by the fluid collections in the subarachnoid cisterns. The basal cisterns are the most important. In basal meningitis, they become filled with purulent exudate which may involve the neighboring cerebral nerves from the second to the eighth, inclusive.   They are in communication with the ventricular system of the brain.

3. **Cerebrospinal Fluid.**—The apparent source of cerebrospinal fluid is the choroid plexuses of the cerebral ventricles.   The cerebrospinal fluid bathes the brain and probably is drained away by the arachnoid villi; their relationship with the superior sagittal sinus has been discussed (p. 29).   Its function is chiefly mechanical—assisting in regulating intracranial pressure and lessening effects of shock to the brain.   Nature's method of combating increased volume from an excess of fluid within the closed cranial chamber is to withdraw the fluid from the ventricular system and the subarachnoid spaces and send it into the blood.   Space compensation, therefore, is the principal function of cerebrospinal fluid.   This explains the large size which brain tumors may attain before causing

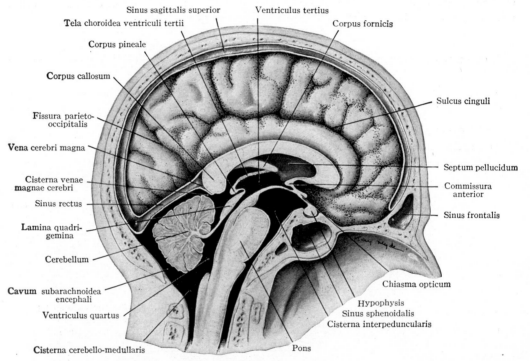

Fig. 24.—Ventricular and Subarachnoid Spaces Viewed in Median Sagittal Section of the Head.

symptoms and, eventually, death.   If the intracranial pressure exceeds the point at which Nature's efforts are exhausted, death must ensue because the cranial chamber is inexpansible.   (Dandy.)

Infection and adhesions in meningitis may obstruct the median aperture of Magendie and the lateral apertures of Luschka in the roof and sides respectively of the fourth ventricle, through which openings cerebrospinal fluid normally passes from the ventricles into the subarachnoid space.

The result is *hydrocephalus*.   The veins of the choroid plexus become congested with increased transudation into the interior of the ventricles.   This condition may be relieved by making a fresh opening into the roof of the fourth ventricle to reestablish the communication between the ventricular system and the subarachnoid space.

SURGICAL CONSIDERATIONS

1. **Leptomeningitis.**—Acute inflammation of the arachnoid and pia may occur as a primary disease and become extensive at an early stage, or be secondary to local or systemic infection and remain localized.

The *cerebrospinal*, or *epidemic form*, caused by meningococcus infection, is a characteristic type of primary meningeal involvement. The exudate thrown off by the infected meninges, in advanced inflammation, covers the cord, brain stem, and cerebral nerves, and sometimes even the cortex, with a dense fibrinopurulent layer. When the exudate occludes the foramina about the roof of the fourth ventricle, hydrocephalus results in the course of, or following, the disease. Infection may extend through the perivascular spaces, or be carried by the blood stream into the brain and cause brain abscess. Basal localization of the effusion accounts for the involvement of the cerebral nerves. The oculomotor nerve is affected most commonly and produces strabismus, diplopia, and pupillary changes. Facial paralysis and auditory disturbances may occur, and the hypoglossal nerve sometimes is involved.

Tuberculous meningitis almost invariably is fatal, probably because of the supervening acute hydrops of the ventricles in the later stages. The basal meninges are those

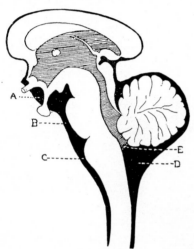

chiefly involved. There may be considerable fibrinous exudate surrounding the nerves; this may extend also into the ventricles along the lateral cerebral fissure and over the hemispheres. Patches of meningo-encephalitis are usual. In the final stage of paralysis caused by ventricular dilation, the patient may remain for days in a semicomatose condition. The signs are muscle rigidity, marked retraction of the neck, choked disks, cerebral nerve palsy, and a subnormal temperature.

Fig. 25.—Diagram Representing the Midsagittal View of the Brain Stem, Showing the Ventricular System (in Cross Lines) and the Subarachnoid System (in Black).
The communication between the two systems is at E (foramen of Magendie); the foramina of Luschka are not shown; A, cisterna interpeduncularis; B, cisterna pontis; C, D, cisterna cerebellomedullaris (cisterna magna). (Dandy and Blackfan.)

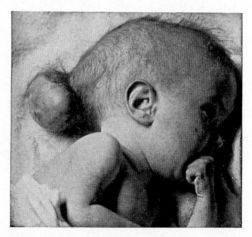

Fig. 26.—Occipital Encephalocele with Hydrocephalus. (Cushing.)

Syphilitic meningitis may be a diffuse process or may occur as single or multiple gummatous tumors. Although the characteristic meningeal lesion arises in the leptomeninges, it may be secondary to syphilis of the cranial vault where the usual focus is in the frontal bone. When the process is primary in the leptomeninges, it is more commonly basal, the cerebral nerves and vessels being involved secondarily by gumma.

2. **Tumors of the Meninges.**—While certain of the pachymeningeal (dural) tumors are of a most malignant nature, lead to absorption of the cranial bones, and commonly appear externally as pulsatile swellings, leptomeningeal tumors generally are less malignant. Their symptoms are caused by pressure on, rather than true invasion of, the brain and nerves. The pia mater acts as a barrier to such extension, a fact which makes enucleation possible without damage to brain structure. Because of the superficial location of these tumors, they are diagnosed accurately from the signs and symptoms. They grow slowly, sometimes over a period of years, and most of them are accessible surgically.

3 Encephalocele.—An encephalocele is a protrusion of the intracranial contents through an area where there is a defective closure of the cranium and meninges It usually is congenital, but may be traumatic in origin.   The contents are brain tissue, meninges, or both, overspread by the scalp.   In some cases, not only the pericranium and bones are absent, but there may be a dural defect; then the pia-arachnoid is covered only by the scalp.

Usually encephalocele is in the median plane in the posterior or anterior part of the head.   The *occipital variety* is more common and has a superior or inferior position with reference to the tentorium.   The inferior occipital variety commonly corresponds to a bony defect which communicates with the foramen magnum.   The *frontal variety* generally occurs through a defect in the longitudinal plate of the ethmoid and may be mistaken for a nasal polyp.   The varieties are naso-orbital, nasofrontal, or naso-ethmoidal, according to the location of the defect and the direction taken by the tumor.

D. BRAIN

(I) Brain in General

Hemorrhages, injuries, and tumors of the brain interfere greatly with motor areas, nerve paths, and special centers, and cause paralysis and sensory disturbances.   For correct diagnosis of these brain conditions and for selection of the proper operative pro-

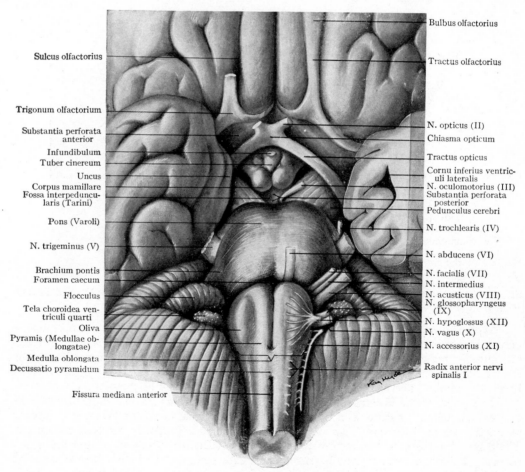

Fig. 27.—Base of the Brain.

Part of the temporal lobe is removed on the left side.   All the nerve roots emerging on the right side, except the trigeminus, are removed.   Part of the olfactory tract is removed to show the olfactory sulcus.

cedures designed for their cure or relief, a thorough working knowledge of the structure and functions, and of the sensory and motor areas of the brain is essential.

In brain surgery, the opening and closing of a wound are a difficult procedure. The approaches are difficult through heavy and resistant structures to vital, delicate, and easily-traumatized organs. The treatment of the lesion itself involves less time and effort than does the exposure of it, and the closure of the wound itself. (Naffziger.)

1. **Vessels.**—The brain is supplied lavishly with **arterial blood** through the two vertebral and the two internal carotid arteries. After entering the cranium, these trunks form an anastomosing *arterial circle* (of Willis) with intercommunicating branches which

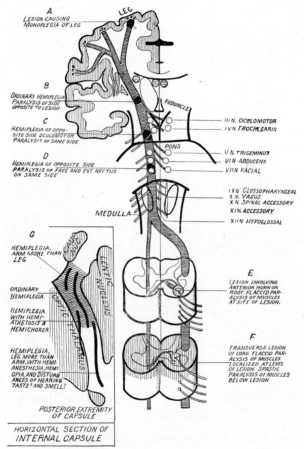

Fig. 28.—Effect of Lesions (Indicated by Circles) of the Motor Path in the Brain and Spinal Cord.

G, Internal capsule lesions and the variation in symptoms caused by lesions in a variety of locations. (Butler.)

equalize the cerebral circulation. The circle is formed in front by the connected anterior cerebral branches of the internal carotid arteries, and behind by the two posterior cerebral arteries, which are the bifurcation of the basilar trunk formed by the two vertebral arteries. The posterior communicating branches between the posterior cerebral arteries and the internal carotid arteries complete the circle. From the vertebral and basilar arteries, there are three branches of considerable size which supply the cerebellum.

The *anterior cerebral artery* supplies the superior and middle frontal convolutions and all of the medial surface of the hemisphere back to the parieto-occipital fissure.

The *middle cerebral artery,* from its size and direction, may be regarded as the continuation of the internal carotid upward and outward to the sylvian fissure—hence its name *sylvian artery*. It supplies the insula, part of the corpus striatum and interna capsule, and most of the exposed surface of the hemisphere. One of its small branches, which runs upward through the lateral zone of the lenticular nucleus of the corpus striatum to the internal capsule, frequently ruptures and has been termed by Charcot the artery of cerebral hemorrhage. From its course, it is evident that the middle cerebral artery supplies the motor areas of the brain, both cortical and central, with the exception of part of the leg center which occupies the paracentral lobule, and the highest point of the precentral convolution. Both of these latter areas lie within the domain of the anterior cerebral artery. It further supplies the cortical center for hearing, part of the center for vision, and the motor speech center in the left hemisphere.

The *posterior cerebral artery* supplies the middle and inferior temporal gyri, the mesia part of the occipital lobe, and the inferior surface of the temporosphenoidal lobe. The vessels which supply the deeper structures emerge directly from the circle or from its main stems. The most important of these vessels penetrate and supply the basal ganglia.

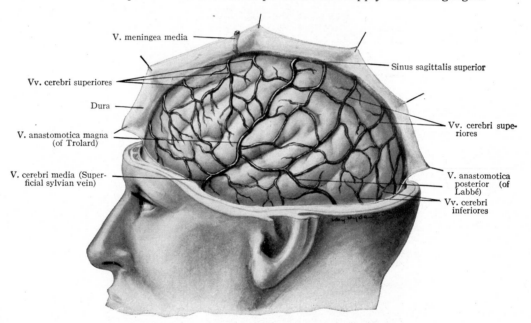

FIG. 29.—LATERAL VIEW OF THE VEINS OF THE CEREBRUM.
The dura is reflected. (After Rouvière.)

When, for any reason, one of the main channels participating in the formation of the circle becomes blocked, the intercommunicating vessels function. If there be no pre-existing vascular disease, ligation of a common carotid artery is not likely to produce deleterious effects upon the brain, as one carotid and two vertebral arteries are sufficient to carry on the circulation. The occlusion of any of these large trunks, however, may be attended by softening of an extensive cerebral area.

Because the cerebral and cerebellar **veins** are thin-walled, unsupported, and without valves, they are injured easily and bleed readily. The superficial veins pierce the arachnoid membrane and the inner layer of the dura and empty into the dural sinuses (p. 29). The veins coursing over the surface of the hemispheres empty, for the most part, into the superior sagittal sinus, whereas the deeper veins converge to the great cerebral vein (of Galen) which enters the straight sinus.

(II) Cerebral Cortex and Cerebellum

1. **Cerebral Cortex.**—The cerebral hemispheres, with their frontal, parietal, occipital, temporal, and insular lobes, occupy the anterior and superior parts of the cranial cavity and rest upon a floor formed by the anterior and middle cranial fossae and the tentorium of the cerebellum. The sagittal falx of the cerebrum and the longitudinal fissure in which it lies divide the cerebrum into right and left hemispheres which are united in the depths of the fissure by a series of interhemospheric connections.

The superolateral surface of the cerebral cortex presents two fissures and one sulcus of major importance; the lateral fissure (of Sylvius), the central sulcus (of Rolando) and the parieto-occipital fissure. These divide the outer surface of the hemisphere into four lobes: frontal, temporal, parietal, and occipital.

The functional centers are located in the gray matter of the cerebral cortex and receive and send impressions which travel to and from them in the white matter. Determination

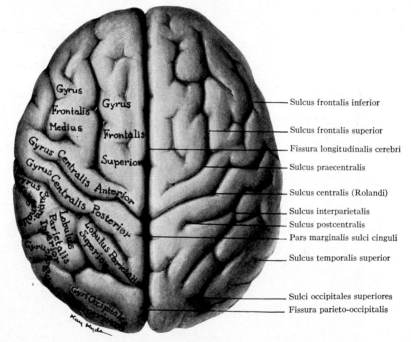

FIG. 30.—GYRI AND SULCI OF THE SUPERIOR SURFACE OF THE CEREBRUM.

of the site of pathologic processes, whether they be tumor, abscess, or hemorrhage, depends on accurate localization of these centers and their nerve paths.

2. **Main and Specialized Motor Areas.**—The **main motor area** is limited to the gray matter of the narrow rolandic strip of the anterior central gyrus. It is a centimeter in width and extends to the depth of the central fissure. Since much of this area lies hidden in the longitudinal fissure, the lesion which actually involves this cortex may lie below the exposed surface of the hemisphere. The inferior boundary of the motor strip falls short of the lateral cerebral fissure (of Sylvius). Generally speaking, the upper part of the area presides over the movements of the lower extremity, the middle region over those of the upper limb, and the lower part over those of the mouth, eyelids, tongue, pharynx, and larynx.

The central sulcus is not straight, but is broken by several well-developed angulations (genua). Above the superior genu, there is exposed only a small triangle of motor cortex, the area for the lower limb, where stimulation results in movements of the hip, knee, and toes. The area for the upper extremity corresponds to the middle third of the precentral gyrus.   The shoulder center is highest, followed by the centers for the elbow, wrist, and fingers.   The area for the neck and face continues downward from the area for the upper limb, the eyelid center occupying the highest position, succeeded below by the mouth and tongue.   The area for the tongue occupies the lower extremity of the precentral gyrus and adjoins that for motor speech which occupies the posterior and inferior part of the

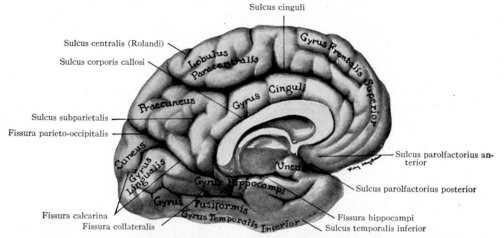

FIG. 31.—SULCI AND GYRI ON THE MEDIAL ASPECT OF THE CEREBRAL HEMISPHERE.

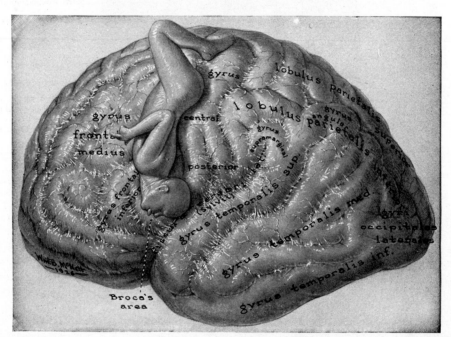

FIG. 32.—DIAGRAM OF THE APPROXIMATE MOTOR REPRESENTATION IN THE CEREBRAL CORTEX.
The figure superimposed on the precentral gyrus suggests the location of motor areas.   (Babcock, "Textbook of Surgery.")

inferior frontal convolution.   The areas for the head and eyes occupy parts of the superior middle, and inferior frontal gyri, in front of the areas for the limbs.

Destruction of these areas leads to complete and permanent loss of movement in proportion to the extent of the lesion and the degree of bilateral representation of the movements concerned, but sensation is not affected.   The motor pathway from the cortical centers is the pyramidal tract, the fibers of which degenerate throughout their full length following injury to the cortical cells.

The **specialized motor areas** are those concerned with speech and writing. The *center for motor speech* is conceded to be in the posterior end of the left inferior frontal

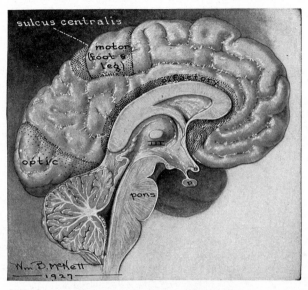

FIG. 33.—CORTICAL CENTERS ON THE MEDIAL ASPECT OF THE CEREBRAL HEMPISHERE. *p*, Hypophysis of the cerebrum (pituitary). (Babcock, "Textbook of Surgery.")

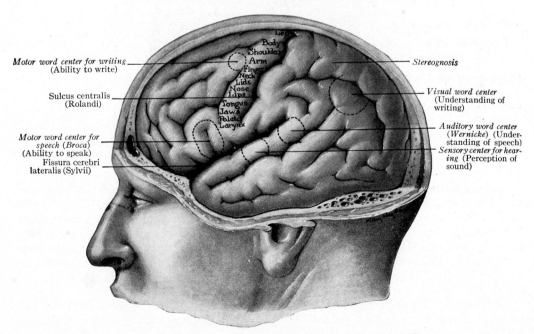

FIG. 34.—MAIN FUNCTIONAL LOCALIZATIONS IN THE CEREBRAL CORTEX.

gyrus (Broca's convolution) in the right handed. A lesion here produces motor aphasia, inability to transform concepts into words, although the vocal cords and tongue are capable of functioning. The *writing center* has been placed at the posterior extremity of the middle frontal gyrus, that is, near the primary cortical centers for movements of the hands and fingers. A lesion here produces agraphia, inability to transfer a concept into written form.

3. **Main and Specialized Sensory Areas.**—The **main sensory area** occupies the postcentral convolution, a position behind the central sulcus analogous to that of motor area in front of it. Similarly, much of it lies hidden on the anterior wall of the gyrus within the central sulcus. The cortical area for *pain and temperature* probably lies a little behind the postcentral cortical sensory area, and that for *stereognosis*, recognition of objects by sense of touch, lies in the parietal lobe.

Specialized sensory pathways terminate in reasonably sharply circumscribed cortical areas which, for the most part, are separated widely from one another by masses of cortical substance.

The *center for reception of visual impressions* has been traced to the occipital lobe. The visual word *center for reading* has been placed definitely in the angular gyrus, and a lesion in it probably causes a loss of ability to read or understand written language, although ordinary sight is not disturbed.

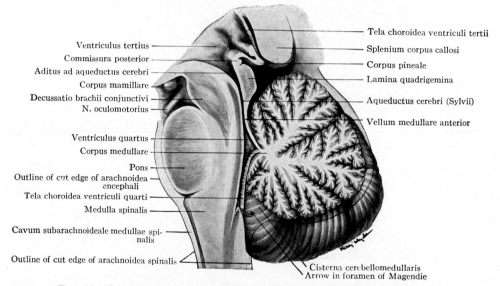

Ventriculus tertius
Commissura posterior
Aditus ad aqueductus cerebri
Corpus mamillare
Decussatio brachii conjunctivi
N. oculomotorius

Ventriculus quartus
Corpus medullare
Pons
Outline of cut edge of arachnoidea encephali
Tela choroidea ventriculi quarti
Medulla spinalis
Cavum subarachnoideale medullae spinalis
Outline of cut edge of arachnoidea spinalis

Tela choroidea ventriculi tertii
Splenium corpus callosi
Corpus pineale
Lamina quadrigemina
Aqueductus cerebri (Sylvii)
Vellum medullare anterior

Cisterna cerebellomedullaris
Arrow in foramen of Magendie

FIG. 35.—SAGITTAL SECTION THROUGH THE FOURTH VENTRICLE AND CEREBELLUM.
The arrow in the foramen of Magendie indicates one of the connections between the fluid in the ventricular system and that in the subarachnoid space.

The *auditory center* is in the superior temporal convolution. Sensations are converted into conscious perceptions in this and adjacent parts of the temporal lobe Those on the left side are bound up particularly with the auditory function of speech mechanism. It is probable that the center for each side is connected with both auditory nerves, so that a paralysis of one side by a unilateral lesion may be compensated by the center on the opposite side. The cortical center for the *recognition of spoken words* lies above the primary area for hearing in the superior temporal gyrus of the left temporal lobe and is the first center developed in the faculty of language.

The centers for smell and taste are not so definite. The center for *smell* is thought to lie in the uncus, and that for *taste* in the hippocampal gyrus. These are important considerations, since lesions in these areas not only give characteristic symptoms, but are accessible surgically.

4. **Cerebellum.**—The cerebellum rests in the posterior cranial fossa below the tentorium and behind the pons and medulla oblongata. It is the largest part of the hindbrain and between it and the pons and medulla lies the fourth ventricle. The cerebellum

consists of three parts, a median, the vermis, and two lateral expansions, the hemispheres The cerebellum is connected to the cerebrum, pons, and medulla oblongata by superior, middle, and inferior peduncles.

SURGICAL CONSIDERATIONS

Although the cerebrum is subject to a great variety of lesions, the symptoms and signs manifested are relatively few and depend more upon the location of the pathologic process than upon the process itself. Any obstructive lesion in the motor path at any point between the cortex and the peripheral end-organ, whether it be neoplasm, hemorrhage, thrombosis, inflammation, injury, or compression, produces paralysis.

While there may be a physiologic interruption of nerve pathways without pressure signs or symptoms, there are certain evidences which frequently accompany increased intracranial pressure. Chief among these are headache, vomiting, choked disks, vertigo, and convulsions. Focal symptoms and signs, when they are present, determine the location of the lesion; they are confined generally to disturbances of motion, common sensation, and the faculties of special sense.

1. **Regional Diagnosis in the Various Areas of the Cerebral Cortex and Cerebellum.**— The surgical accessibility and the fairly definite motor and sensory symptoms of lesions about the central sulcus of Rolando partly account for the success which brain surgery has attained. Lesions in this region involve the sensory receiving stations lying behind the fissure and the motor discharging stations in front of it. The motor neurons from the precentral gyrus comprise the pyramidal tract (p. 43) and pass to the spinal cord, crossing (decussating) in the medulla. The afferent, or sensory, impulses reach the post-central gyrus through relays of neurons, the final of which form a group of radiating fibers which arise from cells in the basal ganglia. Therefore, any motor or sensory disturbance originating in the cortex manifests itself in that half of the body opposite the side involved in the lesion.

An irritative disease in the **motor area** and **pathway,** which is confined to a single group of cells, may cause convulsive movements in the domain of the muscles controlled by these cells, termed attacks of focal or *jacksonian epilepsy.* It is characteristic of such a seizure that convulsive movements spread into groups of muscles, the cortical centers of which immediately adjoin those primarily irritated; in some instances, the entire body musculature may become involved progressively. Any destructive lesion of the motor cortical area or pathway gives rise to loss of motion without accompanying loss of sensory perception.

A postcentral gyrus lesion involves the common **sensory area** and **pathway.** Like lesions in the anterior gyrus, it may be irritative and result only in such forms of paresthesia as numbness and tingling. The lesion may be destructive and lead to hypesthesia or anesthesia. While cortical sensory lesions must be extensive to cause a considerable loss of sensation, subcortical lesions in the sensory pathway produce pronounced anesthesias.

While, anatomically, the **frontal lobe** extends to the central sulcus, clinically, the lobe is limited to that portion of the hemisphere which lies anterior to the precentral sulcus. The forepart of the frontal lobe, from the clinical standpoint, is a silent area. In the postfrontal region are located the centers for the conjugate movements of the head and eyes and the motor part of the mechanism of speech. The left inferior frontal gyrus (Broca's convolution) presides over motor speech, and a lesion here, particularly if sub-cortical, results in *motor aphasia.* A lesion in the posterior extremity of the middle frontal gyrus may result in *agraphia,* inability to write.

Clinically, the **parietal lobe** is the area between the postcentral sulcus and the occipital lobe, and does not include the postcentral gyrus. *Word blindness,* or inability to understand written language, is a characteristic symptom complex which follows a destructive lesion of the angular gyrus of the left side in right-handed individuals. A deep-seated lesion involving the paths radiating from the word-perceiving center also may involve the optic radiation and lead to half-blindness of the corresponding sides of both **retinae.** A lesion of the upper parietal lobe, particularly when subcortical, produces *astereognosis*, or the inability to recognize through contact the form or character of objects.

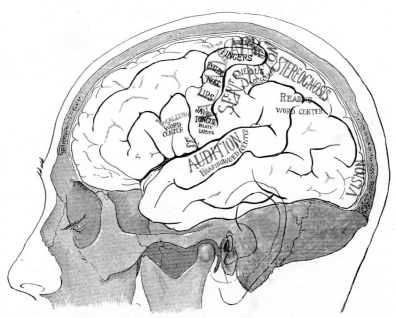

FIG. 36.—DIAGRAM ILLUSTRATING THE MORE DEFINITELY LOCALIZED OF THE CORTICAL CENTERS OF THE EXPOSED SURFACE OF THE CEREBRAL HEMISPHERE IN RELATION TO THE MAIN FISSURES AND CONVOLUTIONS.

The sensory and motor word centers involved in the special mechanism for speech are indicated. (Cushing in "Keen's Surgery.")

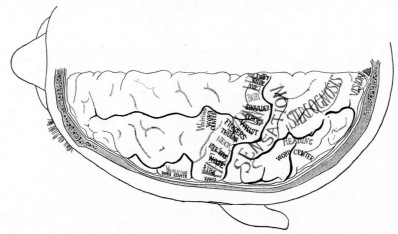

FIG. 37.—DIAGRAM ILLUSTRATING THE MORE DEFINITELY LOCALIZED OF THE CORTICAL CENTERS OF THE EXPOSED SURFACE OF THE CEREBRAL HEMISPHERE IN RELATION TO THE MAIN FISSURES AND CONVOLUTIONS.

This view from above indicates the sensory and motor word centers involved in the special mechanism for speech and shows that the best view of the motor path is obtained from above. (Cushing in "Keen's Surgery.")

The **occipital lobe** includes the posterior extremity of the hemisphere on both its outer and inner aspects. Mesially, it contains the cuneus and the lingual gyri, from which region the *optic radiation* passes by the wall of the posterior end of the internal capsule to the thalamus, whence it runs by way of the optic tracts to the retinae. A destructive lesion of this portion of the occipital cortex causes blindness on the homolateral halves of both retinae, or *homonymous hemianopsia*. The patient then is unable, when looking directly forward, to see objects on the side opposite from the lesion until they are brought across the median plane. In hemianopsia from cortical lesions, the pupils react in the usual manner, as the fibers from the oculomotor nerves are not involved. The location of lesions of other varieties of hemianopsia is indicated in Figure 38.

The main portion of the under surface of the cerebral hemispheres is formed by the **temporal lobes.** They are particularly susceptible to injury in basal fractures; they may

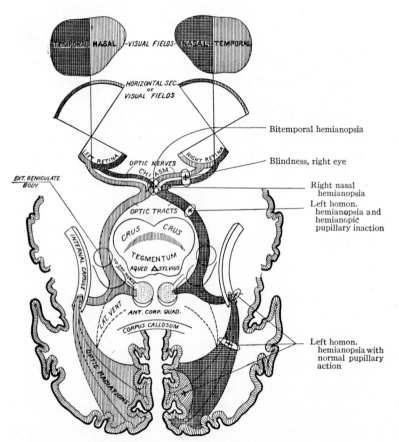

FIG. 38.—DIAGRAM OF THE OPTIC TRACTS AND VISUAL FIELDS.

Lesions at different points in the tract, causing hemianopsia, are indicated by +. (Moorhead, "Traumatic Surgery.")

harbor an extensive latent abscess. *Word deafness,* or the inability to understand spoken language, is pathognomonic of a lesion of the superior temporal gyrus on the left side. The same lesion also may affect the entire speech mechanism so that word blindness and motor aphasia accompany it. The antero-inferior extremity of the lobe, forming the uncus of the hippocampal gyrus (p. 44), is associated with the senses of *taste and smell,* and a destructive lesion here will destroy both.

Cerebellar tumors, cysts, and abscesses may require surgical treatment. The symptoms of these lesions are instability in equilibrium and locomotion, and troublesome vertigo. A coarse ataxia accompanies voluntary movements and nystagmus is a frequent sign. The symptoms are bilateral when the lesion occupies the middle lobe of the cerebellum, and homolateral when a lateral lobe is affected. Rotary movements and a tendency to turn or fall toward the affected side perhaps result from ataxia and weakness of muscle control on that side.

2. **Pineal Body (Gland) and Pineal Shift.**—The pineal body lies in a shallow depression on the dorsal surface of the midbrain. It is a tubular epithelial mass containing a variable amount of calcareous material, opaque to the x-ray. Naffziger has noted that this body is calcified in about 50 per cent of cases. With increased intracranial pressure, this body may be displaced laterally, away from the cerebral hemisphere which contains a tumor. x-Ray examination of pineal shift sometimes yields valuable evidence in lesion localization.

3. **Cerebral Pneumography.**—x-Ray cerebral pneumography (Dandy) marks an important advance in neurosurgical diagnosis. Its value depends on the fact that brain tumors, which cause increased intracranial pressure, produce changes in the size, shape, and position of the cerebral ventricles. Through a small trephine opening, fluid is with-drawn from the ventricle. The amount of fluid removed is replaced by air. The x-ray designates alterations in the ventricles.

4. **Brain Approaches in General.**—Since the pre-antiseptic era, the osteoplastic bone flap for the most part has replaced the measurements of cranio-encephalic topography and the selection of a localizing point for a trephine opening. Similarly, partial craniectomy has given way to bone flap operations on the skull, except in the subtemporal and suboccipital regions. Here, other structures than bone give adequate protection for the brain. In these areas, real openings covered by soft parts possess special decompressive advantages. The temporal and occipital muscles act as protective coverings and, at the same time, restrain excessive or harmful brain herniation. While these craniectomies serve as approaches to nearby structures, the bone flap operations generally are used on the cranial vault.

Parietal, frontoparietal, and frontal osteoplastic flaps are used for operations upon the hemispheres. All have their stalks or bases in the temporal region. With the thin squamous portion of the temporal bone in this location, these flaps break back readily. The temporal muscle and fascia act as a hinge. These flaps permit of wide exposure, and removal of that portion of bone beneath the temporal muscle permits leaving a decompressive opening after the flap has been replaced. Elevation of the frontal and parietal flaps affords access to the chiasmal region, all of the anterior fossa, and the forepart of the middle cranial fossa.

The occipital bone flap (Naffziger) exposes the supra- and infratentorial structures Subtentorial exposure may be gained by wide opening of the tentorium. Access is permitted to the pons, to the entire occipital lobe, to midline structures, and to the superior and anterior surfaces of the cerebellum.

(III) Hypophysis (Pituitary Body) and Its Compartment

The development, structure, and relations of the hypophysis have assumed, in recent years, a position of major importance in brain surgery. Modern physiologic and pathologic research has demonstrated that, in spite of its small size, it occupies a most important position among the endocrine glands and its surgical removal or its destruction by disease is incompatible with life. As it is located among important nerve structures at the base of the brain, its lesions are evidenced by disturbances in function sufficiently localized to permit early clinical recognition and consequent surgical correction. Grave constitutional neighborhood signs and symptoms arise from disordered activity in the gland itself.

1. **Definition and Boundaries.**—The hypophysis of the cerebrum (pituitary body) is a small ovoid mass, located within the hypophyseal fossa in the sella of the sphenoid bone. It is suspended from the cerebrum by a hollow diverticulum, the infundibulum, which grows downward from the floor of the brain from an area corresponding to the floor of the third ventricle. This mushroom-shaped gland, lying between the two cavernous sinuses, measures about 1.5 cm. in its transverse diameter and from 5 to 7 mm. antero-posteriorly.

2. **Relations.**—The hypophysis lies in an osteofibrous compartment within a duplication of the dura, the deep leaf of the dural duplication dipping into the sella to enclose it. Laterally, the deep leaf meets the superficial leaf which passes over the gland and forms the diaphragm for the fossa. The lateral dural walls of the fossa form the mesial walls of the cavernous sinuses (p. 32). The hypophysis is in relation superiorly with the optic chiasm through the intermedium of the dural diaphragm. A tumor of the hypophysis may exert an almost direct pressure against the chiasm and cause eye changes on the nasal halves of both retinae, the condition of *bitemporal hemianopsia*. The intimate relations of the hypophysis with the base of the brain make the intracranial frontal approach hazardous.

Laterally, the cavernous sinuses ramify over the hypophysis and have variable connections with the gland. Through the intermedium of the mesial wall of each sinus, the gland is in relation with the internal carotid artery, the oculomotor, trochlear, and abducens nerves, and the ophthalmic and maxillary divisions of the trigeminal nerve, all

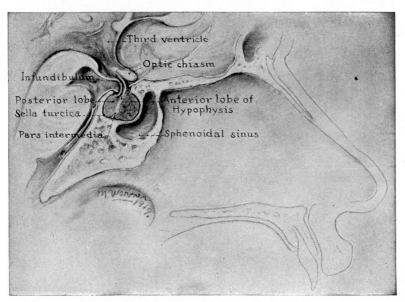

Fig. **39.**—Midsagittal Section of the Hypophysis (Pituitary Gland) with Its Normal Anatomic Relations. (Adson in "Keen's Surgery.")

of which lie within the meshes of the sinus. The complexity of the structures which bound the hypophysis laterally militate against the intracranial temporal approach.

Inferiorly and anteriorly, the hypophysis is in relation with the variable-sized sphenoid sinuses. It is separated from these adnexed nasal cavities, when they are large, only by a thin plate of bone which forms their superior walls. The larger the sinuses, the more extensive are their relations with the gland—an explanation of the tendency of a tumor of the gland to involve the sphenoid sinuses. This involvement indicates that the routes to the gland best adapted to surgical approach are the intranasal, transmaxillary, sphenoid, and transfrontal.

II. SPECIAL SENSES

A. VISUAL APPARATUS

The visual apparatus includes the ocular globe or eyeball and its associated structures: the bony orbits, the palpebrae or eyelids, the lacrimal apparatus, the fascia of the bulb (Tenon's capsule), and the retro-ocular structures.

4

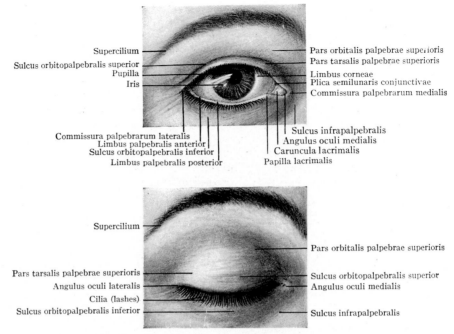

Supercilium
Sulcus orbitopalpebralis superior
Pupilla
Iris

Pars orbitalis palpebrae superioris
Pars tarsalis palpebrae superioris
Limbus corneae
Plica semilunaris conjunctivae
Commissura palpebrarum medialis

Commissura palpebralis lateralis
Limbus palpebralis anterior
Sulcus orbitopalpebralis inferior
Limbus palpebralis posterior

Sulcus infrapalpebralis
Angulus oculi medialis
Caruncula lacrimalis
Papilla lacrimalis

Supercilium

Pars orbitalis palpebrae superioris

Pars tarsalis palpebrae superioris
Angulus oculi lateralis
Cilia (lashes)
Sulcus orbitopalpebralis inferior

Sulcus orbitopalpebralis superior
Angulus oculi medialis

Sulcus infrapalpebralis

FIG. 40.—RIGHT EYE, OPEN AND CLOSED.

(I) ORBITAL REGION

1. Definition and Boundaries.—Each orbit is a deep cavity lateral to the nasal fossae; it is shaped roughly like a quadrilateral pyramid, although its rounded angles liken it somewhat to an irregular cone. The base, measuring about 4 cm. in width and a little less in height, opens on the face; the apex lies at the optic foramen. The orbital capacity more than accommodates the globe and its muscles, vessels, and nerves. The unoccupied intervals contain orbital fat (corpus adiposum orbitae). This fat is differentiated into loculi by fibrous prolongations from the fascia of the bulb (Tenon's capsule) (p. 70).

2. Orbital Margins.—The orbital margins, unlike the fragile and thin walls, are strong and resistant and are not injured easily. The temporal margin recedes too far from the projecting eyeball to afford it adequate protection; hence, eye injuries from blows occur most frequently from the temporal side. The superior margin is prominent and adequately protects the eye above. The mesial rim is less prominent, but protection to the globe is afforded by the bridge of the nose. Knowledge of the minute anatomy of this margin is important in the surgery of the lacrimal sac (p. 60). The entire orbital rim may be likened to a broken circular spring, the broken portion occurring at the mesial edge, where the two ends or crests overlap each other and separate slightly to enclose the lacrimal groove, in which lies the lacrimal sac. The crests are identified readily by palpating along the margins which form them. The anterior lacrimal crest is a continuation of the inferior orbital margin, and is the essential landmark throughout the operation of tear-sac extirpation.

3. Orbital Periosteum.—The lining periosteum, or *periorbita*, is thin but resistant, and is continuous posteriorly with the cranial dura. It is attached loosely to the subjacent bone, from which it may be elevated by pathologic effusions. At the lacrimal groove, the periorbita splits to enclose the lacrimal sac. The layer roofing the groove is the *lacrimal fascia*, and should be recognized in dissection for tear-sac extirpation. About the inferior orbital fissure, a smooth mass of orbital muscle is incorporated into the superficial aspect of the periorbita. This is a vestigial arrangement and is considered an important factor in production of the exophthalmus of Basedow's disease (exophthalmic goiter) (p. 53).

The periosteum at the orbital margin is continued into the eyelids as a membranous septum, fusing in the lower lid with the tarsal plate and in the upper lid with the skin. This *orbital septum* defines the anterior orbital boundary.

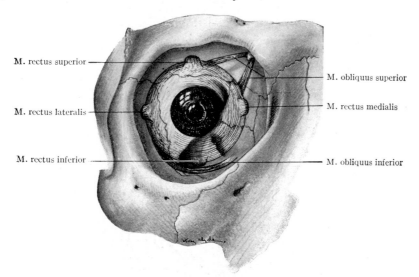

M. rectus superior — — M. obliquus superior

M. rectus lateralis — — M. rectus medialis

M. rectus inferior — — M. obliquus inferior

FIG. 41.—EYEBALL AND ITS RELATION TO THE ORBIT.
The muscles controlling the movements of the globe are indicated; the suture lines in the posterior part of the orbit are projected.

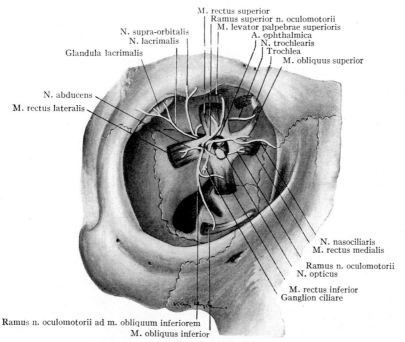

M. rectus superior
Ramus superior n. oculomotorii
M. levator palpebrae superioris
A. ophthalmica
N. trochlearis
Trochlea
M. obliquus superior

N. supra-orbitalis
N. lacrimalis
Glandula lacrimalis

N. abducens
M. rectus lateralis

N. nasociliaris
M. rectus medialis

Ramus n. oculomotorii
N. opticus

M. rectus inferior
Ganglion ciliare

Ramus n. oculomotorii ad m. obliquum inferiorem
M. obliquus inferior

FIG. 42.—POSITION OF THE MUSCLES AND NERVES OF THE ORBIT IN RELATION TO THE OPTIC FORAMEN.

4. Walls of the Orbit.—The *superior wall* or *roof* of the orbit is formed chiefly by the orbital plate of the frontal bone, and posteriorly by the lesser wing of the sphenoid bone. It is part of the floor of the anterior compartment of the cranium and is related to the frontal sinuses. Mesially and anteriorly on the roof is a depression, the trochlear fossa, for the pulley of the superior oblique muscle. The *inferior wall* or *floor* is formed by the orbital plate of the maxilla, the orbital surface of the zygoma, and the orbital process of the palatine bone. Only the thin maxillary wall separates the orbital cavity from the subjacent maxillary sinus. This wall is liable to injury from resection of the maxilla for malignant growths, or to necrosis from inflammation in the underlying sinus. The frail *mesial* wall is in connection with the nasal fossa through the interposed ethmoid labyrinth and sphenoid sinus. Through it, ethmoid disease may extend to the orbit. The mesial wall may be injured by operative manipulation among the ethmoid cells. At the antero-inferior margin of the mesial wall is the lacrimal groove for the lacrimal sac, or dilated end of the nasolacrimal duct, which opens into the inferior nasal meatus (p. 79). The anterosuperior margin of the mesial wall presents the supra-orbital notch or foramen for the transmission of the supra-orbital vessels and nerves. Of the four walls, the *external* is the thickest and most solid, and the only one not in close connection with the paranasal sinuses. By resection of this wall, the contents of the orbit may be approached safely (p. 53).

The *apex* of the orbit is in communication with the cranial cavity through the superior orbital fissure and the optic foramen, the bony channels through which the orbital contents receive their nerve and vascular supply (p. 71). An instrument penetrating the orbit may fracture the walls and be driven into the cranial cavity or into the ethmoid or maxillary sinuses with little external evidence of the seriousness of the lesion.

SURGICAL CONSIDERATIONS

1. **Tumors and Infections of the Orbit.**—*Tumors* of the maxillary sinus readily involve the orbit by invading the superjacent orbital floor. New growths may extend from the nose through the nasolacrimal duct into the orbit or from the brain or cranial cavity through the optic and superior orbital openings. Invasion sometimes occurs by erosion of the bony walls. The retro-ocular space of the orbit may be the site of primary tumor. Failure of the nasal process of the frontal bone to reach that of the maxilla produces a cleft, the site for dermoid tumors which occasionally extend to the dura mater. Either dermoid tumors or meningoceles may occur at the frontonasal suture While removal of a meningocele predisposes to meningitis, excision of a dermoid tumor may be accomplished more safely since it usually has no connection with the cranial meninges.

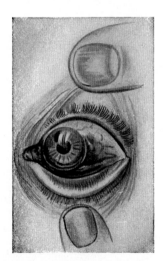

FIG. 43.—SUBCONJUNCTIVAL ECCHYMOSIS.
The hemorrhage in this patient was caused by a slight injury; similar ecchymosis occurs frequently in whooping cough. (Haab.)

The discrepancy between the capacity of the orbit and the bulk of its normal contents accounts for foreign bodies or tumors of an astonishing size remaining unrecognized for long periods of time. Close connection of the orbit with the paranasal sinuses explains orbital infection complicating sinusitis.

2. **Orbital Hemorrhage.**—In violent head contusions with basal skull fractures through the orbital roof, blood may find its way into the orbit and produce subconjunctival pericorneal hemorrhage, which, although not pathognomonic of actual fracture, is an important confirmatory sign. Entrance of blood into the lids is prevented by the intimate attachment of the orbital septum (p. 55).

3. **Orbital Emphysema.**—An orbital fracture which communicates with a paranasal sinus or the nasal fossa allows air to enter the orbit, especially in blowing the nose. The distended lid presents a crackling sensation on palpation (emphysema).

4. **Lateral Temporal Orbital Approach to Retro-ocular Space (Krönlein).**—The greatest diameter of the orbital entrance is transverse and the eyeball, therefore, is farther

from the lateral than from the upper and lower margins of the orbit. Hence, the best mode of approach to the posterior portion of the globe and to the retro-ocular space is through the lateral (temporal) side. After division of the soft parts by a laterally concave incision sufficiently deep to expose the entrance into the orbit, the outer wall is resected. The periosteum is separated from the lateral orbital wall as far as the inferior orbital fissure, which is made the apex for the wedge of orbital wall mobilized. This wedge, with its muscle and cutaneous attachments, is forced backward, giving free access to the contents of the retrobulbar space, still partly covered by periosteum which is split and retracted. If necessary, the external rectus muscle (p. 71) is divided near its tendinous insertion and the dissection is continued to the apex of the orbit. After the surgical maneuvers are carried out, the osteoplastic flap is replaced and the periosteum is sutured.

5. **Intracranial Approach to the Orbit for Orbital Decompression (Naffziger and Jones).**—The operation of decompression of the orbit and the optic foramen was designed to give adequate space for the increased orbital content and the constricted optic nerve in progressive exophthalmus following thyroidectomy. The surgical procedure consists of reflecting bilateral frontal flaps, elevating the dura over the frontal lobe, unroofing the orbit, and removing the superior portion of the optic foramen. Before operation, roentgen studies are made to determine the height and extent of the frontal sinuses and the projection of the ethmoid and the frontal sinuses into the orbital plate. Views of the optic foramina reveal the immediate relationship of the sphenoid sinuses to the orbital plate, so that the operation may be conducted in such a way as not to open these cells.

The frontal bone is exposed by a transverse incision from the temporal fossa on one side, across the frontoparietal region immediately behind the hair line, down to the temporal fossa on the opposite side. The scalp is dissected from the pericranium and is reflected forward, so that the entire frontal bone on both sides is exposed down to the frontal sinus. Bilateral frontal flaps then are fashioned, the hinge of each being the temporal muscle. A small ridge of bone is left in the midline to stabilize these flaps when they are replaced.

Following the reflection of the bone flap, the dura is elevated from the floor of the anterior cranial fossa. The stripping of the dura from the anterior fossa is carried back to the sphenoidal ridge and to the base of the anterior clinoid process. Mesially, the stripping is continued almost to the cribriform plate. The roof of the orbit then is opened and is removed by rongeur. The bone opening is carried anteriorly to the frontal sinus and laterally to the point where the orbital roof merges with the lateral wall of the skull. Posteriorly, it is continued to the sphenoidal ridge. The roof of the optic foramen and its superolateral margin are removed. The orbital contents bulge through the bone opening as it is enlarged. When the bone opening is complete, the orbital fascia is opened.

This approach may be utilized in operative procedures on any of the contents of the retro-ocular space.

(II) PALPEBRAL AND CONJUNCTIVAL REGION

1. **Eyelids.**—The eyelids or palpebrae are upper and lower musculomembranous structures developed in front of the orbit as a protective mechanism to the eyeball. They protect the retina and brain from light which otherwise would create cortical images and maintain cerebral activity. The transverse opening between the free margins of the lids is the palpebral fissure, and the angles formed at the lid junctions are the medial and lateral canthi or commissures. Each lid, in its free margin near the medial canthus, is marked by a small tubercle, the lacrimal papilla, the summit of which presents a punctum, the beginning of the lacrimal drainage system. Both puncta lie in exactly the same vertical line, which relation must be maintained in suturing extensive lacerated wounds of the eyelids. Between the papilla and the rounded margins of the medial canthus is a space, the lacus lacrimalis, on the floor of which is a small, pale-red body, the lacrimal caruncle. The cilia, or eyelashes, are arranged in an irregular line between the lacrimal papilla and the lateral canthus.

The skin of the lids is thin and elastic and is attached loosely to the underlying muscles, partly because of the absence of fat in the subcutaneous tissue. This laxity permits of great distention by effusions, which, however, because of the firm attachment of the skin to the commissures, rarely extend from one lid to the other.

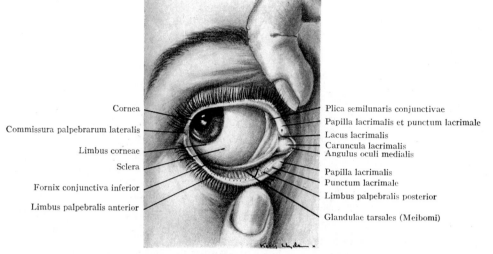

Cornea
Commissura palpebrarum lateralis
Limbus corneae
Sclera
Fornix conjunctiva inferior
Limbus palpebralis anterior

Plica semilunaris conjunctivae
Papilla lacrimalis et punctum lacrimale
Lacus lacrimalis
Caruncula lacrimalis
Angulus oculi medialis
Papilla lacrimalis
Punctum lacrimale
Limbus palpebralis posterior
Glandulae tarsales (Meibomi)

FIG. 44.—SUPERFICIAL STRUCTURES OF THE EYELIDS.

A "black eye" is usually due to local violence causing subcutaneous extravasation of blood into the lids. It also may result from a blow on the skull which causes bleeding into the subepicranial space. The blood, gravitating slowly forward under the frontalis muscle, appears in a day or two in the eyelids, first in the upper lid and then in the lower.

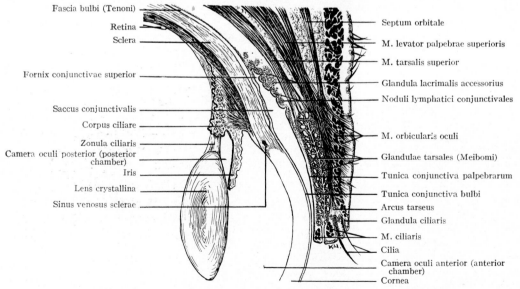

Fascia bulbi (Tenoni)
Retina
Sclera
Fornix conjunctivae superior
Saccus conjunctivalis
Corpus ciliare
Zonula ciliaris
Camera oculi posterior (posterior chamber)
Iris
Lens crystallina
Sinus venosus sclerae

Septum orbitale
M. levator palpebrae superioris
M. tarsalis superior
Glandula lacrimalis accessorius
Noduli lymphatici conjunctivales
M. orbicularis oculi
Glandulae tarsales (Meibomi)
Tunica conjunctiva palpebrarum
Tunica conjunctiva bulbi
Arcus tarseus
Glandula ciliaris
M. ciliaris
Cilia
Camera oculi anterior (anterior chamber)
Cornea

FIG. 45.—PALPEBRAL AND ANTERIOR OCULAR REGIONS IN SAGITTAL SECTION.

Fracture of the orbital plate of the frontal bone causes bleeding into the orbit. The blood tracks forward under the conjunctiva and appears as a triangular flame-shaped hemorrhage, with its apex at the corneal margin.

2. **Structure of the Eyelids.**—The *tarsus* is a thin elongated plate of dense fibrous

tissue which gives each lid its firmness. It is connected with the lateral wall of the orbit by the lateral palpebral raphe or external tarsal ligament, with the medial wall by the medial palpebral or internal tarsal ligament, and with the upper and lower orbital margins by an aponeurotic layer of fibrous tissue known as the orbital septum (orbital ligament, palpebral fascia). In parallel rows in the substance of each tarsus are the tarsal or meibo-

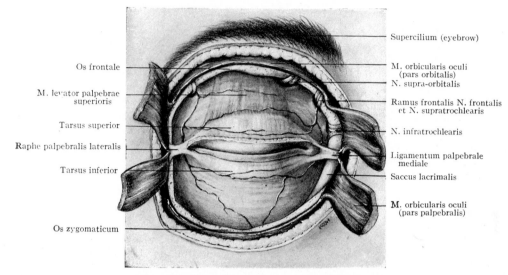

Os frontale

M. levator palpebrae superioris

Tarsus superior

Raphe palpebralis lateralis

Tarsus inferior

Os zygomaticum

Supercilium (eyebrow)

M. orbicularis oculi (pars orbitalis)
N. supra-orbitalis

Ramus frontalis N. frontalis et N. supratrochlearis

N. infratrochlearis

Ligamentum palpebrale mediale

Saccus lacrimalis

M. orbicularis oculi (pars palpebralis)

FIG. 46.—DEEP STRUCTURES OF THE EYELIDS.
The orbicular muscle of the right eyelids is divided and reflected to show the tarsal plates, the orbital septum and the arterial supply.

mian glands, elongated sebaceous glands which open on the free margin of the lid, lubricate it, and prevent the overflow of tears.

The *orbital septum* (p. 51) is a membranous sheet attached peripherally to the periosteum of the orbital margin and centrally to the tarsal plates, thus preventing orbital extravasations from entering the lids. The palpebral portion of the orbicularis muscle overlies it, and to its upper portion, the tendon of the levator palpebrae muscle is fused.

In operations for cataract, the fibers of the lid portion of the orbicularis oculi muscle may be injected with novocain (akinesis), to produce a temporary paresis and prevent "squeezing" of the lids during operation.

The *conjunctiva*, in its tarsal portion, is closely adherent to the tarsal plates, and from them is reflected over the anterior surface of the eyeball to form the bulbar portion. Both above and below, at the point of reflection, there is a loose fold or redundancy forming a culdesac, the conjunctival fornix. The superior fornix sometimes is the seat of trachoma, and always should be examined in trachoma suspects. The bulbar conjunctiva completely covers the eyeball in front and is attached loosely over the sclera. It is so thin that the white of the eye can be seen through it, and because of its elasticity, blood supply, and loose attachment, is ideal for plastic operations.

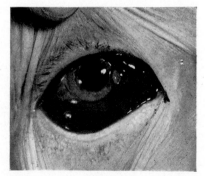

FIG. 47.—SUBCONJUNCTIVAL HEMORRHAGE.
(A. Marfaing, Presbyterian Hospital, New York City.)

3. **Vessels and Nerves.**—The chief *arteries* of the eyelid are the superior and inferior palpebral branches of the ophthalmic artery. They run in loose tissue between the orbicularis muscle and the orbital septum. Laterally, they course from the mesial side of the

orbit, anastomosing with the lacrimal, superficial temporal, and transverse facial arteries, forming an arch in each lid.   The rich vascular anastomoses are of practical importance in the rapid healing of wounds in this region.   The subconjunctival or retrotarsal *veins* drain into the ophthalmic veins.   The *lymphatics* form pretarsal and retrotarsal networks which, for the most part, drain into the pre-auricular and parotid lymph glands.

The chief *motor nerve* of the region is the facial nerve to the orbicularis oculi muscle. It must be preserved since the muscle plays the important sphincter rôle of closing the lids.   In the event of nerve injury, special measures must be taken to prevent desiccation and ulceration of the cornea from nonclosure of the lids.   With central or brain palsy of the nerve root, the orbicularis oculi muscle functions because of its cross-innervation.   The levator palpebrae muscle is supplied by the oculomotor nerve, paralysis of which results in ptosis or inability to lift the lid.

The *sensory innervation* of the lids is derived from the trigeminal nerve through its ophthalmic and maxillary divisions.   The nonstriated fibers of the involuntary palpebral muscle are supplied by the *sympathetic nerves*.   Stimulation of the cervical sympathetic chain causes a contraction in the smooth muscle in the lids, resulting in a slight spreading of the lids or an increase in size of the palpebral fissure.   Resection of the cervical ganglia results in sinking in of the eyeball (enophthalmos), together with a slight ptosis and a contraction of the pupil.   The latter condition is referred to as "Horner's syndrome."

SURGICAL CONSIDERATIONS

1. Common Lid Lesions.—Chronic inflammatory enlargement of the meibomian (tarsal) glands, *chalazion*, is a very common condition which develops in consequence of

Fig. 48.

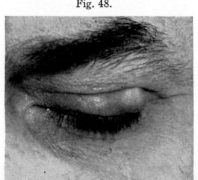

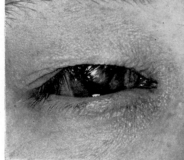
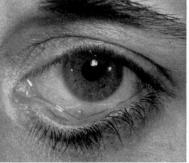

Fig. 49.   Fig. 50.

Fig. 48.—Chalazion of Upper Lid.   (A. Marfaing, Presbyterian Hospital, New York City.)
Fig. 49.—Trichiasis.   (A. Marfaing, Presbyterian Hospital, New York City.)
Fig. 50.—Ectropion.   (A. Marfaing, Presbyterian Hospital, New York City.)

atrophy of the ducts, and often is accompanied by involvement of the surrounding tissues. These lesions show a marked tendency to recurrence in groups.   The affected glands usually are incised and cureted, as complete dissection is difficult.

Drooping of the lid, *ptosis*, is caused by insufficient development or paralysis of the levator palpebrae muscle (p. 71), which, when extreme, disturbs vision by covering the pupil. An attempt is made to raise the lid by forced action of the occipitofrontal muscle, wrinkling the skin of the forehead and raising the brow. When the condition is bilateral, exposure of the pupil is favored by throwing the head backward. Ptosis also occurs in connection with paralysis of other muscles controlled by the oculomotor nerve. Not infrequently, the nerve to the levator palpebrae muscle is injured in removal of tumors from the retro-ocular portion of the orbit (p. 73).

Trichiasis is a distortion of the eyelashes in which they are directed backward instead of forward to the extent that they rub against the cornea, mechanically irritating and injuring it. The condition occurs with contractures of the palpebral conjunctiva and of the tarsal plates in trachoma, and is a complication of entropion.

Entropion is the turning in of the margin of the lid with its lashes, as a result of scar changes in the conjunctiva or tarsal plate or of spasm of the palpebral portion of the orbicular muscle. It occurs usually in the lower lid, and the trichiasis produced irritates and injures the cornea.

Ectropion is an eversion of the lid with more or less exposure and irritation of the palpebral conjunctiva, which becomes hypertrophied and reddened. It results from cicatricial contractions, chronic conjunctivitis, and, in elderly people, from a laxity of the skin and orbicular muscle. An excessive flow of tears (epiphora) aggravates the condition if the eye is wiped downward habitually. In advanced ectropion, the cornea may suffer from exposure occasioned by imperfect approximation of the lids.

Blepharospasm or spasmodic closing of the lids is caused by tonic or clonic contractions of the orbicular sphincter. The tonic form occurs from the irritation of foreign bodies, corneal affections, and local inflammatory conditions, or from any excitation of exposed sensory terminal filaments of the trigeminal nerve. The clonic form is manifested by fibrillary twitching of the palpebral portion of the orbicular muscle, and, although not serious, is annoying and unduly alarming to the patient.

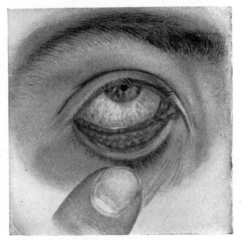

FIG. 51.—TRACHOMA OF THE LOWER LID. There is marked conjunctival congestion. (Haab.)

Bulbar conjunctivitis involves the globe and *tarsal conjunctivitis*, the lids; either may be acute or chronic. The etiology is specific in the gonorrheal and diphtheritic types, but complex and obscure in the chronic type. Treatment is directed largely toward removal of the cause.

Trachoma is a chronic contagious form of conjunctivitis accompanied by conjunctival hypertrophy into follicular masses which undergo cicatricial changes. Adequate and long-continued treatment lessens the menace of conjunctival scar formation. Trachoma in its most chronic form may progress to blindness.

A *symblepharon* is formed by the adherence of two superimposed raw surfaces resulting from destructive change occurring in corresponding parts of the palpebral and ocular conjunctiva. It is caused generally by some caustic substance being introduced into the conjunctival sac between the lid and the globe, but may occur from a postoperative adhesion or from trachoma. It is anterior or partial when it extends like a bridge from the lid to the globe, leaving a free portion of conjunctiva corresponding to the fornix; it is posterior when only the fornix is involved, and complete when all the conjunctiva is affected.

A *pterygium* is a misplaced triangular fold of mucous membrane extending from either the mesial or lateral side of the bulbar conjunctiva to or over the cornea where its apex is attached. The base spreads out and merges with the conjunctiva.

A *hordeolum* or stye is a circumscribed acute inflammation at the margin of the lid, caused by staphylococcic infection of one or more of the sebaceous follicles of the lashes (Zeiss' glands), and usually ends in suppuration.

Fig. 52.

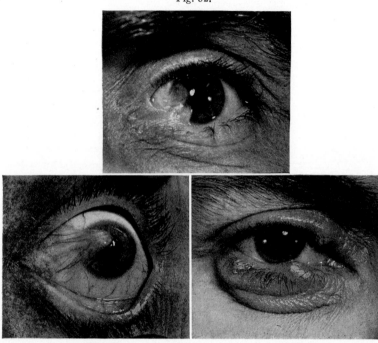

Fig. 53.   Fig. 54.

FIG. 52.—SYMBLEPHARON. (A. Marfaing, Presbyterian Hospital, New York City.)
FIG. 53.—PTERYGIUM. (A. Marfaing, Presbyterian Hospital, New York City.)
FIG 54.—HORDEOLUM (STYE) IN UPPER AND LOWER LIDS. (A. Marfaing, Presbyterian Hospital, New York City.)

Foreign bodies in the conjunctival cavity usually adhere to the subtarsal sulcus of the upper lid and are removed easily after eversion of the lid. Removal of particles striking and lodging in the cornea is more difficult.

(III) LACRIMAL APPARATUS

1. **Definition.**—The lacrimal apparatus is comprised of the lacrimal gland and its intrinsic ducts, the two lacrimal ducts, the lacrimal sac, and the nasolacrimal duct.

2. **Lacrimal Glands and Their Ducts.**—The lacrimal gland is a small oblong body situated in the upper lateral part of the orbit, deep to the upper lid and adherent to the orbital fat lying behind it. The aponeurosis of the levator palpebrae muscle divides it into two parts or lobes, orbital and palpebral.

The *orbital portion* or *superior lacrimal lobe* is the longer and is located in and fixed to a depression in the orbital plate of the frontal bone. Behind, it rests on the outer part of the tendon of the levator palpebrae muscle; in front, it lies against the orbital septum, through which easy access is gained for removal of this portion of the gland.

The *palpebral portion* or *accessory lobe* is much smaller and joins the superior lobe behind. It extends beyond the orbital margin, where it lies mainly on the palpebral conjunctiva to which it is adherent and through which its ducts open. The openings of the ducts of both lobes may be seen by everting the upper lid. The lacrimal secretion is a clear, salty, alkaline fluid, and the gland usually secretes just enough to moisten the eyeball. Psychic stimulation or irritation of the eye or nose increases the flow. The lubrication of the margins of the lids prevents the escape of tears from the conjunctival cavity.

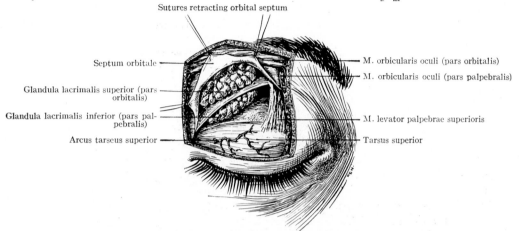

FIG. 55.—DIVISIONS OF THE RIGHT LACRIMAL GLAND.
The right upper lid is dissected and the orbital septum is retracted upward and laterally.

3. Tear Passages.—By movements of the lids, tears are collected into the lacus lacrimalis at the medial angle of the eye. From here, by capillarity, they pass through the two small lacrimal puncta into the lacrimal ducts, and thence into the lacrimal sac. From the sac, they are conveyed into the nasal fossa by the nasolacrimal duct. A lesion in any segment of the lacrimal paths may produce excessive flow of tears (epiphora).

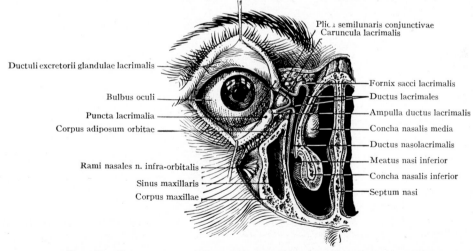

FIG. 56.—DIAGRAM OF THE LACRIMAL PASSAGES EXPOSED FROM THE FRONT.

The *lacrimal puncta*, one on each lid, are minute orifices leading into the two small *lacrimal ducts* or canals. These canals, each about 1 cm. long, run in the skin mesial to the posterior external wall of the lacrimal sac, into which they empty through a common canal which is covered by the mesial palpebral ligament.

The *lacrimal sac*, 1 to 1.5 cm. in length, is the expanded upper part of the tear passage lying at the medial margin of the orbital septum. It is roofed completely by a specialized layer of periorbita, the fascia lacrimalis. The mesial palpebral ligament and the inner tendon of the orbicularis oculi muscle lie in front of and against it, dividing it into two portions, one above and one below. The lower part, which is accessible surgically, may become distended and bulge forward. The landmarks for the location of the sac are the mesial palpebral ligament and the anterior lacrimal crest, which are brought into relief by drawing the lids laterally. Since the sac lies in a fossa of the lacrimal bone in intimate relation with the anterior ethmoid cells, inflammation of the sac, dacryocystitis, may follow upon or cause ethmoiditis.

The *nasolacrimal duct* is the downward continuation of the lacrimal sac, draining the tears into the inferior nasal meatus about 1 cm. behind the anterior tip of the inferior turbinate bone (p. 79). It is contained in a bony canal formed largely by the maxilla, which brings it into close relation with the maxillary sinus. Continuity of the duct and nasal mucous membrane explains the frequency of disease extending from the nose to the lacrimal passages.

Surgical Considerations

1. Dacryocystitis.—Disease of the lacrimal gland itself is rare, but involvement of the tear-conducting passages (dacryocystitis) is common. The cause of inflammation of the tear sac usually is obstruction in the nasolacrimal duct, the consequence of infection in the nasal fossa or paranasal sinuses. Epiphora or increased lacrimation is a prominent symptom in all diseases of the tear-conducting apparatus. It may be caused by foreign bodies, conjunctivitis, irritating vapors, or nasal disease.

2. Probing of the Lacrimal Passages; Extirpation of the Sac.—The normal lacrimal duct admits a probe, 3.5 mm. in diameter, which is passed mesially through the lower punctum. When it reaches the medial wall of the sac, which is recognized by the resistance offered by the lacrimal bone, the probe is raised so that its lower end is directed toward the sulcus between the nose and the cheek, and is pushed gently downward until it enters the nose. Should this measure fail to relieve long-standing obstruction, a more radical course is advised, such as extirpation of the lacrimal sac, or establishment of a communication between the sac and the middle nasal meatus (dacryocystorhinostomia or Toti's operation).

For the extirpation of the lacrimal sac, an incision about 2 cm. long is made through the skin and underlying tissue along the anterior orbital margin inferior to the mesial palpebral ligament. When the sac is exposed, it is separated from the periosteum of the lacrimal fossa, the upper extremity is freed, the ducts are divided, and the sac is excised as low as possible in the nasolacrimal duct.

(IV) Ocular Globe

The ocular globe or eyeball, with its wall and contents, occupies that part of the orbit anterior to Tenon's capsule (fascia of the bulb). The wall is made up of three concentric membranes. The external or fibrous membrane is the sclera, transformed in front into the transparent cornea. The middle or vascular layer is the choroid, differentiated anteriorly into the ciliary body and a muscular diaphragm, the iris. The inner or nerve layer, the retina, is differentiated highly over the posterior part of the globe.

The contents of the globe are the transparent media of the eye, which are: the crystalline lens directly behind the iris, the cornea, the aqueous humor filling the space between the lens and the cornea, and the vitreous humor between the lens and the retina. These refracting media are so constituted and placed that normally they converge rays to a focus on the retina.

Focusing depends upon the depth of the anteroposterior diameter of the eyeball and the distance traveled by the rays reaching the retina. Under abnormal conditions, the anteroposterior diameter of the eye may be lengthened or shortened. When shortened, the refractive media are incapable of sufficient convergence and the rays reach a focus behind the retina. This constitutes the hypermetropic eye. To bring about a retinal focus, the converging apparatus must be supplemented by a convex lens. When the antero-posterior diameter is greater than normal, the rays come to focus in front of the retina, constituting the myopic eye. The refractive media in this condition overconverge and require a concave lens to lessen the convergence and to bring the focus on the retina.

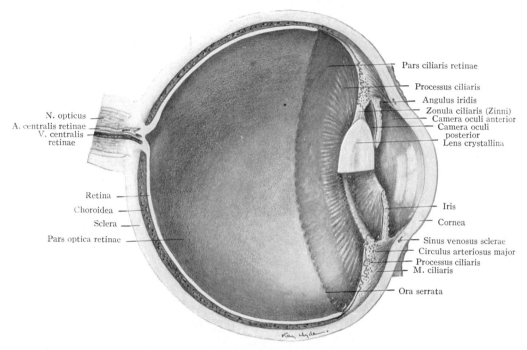

FIG. 57.—OCULAR GLOBE IN SAGITTAL SECTION.

(A) WALLS OR TUNICS OF THE GLOBE

1. **Fibrous or Sclerocorneal Tunic.**—The sclera behind and its specialized cornea in front constitute the outer tunic of the globe. The **sclera** is a thick, resistant, nondistensible membrane, thickest posteriorly, giving form to the eye and affording attachment to the ocular muscles. The "white of the eye" is the anterior portion of the sclera seen through the transparent ocular conjunctiva. Rupture of the eyeball usually occurs where the sclera is thinnest, near the sclerocorneal junction.

Where the optic nerve penetrates the globe, the fibrous sheath of the nerve blends with the outer part of the sclera. The sclera is pierced for the passage of the nerve bundles, creating a sievelike portion designated the *lamina cribrosa*. About the entrance of the nerve are several minute openings carrying the ciliary nerves and arteries. The *ciliary arteries* are derived from the numerous posterior ciliary branches of the ophthalmic artery. The long ciliary branches run forward between the choroid and the sclera to supply the iris and ciliary region, and the short ciliary arteries terminate in the choroid. The *veins* converge to form four or five main trunks, the venae vorticosae, which pierce and leave the sclera midway between the cornea and the optic nerve to join the ophthalmic veins.

The **cornea** is continuous with the opaque sclera and, although made up of the same connective tissue, is transparent. It forms the anterior fifth or sixth of the fibrous tunic of the globe and is thinnest in the center and thickest at the periphery. It contains no trace of blood vessels save at its extreme periphery, and, when inflamed, becomes opaque. Vascularizations, such as occur after the healing of ulcers or wounds, are likely to cause opacity. The line of junction between the cornea and sclera is the *limbus*, close to which incisions are made for operations on the structures directly posterior, the iris and lens. The *posterior lamina* of the cornea (Descemet's membrane) is a thin, highly elastic layer behind the proper substance of the cornea.   At the sclerocorneal junction, this membrane splits into bundles of fine interlacing fibers which form the *pectinate ligament*, connecting the sclera with the root of the iris.   The spaces between these trabeculated bundles are known as the *spaces of the angle of the iris* (spaces of Fontana).   They are lined with endothelium prolonged from the endothelium of the anterior chamber of the globe (Descemet's membrane).   Anterior to the sclerocorneal junction in the sclerocorneal layer is the *venous sinus of the sclera* (canal of Schlemm).

That area of the anterior chamber, where the sclerocorneal margin, iris, and pectinate ligament meet, is the filtration angle of the iris, often called the *iris angle* or *iridocorneal*

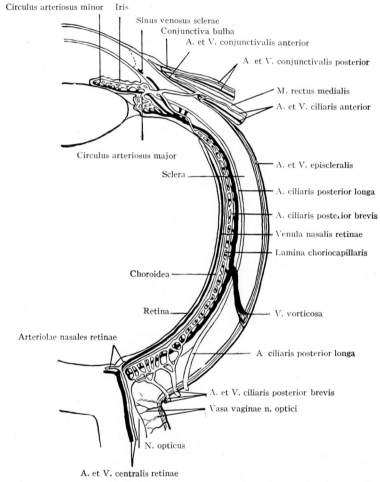

Circulus arteriosus minor   Iris
Sinus venosus sclerae
Conjunctiva bulba
A. et V. conjunctivalis anterior
A et V. conjunctivalis posterior
M. rectus medialis
A. et V. ciliaris anterior
Circulus arteriosus major
Sclera
A. et V. episcleralis
A. ciliaris posterior longa
A. ciliaris posterior brevis
Venula nasalis retinae
Lamina choriocapillaris
Choroidea
Retina
V. vorticosa
Arteriolae nasales retinae
A ciliaris posterior longa
A. et V. ciliaris posterior brevis
Vasa vaginae n. optici
N. opticus
A. et V. centralis retinae

Fig. 58.—Vascular Supply of the Ocular Globe.   (After Th. Leber.)

angle.   It forms the principal exit for the intra-ocular fluids, and its blockage causes their retention.   The normal flow of intra-ocular fluid is from the anterior chamber to the venous sinus of the sclera by filtration through the spaces of the iris angle and thence into the anterior ciliary veins.   Blockage of the iris angle is a consequence of embarrassment in the circulation between the anterior and posterior aqueous chambers or of pushing forward of the vitreous chamber and lens with venous congestion, subsequent swelling of the ciliary body, and pushing of the periphery of the iris against the sclerocorneal junction.

In *glaucoma*, a condition marked by increased intra-ocular pressure, the added tension depends upon a disturbed relationship between intra-ocular secretion and excretion. The obstruction to the escape of intra-ocular fluid is thought to be effected at the angle of the anterior chamber (iris angle) by pressure of the peripheral portion of the iris and of the congested and swollen ciliary processes against the sclerocorneal junction. Later, it may be caused by an adhesive inflammation of the opposed surfaces with proliferation of the endothelium of Descemet's membrane and that of the iris.

2. **Vascular or Irido-ciliary-choroidal Tunic (Uveal Tract).**—The irido-ciliary-choroidal layer is composed of the iris, ciliary body, and choroid, and extends from the pupil to the optic nerve. The choroid and ciliary portions are in contact with the sclera, while their termination, the iris, turns sharply inward and floats in the aqueous humor between the cornea and lens. It divides the space in front of the lens unequally into the anterior and posterior chambers (cameras) of the eye.

The **choroid** is the part of the uveal tract lining the posterior portion of the eye. It is the nourishing tunic, comprised essentially of blood vessels. These vessels are visible in ophthalmoscopic examination in very blond individuals with transparent retinae. They produce the red background in the fundus of the eye, against which the retinal vessels stand out in bold relief. Diseases of the circulatory system, particularly syphilis and arteriosclerosis, often are manifested in the choroid. The presence of pigment cells in this layer gives rise to the pigmented melanosarcoma.

The **ciliary body** connects the choroid to the circumference of the iris. The line of junction between it and the retina anteriorly is the *ora serrata*, in front of which arise the ciliary processes, about 70 in number. Suspensory ligaments are attached to these meridional processes and to the periphery of the lens. When the ciliary muscle contracts, it draws its processes and the choroid forward, thus relaxing the ligament suspending the lens, allowing the lens to bulge and assume a more convex shape. This relaxation and contraction controls the convexity of the lens and, therefore, its refracting power, making it the chief agent in accommodation.

The **iris** is the anterior segment of the vascular tunic and is visible through the cornea. It is a thin, delicate, contractile membrane placed as a circular diaphragm in front of the lens, presenting an aperture of variable size called the *pupil*. This membrane partially divides the space between the lens and cornea into two parts, the *anterior* and *posterior chambers* (cameras) of the eye, which are filled by aqueous humor. The unstriped muscle fibers of the iris are arranged in two sets, a circular sphincter set, contraction of which narrows the pupil, and a radial set which dilates it. The pupillary margin of the iris lies on the anterior capsule of the lens, from which it derives much support.

When completely dilated, the iris hangs free in the space in front of the lens. Action of the dilator and sphincter muscles regulates the amount of light admitted to the interior of the eye and cuts off the marginal rays which otherwise interfere with the sharpness of the retinal image. The sphincters are supplied by the *oculomotor nerve* and the dilators by the *sympathetic nerves*. The pigment cells of the iris give it color.

The peripheral margin of the iris is derived from the anterolateral portion of the ciliary body, and is attached in front to the cornea by the pectinate ligament. The iris is torn easily from this origin and attachment (*iridodialysis*) by trauma to the globe. The iris frequently protrudes through perforating wounds of the cornea and excision of the prolapsed piece (*iridectomy*) is necessary.

The vascularity of the iris renders it peculiarly liable to inflammatory changes, and infection readily spreads to it through its attachments. Since the iris and choroid are part of the same vascular membrane, inflammation set up in the choroid tends to involve the iris. Inflammatory changes cause the membrane to become swollen and the pupil small and sometimes covered by exudate (*occlusio pupillae*). With the pupillary margins in actual contact with the lens capsule, and especially in severe iritis, adhesions may form between the opposed parts (*posterior synechia*). If the synechia formation is extensive, it may seal the pupil completely posteriorly, thereby blocking the only communication between the posterior and anterior chambers and leading directly to a rise in intra-ocular tension (*secondary glaucoma*). An adhesion between the iris and the cornea is an *anterior synechia*.

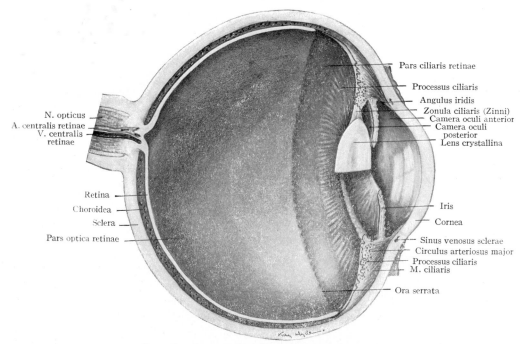

Pars ciliaris retinae

Processus ciliaris

Angulus iridis

Zonula ciliaris (Zinni)

Camera oculi anterior

Camera oculi posterior

Lens crystallina

N. opticus

A. centralis retinae

V. centralis retinae

Iris

Cornea

Sinus venosus sclerae

Circulus arteriosus major

Processus ciliaris

M. ciliaris

Retina

Choroidea

Sclera

Pars optica retinae

Ora serrata

FIG. 59.—OCULAR GLOBE IN SAGITTAL SECTION.

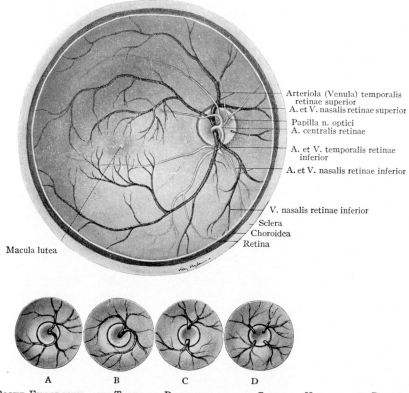

Arteriola (Venula) temporalis retinae superior

A. et V. nasalis retinae superior

Papilla n. optici

A. centralis retinae

A. et V. temporalis retinae inferior

A. et V. nasalis retinae inferior

V. nasalis retinae inferior

Sclera

Choroidea

Retina

Macula lutea

A   B   C   D

FIG. 60.—NORMAL RIGHT EYEGROUND AND TYPES OF BRANCHES OF THE CENTRAL VEIN OF THE RETINA.
A, Bifurcation of the retinal vein at the center of the optic disk. B, Bifurcation at the margin of the disk. C, Bifurcation before emerging from the disk. D, Branching of the central vein of the retina before emerging from the optic disk. (After Testut and Jacob.)

3. Retinal or Nerve Tunic.—The retina is an extension and expansion of the fibers of the optic nerve into a specialized apparatus for the reception of visual stimuli. It lies between the membrane containing the vitreous humor (hyaloid membrane) internally and the choroid externally, and extends forward almost to the ciliary body where it presents a wavy line, the *ora serrata*. Beyond this line, the membrane loses its nerve cells, becomes thin, and is extended to the ciliary body. It is unattached to the choroid save at the entrance of the optic nerve and at the ora serrata, which accounts for its easy separation from the choroid in severe trauma to the head, in intra-ocular tumors, and in diseases of the vitreous body. The retina is transparent under normal conditions because the optic nerve fibers composing it lose their opaque myelin coverings on entering the ocular globe. This transparency prevents its visibility, but renders visible the subjacent vascular choroid, seen as the red background of the eye in ophthalmoscopic examination.

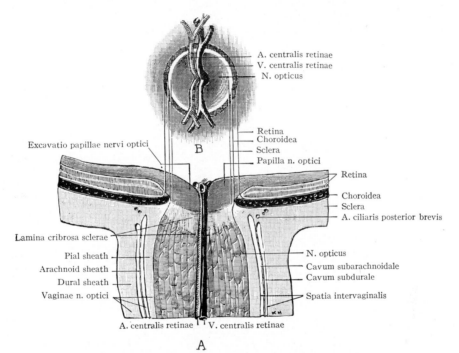

Fig. 61.—Diagram of the Optic Disk or Papilla to Correlate Its Structures with Ophthalmoscopic Findings.

A, Sagittal section through the optic nerve at its entrance into the eyeball; B, structures seen on sagittal section projected on the disk as viewed ophthalmoscopically. (After Testut and Jacob.)

In the retina, there are three intrinsic elements of the greatest clinical and pathologic importance, since in and about them the most important lesions in the background of the eye develop. These are the vessels of the retina, the point of entrance of the optic nerve (optic disk), and the point of clearest vision (macula). Their observation is the cardinal object of ophthalmoscopic examination.

The *central artery* of the *retina*, a branch of the ophthalmic artery, is not in direct communication with collateral vessels except at the entrance of the optic nerve. Accompanied by corresponding veins, it pierces the optic nerve about 2 cm. from the globe and runs within it to enter the retina about the middle of the optic disk. The branches of the artery are terminal, and permanent plugging of the parent trunk brings about extinction of the retinal arterial system, resulting in complete blindness. On reaching the retina, the artery divides into ascending and descending branches of variable number, shape, and location. These vessels, on account of the transparency of the retina, are perfectly

5

visible through the ophthalmoscope.   The opportunity of studying blood vessels *in situ* with adequate illumination under ideal optical conditions is offered nowhere else in the body.   Each artery presents a double outline, appearing as two bold red lines separated by a lighter interval.

The *veins* are broader and more homogeneous than the arteries.   They empty into the ophthalmic veins which, in the retro-orbital region, form the cavernous sinus (p. 32). Engorgement of these veins naturally occurs in venous stasis accompanying increased intracranial pressure.   Lesions of the retinal vessels are manifested by retinal hemorrhages and sclerotic changes in the vessels themselves.

About 3 mm. to the inner side of the posterior part of the eye is a conspicuous, pale, round, opaque area, the *optic disk* or *papilla*, which marks the entrance of the optic nerve into the eyeball.   The term "papilla" was given by early authors under the erroneous impression that it represented a projection into the interior of the eye.   In the normal state, it is flat, lying in the same plane as the retina, or having a central or eccentric depression.   This depression, the *physiologic cup* or excavation, marks the point of divergence

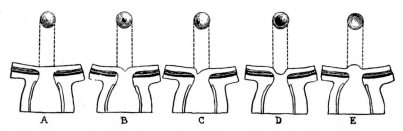

Fig. 62.—Variations in the Contour of the Optic Disk as Seen in Sagittal Sections.

The variations in contour are projected into ophthalmoscopic images. A, Flat disk (within physiologic limits). B, Central depression or cupping (within physiologic limits). C, Eccentric depression (within physiologic limits). D, Excavation (seen in glaucomatous conditions). E, Protrusion (seen in increased intracranial pressure). (Testut and Jacob.)

of the entering optic nerve fibers and is the common entry of the retinal vessels.   Gray dots in its depth indicate lacunae in the lamina cribrosa (p. 61), through which the separate funiculi of the optic nerve enter.   While the nerve fibers normally lose their myelin sheaths before passing through the lamina cribrosa, the presence of myelinated fibers about the disk is not unusual.   They have the appearance of glaring white tufts of cotton   The normal level of the optic disk is swollen and elevated in choked disk and optic neuritis, and depressed in nerve atrophy and glaucoma.

In the axis of the globe, the surface of the retina presents a yellow spot, the *macula lutea*, or area of most distinct vision.   It is about 1 to 2 mm. in diameter and has in its center a small depression, the *fovea centralis*, or spot of most distinct vision.   Lesions in this locality are serious, bringing about loss of central vision.

SURGICAL CONSIDERATIONS

1. **Inflammation, Staphyloma, and Rupture of the Sclera.**—Inflammation of the sclera may be superficial or deep.   If deep, it may extend to subjacent and contiguous parts and cause a thinning of the wall and bulging of the sclera, resulting in *scleral staphyloma*.   When the globe is *ruptured* by violence, the scleral coat usually yields and rents occur in the thinnest portion a little behind the cornea.   The sclera sometimes is ruptured when the conjunctiva remains intact, and the lens may escape through the subconjunctival rent.

2. **Diseases of the Cornea.**—Inflammation of the cornea, *keratitis*, may be superficial or deep, involving only the epithelium on the anterior or free surface, or involving the corneal tissue proper.   In interstitial keratitis, the numerous laminae of the cornea and their freely anastomosing lymph channels are affected, with resulting effusion into the

lymph vessels and consequent haziness and loss of transparency. This haziness may or may not be followed by complete resorption; permanent opacity results when resorption fails.

A *corneal ulcer* is caused by infection of a portion of the cornea followed by suppuration and loss of substance of the tissue involved. Connective tissue repair of deep ulcers produces a scar and consequent *opacity*. The opacity following corneal ulcers or wounds may resemble a puff of smoke (*nebula*), or be pearly-white (*leukoma*). A deep ulcer sometimes gives rise to inflammation in the conjunctiva and iris; a virulent process may destroy the eye.

Arcus senilis is an opaque, whitish ring or crescent, appearing at the periphery of the cornea within the sclerocorneal junction, usually in people of advanced age. It results probably from fatty degeneration of the corneal tissue, the changes occurring in the layers just deep to the anterior elastic membrane.

Since the cornea is a segment of a flattened sphere (ellipsoid), there is a slight difference in the refraction of the two principal meridians, the vertical curvature being greater than the horizontal. *Astigmatism* is a condition of the eye in which the refraction from these diameters or meridians varies considerably because of changes or differences in the curvature of the cornea, with or without shortening or lengthening of the anteroposterior diameter of the eyeball. It is, as a rule, congenital, but may be acquired from corneal changes produced by inflammation, injury, or operation.

3. **Diseases of the Iris.**—Inflammation of the iris from any one of a variety of infections, including syphilis and tuberculosis, is associated so frequently with inflammation of the ciliary body that most cases called iritis really are *iridocyclitis*. The iris, when inflamed, appears dull and swollen, and the pupil small, irregular, and sluggish in its reaction to light; there may be pus in the aqueous chamber, a lesion which is called *hypopyon*. As a consequence of this infection, adhesions between the iris and the lens capsule (synechia) (p. 63) may develop.

4. **Lesions of the Ciliary Body and Uveitis.**—The conception of the choroid, ciliary body, and iris constituting a continuous vascular tunic, the uveal tract, explains why an inflammation of the individual elements frequently involves the whole tract, *uveitis*. Inflammation of the ciliary body, *cyclitis*, when combined with infection of the iris, is *iridocyclitis*.

Since the ciliary region is an extensive vascular anastomotic area about the cornea, infections can pass directly from the ciliary region to the other elements of the eye, particularly the vitreous humor. An acute purulent cyclitis occurring immediately after injury may involve all the structures of the eye (*panophthalmitis*), and the eye must be enucleated at once so that the other eye may not become infected. Chronic plastic iridocyclitis in one eye sometimes causes destructive inflammation in the sound eye (*sympathetic ophthalmia*). A blind, shrunken eye, resulting either from injury or operation, should be enucleated to preclude the development of the same dread complication.

5. **Diseases of the Choroid.**—In many instances, disease involving the choroid affects the retinal coats, *chorioretinitis*. In exudative *choroiditis*, the decrease in the field of vision is in proportion to the extent of the exudative process. Absorption of the exudate leaves patches of choroidal atrophy, evidenced by white areas where the sclera shows through. Central vision is unimpaired if the macula escapes. If a retinal vessel passes unchanged through a patch of exudate, the destructive process probably has occurred in the choroid; if the outline of the vessel is blurred, the lesion is in the retina, *retinitis*.

6. **Inflammation of the Retina.**—All the objective evidences of inflammation of the retina are ophthalmoscopic; there are no external signs. Diminished visual acuity may result and perception be inaccurate as to the size and shape of objects, things appearing smaller than they really are, *micropsia*, or larger than normal, *macropsia*. Ophthalmoscopic examination reveals whitish or pigmented patches which represent retinal exudate and hemorrhage.

The optic disk, the extension and only exposed region of the brain, is studied ophthal moscopically for evidence of pathologic change in the brain proper. In inflammation of the disk, *optic neuritis* or *papillitis*, the nerve head presents characteristic signs. In addition to or independent of inflammatory signs, a marked edema of the disk may appear so that the swollen nerve head protrudes into the vitreous, a condition of *choked disk*, or *papilledema*. Full-blown papilledema, and the gradations leading to this condition, offer important evidence of increased intracranial pressure and are present in such intracranial disturbances as abscess, hydrocephalus, aneurysm, and brain tumor. The recognition of optic atrophy is important from the visual standpoint and from the underlying systemic disease. Frequently, glaucoma is unsuspected until discovered by ophthalmoscopic examination.

7. **Detachment of the Retina.**—The retina not infrequently is torn as a result of trauma, and the resulting detachment causes blindness in the corresponding field of vision. The operation to reattach the retina opens a new field in ophthalmic surgery, and offers a chance for permanent cure of a condition heretofore incurable. Multiple electropunctures of the sclera are made, each of which results in a minute focus of exudative choroiditis. Adhesions then develop which bind the previously separated retina to the choroid. The amount of restitution of vision depends on the condition of the retina before detachment, and upon the duration of the detachment.

(B) TRANSPARENT OR REFRACTING MEDIA

In addition to the cornea, the media which focus the rays entering the pupil are the aqueous and vitreous humors and the muscle-controlled lens suspended between them.

1. **Anterior or Aqueous Chamber and the Aqueous Humor.**—The space between the cornea and lens, the anterior compartment of the eye, is filled with transparent aqueous humor. The iris diaphragm subdivides this space into anterior and posterior cameras: that between the iris and cornea, the anterior; that between the iris and lens with its suspensory ligament, the posterior. With the iris in actual contact with the lens, the posterior camera is only an angular interval, triangular in cross section, between the iris, ciliary processes, suspensory ligament of the lens, and the lens periphery. The chambers communicate by the pupillary orifice.

The mode of formation of the aqueous humor and its manner of filtration are exceedingly important in relation to ocular tension (p. 62). This transparent fluid is secreted into the aqueous space by blood vessels of the ciliary processes. The collection of excess aqueous fluid is absorbed into the *iris angle spaces* (of Fontana) in the pectinate ligament, and from there filters into the circular venous sinus of the sclera (*canal of Schlemm*) (p. 62). Through the canal of Schlemm and the ciliary veins anastomosing with it, the aqueous humor leaves the eye. The required or physiologic tension in the globe probably is maintained by regulation of secretion and absorption of the fluid.

Obstruction to the filtration space about this angle renders escape of fluid difficult and brings about the grave accidents consequent upon increased intra-ocular tension. When the pupil is dilated, the periphery of the iris tends to encroach on the iris angle and render fluid passage difficult. Giving a pupil-dilating drug, such as atropine, in conditions of increased tension may precipitate glaucoma.

2. **Posterior or Vitreous Chamber and the Vitreous Humor.**—The vitreous body is a transparent substance composed of semisolid connective tissue which occupies the vitreous compartment of the eye, the posterior four-fifths of the bulb. The vitreous body rarely is involved by ocular disease, but may be affected secondarily by inflammation in adjacent parts. Its connective tissue cells occasionally produce shadows on the retina, *muscae volitantes*.

3. **Crystalline Lens.**—The most important refracting medium of the eye, the crystalline lens, lies between the iris and the vitreous body, and separates the aqueous and vitreous cavities. It is a biconvex, transparent, colorless body enclosed by a thin, transparent hyaloid capsule, and lies within the circle formed by the ciliary processes, where it is held in position by its suspensory ligament. The convex surfaces, particularly the anterior,

are constantly changing to aid in the focusing of rays from near or distant objects upon the retina.

The substance of the lens is seen best in elderly subjects in whom the lens nucleus takes on a change of color and consistency, clearly differentiating it from the cortical substance. The resulting gray reflex must not be confused with cataract. The sclerosing process begins in childhood, and, at about the age of twenty-five, a distinct nucleus is visible. After sixty years, the lens becomes almost entirely nucleus. The inability of the sclerotic lens of middle life to change its shape accounts for the loss of the power of accommodation.

The circumference of the lens is fixed to the extremities of the ciliary processes by a system of fine transparent radial fibers, the *suspensory ligament* or *ciliary zonule*. The lens is subject to injuries, dislocations, and senile changes.

The function of the lens is performed by virtue of its elastic structure, whereby the convexity of its surfaces is changed promptly so that the rays are focused to form a perfect image on the retina. The ability of a lens to change its refractive power for objects at

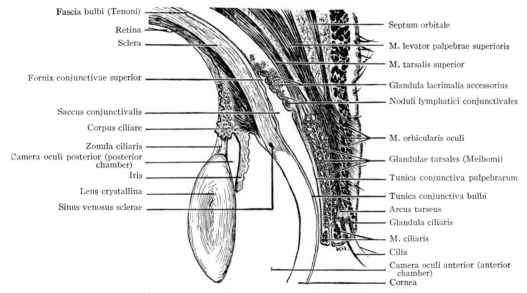

FIG. 63.—PALPEBRAL AND ANTERIOR OCULAR REGIONS IN SAGITTAL SECTION.

various distances is the *power of accommodation*. The change in the shape of the lens, affecting its anterior curvature chiefly, is produced by the action of the ciliary muscle tensing or relaxing the ciliary processes to which the suspensory ligament is attached. The ciliary muscle, by pulling the ciliary processes and the attached ciliary zonule forward, relaxes the ligament and allows the lens to become more convex. Loss of elasticity in the lens reduces the power of accommodation, a condition termed *presbyopia*. With changes in the lens in middle age, power of accommodation is insufficient to permit of exact vision, and the patient is obliged to supplement the diminished power with convex lenses. In *hypermetropia*, in which the eyeball is short and rays attain their natural focus behind the retina, effort of accommodation of the lens must be exerted continually to bring about retinal focus and clear vision. This accounts for the symptoms of eye strain so prevalent in uncorrected hyperopia.

Errors in refraction, particularly astigmatism, are responsible for a great variety of symptoms usually referred to the head. They are relieved, for the most part, by corrective lenses, together with suitable medical measures. It cannot be emphasized too strongly that refraction is essentially a medical problem.

Surgical Considerations

1. Injuries to the Lens.—The lens is loosened and displaced easily from the suspensory ligament and may make its way anteriorly into the aqueous compartment or posteriorly into the vitreous. The lens, if displaced into the aqueous humor, may be removed through a corneal incision. If dislocation takes place into the vitreous humor, glaucoma usually ensues. In scleral rupture, the lens may escape from the globe and lie just deep to the conjunctiva.

2. Cataract.—When the lens capsule is wounded, aqueous humor is imbibed by the lens fibers which, in consequence, swell and become opaque, forming a traumatic cataract. In cataract of any etiology, some portion of the lens or all of it becomes the seat of opacity. Location of the opacity in either the *cortical* or *nuclear* substance establishes one basis for cataract classification.

(V) Tenon's Capsule (Fascia of the Bulb)

1. Fascia of the Bulb.—The fascia of the bulb, or Tenon's capsule, is a loose frontally disposed membrane, surrounding the posterior part of the eyeball, so placed as to partition the globe from the rest of the orbit. It is derived from the connective tissue of the structures of the orbit and from the periosteum about the orbital margin. It furnishes tubular sheaths to the orbital muscles as they attach to the globe, separates the globe from the orbital fat, and forms an articular socket which permits free movement of the eyeball.

The surgical importance of the fascia lies in its action as a barrier to the spread of infection or hemorrhage between the eyeball and the retro-ocular space, and its efficacy as a socket for a prosthesis (artificial eye) after enucleation of the eyeball.

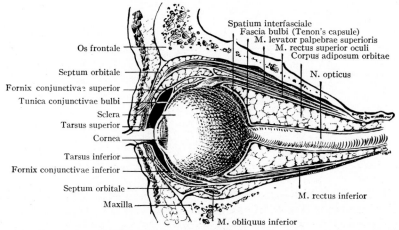

FIG. 64.—Diagrammatic Sagittal Section Through the Orbit to Show the Fascia of the Bulb (Tenon's Capsule).

2. Fascial Expansions.—Where the internal and external rectus muscles perforate the fascia, strong capsular expansions spread to the inner and outer walls of the orbit, limiting the play of the recti muscles and acting as *inner* and *outer check ligaments*. The check ligaments are important surgically in that they limit the retraction of the muscles after tenotomy, or after section in enucleation of the eyeball. That part of the fascia below the bulb is slung like a hammock from side to side of the orbit as a *suspensory ligament;* its extremities are fixed to the lacrimal and zygomatic bones. In resection of the maxilla, the attachments of the suspensory ligament should be maintained to keep the eyeball in position.

The intimate relation between Tenon's capsule and the ocular muscles must be borne in mind in muscle operations to correct *strabismus* (squint). Even when an ocular muscle tendon is severed at the scleral attachment, it still exerts an action on the globe through its attachment to Tenon's capsule and its capsular prolongation.

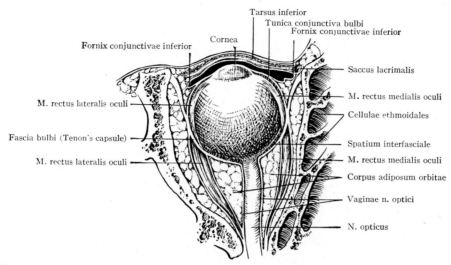

FIG. 65.—DIAGRAMMATIC CROSS SECTION THROUGH THE ORBIT TO SHOW TENON'S CAPSULE.

(VI) RETROBULBAR OR RETRO-OCULAR SPACE

The retrobulbar space lies behind the fascia of the bulb and contains the eye muscles which, with the exception of the inferior oblique, take their origin from the orbital bone and the periosteum near the optic foramen. It also contains the ocular vessels and nerves lying close together in the semifluid fat and the connective tissue which abounds here.

1. **Action of the Eye Muscles.**—The eye is *adducted* by the action of the internal rectus muscle, assisted toward the end of its course by the superior and inferior recti. It is *abducted* by the external rectus muscle, reinforced toward the end of the course by the two oblique muscles, and *elevated* by the superior rectus and inferior oblique. The superior rectus muscle acting alone carries the eye upward and a little medially. The inferior rectus muscle acting alone *depresses* the globe and carries it a little inward; the superior oblique muscle acting alone carries it downward and a little outward; their combined action carries the globe straight downward. The main purpose of the neuromuscular mechanism of the eye is to secure binocular fixation, and actions of the eyes therefore are correlated so that there are no interfering movements.

The *levator palpebrae muscle* inserts mainly into the tarsal plate of the upper lid. This muscle raises the lid, thereby widening the palpebral fissure, and acts in apposition to the orbicularis oculi muscle which closes it.

The four *recti muscles* attach to the sclera behind the cornea and are fused to the fascia of the bulb, which they pierce. Advancement and resection of the muscles are practiced commonly to cure strabismus, section of the scleral and fascial attachments being complete or incomplete according to the degree of muscle action required.

2. **Vessels and Nerves of the Orbit.**—The **ophthalmic artery,** a branch of the internal carotid, supplies all the contents of the orbit. The terminal ophthalmic branches, the *supra-orbital, frontal,* and *nasociliary arteries,* supply the palpebral and nasal regions of the face. The ophthalmic artery emerges from the cranial cavity through the optic foramen. Early in its course, it gives off the *central artery of the retina,* and later, the two posterior long and several short *ciliary arteries* near the entrance of the nerve into the sclera (p. 61).

The **orbital veins** gradually converge as they pass backward into the orbit where they form the *superior* and *inferior ophthalmic trunks,* which usually unite before leaving the orbit by way of the superior orbital fissure to empty into the cavernous sinus (p 32). The anastomoses which the superior orbital vein forms with the supra-orbital and angular veins of the face are of great practical importance because through them infections of the face, especially about the upper lip and nose, are carried readily to the orbit, cavernous sinus, and brain.

The **orbital nerves** include the optic nerve, the motor nerves to the eye muscles, and the sensory nerves to the orbital contents. The *optic nerve*, after piercing the fibrous sclera and the vascular coat of the globe, spreads out to form the nerve fiber layer of the retina (p. 66). The *oculomotor nerve* innervates all the muscles of the eyeball except the superior oblique and the lateral rectus, which are supplied by the trochlear and abducens nerves, respectively.

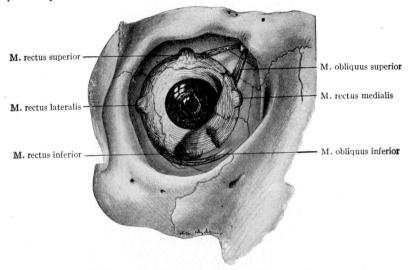

M. rectus superior

M. rectus lateralis

M. rectus inferior

M. obliquus superior

M. rectus medialis

M. obliquus inferior

Fig. 66.—Eyeball and Its Relation to the Orbit.
The muscles controlling the movements of the globe are indicated; the suture lines in the posterior part of the orbit are projected.

The *ciliary ganglion* has a sensory supply from the nasociliary branch of the ophthalmic nerve, a motor supply from the inferior division of the oculomotor nerve, and sympathetic fibers from the cavernous plexus on the internal carotid artery The *short ciliary nerves* leave the ganglion to supply the coats of the eyeball, the iris, and the ciliary muscles. It is possible to inject an anesthetic into the region of the ciliary ganglion and thereby obtain complete regional anesthesia during operations on the ocular globe.

SURGICAL CONSIDERATIONS

1. **Retrobulbar Abscess.**—Retrobulbar infection develops and spreads rapidly in the abundant fat of the orbital compartment. It may complicate disease of the nasal accessory sinuses, particularly ethmoiditis, follow orbital periostitis or operative infection of the orbit, or be a sequel to facial erysipelas. The abscess sometimes occupies almost the entire orbit, pushing the globe forward and greatly embarrassing its movements and circulation. Thrombosis in the ophthalmic veins, following an abscess in the orbit or secondary to some neighboring suppurative focus, may lead to cavernous sinus thrombosis, which is often fatal. Antibiotics may be successful in some cases.

2. **Strabismus or Squint.**—Squint is a manifest deviation of one of the visual axes. It may be a result of deficiency in the fusion sense in the brain (concomitant squint), or be caused by paralysis of one or more of the ocular muscles (paralytic squint). In normal binocular vision, the image is projected on corresponding points of both retinae and a single image results. Injury or paralysis of one of the eye muscles disturbs the delicate balance

necessary for normality and the images fall on dissimilar points of the retina, resulting in double vision or *diplopia*. In concomitant squint, diplopia does not ensue, owing to the voluntary suppression of one image. In paralytic squint, the eye deviates to the side of the stronger muscle pull, with a resulting squint or strabismus. If the eye be turned laterally, the squint is *divergent* (external strabismus); if mesially, *convergent* (internal strabismus). All the recti muscles, save the external, are supplied by the oculomotor nerve, paralysis of which leads to lateral deviation or divergent squint. Paralysis of the sixth nerve, the abducens, which supplies the lateral rectus muscle, causes internal strabismus, a condition sometimes seen in skull injuries and brain tumors.

3. **Nerve Paralysis.**—*Complete paralysis* of the oculomotor nerve presents a complex picture. There is a drooping of the upper lid (ptosis) and the almost immobile eye has a divergent squint caused by the unopposed action of the lateral rectus muscle. The pupil is dilated because of the paralysis of the circular fibers of the iris, and the accommodation is impaired as a result of ciliary paralysis. There is a slight exophthalmos from the paralysis of all but one of the recti muscles. *Partial paralysis* of this nerve is more common than complete paralysis. *Paralysis of the fourth or trochlear nerve* is an uncommon type of isolated muscle palsy and frequently is congenital. Paralysis of a single muscle, if acquired, usually affects the external rectus, innervated by the *abducens nerve*, and is evidenced by internal strabismus and an inability to turn the eyeball outward.

Paralysis or section of the cervical sympathetic chain results in a narrowing of the palpebral fissure because of the drooping of the upper lid, following paralysis of the superior palpebral muscles (of Müller). There also is a contraction of the pupil from paralysis of the dilating radial muscle fibers of the iris, and a slight retraction of the globe, enophthalmos. This symptom complex is called *Horner's syndrome*, and may be caused by tumors in the neck, goiter, or enlarged lymphatic glands, as well as by trauma, surgical or otherwise.

4. **Orbital Tumors and Foreign Bodies.**—Orbital tumors may originate in the contiguous cavities and invade the orbit secondarily. The outstanding symptom is protrusion of the eye, or exophthalmos. Foreign bodies have been embedded in the orbit over a period of years without causing trouble.

5. **Pulsating Exophthalmos.**—Protrusion of the eyeball, pulsation in the globe and surrounding parts, a bruit heard over the regions about the eye, and marked distention of the vessels of the conjunctiva and lids, constitute the clinical picture of pulsating exophthalmos. Its cause usually is an arteriovenous aneurysm resulting from rupture of the internal carotid artery into the cavernous sinus, the arterial blood being forced under pressure into the veins of the globe and associated structures. The rupture of the carotid artery usually is the result of trauma, particularly fracture of the base of the skull. Spontaneous ruptures caused by degeneration of the vessel wall may occur. Compression of the carotid artery on the same side as the exophthalmos diminishes the pulsation and the bruit.

B. OLFACTORY APPARATUS

The olfactory apparatus may be divided topographically into the external nose, nasal fossae, and paranasal sinuses.

(I) EXTERNAL NOSE

The external nose is pyramidal in shape. Its open posterior wall is applied directly to and communicates with the nasal fossae. The free anterior margin or bridge runs to its root at the forehead and terminates below at the apex or lobule of the nose. The lateral walls of the pyramid expand into the mobile alae (wings) of the nose. The base presents two apertures or nares separated by a median column or septum. Because of the cosmetic importance of the nose and the high incidence of deformity from disease and injury, many devices have been developed to improve its appearance or to repair its loss.

1. **Superficial Structures.**—The skin is thin and movable over the root of the nose, but is thick and adherent over the apex where inflammation is exceedingly painful because

of the tenseness of the parts and the consequent pressure on the nerves.   The skin of the nose is a favorite site for tuberculosis (lupus) and for rodent (carcinomatous) ulcer.   About the apex, comedos or blackheads and subcutaneous cysts are very common.   When acne

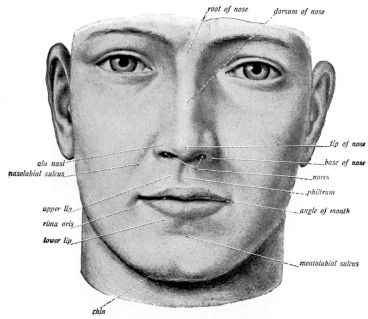

FIG. 67.—MOUTH, CHIN, AND EXTERNAL NOSE.   (Sobotta and McMurrich.)

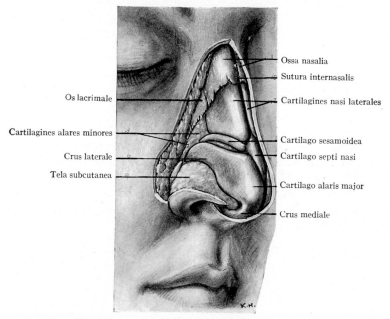

FIG. 68.—SKELETAL STRUCTURES OF THE EXTERNAL NOSE.

rosacea becomes exaggerated to the degree that an increase in the connective tissue takes place, the base and sides of the nose are converted into a lobulated mass.   This condition is known as *rhinophyma*.

2. **Skeletal Structures.**—The lateral, greater, and lesser alar cartilages, the cartilage of the septum, and the nasal bones make up the skeletal framework of the external nose. At their upper extremities at the root of the nose, the nasal bones articulate with the frontal bone and the perpendicular plate of the ethmoid bone, and with the frontal processes of the maxillae, and are narrow, thick, and well protected from injury. At their lower extremities, they are broad, thin, much exposed to trauma, and frequently are fractured. Nasal bone fracture almost always is compound because of the rupture of the closely adherent mucous membrane and therefore is accompanied by epistaxis. Fractured nasal bones heal readily because of their great vascularity.

The lacrimal bones form part of the mesial wall of the orbit and articulate with the frontal processes of the maxillae, for which they act as shock absorbers so that a blow on the nose, with or without nasal fracture, may cause fracture of the lacrimal bones. A blow directed against the base of the nose may break the cribriform plate of the ethmoid or the anterior wall of the frontal sinuses. Fracture of the cribriform plate of the ethmoid is a compound fracture of a portion of the root of the skull. The dura is exposed to injury and infection from the nasal fossae. If there is associated fracture of the nasal bones with epistaxis, it is difficult to know whether or not cerebrospinal fluid has escaped.

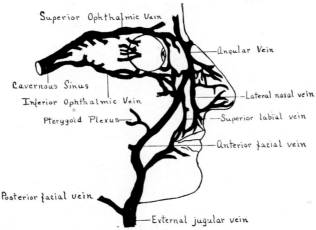

FIG. 69.—ANASTOMOSES OF THE SUPERFICIAL VEINS OF THE NOSE AND LIPS WITH THE OPHTHALMIC VEINS AND THE CAVERNOUS SINUS. (Ingersoll in Jackson and Coates, "The Nose, Throat, and Ear and Their Diseases.")

Ulcerating syphilis in the cartilaginous septum causes the bridge of the nose to become depressed and to present a characteristic saddle-like appearance.

3. **Anterior Nares or Nostrils.**—Each nostril opens directly into the vestibule, the slightly expanded forward portion of the nasal cavity. The vestibule is lined with skin, and in its lower half are hairs and sebaceous glands, frequent seats of annoying and distressing infection. Since the floor of the nose is on a lower level than the plane of the nasal fossae, the apex should be elevated with the nasal speculum in examination of the nasal cavities.

4. **Vessels and Nerves.**—The external nose has an abundant vascular supply and, for this reason, responds to the many plastic operations performed upon it. The lateral and angular terminations of the external maxillary artery form the main arterial supply. The veins empty into the anterior facial vein, and establish a communication through the ophthalmic vein with the cavernous sinus. Even slight infections about the nose and upper lip must be considered as potential of serious extension to the cerebral meninges; an abscess should be allowed to localize under hot compresses and should not be opened by untimely incision. The lymphatics drain to the submaxillary and deep cervical lymph glands, and their network over the nose communicates with that over the inner part of the vestibule and the nasal mucous membrane.

(II) Nasal Fossae

The anterior portion of the external nose, the vestibule, expands above and behind into triangular spaces or fossae which are separated from each other by the septum, which lies between the base of the skull and the hard palate. The fossae communicate more or less freely with the nasal accessory or paranasal air sinuses in the bodies of the frontal, sphenoid, ethmoid, and maxillary bones. They open on the face by the vestibule and the anterior nares, and into the pharynx by the posterior nares or choanae.

Each fossa has a mesial, lateral, superior, and inferior wall, consisting essentially of a bony and cartilaginous framework covered by mucous membrane. The maxillae and ethmoid bones form the bulk of the bony skeleton and furnish the cavities of the larger accessory sinuses. The mucous membrane is attached closely to the periosteum and cartilage, so that any inflammation of its surface is propagated to the underlying structure. The horizontal portion of the maxilla (palatine process) forms the floor of the fossa, and the mesial portion forms part of the lateral wall. The mesial surface of the ethmoid

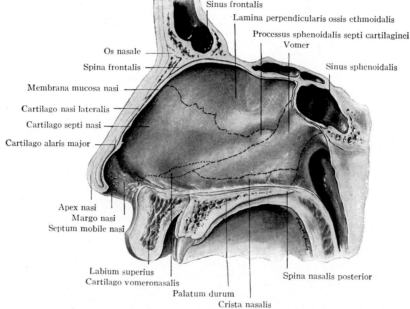

FIG. 70.—PARAMEDIAN SAGITTAL SECTION THROUGH THE LEFT NASAL FOSSA TO SHOW THE NASAL SEPTUM
The component elements of the septum are mapped out by dotted lines.

bone forms the upper half of the lateral wall, the cribriform plate, the roof of the fossa, and the perpendicular plate, the upper half of the bony septum. The vomer is the bony framework of the septum in its lower portion (Fig. 79).

1. **Mesial Wall of the Nasal Fossa, the Septum.**—The mesial wall of each fossa is a midsagittal partition, the nasal septum, formed by the perpendicular plate of the ethmoid, the vomer, and the septal cartilages, and covered by mucous membrane. The extreme antero-inferior part of the septum is membranous and flexible. In most adults, the septum presents a considerable amount of deviation, usually most marked at the union of the ethmoid and vomer, or along the union of the vomer and the septal cartilage, but it may occur in any part of the septum and ranges from a small bulge to a sharp ridge or spur. The deviation may be sufficient to block one nostril, with obstruction of the openings of the paranasal sinuses, leading to congestive reaction and inflammation in their cavities.

2. **Lateral Wall of the Nasal Fossa; the Conchae (Turbinates).**—The lateral walls of the nasal fossae are modeled characteristically by three turbinate scrolls or nasal conchae, placed one above the other. The scrolls project as more or less horizontally disposed ledges

from the lateral walls and have their free margins directed downward and inward. The bony framework of the superior and middle conchae is furnished by the ethmoid bone, but that of the inferior or maxillary concha is an independent bone. The spaces which the ledges overlie and partially shut off from the nasal cavity are the superior, middle, and inferior meatuses.

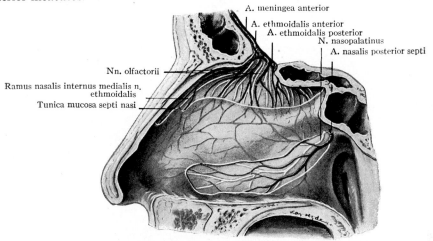

FIG. 71.—ARTERY AND NERVE SUPPLY OF THE SEPTUM.

The *superior concha* is much the smallest and its anterior extremity usually lies beneath the middle of the cribriform plate. The depression above and behind the superior concha is the spheno-ethmoidal recess; it communicates with the sphenoid sinus.

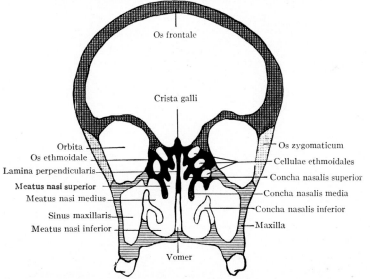

FIG. 72.—FRONTAL SECTION THROUGH THE SKULL, ORBITS, NASAL FOSSAE, AND PARANASAL SINUSES TO SHOW THE BONES WHICH FORM THE NASAL FOSSAE AND PARANASAL SINUSES.
Variations in shading denote the individual bones. (After Corning.)

The *middle concha* extends forward much farther than the superior and reaches the level of the anterior extremity of the cribriform plate. Its free margin descends almost vertically and then extends backward and downward to the posterior aperture of the fossa. On the outer wall of the nasal fossa, just anterior to the middle turbinate, is a moundlike elevation, known as the agger nasi.

The *inferior concha*, lying along the lower part of the lateral wall of the nasal cavity, is on the functional respiratory pathway of the nose. It reaches to within 2 cm. of the middle of the anterior naris, and its posterior tip lies 1 cm. in front of the pharyngeal orifice of the auditory (eustachian) tube. This last relation is responsible for the symptoms of middle ear disease consequent upon hypertrophy of the posterior extremity of the inferior turbinate. Swelling of the inferior turbinate usually indicates sinus disease, mainly that of the antrum, since pus from the antrum runs over it; at times, at its posterior extremity is a large polypoid mass almost filling the choana.

3. **Nasal Meatuses.**—The *superior meatus* presents anteriorly the openings of most of the posterior ethmoid cells; in the spheno-ethmoidal recess is the entrance into the sphenoid sinus.

The *middle meatus* presents the orifices of the frontal and maxillary sinuses and of the anterior and middle ethmoid cells. The middle ethmoid cells project into the meatus, forming a rounded elevation, the *ethmoidal bulla*. This conspicuous, bleblike, cell-containing structure is revealed by turning the middle nasal concha upward. Hypertrophy of the

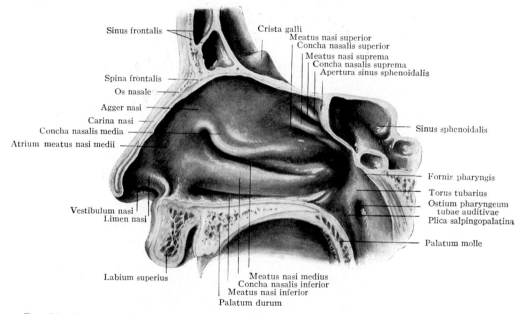

FIG. 73.—CONCHAE (TURBINATE BONES) ON THE LATERAL WALL OF THE RIGHT NASAL FOSSA.

ethmoid bulla may be sufficient to obstruct the nasal fossa. The middle turbinate overlying the meatus yields before the expanding cells, and may press against the septum, sometimes to the degree of obstructing the nasal fossa on the opposite side. Below the bulla is a sharp crescentic lamella, the *uncinate process*. Between the free border of this process and the ethmoid bulla is the cleftlike *semilunar hiatus*, which leads from the middle meatus into a groove of variable depth and dimensions, the *ethmoidal infundibulum*.

Generally, the ethmoidal infundibulum ends blindly as one or more anterior infundibular ethmoid cells. Posteriorly, it ends in a pocket or merges gradually with the middle meatus. Occasionally, it is continuous anatomically with the *nasofrontal* duct, the infundibulum of the frontal sinus, or, where the nasofrontal duct is absent, with the frontal sinus proper. In the depth of the ethmoidal infundibulum are the aperture of the frontal sinus and the openings of the infundibular group of the anterior ethmoid cells.

The *orifice of the maxillary sinus* ordinarily is posterior to that of the frontal sinus, which frequently lies in such a position that discharge from the frontal and ethmoidal cells crosses indirectly through the infundibulum into the ostium of the maxillary sinus.

The opening of the maxillary sinus into the middle meatus may be single or there may be a number of accessory orifices. The middle turbinate bone, when congested, may block drainage of the whole region. Attempt to rectify this obstruction formerly constituted indiscriminate removal of the turbinate; at present, a submucous resection of the nasal septum is performed. This allows the turbinate to swell without preventing adequate sinus drainage. If the turbinate is cystic, polypoid, or otherwise diseased, the affected part is trimmed away.

Between the attached border of the uncinate process and the inferior nasal concha, the lateral wall of the middle meatus is wholly membranous. It may present the *accessory maxillary ostium*, a direct communication between the middle meatus and the maxillary sinus. The *suprabullar furrow* or recess, located between the ethmoidal bulla and the

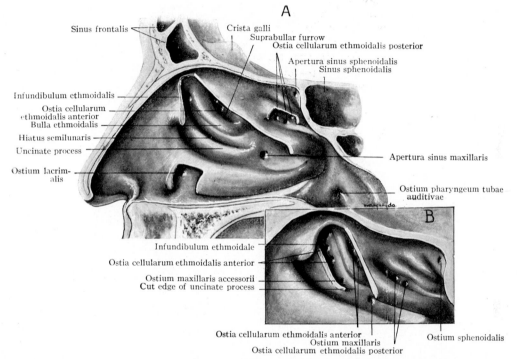

FIG. 74.—LATERAL WALL OF THE RIGHT NASAL FOSSA WITH PARTS OF THE TURBINATES REMOVED TO SHOW DIAGRAMMATICALLY THE OPENINGS INTO THE PARANASAL SINUSES.

In A, portions of the superior, middle, and inferior turbinates have been removed; the openings into the frontal and ethmoid sinuses are strictly diagrammatic as they are too small to locate accurately.

In B, the anterior portion of the middle turbinate is removed to show the sinus openings in the semilunar hiatus of the middle meatus; part of the uncinate process has been cut away.

attached border of the middle turbinate, contains the ostia of most of the bullar group of anterior ethmoid cells, usually classed as middle ethmoid cells.

The *frontal recess* is the frontal portion of the middle meatus and is a pouchlike extension with which the frontal sinus communicates by way of the nasofrontal duct. Usually, the ethmoidal infundibulum and the nasofrontal duct are separate channels, but occasionally they are united.

The *interior meatus,* bounded by the concave surface of the inferior turbinate and the lateral wall of the fossa, is funnel-shaped and varies in size with the degree of projection of the turbinate from the wall. The nasal ostium of the nasolacrimal duct is concealed in the forward portion of the meatus. Resection of a part of the turbinate may be required to expose properly the meatus and the opening of the *nasolacrimal duct.*

4. **Superior Wall or Roof of the Fossa.**—The roof of each nasal fossa is but 3 to 4

mm. wide and is coextensive with the cribriform plate of the ethmoid. Considering the roof as cranially arched, the cribriform plate forms the horizontal or middle portion; the body of the ethmoid with the wing of the vomer and the sphenoid process of the palate bone forms the curved posterior portion; and the frontal and nasal bones form the curved anterior portion. The roof is an anteroposterior groove with its concavity inferior because of the approximation of the lateral and mesial walls of the fossa. It extends to the naso-pharynx with no line of demarcation. The region may be divided into anterior or nasal, superior or fronto-ethmoidal, and posterior or sphenoid portions.

The thin, but compact, cribriform plate supports the olfactory lobe of the brain and separates the nasal from the cranial cavity. The plate is fragile because it is pierced by numerous orifices for the passage of the fibers of the olfactory nerve and their meningeal investments. In the angle between the sphenoid and ethmoid bones is the *spheno-ethmoidal recess*, which receives the opening of the sphenoid sinus. After resection of the superior turbinate bone, a probe, with its tip dipped a little downward and passed backward along the roof of the spheno-ethmoidal recess, will enter the sphenoid sinus.

A *meningocele*, projecting through the roof of the nasal fossa into the nasal cavity, has been mistaken for a nasal polyp and removed with fatal outcome from meningeal com-plications. Fracture of the cribriform plate is exceedingly serious since the meninges are exposed to the infected areas of the nasal fossae. The abundant epistaxis accompanying cribriform plate fracture may mask a considerable flow of spinal fluid through the nose. *Meningitis* sometimes complicates infection of the nasal fossae. The inflammation extends through the cribriform plate which, through the perineural and perivascular sheaths, brings the venous drainage of the nose into continuity with the meninges.

5. **Inferior Wall or Floor of the Nasal Fossa.**—The floor of the nasal fossa is much wider than the roof. The mucous membrane is supported by the palatal processes of the maxillary bones and the horizontal plates of the palate bones. While almost horizontal, it presents a gentle slope backward. Along this floor, a probe can be passed into the nasal portion of the pharynx and into the auditory (eustachian) tube. A nasal tube can be passed with ease along this pathway.

6 **Posterior Openings of the Nasal Fossae, the Choanae.**—By the method of nasal examination known as *posterior rhinoscopy*, the posterior orifices of the nasal fossae may be seen. Their osseous boundaries keep them permanently open for the ingress and egress of air. They are limited above by the body of the sphenoid bone and the alae of the vomer, below by the line of junction of the hard and soft palates, and laterally by the medial plates of the pterygoid processes of the sphenoid bone.

In posterior rhinoscopy, a mirror is introduced through the mouth behind the soft palate, and is illuminated through the mouth. Under favorable circumstances, there may be seen on each side the nasal opening, middle meatus, auditory tube, mucous membrane of the upper nasopharynx, the septum, and part of the inferior meatus. These structures also can be made out with the examining finger thrust behind and above the soft palate. Each adult posterior aperture (choana) is an oval orifice about 2.5 cm. in vertical diam-eter and 1 cm. in transverse diameter. The size of the openings must be appreciated when fitting plugs for them in the attempt to arrest severe hemorrhage from the nose. Hypertrophy of the posterior extremity of the turbinates, pharyngeal adenoid growths, polyps, and tumors obstruct the posterior nares, and may be as efficient obstacles to nasal breathing as any intranasal obstruction.

7. **Nasal Mucous Membrane.**—The nasal cavities are lined by mucous membrane which is continuous with that of the pharynx, paranasal sinuses, and lacrimal sac; this continuity is important because of the interrelationship of the diseases of these areas. The mucosa may be divided into respiratory and olfactory areas since it not only lines the tracts followed by the respired air but also covers the cells which receive the impressions for smell. The *respiratory mucosal tract* occupies the lower two-thirds of the region, is covered with ciliated epithelium, and is supplied richly with glands which are capable of producing a copious secretion, sometimes so free as to be mistaken for a flow of cerebro-

spinal fluid.   The thickness of the mucosa varies greatly, reaching a thickness of several millimeters over the inferior turbinate; it is hardly a millimeter thick on the lateral wall. The mucosa is bound down closely to the underlying bone so as to constitute a muco-periosteum.   On both lower turbinate bones, the vessels form a sort of erectile tissue, developed in cavernous spaces, which plays an important rôle in the physiology and pathology of the nasal cavity.   In chronic catarrhal inflammation, these cavernous spaces are distended with blood until the nasal cavity is occluded and breathing is obstructed.   The

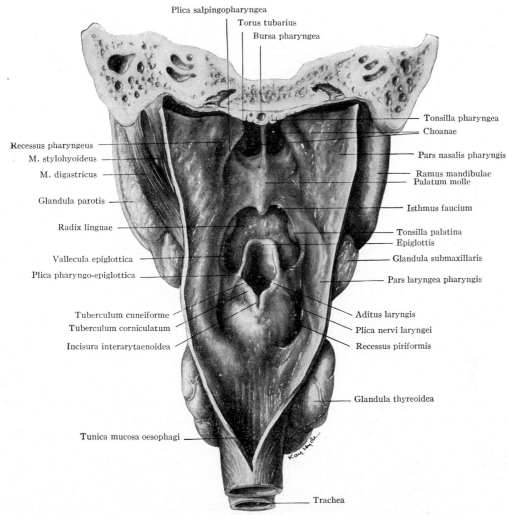

Plica salpingopharyngea
Torus tubarius
Bursa pharyngea

Tonsilla pharyngea
Choanae
Recessus pharyngeus
M. stylohyoideus
M. digastricus
Pars nasalis pharyngis
Ramus mandibulae
Palatum molle
Glandula parotis
Isthmus faucium
Radix linguae
Tonsilla palatina
Epiglottis
Vallecula epiglottica
Glandula submaxillaris
Plica pharyngo-epiglottica
Pars laryngea pharyngis
Tuberculum cuneiforme
Tuberculum corniculatum
Aditus laryngis
Incisura interarytaenoidea
Plica nervi laryngei
Recessus piriformis
Glandula thyreoidea
Tunica mucosa oesophagi
Trachea

FIG. 75.—POSTERIOR VIEW OF THE PHARYNX AND ESOPHAGUS.
The posterior wall of the pharynx is opened.

mucous membrane over the turbinates, when the seat of chronic inflammation, may undergo polypoid degeneration.   The *olfactory mucosal region* is limited in extent and is highly specialized.   It embraces an area situated above the center of the middle turbinate bone and the corresponding part of the septum.

8. **Vessels and Nerves.**—The principal *arterial* supply of the nasal fossae comes from the ophthalmic arteries through the anterior and posterior ethmoid branches, and from the internal maxillary artery through the sphenopalatine arteries.   The *veins* accompany the arteries and form a rich network beneath the mucous membrane of the middle and

6

inferior turbinate bones. The ethmoidal veins open into the superior sagittal sinus, and the nasal veins into the ophthalmic veins and thence into the cavernous sinuses. These venous communications between the intracranial and intranasal circulations explain the danger to the meninges and the brain of infective processes in the nose. The *lymph drainage* from the cavities of the nose is by way of the deep cervical lymph glands along the internal jugular vein.

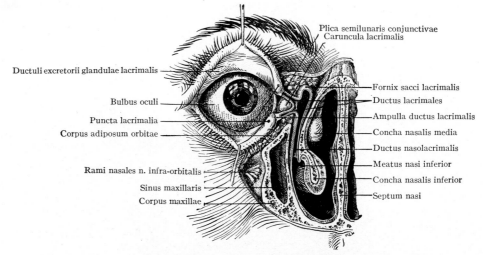

Plica semilunaris conjunctivae
Caruncula lacrimalis
Ductuli excretorii glandulae lacrimalis
Fornix sacci lacrimalis
Ductus lacrimales
Bulbus oculi
Ampulla ductus lacrimalis
Puncta lacrimalia
Concha nasalis media
Corpus adiposum orbitae
Ductus nasolacrimalis
Meatus nasi inferior
Rami nasales n. infra-orbitalis
Concha nasalis inferior
Sinus maxillaris
Septum nasi
Corpus maxillae

FIG. 76.—DIAGRAM OF THE LACRIMAL PASSAGES EXPOSED FROM THE FRONT.
The submucosal cavernous tissue on the inferior turbinate is indicated.

The fibers of the *olfactory nerves* pierce the openings of the cribriform plate of the ethmoid to supply the mucous membrane of the superior third or olfactory part of the nasal fossae.

The *sensory nerves* for the respiratory tract of the nasal fossae come from the ophthalmic nerve through the ethmoidal branch and from the maxillary nerve through the branches of the sphenopalatine ganglion.

SURGICAL CONSIDERATIONS

1. **Complications of Nasal Mucous Membrane Inflammation.**—The pivotal position which the nasal chambers occupy with reference to the paranasal sinuses, the tear apparatus, conjunctiva, pharynx and auditory (eustachian) tubes, explains the importance of the mucous membrane which lines these cavities in common. Inflammation of the lining membranes extends up the auditory tubes by way of the posterior nares and the pharynx. Aching of the face and frontal headache may occur from involvement of the maxillary and frontal sinuses. Serious intra-orbital or intracranial disease may follow ethmoid or sphenoid sinus involvement. Meningitis may arise when infection extends through the cribriform foramina along the neural and vascular sheaths. The severer forms of rhinitis and complicating pharyngitis may involve the retropharyngeal lymph glands and cause retropharyngeal abscess and even, although rarely, involve the deep cervical lymph glands.

The mucous membrane, in spite of an abundant blood supply, has no submucous areolar tissue between it and the underlying periosteum and perichondrium, and is slow to heal. Mucous membrane involvement is caused by mechanical or bacterial irritation. The accompanying congestion causes swelling of the nasal and allied mucous membranes, producing closure of the orifices communicating with the paranasal sinuses. Closure results in retention of inflammatory products. The subsequent infection and thrombosis destroys the sinus lining. Reaction to inflammation results in the formation of granulation tissue, and reparative processes result in polypoid degeneration or scar formation.

2. **Nosebleed (Epistaxis).**—The general vascularity of the nose, and the presence of a rich venous plexus deep to the turbinate mucous membrane, together with exposure to trauma, explain the great frequency of nosebleeding. When the bleeding point is in the anterior portion of the septum, as it most frequently is, it is arrested easily by plugging the anterior nares. When the bleeding point is posterior and cannot be found, or when a sinus is the source of hemorrhage, bleeding must be checked by plugging both the anterior and posterior nares. To plug the posterior nares, a ligature is threaded through the nose to the pharynx and out through the mouth. To the middle of the ligature is attached a plug of gauze the size of a walnut. This plug is drawn by the upper end of the ligature into the posterior nares. The two ends of the ligature are tied together so that the plug can be pulled against the posterior nares or withdrawn and reapplied if necessary. One or both nasal fossae then are plugged from before backward.

3. **Septum Deviations.**—The septum usually is deviated. The deviation most commonly occurs at the junction of the bony with the cartilaginous portion. The dorsum or free border of the septum almost always is in the median plane. It must be remembered that the septum may be essentially straight, yet a marked ridge or spur occurs on one or the other side and produces asymmetry.

Trauma, which often is unrecognized, and disturbances in development are the commonest and most important etiologic factors in septum deviation. Septal deviation does not mean that the breathing space of the narrowed nasal fossa is encroached upon seriously, but frequently the septum is forced against the jutting middle or inferior turbinate, setting up irritation and inflammation. This inflammation and its resultant congestion may obstruct the orifices of the paranasal sinuses and bring about sinus disease; this is the anatomical reason for septum resection in cases of sinus and turbinate disease. Septal spurs are found on the anterior edge of the vomer, and sometimes form a distinct ridge of bone running upward and backward. Infection of the septum is exceedingly dangerous since the septal veins may carry the infection through the cribriform plate of the ethmoid to the meninges.

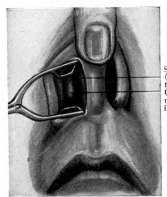

Septum nas (deviated to right)
Concha nasalis inferior

FIG. 77.—ANTERIOR RHINOSCOPIC EXAMINATION.

4. **Methods of Examination.**—Since the anterior nares are directed downward and are on a lower plane than the floor of the nose, an *anterior rhinoscopic examination* of the nasal cavities can be made best with the head thrown slightly backward and the nose lifted up. The dilating speculum introduced into the anterior nares should not be inserted beyond the cartilaginous portion of the nose because of the pain produced by pressure against the unyielding bony structure. The anterior part of the middle concha, a considerable portion of the inferior concha, a small portion of the middle meatus, and part of the inferior meatus may be seen under favorable conditions. The opening of the nasolacrimal duct cannot be seen, although it is but 2.5 cm. from the nostril and 2 cm. from the nasal floor, since it lies concealed beneath the depressed anterior extremity of the inferior concha.

Posterior (pharyngeal) rhinoscopic examination is done with difficulty because of the sensitiveness of the pharynx, but with some practice it can be done readily. While the patient breathes through the nose, the tongue is depressed by the examiner and a small mirror, similar to that of a laryngoscope, is carried through the mouth into the pharynx behind the soft palate. With light reflected through the mouth, the posterior nares, the posterior extremity of the nasal septum, the conchae and the corresponding meatuses, especially the middle conchae and middle meatuses, may be seen. The roof of the nasopharynx and the pharyngeal orifices of the auditory tubes usually can be made out. With a finger introduced through the mouth, the same structures can be differentiated, and such outgrowths as pharyngeal adenoids, tumors, and abscesses can be felt.

(III) Paranasal Sinuses

Of recent years, knowledge of the sinuses adnexed to the nasal fossae has assumed an increasingly important rôle to clinicians and surgeons, as sinus disease is much more common than formerly was supposed; attempts to deal with it have developed a special field in surgery. The air-containing, irregularly shaped diverticula of the nasal fossae are included in the "upper respiratory tract." Their communications with the nasal fossae are more or less narrow orifices which may be occluded by the congestion arising from swelling of their lining mucous membrane.

In the third or fourth month of fetal life, the sinuses form as outpocketings or evaginations of areas of the mucous membrane of the nasal meatuses. The sphenoid sinus arises

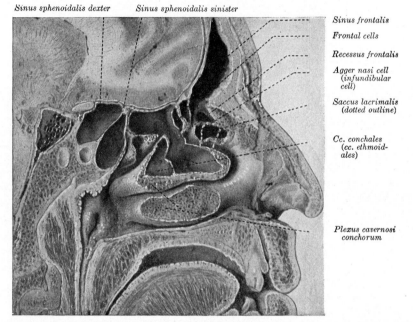

Sinus sphenoidalis dexter   *Sinus sphenoidalis sinister*

Sinus frontalis

Frontal cells

Recessus frontalis

Agger nasi cell (infundibular cell)

Saccus lacrimalis (dotted outline)

Cc. conchales (cc. ethmoidales)

Plexus cavernosi conchorum

Fig. 78.—Lateral Nasal Wall with the Paranasal Sinuses Exposed (the Maxillary Sinus Excepted).

Note the extension of the posterior ethmoid cells into the middle nasal concha, forming conchal cells; an agger nasi cell (infundibular anterior ethmoid cell) overlies the lacrimal sac: in the endonasal approach to the lacrimal sac and to the nasolacrimal duct, ethmoidal cells of this type would be opened before the sac is reached. (After J. Parsons Schaeffer, "The Nose, Olfactory Organ, and Accessory Sinuses.")

as a constriction of the posterosuperior region of the nasal fossa. The points of outgrowth are the ostia or orifices of communication between the sinuses and the nasal fossae. These mucous membrane sacs expand into the bones related to the nasal walls, with absorption of the bone, pneumatizing large portions of the frontal, ethmoid, and maxillary bones and forming frontal, ethmoidal, and maxillary sinuses.

There is no constancy in the anatomy of the paranasal sinuses, and great variations in elaboration, size, and type are common. A conventional type of sinus should not be visualized. Under normal conditions, there is an interchange of air in the paranasal sinuses during respiration, and good ventilation in them is essential to health. Although the nasal cavities exert an important influence over vocalization, the paranasal sinuses apparently do not.

1. **Frontal Sinuses.**—The frontal sinuses, formed bilaterally at the expense of the

frontal bones, are the most anteriorly placed of the nasal accessory sinuses and may be considered as extensions of the anterior ethmoid cells. Each may develop as a direct extension of the whole frontal recess of the middle meatus from one or more anterior ethmoid cells which originate in the frontal recess, or, occasionally, from the anterior extremity of the ethmoid infundibulum. At the age of six years, they are but a bud of mucous membrane in the vicinity of the anterior extremity of the semilunar hiatus; at the age of eight years, the frontal sinuses insinuate their way between the two plates of the frontal bones, and develop to their maximum size by about the twenty-fifth year.

The anterior wall of each sinus forms the prominence of the forehead above the eyebrow. Its upper wall separates the sinus from the frontal lobe of the brain, a relation which explains the endocranial and orbital complications of severe frontal sinus disease. The nasal part of the inferior wall is in relation with the ethmoid cells and the roof of the nasal fossa.

Occasionally, cells extend beyond the confines of the frontal bone into the sphenoid, nasal, and parietal bones, and, by way of the crista galli, into the ethmoid bone. Supernumerary sinuses are common, and each has its own connection with the nasal fossa. One sinus may develop at the expense of the other and cause the septum between them to be displaced from the median line. Subdivision or pocketing by more or less complete septa makes irregular what otherwise would be a smooth cavity. The sinus most commonly opens into the middle meatus by the frontonasal duct, or infundibulum of the frontal sinus. This duct is about 2 cm. long, runs downward and slightly backward from the posterior wall of the sinus, and opens at or near the anterior end or frontal recess of the semilunar hiatus. It is usual for one or more of the anterior ethmoid cells to open with the frontonasal duct into the semilunar hiatus. A frontonasal duct directly continuous with the ethmoid infundibulum is not unusual.

In about 50 per cent of cases, the relationship between the nasal end of the frontonasal duct and the frontal end of the ethmoid infundibulum is so intimate and of such a character that some of the secretion from the frontal sinus drains readily toward and into the ethmoid infundibulum. The opening of the maxillary sinus into the middle meatus may be placed so that it receives the pus from the frontal sinus and anterior ethmoid cells as the pus gravitates along the groove of the semilunar hiatus. The maxillary antrum thus may be converted into a cesspool, giving symptoms which divert attention from the true focus, which is frontal and anterior ethmoid sinus disease.

2. **Maxillary Sinuses.**—The maxillary sinuses (antra of Highmore) are paired cavities occupying the interior of the maxillary bones and conforming, in the main, to their shape. Extensive pneumatization of the alveolar, palatal, frontal, and zygomatic processes of the maxilla affords the sinuses an increased volume. The volume may be augmented by a marked encroachment of the mesial wall on the cavity of the nasal fossa. The capacity of the sinus is diminished by thickening of the sinus walls, retention of teeth, diminished pneumatization of the body and outlying processes of the maxilla, and by a deep anterior cranial fossa.

By the oval or elongated *maxillary ostium*, the sinus communicates with the deep aspect of the posterior half of the ethmoid infundibulum. The ostium may vary from a minute opening to a complete replacement of the floor of the infundibulum. The slitlike space between the free border of the uncinate process and the ethmoidal bulla is the semilunar hiatus, which connects the middle meatus with the ethmoid infundibulum. The maxillary opening is placed disadvantageously as a drainage aperture because it is located at the upper part of the sinus and drains into the narrow, deep, and much restricted ethmoid infundibulum. In about one third of adults, there is an *accessory maxillary ostium* which communicates directly between the middle meatus and the maxillary sinus. The opening lies behind the ethmoid infundibulum or projects into it between the posterior third of the uncinate process and the related part of the inferior turbinate. The accessory ostium is placed more advantageously for drainage purposes than is the maxillary ostium because it is lower and frequently is larger.

The fossa of the maxillary sinus is of a quadrangular pyramidal shape, with its base lying mesially and its apex extending laterally toward the zygomatic (malar) bone. The nasal or mesial wall is divided for practical purposes into an upper and lower part, the junction line being along the attachment of the inferior concha. The upper part is in relation with the middle meatus and the lower with the inferior meatus where it extends below the level of the palate.

The orbital or superior wall presents a longitudinal bulge which runs backward and contains the infra-orbital nerve. To this nerve relationship is attributed the infra-orbital face pain accompanying maxillary sinus involvement. The anterior wall extends from the alveolar border to the margin of the orbit. Most maxillary sinuses have their floor below the floor of the nasal fossa and markedly below the lowest usual point of surgical entrance, the inferior meatus. At times, half of the vertical extent of the sinus is posterior to the point of perforation. It is obvious that pus cannot be removed by dependent drainage with an opening above the palatal level. Pus present in quantity in the maxillary sinus

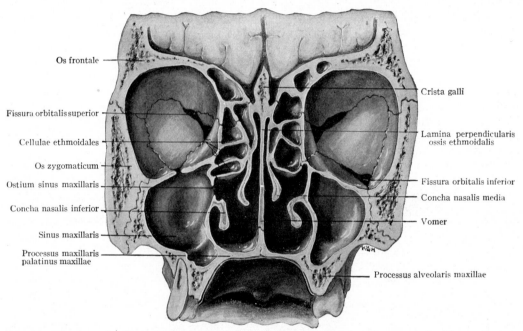

Os frontale

Fissura orbitalis superior

Cellulae ethmoidales

Os zygomaticum

Ostium sinus maxillaris

Concha nasalis inferior

Sinus maxillaris

Processus maxillaris palatinus maxillae

Crista galli

Lamina perpendicularis ossis ethmoidalis

Fissura orbitalis inferior

Concha nasalis media

Vomer

Processus alveolaris maxillae

Fig. 79.—Frontal Section Through the Brain, Orbits, Paranasal Sinuses, and Nasal Fossae to Show Their Interrelations.

empties with the head turned so that the affected cavity is uppermost; the sphenoid empties most easily with the head bent forward, and the frontal, with the head thrown backward.

The roots of the upper three molar and two bicuspid teeth ordinarily make a bulge into the floor of the sinus, and are separated from the cavity by a thin layer of spongy bone. Not infrequently, this spongy tissue is deficient and the uncovered roots project into the sinus, a matter of great surgical importance, as it explains the production of maxillary sinusitis by dental caries and the establishment of drainage for empyema of the antrum by accidental or intentional removal of one of these teeth. The floor of the sinus is not smooth or regular, and often presents incomplete septa, forming divisions into which inflammatory products tend to seep; these may be inaccessible to treatment by antrum puncture. These divisions may be of such size as to require individual attention and should be considered in cases resistant to ordinary treatment.

3. Ethmoid Labyrinth.—The ethmoid cells, 8 to 10 in number, are cavities with paper-thin walls, lying in the thickness of the lateral masses of the ethmoid bone between

the upper parts of the nasal fossae and the orbits, between the frontal and sphenoid sinuses, and between the floor of the cranial cavity and the middle turbinate. The cells as a whole constitute the ethmoid labyrinth, which occupies the entire ethmoidal field; hence, the individual cells are many if small and few if large. The cells open into the superior and middle meatuses of the nasal fossae and their mucosa is continuous with the nasal mucosa. An ethmoid cell usually extends into the middle meatus and forms the ethmoid bulla.

An anterior and posterior group of ethmoid cells may be differentiated. The *anterior* or *middle meatus cells* generally are about 5 in number and open into the semilunar hiatus. They may be divided into frontal anterior cells, opening into the ethmoidal infundibulum, and bullar anterior cells, opening into the middle meatus below, above, or upon the ethmoid bulla. In the last arrangement, the bulla is made pneumatocystic by the cells. The frontal sinus may be considered an anterior ethmoid cell, opening as it does on the infundibular portion of the semilunar hiatus. The posterior cells lie in the posterior portion of the lateral mass of the ethmoid. Their orifices open above the attached border of the concha and communicate with the superior and middle meatuses.

The relations of the ethmoid air cells to the cranial cavity are more extensive than are those of the frontal and sphenoid sinuses. The bone separating these cells from the cranial meninges is compact, save at the level of the shallow olfactory grooves, where the

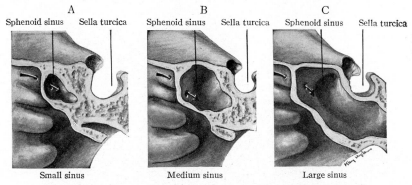

A | B | C
Sphenoid sinus Sella turcica | Sphenoid sinus Sella turcica | Sphenoid sinus Sella turcica

Small sinus | Medium sinus | Large sinus

FIG. 80.—RIGHT PARAMEDIAN SAGITTAL SECTIONS THROUGH NORMAL SPHENOID SINUSES TO SHOW VARIATIONS IN SIZE.
Note the possibility, in the large sinus, of perforation of the walls by erosion; arrow indicates the opening from the spheno-ethmoidal recess into the sphenoid sinus. (After Testut and Jacob.)

cells bulge upward lateral to the crista galli. The bony wall here may be paper-thin and sometimes is lacking. This relation explains the meningeal and cerebral extensions, meningitis, cerebral abscess, subdural abscess, and sinus thrombosis which may complicate ethmoiditis.

4. Sphenoid Sinuses.—The sphenoid sinuses are two paramedian cavities of irregular cube-shape which lie within the body of the sphenoid bone, and not infrequently extend into the great wing, pterygoid process, and rostrum of the sphenoid, and into the basilar process of the occipital bone. The sinuses are separated by a thin and often much deviated septum. Rather commonly, they replace certain posterior ethmoid cells and, occasionally, come far enough forward to establish communication with the maxillary sinus. The reverse may occur and one or more posterior ethmoid cells grow posteriorly into the body of the sphenoid bone, restricting its contained sinuses.

Extremely rudimentary or very large sinuses may be encountered; their capacity varies from 0.5 to 30 cc. They are largest toward the age of twenty to twenty-five years. A sinus may be only a small cavity behind the sphenoid orifice in the anterior part of the body of the sphenoid bone, or a large, irregular cavity encroaching extensively upon the opposite sinus.

Since the symptoms of sphenoid sinusitis are vague and overshadowed by the symptoms of other sinus involvement, the prognosis as to operative results should be guarded

SURGICAL CONSIDERATIONS

1. Frontal Sinus Disease and Drainage.—Congestion of the mucous membrane lining the frontal sinuses, so frequent in acute coryza, produces a dull ache over the glabella and superciliary arches. When drainage from the sinus is blocked, purulent fluid collects, producing an *empyema*. With the frontal duct open, pus is conveyed along the semilunar hiatus to the opening of the maxillary sinus, infecting the maxillary cavity. Since the anterior ethmoid cells open with the frontal duct into the infundibulum of the semilunar hiatus, these cells may be involved easily in frontal sinus disease. Infection of the frontal bone may result from frontal sinus suppuration by the development of an osteitis which may terminate in frontal lobe abscess and meningitis.

The aim of all *intranasal surgery* for frontal sinus disease is improved drainage. Removing obstructions within the nose, clearing the frontonasal opening, resection of the

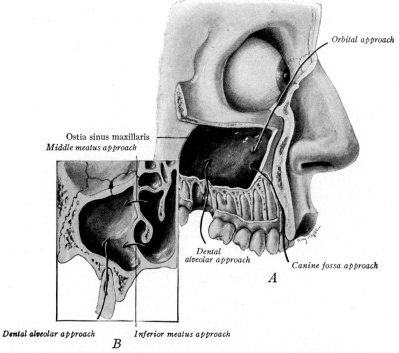

FIG. 81.—SURGICAL APPROACHES TO THE MAXILLARY SINUSES.
A is a diagrammatic lateral view. *B* is a frontal section.

anterior end of the middle turbinate, and curettement of the anterior ethmoid cells are followed so frequently by relief of frontal suppuration that they always should be performed before resorting to frontal sinus operation. Where operation is indicated, the usual resection of the middle turbinate is followed by removal of the nasal wall above the anterior end of the resected bone, thus eliminating the anterior ethmoid cells. A sound now passes readily into the frontal sinus, so that its passage can be enlarged and cleared.

Originally, frontal empyema was treated by *extranasal operation*. A trephine or chisel opening was made in the bone of the front wall of the sinus. Since an anterior opening could not drain the sinus in its most dependent portion, and the drainage of the irregularly shaped and loculated cavity was difficult at best, this simple method often failed. Both curative and cosmetic results are attained by the Killian operation, which involves the removal of the anterior and inferior walls of the sinus, frontal process of the maxilla, upper portion of the lacrimal bone, and adjacent ethmoid cells, with preservation of a rim of bone at the supra-orbital margin for cosmetic reasons. Curettement of the mucous lining of the sinuses completes the operation.

The *combined intranasal* and *extranasal approach* effects an efficient and permanent drainage. Curved incisions are made over the mesial portion of each eyebrow avoiding, if possible, the supra-orbital nerve. The bone is removed, the cavities are explored, and granulations and pus cleared away. Intranasally, the bone surrounding the nasal opening of the frontonasal duct is removed.

2. Maxillary Sinus Disease and Drainage.—Infection of the maxillary antrum may occur from the carious fangs of teeth which present in its cavity; also, from the infection of adjacent frontal, sphenoid, and ethmoid air cells. Since the frontal and anterior ethmoid cells open into the infundibulum, seepage along the infundibular groove is directed into the maxillary antrum If the maxillary orifice is not occluded, pus from the sinus may overflow and escape into the middle meatus; the drainage is facilitated by placing the affected sinus uppermost. Pus flowing from beneath the middle turbinate is an important diagnostic sign

The sinus can be approached surgically through the lateral wall of the inferior meatus, through a dental alveolus, or through the canine fossa. For years, the dental alveolar

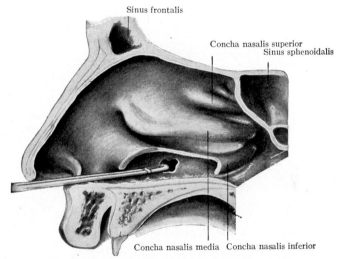

Sinus frontalis

Concha nasalis superior
Sinus sphenoidalis

Concha nasalis media   Concha nasalis inferior

FIG. 82.—APPROACH TO THE MAXILLARY SINUS THROUGH THE INFERIOR MEATUS.
A part of the inferior concha need or need not be removed.

approach was the one used for empyema of the antrum, and was commended for its simplicity and the quick relief it occasioned. Unfortunately, reinfection from the mouth was common, and the tendency for the trocar opening to close was great. Should a diseased tooth project into the antrum, it now is deemed best to remove the tooth, and curet the socket without establishing communication with the sinus and to develop, instead, a naso-antral window for drainage. To prevent sacrifice of a healthy tooth, the sinus can be drained through the mouth by everting the upper lip and drilling or trephining the canine fossa just above the second bicuspid tooth. If bone here is thin, the antrum is reached conveniently. As extensive an opening as desired may be made but the roots of the teeth should not be exposed.

For permanent communication, the removal of a section of the lateral wall of the nasal fossa is of great value. This may be accomplished with or without removal of the inferior concha. An extensive resection is advisable to attain free drainage and to compensate for the tendency of the opening to close over. Resection, extended to include a portion of the lateral wall of the inferior meatus and necessitating partial resection of the inferior concha, should remove as little of the inferior concha as is consistent with adequate drainage.

Examination of the maxillary sinus is made with the patient in a dark room and with an electric light placed in the mouth. The outlines of each maxillary antrum, if empty, are clearly made out. If a sinus is inflamed, that side of the face will appear darker, the shadow being produced by accumulated pus or mucous membrane thickening. This examination gives valuable information as to the size of the sinus and the presence or absence of disease. Pathologic changes can be demonstrated with absolute certainty only when the sinus is opened, although the x-ray affords valuable information.

Benign or malignant tumors may originate in the antrum. The tumor invades the nose by rupturing the thin mesial wall, the orbit by pushing up the roof of the cavity, the mouth by eroding the floor of the sinus, and the cheek by eroding the thin anterior maxillary wall. The dense malar bones do not yield to invasion, and there is little tendency for the growth to spread backward. As the infra-orbital nerve runs along the roof of the sinus, and the nerves to the upper teeth run in its walls, they may be pressed upon by growths, producing neuralgia of the face and teeth.

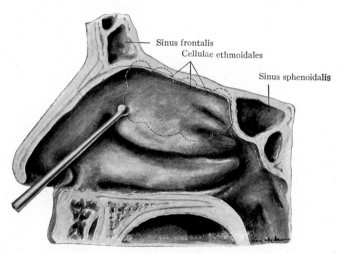

FIG. 83.—DIAGRAMMATIC PROJECTION OF THE ETHMOID CELLS ON THE LATERAL WALL OF THE NASAL FOSSA.
The curet indicates the ethmoid area to be removed first.

3. **Ethmoid Disease and Drainage.**—The cells of the ethmoid labyrinth usually are involved when the other paranasal sinuses are infected seriously. Conversely, their infection will cause suppuration in the other sinuses, as evidenced by the fact that suppuration in the adjacent sinuses often ceases when ethmoid cells are drained properly. Repeated attacks of infection lead to changes in the ethmoid mucosa, which contribute to the ultimate formation of polypoid tissue. Once polyps are formed, the mucosa shows a tendency to hyperplasia in adjoining cells. The more chronic the process, the greater is the amount of polypoid infiltration. When ethmoid cells are subject to a chronic suppurative process, there is no hope of their being restored, as they are so small that nothing short of exenteration effects a cure. A definite relationship seems to exist between sinus disease and the common bronchial affections such as asthma, chronic bronchitis, and bronchiectasis. These complications are an additional indication for sinus surgery.

Operation on the ethmoid cells involves the removal of the diseased cells and some of the adjacent normal tissue. According to the extent of involvement of the ethmoid cells, a greater or less amount of the middle turbinate bone is resected. The anteriorly placed cells are the most accessible. Safety lies in keeping below the roof of the nose and following the cells backward to the outer walls, appreciating that the lateral boundary of the cells is the mesial orbital wall.   The ethmoid bulla is opened and polypi, if present, are removed.

4. **Routes to the Sphenoid Sinus; Transsphenoid Approach to the Hypophysis.**—Operation on an infected sphenoid sinus, by whatever route, entails as complete a removal of the anterior wall of the sinus as possible, in the ethmoid as well as in the nasal portion. Removal of this wall is necessary because of the tendency to prolonged discharge of pus. The region deserves a wholesome respect because of the close association of the cavernous sinuses with their enclosed internal carotid arteries, and the optic nerves. The sphenoid is exposed readily in any of the extranasal operations on the frontal sinus. After the removal of the ethmoid labyrinth, the next procedure is the removal of the anterior wall of the sphenoid sinus.

An exposure of the hypophysis is effected by removing the front wall and roof of the sphenoid. The mucous membrane is elevated from both sides of the septum as in submu-

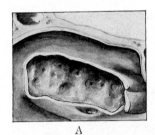 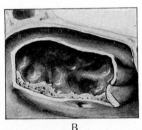

A   B

FIG. 84.—OPERATIVE STEPS IN INTRANASAL EXENTERATION OF THE ETHMOID CELLS.
The lateral and most superior cells cannot be removed safely through this approach.

cous resection, and a portion of the bone and cartilage is removed, including the inferior end of the perpendicular plate of the ethmoid, together with most of the vomer. The turbinates on each side are flattened against the lateral nasal walls. The anterior wall and bony roof of both the sphenoids are removed, exposing the hypophysis (p. 48).

C. AUDITORY APPARATUS

The auditory apparatus should be considered with full appreciation of the significance of its connection through the auditory tube with the mucous membrane of the nasopharyngeal tract. The continuity of mucous membrane throughout the correlated mechanisms of this tract makes possible the extension of a localized infection or irritation and congestion of the upper air tract to the lungs through the trachea, to the mucous membrane of the head in general, and to the ear through the auditory tube. For this reason, aural conditions are dependent, to a great extent, upon the condition of the mucous membrane of the upper air passages. An exact knowledge of the accessory spaces associated with the tympanic cavity is as important in the interpretation of auricular pathologic change as is that of the accessory sinuses in pathologic change of the nasal passages.

The hearing apparatus is comprised of a central and a peripheral portion. The central portion, lying within the cranial cavity, is made up of the central pathways of the eighth nerve and the cortical area in the superior temporal gyrus. The peripheral portion, which is described in this section, is located, for the most part, within the temporal bone.

The peripheral hearing apparatus embraces the external, the middle, and the internal ear. The external ear may be studied with reference to its main structures, the auricle or pinna, and the external auditory (acoustic) canal. For convenience of description, the middle ear is divided into its more or less clinical divisions: tympanic membrane, tympanic cavity, mastoid antrum, mastoid air cells, and auditory tube. Each of these regions, n addition to being correlated, has a physiology, pathology, and field of surgery of its own.

(I) External Ear

1. Auricle or Pinna.—The auricle is attached to the side of the head behind the temporomandibular joint and in front of the mastoid process, on a line from the eye to the external occipital protuberance. The lateral surface looks slightly forward and is irregularly concave. The largest and deepest of its concavities is the funnel-like fossa which surrounds the opening of the external auditory meatus.

Fibrocartilages, ligaments, rudimentary musculature, and a skin-covering compose the auricle. The fibrocartilages are thin flexible structures which are the supporting framework for all the pinna save the lobule, and permit free movement of the body of the ear. Extrinsic ligaments attach the auricle to the temporal bone, while intrinsic ligaments maintain the cartilages in position. There are both extrinsic and intrinsic muscles which have very little action. The skin is more closely adherent to the anterior than to the posterior surface of the auricle, and in an inflammatory disease, such as erysipelas, the skin over the ear may become extremely swollen and exquisitely tender from perichondrial inflammation.

A fairly rich *arterial supply* for the auricle (pinna) arises from the external carotid artery by way of the superficial temporal artery in front and the posterior auricular artery behind.

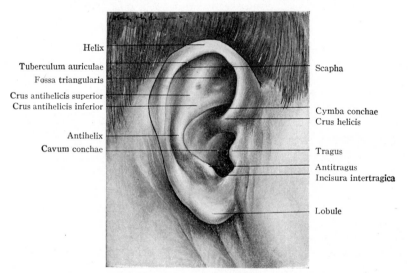

Helix

Tuberculum auriculae

Fossa triangularis

Crus antihelicis superior
Crus antihelicis inferior

Antihelix
Cavum conchae

Scapha

Cymba conchae
Crus helicis

Tragus

Antitragus
Incisura intertragica

Lobule

Fig. 85.—External Ear.

The *venous drainage* enters the superficial temporal vein in front and the external jugular vein below. From the mesial aspect of the ear and the posterior aspect of the auditory meatus, the *lymphatic vessels* collect into the mastoid glands at the mastoid tip. They seldom drain into the retro-auricular glands, which commonly are involved in scalp infections. The swelling of enlarged retro-auricular glands from infection of some small scalp area frequently has been confused with the edema of mastoid disease. The efferent lymphatic trunks pierce the sternocleidomastoid muscle near its origin and enter the deep cervical chain. The lymphatics of the external aspect of the pinna drain to the anterior or preauricular glands, and to some extent to the glands about the parotid, and eventually drain into the deep cervical chain. The pinna frequently is frost-bitten because its vessels lie superficially in scant subcutaneous tissue.

2 External Auditory Meatus or Canal.—An external fibrocartilaginous and an internal bony portion make up the canal, which runs about 3.5 cm., from the concha to the tympanic membrane. The outer third of the wall of this canal is fibrocartilage and the inner two thirds is bone. The *fibrous portion* of the fibrocartilaginous part of the canal is concave and makes up the superior and posterior walls. The *cartilaginous portion* is formed from the tonguelike cartilage which makes up the auricle, and which is split by two horizontal breaks or incisurae to give mobility to the auricle. Through these incisurae, an abscess in the parotid may discharge into the external meatus, or a deep-lying furuncle of the meatus may open and discharge into the parotid.

The *bony portion* is derived from the temporal bone. The upper wall is formed from the squamous portion, and the upper part of the posterior wall from the petrous portion as it expands to form the mastoid process. Cholesteatomata of the antrum often break through this wall into the external meatus. A periostitis along this segment of the meatus may complicate mastoiditis. In the newborn, the osseous portion is absent. It is not formed until the temporal bone is developed fully. Because of the mesial obliquity of the drum, which may be seen in frontal section, the inferior wall of the canal is longer than the superior wall. In a general way, the tube is flattened anteroposteriorly and undergoes a sort of torsion from without inward until gradually its anterior wall becomes antero-inferior. The result is that the ellipse representing the section of the tube, while vertical in its external portion, has its greater diameter in the more mesial portion rather inclined toward the horizontal.

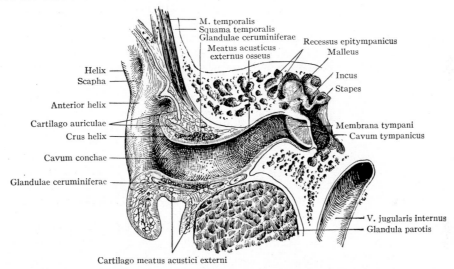

FIG. 86.—FRONTAL SECTION THROUGH THE RIGHT EXTERNAL AUDITORY MEATUS.

The direction of the canal in the cartilaginous portion is upward, inward, and forward; that in the bony portion is inward, downward, and forward. Thus, there is a convex curve near the middle of the canal. To facilitate examination of the canal, the pinna should be drawn upward and backward, which places the cartilaginous and bony portions of the tube in line, and eliminates the curve.

A conspicuous landmark, the *suprameatal spine*, lies at the upper, posterior part of the margin of the bony meatus (p. 109). To it attaches the superior ligament of the auricle.

The skin adheres closely to the wall it covers, and is continuous with the skin over the concha and over the external wall of the tympanic membrane to which it furnishes the external layer.

The *anterior* wall of the canal is in such intimate relation with the temporomandibular joint that the condyle of the mandible pushes into the membranous and cartilaginous portion sufficiently to produce a constriction. The constriction disappears when the jaws are opened. Areolar tissue separates a prolongation of the parotid gland from the anterior wall of the canal. A fall or blow upon the chin may break the wall, and the ensuing hemorrhage may be interpreted as bleeding from cranial fracture. The *posterior* wall is a bony partition, separating the canal from the mastoid air cavities with which it has a fairly intimate relationship. The canal is tender, swollen, and even is invaded by pus in certain types of mastoid disease. When a radical mastoid operation is performed in serious middle ear disease, the entire posterior wall of the external meatus is removed. In relation with the middle cranial fossa is the *superior wall*, formed from the squamous portion of the temporal bone. This wall may be permeated with air cells which are in communication with the cavities of the middle ear. These cells are susceptible to purulent disease of the middle ear and their presence explains the path by which pus from an otitis media may invade the external canal without perforating the drum membrane. Bone disease in the wall may lead to cranial meningitis. Through the intermedium of the parotid fascia, the *inferior wall* is in relation with the contents of the parotid compartment. Defects in the cartilage, loosely filled with connective tissue, afford a path of infection from a parotid abscess to the external canal. The drum membrane closing the inner extremity of the canal is of such surgical importance that it merits description under its own caption (see below).

Surgical Considerations

1. Infections and Ear Wax Deposits in the External Auditory Meatus (Canal).—The sebaceous glands in the skin of the canal frequently are the foci for small abscesses which are exquisitely painful because of the indistensibility of the skin in the region. The skin of the meatus, when infected, may seep a mucopurulent discharge justifying the term *otitis externa*. The skin of the canal, as well as that of the auricle, suffers from varying types and degrees of eczema, the most severe of which penetrate to, but rarely through, the drum. Reciprocally, an otitis media, discharging through the drum may inflame the skin of the canal, setting up an eczema. Excessive secretion of the ceruminous glands often plugs the meatus, causing temporary deafness. Forcible effort to remove wax frequently results in impaction and possible infection.

2. Foreign Bodies in the Canal.—Foreign bodies may remain for some time in the external auditory canal without causing serious damage or much inconvenience. They often are exceedingly difficult to extract, and more damage has been done by ill-advised attempts at removal with hairpins and matches than has been caused by their presence. Insects, small foreign bodies, or wax may be removed by syringing the canal gently with a stream of warm water. Instrumental removal should be attempted only with the instrument and foreign body well in view, and by one skilled in ear manipulation. Should the walls of the canal be swollen, the removal of the foreign body should be deferred until the swelling has subsided.

3. Cholesteatoma Externa.—In this form of dermatitis which occurs in the external auditory meatus, the epithelium desquamates very rapidly, accumulates, and mixes with wax, sebum, and other foreign material. The mass created irritates the underlying skin, which may become infected and even ulcerated. The condition is known as cholesteatoma externa. The process may progress to such an extent as to perforate the tympanic membrane or even cause necrosis and sequestration of part of the external canal. Healing after cholesteatoma may result in a narrowing or constriction of the canal.

(II) Middle Ear

The middle ear, for purposes of topographic discussion, consists of the tympanic membrane, the tympanic cavity, the auditory tube, and the mastoid air cells.

(A) TYMPANIC MEMBRANE

1. Definition and External Characteristics.—The tympanic membrane, or drumhead, is the thin, opaque, concave disk separating the external auditory canal from the tympanic cavity. It is resistant, and protects the tympanic cavity, of which it is part of the lateral wall. It also functions as a highly specialized part of the hearing mechanism, and vibrates with sound waves and transmits them along the ossicle chain to the labyrinth. It is developed fully at birth.

From external or otoscopic examination of this membrane, valuable information may be derived as to conditions within the tympanic cavity. An exact knowledge of the main physical characteristics of the membrane and of the changes caused by disease is a valuable diagnostic and therapeutic adjunct.

In the development of acute middle ear disease, its thickness may be increased greatly by edema; this should be considered in paracentesis when a large opening is demanded. In chronic disease of the drum (myringitis) the membrane may be thickened irregularly and permanently. The color of the normal ear drum is a lustrous pearl gray, which is modified by the color of the light used and by the reflection from the inner wall and contents of the tympanic cavity. It undergoes great changes in color during ear disease, becoming reddened in otitis media and pale in sclerotic otitis. Its strength is the obstacle to the exit of pent-up pus in the tympanic cavity in acute middle ear disease. Paracentesis in this condition affords immediate, but sometimes only temporary, relief.

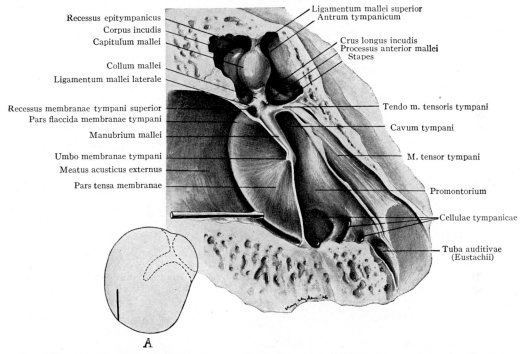

FIG. 87.—FRONTAL SECTION THROUGH THE RIGHT TYMPANIC MEMBRANE AND TYMPANIC CAVITY. A is a diagram of the ear drum with the position of the incision indicated.

2. Bony Insertion of the Tympanic Membrane.—The periphery of the membrane save at the anterosuperior region, is inserted into the *tympanic sulcus* or groove in the tympanic part of the temporal bone, from which the strong fibrous portion of the membrane develops. The sulcus is absent for a distance of 5 mm. in the anterosuperior area, and the gap so formed is called the *tympanic incisura* (Rivini). Over this region, the membrane has no strong fibrous constituent, but is represented simply by a thickened continuation of the covering of the auditory canal overlying the bulging mucosa which lines the tympanic cavity.

3. Topographic Division of the Drum.—From the surgical and structural points of view, the drum membrane is divided into two areas, one flaccid, and the other tense or vibrating.

A very small part of the drumhead is occupied by *pars flaccida (Shrapnell's membrane)* which, in general, is in relation with the epitympanic recess and its contents, the ear ossicles. This portion of the membrane is within the area of the tympanic incisura, and its triangular outline is encompassed by the shorter anterior and the longer, more prominent posterior mucous folds or ligamentous bands which converge from the incisura to the button-like prominence of the lateral or short process of the malleus. The area demarcated is loose and flaccid, and lacks the fibrous-tissue framework of the remainder of the membrane. Its looseness allows it to bulge outward into the meatus as a pouch (of Prussak). Perforation here is common, as the pouch often harbors a chronic purulent collection of fluid from ossicle osteitis. During an acute attack of middle ear disease, this pouch, along with involvement of the tense portion of the drum, may become distended with pus.

The larger *vibratory* or *tense portion* of the tympanic membrane is stretched tightly on a framework of fibrous and elastic tissue, to which the handle of the malleus is attached firmly. The tip of the hammer draws the membrane inward, forming a concavity, the

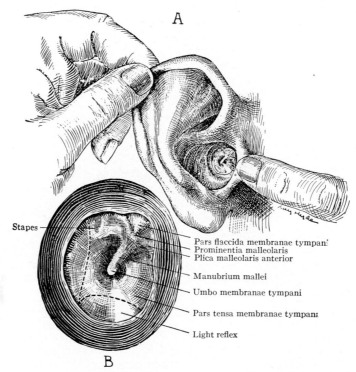

Stapes

Pars flaccida membranae tympani
Prominentia malleolaris
Plica malleolaris anterior

Manubrium mallei

Umbo membranae tympani

Pars tensa membranae tympani

Light reflex

Fig. 88.—Lateral View of the Right Tympanic Membrane. The Size and Visibility of the Membrane Are Much Exaggerated.

B is a detailed drawing of the membrane; the dotted lines enclose areas through which paracentesis can be done safely.

apex of which is a depression known as the umbo. The segment of membrane above the umbo is supplied very freely with vessels and nerves while that below it is less vascular and less sensitive.

4. External Configuration and Quadrant Formation.—Otoscopic examination reveals the membrane as concave at its center, or the *umbo*. The attachment of the tip of the handle of the malleus is a little below and behind the center of the diaphragm. An essential and constant landmark, found when others are obliterated, is a small but distinct bulge, the *malleolar prominence*, lying in the anterosuperior region and pushed forward by the short process of the malleus. From this bulge, a distinct line, the *anterior tympanic* or *malleolar fold*, runs forward to the periphery of the drum. Behind the malleolar prominence is a longer line, the *posterior malleolar fold*, which, with the anterior fold, the prominence, and the periphery of the drum, bounds the flaccid portion of the membrane. From the malleolar prominence, a broad grayish-white line is directed downward and backward as far as the umbo. This line or bulge corresponds to the *handle of the malleus* which is included within the thickness of the membrane. A small, conspicuous, triangular, luminous region fans out in the antero-inferior portion of the membrane from its apex at the umbo to the periphery. This is the cone of *light reflex*, a direct reflection to the examiner's eye of those light rays falling upon that segment of the membrane perpendicular to the line of vision. The light reflex varies with varying degrees of concavity and obliquity of the drum.

Normally, the malleolar prominence, short process, handle of the malleus, and cone of light should be seen. In a particularly transparent drum, occasionally there is seen a broad grayish line which marks the long process of the incus, showing through the drum-

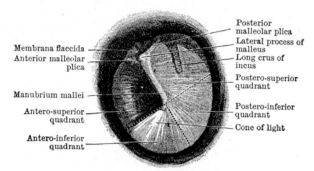

FIG. 89.—NORMAL LEFT DRUMHEAD SHOWING LIGHT TRIANGLE, MALLEUS HANDLE, AND FOLDS ABOUT THE SHORT PROCESS.

head, approximately parallel with, and posterior to, the handle of the malleus. Farther back, the stapes, the tendon of the stapedius muscle, and the niche of the round window sometimes are visible.

For topographic and surgical purposes, the drum may be divided by two imaginary oblique lines. One is drawn downward and backward along the line of the handle of the malleus, the other at right angles to the first, downward and forward through the umbo, forming two supra-umbilical and two infra-umbilical quadrants.

In the anterosuperior quadrant is the flaccid membrane (of Shrapnell) which forms the outer wall of Prussak's space and protects the ossicles in the tympanic cavity. It is the danger zone of the tympanum and must be avoided in paracentesis.

SURGICAL CONSIDERATIONS

1. **Curvature Changes in the Membrane.**—While the normal curvature of the tympanic membrane depends largely upon the tension of the tensor tympani muscle, it may be depressed unduly as a consequence of unequal air pressure upon its surfaces. The depression may result from absorption of the air within the tympanum, closed by obstruction in the auditory tube, producing a partial vacuum. Changes in curvature are indicated by disturbance in the light reflex, the base of the cone, in some instances, narrowing to a line or disappearing. There may be an increase in prominence of the short process of the malleus and of the anterior and particularly the posterior tympanic folds. The handle of the malleus often is fore-shortened and more horizontal than normal as it is drawn inward, backward, and upward.

The tympanic membrane as a whole may bulge outward from fluid within the tympanum or there may be a localized pointing of pus over any area of the membrane.

2. **Otoscopic Examination.**—The meatus should be examined through an illuminated speculum for obstruction or occlusion resulting from acute inflammatory swelling. Pus, wax, or foreign bodies may be present in the canal. The drum membrane should be examined carefully for luster, color, mobility, hyperemia, retraction, thickening, or perforation. Attention should be directed along the handle of the malleus until the flaccid portion

7

of the membrane is brought into view, and then to the anterior and posterior malleolar folds, after which the remainder of the circumference of the membrane should be inspected Particular care must be exercised in examining the size, shape, and position of the light reflex, or "luminous cone," and the degree of prominence of the short process of the malleus.

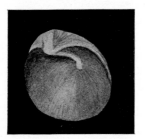

FIG. 90.—INDRAWN TYMPANIC MEMBRANE. (Dickie in Jackson and Coates, "The Nose, Throat, and Ear and Their Diseases.")

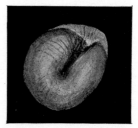

FIG. 91.—APPEARANCE OF THE TYMPANIC MEM· BRANE IN ACUTE OTITIS MEDIA.

There is marked bulging of the drum. (Dickie in Jackson and Coates, "The Nose, Throat, and Ear and Their Diseases.")

Alterations in the color, luster, apparent thickness, and curvature of the drum, as well as any abnormal areas on its surface, should be noted.

3. **Inflammation of the Tympanic Membrane, Myringitis.**—Inflammation of the drum is present nearly always in acute inflammation in the tympanic cavity. The ear drum may be swollen and congested, even ulcerated, without impairing the hearing seriously, unless the inflammation involves the entire tympanic cavity. As the largest vessels lie in the plexus which follows the malleus handle, redness is most frequent in that area. It is well to remember that the redness, as well as the luster, of an acutely inflamed drumhead may be

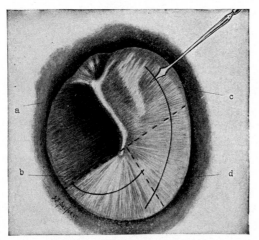

FIG. 92.—INCISION (PARACENTESIS) OF THE LEFT TYM PANIC MEMBRANE.

The quadrants of the left tympanic membrane are shown: *a*, Anterosuperior quadrant; *b*, antero-inferior; *c*, posterosuperior; *d*, postero-inferior; the two most usual sites in which the ear drum is incised are shown; a paracentesis knife is making a long incision, parallel with, and a short distance in front of, the posterior border of the membrane, extending through one or more quadrants; a shorter, curved incision is seen in the antero-inferior quadrant. (Bickham, "Operative Surgery.")

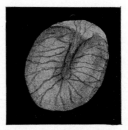

FIG. 93.—ACUTE CATARRHAL INFLAMMATION OF THE TYMPANIC MEMBRANE.

Dilated vessels are seen running across the drumhead, and the membrane has lost its gloss. (Dickie in Jackson and Coates, "The Nose, Throat, and Ear and Their Diseases.")

obscured by exfoliating epithelium, and that marked swelling may obscure all landmarks. The inflammation generally subsides after the otitis media has cleared up. If the disease becomes chronic, deposits of chalk may occur within the membrane, thickening it, rendering it rigid, and interfering with its mobility, elasticity, and vibrating function

4. **Incision of the Ear Drum.**—Paracentesis, or simple puncture, of the drum should

not be confused with incision of the drum. It is agreed that simple puncture is not sufficient to secure adequate drainage, and that a free incision is attended by more immediate and more favorable results. No harm can come from free incision since healing takes place quickly, sometimes before desired. If the drumhead is bulging, the incision should be made through the most prominent part. If not, the most suitable place on the drum for incision is its postero-inferior quadrant midway between the handle of the malleus and the posterior periphery of the drumhead. The incision always should be made downward, carrying the knife away from the ossicles and affording the freest and most dependent drainage.

Supra-umbilical incision may sever the attachment of the incus to the malleus, or may cut the chorda tympani nerve, causing a cessation of salivary secretion.

Early incision in otitis media is accompanied by very favorable results, often shortening the course of the disease and preventing extension of the purulent infection into the mastoid cells.

5. **Rupture of the Membrane.**—The tympanic membrane may be ruptured by direct or indirect violence. The commonest forms of direct violence are scratching the drum with a sharp instrument, or attempts to remove a foreign body. Many ruptures result from sudden compression of the air in the external auditory canal, which follows a fall or blow upon the ear. Rupture by indirect violence occurs commonly in skull fracture. The fracture may be transverse, running along the line of the external auditory canal through the labyrinth and across the tympanum. In this fracture, there is discharge of blood and cerebrospinal fluid through the meatus. When the fracture line is sagittal, it follows the roof of the middle ear cavity and may not open the labyrinth. There then will be blood, but no cerebrospinal fluid, in the external meatus.

The membrane may burst outward following violent sneezing, coughing, or vomiting. acts which transmit air under increased pressure through the auditory tube to the tympanic cavity.

When the membrane ruptures from concussion from violent pressure transmitted through the air, it usually gives way in the antero-inferior quadrants or around the malleus. Perforations which take place near the attachment of the drum are exceedingly slow in healing.

Perforation of the membrane, which occurs usually in the inferior quadrants, generally is caused by the ulceration of purulent otitis media.

(B) TYMPANIC CAVITY

1. **Definition and Topographic Divisions.**—The tympanic cavity lies between the drum membrane and the promontory of the labyrinth of the inner ear. In the upper reaches of the tympanic cavity, above the level of the drum membrane, is an extremely important vault-shaped compartment, the *superior tympanic cavity*, or the *epitympanic recess (attic)*. It contains the head of the malleus and the body of the incus. This recess is continuous, posteriorly, with the mastoid antrum and, anteriorly, with the tympanic cavity at a level somewhat above the entrance of the auditory tube. The attic is divided into mesial and lateral secondary cavities by the ossicles and the ligaments holding them to its walls The mesial compartment communicates with the tympanic cavity proper, interrupted only by the tendon of the tensor muscle of the drum and its folds of mucous membrane. The lateral space is compressed between the flaccid portion of the drum membrane laterally, and the head of the malleus and the body of the incus mesially. It terminates below in a depression in the flaccid part of the membrane known as "Prussak's pouch." This pouch is the natural path of egress for pus in the outer compartment of the attic through the drum into the external auditory meatus. Infection in this pouch may be reached by curetting the lateral wall of the attic above the drum membrane. It frequently is complicated by osteitis of the ossicles.

On the floor of the main cavity is a deep groove, the *inferior tympanic cavity (hypotympanic recess)*. A thin layer of bone separates it from the bulb of the jugular vein inferiorly, and from the internal carotid artery anteriorly. Suppuration within the tympanic cavity proper may cause pus to settle in this recess and result in secondary osteitis of the floor, which, in turn, may cause a thrombosis of the internal jugular vein or an ulceration of the internal carotid artery.

2. **Chain of Ossicles.**—The three ossicles of the tympanic cavity, the malleus (hammer), incus (anvil), and stapes (stirrup), are arranged in a movable chain which connects the tympanic membrane with the oval window in the vestibule of the labyrinth. The malleus, or outer bone of this chain, is embedded in the substance of the tympanic membrane. It articulates with the second ossicle, the incus, which contacts the stapes, the foot plate of which is engaged in the oval window of the vestibule. The head of the malleus and the body of the incus lie in the epitympanic recess above the upper margin of the tympanic membrane. The handle of the malleus is an important landmark, observed readily in otoscopic examination.

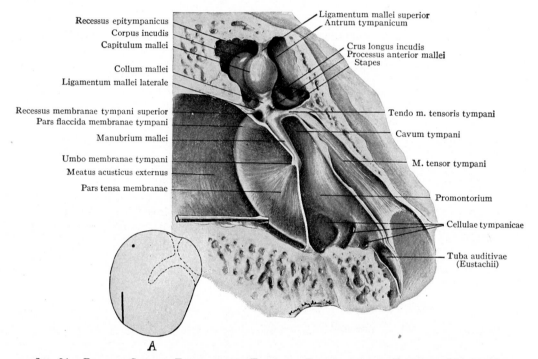

Recessus epitympanicus
Corpus incudis
Capitulum mallei

Collum mallei
Ligamentum mallei laterale

Recessus membranae tympani superior
Pars flaccida membranae tympani
Manubrium mallei

Umbo membranae tympani
Meatus acusticus externus
Pars tensa membranae

Ligamentum mallei superior
Antrum tympanicum

Crus longus incudis
Processus anterior mallei
Stapes

Tendo m. tensoris tympani

Cavum tympani

M. tensor tympani

Promontorium

Cellulae tympanicae

Tuba auditivae
(Eustachii)

A

Fig. 94.—Frontal Section Through the Tympanic Cavity and the Tympanic Membrane.
The arrow indicates the position for paracentesis of the drum; A is a diagram of the ear drum with the position of the incision indicated.

The bones are connected by true joints, lined by synovia. They are bound together with intrinsic ligaments and are secured to the walls of the cavity by extrinsic ligaments covered with mucous membrane. The chain of jointed ossicles constitutes a series of levers by means of which the movements of the drum membrane are transmitted through the foot plate of the stapes to the labyrinth. The resulting excursions of the stapes are less extensive and, therefore, more forcible than are the movements imparted to the handle of the malleus. Sclerosis and ankylosis of these small bones cause immobilization of the chain and impaired hearing, ever-present dangers in inflammatory lesions of the middle ear.

Two small muscles regulate the tension between the ossicles, one attached to the handle of the malleus, the other to the stapes. The *tensor muscle* of the tympanum draws the membrane mesially and tenses it, simultaneously pulling the handle of the malleus winard. The foot plate of the stapes is forced into the oval window and increases the intralabyrinthine pressure Contraction of the *stapedius muscle* tilts the stapes out of the oval window, decreases intralabyrinthine pressure, and relieves tension on the drum membrane.

This disposition of a mucous membrane sheath over the ossicles, continuous with that lining the tympanic cavity, explains the imminent possibilities of pharyngeal infection involving the tympanic cavity, the associated air spaces, and the tiny ear bones and their delicate joints. The folds of mucous membrane, which extend from the inner wall of the tympanic cavity to the ossicles, often form stiffened adhesive bands after inflammatory conditions in the tympanum; these bands constitute the basis for a serious impairment of hearing. In chronic middle ear disease, involvement of the mucous membrane on the ossicles requires removal of the ossicles themselves as well as the drum.

3. **Walls of the General Tympanic Cavity.**—The tympanic cavity, a cuboid space, presents a lateral or drum membrane wall, a mesial or labyrinthine wall, an inferior or jugular wall, an anterior or carotid wall, a posterior or mastoid wall, and a superior or cranial wall.

The *lateral wall* of the tympanum is formed partly by the tympanic membrane and partly by the segment of the squamous portion of the temporal bone which forms the upper wall of the external auditory meatus. The drum membrane, constituting the main

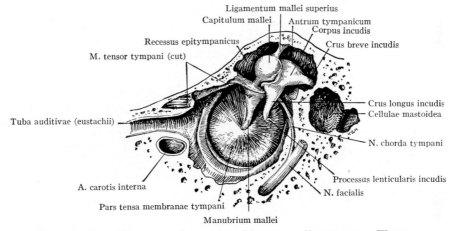

FIG. 95.—RIGHT TYMPANIC CAVITY AND MEMBRANE VIEWED FROM WITHIN.

component of the lateral wall, is of such surgical import that it merits separate regional discussion (p. 94).

The *mesial (labyrinthine) wall* separates the tympanic cavity from the inner ear and presents a point of orientation, the bony capsule of the labyrinth, consisting of the conspicuous rounded *promontory*, formed by the first turn or basal whorl of the cochlea (p. 112) and occupying the middle of the wall. The slightly concave tympanic membrane encroaches on the lumen of the main cavity to within 2 mm. of the promontory. Two openings in the mesial wall lead to the labyrinth. The upper opening lies opposite the upper posterior quadrant of the tympanic membrane and is the oval window (fenestra ovalis) into which fits the foot plate of the stapes. Directly below, separated from the upper opening by only a few millimeters, is the lower opening, the round window (fenestra rotunda). This is closed by a strong membrane, the secondary tympanic membrane, separating the tympanum from the cochlea.

Just above the oval window lies the canal for the facial nerve, which passes downward and backward in the posterior portion of the mesial wall. The thin bony lamella which forms the wall of this canal (aqueduct of Fallopius) sometimes presents a defect which leaves the nerve sheath directly in contact with the mucous membrane of the tympanic cavity. Chronic inflammation of the overlying mucous membrane or mechanical injury from an ill-directed curet may result in paralysis of the facial nerve. Above and behind the canal for this nerve is the entrance (aditus) to the mastoid (tympanic) antrum.

The *inferior wall* or floor of the cavity is a thin-walled groove which sinks below the level of the tympanic membrane and the opening of the auditory tube, forming the hypotympanic recess. This cavity favors the collection of pus from middle ear disease. Pneumatic spaces frequently lead off from this region, forming the cells of the tympanum. The bulb of the jugular vein may encroach on the floor of the tympanum and produce a dome-like elevation in which dehiscence occasionally occurs.

The large, bell-like opening of the auditory tube is located in the *anterior wall*. The internal carotid artery encroaches on the tympanum in this region, from which it is separated by a thin plate of bone. The thinness of this bony interval accounts for the distressing auditory symptoms of which patients with carotid aneurysm complain. Infection here may extend to the adjoining cavernous sinus and cause thrombosis. Fractures frequently occur through this wall.

The *posterior* or *mastoid wall* in the upper or epitympanic portions leads into the mastoid antrum by way of the aditus.

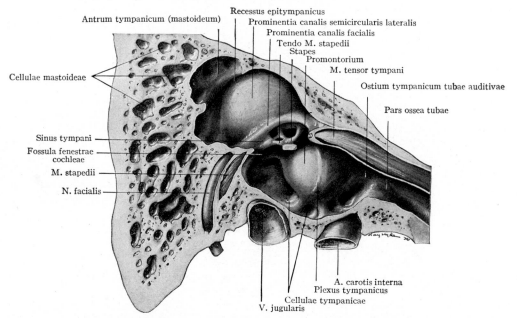

FIG. 96.—MEDIAL WALL OF THE RIGHT TYMPANIC CAVITY AND ANTRUM.

A thin plate from the squamous portion of the temporal bone, which itself is often paper-thin, separates the *superior wall* of the cavity from the temporal lobe of the brain and its enveloping meninges. This plate, called the tegmen, continues posteriorly as the roof of the antrum. The petrosquamosal suture passes diagonally through the tegmen. This, in the young, transmits blood vessels and lymphatics from the middle ear to the middle cerebral fossa. It may be so broad as to present an extensive dehiscence in the wall, where the mucosa of the cavity is in direct contact with the dura. Certain meningeal and cerebral complications of otitis media may be accounted for in this way.

SURGICAL CONSIDERATIONS

The hearing disturbances which complicate disease of the tympanic cavity, in all or any of the divisions, are the result of sclerosis of the drumhead with ankylosis of the ossicle joints. The utmost in hearing is attainable only with normal play in the ligaments and joints and absolute integrity of the muscles which control them. Treatment for the loss of hearing is directed toward restoration of mobility resulting from the sclerosis and ankylosis. Restoration of mobility is attempted by such mechanical procedures as pneumatic massage of the tympanic membrane and inflation of the tympanic cavity through the auditory tube.

1. **Acute Middle Ear Disease.**—Acute catarrhal middle ear disease is caused in most instances by spread of a catarrhal condition from the nose or nasopharynx along the auditory (eustachian) tube into the middle ear. A hypertrophied pharyngeal tonsil or adenoid vegetations are by far the most important predisposing causes. These growths, by occluding the auditory tube, interfere with the ventilation of the middle ear. There is first a hyperemia and swelling of the mucous membrane of the middle ear, followed by the secretion of an exudate. The tympanic cavity becomes filled, partially or completely with this fluid and, as the auditory tube also is swollen and congested, leakage of the fluid into the throat is not possible. The condition may persist and pass imperceptibly into subacute and chronic forms. On the other hand, the infection may become more severe and develop into acute middle ear suppuration. As regards functional disability, congestion alone scarcely affects the hearing. If the ear is filled only partially with exudate

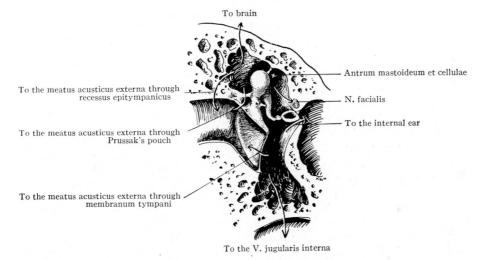

FIG. 97.—FRONTAL SECTION THROUGH THE RIGHT MIDDLE EAR TO SHOW THE PATHS OF INFECTION FROM THE TYMPANIC CAVITY.

the hearing may be almost normal, but if the exudate fills the tympanic cavity completely there is considerable deafness.

Pathologic changes which occur in acute middle ear disease are essentially similar to those occurring in catarrhal disease, and vary only in degree. In all but the rarest instances, infection reaches the tympanic cavity by way of the tube. With increasing formation of purulent exudate, the tympanic membrane bulges outward, either to give way and allow a copious discharge of pus, or, if not rupturing early, to cause the purulent exudate to be forced back into the mastoid cells and perhaps to fill them completely. Drum perforation is not merely a mechanical process, but is preceded by pathologic infiltration of its layers with destruction of part of the fibrous tissue framework. Perforation generally occurs before the mastoid cells are involved to any serious degree, and the discharge of pus is followed by a gradual recession of the inflammation. In most instances, the discharge lessens, the drum perforation heals, and conditions in the tympanic cavity return to normal. If, as frequently occurs, the perforation is too small or the pus is too thick for free and adequate drainage, the healing process is delayed and there is great danger of the pus being forced into the mastoid cells. When the perforation becomes free, the infection in the mastoid cells may clear up, although the complexity of their arrangement must make drainage of the more distant cells imperfect, at best. If drainage is inadequate, infection in the mastoid cells becomes more acute. Mucous membrane necrosis takes place and the bony framework is broken down and absorbed, with consequent abscess formation (acute mastoiditis). In time, the pus may work its way to the surface by perforating the cortex, or it may burrow through the inner table of the skull and produce a subperiosteal or an intracranial abscess.

2. **Chronic Middle Ear Disease and Cholesteatoma Formation.**—Chronic middle ear suppuration is the result of an unhealed or recurrent otitis media. A factor delaying cure in otitis media is the presence of adenoid vegetation in the nasopharynx, which causes continual re-infection of the tympanic cavity through the tube.

In the milder cases, the mucous membrane is thickened and fibrous to the degree that the contours of the cavity are smoothed out. The bone may show signs of caries in certain areas, and the condition is fraught with considerable danger if the caries appears on the inner or upper walls of the tympanum.

In certain cases, the epithelium of the meatus or of the outer surface of the drumhead may grow into the middle ear and spread over the inside, replacing the mucous membrane. With a very large perforation, the whole of the tympanum may be lined with dry skin upon cessation of the discharge. In other cases, especially where the epitympanic recess or the antrum is the seat of chronic suppuration, the course is not so favorable. The skin grows in through a marginal drum perforation and spreads into a cavity where pus and granulations are present and are obstacles to the complete epidermization and drying up of the cavity. The result is the formation of a lamellated mass of material full of micro-organisms of various varieties—*cholesteatoma*. This gradually increases from deposition of fresh layers until it fills the cavity completely. Slow erosion of the bone occurs, particularly in the projecting spots. The projection of the external semicircular canal is particularly likely to become eroded, resulting in the invasion of the labyrinth with a cystic process. The bone erosion may be extensive in all directions and lay bare the dura mater over the roof to the tympanum, or the lateral sinus posterior to it. The consequences may be of the utmost gravity.

(C) AUDITORY (EUSTACHIAN) TUBE

1. **Definition, Boundaries, and Physiology.**—The auditory (eustachian) tube, commonly considered to be a portion of the middle ear, is an osteocartilaginous duct connecting the tympanic cavity with the nasal portion of the pharynx. Its mucous membrane lining is continuous with that of the communicating tympanum and pharynx. Through this passage, the air pressure on both sides of the tympanic membrane is equalized, a factor essential to proper function of the membrane. Obstruction to the entrance of air into the tube results in a negative pressure in the tympanic cavity, which, with the atmospheric pressure on the outer side of the drum, causes the membrane to be retracted into the cavity. Otoscopic examination in this condition reveals foreshortening of the long process, prominence of the short process, thickening of the drum, and distortion or absence of the light reflex. If the obstruction persists, the sensation of fullness of the ear results. Permanent changes in the drum occur from hyperemia and fibrosis with scar formation. The scar formation involves the ligamentous structures of the ossicles, causing a semi-ankylosis of the bones, which is, by far, the most common cause of deafness. This is the so-called "catarrhal deafness."

2. **Anatomic Summary.**—The auditory tube is about 3.5 cm. long, and is directed downward mesially, and forward from the tympanic cavity. Structurally, the wall is divided into bony and cartilaginous portions. The bony wall extends about a third of the length of the tube from the tympanic orifice to the pharynx. Its shape is that of two elongated cones, a pharyngeal and a tympanic, placed together at their truncated summits. The lumen of the duct, therefore, is widest at the two orifices and is narrowed at the junction of the bony and cartilaginous portions. This narrowing is known as the *isthmus* and is from 1 to 2 mm. in diameter, a fact which predisposes to obstruction from

congestive swelling of its mucous membrane lining. A long-standing infection may produce scar formation with permanent constriction, so that the tube will not admit a catheter or bougie much larger than 1 mm. in diameter. It is a question, however, whether such a procedure, because of the trauma produced, does not aggravate the condition toward which therapy is directed.

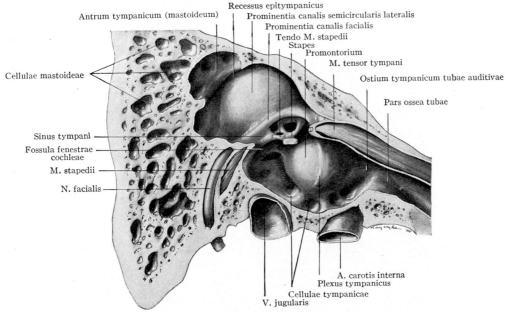

FIG. 98.—MEDIAL WALL OF THE RIGHT TYMPANIC CAVITY AND ANTRUM.
The relations of the tympanic opening of the auditory tube are emphasized.

The *pharyngeal orifice* (p. 150) is located on the lateral wall of the nasopharynx about 1 cm. behind the posterior extremity of the inferior concha.

SURGICAL CONSIDERATIONS

1. **Obstruction of the Auditory Tube.**—Auditory tube obstruction is caused primarily by inflammation of the lymphoid ring under the mucous membrane lining its pharyngeal orifice. Generally, the edema results from an inflammatory extension along the mucous membrane from some focus in the nasopharyngeal tract. The mucous membrane of the pharyngeal orifice of the tube may be involved by adjacent adenoid tissue. The occlusion which follows produces negative pressure within the tympanum, passive congestion, and connective tissue formation. It may bring about deafness by causing scar tissue to be formed over the joints of the ossicles, which cuts off the innervation and blood supply and limits mobility.

The pharyngeal orifice may be injured during operations in the nasopharynx or on the posterior ends of the turbinate bones, mainly in the unguarded curettage of adenoids, so as to result in scar formation which brings about occlusion of the orifice. This scar formation may be so extensive, or be so located, as to involve the superior and middle constricting muscles, contracting the tubal opening and leaving the orifice permanently open. The scar has little resistance to infection.

2. **Inflation of the Tympanic Cavity.**—Inflation of the tympanic cavity for diagnostic, prognostic, or therapeutic purposes can be accomplished only through the auditory tube. A variety of methods may be used. Valsalva's procedure consists of a vigorous expiratory effort with the nose and mouth held closed. The contained air, having no other means of escape, is distributed into the open auditory tubes and into the tympanic cavities. A

sense of pressure is produced in both ears, with a distinct click of air against the drum. The hearing at the same time is dulled, the change being caused by the bulging outward of the tympanic membrane by the air forced through the tubes into the tympanum. Any catheterization procedure should be done only under the direction of a skilled otologist (p. 153).

(D) MASTOID ANTRUM AND MASTOID AIR CELLS

The mastoid (tympanic) antrum and the mastoid air cells are the second division of the air-containing compartments of the middle ear. By the antrum and mastoid air cells are meant the diverticula of the tympanic cavity formed at the expense of the mastoid portion of the temporal bone. Extending backward from the epitympanic recess of the tympanic cavity are: first, a narrow bony opening called the aditus ad antrum; second, a cavity usually more extensive than those behind it, called the mastoid antrum; and third, small diverticula of the antrum, the mastoid air cells proper. The mastoid antrum

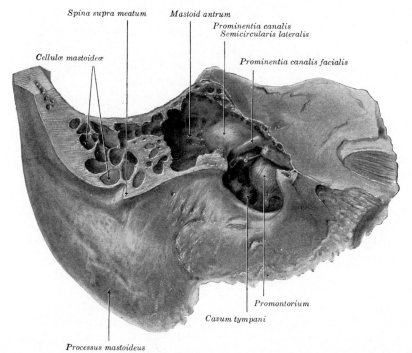

Spina supra meatum   *Mastoid antrum*
                          Prominentia canalis
                          Semicircularis lateralis

Cellulæ mastoideæ   *Prominentia canalis facialis*

Promontorium

Cavum tympani

Processus mastoideus

FIG. 99.—LATERAL VIEW OF THE RIGHT TYMPANIC CAVITY AND ITS MASTOID EXTENSIONS.
These are exposed by removing their outer wall and contiguous portions of the anterior and superior walls.
(Shambaugh in Jackson and Coates, "The Nose, Throat, and Ear and Their Diseases.")

or original mastoid cell is present at birth and the remaining mastoid cells evaginate from it in early life. These appendages of the tympanic cavity are lined by mucous membrane.

1. Aditus ad Antrum.—The aditus ad antrum, or entrance into the antrum, is a relatively broad, short canal of variable dimensions, which places the mastoid antrum and air cells in communication with the tympanic cavity. The shallowness of this communication is accounted for in large part by the lifting up of the floor of the antrum by the facial ridge, which contains the seventh (facial) nerve and a small artery. On the *medial wall* of the aditus (Fig. 100), above and behind the facial ridge, is a smooth convex area of bone, marking the position of the lateral semicircular canal of the inner ear. Any obstruction of the narrow entrance favors the retention of inflammatory products in the mastoid air cells. For this reason, removal of the *external wall* of the aditus is one of the most important steps in the procedure designed to place the mastoid air cells and antrum into broad and open communication with the tympanic cavity.

2 **Mastoid (Tympanic) Antrum.**—The mastoid antrum is a large mastoid air cell, formed before birth by upward and posterior extension of the tympanic cavity. The remaining cells of the mastoid cavity develop from this cell and remain in communication with it by orifices in the antral walls. In general, the antrum lies behind and above the bony portion of the external auditory meatus, but its location and size vary between wide limits; these variations are of the greatest surgical importance. In the newborn, the antrum lies higher than in the adult, being almost directly above the bony auditory meatus, on a level with its upper margin. As the mastoid bone develops, the antrum moves progressively backward and downward. It holds a fairly constant relationship to the suprameatal spine (of Henle). In the infant, the bony wall separating the antrum from the exterior is not more than from 2 to 4 mm. in thickness; as age advances, the lateral plate may attain a thickness of 1 to 1.5 cm.

The *lateral (external) wall* of the antrum is the wall of surgical approach, which, projected externally, is that part of the temporal bone overlain by the auricle. In the adult, it is about 1 to 1.5 cm. thick. The *posterior wall* opens into mastoid air cells separating

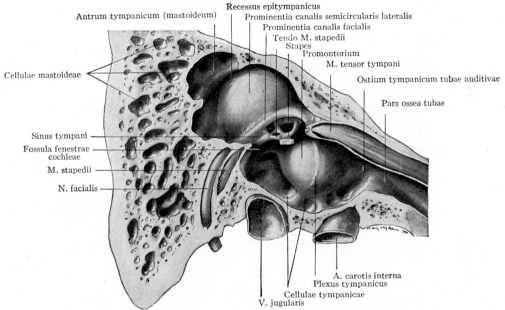

FIG. 100.—MEDIAL WALL OF THE RIGHT TYMPANIC CAVITY AND ANTRUM.
Section shows the thin layer of bone between the mastoid antrum and the middle cranial fossa.

it from the lateral sinus which is slightly inferior, as well as posterior, to it. The *mesial wall* is composed of the mastoid cells in the sclerosed portion of the petrous part of the temporal bone. On this mesial wall, deep in and a little anterior, lie the lateral (horizontal) semicircular canal and the canal for the facial nerve. The mesial wall of the antrum is well anterior to a normally placed lateral sinus. The *superior wall* or *roof* of the antrum lies against the middle cerebral compartment; osteitis of this wall may cause a subtemporal abscess. An incision above the line of the roof or above the line of the suprameatal spine (of Henle), projected internally, enters the cranial cavity. The anterior portion of the *inferior wall* is in close relation with the seventh (facial) nerve, which, in its bony canal, descends vertically through the mastoid bone; the nerve leaves the stylomastoid foramen, after having wound about the posterosuperior margin of the tympanic cavity and around the lateral semicircular canal into the floor of the antrum. The *anterior wall* presents an opening into the tympanic cavity through the aditus.

3. **Mastoid Air Cavities.**—The air spaces of the mastoid process do not exist in the newborn. Toward the end of fetal life, the antrum sends out buds or trabeculae into the

spongy tissue between its two bony tables; these are the progenitors of the mastoid air cells. These buds enlarge and divide secondarily until they ramify, with great individual variation, throughout the mastoid portion of the temporal bone, even into the squamous part of the temporal bone and into the occipital bone and the zygomatic process. As the margin of the mastoid process is approached, the cells tend to become larger, the tip usually being occupied by one or several large cells.

Infection from the tympanic cavity invades these cells and spreads down to the mastoid tip cell by way of the deep-lying cells. This causes tenderness in the tip, which in adults may be one of the earliest symptoms in mastoid disease, but in children tenderness is found more often over the antrum. Infection may spread to the tip cell and subside because of the channel of drainage through the chain of cells from the tip to the antrum direct.

4. **Types of Mastoid Structure.**—Four types of mastoid bone may be differentiated: pneumatic, diploic, sclerotic, and mixed. In the *pneumatic* type there is complete development of cell structure and the whole mastoid process is composed of large air spaces communicating with each other and with the antrum. The cortex is relatively thin and

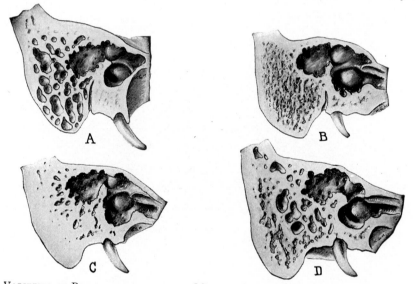

Fig. 101.—Varieties of Pneumatization of the Mastoid Process and Types of Mastoid Air Cells. A, Pneumatic type; B, diploic type; C, sclerotic type; D, mixed type.

perforates early in disease, especially in children. Danger of intracranial complication, particularly if the location of the inflammation is external, is reduced to a minimum. In the *diploic* type the mastoid process conforms to the structures of the other cranial bones, having an outer and an inner table with diploë between. The antrum usually is the only cell present. The cortex is thick and does not present localizing symptoms of mastoid disease. The *sclerotic* type is that in which the mastoid process is composed of compact bone of extreme density, the result of chronic infection which has interfered with the usual absorption of diploë and subsequent pneumatization and has brought about a condensing osteitis resulting in nondevelopment or complete obliteration of the cell system. The antrum remains, although frequently reduced in size. The almost acellular mastoid bone usually is of the consistency of ivory. The improbability of localizing symptoms of mastoid disease, presenting themselves in such circumstances, is evident. Infection follows the line of least resistance and may invade the middle or posterior cranial fossa, lateral sinus, or lateral semicircular canal. The *mixed* type represents a combination of the diploic and sclerotic types with perhaps a few pneumatic cells present. An index of the type of mastoid upon which operation is contemplated may be obtained by roentgenologic examination.

5 Suprameatal Triangle, Spine, and Fossa; Relations to the Mastoid Antrum.—
The outer surface of the mastoid process has few conspicuous landmarks. The *postero-superior margin* of the opening of the bony meatus usually is a conspicuous marking. Within its border, or just adjacent to it, is the more or less prominent *suprameatal spine* (of Henle) to which the superior ligament of the auricle is attached.

The outer opening of the bony meatus is oval in outline with its long diameter vertical. At the level of the superior margin of the opening, the posterior root of the zygoma, the *suprameatal crest*, runs horizontally backward. The original *suprameatal triangle*, as described by Macewen, has, as one side, the posterior root of the zygoma, as a second, the posterosuperior margin of the opening of the bony meatus with its contained suprameatal spine, and, as a third, a line joining the two other sides. In the floor of the triangle lies the *suprameatal fossa*. These landmarks are not always easy to outline definitely in an operative field.

Another description gives as one side of the suprameatal triangle a horizontal line tangent to the superior margin of the bony meatus, as a second, a vertical line passing

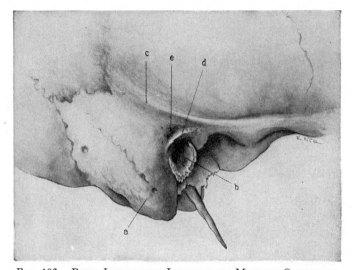

FIG. 102.—BONY LANDMARKS INVOLVED IN MASTOID OPERATION.
a, Mastoid process of the temporal bone; *b,* the bony part of the external auditory canal; *c,* suprameata crest; *d,* suprameatal spine; *e,* suprameatal fossa. (Bickham, "Operative Surgery.")

tangent to the posterior margin of the bony meatus, and as a third, a line formed by the posterosuperior margin of the canal wall. This triangle, while actual, calls for considerable dissection if it is to be determined accurately.

Since the posterosuperior margin of the canal wall can be determined readily, it may be used as a base for an equilateral triangle which may be constructed in the imagination, no other landmark being necessary.

The *mastoid antrum* lies deep to the suprameatal fossa and, therefore, directly within the suprameatal triangle or just behind it; in other words, it lies half way up the posterior wall of the meatus between the suprameatal spine and the posterior portion of the horizontal suprameatal crest: The suprameatal crest marks the inferior edge of the dura, the roof of the antrum, and the middle cerebral fossa. Incisions must be kept below this crest to avoid injury to the middle cerebral fossa which sometimes dips to an extremely low level. When the suprameatal crest cannot be felt, incisions should be kept below a horizontal line running backward from the upper edge of the bony external meatus or its most prominent part, the suprameatal spine (of Henle). An instrument in the antrum must be checked from going deeper to avoid injury to the lateral semicircular canal and the facial nerve.

Surgical Considerations

1. **Mastoiditis.**—True mastoiditis almost always is subsequent to an extension of acute disease of the tympanic cavity by mucous membrane continuity, a part of the complex of suppuration of the middle ear. The secondary type of mastoiditis is of common occurrence, whereas primary inflammatory mastoid disease is rare. Chronic mastoiditis usually is the result of neglect of the acute form. True clinical mastoiditis seldom, if ever, develops under from five to seven days following the onset of the acute middle ear disease, but in all acute suppurative inflammations of the middle ear the mastoid antrum is involved to some degree. Empyema of the mastoid cavities is restricted to suppuration of the cell spaces without bony wall involvement. If the bony septa between the tiny cavities are involved seriously, there is softening and disintegration at the expense of the bony tissue. This process may go on until the lateral sinus wall is destroyed. The most definite and important symptoms of mastoid involvement are subperiosteal edema and post-auditory canal edema with mastoid tip tenderness. The pain probably results from periosteal stretching.

2. **Paths of Extension of Mastoid Infection.**—Although infection of the *lateral sinus* may arise from infection of the superior petrosal sinus as a result of inflammation of the attic of the tympanic cavity, or, in children, by involvement of the jugular bulb from infection through the floor of the tympanic cavity, it usually arises from suppurating mastoid cells. It is the sinus most commonly involved because of its relations to so large a series of diseased cavities. Extension occurs by way of the numerous small veins that reach the sinus through the bone, and by direct infection arising from perisinus abscess. With the lateral sinus involved, extension may occur to associated venous channels, especially the internal jugular vein, or to the other side of the skull by way of the confluens sinuum. The lateral sinus runs horizontally forward from the confluens to a point 1.5 cm. behind, and slightly inferior to, the antrum, at which point it turns downward and forward forming what is known as the elbow of the sinus. It ends atthe jugular foramen as the internal jugular vein. Its descending portion has relations with the posterosuperior angle of the suprameatal triangle. In the pneumatic type of mastoid, the sinus runs in a shallow groove on the mesial aspect of the temporal bone, and is more mesial and more posterior than in sclerosed and allied types of mastoid bone. In the sclerosed type, the sinus almost canalizes the bone and runs near the antrum and the posterior wall of the external auditory meatus.

Mastoid disease may extend to the *meninges* and *brain*. Inflammation may extend upward through the roof of the antrum and the superior mastoid cells contained in that wall By this route, it may extend through the small vascular channels and cause extra-dural abscess, localized or general meningitis, or brain abscess. Most of this disturbance is seen in the posterior cranial fossa.

It should be borne in mind that the facial canal with the enclosed *facial nerve* arches backward over the oval window and descends almost perpendicularly, in relation to the lateral semicircular canal and the floor of the antrum. Cholesteatoma following chronic middle ear disease may cause destruction of this nerve with resultant facial palsy. This results in complete immobility of the muscles of expression on the affected side of the face.

In the pneumatic mastoid, infection readily finds its way into the contiguous cells causing early *perforation of the cortex*. It may penetrate the inner aspect of the mastoid tip, burst through the sternomastoid muscle, and break into the submaxillary region of the neck producing what is known as Bezold's type of mastoiditis, which may be confused with involvement of the glands of the posterior cervical triangle in so far as swelling and tenderness are concerned.

3. **Simple Mastoid Operation.**—The simple mastoid operation consists in opening and draining the mastoid antrum and air cells, and clearing a passage to the middle ear. A single incision about 0.5 cm. behind the attachment of the auricle is made through the overlying tissues and periosteum. The auricle and the membranous meatus are pushed

forward and the periosteum is stripped backward from the mastoid bone. In the antero-superior part of the wound, the suprameatal spine (of Henle) and the posterior boundary of the external auditory meatus are exposed and the cortex of the mastoid is removed below the posterior continuation of the suprameatal spine. The spine should be allowed to remain intact to serve as a landmark for any later work on the mastoid area which may be required. The cells overlying the antrum are sought, the antrum is entered, and the mastoid cells are curetted, with the antrum as a center of operation.

4. **Radical Mastoid Operation.**—The radical mastoid operation resolves the mastoid antrum and cells and the middle ear into a single cavity. It is performed for chronic mastoiditis and otitis media with diseased ossicles, and to relieve or prevent serious complications from middle ear disease. Hearing is not lost completely, and sometimes actually is improved. All the ossicles except the stapes are removed, and later, a skin graft is used for epithelization of the denuded area. In this procedure, the posterosuperior portion of the bony meatus is removed to give access to the tympanic cavity. The bone which

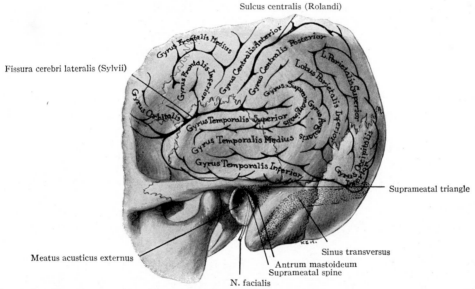

FIG. 103.—RELATIONS OF THE MASTOID ANTRUM TO THE TEMPORAL LOBE AND THE TRANSVERSE SINUS.

separates the epitympanic cavity from the roof of the bony meatus and drumhead and the ossicles are removed. As many of the mastoid air cells as are involved are cleared away. When the deep portion of the posterior wall of the meatus is chiseled away just below the antrum, the facial nerve is in danger, since only a thin, hard, bony covering protects it.

(III) INTERNAL EAR

In the petrous portion of the temporal bone, mesial and posterior to the tympanic cavity, lies the internal ear or labyrinth; this has two distinct functions, cochlear or sound perception, and vestibular or equilibration and orientation. The internal ear consists of a bony labyrinth which encloses the highly complex membranous labyrinth. In most areas, the membranous labyrinth is not in contact with its bony case, but is surrounded by fluid known as perilymph. The membranous labyrinth is filled with a fluid known as endolymph, which is not in communication with the perilymph. Both the acoustic and the equilibratory nerve paths arise from the membranous labyrinth. Exact knowledge of the labyrinth and its projection on the tympanic cavity is clinically important because of the possibility of its injury in operations upon the tympanic cavity and antrum. The walls of the cavity may be eroded by cholesteatoma, and occasionally they are injured by the curetting of granulations.

1. Osseous Labyrinth.—The bony capsule of the labyrinth, 2 to 3 mm. thick, is a hard, ivory-like structure, embedded in the petrous pyramid of the temporal bone. It is long resistant to pus in suppurative otitis media. In this labyrinth are distinguished four portions: a middle or vestibular portion, a posterosuperior or semicircular canal portion, an anterior or cochlear portion, and the internal auditory canal.

The *vestibule* is an irregularly elliptical cavity which communicates with the cochlea in front and the semicircular canals behind. It lies between the tympanic cavity laterally and the internal auditory canal mesially. The lateral wall contains the oval window for the reception of the foot plate of the stapes. The secondary tympanic membrane of this wall closes the fenestra of the cochlea (fenestra rotunda) and separates the perilymphatic space from the tympanic cavity. In the posterior portion of the vestibule are the five openings of the semicircular canals.

The *semicircular canals* are elliptical, horseshoe-shaped tubes which open at both their extremities into the vestibule. Each canal has a dilation called the ampulla. The

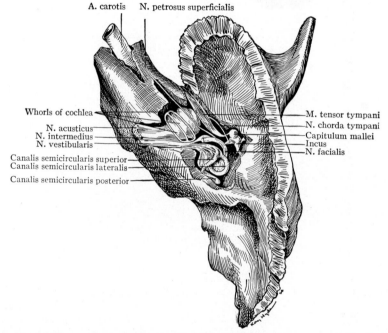

FIG 104.—AUDITORY NERVE, LABYRINTH, AND EAR OSSICLES PROJECTED ON THE PETROUS PORTION OF THE TEMPORAL BONE. (After Rouvière.)

three canals are disposed so that their planes correspond with the corners of a cube, and they are distinguished according to their direction into superior, posterior, and lateral or horizontal. The plane of the superior canal is perpendicular to the long axis of the petrous portion of the temporal bone, and its convexity looks upward. The plane of the posterior canal is parallel to the long axis of the petrous bone and to the superior canal of the opposite side. Its convexity looks backward, a little laterally, and pushes laterally the mesial wall of the aditus ad antrum. The arch of the horizontal or lateral canal is projected horizontally backward and laterally, and forms a conspicuous prominence in the floor of the aditus.

The promontory on the mesial wall of the tympanic cavity is formed by the first coil of the *cochlea*, which forms the anterior part of the bony labyrinth and lies between the vestibule and the internal carotid artery. The *internal auditory meatus* is a bony canal, running from the posterior surface of the petrous pyramid laterally and posteriorly to the vestibule. Its external bony orifice on the mesial wall of the vestibule is closed by a cribriform wall with orifices for the passage of the cochlear division of the eighth nerve and for the vestibular branches of the eighth nerve which run to the semicircular canals. Near it is the opening for the aqueduct of the vestibule which transmits from the membranous labyrinth a tube known as the endolymphatic duct.

2. Perilymphatic Space and Membranous Labyrinth.—The membranous labyrinth lies within the bony labyrinth and, save where it is attached to the bony walls by fibrous bands, especially at the exit of the nerve fibers, is surrounded on all sides by fluid, the perilymph.

The perilymph within the *perilymphatic space* conducts the least modification of pressure to all parts of the stream, and possibly has a direct communication with the subarachnoid spaces of the brain, both by way of the aqueduct of the cochlea and by the sheaths of the auditory nerves. The membranous labyrinth contains fluid known as the endolymph. Since pressure in this space is equalized, changes in position in different movements of the head are transmitted at once to the sensory cells in connection with the vestibular branch of the auditory nerve.

3. Blood Supply of the Labyrinth.—An interest in the blood supply of the labyrinth has arisen because of its bearing on clinical otology. The Ménière syndrome, sudden occurrence of deafness and vertigo, is probably dependent upon some circulatory disturbance, possibly hemorrhage into the labyrinth. The question of extension of infection from the middle ear to the labyrinth and of extension of labyrinthine infection into the cranial cavity deal, in large measure, with vascular complications.

The sole arterial supply of the internal ear is the *internal auditory artery*, a branch of the basilar artery, which enters the labyrinth through the internal acoustic canal. Its branches are end-arteries and constitute the sole supply for definite areas. The first branch is given off in the internal acoustic canal. It is the cochleovestibular artery, supplying part of the cochlea and part of the vestibular apparatus. This branch divides into two trunks, one supplying the proximal two thirds of the basal whorl of the cochlea, and the other running backward as the posterior vestibular artery.

The continuation of the internal auditory artery divides again into two trunks, one of which penetrates the modiolus and furnishes the arterial supply for all of the cochlea save the proximal two thirds of the basal whorl, the other of which runs backward as the anterior artery of the vestibule. Continuation of the anterior cochlear artery supplies portions of the semicircular canals.

Shambaugh points out the clinical bearing which attaches to the branching of the labyrinthine artery. Recognizing that the organ of Corti, throughout the entire length of the basal whorl, is supplied by minute terminal end-arteries, it becomes apparent that disturbances in these separate terminal twigs should be capable of disturbing the function of definite circumscribed areas of Corti's organ It is possible for an embolus to lodge in the main trunk and to destroy completely the function of the vestibular and cochlear mechanisms. An embolus which lodges in the cochleovestibular vessels disturbs the function which resides in the proximal two thirds of the basal coil of the cochlea, that portion which has to do with the perception of tones toward the upper end of the tone scale. At the same time, there occur disturbances of equilibrium in the domain of the semicircular canals. An embolus lodging in a continuation of the labyrinthine artery should suppress perception of the lower tones, which are taken up by the nerve cells in the upper coils of the cochlea. This embolus should produce a profound derangement in equilibrium through disturbance of portions of the superior and lateral semicircular canals.

4. Sensory Paths of the Auditory Nerve.—The eighth (auditory) nerve, with its meningeal coverings, extends into the internal auditory canal and divides into its terminal branches. The *anterior (cochlear)* branch transmits to the brain the auditory impressions from the organ of Corti. The *posterior (vestibular)* division of the eighth nerve is concerned with transmission of the sensations of equilibrium, which originate in the membranous semicircular canals and in other constituent elements of the membranous labyrinth. In its course through the internal auditory canal, the eighth nerve may be injured by skull

8

fracture or it may be compressed from hyperostosis to the extent that the functions of both divisions are impaired. Within the cranial cavity, the nerve or its sheath may be the point of origin for tumors arising at the cerebellopontine angle.

Surgical Considerations

Equilibrium depends not only upon impressions sent to the brain from the labyrinth but also upon those sent from the eyes and from the muscles. If one set of impressions be destroyed, the resulting vertigo gradually is compensated for by the remaining two sets which are sufficient to maintain balance properly. This compensation will not take place while infection in the labyrinth is active.

1. Sources of Labyrinthine Infection.—Inflammation of the labyrinth is of mastoid, meningeal, tympanic, or metastatic origin. The mastoid origin from erosion by cholesteatoma is by far the most common. The lateral semicircular canal is the commonest seat of localized labyrinthitis, since it is the one most immediately adjacent to the mastoid cells. Inflammation of the cochlea in its basal whorl may occur by infection through the oval window, following acute osteomyelitis of the stapes which fits into this window. A localized infection may spread to other portions of the perilymphatic space without involving the endolymph.

Infection may follow traumatic opening of the labyrinth in the course of a middle ear operation in which the stapes has been dislocated. This infection may complicate the removal of foreign bodies from the tympanic cavity, ill-performed paracentesis of the drum membrane, or radical mastoid operation where the labyrinth at the level of the lateral or horizontal circular canal or the oval window is exposed to trauma.

2. Paths of Spread of Labyrinthine Infection.—While the labyrinth lies largely within the bony mass of the petrous pyramid, connections possibly exist between it and the base of the brain. Over the convexity of the superior semicircular canal, a thin area of extremely hard bone underlies the brain. In this area, localized abscess rarely occurs. Labyrinthine propagation of infection may cause abscess or meningitis in the posterior fossa, but periantral and perisinus cell extension of infection is a much more common cause. The roof of the petrous bone is so dense that its erosion, save by cholesteatoma, is not likely to take place.

III. Regions about the Mouth

For anatomic and clinical consideration, the regions about the mouth are divided into the labial, buccal, masseter-mandibular, zygomatico-pterygo-maxillary, and parotid. These regions, as well as those within the mouth, and the problems they present will be understood most clearly in the light of embryologic study.

The soft parts and the skeleton of the face are formed by the outgrowth of three buds, a median premaxillary and two lateral maxillomandibular. Partial or total failure of one or more of these components to unite, form, and differentiate the nasal and buccal cavities gives rise to the various types of deformity about the nose and mouth.

The lateral buds grow toward the median line and divide to produce two processes, an inferior or mandibular, and a superior or maxillary. The mandibular processes unite in the midline to form the lower jaw or mandible. Absence of union here is rare but, when present, is manifested by a fissure of the lower lip.

The maxillary processes grow toward the midline to unite with the premaxillary bud or frontonasal process, which is a downgrowth from the cranium. Union of these three processes forms the superior or maxillary arch. Defective union gives rise to a variety of anomalies. The premaxillary bud may unite with only one maxillary bud, producing a unilateral cleft on the side where fusion does not take place; it may unite with neither maxillary bud and extend downward and forward as a proboscis, in which case a bilateral cleft results. The deformity is designated as simple or complex, depending upon whether the lip alone is involved or the hard and soft palates as well are affected. In the complex type, the buccal and nasal cavities are in broad communication

The maxillary processes form the zygomatic bones, the maxillae, and the lateral parts of the lips. The descending median or premaxillary bud contributes to the formation of the nasal fossae and forms the incisor teeth and the intermaxillary portion of the upper lip and jaw.

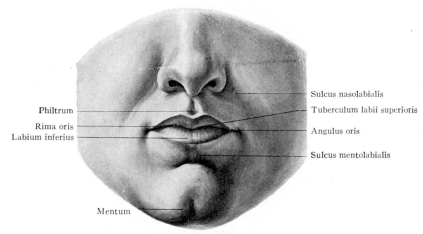

Philtrum

Rima oris
Labium inferius

Sulcus nasolabialis

Tuberculum labii superioris

Angulus oris

Sulcus mentolabialis

Mentum

FIG. 105.—STRUCTURES ABOUT THE NOSE AND MOUTH.

The nasal areas presenting between the maxillary and premaxillary buds in the fourth week of embryonic life form the nasal pits which, at this stage, are continuous with the mouth. They later become separated from it by the union of the maxillary and premaxillary processes. The pits establish secondary connections with the roof of the early

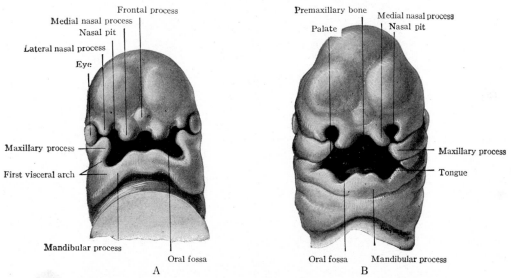

Frontal process
Medial nasal process
Nasal pit
Lateral nasal process
Eye

Maxillary process

First visceral arch

Mandibular process

Oral fossa
A

Premaxillary bone
Palate

Medial nasal process
Nasal pit

Maxillary process

Tongue

Oral fossa   Mandibular process
B

FIG. 106.—STAGES IN THE DEVELOPMENT OF THE NOSE AND MOUTH.

A, Face of an 8-mm. embryo (nineteen days). B, Face of an 11-mm. embryo (thirty-five days).

mouth cavity, and, by a thinning out and rupture of the bucconasal membranes, form the primitive choanae or posterior nares. At a later stage, the more cranial portion of the mouth cavity becomes a part of the nasal cavity by the formation, growth, and fusion in the median plane of the paired palatal processes of the maxillary and palate bones. This constitutes the formation of the palate and the establishment of communication between the nasal cavity and the nasopharynx. The septum between the nasal pits narrows and becomes the nasal septum proper, dividing the nasal cavity into paired nasal fossae.

In the eighth week of development, the smooth lateral wall of each nasal fossa presents grooves or furrows which are the forerunners of the nasal meatuses. The furrows delimit folds which are the precursors of the nasal conchae, in which cartilage later develops. This cartilage, together with that of the septum and lateral nasal walls, largely undergoes ossification. The nasal mucous membrane evaginates into neighboring bones and leads to the formation of maxillary, sphenoid, and frontal sinuses, and ethmoid cells. The initial points of evagination remain as the ostia of the adult sinuses and cells.

A. LIP REGION

1. **Definition, Boundaries, and Landmarks.**—The lip region includes an upper and a lower fleshy fold which converge at lateral commissures, circumscribe the buccal orifice, and, when closed, form the anterior wall of the buccal cavity. The upper lip is marked in the median line by the infranasal groove, which ends at the free border in a tubercle.

2. **Deep Structures of the Lip.**—The essential muscle of the lip is the *orbicularis oris*, which is disposed in an elliptical manner about the buccal aperture, with the extremities

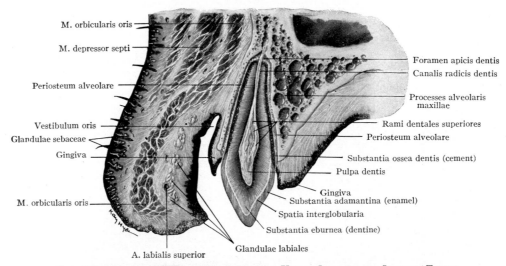

FIG. 107.—SAGITTAL SECTION THROUGH THE UPPER LIP AND AN INCISOR TOOTH.

of its upper and lower portions meeting at the lip commissures. To these commissures, the bilateral facial muscles converge and are attached. These muscles physiologically are dilators of the orifice.

The orbicularis oris muscle closes the mouth. It is supplied by the facial nerve, paralysis of which interferes with articulation, particularly that of the labial consonants, prevents tight closing of the mouth, and allows saliva to drip from the drooping corner.

The *glands* are labial, buccal, or molar, according to their location, and are most numerous between the musculature and the mucosa. Tumors arising from these glands bulge through the mucous membrane.

3. **Vessels and Nerves.**—A rich blood supply to the lips is afforded by the labial branches of the *external maxillary (facial) artery*, which have a coronary distribution deep to the orbicular muscle, therefore, nearer to the mucous membrane than to the skin. The labial arteries are large and their pulsation sometimes can be felt. In trauma of the lips against the teeth, the lips may be cut and free bleeding result. The *veins* lie to the outer side of the muscle. The *lymphatics* are arranged in plexuses lying within the mucous

membrane and skin; they follow the facial vein and empty into the submaxillary nodes. Those originating in the median portion of the lower lip drain into the submental glands, while those in the lateral portions drain directly into the submaxillary glands.

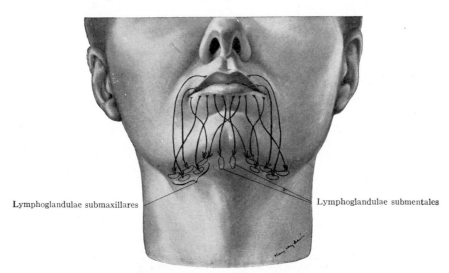

Lymphoglandulae submaxillares   Lymphoglandulae submentales

FIG. 108.—LYMPHATIC DRAINAGE FROM THE LIPS.

Certain of the channels decussate and empty into the glands of the opposite side. The lymphatic drainage in and about the lips has great surgical significance because of its rôle in carcinoma of the lip. Metastatic involvement continues from the submental and submaxillary nodes to the superior and inferior chains of the deep cervical glands.

SURGICAL CONSIDERATIONS

Because the lips have no bony attachment, the healing of a severe injury or of a destructive infection, with consequent contracture of muscle and scar tissue, is likely to result in mouth deformity and even serious distortion of neighboring structures. The great vascularity of the lips and their freedom from bony attachment partly account for the success of the many plastic operations devised for the relief of deformities.

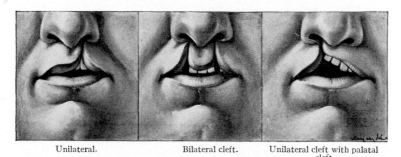

Unilateral.   Bilateral cleft.   Unilateral cleft with palatal
                                                          cleft.

FIG. 109.—TYPES OF HARELIP.

1. **Carcinoma of the Lip.**—Squamous-cell carcinoma occurs rarely on the upper lip but commonly on the lower. The complication of this lesion is the metastases which pass into the submental and submaxillary regions and thence into the deep cervical chain of glands. The involvement of the glands of both sides of the neck by decussation of the lymphatic drainage requires bilateral excision of these glands, with thorough removal of the growth itself, usually by a V-shaped incision. Palpable involvement of the submax-

illary glands presupposes involvement of those of the corresponding deep cervical chain. Because metastasis is by embolus rather than by direct extension, the operation for the primary growth and that for the removal of metastases may be performed at two different times, but removal of the glands must be complete.

2. Harelip.—The common congenital deformity of harelip results from the nonfusion of the embryonic elements which make up the lip and differentiate the nasal from the buccal cavity. Harelip frequently is complicated by a corresponding cleft in the hard and soft palates (p. 91). The degree of deformity may vary from a simple fissure to a complete cleft in the lip and in the alveolar portion of the palate (p. 137). In the repair of extensive clefts, the importance of the frontonasal process must be recognized fully. Should it be removed, there would result a loss of the intermaxillary portion of the upper jaw and its central incisor teeth. This subject is continued in the palatal region (p. 135).

B. BUCCAL (CHEEK) REGION

1. Definition.—The buccal region is the area between the inferior margin of the orbit and the lower jaw, extending from the anterior border of the masseter muscle to the fold of the nose and the commissure of the lip.

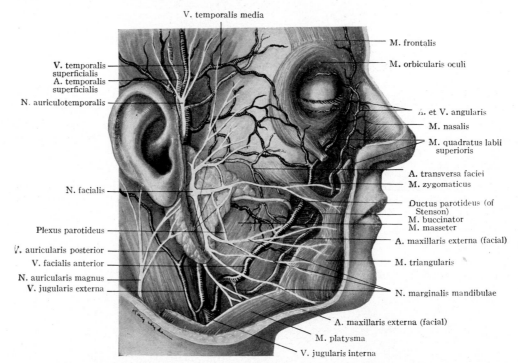

Fig. 110.—Structures on the Side of the Face.

2. Structures.—The *fat (suctorial) pad* of the cheek is a collection of the fat of the subcutaneous tissue in the space between the buccinator and masseter muscles. This fatty tissue is continuous with that of the temporal and deep lateral regions of the face, and explains the ready spread of infection or of carcinoma to these regions.

The superficial muscle layer is made up of many small *muscles* adjacent to the mouth; these have the common characteristic of being attached to the skin and orbicularis oris muscle, thereby controlling facial expression. For the most part, they converge to the labial commissures. Extending from the alveolar arch of the maxilla to that of the mandible is the more deeply placed buccinator muscle, which forms the lateral wall of the mouth.

The *parotid duct* (of Stensen), after passing forward from the surface of the masseter muscle, perforates the buccinator muscle obliquely, and courses anteriorly on the buccal mucous membrane. Its course is represented by the middle third of a line drawn from the inferior edge of the external acoustic meatus to a point midway between the ala of

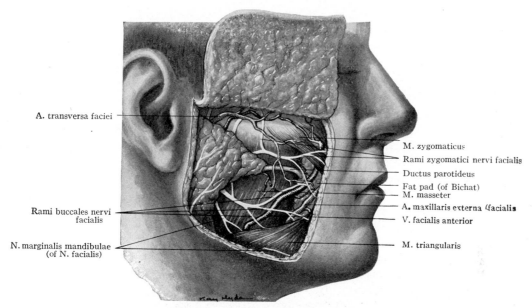

A. transversa faciei

M. zygomaticus
Rami zygomatici nervi facialis
Ductus parotideus
Fat pad (of Bichat)
M. masseter
A. maxillaris externa (facialis
V. facialis anterior

Rami buccales nervi facialis

M. triangularis

N. marginalis mandibulae (of N. facialis)

FIG. 111.—SUPERFICIAL STRUCTURES OF THE MASSETER REGION AND PART OF THE CHEEK.

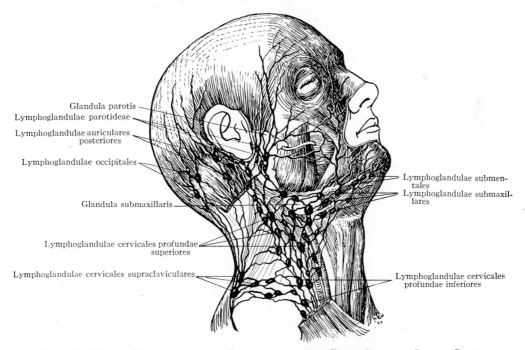

Glandula parotis
Lymphoglandulae parotideae
Lymphoglandulae auriculares posteriores

Lymphoglandulae occipitales

Lymphoglandulae submentales
Lymphoglandulae submaxillares

Glandula submaxillaris

Lymphoglandulae cervicales profundae superiores

Lymphoglandulae cervicales supraclaviculares

Lymphoglandulae cervicales profundae inferiores

FIG. 112.—LYMPH DRAINAGE TO THE SUBMAXILLARY AND DEEP CERVICAL LYMPH GLANDS.

the nose and the commissure of the lip. It penetrates the buccal mucosa, and opens into the vestibule of the mouth by a slitlike orifice on a variably developed papilla opposite the second upper molar tooth; through this orifice, the duct may be catheterized. The duct furnishes a path for infection from the mouth to the parotid gland. When the duct is severed, its proximal end may grow fast to the skin surface, forming a fistula which is difficult to heal. To repair this condition, the cut ends of the duct should be approximated by sutures which do not enter the lumen of the duct.

The *external maxillary (facial) artery*, the only important artery to the cheek, enters at the antero-inferior angle of the masseter muscle, courses forward on the buccinator muscle, and becomes the angular artery at the corner of the mouth. It is accompanied by the anterior facial *vein* which, at its origin, has direct communication with the ophthalmic

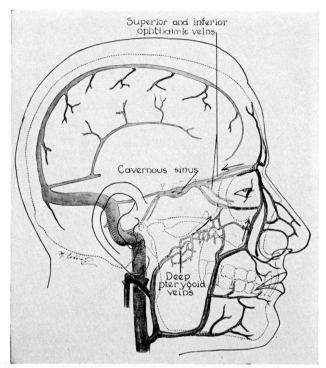

FIG. 113.—ANASTOMOSES BETWEEN THE SUPERFICIAL AND DEEP VEINS OF THE FACE AND THE OPHTHALMIC TRIBUTARIES OF THE CAVERNOUS SINUS. (E. C. Cutler in Coller and Yglesias, Surg., Gynec. and Obst Feb. 15, 1935.)

veins and through them with the cavernous sinus. Infections in this region, particularly of the upper lip and nose which may result in facial phlebitis, are exceedingly grave since they may be propagated by this direct route to the cavernous sinus and cerebral meninges (p. 32).

The *lymph drainage* is to the submaxillary and deep cervical lymph nodes. The muscles of the cheek are innervated by the facial *nerve*.

C. MASSETER-MANDIBULAR-TEMPORAL REGION

The masseter-mandibular-temporal region is the pivotal region in which the mandible, the only movable bone of the face, is controlled in its relations with the superior maxilla at the temporomandibular joint. Within the area are the ramus and body of the mandible, the overlying masseter muscle, its fascia, a portion of the parotid gland and duct, the dense parotid fascia, and the vessels and nerves coursing anteriorly over the masseter muscle.

1. **Landmarks.**—At the antero-inferior border of the region, the external maxillary (facial) artery winds about the body of the mandible, where it can be palpated and its pulsations felt. By clenching the jaws tightly, the thickness of the masseter muscle over the angle of the jaw may be brought into prominence.

2. **Superficial Structures.**—The bulk of the *parotid gland* lies on the side of the face posterior to the angle of the jaw (p. 128), but its anterior facial prolongation and duct are superficial structures within this region. From the deep cervical fascia is derived the *parotid fascia* which divides to embrace the gland (p. 129). The fascia over the anterior

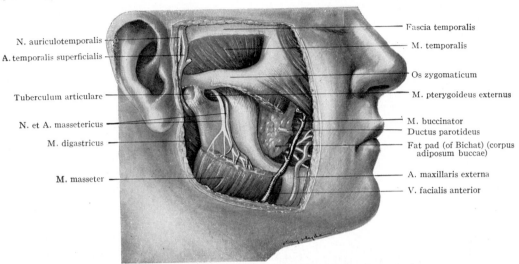

N. auriculotemporalis
A. temporalis superficialis
Tuberculum articulare
N. et A. massetericus
M. digastricus
M. masseter

Fascia temporalis
M. temporalis
Os zygomaticum
M. pterygoideus externus
M. buccinator
Ductus parotideus
Fat pad (of Bichat) (corpus adiposum buccae)
A. maxillaris externa
V. facialis anterior

FIG. 114.—DEEP STRUCTURES OF THE MASSETER REGION.

prolongation of the parotid blends with the fascia on the masseter muscle. The *parotid duct* emerges through the masseter fascia, winds around the anterior border of the masseter muscle and enters the buccinator muscle in the cheek region (p. 118). In their course to the anterior regions of the face, the *transverse facial artery* and the zygomatic and buccal

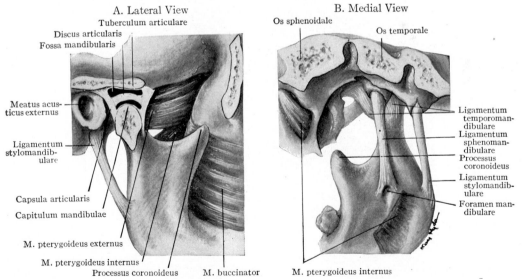

A. Lateral View
Tuberculum articulare
Discus articularis
Fossa mandibularis

B. Medial View
Os sphenoidale
Os temporale

Meatus acus-
ticus externus

Ligamentum
stylomandib-
ulare

Capsula articularis
Capitulum mandibulae

M. pterygoideus externus
M. pterygoideus internus
Processus coronoideus   M. buccinator

Ligamentum
temporoman-
dibulare
Ligamentum
sphenoman-
dibulare
Processus
coronoideus
Ligamentum
stylomandib-
ulare
Foramen man-
dibulare

M. pterygoideus internus

FIG. 115.—LATERAL AND MEDIAL VIEWS OF THE REGION ABOUT THE TEMPOROMANDIBULAR JOINT.

branches of the *facial nerve* traverse this region. Vertical incisions, therefore, are ill-advised, as they sever these structures. An incision from the tragus of the ear to the commissure of the lip uncovers the duct in its course over the masseter. Injury to the duct where it lies on the masseter muscle may result in a salivary fistula, which is difficult to cure.

The *masseter fascia* binds the underlying muscle to the margin of the ramus and the body of the mandible.   An expansion of this fascia overlies and secures the fat pad of the cheek to the buccinator muscle (p. 118).   The parotid duct lies within the fascia and, in a measure, is protected by it.

3. **Masseter Muscle.**—The masseter muscle runs from the zygomatic arch to the angle of the mandible and covers the lateral surface of the ramus.   In tetanus, it goes into contracture early.   Inflammatory lesions about the mandibular joint may produce a chronic masseter myositis with subsequent fibrosis, which may restrict the play of the muscle and limit movement of the jaws.

4. **Temporal Muscle and Fascia.**—The broad radiating temporal muscle arises from the temporal fossa and the temporal fascia.   Its fibers converge into a tendon which

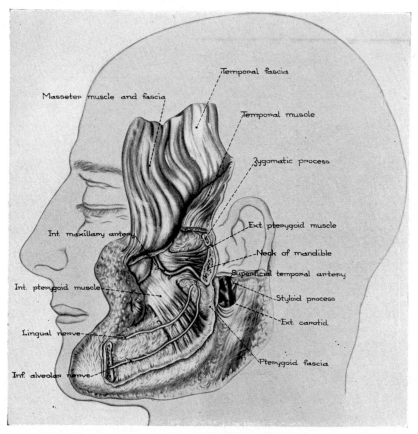

FIG. 116.—THE MASTICATOR SPACE.
The mandible has been removed.   (Coller and Yglesias, Surg., Gynec. and Obst., Feb. 15, 1935.)

passes deep to the zygomatic arch and inserts into the coronoid process of the mandible. The temporal fascia covers the temporal muscle and is attached below to the zygomatic arch.

5. **Skeletal Framework.**—The framework is the zygomatic process and the mandibular fossa of the temporal bone, and the ramus and angle of the mandible.   One of the most important landmarks in cranio-encephalic topography is the zygomatic arch, formed from the horizontal processes of the malar and temporal bones.   On the upper margin of the ramus of the mandible are two processes, the coronoid and the condyloid.   The coronoid process is the upward continuation of the anterior border of the ramus of the mandible; it affords insertion mainly to the temporal muscle.   The condyloid process is the upward continuation of the posterior border of the ramus.

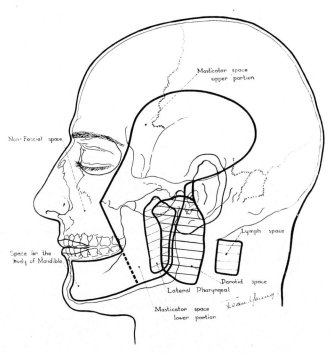

Fig. 117.—Surface Projection of Masticator and Related Spaces. (Coller and Yglesias, Surg., Gynec. and Obst., Feb. 15, 1935.)

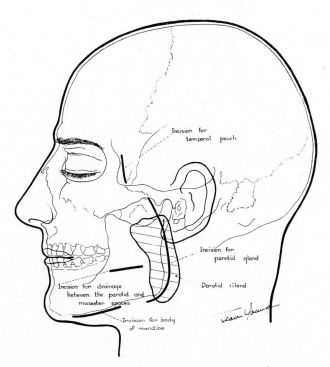

Fig. 118.—Drainage Incisions for Facial Spaces. (Coller and Yglesias, Surg., Gynec. and Obst., Feb. 15, 1935.)

6. **Temporomandibular Joint.**—The temporomandibular joint is compound, with its socket in the temporal bone and its condyle surmounting the ramus of the mandible. Within the joint is an interarticular disk which divides the joint cavity into upper and lower divisions. The posterior wall of the temporal glenoid fossa is the anterior wall of the external auditory meatus, which explains how trauma to the chin may thrust the condyle far enough upward and backward to injure the meatus and even penetrate its cavity (p. 93) Since only a thin bony plate separates the temporal glenoid fossa from the brain, a suppurative joint lesion may invade the intervening bone and result in subdural abscess or meningitis.

The very strong lateral or temporomandibular ligament protects the joint laterally. The reinforced capsule is sufficiently strong to maintain the articular contents in apposition without the aid of accessory ligaments. The external pterygoid muscle is a powerful reinforcement to the joint. It arises from the base of the skull, runs horizontally backward, and inserts into the neck of the condyle of the mandible and into the disk and capsule of the joint.

7. **Masseter-mandibulo-pterygoid (Masticator) Space and Prolongations.**—Attention has been called by Coller and Yglesias to a space occupied by the masseter muscle, the ramus, and posterior part of the body of the mandible and the pterygoid muscles. This space extends superiorly to the level of the insertion of the temporal muscle. It is difficult for enclosed infection here to spread inferiorly, superficially, or medially. However, it can pass upward into the temporal prolongations of this space, areas superficial and deep to the temporal muscle insertion on the coronoid process (temporal pouches).

Abscess within the space may point at the anterior border of the masseter muscle or internally into the mouth. These sites may be used for drainage. Infection may point posteriorly deep to the parotid gland, simulating a deep parotid abscess. Osteomyelitis of the zygomatic arch involves the superficial temporal pouch. Infection of the squama of the temporal bone invades the deep pouch.

The temporal spaces can be drained by a vertical incision posterior to the lateral rim of the orbit, developed through the temporal fascia.

Surgical Considerations

1. **Dislocation of the Mandible and Its Reduction.**—The mandibular joints are strengthened by muscle and ligament supports so that they permit anterior dislocation only. Dislocation ordinarily occurs when the mouth is wide open and the condyles and the interarticular disks are forward on the upper joint eminences. With the jaws in this position, a spasmodic muscle effort, or a downward blow on the chin, throws the condyles forward out of their sockets. After dislocation, the combined contraction of the temporal, masseter, and pterygoid muscles holds the condyles in this forward position and wedges the coronoid processes firmly in the zygomatic fossae.

To reduce this dislocation, the condyles must be depressed and pushed back to their proper articular surfaces. The padded thumbs are placed against the last molar teeth, and, with the fingers about the jaws, pressure is exerted downward and backward on the jaw until the condyles are loosened and lowered. The jaws then can be closed over the thumbs by pulling up the chin; the thumbs are used as levers. If manual reduction fails, a wedge may be placed between the upper and lower molars and the chin be pressed upward and forward.

2. **Fracture of the Mandible.**—Fracture of the mandible usually occurs in the body of the bone near the canine tooth, or a little lateral to the symphysis. It generally is compound into the mouth because the alveolar periosteum and buccal mucous membrane are torn at the line of fracture. The posterior fragment tends to override the anterior. If the fracture is anterior to the masseter muscle, any deformity present is shown by malalignment of the teeth. The anterior (distal) fragment is drawn downward and backward by the action of the geniohyoid, digastric, and genioglossus muscles. The temporal, internal

pterygoid, and masseter muscles draw the overriding posterior (proximal) fragment upward and forward.

Unless early immobilization of the fracture is effected, infection from the compounding into the mouth involves the submaxillary and deep cervical lymph glands. Osteomyelitis of the jaw also may result. The deformity must be corrected carefully and the teeth be brought into perfect alignment. To secure and maintain apposition, it is necessary to wire the teeth or fragments together, or to apply an interdental splint.

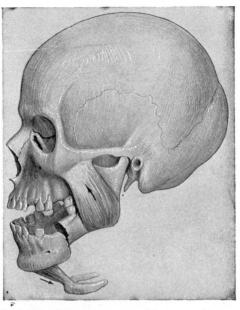

Fig. 120.—Fracture of the Mandible Anterior to the Masseter Muscle.

There is displacement of the proximal fragment upward by the masseter and temporal muscles; the anterior fragment is displaced downward and backward by the geniohyoid, genioglossus, anterior part of the mylohyoid, digastric, and platysma muscles. (Babcock, "Textbook of Surgery.")

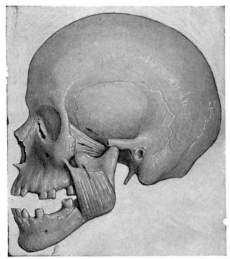

Fig. 119.—Anterior Dislocation of the Mandible, Showing the Action of the External Pterygoid and Masseter Muscles in Fixing the Deformity. (Babcock, "Textbook of Surgery.")

D. ZYGOMATICO-PTERYGO-MAXILLARY (DEEP LATERAL) REGION OF THE FACE

1. **Definition, Boundaries, and Landmarks.**—The zygomatico-pterygo-maxillary region lies deep to the masseter-mandibular region, and extends from the parotid gland forward to the cheek. It offers surgical approach to the trigeminal nerve and its semilunar and sphenopalatine ganglia. Accurate diagnosis of facial neuralgia calls for an intimate knowledge of the trigeminal nerve distribution. Severe neuralgia requires severing the sensory roots. The peripharyngeal space alone separates the region from the pharynx. Clinical examination and surgery in this region are hindered by the overlying masseter muscle and mandible, but a limited exploration can be made through the mouth and pharynx.

2. **Walls of the Space.**—The *lateral wall* of this irregular and ill-defined space is the medial surface of the ramus of the mandible. The only outward communication with the masseter compartment is through the notch in the superior border of the ramus between the coronoid and condyloid processes. The bony portion of its *superior wall* is composed of parts of the great wing of the sphenoid and the temporal bone. The remainder of the superior wall is occupied by the large opening between the zygomatic arch and the skull. Through this wide space, the region is in communication with the temporal region. The *anterior wall* above is the tuberosity of the maxilla; below it are the bulging fibers of the buccinator muscle and part of the superior constrictor muscle of the pharynx. The bony elements of the *medial wall* form the zygomatic and pterygomaxillary fossae, within which lie the two pterygoid muscles, the interpterygoid fascia, the internal maxillary vessels, and the maxillary and mandibular nerves.

3 **Muscles.**—The *internal pterygoid muscle* arises from the walls of the pterygo-maxillary fossa, and is directed downward, outward, and backward to the angle of the jaw. As a levator of the jaw, it is almost as powerful as the masseter muscle. The dense *interpterygoid fascia*, fixed above to the base of the skull, covers the lateral surface of the internal pterygoid muscle and is attached to the ramus and angle of the jaw. The inferior alveolar and lingual vessels and nerves course over its lower lateral surface. The *external pterygoid muscle* arises from the walls of the zygomatic and pterygomaxillary fossae and inserts mainly into the neck of the mandible. Its action is to draw the jaw forward.

4. **Vessels and Nerves.**—The main artery, a terminal branch of the external carotid, is the *internal maxillary artery* which enters the region by winding around the condyle of the mandible

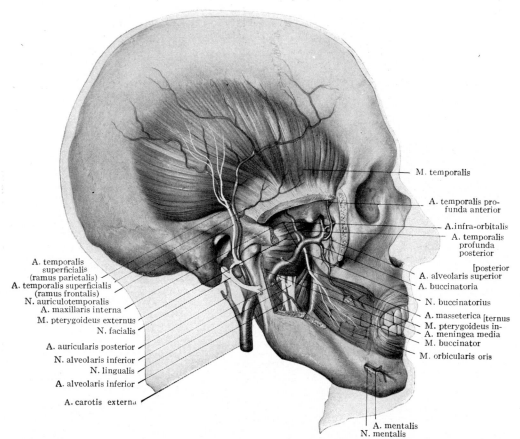

M. temporalis

A. temporalis pro-
funda anterior

A. infra-orbitalis

A. temporalis
profunda
posterior

[posterior
A. alveolaris superior
A. buccinatoria

N. buccinatorius

A. masseterica [ternus
M. pterygoideus in-
A. meningea media
M. buccinator

M. orbicularis oris

A. temporalis
superficialis
(ramus parietalis)
A. temporalis superficialis
(ramus frontalis)
N. auriculotemporalis
A. maxillaris interna
M. pterygoideus externus
N. facialis

A. auricularis posterior

N. alveolaris inferior
N. lingualis

A. alveolaris inferior

A. carotis externa

A. mentalis
N. mentalis

Fig. 121.—Deep Structures in the Zygomatico-pterygo-maxillary Regions.

The *trigeminal nerve* has a wide distribution through the semilunar ganglion and its three large trunks, the mandibular, maxillary, and ophthalmic nerves. The first two nerves are important structures in this region. The *mandibular nerve*, the most inferior of the three divisions, has a large, superficial, sensory root and a smaller, more deeply placed motor root, both of which leave the middle fossa of the skull through the foramen ovale and enter this region. Outside the skull, they combine to form a single trunk which separates into an anterior or lingual, and a posterior or inferior alveolar division. The lingual nerve sweeps forward to the side of the tongue, to the anterior two thirds of which it is distributed. The inferior alveolar nerve is larger than the lingual nerve and passes from beneath the inferior border of the external pterygoid muscle to enter the mandibular canal through the mandibular foramen. It traverses the ramus and body of the mandible and distributes branches to the teeth.

The *maxillary nerve* or middle branch of the trigeminal is a sensory nerve. After leaving the semilunar ganglion, it passes horizontally forward and leaves the skull through

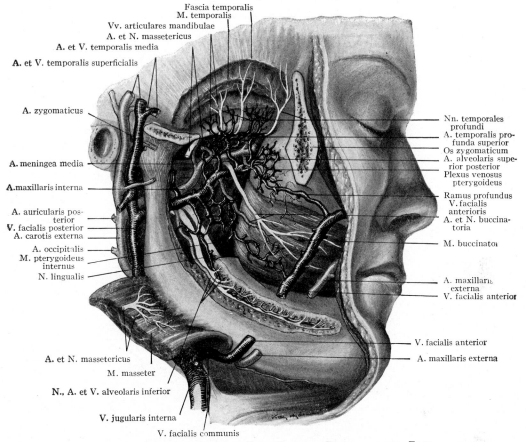

FIG. 122.—STRUCTURES IN THE DEEP LATERAL REGION OF THE FACE.

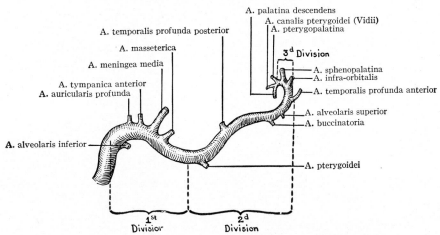

FIG. 123.—DIVISIONS AND BRANCHES OF THE INTERNAL MAXILLARY ARTERY.

the foramen rotundum. It crosses the pterygopalatine fossa, neters the orbit through the inferior orbital fissure, and traverses the floor of the orbit to appear on the face at the infra-orbital foramen

Surgical Considerations

The areolar tissue of the deep lateral region of the face is continuous with that of the tongue, cheek, and temporal regions. This continuity explains the spread of infection from one region to another. Tumors arising in the area may invade the orbit and the nasal fossae. Lymph drainage is to the upper deep cervical lymph nodes.

1. **Facial Neuralgia.**—The trigeminal nerve is sensory to the face and motor to the muscles of mastication; more than any other nerve of the body, it is subject to neuralgia. Pain may be present over the distribution of any, or all, of its divisions, but the ophthalmic and maxillary divisions are involved most frequently. When the ophthalmic division is involved, pain is confined usually to the supra-orbital branch. If the maxillary division is affected, there is pain in the cheek and in the ala of the nose over the distribution of the infra-orbital branch. Resection of the infra-orbital nerve often gives great relief. Should disease involve the inferior alveolar branch of the mandibular division, relief sometimes follows excision of the mental branch at the mental foramen. When peripheral resection of the terminations of the main trigeminal divisions fails to cure, or when pain shifts from the territory of one division to that of another, the indication is that the semilunar ganglion is involved extensively and its sensory portion must be destroyed to give relief.

2. **Routes to the Maxillary Nerve and Sphenopalatine Ganglion (of Meckel).**—The maxillary nerve lies in the highest and most inaccessible portion of the pterygomaxillary fossa. Suspended from the nerve and lying mesial to it is the sphenopalatine ganglion (of Meckel). Sensory nerves from this ganglion are distributed, in part, to the mucous membrane of the nose, to the soft palate, tonsils, roof of the mouth, and upper part of the pharynx. Resection of the zygomatic bone and the lateral wall of the orbit exposes the nerve in its course from the infra-orbital groove to the foramen rotundum. Since this approach is below the internal maxillary artery, the operation may be performed without vessel injury. The nerve also may be approached and reached through the maxillary sinus.

3. **Routes to the Inferior Alveolar Branch of the Mandibular Nerve.**—The mental branch of the inferior alveolar nerve can be excised at the mental foramen through the mucosa of the mouth. Excision of the inferior alveolar trunk for more extensive neuralgia may be accomplished through a trephine opening in the ramus of the mandible, after incision of the overlying masseter muscle. The inferior alveolar nerve can be reached with great difficulty through the mouth (buccal approach) by an incision along the anterior margin of the ramus to the mandibular foramen, where it enters the canal with its corresponding artery.

4. **Approach to the Semilunar (Gasserian) Ganglion.**—The true anatomic approach to the semilunar ganglion is a temporal-subdural route which does not involve the deep lateral region of the face. In the transtemporal approach, the dura is separated from the temporal bone and base of the skull until the middle meningeal artery is seen emerging from the foramen spinosum. The artery is ligated, and cleavage is continued until the ganglion is reached. Section of the sensory root of the ganglion with conservation of the motor roots can be accomplished.

E. PAROTID REGION

1. **Definition and Boundaries.**—The recess, or vertical depression which holds the parotid gland, lies behind the ramus of the lower jaw and below the base of the cranium. It has been considered a constituent element of the neck, but its relations place it rather as one of the regions of the face. The parotid region is bounded anteriorly by the ramus of the mandible, posteriorly by the mastoid process and anterior margin of the sternocleidomastoid muscle, and superiorly by the external auditory meatus and the zygomatic arch. The inferior margin of the recess extends to the angle of the mandible, and its mesial wall reaches to the styloid process and the lateral wall of the pharynx.

2. **Landmarks.**—The capacity of the space is increased when the mandible is moved forward, as in protruding the chin or extending the head, and is decreased when the head is flexed. This observation is significant in clinical examination and in operations in the region. The gland cannot be felt under normal conditions, but is palpable when inflamed, enlarged by a new growth, or swollen by back pressure through its duct. Under such circumstances there is a change of contour in the upper neck and face, and any movement restricting the capacity of the space or pressing on the gland causes pain.

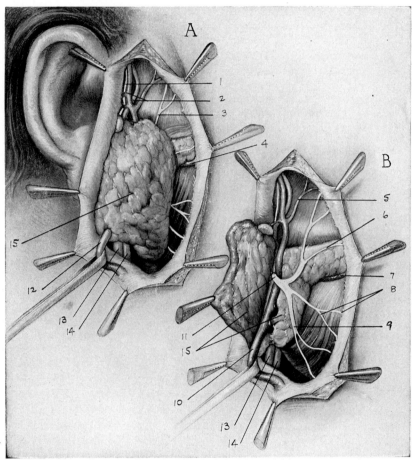

FIG. 124.—SUPERFICIAL AND DEEP DISSECTIONS OF THE PAROTID REGION.
(In B, the outer part of the parotid gland is retracted to show the vessels and nerve which traverse it.)

1, N. auriculotemporalis; 2, A. et V. temporalis superficialis; 3, ramus temporalis N. facialis; 4, ductus parotideus; 5, V. temporalis media; 6, ramus zygomaticus N. facialis; 7, ductus parotideus; 8, rami buccales N. facialis; 9, ramus marginalis mandibulae N. facialis; 10, B. jugularis externa; 11, N. facialis; 12, V. jugularis externa; 13, A. carotis externa; 14, V. facialis posterior; 15, glandula parotis.

The region varies in appearance in different individuals. In children, young adults, and those possessing abundant adipose tissue, it is smoothly rounded and full. In thin persons, the gland has very little supporting tissue on its deep aspect and sinks inward, leaving a noticeable depression behind the jaw.

3. **Fibrous Capsule of the Parotid.**—The subcutaneous tissue contains vessels and nerves of little importance. The gland is invested closely with a dense fascia derived from the enveloping fascia of the neck. The outer layer, continuous with the fibrous sheath about the sternocleidomastoid and masseter muscles, is particularly strong, and is attached above to the zygomatic arch. The deep layer, derived from the same sheath,

9

runs deep to the parotid gland toward the pharynx. This dense sac of fascia encasing the gland is closed below but is open above. In the deep wall of the fascia, there is a gap between the styloid process and the internal pterygoid muscle through which the parotid space communicates with the connective tissue about the pharynx. Because of this communication, a retropharyngeal or parapharyngeal abscess may push the parotid gland outward. In some instances, these abscesses have been evacuated into the parotid space.

The sensory nerves of the gland, the auriculotemporal and major auricular, are bound up in the unyielding parotid fascia, which accounts for the excessive pain in acute inflammation and in rapidly growing tumors of the gland.

4. **Parotid Gland, Its Processes and Its Duct.**—The *parotid* is the largest of the salivary glands, and completely fills the irregular parotid fascial space, being molded and

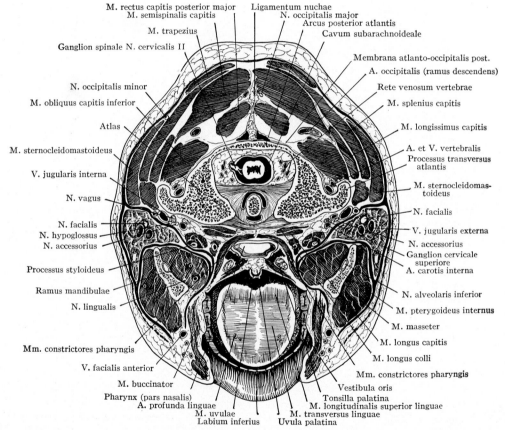

Fig. 125.—Cross Section of the Head at the Level of the Atlas to Show the Fascial and Vascular Relations of the Parotid Gland.

adherent to its walls. The fibrous capsule sends into the interior of the gland processes which divide it into lobes and lobules, and which, in removal of the gland, necessitate a piecemeal procedure. In this respect, the parotid differs from the submaxillary gland, which is enveloped loosely by its sheath and may be shelled from it easily. From the mesial surface of the gland, in front of the styloid process, there arises a *pharyngeal prolongation* which is related intimately to the wall of the pharynx and to the great vessels in the parapharyngeal space. This is seen well in a cross section through the parotid region. The fascial barrier separating it from the carotid sheath may be broken through by sharp instruments, the erosion of an abscess, or the invasion of a malignant growth.

The principal or *facial process* tapers like a wedge as it advances forward over the masseter muscle. In connection with it, a detached portion of the gland sometimes is found lying upon the masseter muscle above the parotid duct. A *cervical process* usually is present, directed downward toward the neck between the outer aspect of the posterior belly of the digastric muscle and the deep cervical fascia. The upper border of the gland is grooved deeply, and is applied closely to the capsule of the temporomandibular joint.

The *parotid duct*, about 5 cm. in length, lies one fingerbreadth below the zygomatic arch and, when the teeth are clenched, may be rolled up and down against the tense masseter muscle. It emerges from the most anterior part of the gland and runs forward on the masseter muscle to its anterior margin. The duct then passes mesially, piercing the buccinator muscle obliquely to reach the mucous membrane of the cheek. Opposite the second molar tooth, the duct opens into the mouth. The course of the duct on the masseter muscle is represented by a line drawn from the lower margin of the concha of the ear to the commissure of the lips. Injury to the duct may produce a salivary fistula. Inflammatory lesions in the mouth may spread backward along the duct and involve the gland.

Infection in the parotid gland, *parotitis*, may be blood-borne, or it may occur by direct extension from the buccal cavity or from duct obstruction. In nonsuppurative parotitis or mumps, the painful tender tumor disappears after a few days, but in septic or metastatic parotitis the swelling persists. Abscess may set in with the alarming symptoms of bacteremia. Early incision is demanded only after intensive radiotherapy (x-ray and radium) has failed to abort the infection.

5. **Surgical Approach to Parotid Abscess** (Fig. 118).—Infection in the parotid space may be drained through an incision (Blair) which begins 2 cm. anterior to the ear and is carried downward to a point behind and below the angle of the jaw. The incision is developed through the capsule of the gland. The parenchyma can be opened by blunt dissection. The lateral surface of the parotid gland can be exposed throughout its extent without injuring the facial nerve if the dissection is kept external to the parotid substance. The deep part of the gland can be drained by lifting forward the lower pole of the gland, carefully guarding the external jugular vein and the great auricular nerve. Continuing the deep dissection in front of the external carotid artery opens the parapharyngeal space (p. 146).

If it is necessary to drain the space between the masseter muscle and the superficial division (facial process) of the parotid gland, a horizontal incision can be made safely. This should be located at the body of the mandible, and can be joined to the vertical incision before mentioned.

6. **Vessels and Nerves in and about the Parotid Gland.**—The most important structures entering and leaving the gland are the facial nerve and its branches, the posterior facial vein, and the external carotid artery with its terminals, the superficial temporal and internal maxillary arteries.

The *external carotid artery* does not run in the inferior portion of the gland, but enters higher up, on a level with the junction of the middle and lower thirds of the ramus of the mandible. It traverses the substance of the gland from this point upward and gives off its terminal branches at the level of the neck of the mandible. Within the gland, the external carotid artery is deep to the posterior facial vein which, in turn, is deep to and crossed by the facial nerve. Occasionally, the external carotid artery runs between the parotid gland and the pharynx.

The *lymph glands* of the parotid region are divisible into two groups. Superficial to the parotid sheath lie the glands of the anterior auricular (preauricular) group which drain the temporal and frontal regions of the scalp, the outer portions of the lids, and the outer ear. Scattered through the gland substance, although chiefly situated near its surface, lie the glands of the parotid group, which drain the upper and posterior part of the nasopharynx, the soft palate, and the middle ear. Because of the frequency of inflammation in the areas drained, a parotitis must not be considered as primary (mumps) until secondary lesions in tributary parts have been ruled out, as, for instance, the parotitis of otitis media.

An abscess arising in connection with the preauricular lymph glands points superficially. The density of the outer sheath of the parotid gland resists the outward progress of an abscess occurring in the parotid lymph glands. The abscess tends to advance upward in the line of least resistance, although such progress is resisted by gravity. It is much more likely to invade the thinner mesial wall of the parotid space and to point in the pharynx or buccal cavity, or burst through the lower confines of the parotid space and enter the neck. Infections may invade the external auditory meatus and the temporomandibular joint.

The auriculotemporal and facial nerves traverse the upper portion of the parotid. The *auriculotemporal nerve* is a sensory branch of the mandibular nerve, supplying the skin in front of the ear, and extending upward through the temporal region to the vertex of the skull. Its compression in tumors of the parotid gland causes exquisite pain, which radiates over the temple and associated scalp, even to the vertex of the skull.

The *facial nerve* leaves the base of the skull through the stylomastoid foramen and runs forward, laterally, and slightly downward. It then begins its intraglandular course by entering the posterosuperior margin of the parotid gland at a deep level. It is superficial to the external carotid artery and the posterior facial vein, and may be injured in any operation on the parotid gland. Within the parotid gland, the nerve at once breaks up into its main branches, which diverge on leaving the gland and terminate by supplying the muscles of expression.

IV. REGIONS WITHIN THE BUCCAL CAVITY

The buccal cavity and its contents are divided conveniently into: vestibule and gingivodental region, palate region, sublingual region, and tongue. As a whole, it includes the space between the nasal cavities above, the neck below, the lips in front, and the pharynx behind.

A. VESTIBULE OF THE BUCCAL CAVITY AND GINGIVODENTAL ARCHES

The gingivodental arches divide the buccal cavity into the vestibule and the buccal cavity proper.

1. Vestibule.—The vestibule is lined by the mucous membrane from the lips, the cheeks and from the outer alveolar surface of the jaws. Where the mucous membrane of the lip is reflected to the alveolar processes of the jaws, horseshoe-shaped grooves are formed, known as the superior and inferior vestibular fornices. The maxillary sinuses do not descend to the upper fornix, but can be reached surgically through an opening at this point (p. 88). At the level of the first or second upper molar tooth, the buccal orifice of the parotid duct opens upon the lateral wall of the vestibule (p. 131).

The vestibule communicates with the buccal cavity proper through the interdental spaces and through the openings between the rami of the mandible and the last molar teeth. The latter communication can be utilized for the introduction of food into the buccal cavity proper when there is a locking of the jaws, as in tetanus, or in ankylosis of the temporomandibular joint.

2. Gingivae or Gums.—The term "gingiva" is used to indicate the composite mucous membrane and submucous tissue which is attached firmly to the alveolar processes and to the dental arches. In the newborn, it covers the toothless borders of the jaws. Its submucous base is directly continuous with the alveolar periosteum, which dips down into each tooth socket to form the root membrane, or pericementum. The gingiva is fairly vascular and not very sensitive. A portion of the gingiva projects into each interdental space and surrounds the necks of the teeth.

3. Alveolar Processes of the Jaws and the Alveolar or Tooth Sockets.—The teeth are rooted in the alveolar cavities or sockets. The divergence of the roots and their twisted character serve to maintain them mechanically in their beds. Inflammation of the root membrane, or pericementum, early follows root caries and dental periostitis. The alveolar cavities, particularly in the lower jaw, are much nearer the outer than the inner table, as evidenced by their palpable bulging into the vestibule. The thinness of this outer plate explains the easy perforation of root abscesses to the vestibular surfaces of the gums

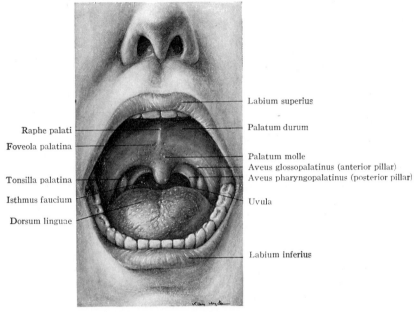

Raphe palati

Foveola palatina

Tonsilla palatina

Isthmus faucium

Dorsum linguae

Labium superius

Palatum durum

Palatum molle
Aveus glossopalatinus (anterior pillar)
Aveus pharyngopalatinus (posterior pillar)

Uvula

Labium inferius

FIG. 126.—BUCCAL CAVITY.

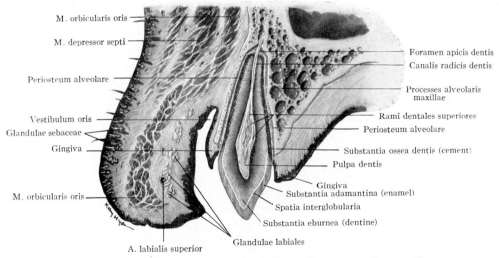

M. orbicularis oris

M. depressor septi

Periosteum alveolare

Vestibulum oris

Glandulae sebaceae

Gingiva

M. orbicularis oris

A. labialis superior

Glandulae labiales

Foramen apicis dentis

Canalis radicis dentis

Processes alveolaris maxillae

Rami dentales superiores

Periosteum alveolare

Substantia ossea dentis (cement)

Pulpa dentis

Gingiva
Substantia adamantina (enamel)

Spatia interglobularia

Substantia eburnea (dentine)

FIG. 127.—SAGITTAL SECTION THROUGH THE UPPER LIP AND AN INCISOR TOOTH.

This also is the cause of frequent fracture of the outer plate in tooth extraction. The alveolar process is the point of origin of the tumor, *epulis.*

SURGICAL CONSIDERATIONS

1. **Alveolar or Alveolodental Abscesses.**—An alveolodental abscess is a circumscribed pus cavity located at the apex of a tooth, and usually is caused by the death of the pulp. The infection in the pulp cavity invades the space between the root and the socket and may progress until it reaches the compact tissue on the alveolar surface of the jaw. The pus

from the abscess generally escapes through the surface offering least resistance, namely the external alveolar plate, lateral to the apex of the affected tooth. In doing so, it may lift up the periosteum for a sufficient distance to cause considerable necrosis of underlying

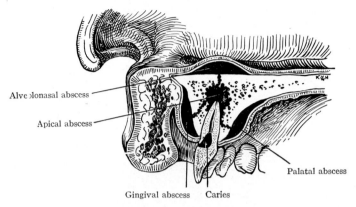

Alveolonasal abscess

Apical abscess

Palatal abscess

Gingival abscess   Caries

FIG. 128.—PERIAPICAL ABSCESS IN THE MAXILLA AND ITS EXTENSIONS.

bone The pus finally may escape through a sinus remote from the point of origin In the lower jaw, the force of gravity and the pressure of accumulating pus may make a path between the periosteum and soft tissues, or between the periosteum and bone, with final discharge on the neck beneath the chin or jaw. An abscess in connection with the third

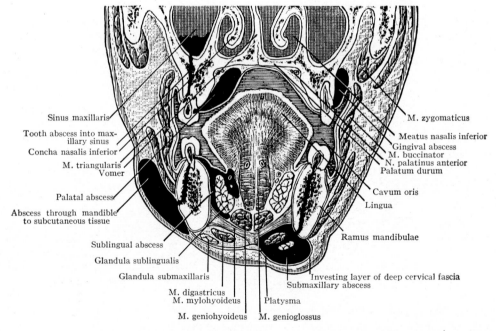

Sinus maxillaris

Tooth abscess into max-
illary sinus

Concha nasalis inferior

M. triangularis
Vomer

Palatal abscess

Abscess through mandible
to subcutaneous tissue

Sublingual abscess

Glandula sublingualis

Glandula submaxillaris

M. digastricus
M. mylohyoideus

M. geniohyoideus   M. genioglossus

M. zygomaticus

Meatus nasalis inferior

Gingival abscess
M. buccinator
N. palatinus anterior
Palatum durum

Cavum oris

Lingua

Ramus mandibulae

Investing layer of deep cervical fascia
Submaxillary abscess

Platysma

FIG. 129.—FRONTAL SECTION THROUGH THE FACE AND UPPER NECK TO SHOW THE VARIETIES OF ALVEOLAR ABSCESS.

lower molar (wisdom tooth) may penetrate the lateral tissues at the angle of the jaw, or occasionally may burrow downward into the neck, forming large pus cavities in the submaxillary region. The pus may take a mesial course and discharge through the buccal surface of the gum.

Abscesses are less likely to occur in the upper jaw where there is an abundant blood supply. The pus from abscesses in the upper jaw may extend into the nasal cavity or perforate the maxillary sinus and establish an empyema. However, the pus may pass directly through the external alveolar plate and form a sinus on the cheek, or discharge around the root socket.

The underlying principle of treatment is the opening and draining of the pus cavity with the least sacrifice of normal tissue. Simple removal of gangrenous dental pulp, which frequently is the origin of the abscess, may suffice in those cases where there has not been serious bone destruction. This usually is impractical, and it becomes necessary to limit the destruction of tissue and reach the focus by surgical means, either by trephine of the alveolar plate or by extraction of the tooth. Tooth extraction in acute abscess may develop into an extensive sepsis, absorption taking place at the extracted tooth socket. Treatment of abscesses which have burrowed downward into the neck is evacuation by external incision.

2. **Dental Caries.**—A breaking down of the enamel exposes the dentin to the destructive action of micro-organisms, which cause progressive destruction of the teeth, advancing from the exterior to the interior. A tooth may undergo disintegration in part or entirely.

3. **Pyorrhea Alveolaris.**—Pyorrhea alveolaris is an exuding of pus from the dental alveoli. It is primarily a disease of the bony substance, the pericementum, and usually manifests itself as a chronic suppurative inflammation. Secondarily, the process involves the gingiva and the walls of the alveoli. It causes loosening and extrusion of the teeth, a discharge of pus from their alveolar margins. and caries of the alveolar process. Recession of the gums takes place until the teeth lose their gingival and alveolar connections and fall out. Upon the loss of the teeth, the inflammatory symptoms subside immediately. The point of greatest clinical importance is prevention, which is based on unremitting care of the teeth, to keep the gums free from inflammatory change.

4. **Epulis.**—Epulis usually implies any tumor of the gum, but is specifically that growth which originates from the periosteum at the border of the alveolar process. It occurs most frequently anterior to the molar teeth. The gum tissue is involved secondarily as the tumor develops. This common oral tumor primarily is benign, but, subjected to continuous irritation, may present malignant characteristics.

5. **Syphilis of the Teeth.**—The temporary teeth in hereditary syphilis show malformations dependent upon perversion of nutrition. The enamel may be lacking or chalky, the dentin soft, or the teeth irregular in shape and position. The permanent central incisors in hereditary syphilis are known as *hutchinsonian teeth*. They are shorter than normal teeth, and their free borders are narrow, notched, and bevelled. The first molar teeth often are reduced in size.

B. PALATE REGION

The embryology of the palate is bound up intimately with the developmental changes about the lip, the details of which are described elsewhere (p. 114).

1. **Definition and Boundaries.**—The roof of the mouth, or the palate, separates the main buccal cavity from the nasal cavity and from the nasal portion of the pharynx. Its anterior two thirds comprises the hard palate and its posterior third, the soft palate.

2. **Landmarks.**—The hard palate is vault-shaped, the soft palate veil-like, and the whole is designed for the rôle it plays in deglutition and phonation. In a person breathing normally, the soft palate hangs semivertically between the buccal and pharyngeal cavities. In the act of sucking, it is brought into contact with the base of the tongue, thereby stopping all communication between the mouth and pharynx. Swallowing lifts it out of its vertical position and spreads it as a horizontal septum between the buccal and nasal portions of the pharynx, thus preventing food entering the nose by way of the posterior nares. This action is lost in diphtheritic and other paralyses of the muscles controlling the soft palate. The free margin of the soft palate forms an arch, extending from one side of the pharynx to the other, from the middle and highest point of which projects the variable-

sized, pendant *uvula*. Laterally, the free margin continues into the posterior or *pharyngo-palatine arch* (posterior pillar of the fauces), and forward into the *glossopalatine arch* (anterior pillar of the fauces) (p. 144).

3. **Structures of the Hard Palate.**—The hard palate is a horizontal plate, covered by a dense structure formed by the periosteum and mucous membrane of the mouth. The tissue contains a large number of palatine glands, intrinsic nerves, and blood vessels. The hard palate is a frequent site of disease in tertiary syphilis.

The buccal palatine mucosa is remarkably thick, especially at the alveolar margin where it is continuous with the gingiva. This relationship explains the extension of dento-alveolar abscesses to the palatal vault. The soft tissues covering the buccal surface of the hard palate are fused into a closely knit layer, but in cleft palate surgery, the whole (muco-periosteum) may be detached readily from the bone. A ridge running sagittally on the

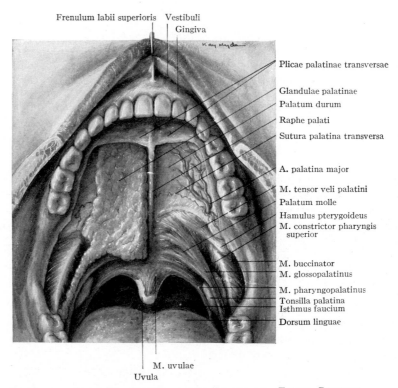

Frenulum labii superioris   Vestibuli
                            Gingiva

Plicae palatinae transversae

Glandulae palatinae
Palatum durum
Raphe palati
Sutura palatina transversa

A. palatina major

M. tensor veli palatini
Palatum molle
Hamulus pterygoideus
M. constrictor pharyngis superior

M. buccinator
M. glossopalatinus

M. pharyngopalatinus
Tonsilla palatina
Isthmus faucium
Dorsum linguae

M. uvulae
Uvula

Fig. 130.—Superficial and Deep Structures of the Palate and Tonsil Regions.
The palatine glands have been removed on the left side.

hard palate, often mistaken for a tumor, is an excessive developmental heaping up of bone along the suture between the palatine processes of the maxillae.

4. **Structures of the Soft Palate.**—The soft palate is a mobile, musculomembranous septum about 1 cm. thick, attached to and extending backward from the hard palate. The palatine mucosa covers its superior and inferior surface and winds about its free border. Deep to the mucosa is the submucosa, so loosely attached to the underlying structures, especially at the uvula and pillars, that edema may develop easily. The dense palatine aponeurosis, to which the several muscles of the palate are attached, forms the framework of the soft palate. The anterior part of the soft palate is made up almost exclusively of this aponeurosis, covered on its buccal surface by an extremely thick layer of glands; it contains no muscle fibers.

The muscles which help form the soft palate are the pharyngopalatine, glossopalatine and uvular muscles, and the levators and tensors of the palate. The pharyngopalatine and glossopalatine muscles, which form the pillars or arches of the tonsil, are important in tonsillectomy (p. 149). In cleft palate operations for complete fissure, these muscles have a strong tendency to retract laterally the parts of the soft palate into which they insert. The tensor veli palatini muscle also is important in postoperative retraction, and may require division to reduce the strain on the repaired soft palate.

5. **Vessels and Nerves.**—The arteries to both the hard and soft palate come chiefly from the internal maxillary through the descending palatine branches, which run down through the pterygopalatine canal and forward in the angle between the vertical and horizontal processes of the maxillae, almost in contact with the bone. In repair of the cleft palate (uranoplasty), these arteries must be protected to nourish the flaps of tissue used in closing the cleft. This may be done by making the incisions of the mucous membrane as close as possible to the gingival border. As the incision is carried posteriorly, it should wind about the last molar tooth to avoid injury to the major palatine artery where it leaves the palatine canal. No vessels are endangered in division of the tendon of the tensor veli palatini muscle.

Surgical Considerations

1. **Cleft Palate.**—Harelip and cleft palate occur with such frequency, cause such faulty articulation, and affect the spirit of the patient to such an extent, that any measure promising relief should be instituted as early as possible. Cleft palate, which may or may

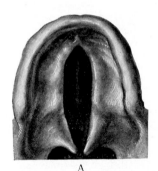 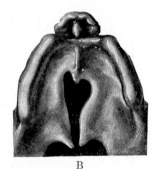

A   B

FIG. 131.—VARIETIES OF CLEFT PALATE.

A shows a cleft extending through the soft and hard palate. In B, there is a cleft in the soft palate, extending into the hard palate; the premaxillary process is entirely separate from the maxillary bones, a condition usually coexisting with double harelip.

not be accompanied by harelip, single or double, invariably is congenital. The fissure or fissures so formed are brought about by an arrest in normal development. In any case, there is not absence of tissue, but failure of union of tissue.

If the maxillary bud fails to unite with the frontonasal process, there is a cleft extending from the mouth to the lateral part of the upper lip or even to the eye and beyond. If failure to unite occurs only at the extremity of the frontonasal process, the cleft extends from the lateral part of the lip toward, or into the nostril, and a simple harelip results. If, as rarely occurs, the two globular tips of the frontonasal process fail to unite, there is a median fissure Should the mandibular processes fail to unite, a median cleft of the lower lip, and even of the jaw and tongue, may result.

2. **Cleft Palate Operations.**—The object in the treatment of cleft palate is to establish normality. The procedure is mechanical closure of the gap or fissure. *Staphylorrhaphy* is the name given to the operation which approximates and unites a cleft in the soft tissue, and *uranoplasty* to that which remedies a defect in the bone. The features common to operations designed to close the fissure by the suture method are: freshening of the margins of the cleft, mobilizing and approximating the soft parts to close the cleft, and suturing of the apposed margins.

It may be necessary to adopt measures to eliminate countertraction, which tends to cut out sutures and pull apart the newly apposed margins. This may be accomplished by cutting the levators of the soft palate and the pharyngopalatine and glossopalatine muscles or sectioning the tensor veli palatini muscles. The approximation operation

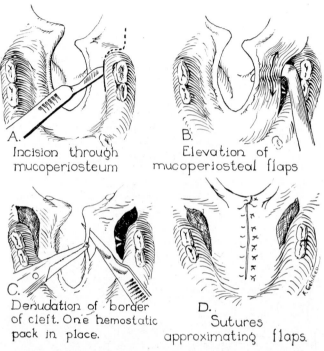

A. Incision through mucoperiosteum

B. Elevation of mucoperiosteal flaps

C. Denudation of border of cleft. One hemostatic pack in place.

D. Sutures approximating flaps.

Fig. 132.—Operative Closure of Cleft Palate. (After Blair.)

can be done only early in infancy, preferably within the first three months. After this period, ossification has progressed so far that lateral incisions in the mucoperiosteum do not permit sufficient flap mobilization.

C. FLOOR OF THE MOUTH OR SUBLINGUAL REGION

1. **Definition and Boundaries.**—Each sublingual region is a deep groove in the floor of the mouth, and lies between the mandible and the root of the tongue on the mylohyoid and hyoglossus muscles. Its posterior boundary is the glossopalatine arch, or the anterior pillar of the tonsil. The sublingual region is separated from the submaxillary region by the mylohyoid and hyoglossus diaphragm.

2. **Landmarks.**—The middle fold or frenum of the tongue is seen best by elevating the tongue. If, in the newborn, the frenum interferes with proper movements of the tongue because of its extensive attachment, it may be divided. At the base of the frenum is the salivary caruncle with the openings of the submaxillary ducts and the principal duct for the sublingual gland. Beginning at the caruncle and running backward on both sides of the base of the tongue is an elevated crest of mucous membrane, the sublingual fold. The minor sublingual ducts (of Rivinus) open by orifices on this ridge and are scarcely visible. The sublingual salivary gland is the most important structure in the area. Sublingual adenomas, carcinoma, or diffuse sublingual abscess may distort the area.

3. **Contents of the Sublingual Region.**—Each compartment encloses the sublingual gland, the anterior prolongation of the submaxillary gland, the submaxillary duct, the lingual and hypoglossal nerves, and the sublingual vessels.

The *sublingual gland* is the smallest of the salivary glands and rests against the sublingual fossa of the mandible, close to the symphysis, on the mylohyoid muscle. Its posterior extremity is in contact with the anterior prolongation of the submaxillary gland. Thus, both salivary glands form an almost continuous mass, lying partly in the submaxillary region and partly in the sublingual region. Between the sublingual gland and the root of the tongue run the submaxillary duct, the lingual and hypoglossal nerves, and the sublingual vessels.

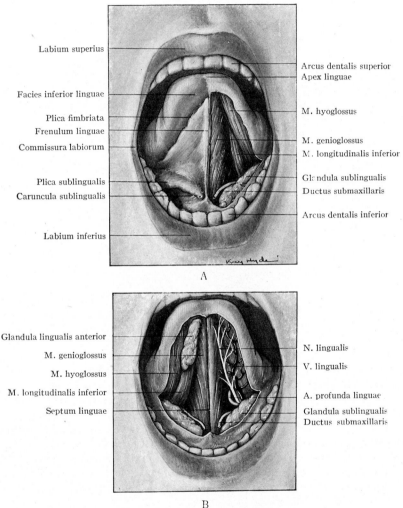

FIG. 133.—SUPERFICIAL AND DEEP STRUCTURES IN THE SUBLINGUAL REGION.

A, The mucosa is left intact on the right side; on the left, the region has been cleared of the vessels and nerves.

B, The vessels and nerves have been removed on the right side, and on the left the vessels and nerves are *in situ*.

The *anterior prolongation of the submaxillary gland* is wedged between the mylohyoid and hyoglossus muscles and contains the submaxillary duct.

The *submaxillary duct* is not difficult to catheterize at its orifice at the sublingual caruncle; this duct, despite its thinness, is very resistant. Its canal occasionally is obstructed by a calculus, which can be felt through the buccal mucosa and can be removed easily. The structures of the space lie in the midst of areolar tissue, designed to allow free movement of the tongue. Infection readily develops and spreads within this tissue.

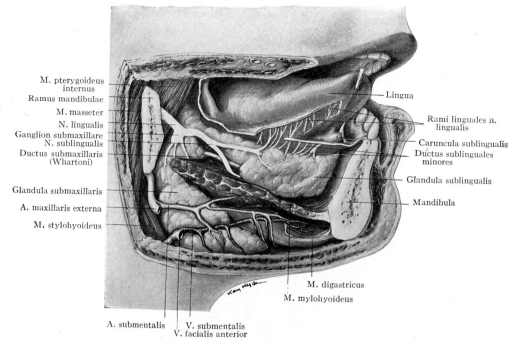

M. pterygoideus internus
Ramus mandibulae
M. masseter
N. lingualis
Ganglion submaxillare
N. sublingualis
Ductus submaxillaris (Whartoni)

Glandula submaxillaris

A. maxillaris externa

M. stylohyoideus

Lingua

Rami linguales n. lingualis

Caruncula sublingualis
Ductus sublinguales minores

Glandula sublingualis

Mandibula

M. digastricus
M. mylohyoideus

A. submentalis   V. submentalis
               V. facialis anterior

FIG. 134.—LATERAL VIEW OF THE SUBLINGUAL REGION.
The body of the mandible has been removed.

SURGICAL CONSIDERATIONS

1. Ludwig's Angina.—Ludwig's angina is a fulminating streptococcic infection, which usually manifests itself about the submaxillary gland, but occasionally about the sublingual gland.   This infection is virulent from the beginning and spreads rapidly along fascial planes to the sublingual region and pharynx.   Though it begins as a painful and indurated swelling beneath the body of the jaw, the infection may extend into the neck and reach the sternum.   Prompt and free incision under local anesthesia should be made through the submaxillary swelling.   The mylohyoid muscles should be divided and the fingers passed through the wound into the sublingual region as far as the mucous membrane of the mouth.

The origin of the infection usually is within the lower gingival borders, especially around the molar teeth.   The process is essentially a cellulitis, the submaxillary glands and associated lymph nodes lying more or less intact in the midst of necrotic cellular tissue. Elevation of the tongue, with redness and edema of the mucous membrane over the involved area, is characteristic.   The presence or absence of pus depends upon the stage of the process at the time of incision.   The fact that many deaths result from edema of the larynx emphasizes the danger of delaying tracheotomy, which is a justifiable procedure when dyspnea and edema of the glottis prove alarming.

2. Ranula.—A ranula is a retention cyst of the submaxillary or sublingual ducts. When first formed, it contains saliva which later degenerates into a mucus-like substance. A true ranula may appear on either side of the floor of the mouth.   True mucous cysts do not occur in the mucous glands of the floor of the mouth.   In true ranula, it usually is advisable to remove both the cyst and the sublingual gland.   A portion of the cyst wall, however, may be removed and the interior of the cyst cauterized.

3. Calculus in the Sublingual Gland and Ducts.—The sublingual gland may require removal because of an embedded calculus.   The calculus can be palpated between a finger in the mouth and the thumb below the angle of the jaw.   A simple incision through the mucous membrane suffices for removal of the calculus.

A

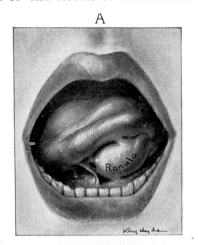

B

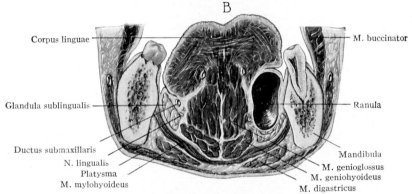

Corpus linguae — M. buccinator

Glandula sublingualis — Ranula

Ductus submaxillaris
N. lingualis
Platysma
M. mylohyoideus
Mandibula
M. genioglossus
M. geniohyoideus
M. digastricus

FIG 135.—RANULA.

A, The ranula is seen bulging upward from the sublingual area.   B, The ranula in frontal section.

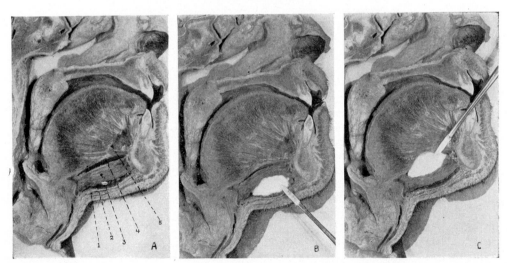

FIG. 136.—SAGITTAL SECTIONS THROUGH THE SUBLINGUAL AREA TO SHOW THE LOCATION OF SUBLINGUAL ABSCESSES.

A, Muscles and spaces in the floor of the mouth. 1, Mylohyoid muscle; 2, space between geniohyoid and mylohyoid muscles; 3, geniohyoid muscle; 4, space between geniohyoid and genioglossus muscles; 5, genioglossus muscle.

B, External approach to space between the mylohyoid and geniohyoid muscles.

C, Approach through the mouth to space between geniohyoid and genioglossus muscles. (Courtesy of Dr. A. C. Furstenburg, from Coller and Yglesias, Surg., Gynec. and Obst., Feb. 15, 1935.)

D. REGION OF THE TONGUE

1. Definition and Boundaries.—The tongue is attached to the floor of the mouth, the mandible, and the hyoid bone, so as almost to fill the mouth cavity. It lies below the palate region, above the floor of the mouth, and in front of the pharynx. The superior portion is free, mobile, and covered by mucosa.

There are two divisions of the mobile portion: an anterior, or buccal, and a posterior, or pharyngeal. The buccal part of the tongue is disposed almost horizontally, and the pharyngeal base vertically, forming part of the anterior wall of the pharynx.

The buccal part is demarcated from the pharyngeal part by a distinct V-shaped groove, the terminal sulcus, the apex of which corresponds to a depression on the posterior surface of the tongue, the *foramen caecum*.

2 Structures.—The main substance of the tongue is composed of *intrinsic lingual muscles*. The *extrinsic lingual muscles*, arising from the mandible, hyoid bone, styloid process, and soft palate, are inserted into the main intrinsic muscle mass of the tongue.

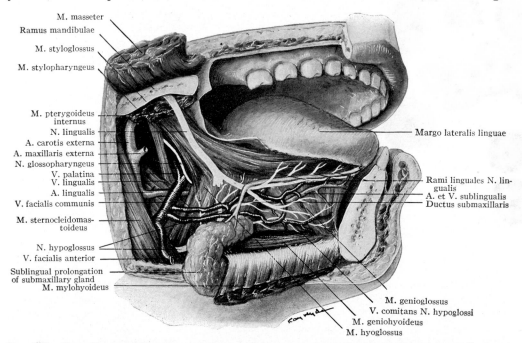

FIG. 137.—DEEP LATERAL VIEW OF THE LINGUAL REGION WITH THE BODY AND PART OF THE RAMUS OF THE MANDIBLE CUT AWAY AND THE SUBLINGUAL GLAND REMOVED.
The mylohyoid muscle has been reflected downward.

The *mucous membrane* over the anterior two thirds of the tongue is closely adherent to the underlying musculature. These muscles elevate, depress, protrude, or retract the tongue. The muscle mass of the tongue is kept from falling backward by its attachment to the symphysis of the jaw. Profound anesthesia which relaxes all muscles of the tongue is likely to allow the organ to fall back and obstruct the larynx by depressing the epiglottis. During anesthesia, therefore, the lower jaw should be carried well forward to advance the base of the tongue and keep it from interfering with the epiglottis. When this procedure is not sufficient to prevent suffocation direct traction on the tongue is necessary.

Below the tip, it forms a fold in the median line, the *frenum*.

At the apex of a V-shaped row of circumvallate papillae is a small depression, the *foramen caecum*, the remains of an embryonic tubular downgrowth in the floor of the primitive pharynx. It is the beginning of the fetal thyroglossal duct, from which the thyroid gland is developed.

The surface of the pharyngeal portion of the tongue is studded with masses of lymphoid tissue which make numerous elevations, called in aggregate, the lingual tonsil. This is a part of the general peribuccal ring of lymphatic tissue (of Waldeyer) (p. 146). The mucous membrane on the pharyngeal part of the tongue is continuous with that covering the epiglottis and forms the glosso-epiglottic folds and fossae.

3. **Vessels and Nerves.**—The principal *arteries* supplying the tongue are branches of the lingual artery which pass forward mesial to the hyoglossal muscle and then continue to the apex of the tongue as the deep lingual artery.

The *lymphatics* are very numerous and originate in an extensive network in the submucosa and in a smaller network in the muscle substance. The lymph vessels of the anterior portion of the tongue drain into the submental and submaxillary glands and into the upper deep cervical chain. From the margins and dorsum of the tongue behind the apex

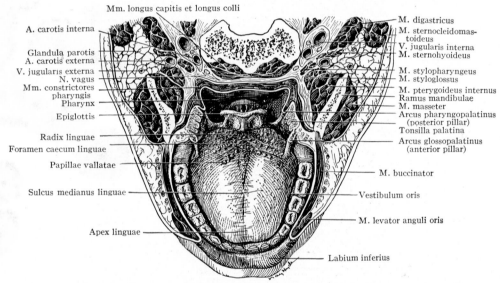

Mm. longus capitis et longus colli

A. carotis interna

Glandula parotis
A. carotis externa
V. jugularis externa
N. vagus
Mm. constrictores
pharyngis
Pharynx
Epiglottis

Radix linguae
Foramen caecum linguae

Papillae vallatae

Sulcus medianus linguae

Apex linguae

M. digastricus
M. sternocleidomas-
toideus
V. jugularis interna
M. sternohyoideus

M. stylopharyngeus
M. styloglossus
M. pterygoideus internus
Ramus mandibulae
M. masseter
Arcus pharyngopalatinus
(posterior pillar)
Tonsilla palatina
Arcus glossopalatinus
(anterior pillar)

M. buccinator

Vestibulum oris

M. levator anguli oris

Labium inferius

FIG. 138.—Cross Section Through the Buccal Cavity and the Oral Division of the Pharynx.

and extending back to the vallate papillae, the lymph vessels pass to the submaxillary and upper deep cervical glands. The lymphatic system from the base of the tongue drains into the deep cervical group. Carcinoma of the tongue, when confined to the lip or to the posterior one third of the organ, involves glands of both sides because of the decussation of the lymph paths. The motor *nerve* to the tongue is the hypoglossal.

SURGICAL CONSIDERATIONS

From time immemorial, the dorsum of the tongue has been an area of special observation in disease. Although there may be little of practical value in many of these observations, nevertheless, the appearance of the tongue is of some import in the diagnosis of febrile and digestive disturbances.

1. **Macroglossia and Ankyloglossia (Tongue-tie).**—*Macroglossia* is a term applied to a more or less uniform enlargement of the tongue, in contradistinction to true tumor formation. The superabundance of tissue frequently is congenital, and in this form may show an excess of fibrous, glandular, or lymphatic elements. The enlargement occurs mainly in the base of the tongue where the lymphatic elements are most numerous. The tongue may attain extraordinary dimensions and be forced outside the mouth, even causing deformities of the teeth.

Ankyloglossia (tongue-tie) is the result of a congenital shortening of the frenum which holds the tongue to the floor of the mouth. Protrusion of the tongue is hampered and the frenum may require division lest articulation be impaired.

2. **Thyroglossal Duct Remains.**—The thyroglossal duct is an early embryonic structure which passes from the posterior part of the dorsum of the tongue to the isthmus of the thyroid gland. It is composed of several layers of epithelium derived from the mucous membrane of the tongue. The caudal portion of the duct may persist as the pyramidal thyroid lobe. Under normal conditions, the duct atrophies early and its adult vestige is the *foramen caecum*. Between the foramen caecum and the hyoid bone, a portion of duct may remain and develop into a *sublingual cyst* (p. 184).

3. **Leukoplakia.**—The superficial epithelium of the tongue, in a condition known as superficial glossitis or leukoplakia, may be heaped up into whitish areas which are difficult to heal; they are considered precancerous. The constant exposure of such areas to the bacterial flora of the warm mouth cavity, together with frequent trauma and the inability to maintain immobilization, are causes of delayed healing of the lesion.

4. **Carcinoma.**—Carcinoma of the tongue is fairly common; it begins usually in the anterior two thirds or at the tip. It may start as a warty growth, an ulcer, a fissure which later indurates, or an indurated area which ulcerates. Syphilis and trauma, such as irritation from a jagged tooth, a pipe stem, or from holding articles such as nails in the mouth, are considered etiologic. One factor in rapid growth of the lesion is the repeated contraction of the lingual musculature which carries cancer cells into the numerous lymphatics. When the lesion is differentiated from a syphilitic lesion, it should be removed radically at the earliest possible moment, a truly mutilating operation and one now rarely performed, or it should be treated by radium. Whatever treatment is given the involved area, the lymphatic glands to which the area drains must be removed completely (p. 202).

Carcinoma of the tip of the tongue early involves the lingual, submental, and submaxillary glands; that farther back on the anterior two thirds of the tongue involves the sublingual, submaxillary, and upper deep cervical lymph glands. A carcinoma on the tip of the tongue, in rare instances, may spread directly to the inferior group of deep cervical lymph glands. A growth in the inferior surface or in the base of the tongue metastasizes to the submaxillary and deep cervical glands.

V. Tonsillar Region and Pharynx

A. PALATINE TONSIL REGION OR FOSSA

1. **Definition and Boundaries.**—Although anatomically located in the anterolateral pharynx and properly belonging to it, the faucial tonsillar region is more particularly an intermediate area between the buccal cavity and the oral division of the pharynx. The anterior and posterior boundaries of the fossa are its two pillars or arches. These diverge downward from the soft palate, the anterior pillar to fuse with the lateral wall of the tongue, and the posterior pillar to spread out on the side wall of the oral division of the pharynx. The glossopalatine muscle is the essential muscle of the anterior pillar or arch, and the pharyngopalatine muscle that of the posterior pillar or arch. The deep tonsillar recess between the pillars has as its apex the soft palate, as its base the lateral wall of the oral division of the pharynx, and as its floor the intrapharyngeal aponeurosis of the side wall of the pharynx.

2. **Palatine Tonsil.**—The palatine tonsil, like the lingual and pharyngeal tonsils, varies considerably in size and in shape. A study of its development serves to explain this variation.

Soon after birth, the tonsil undergoes a characteristic irregularity of growth, the ultimate shape and size of the organ depending on the amount of lymphoid tissue present. The maximum growth generally takes place in the two lower lobes, which project into the pharynx and obscure the smaller upper lobes lying deep in the *supratonsillar recess*. The recess might be termed the "intratonsillar fossa," since the tonsillar tissue extends upward, beneath, and around it into the soft palate.

On drawing the anterior pillar of the fauces forward and outward, a triangular fold can be seen passing backward to the tonsil. This fold is the posterior and inferior prolongation of the mucous membrane from the anterior pillar. It covers a thin layer of fibrous tissue which is continuous with the capsule of the tonsil. The upper or supratonsillar part of the fold extends across the intratonsillar recess as the *semilunar fold* and forms the mesial fold of the recess. The remainder of the fold is known as the *triangular plica*.

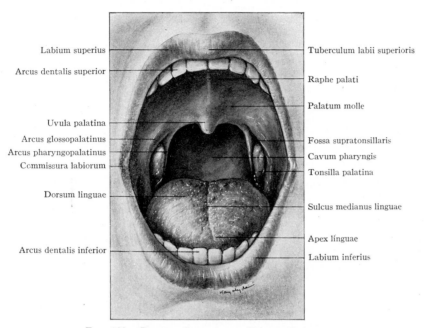

Labium superius — Tuberculum labii superioris
Arcus dentalis superior — Raphe palati
— Palatum molle
Uvula palatina
Arcus glossopalatinus — Fossa supratonsillaris
Arcus pharyngopalatinus — Cavum pharyngis
Commissura labiorum — Tonsilla palatina
Dorsum linguae — Sulcus medianus linguae
— Apex linguae
Arcus dentalis inferior — Labium inferius

FIG. 139.—BUCCAL CAVITY AND TONSIL REGION.

There are numerous *varieties of tonsils*, from the type deeply embedded between the pillars, to that enlarged so as almost to reach the median line. From the surgical stand-

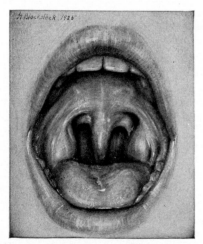

FIG. 140.—BURIED TONSILS. (Birkett in Jackson and Coates, "The Nose, Throat, and Ear and Their Diseases.")

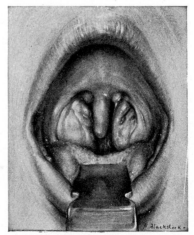

FIG. 141.—PEDUNCULATED TONSILS. (Birkett in Jackson and Coates, "The Nose, Throat, and Ear and Their Diseases.")

point, the embedded tonsil is much more difficult to enucleate than is the pedunculated tonsil, most of which is exposed and easy of access. The greater part of the "buried tonsil" can be made prominent by pressing on the anterior pillar, or by the patient's gagging during the examination. Much of the hidden tonsil extends upward into the soft palate.

10

above and deep to the intratonsillar recess. A large part may extend downward to the tongue in the form of infratonsillar lymphoid nodules, and frequently a portion extends forward for a variable distance beneath the triangular fold and the anterior pillar. Like all lymphoid structures, tonsils diminish in size after puberty and atrophy in old age.

The *tonsillar crypts* are ingrowths of the surface epithelium and vary greatly in number and size. They extend varying distances into the lymphoid tissue of the tonsil. The tonsil is separated from the pharynx by its *capsule*, a specialized portion of the intra-pharyngeal aponeurosis. The capsule covers all but the mesial surface of the gland and sends strong fibrous trabeculae into the lobular substance, affording paths to blood vessels and nerves. The tonsil capsule is separated from the superior constrictor muscle of the pharynx by lax connective tissue. When the tonsil is pulled forcibly into the oropharynx by a volsella during tonsillectomy, the pharyngeal muscle is not drawn out with it. A cleavage plane for enucleation of the gland thus is afforded, and the tonsil is removed with the part of the pharyngeal aponeurosis which forms the tonsil capsule. After repeated attacks of peritonsillar infection (quinsy), the tonsil capsule may become so densely adherent to the constrictor muscle that the tonsil can be removed only by sharp dissection.

3. **Infratonsillar Lymphoid Nodules.**—The palatine tonsil has been described. Lying on the lateral wall of the pharynx and tapering down to a free end is a *pharyngeal branch of the tonsil*. The upper extremity of this branch may be disclosed directly by deep depression of the tongue, and indirectly by the laryngeal mirror or by palpation. The *lingual branch of the tonsil*, in reality, is a continuous structure, extending from one side to the other with but a notch to mark the median raphe. The *lymphoid apron* perhaps is the most important division of the infratonsillar nodules. It is a wide, thick band of lymphoid tissue partially framed by the lingual branches of the tonsils. It overlies nearly the entire base of the tongue and supports the *lingual tonsil* near its center.

It is interesting to note that the lymphoid masses, commonly known as *recurrent tonsils*, really are only the upper parts of the trunks which unite the tonsillar branches. Even when the palatine tonsils have been enucleated perfectly, large segments of the branches may, in the course of time, work their way upward into the empty fossa where, particularly during attacks of acute inflammation, they appear to be parts of the original tonsils. To the uninitiated, such apparent postoperative defects reflect discredit on the surgeon's skill and prompt unjustifiable criticism.

The palatine tonsil, with this scattered circular band of lymphoid tissue and the tubal and pharyngeal tonsils, forms the *lymphoid ring* (of Waldeyer). This peribuccal ring acts possibly as a first line of defense against bacterial invasion of the nasal and buccal passages; the second line is the lymph nodes draining the area.

4. **Relations of the Palatine Tonsil.**—The lateral surface, or hilus of the tonsil, is applied through its capsule to the constrictor muscle of the pharynx. The vessels and nerves enter the gland in the areolar tissue around the gland. In this potential space, peritonsillar abscess (quinsy) develops. The pharyngeal wall separates the tonsil from the parapharyngeal space.

The major part of the *parapharyngeal* or *mandibulopharyngeal space* is occupied by the vagus, hypoglossal, glossopharyngeal, and spinal accessory nerves, the internal carotid artery, and the internal jugular vein. The relations of the tonsil differ in the prestyloid and retrostyloid divisions of the parapharyngeal space.

In the anterior (prestyloid) area, the tonsil is related to the areolar tissue between the pharyngeal wall and the internal pterygoid muscle. It is only over the retrostyloid portion that the tonsil has any possible relationship to the internal carotid artery and internal jugular vein. Only under most abnormal conditions does the *internal carotid artery* lie immediately lateral to the tonsil. Ordinarily, it is on a plane well posterior to the tonsil and is separated from it by the stylopharyngeus muscle. Moreover, there is an interval of 1.5 cm. or more separating the tonsil from these structures. The interval between the artery and tonsil is such that the gland may be removed for carcinoma through a posterior incision in the neck without injury to the vessels, provided the operative field is kept well forward of the styloid muscles and the posterior belly of the digastric muscle.

The *external carotid artery* lies about 2 cm. from the lateral pharyngeal wall, and is separated from it by a portion of the parotid gland and the musculature about the styloid process. It must be borne in mind, however, that a deeply embedded and enlarged tonsil is on a more lateral plane than is the remainder of the pharyngeal wall and, as such, is more closely related to the large vascular trunks than a description of the relations of a normal tonsil implies (Fig. 148).

It is important to realize that the *external maxillary (facial) artery* occasionally has an important relation to the postero-inferior portion of the gland. This artery, after branching from the external carotid artery, very frequently takes an upward bend deep to the ramus of the mandible. When this bending is marked, the arterial loop thus formed

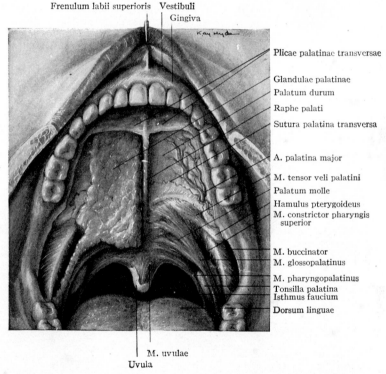

Frenulum labii superioris Vestibuli
Gingiva

Plicae palatinae transversae

Glandulae palatinae
Palatum durum
Raphe palati
Sutura palatina transversa

A. palatina major

M. tensor veli palatini
Palatum molle
Hamulus pterygoideus
M. constrictor pharyngis superior

M. buccinator
M. glossopalatinus

M. pharyngopalatinus
Tonsilla palatina
Isthmus faucium
Dorsum linguae

M. uvulae
Uvula

FIG. 142.—SUPERFICIAL AND DEEP STRUCTURES OF THE PALATE AND TONSIL REGIONS.
The palatine glands have been removed on one side; the pillars are denuded of their mucosa.

may come into close relation with the inferior portion of the tonsil, permitting possible injury to it in tonsil enucleation. The superior constrictor muscle of the pharynx is the only muscle interposed between this artery and the tonsil. When hemorrhage occurs in this region, it almost always comes from injury either to the ascending palatine or tonsillar branches of the external maxillary artery where they pierce the superior constrictor muscle of the pharynx and supply the palatine tonsil.

Tonsil relations to the parapharyngeal space show that anterior peritonsillar abscesses may invade the anterior or prestyloid portion of the space. Early evacuation of the abscess lessens the chance of parapharyngeal involvement and possible invasion of the posterior vascular structures of the space.

5. **Vessels and Nerves.**—The *arterial supply* to the palatine tonsil, while derived from several sources, comes ultimately from the external carotid trunk. The ascending palatine and tonsillar branches of the external maxillary artery enter the gland from below.

The gland receives a supply posteriorly from the ascending pharyngeal branch of the external carotid artery and anteriorly from small branches of the lingual artery. The supply from above is from the descending palatine branch of the internal maxillary artery. These vessels ordinarily are small, but occasionally are sufficiently large to cause troublesome hemorrhage. The tonsillar branch of the external maxillary artery usually is the largest vessel and passes upward on the outer wall of the pharynx, traversing it to supply the tonsil and soft palate. When the branches are cut as they enter the capsule of the tonsil, the hemorrhage usually is of little consequence, but when a vessel is severed in the pharyngeal wall before it breaks into its small branches, the hemorrhage may be alarming. Tonsillectomy hemorrhage is most severe when tags of tonsils are left in place, the explanation possibly being that the severed vessel cannot retract and thrombose.

The *lymph supply* to the tonsil is particularly abundant. From the collecting vessels over the lateral tonsillar surface, the drainage is through the wall of the pharynx to the deep cervical glands a little below the angle of the jaw. Consequently, these glands are enlarged in inflammatory or carcinomatous lesions of the tonsil. One of these glands, situated just behind the angle of the jaw beneath the anterior edge of the sternocleidomastoid muscle, is enlarged so constantly in tonsillar infection as to be termed the "tonsillar lymph node."

SURGICAL CONSIDERATIONS

1. **Peritonsillar Abscess and Its Incision.**—An abscess may arise in the peritonsillar connective tissue (outside the capsule of the tonsil) following acute suppurative tonsillitis. This abscess (quinsy) commonly occurs in the anterior portion of the peritonsillar space

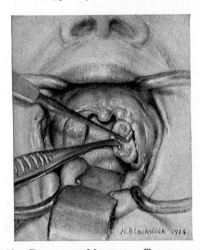

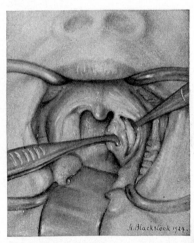

FIG. 143.—DISSECTION METHOD OF TONSILLECTOMY. The tonsil is grasped by the forceps and the knife is inserted behind the anterior pillar, releasing it from the attachment to the tonsil. (Birkett in Jackson and Coates, "The Nose, Throat, and Ear and Their Diseases.")

FIG. 144.—DISSECTION METHOD OF TONSILLECTOMY. That part of the capsule of the tonsil is exposed which lies behind the anterior pillar. (Birkett in Jackson and Coates, "The Nose, Throat, and Ear and Their Diseases.")

and probably results from direct extension from suppurative foci in the tonsillar crypts. The abscess may invade the pharyngeal wall and the structures of the parapharyngeal space.

Peritonsillar abscess usually is opened through the mouth by a stab incision about 1 cm. lateral to the free border of the anterior pillar at its upper attachment, and sufficiently deep to enter the peritonsillar space. Vessels encountered here are small and hemorrhage from them usually stops spontaneously or can be arrested easily by pressure. The incision sometimes is made midway on a line which unites the base of the uvula to the last upper wisdom tooth. In many instances, the abscess seems to point mesially where it can be evacuated by plunging a hemostat between the tonsil and one or the other of its pillars. The use of the anatomic route employed in tonsillectomy encounters no essential structures.

2. **Tonsillectomy by Dissection.**—The main feature in any removal of the tonsil is total excision of the gland with its capsule. To accomplish this, the mucous membrane folds uniting the tonsil to the anterior and posterior pillars must be incised. The tonsil is grasped by a tenaculum and is drawn mesially into the pharynx, so that the interval between the tonsil and its anterior pillar can be recognized clearly. A sharp dissector then is carried through this interval along the anterior pillar just beneath the mucous membrane covering the tonsil. Retraction of the anterior pillar and blunt dissection expose the bluish-white capsule. In continuing the enucleation, close contact with the capsule must be maintained. By pushing the areolar tissue outward, the upper pole is exposed readily and is drawn downward with grasping forceps. At this stage, the tonsil is freed by sharp or blunt dissection from its attachment to the posterior pillar, leaving it attached only to the inferior part of the fossa. The tonsil, with its capsule intact, then can be separated, either by scissors or snare, from the fascia holding it in its fossa. The snare is in common usage because its crushing action tends to thrombose the vessels. It has the added advantage

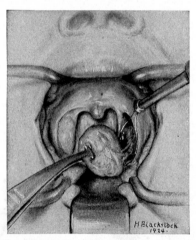

FIG. 145.—DISSECTION METHOD OF TONSILLECTOMY.

The wire loop of the snare is applied to the pedicle of the tonsil. (Birkett in Jackson and Coates, "The Nose, Throat, and Ear and Their Diseases.")

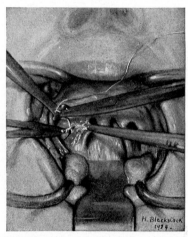

FIG. 146.—METHOD OF EXPOSING THE FLOOR OF THE TONSILLAR FOSSA IN THE SEARCH FOR BLEEDING POINTS. (Birkett in Jackson and Coates, "The Nose, Throat, and Ear and Their Diseases.")

that, when applied about a partially enucleated tonsil, it tends to follow the tonsillar capsule, removing it more satisfactorily than the tonsillotome, which cuts through a resistant mass rather than follows its irregularities. Finger dissection or enucleation, while successful in the hands of those accustomed to it, is likely to be attended by considerable trauma. It is difficult to separate the tonsillar capsule from the pharyngeal bed when repeated attacks of inflammation have made their union almost fibrous.

B. REGION OF THE PHARYNX

1. **Definition and Boundaries.**—The pharynx is a vertically placed musculomembranous tube situated behind the nasal fossae, the mouth, and the larynx. It is roofed by the base of the skull and is continued below into the esophagus opposite the sixth cervical vertebra. Its lateral and posterior walls are formed by the three constrictor muscles, which are arranged like three flower pots fitted into one another. The continuity of the anterior wall is interrupted by the choanae (posterior nares), the entrance into the buccal cavity, and the superior orifice of the larynx. Lesions are manifested clinically by disturbances in breathing, swallowing, and phonation.

2. **Divisions of the Pharynx.**—The pharynx is divided into three divisions: nasopharynx, oropharynx, and laryngopharynx.

The *nasopharynx* is roughly cube-shaped and is the direct posterior continuation of the nasal fossae. The posterior nares form the boundary between the two areas. The nasopharynx is bounded below by the soft palate, and the region can be examined by a finger introduced through the mouth and carried upward behind that structure. In swallowing, the soft palate (p. 135) is applied against the posterior pharyngeal wall, and ef-

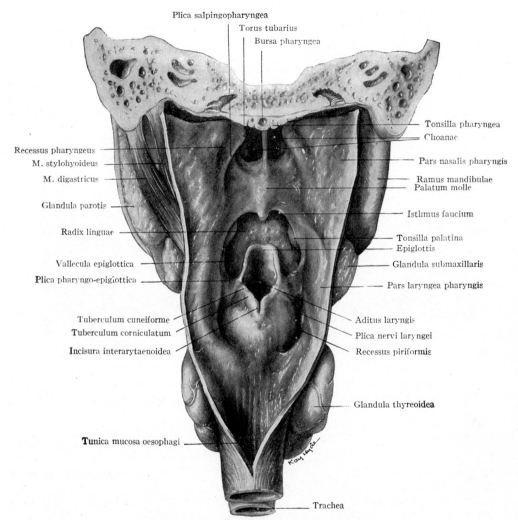

FIG. 147.—POSTERIOR VIEW OF THE PHARYNX AND ESOPHAGUS.
The posterior wall of the pharynx is opened.

fectively partitions the nasopharynx from the oropharynx. This arrangement keeps food from entering the nasopharynx and nose. During respiration, the soft palate hangs vertically downward, placing the nasal and oral divisions in broad communication.

In the anterior wall of the nasopharynx, the posterior border of the nasal septum (p. 80) can be felt, and, on each side of it, the finger can be passed through the choanae to touch the posterior extremities of the middle and inferior conchae. The basilar part of the occipital bone forms the roof of the nasopharynx; the regularity of the sinus varies with the shape and size of the sphenoid sinuses. A little below the roof of the posterior wall, the anterior arch of the atlas may be palpated. The *pharyngeal tonsil* lies on this wall, and overgrowth of its lymphoid tissue (adenoids) may fill up the nasopharynx and hinder or completely obstruct nasal breathing.

On the lateral wall, the bulging orifice of the auditory (eustachian) tube leads upward, backward, and laterally to the tympanic cavity (p. 104). The posterior lip of the opening is a prominent elevation (eustachian cushion) derived from the cartilaginous portion of the tube, behind which lies the pharyngeal recess (fossa of Rosenmüller). Beneath the mucous membrane of the pharyngeal opening of the tube is a considerable amount of lymphoid tissue, the *tubal tonsil* (of Gerlach). When the orifice of the tube is occluded, as by adenoids, the air in the tympanic cavity is absorbed gradually and deafness results. The unyielding character of the walls of the nasopharynx favors packing of the cavity for the arrest of nasal hemorrhage (p. 83).

The *oropharynx* is the posterior continuation of the mouth cavity. Although anatomically the tonsillar region is a part of the lateral wall of the oropharynx, the tonsils are of such clinical importance as to have been discussed as a separate region. When the mouth is closed, the anterior wall of the oropharynx consists of the posterior vertical part of the tongue. A retropharyngeal abscess causes a forward bulging of the posterior

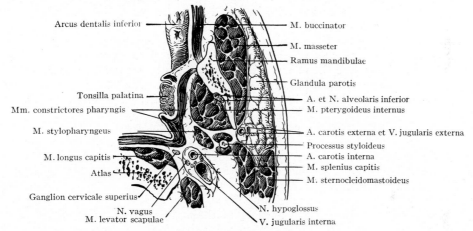

Arcus dentalis inferior —
M. buccinator
M. masseter
Ramus mandibulae
Glandula parotis
Tonsilla palatina —
A. et N. alveolaris inferior
Mm. constrictores pharyngis —
M. pterygoideus internus
M. stylopharyngeus —
A. carotis externa et V. jugularis externa
Processus styloideus
M. longus capitis —
A. carotis interna
Atlas —
M. splenius capitis
M. sternocleidomastoideus
Ganglion cervicale superius —
N. vagus
N. hypoglossus
M. levator scapulae
V. jugularis interna

Fig. 148.—Cross Section Through the Middle of the Tonsil to Show the Relations about the Peripharyngeal Spaces.

pharyngeal wall, which may interfere with respiration and cause symptoms not unlike those associated with adenoids and enlarged palatine tonsils.

The *laryngopharynx* is the lowermost division of the pharynx, and is separated from the oropharynx by the pharyngo-epiglottic fold. It lies below the level of the hyoid bone. At the center of the laryngopharynx is the raised opening of the larynx below the epiglottis, on each side of which is the piriform sinus. Behind the laryngeal opening, the laryngopharynx narrows down to join the cervical esophagus. The relation of the pharynx to the laryngeal orifice explains how foreign bodies in the pharyngeal recesses cause laryngeal symptoms.

3. **Structure of the Pharyngeal Wall.**—The pharyngeal walls present mucosal, submucosal (intrapharyngeal aponeurosis), and muscle layers.

The *mucous membrane* is vascular and readily inflamed, and, in acute or chronic catarrhal disease, secretes an obnoxious discharge from its many glands. It may present tuberculous or syphilitic ulceration or be the point of origin of an epithelioma. Within it lie the masses of lymphoid tissue which play so important a rôle in the nasopharynx, from both the infective and obstructive standpoints.

In the posterior and lateral walls of the pharynx, the cellular tissue between the mucosa and muscularis is differentiated into an *intrapharyngeal aponeurosis*. This layer is strongest and densest in the floor of the tonsillar fossa. From it is derived the capsule of the tonsil.

The *pharyngeal muscles* are divided into constricting and elevating groups. The superior, middle, and inferior constrictors overlap one another from below upward and contract the cavity of the pharynx. The elevating muscles run longitudinally and raise the pharynx and larynx. The pharyngeal musculature may be paralyzed in bulbar brain lesions or in diphtheria. Since these muscles are concerned vitally in swallowing, their paralysis allows food to be forced upward into the nasal fossae or downward through the larynx.

4. **Peripharyngeal Spaces.**—The upper pharynx is separated from the surrounding structures by lateral and retropharyngeal spaces.

Each *lateral space*, roughly defined between the internal pterygoid muscle and the sagittal septum which relates the pharynx to the prevertebral fascia, contains the internal carotid artery and internal jugular vein.

The *retropharyngeal space* lies between the pharynx and prevertebral fascia and is continuous below with the retro-esophageal and mediastinal connective tissue. The cellular tissue behind the pharynx contains small unimportant vessels, as well as several lymph glands. These glands drain, to some extent, the nasal mucous membrane, the tonsils, the auditory tube region, and the middle ear. They may become inflamed acutely with abscess formation, especially in the young. Acute pyogenic suppuration must not be confused with tuberculous retropharyngeal abscess which arises from caries of the bodies of the cervical vertebrae and which rarely breaks through the prevertebral fascia. Pyogenic abscesses bulge into the pharynx where they may be seen and palpated readily, and may be opened without fear of injury to the great vessels which lie far to the lateral side Extreme care must be observed lest there be aspiration of the septic contents.

Surgical Considerations

1. **Nasopharyngeal Examination.**—Examination of the nasopharynx is made by reflecting light directly upon a rhinoscopic mirror held behind the soft palate while the patient breathes quietly through his nose. The mirrored image reflects the posterior nares, the septum, and the posterior extremities of the superior, middle, and inferior conchae. On each side is seen the pharyngeal opening of the auditory tube, the auditory eminence, and the pharyngeal fossa (of Rosenmüller). Examination may be made with the pharyngoscope passed into the nasopharynx through the nose.

2. **Pharyngeal Tonsil (Adenoids).**—Adenoids appear as simple enlargement of the pharyngeal tonsil. The term usually is applied to lymphoid tissue of sufficient amount to cause obstruction to normal breathing. Adenoids of moderate size appear as rounded masses on the posterior walls of the nasopharynx. When large, they cover the upper part of the septum, as may be seen in the rhinoscopic mirror. Their size may be such as to fill the nasopharynx and extend below the level of the soft palate, making posterior rhinoscopic examination impossible. When acutely inflamed, they become considerably enlarged, and contain exudate similar to that found in the crypts of the palatine tonsils in the course of a follicular tonsillitis.

The symptoms of excessive adenoid vegetation are caused by auditory tube and nasal obstruction and by the extension of the inflammation to contiguous structures. With a virulent infection, there may be an acute adenoiditis with marked systemic reaction. The infection may extend up the auditory tube into the middle ear (otitis media) (p. 103). Surgical removal is the only treatment for adenoid obstruction, and the whole of the nasopharyngeal vault should be cleared of lymphoid tissue.

Adenoids may be confused with pedunculated nasopharyngeal polyps, which originate in the maxillary antrum, on the middle turbinate, or on the posterior portion of the nasal septum. Polyps usually undergo cystic degeneration before attaining any considerable size.

In the rhinoscopic mirror, a polyp is seen as a bluish-white tumor which may fill the nasopharynx. It usually is removed with a nasal snare.

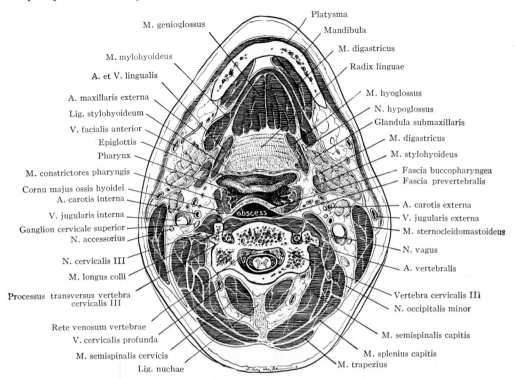

M. genioglossus
Platysma
Mandibula
M. mylohyoideus
M. digastricus
A. et V. lingualis
Radix linguae
A. maxillaris externa
Lig. stylohyoideum
V. facialis anterior
Epiglottis
Pharynx
M. constrictores pharyngis
Cornu majus ossis hyoidei
A. carotis interna
V. jugularis interna
Ganglion cervicale superior
N. accessorius
N. cervicalis III
M. longus colli
Processus transversus vertebra cervicalis III
Rete venosum vertebrae
V. cervicalis profunda
M. semispinalis cervicis
Lig. nuchae
M. hyoglossus
N. hypoglossus
Glandula submaxillaris
M. digastricus
M. stylohyoideus
Fascia buccopharyngea
Fascia prevertebralis
A. carotis externa
V. jugularis externa
M. sternocleidomastoideus
N. vagus
A. vertebralis
Vertebra cervicalis III
N. occipitalis minor
M. semispinalis capitis
M. splenius capitis
M. trapezius

abscess

FIG. 149.—CROSS SECTION AT THE LEVEL OF THE THIRD CERVICAL VERTEBRA TO SHOW THE BULGING OF A RETROPHARYNGEAL ABSCESS INTO THE PHARYNX.
The abscess has arisen from infection of the retropharyngeal lymph glands and is in contradistinction to retropharyngeal abscess of spinal tuberculous origin.

Primary sarcoma may occur in the nasopharynx at any age, and usually arises on the posterosuperior wall. Its rapid growth early leads to nasal obstruction.

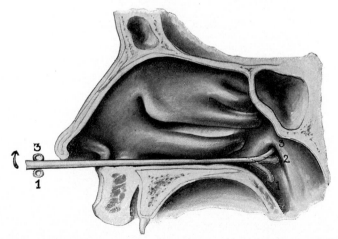

FIG. 150.—CATHETERIZATION OF THE RIGHT AUDITORY (EUSTACHIAN) TUBE.

3. **Inflation of the Tympanic Cavity.**—The tympanic cavity may be inflated through the pharyngeal orifice of the auditory tube by means of a eustachian catheter. This in-

strument is passed backward along the floor of the inferior meatus until its down-turned beak reaches the posterior wall of the nasopharynx.   The catheter is rotated laterally through a right angle until its point is lodged in the pharyngeal recess.   It then is withdrawn slowly until the point is felt to catch on the tubal eminence.   Partial withdrawal and slight upward rotation of the beak then conducts it past the obstruction.   The instrument, when directed laterally again, enters the orifice of the auditory tube.

THE NECK

I. General Considerations; Fascias of the Neck

THE neck provides passage for the many structures communicating between the head and trunk, and permits a wide range of movements of the head. The great number and variety of surgical conditions which present in this region make it one of considerable practical interest and importance.

1. **Boundaries of the Neck.**—The superior boundary of the neck is the line of the inferior margin of the body of the mandible, continued from the angle of the jaw through the mastoid process joining the *superior* nuchal line. The *inferior* boundary is marked

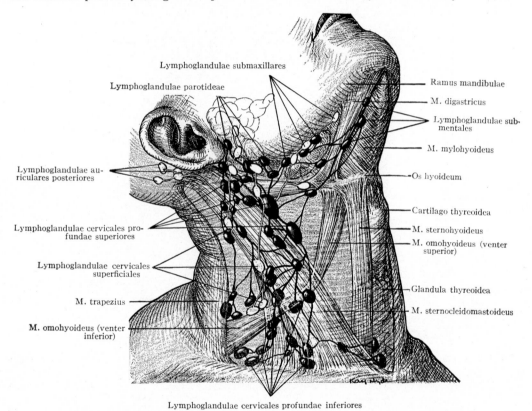

Lymphoglandulae submaxillares

Lymphoglandulae parotideae

Ramus mandibulae

M. digastricus

Lymphoglandulae submentales

M. mylohyoideus

Lymphoglandulae auriculares posteriores

Os hyoideum

Cartilago thyreoidea

M. sternohyoideus

M. omohyoideus (venter superior)

Lymphoglandulae cervicales profundae superiores

Lymphoglandulae cervicales superficiales

Glandula thyreoidea

M. sternocleidomastoideus

M. trapezius

M. omohyoideus (venter inferior)

Lymphoglandulae cervicales profundae inferiores

FIG. 151.—SURFACE ANATOMY OF THE LATERAL REGION OF THE NECK SHOWING THE DISTRIBUTION OF THE SUPERFICIAL AND DEEP CERVICAL LYMPH GLANDS.

by the suprasternal notch, the superior margin of the clavicle, and a line drawn from the acromioclavicular joint to the spinous process of the seventh cervical vertebra (vertebra prominens).

2. **Surface Anatomy.**—The surface anatomy of the neck presents marked age, sex, and individual variations. In children and women, the contour is well rounded; in men, the landmarks are very prominent. The most important single landmark is the *sternocleidomastoid muscle*, which forms a broad relief between the anterior and lateral regions. In the midanterior region, particularly in men, the *thyroid cartilage* (*Adam's apple*) projects prominently. About 2.5 cm. above the margin of the thyroid cartilage lies the body of the *hyoid bone*, which, because of its mobility, must be steadied on both sides to render

it palpable. The greater horn of the hyoid bone lies about midway between the mastoid process and the thyroid prominence. Just inferior to the thyroid prominence, the arch of the *cricoid cartilage* may be felt. Pressure at the anterior margin of the sternocleido-mastoid muscle at the level of the cricoid cartilage compresses the common carotid artery against the anterior tuberosity of the transverse process of the sixth cervical vertebra. This palpable process is the *carotid tubercle* (of Chassaignac), and is the landmark in liga-tion of the common carotid artery. The anterior edge of the *trapezius muscle* may be traced from its origin along the superior nuchal line down the lateral region of the neck to its insertion on the clavicle. The prominent *spinous process* of the *seventh cervical vertebra* is an important landmark in the inferior portion of the nuchal furrow.

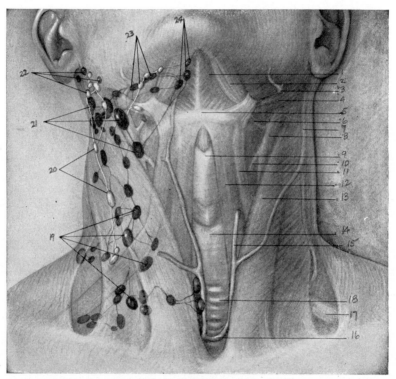

Fig 152.—Surface Anatomy of the Neck and Distribution of the Superficial and Deep Cervical Lymph Glands.

1, M. mylohyoideus; 2, M. digastricus (venter anterior); 3, V. facialis communis; 4, M. digastricus (venter posterior); 5, os hyoideum; 6, V. lingualis; 7, V. jugularis externa; 8, V. jugularis interna; 9, cartilago thyreoidea; 10, V. thyreoidea superior; 11, M. omohyoideus (venter superior); 12, M. sternohyoideus; 13, M. sternocleidomastoideus; 14, isthmus glandulae thyreoideae; 15, V. jugularis anterior; 16, arcus venosus juguli; 17, M. omohyoideus (venter posterior); 18, trachea; 19, lymphoglandulae cervicales profundae inferiores; 20, lymphoglandulae cervicales superficiales; 21, lymphoglandulae cervicales profundae superiores; 22, lymphoglandulae parotideae; 23, lymphoglandulae submaxillares; 24, lymphoglandulae submentales.

3. **Topographic Division of the Neck.**—The neck may be divided topographically into three general regions: anterior, lateral, and posterior. The *anterior* region comprises the structures between the sternocleidomastoid muscles, and is divided into suprahyoid and infrahyoid areas. The suprahyoid area has two subdivisions: submental and sub-maxillary. The infrahyoid area has several subdivisions: superficial infrahyoid, laryngo-tracheal, thyroid, cervical esophageal, and prevertebral. The *lateral* region is differentiated into the sternocleidomastoid (carotid) and the supraclavicular areas. To these general divisions is added the region of the root of the neck, the *thoracocervical* boundary between the neck and chest.

4. Divisions of Cervical Fascia and Fascial Spaces.—The fascias of the neck are superficial and deep.   The **superficial fascia,** carrying the superficial vessels and nerves, is separated from the investing or enveloping layer of deep cervical fascia by the thin sheet of *platysma* muscle extending over the front of the neck.   Inferiorly, this muscle arises from the deep fascia of the pectoral region and from the clavicle; superiorly, it is attached to the inferior border of the mandible and extends to and blends with some of the muscles of the face.   Closure of lacerations and operative incisions require careful approximation of the skin-platysma layer to avoid unsightly scars.

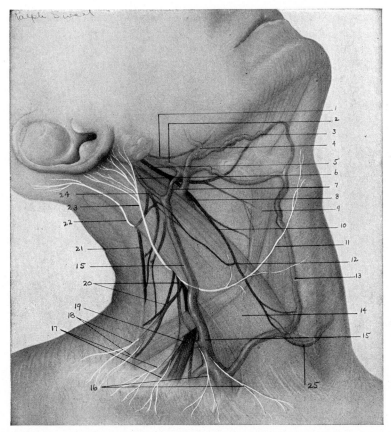

Fig. 153.—Surface Anatomy of the Lateral Region of the Neck and the Distribution of the Superficial Veins and Nerves.

1, Ramus marginalis mandibulae n. facialis; 2, V. facialis posterior; 3, V. submentalis; 4, V. facialis anterior; 5, N. hypoglossus; 6, V. jugularis externa; 7, V. facialis communis; 8, V. jugularis interna; 9, M. omohyoideus; 10, ramus descendens n. hypoglossi; 11, N. cutaneus colli; 12, N. ansa hypoglossi; 13, V. jugularis anterior; 14, M. sternocleidomastoideus; 15, V. jugularis externa; 16, Nn. supraclaviculares anteriores; 17, Nn. supraclaviculares medii; 18, Nn. supraclaviculares posteriores; 19, plexus brachialis; 20, trunks of supraclavicular nerves; 21, ramus externus nervi accessorii; 22, N. occipitalis minor; 23, N. auricularis magnus; 24, N. cervicalis III; 25, arcus venosus jugularis.

The **deep fascia** comprises an investing layer, with prevertebral and pretracheal divisions; these invest and support the muscles, pharynx, trachea, esophagus, lymph glands, large vessels and nerves.   A complete envelope for all the cervical structures in the neck, save the platysma and the superficial vessels and nerves, is formed by the *investing layer of deep cervical fascia.*   It is attached above to the inferior margin of the mandible, and behind the angle of the jaw is carried up to enclose the parotid gland and attach to the zygomatic arch, mastoid process, superior nuchal line, and external occipital protuberance. Posteriorly, this investing layer is attached over the spinous processes of the cervical vertebrae, and its lamellae sheathe the trapezius muscle. At the anterior margin of the trapezius and over the supraclavicular triangle, it appears as a single layer, dividing at the posterior edge of the sternocleidomastoid muscle, which it sheathes. Over the front of the neck superiorly, the fascia appears again as a single layer to meet the corresponding layer of the opposite side in the midline. It is attached to the hyoid bone, and below this level, it splits to form a superficial and a deep layer. These layers are applied to the

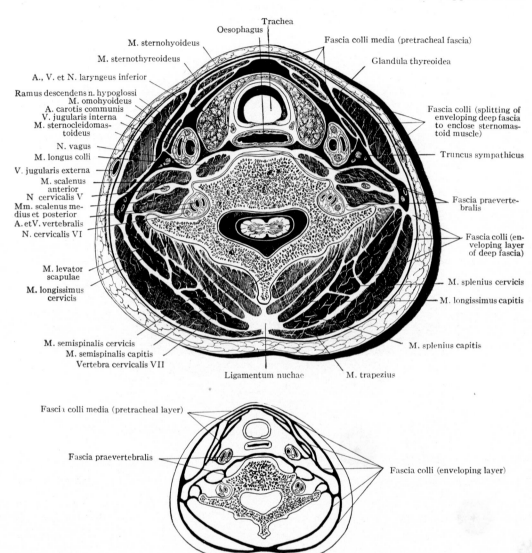

FIG. 154.—CROSS SECTION THROUGH THE NECK AT THE LEVEL OF THE SEVENTH CERVICAL VERTEBRA
TO SHOW THE LAYERS OF DEEP CERVICAL FASCIA.
Inset delineates the fascial layers without reference to the structures they enclose.

anterior and posterior borders of the sternum (p. 215). Between them lie the sternal heads of the sternocleidomastoid muscles and the anterior jugular veins in their course toward the external jugular veins. In the interval between the angle of the jaw and the greater horn of the hyoid bone, the enveloping layer fuses with the fascial covering of the posterior belly of the digastric muscle. Similar fusion takes place between the enveloping fascia and that covering the anterior belly of the digastric muscle. Thus, the submaxillary and submental areas, to a great extent, are shut off from one another and from the other regions of the neck.

The *prevertebral fascia* is the more posterior septum derived from the enveloping layer. It extends over the prevertebral musculature across the neck behind the pharyngo-esophageal tube. It lies behind the great vessels of the neck and covers the muscles on which they lie. The prevertebral fascia forms the floor of the supraclavicular triangle where it overlies the cervical and the subclavian vessels. These structures, on leaving the supraclavicular area, invaginate the prevertebral fascia and thus carry with them a fascial tubular prolongation, known as the axillary sheath. Thus, a collection of fluid under the prevertebral fascia may extend down this fascial tube along the axillary vessels and appear as a swelling on the lateral wall of the axilla along the course of the artery. It may appear as far down as the elbow. Superficial branches of the cervical plexus pierce the prevertebral layer, but the phrenic nerve remains deep to it (p. 191). Pus from tuberculosis of

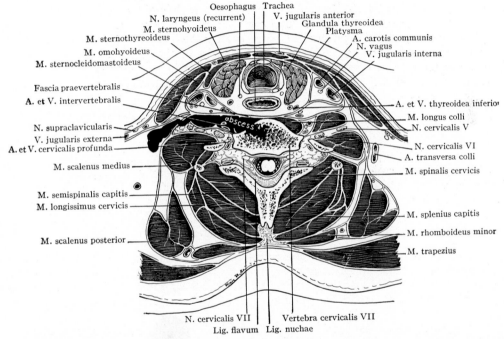

FIG. 155.—CROSS SECTION THROUGH THE NECK AT THE LEVEL OF THE SEVENTH CERVICAL VERTEBRA TO SHOW TUBERCULOUS EROSION OF THE VERTEBRAL BODY AND THE LATERAL EXTENSION OF THE RESULTING TUBERCULOUS ABSCESS INTO THE SUPRACLAVICULAR REGION BEHIND THE PREVERTEBRAL FASCIA.

the cervical vertebrae lies behind the fascia, and may bulge into the posterior wall of the pharynx (retropharyngeal abscess). Owing to the strength of the fascia, perforation does not occur, and the pus usually passes downward and laterally to escape behind the sterno-cleidomastoid muscle into the supraclavicular triangle where the fascial layer is weaker. Here it can be evacuated through an incision behind the muscle with retraction forward of the carotid sheath. Occasionally, pus may pass downward behind the fascia into the posterior mediastinum.

The *pretracheal* or *middle layer of cervical fascia* is derived from the enveloping layer deep to the sternocleidomastoid muscle. It lies in front of the laryngotracheal tube and the infrahyoid muscles and descends behind the enveloping layer into the root of the neck and mediastinum to blend with the covering of the aorta and pericardium. It is much more delicate than the prevertebral fascia, and its densest and most differentiated portion covers the area below the hyoid bone between the omohyoid muscles, the sternal halves of the clavicles, and the suprasternal notch. Laterally, it forms the carotid sheath. The anterior fascial layer of the pretracheal division sheathes the omohyoid and sternohyoid muscles; the posterior layer sheathes the sternothyroid muscle. In the root of the neck, fibrous expansions are thrown over the large vascular trunks, tending to hold them open, so that a sectioned vessel in the region will not close readily and entrance of air (air embolus) may occur with a fatal result.

Three **spaces** are delimited by these fascias. The *visceral space*, lying between the pretracheal and prevertebral fascias, contains the laryngotracheal tube, lower pharynx, cervical esophagus, thyroid gland, and great vessels. These structures are surrounded by areolar connective tissue which is sufficiently lax to permit great distention. Fluid collections in this compartment may spread behind the clavicle into the mediastinum or may follow the subclavian vessels into the axillary space. Migrating abscesses within this space may burrow laterally into the posterior cervical triangles or upward through the submaxillary areas into the retromandibular spaces. The *suprahyoid space* lies between the enveloping fascia and the fascial covering of the mylohyoid muscles. Fluids may collect either in the submaxillary or submental divisions of this space and invade the visceral compartment. The *prevertebral space* lies on the vertebral bodies and muscles behind the prevertebral fascia. The products of caries of the cervical vertebrae invade this musculofibro-osseous compartment and either migrate laterally, or burrow along the cervical column through the thoracic inlet and into the posterior mediastinum.

II. ANTERIOR REGIONS OF NECK

A. SUPRAHYOID AREAS

The suprahyoid region has three divisions: a median submental and two lateral submaxillary. For purposes of topography, the submaxillary areas are understood to extend to the anterior margins of the sternocleidomastoid muscles.

(I) MEDIAN SUPRAHYOID OR SUBMENTAL REGION

1. **Location and Boundaries.**—The submental region is a triangle, having as its base the body of the hyoid bone, as its apex the symphysis of the mandible, and as its lateral margins the anterior bellies of the digastric muscles. Its floor consists of the mylohyoid muscles which separate it from the sublingual compartment. The roof or outer covering is the investing layer of the deep cervical fascia.

2. **Contents.**—The submental group of pea-sized *lymph glands* receives afferents from the chin, central portion of the lower lip, centrally placed teeth, gums, floor of the mouth, and tip of the tongue. *Abscess* of these glands produces a swelling which bulges downward below the chin, but is hindered from rising into the mouth by the mylohyoid muscles.

Ranulas and other tumors in the sublingual space (p. 140) usually present in the floor of the mouth, but may bulge downward into the submental space. The efferents of the submental glands pass to the submaxillary group. That portion of the thyroglossal duct (p. 144) which traverses the region may give rise to a *cyst* which presents in the median line above the hyoid bone.

3. **Surgical Access.**—Access to the contents of this region is obtained by a horizontal incision just above the hyoid bone. After the investing layer of deep fascia is penetrated, the digastric muscles and mylohyoid floor are guides to lateral and deeper structures. Wide incision can be made because there are no important contents. Because of the edema of the overlying and surrounding structures, abscesses which seem superficial are found to be deep. Infection in the adjoining submaxillary areas is reached by blunt dissection and drained into the submental incision. A sublingual cyst is accessible through a horizontal incision, splitting the mylohyoid raphe.

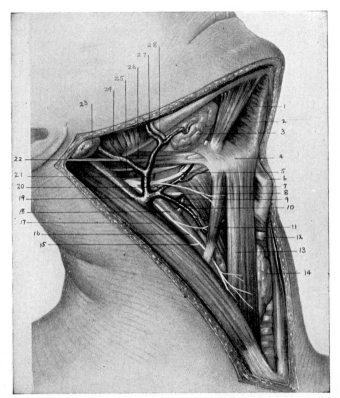

FIG. 156.—RELATIONS BETWEEN THE SUBMAXILLARY, SUBMENTAL, AND UPPER STERNOMASTOID REGIONS
Attention is directed to the continuity of the regions in the spread of infection.

1, M. mylohyoideus; 2, M. digastricus (venter anterior); 3, glandula submaxillaris; 4, os hyoideum;
5, N. hypoglossus; 6, cartilago thyreoidea; 7, ramus thyreohyoideus n. hypoglossi; 8, N. laryngeus superior;
9, A. et V. laryngea superior; 10, A. et V. thyreoidea superior; 11, M. omohyoideus (venter superior);
12, cartilago cricoidea; 13, M. sternohyoideus; 14, isthmus glandulae thyreoideae; 15, N. ansa hypoglossi;
16, ramus descendens n. hypoglossi; 17, M. sternocleidomastoideus; 18, A. carotis communis; 19, V. jugularis
interna; 20, A. et V. lingualis; 21, V. facialis communis; 22, V. facialis posterior; 23, glandula parotis; 24, M.
masseter; 25, M. digastricus (venter posterior); 26, M. stylohyoideus; 27, V. facialis anterior; 28, A. maxillaris externa.

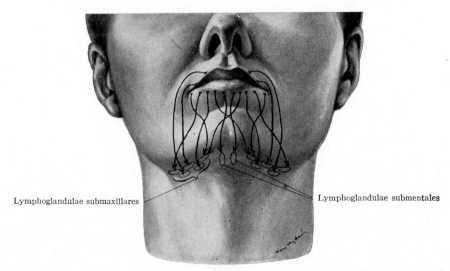

Lymphoglandulae submaxillares   Lymphoglandulae submentales

FIG. 157.—LYMPHATIC DRAINAGE FROM THE LIPS TO THE SUBMENTAL AND SUBMAXILLARY GLANDS
11

(II) Lateral Suprahyoid or Submaxillary Region

1. Definition and Boundaries.—The lateral suprahyoid or submaxillary region is comprised essentially of the digastric triangle and its submaxillary contents; for topographic purposes, the region extends *laterally* to the sternocleidomastoid muscle. The *inferior* boundary is a line from the point of attachment of the digastric tendons along the body of the hyoid bone to the sternocleidomastoid muscle; the *superior* boundary is the inferior margin of the mandible, projected to the sternocleidomastoid muscle; and the *anterior* limit is the anterior belly of the digastric muscle.

The *outer wall* or *roof* of the area is the investing layer of the deep cervical fascia connecting the inferior margin of the mandible and the hyoid bone. Through it are visible

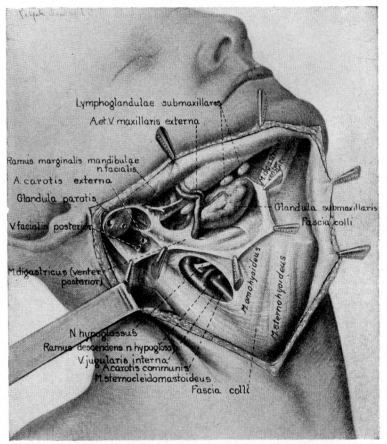

Lymphoglandulae submaxillares
A.et.V. maxillaris externa
Ramus marginalis mandibulae
n.facialis
A. carotis externa
Glandula parotis
V.facialis posterior
M.digastricus (venter posterior)
M.digastricus (venter posterior)
Glandula submaxillaris
Fascia colli
M.omohyoideus
M.sternohyoideus
N.hypoglossus
Ramus descendens n. hypoglossi
V.jugularis interna
A. carotis communis
M.sternocleidomastoideus
Fascia colli

Fig. 158.—Dissection of the Submaxillary Area Carried Down Through the Investing Layer of Deep Cervical Fascia. (Bartlett and Callander.)
The parotid space and part of the sternomastoid region are opened.

the digastric bellies and the submaxillary gland. The *deep wall* or *floor* is formed by the mylohyoid muscle, the posterior part of the hyoglossal muscle, and the lateral surface of the middle constrictor muscle of the pharynx. Between the posterior border of the mylohyoid and the superjacent hyoglossus is a cleft which forms a communication with the sublingual region (p. 138).

The tri-muscle floor of the suprahyoid region may be divided into three areas: a predigastric, the floor of the submental area; an interdigastric, the floor of the submaxillary area; and a retrodigastric, extending to the margin of the sternocleidomastoid muscle. The retrodigastric area is the lowermost part of the parapharyngeal space and its posterior extremity is separated from the contents of the parotid compartment by a septum.

2. **Contents.**—Incision through the deep fascia reveals the *submaxillary salivary gland,* which can be separated easily from the cellular tissue surrounding it.   The gland may be retracted without injury to adjacent structures, an important fact in ligation of the lingual artery.   The normal gland is about the size of a large almond, but it is enlarged by infection, malignancy, or involvement of the lymph glands about it.   Malignancy may be primary; more commonly it is secondary, the extension of a tumor process from an adjacent structure such as: the tongue, floor of the mouth, jaw, or lymph glands.   In malignancy, the gland may become fixed to the mandible.

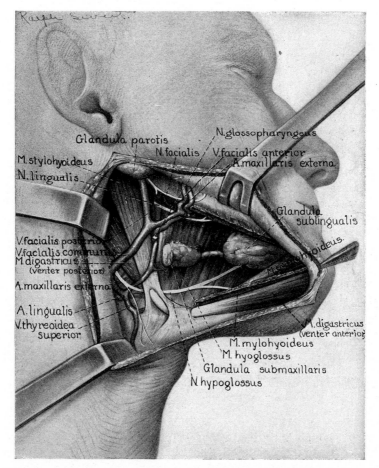

FIG. 159.—DISSECTION OF THE SUBMAXILLARY AREA, CARRIED THROUGH THE MYLOHYOID MUSCLE.
The submaxillary gland and the mylohyoid muscle have been removed to show the prolongation of the submaxillary gland and its relation with the sublingual gland.

The inferior border of the submaxillary salivary gland often extends below the great horn of the hyoid bone.   A portion of it may overlie and extend beyond the posterior digastric belly, reaching almost to the sternocleidomastoid muscle.   A deep prolongation penetrates the sublingual region through the cleft between the mylohyoid and hyoglossal muscles.   This prolongation and its duct (of Wharton) have immediate relations with the sublingual gland (p. 139).   The posterior extremity of the submaxillary gland presents intimate and important surgical relations with the parotid gland, external maxillary artery, and the thyroid, hypoglossal, and facial trunks of the common facial vein.

The *external maxillary (facial) artery* arises from the external carotid artery on a level with the great horn of the hyoid bone, and enters this compartment under the stylohyoid muscle and the posterior belly of the digastric muscle. It continues upward and forward in a groove in the posterior surface of the gland, emerges from the deep fascia, winds around the inferior border of the body of the mandible, and reaches the face at the anterior margin of the masseter muscle. In contrast to the deep-lying artery are the superficially coursing *facial veins*. These run over the submaxillary gland just beneath the fascial covering of the space and empty into the common facial (thyro-facial-lingual) vein, which drains into the external jugular. The *lingual artery* is the only other large arterial trunk in the region From its external carotid origin, it runs a short stretch in the lateral suprahyoid region above the hyoid bone and runs deep to the posterior margin of the hyoglossal muscle. It runs forward on the mesial aspect of this muscle, into the sublingual compartment.

Three to six *lymph nodes* are disposed about the submaxillary salivary gland; the greater number lie immediately under the deep cervical fascia, and the remainder lie between the gland and the mylohyoid muscle. They are regional nodes for lymph vessels from the nose, lips, and anterior and lateral portions of the tongue. Their efferents lead into the deep cervical lymph nodes in the sternomastoid region. The numerous infections in the regions tributary to the glands explain the great frequency of suprahyoid abscess formation. These nodes are involved secondarily in cancer within the drainage territory, and are closely attached to, and sometimes incorporated in, the substance of the submaxillary gland; their removal necessitates clearing the compartment of its glandular content.

The *hypoglossal nerve* enters the submaxillary space between the hyoglossal muscle and the posterior belly of the digastric muscle and runs through the greater portion of the suprahyoid space before entering the sublingual compartment through the cleft between the hyoglossal and mylohyoid muscles. The *lingual nerve* lies at a much higher level on the lateral surface of the hyoglossal muscle. It supplies a branch to the submaxillary gland which must be severed in suprahyoid dissection before the gland can be mobilized.

Surgical Considerations

1. Submaxillary Abscess.—Submaxillary abscesses arise from lymphatic involvement incident to infections in the tributary areas. The infection may settle in the lymph glands as adenitis, or manifest itself as lymphangitis or cellulitis. The buccal cavity, teeth, tongue, gums, and pharynx drain directly to the space, and the afferent vessels also drain the upper forehead, inner eyebrow, and anterior face.

One of the commonest sources of infection is an alveolar abscess which gravitates into the compartment from a carious tooth. The acute and exceedingly grave infection, known as *Ludwig's angina,* begins in the sublingual region and rapidly involves the submaxillary region since the cellular tissue is in continuity (Fig. 129). This fulminating cellulitis may spread rapidly into the neck, up on the face or into the pharynx, and often proves fatal. It calls for immediate wide incision for adequate drainage, and often for tracheotomy.

Fractures of the mandible, especially when immediate immobilization has not been attained, are likely to be complicated by infection. The purulent collection about the dependent area of the fracture line, finding no ready access to the mouth, may gravitate into the submaxillary space or follow the deeper planes down the neck. The removal of a sequestrum may be necessary in addition to adequate drainage of the abscess.

2. Suprahyoid Gland Dissection.—Suprahyoid lymph gland and submaxillary salivary gland dissection is performed independently of deep lateral neck dissection in the attempt to eradicate metastases from carcinoma of the lip. Suprahyoid dissection alone is made only if gross examination of the submental and submaxillary glands shows no evidence of metastasis. Gross involvement of these glands is an indication for a combined (complete) neck dissection (p. 202).

Suprahyoid dissection is a bilateral procedure for lip carcinoma near or at the midline. The cut-throat incision employed extends from one anterior margin of the sternocleidomastoid muscle to the other, and passes across the front of the neck just above the hyoid bone.   The inferior flap is undisturbed and the superior flap is dissected upward, taking skin, subcutaneous tissue, and platysma; the contents of the entire suprahyoid area are exposed through the enveloping layer of deep fascia.   The fascial layer is divided along the inferior border of the mandible as far as the anterior margin of the sternocleidomastoid muscles, but no structures below the level of the posterior belly of the digastric are disturbed.   By a peeling-down process of blunt dissection, this fascial flap is removed and the glandular and areolar elements are separated from the mandible, parotid gland, and outer surface of the mylohyoid and hyoglossal muscles.   Ligation of the external maxillary vessels is necessary where they pass over the jaw.   Section of the branch of the lingual nerve to the submaxillary gland and of the submaxillary duct then is performed.   Lest a permanent paralysis of the angle of the mouth occur, the marginal mandibular branch of the seventh (facial) nerve must be isolated and retracted from danger.   The lingual nerve also is retracted and the hypoglossal nerve is saved when practicable.   The tissues removed

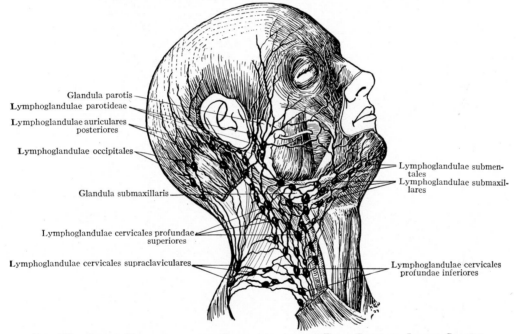

Glandula parotis
Lymphoglandulae parotideae
Lymphoglandulae auriculares posteriores
Lymphoglandulae occipitales
Glandula submaxillaris
Lymphoglandulae cervicales profundae superiores
Lymphoglandulae cervicales supraclaviculares
Lymphoglandulae submentales
Lymphoglandulae submaxillares
Lymphoglandulae cervicales profundae inferiores

FIG. 160.—LYMPH DRAINAGE TO THE SUBMAXILLARY AND DEEP CERVICAL LYMPH GLANDS.

should include the submaxillary salivary glands, the portions of the external maxillary vessels traversing the space, and all the lymph glands and areolar tissue.   Dissection is completed by clearing the mylohyoid and hyoglossal muscles as far as the stylohyoid muscle and the posterior belly of the digastric muscle.

B. INFRAHYOID AREAS

The infrahyoid region is described as the mesial triangle (trigonum) of the neck. It has as its base the hyoid bone, and as its sides the mesial borders of the sternocleidomastoid muscles.   Layer by layer, it is made up of several subregions: superficial infrahyoid, thyroid gland. laryngotracheal tube, cervical esophagus, and prevertebral region.

(I) SUPERFICIAL INFRAHYOID REGION

1. **Definition and Boundaries.**—The superficial infrahyoid region extends from the hyoid bone to the suprasternal notch and embraces the superficial structures anterior to the thyroid gland and the laryngotracheal tube.

2. **Surface Anatomy.**—When the head is thrown back, the infrahyoid region is well outlined. The laryngotracheal tube and the thyroid gland form a median bulge. On each side, mesial to the sternocleidomastoid muscle, the carotid groove can be seen and palpated. In the depth of each gutter, the pulsations of the carotid artery can be felt and even seen. With the head flexed, landmarks are palpated more readily. The bulge of the thyroid cartilage is felt below the hyoid bone, and below it, the transverse bulge of the cricoid cartilage. The interval between the two cartilages is occupied by the cricothyroid membrane.

3. **Superficial Structures.**—The veins in the region are small and irregularly placed, and empty, for the most part, into the external jugular vein. The *anterior jugular veins*

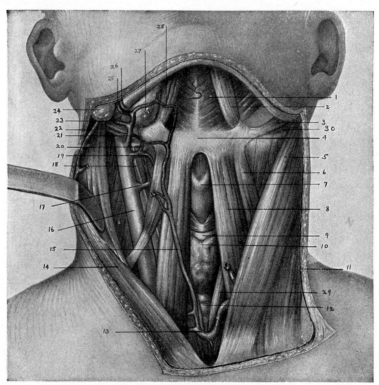

FIG. 161.—THE STRUCTURES IN THE SUPRAHYOID AND INFRAHYOID REGIONS.

1, M. mylohyoideus; 2, M. digastricus (venter anterior); 3, M. stylohyoideus; 4, os hyoideum; 5, M. sternocleidomastoideus; 6, M. omohyoideus; 7, cartilago thyreoidea; 8, M. sternohyoideus; 9, cartilago cricoidea; 10, isthmus glandulae thyreoideae; 11, platysma; 12, trachea; 13, arcus venosus juguli; 14, M. sternocleidomastoideus; 15, V. jugularis anterior; 16, V. jugularis interna; 17, V. thyreoidea superior; 18, ramus descendens n. hypoglossi; 19, V. laryngea superior; 20, V. lingualis; 21, V. facialis communis; 22, V. jugularis externa; 23, V. facialis posterior; 24, glandula parotis; 25, V. facialis anterior; 26, A. maxillaris externa (facial); 27, glandula submaxillaris; 28, V. submentalis; 29, M. sternothyreoideus; 30, M. digastricus (venter posterior).

are important in any transverse incision in this region. They arise from the superficial submental veins by anastomosis with the facial veins, descend paramedially to within a few centimeters of the suprasternal fossa, engage under the sternocleidomastoid muscles, parallel the upper margins of the clavicles, and empty into the termination of the external jugulars. In the superior portion of their course, they lie superficial to the platysma muscle; more inferiorly, they are covered by it; and near the sternum, they are held intimately within the meshes of, or deep to, the enveloping fascia. This arrangement makes it possible in a transverse incision in the lower neck to reflect the skin and the platysma layer upward and downward without involving these veins. A thyroglossal duct sinus or fistula (p. 144) sometimes presents in this region.

4. **Enveloping Fascia and the Suprasternal Fossa.**—Over all the region, the *enveloping fascia* lies immediately subjacent to the skin-platysma layer, covering the areas as with a veil. The fascia divides at the mesial border of the sternocleidomastoid muscles to enclose them, forming their sheaths. Lower down in the neck, the enveloping fascia splits into two layers, an anterior layer attached to the anterior superior margin of the manubrium, and a posterior layer attached to the posterior superior margin. Between them is the *suprasternal fossa* (of Burns, Gruber) (p. 215) which has premanubrial and retromanubrial culdesac whose lateral projections insinuate themselves under the sternocleidomastoid muscles. The posterior wall of the space is reinforced by the deeper (pretracheal) fascia investing the infrahyoid muscles. The anterior jugular veins and their transverse anastomosis (arcus venosus juguli) traverse the space, which holds also suprasternal lymphatic glands and areolar tissue.

5. **Infrahyoid Muscles and Their Fascial Connections.**—Deep to the enveloping fascia are two muscle layers, enclosed within the pretracheal fascia. The superficial layer includes the omohyoid muscle laterally and the sternohyoid muscle mesially. Only the upper part of the *omohyoid* belongs to this region; its posterior belly traverses the lateral portion of the neck in its course to the scapula. The *sternohyoid* is entirely within the region. The triangular interval, formed by the divergence of the omohyoid and sternohyoid, is occupied by pretracheal fascia

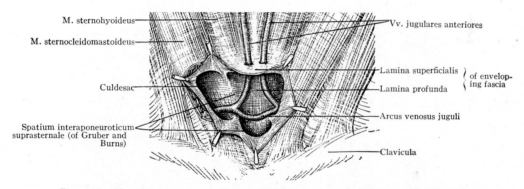

Fig. 162.—The Vascular and Fascial Relation in the Suprasternal Fossa.

The deep layer consists of the sternothyroid and thyrohyoid muscles. The *sternothyroid* arises deep to the sternohyoid from the posterior surface of the sternum and inserts into the thyroid cartilage. The *thyrohyoid* continues the line of the sternothyroid, running from the thyroid cartilage to the great cornu of the hyoid bone. The sternothyroid muscles diverge upward. Within the interval thus formed, the superficial and deep layers of the middle cervical or pretracheal fascia unite in one layer directly overlying the trachea and thyroid gland. This layer is fused to the overlying enveloping layer to form the aponeurotic *linea alba of the neck*, through which access to the thyroid gland is gained.

Spreading aside of the musculo-aponeurotic layers of the infrahyoid region reveals the laryngotracheal tube, thyroid, and esophagus in their common fascial casing, the *visceral sheath*. These structures are designated the visceral mass. This is attached to the vertebral column by sagittal septa.

(II) Laryngotracheal Region

The laryngotracheal tube or median air passage is made up of the larynx and the cervical trachea.

1. **Larynx.**—The larynx is a series of cartilages adapted for phonation. The thyroid and cricoid cartilages constitute the principal part of its framework, and the epiglottis guards its entrance. There are, also, three sets of paired cartilages: the arytenoids, corniculates, and cuneiforms. The arytenoids furnish attachment to the intrinsic muscles

of the larynx which govern the tension of the vocal cords. The whole larynx is capable of a considerable range of mobility. It moves up and down with each effort of swallowing, and laterally with passive movement produced by palpation or by the pressure of a neighboring mass.

2. **Hyoid Bone and Cartilages of the Larynx.**—The *hyoid* bone, the chief support for the true laryngotracheal tube, is elevated, depressed, and moved forward in speech, mastication, and swallowing. The anterior aspect of the bone is superficial and accessible to palpation. With the chin elevated, it may be grasped between the thumb and forefinger and moved from side to side. It forms a stable, yet flexible, fixation center, slung above from the styloid process of the temporal bone and from the mandible and tongue, and secured below by its attachment to the larynx. The genioglossal and hyoglossal muscles attach the hyoid bone to the tongue, and the mylohyoid, geniohyoid, and digastric muscles connect it with the lower jaw. It supports the larynx by means of the thyrohyoid muscles and thyrohyoid membrane. It is fixed to the sternum by the sternohyoid muscles, and to the scapulae by the omohyoid muscles. Its mobility, pliability, and protection explain the infrequency of fracture.

The leaflike *epiglottic cartilage* lies dorsal to the root of the tongue and ventral to the opening into the larynx. It is attached by the thyro-epiglottic ligament to the body of

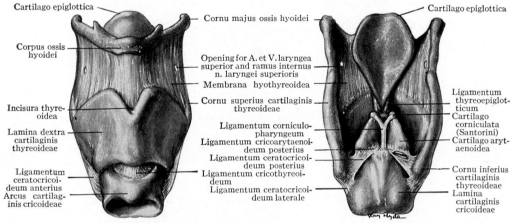

FIG. 163.—ANTERIOR AND POSTERIOR VIEWS OF THE LARYNX, ITS CONNECTING LIGAMENTS, AND THE HYOID BONE.

the thyroid cartilage just above the vocal cords, and is connected to the base of the tongue by the glosso-epiglottic folds. During respiration, the epiglottis is semivertical. In the act of swallowing (deglutition), the epiglottis does not fall, valvelike, over the laryngeal opening, but maintains its upright position. Solid food is swept beyond it by the base of the tongue into the grasp of the constrictor musculature of the pharynx. The pharyngeal muscles direct the food into the esophagus. Liquids are diverted around the epiglottis into the piriform sinuses of the pharynx and thence into the esophagus.

The *thyroid cartilage*, because of its strength and power of resistance, affords valuable protection to the structures in the larynx, most important of which are the vocal cords. Its two quadrangular lateral plates (laminae) unite in the midline of the neck to form a prominent angle, the Adam's apple, which is palpable and is the principal landmark of the larynx. During early adult years, the thyroid cartilage is hyaline, but, as a rule, by the twentieth year it begins to ossify. Ossification may progress to such a state that in older people the cartilage sometimes fractures on lateral compression of the two wings, or compression backward against the vertebral column, as in strangling or hanging. Injury to this cartilage may be serious because of subsequent edema of the laryngeal mucous membrane, with impairment of respiration.

The *cricoid cartilage* is the palpable landmark indicating the beginning of the trachea, and corresponding in level to the superior border of the esophagus. It is a modified tracheal cartilage shaped like a signet ring with the seal placed posteriorly, and is adapted to support the larynx. In front, its narrow arch is attached to the thyroid cartilage by the conus elasticus (cricothyroid membrane).

The upper angles of the signet part of the cricoid cartilage support the *arytenoid cartilages*, to the anterior angles of which the vocal cords are attached.

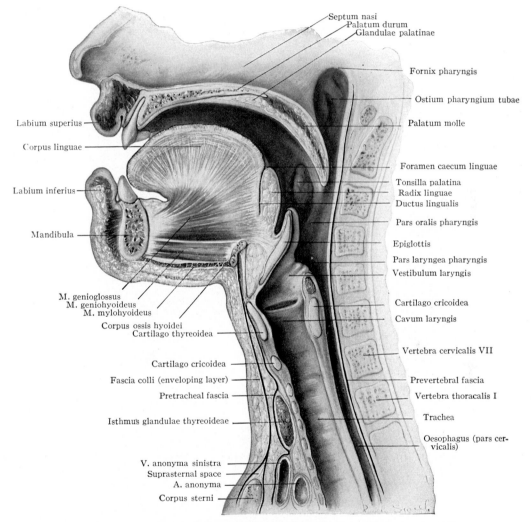

FIG. 164.—SAGITTAL SECTION THROUGH THE UPPER AIR PASSAGES, PHARYNX, AND ESOPHAGUS.

3. **Membranes of the Larynx.**—The uniformly resistant *thyrohyoid membrane* suspends the larynx from the hyoid bone by extending from its posterosuperior margin to the upper margin of the thyroid cartilage. The bursa located between the superior portion of the membrane and the body of the hyoid bone may become inflamed and cystic. Posteriorly, the membrane is separated from the epiglottis by a wedge-shaped mass of fatty tissue which occupies the thyro-epiglottic space.

The *conus elasticus (cricothyroid membrane)* closes the interval between the cricoid and thyroid cartilages. Through it the easiest and most rapid laryngotomy can be performed for the urgent relief of suffocation (p. 177).

4. Interior of the Larynx, or Endolarynx.—The cavity of the larynx is divided into three compartments by two paired folds of mucous membrane stretched anteroposteriorly across it.   These folds project medially from the lateral walls and extend from the arytenoid cartilages to the thyroid cartilage below the attachment of the epiglottis.   The superior

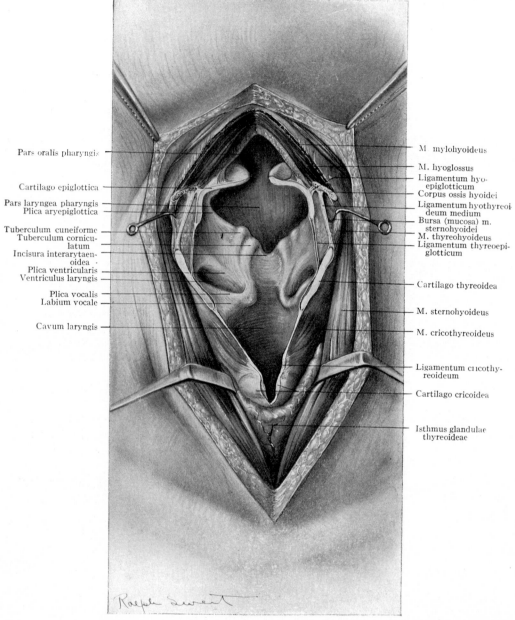

Pars oralis pharyngis

Cartilago epiglottica

Pars laryngea pharyngis
Plica aryepiglottica

Tuberculum cuneiforme
Tuberculum cornicu-
        latum
Incisura interarytaen-
        oidea
Plica ventricularis
Ventriculus laryngis

Plica vocalis
Labium vocale

Cavum laryngis

M mylohyoideus

M. hyoglossus
Ligamentum hyo-
    epiglotticum
Corpus ossis hyoidei
Ligamentum hyothyreoi
    deum medium
Bursa (mucosa) m.
    sternohyoidei
M. thyreohyoideus
Ligamentum thyreoepi-
    glotticum

Cartilago thyreoidea

M. sternohyoideus

M. cricothyreoideus

Ligamentum cricothy-
    reoideum

Cartilago cricoidea

Isthmus glandulae
    thyreoideae

Fig. 165.—Front View of a Partial Midsagittal Section Through the Pharynx, Larynx, and
Upper Trachea.
The cricothyroid ligament is elongated greatly to show the interior of the subglottic area.

folds are the false vocal cords and the inferior the true.   The compartments are: the upper supraglottic area (vestibule); the middle, more constricted glottic area, and the broad, **infraglottic** area.   The **entrance** (aditus) into the **larynx** is triangular in shape.   The base of the triangle, directed forward, is formed by the epiglottis; its lateral boundaries are the aryepiglottic muscles in the aryepiglottic folds. On either side of the laryngeal opening is a pharyngeal recess, termed the *piriform sinus*. This recess is likely to be the lodging place of foreign bodies entering the pharynx.

The **vestibule** or **supraglottic compartment** extends from the laryngeal inlet to the level of the false vocal cords (plicae ventriculares). Its walls may be the seat of localized

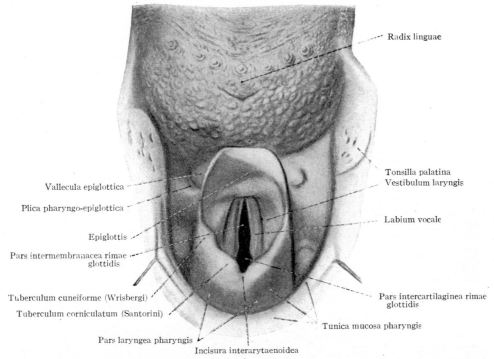

Radix linguae

Tonsilla palatina
Vestibulum laryngis

Labium vocale

Vallecula epiglottica

Plica pharyngo-epiglottica

Epiglottis

Pars intermembranacea rimae
glottidis

Pars intercartilaginea rimae
glottidis

Tuberculum cuneiforme (Wrisbergi)

Tuberculum corniculatum (Santorini)

Tunica mucosa pharyngis

Pars laryngea pharyngis

Incisura interarytaenoidea

FIG. 166.—THE POSTERIOR PORTION OF THE TONGUE AND ITS RELATION TO THE ADITUS OF THE LARYNX. (After Sobotta.)

edema, infiltration, tumors, and ulceration. Cancer rarely involves it, and when it does, is secondary, extending from the base of the tongue, and pharynx. The two membranous

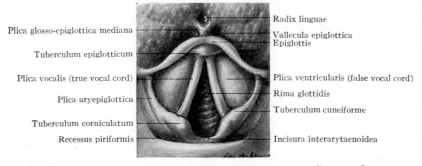

Plica glosso-epiglottica mediana

Tuberculum epiglotticum

Plica vocalis (true vocal cord)

Plica aryepiglottica

Tuberculum corniculatum

Recessus piriformis

Radix linguae

Vallecula epiglottica
Epiglottis

Plica ventricularis (false vocal cord)

Rima glottidis

Tuberculum cuneiforme

Incisura interarytaenoidea

FIG. 167.—A MIRROR LARYNGOSCOPIC IMAGE WITH THE GLOTTIS OPEN.

folds known as the *false vocal cords* play no rôle in phonation. In laryngoscopic examination, they appear as horizontal projections from the inner surfaces of the aryepiglottic folds.

The **glottis** or **middle compartment** of the larynx corresponds to the recess or ventricle between the true and false cords. It contains the arytenoid cartilages behind, which are separated by the interarytenoid notch. The mucosa uniting them is the posterior commissure, the seat of election of early tuberculosis of the larynx.   The *true vocal cords* are contiguous at the anterior commissure and diverge behind, separated by the breadth of the posterior commissure.   In the laryngoscopic mirror, the cords appear as thin, brilliant bands, converging anteriorly.   In contrast to the mucosa of the vestibule of the larynx, that of the true cords adheres so intimately that these cords rarely are the seat of edema. In acute or chronic inflammatory conditions, the cords lose their brilliant color and take on reddish and violet colorations.   They frequently are the seat of intrinsic carcinoma of the larynx.

The *rima glottidis* (*glottic slit*) is the fissure which separates the true vocal cords and the arytenoid cartilages.   The vocal or ligamentous glottis is in front, and the respiratory

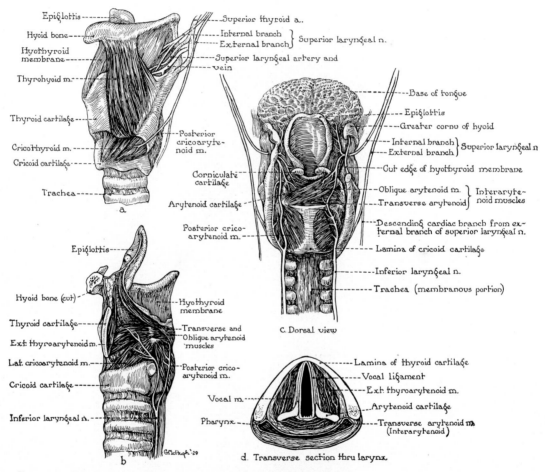

FIG. 168.—DISSECTION OF THE LARYNX TO SHOW THE INTRINSIC LARYNGEAL MUSCLES AND THE DISTRI-
BUTION OF THE LARYNGEAL NERVES.

Note the muscular distribution of the internal branch of the superior laryngeal nerve.   (Modified from Jackson from Nordland, Surg., Gynec. and Obst., Oct., 1930.)

or cartilaginous glottis behind.   The fissure is triangular at rest, linear in phonation, and lozenge-shaped in respiration.   When a diphtheritic membrane threatens to embarrass respiration, the glottic slit may be kept open by the introduction of an intubation tube. The tube holder and tube are introduced along the base of the tongue until the epiglottis is reached.   The epiglottis is raised with the index finger, and the tube is introduced into the glottis posterior to the vocal cords and is released from the holder.

The **infraglottic compartment** of the larynx extends from the true vocal cords to the first tracheal ring. Inflammatory processes cause swelling of the mucosa, manifest particularly in the infant by symptoms of spasmodic croup (stridulus laryngismus).

5. **Cervical Trachea.**—The cervical trachea, measuring about 6.5 cm. in length, is flattened on its posterior surface because of the deficiency in the cartilaginous rings. The cartilage arrangement keeps the trachea distended and permits a certain degree of elasticity. Mobility is enhanced by the loose cellular tissue which surrounds the tube, so that it may be deviated from one side to the other with little difficulty.

6. **Vessels and Nerves.**—The **arterial** supply to the larynx is derived from two sources. The *superior laryngeal artery*, a branch of the superior thyroid, perforates the thyrohyoid membrane in company with the internal laryngeal veins. The inferior laryngeal branch

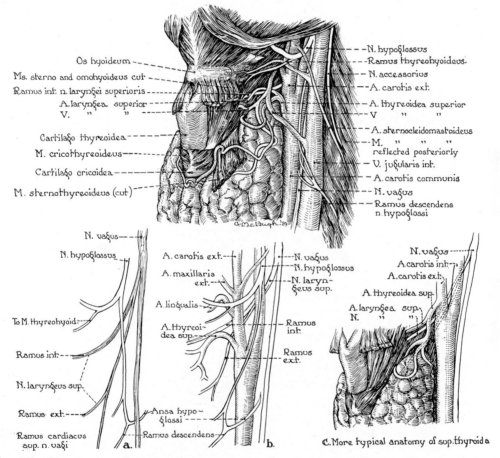

FIG. 169.—DISSECTION TO SHOW THE EXTRALARYNGEAL RELATIONS OF THE SUPERIOR LARYNGEAL NERVE. (Martin Nordland, Surg., Gynec. and Obst., Oct., 1930.)

of the *inferior thyroid artery* accompanies the recurrent laryngeal nerve to the lower part of the larynx.

Study of the **lymphatic drainage** of the larynx is extremely important because of the incidence of cancer in this region and the extent of operative intervention required to remove it. The lymphatics are most numerous about the supraglottic area and communicate with the lymph vessels of the pharynx. There are few lymph vessels in the infraglottic area and exceedingly few at the level of the glottis. The group from the supraglottic area drains to the superior deep cervical lymph nodes. Vessels from the anterior part of the lower larynx drain to several small prelaryngeal and pretracheal glands. The group draining the posterior segment of the infraglottic compartment empties through the recurrent glands to the inferior deep cervical lymph chain. The cervical-tracheal lymphatics drain posteriorly to the deep cervical glands.

The **nerve mechanism,** by means of which the laryngeal muscles are coordinated and their mucous membranes sensitized, involves motor and sensory nerves. These nerves are the superior and inferior laryngeal branches of the vagus. The *superior laryngeal nerve* arises from the ganglion nodosum and, after a short course, divides into two branches, a small external and a large internal. The external branch passes downward, gives a branch to the inferior constrictor muscle of the pharynx and is distributed finally to the crico-thyroid muscle. These muscles change the position of the cricoid and thyroid cartilages, and by so doing lengthen, or tense, the vocal cords. Paralysis of the cricothyroid muscles causes the voice to become weak, rough, and easily fatigued. Laryngoscopic examination shows the cords to have a wavy outline. The internal branch passes mesially and enters

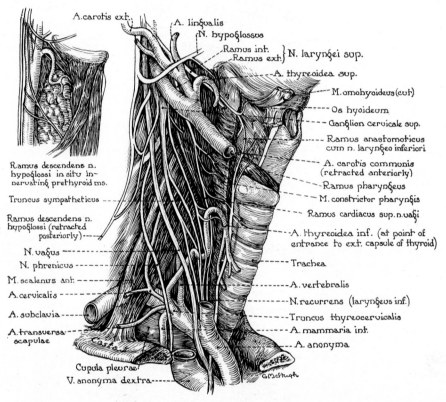

Fig 170.—Dissection of the Right Side of the Neck to Show Relations of the Superior and Inferior Laryngeal Nerves. (Martin Nordland, Surg., Gynec. and Obst., Oct., 1930.)

the larynx through the thyrohyoid membrane. It is distributed to the mucous membranes of the larynx and epiglottis, accounting for the extreme sensitiveness of the laryngeal mucosa. A branch of this nerve passes downward and anastomoses with ramifications of the inferior laryngeal nerve. Recent investigations (Nordland, Berlin and Schley) indicate that the internal branch of the superior laryngeal nerve innervates the interarytenoid muscle in the majority of cases. Since these muscles approximate the posterior portions of the vocal cords and are important in phonation, it is essential that their nerve supply, the superior laryngeal nerves, be spared in thyroid surgery. The superior laryngeal nerve from its origin lies parallel to, and in close proximity with, the superior thyroid artery (p. 181).

The *inferior* or *recurrent laryngeal* nerves arise from the vagus at different levels on the two sides. On the right, the nerve is given off where the vagus crosses the first portion of the subclavian artery, and usually ascends in a groove between the esophagus and larynx. At the thyrocricoid articulation, it divides into branches which supply the main motor muscles of the larynx.

At the lower pole, the recurrent nerve often lies 1 to 2 cm. lateral to the trachea. Here, it meshes among the branches of the inferior thyroid artery. The most intimate relations the nerve bears to the thyroid gland are on its posterolateral surface at the junction of the middle and lower thirds; namely at that place, or just above, where the main branches of the inferior thyroid artery enter the gland. The possibility that the nerve may penetrate

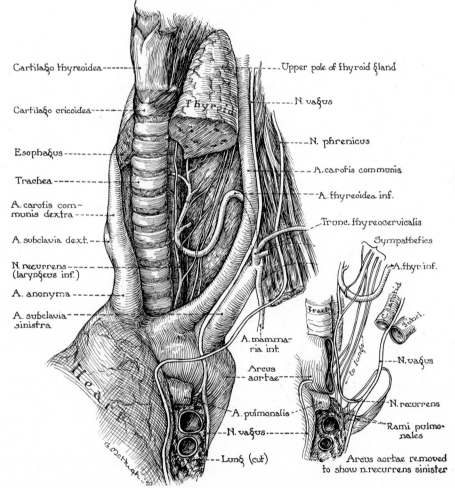

FIG. 171.—DISSECTION OF THE LEFT SIDE OF THE NECK TO SHOW RELATIONS OF THE INFERIOR (RECURRENT) LARYNGEAL NERVE. (Martin Nordland, Surg., Gynec. and Obst., Oct., 1930.)

the gland, or that it may lie between the trachea and that part of the thyroid which adheres to the trachea, must be remembered (Berlin).

Section of the superior laryngeal nerves is followed at once by a loss of sensation in the laryngeal mucous membrane and a paralysis or relaxation of the cricothyroid muscles. This results in a lowering of the pitch and a diminution in the clearness of the voice. From the loss of sensation there is an inability to perceive the entrance of foreign bodies into the larynx. Transverse section of both inferior laryngeal nerves is followed by complete paralysis of the vocal cords.

Surgical Considerations

1. **Laryngoscopy.**—Indirect or direct examinations of the larynx may be made through the mouth. The *indirect*, or mirror, method offers a reflected image of the larynx by use of the principle that in the reflection of a ray of light, the angle of incidence is equal to the angle of reflection. With good illumination and the tongue drawn downward and forward over the lower incisor teeth, a small mirror is introduced into the mouth, mirror downward. It presses the lower surface of the soft palate backward and upward. In this view, the parts which are reflected first in the mirror are the epiglottis, aryepiglottic folds, and posterior part of the base of the tongue. By tilting the mirror backward, the entrance to the larynx may be seen. The curved outline of the unattached margin of the epiglottis is visible. The anterior extremities of the aryepiglottic folds are hidden by the epiglottis, but the posterior extremities present two rounded elevations. The more medial and posterior elevation is the corniculate cartilage (of Santorini) which surmounts the arytenoid cartilage. The lateral and anterior elevation is the cuneiform cartilage (of Wrisberg). The posterior commissure, an interarytenoid fold of mucous membrane between the corniculate cartilages, varies in width as the summits of the arytenoid cartilages converge toward or diverge from each other.

The false cords are much wider apart than the true, are redder, and have but a slight range of movement. The true cords are pearly white in color and move freely during phonation. Their direction varies with the production of the different tones of the voice,

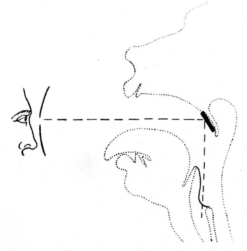

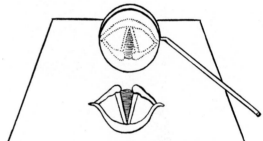

FIG. 172.—INDIRECT OR MIRROR LARYNGOSCOPY.

This method utilizes the principle of optics which states that the angle of incidence is equal to the angle of reflection. (After Laurens.)

FIG. 173.—MIRROR LARYNGOSCOPY.

Reflection in the mirror of the drawn diagram of the larynx. (After Laurens.)

and in variations of respiration. To produce high-pitched notes, the cords are adducted until the chink which separates them is reduced to a linear slit, and only that part of the glottic slit between the arytenoid cartilages (respiratory portion) remains open. In quiet respiration and, to a less degree, in the formation of low-pitched sounds, the slit of the glottis is triangular, with the apex in front. On each side of the laryngeal inlet, the laryngoscope reveals the piriform recess. Foreign bodies may be detected in these recesses or in the valleculate depressions between the epiglottis and the root of the tongue.

Direct laryngoscopy consists of examination of the larynx through the mouth, using a speculum to displace the tissues that otherwise would obstruct the view. It is required often for inspection supplementary to the mirror examination, and is the only method applicable to children under four or five years of age, since they will not tolerate the use of a mirror. With its use, foreign bodies, new growths, and biopsy specimen can be removed.

2. **Laryngotomy.**—Incision into the cavity of the larynx is accomplished in a number of ways and is necessitated by a number of conditions, chiefly the presence of foreign bodies lodged in the larynx, or as a preliminary step to extensive operations on the mouth. The

entrance to the larynx and supraglottic area may be exposed by the infrahyoid pharyngotomy incision; the glottis by median longitudinal section of the thyroid cartilage, thyrotomy; and the infraglottic area by the intercricothyroid laryngotomy incision.

The *infrahyoid laryngotomy*, or better, *pharyngotomy* is accomplished by a transverse incision along the inferior margin of the hyoid bone. The infrahyoid muscles and thyrohyoid membrane are incised and the pharynx is opened. The operation affords exposure of the entrance to the larynx, the lower end of the pharynx, and the beginning of the esophagus.

Thyrotomy is the type of laryngotomy which contemplates midsagittal splitting of the thyroid cartilage, thereby avoiding the insertion of the vocal cords. When the two plates of the cartilage are retracted laterally, the excellent exposure afforded the interior of the larynx makes possible the removal of new growths or foreign bodies. Increased exposure may be obtained by extending the thyrotomy incision upward through the

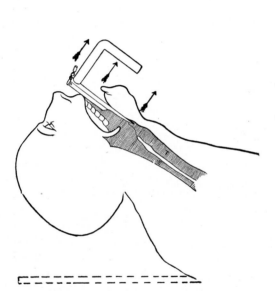

FIG. 174.—SCHEMA ILLUSTRATING DIRECT LARYN-
GOSCOPY ON THE RECUMBENT PATIENT.

The motion is imparted to the tip of the laryngoscope as if to lift the patient by his hyoid bone. (Jackson in Jackson and Coates, "The Nose, Throat, and Ear and Their Diseases.")

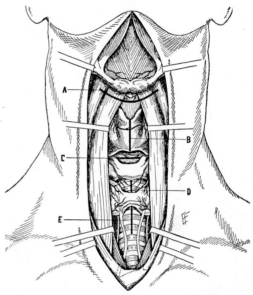

FIG. 175.—THE POSITION OF INCISION FOR OPENING.
THE LARYNGOTRACHEAL TUBE. (Bickham.)

A, Infrahyoid laryngotomy (subhyoid pharyngotomy); B, thyrotomy; C, intercricothyroid laryngotomy; D, high tracheotomy; E, low tracheotomy. (Keen.)

thyrohyoid membrane and downward through the cricoid cartilage and the first tracheal ring (Fig. 165).

The *intercricothyroid* incision, made transversely above the cricoid cartilage, avoids section of the cricothyroid artery, approaches the larynx in its most accessible, superficial, and bloodless area, and, except in children, opens a sufficient interval to admit the introduction of a laryngotomy tube. This incision, so long taught as an emergency measure, should be abandoned in almost all instances because it predisposes to laryngeal stenosis. The preferable location for operative intervention is the trachea at a level well below the larynx.

3. **Tracheotomy.**—Incision into the trachea is undertaken for the relief of menacing asphyxia or as a procedure preliminary to operations on the larynx. Obstructive laryngeal dyspnea arises in the course of many different diseases; when indicated, tracheotomy should be done before the emergency arises, as hasty tracheotomy may be done too high, with increased likelihood of laryngeal stenosis.

12

An anatomic picture of all the blood vessels and structures in front of the neck is likely to devastate the confidence of one confronted with performing an emergency tracheotomy. Essentially, only these facts merit consideration: the thyroid cartilage is easy to find; the trachea extends down the median line of the neck to the suprasternal notch; incision can be carried down the midline without endangering any important structure; all the structures that must not be cut are at the sides; and the cricoid cartilage is the only complete ring in the lower air passages and should not be cut unnecessarily. These facts are the fundamentals incorporated in the "tracheotomy triangle of Jackson."

Under favorable operative conditions the technic of tracheotomy is as follows: a midline incision dividing the skin and fascia is made from the thyroid notch to the suprasternal fossa, the cricoid cartilage is located, and the deeper dissection is continued below it, after the infrahyoid (ribbon) muscles are separated. If the thyroid isthmus is in the way, it may be retracted upward; if large, it should be ligated and divided, lest it slip over and interfere with the availability of the tracheal incision in postoperative care. The corrugated surface of the trachea can be located accurately by palpation, and incision into it should be as low as possible. The cricoid cartilage should not be cut, as stenosis is almost sure to follow wearing a cannula in this position.

4. **Cut-throat Wounds.**—The cut-throat incision, either suicidal or homicidal, most frequently involves the thyrohyoid interval of the infrahyoid space. Throwing back the head to inflict the wound often retracts the carotid sheath and its structures to a protected position under the sternocleidomastoid muscles. When a wound occurs *across the thyrohyoid space*, the anterior jugular veins, superior laryngeal nerve, superior thyroid artery, sternohyoid and omohyoid muscles, and the thyrohyoid membrane are divided. The inferior constrictor muscle also is cut, and its upper portion may drop back and cause respiratory obstruction.

When the incision is *above the hyoid bone*, the anterior jugular vein, the mylohyoid, hyoglossal, genioglossal, and geniohyoid muscles are divided. The lingual vessels and hypoglossal nerves are severed, but the lingual nerve usually lies above the level of the wound. The external maxillary vessels are the first large vessels severed; the elements in the carotid sheath are uninjured save when the wound is very extensive. The substance of the tongue may be cut and the floor of the mouth be opened. When the anterior attachment of the tongue is severed, the tongue is likely to fall backward, push down the epiglottis, and produce suffocation.

Wounds occasionally are low and *involve the trachea and cricothyroid space*. These wounds reach the carotid sheath vessels more readily than do transverse wounds in any other part of the neck. Many instances, however, have been reported in which the trachea and esophagus have been divided without injury to any of the great vessels.

(III) THYROID REGION

1. **Thyroid Gland and Its Divisions.**—The thyroid gland, with its parathyroid bodies, occupies an exceedingly important place in surgical physiology and pathology. It consists of two somewhat conical or pyramidal lateral lobes united by an isthmus, and is firmly bound by fibrous tissue to the anterior and lateral aspects of the larynx and to the upper trachea. There are many variations in the size, shape, and relative level of the gland. A vertical prolongation known as the *pyramidal lobe* occasionally arises from the isthmus. This lobe may extend in front of the cricoid and thyroid cartilages toward the hyoid bone, to which it may be attached by a fibromuscular flap or slip. The thyroid is surrounded by a sheath formed by extensions from the pretracheal fascia. This sheath is separated from the true capsule of the gland by areolar tissue, in which run vessels and nerves.

The upper extremity of each *lateral lobe* lies against the posterosuperior portions of the wings of the thyroid cartilage and the walls of the pharynx. The superior thyroid vessels which reach it at this level constitute its upper vascular or superior thyroid pedicle. The rounded lower extremity of each lobe extends to the level of the fifth or sixth tracheal ring, and is related to the inferior thyroid pedicle, in which the veins lie more superficially than the arteries. The inferior extension of this pole may reach to the level of or below the suprasternal fossa (*substernal thyroid*). Its intimate vascular connections make dislocation of the lower pole the dangerous part of operations on the thyroid gland.

The convex surface of the gland is in relation with the infrahyoid muscles; only the pretracheal fascia intervenes. An enlarged lateral lobe may press upon and thin out these muscles until they are almost unrecognizable. The posterolateral surface is grooved by contact with the common carotid artery, and is related to the prevertebral muscles and the sympathetic gangliated chain. The most important surgical relation is with the recurrent laryngeal nerve as it ascends in the tracheo-esophageal sulcus. The mesial surfaces of the thyroid lobes embrace the lateral surface of the tracheal and cricoid cartilages and the inferior and lateral parts of the pharynx and esophagus. These relations explain the difficulties in respiration, deglutition, and phonation caused by large goiters.

The *thyroid isthmus* occupies a variable level, and occasionally is absent. In the adult, it usually overlies the second, third, and fourth tracheal rings. An enlargement of the substance of the pyramidal lobe may penetrate into the mediastinum as a retrosternal or plunging goiter. If interposed between the sternum and trachea, it may cause pressure suffocation.

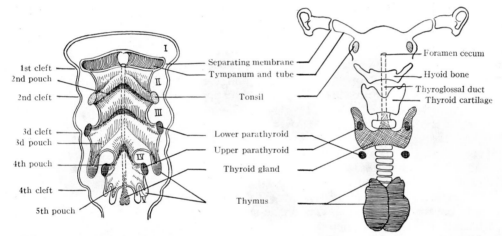

FIG. 176.—DIAGRAM OF THE BRANCHIAL CLEFTS, ARCHES, AND POUCHES AND SOME OF THEIR DERIVATIVES. Roman numerals indicate branchial arches. (After Beesley and Johnson.)

2. **Development.**—The thyroid gland makes its appearance as an evaginating bud from the entodermic lining of the anterior pharyngeal wall. This bud has its origin at a point which later becomes the foramen cecum of the tongue. It takes on a tubular growth (thyroglossal duct) which extends downward and forward, and it widens laterally at its inferior extremity to become the lateral thyroid lobes. Usually nothing remains of this median segment but the thyroid isthmus. In many cases, the existence of the duct is shown by the form of the pyramidal lobe.

In the vicinity of the thyroid gland, and particularly along the thyroglossal duct, small glandular masses frequently are found which present the same structure as the thyroid. In incomplete obliteration of the thyroglossal duct, these masses may be found at any or all levels from the foramen cecum to the thyroid isthmus. They may be located within the thickness of the base of the tongue, in front of, within, or behind the hyoid bone, or, as is most usual, below the hyoid bone and above the thyroid isthmus. They may replace the pyramidal lobe wholly or in part, and occasionally are found inferior to the thyroid gland.

3. **Perithyroid Sheath and Thyroid Capsule.**—The pretracheal fascia loosely invests the thyroid gland with a variable fascial covering which is thickest and densest over the lateral surface of the thyroid cartilage where it holds the superior pole of the gland firmly

in place. This so-called *sheath* or false capsule usually is thin, transparent, and easy to separate; it allows dislocation of the gland to expose the thyroid vessels.

When freed from the perithyroid sheath, the thyroid parenchyma is bound by its *capsule*, a densely adherent peripheral condensation of the connective tissue of the gland, wherein the thyroid vessels anastomose in a rich network. Large vessels lie in the capsule, but the branches which leave it to supply the substance of the gland are of small caliber. The capsular arrangement of vessels makes partial thyroid excision or removal of an adenoma a relatively bloodless procedure when the vessels are clamped severally in the supporting structure of the gland.

4. **Parathyroid Bodies.**—The parathyroids, ordinarily four in number, are small, oval or bean-shaped bodies ranging from 3 to 8 mm. in length, 2 to 4 mm. in width, and 1 to 3 mm. in thickness. Accessory fragments of parathyroid tissue generally are present about the thyroid gland or along the trachea. Parathyroid tissue varies in color from

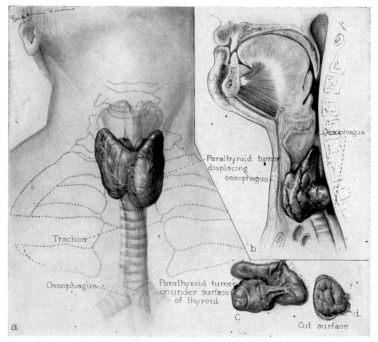

FIG. 177.—PARATHYROID ADENOMA.

a, Anteroposterior view shows the deflection of the esophagus, to the right; *b,* left lateral view demonstrates the retrotracheal position of the adenoma; *c,* comparative size of the adenoma and that of the thyroid gland. (Goldman and Smyth, Annals of Surgery, Dec., 1936, J. B. Lippincott Co., Publishers.)

yellowish-orange to pinkish-brown or brownish-red, according to the degree of vascularity and the amount of fat present beneath the parathyroid capsule. Microscopic examination reveals a structure resembling that of the medulla of the suprarenal glands. The parathyroids are not likely to be removed if intracapsular resection of the thyroid is performed. Their excision causes death by tetany unless their secretion is supplied artificially.

The *superior parathyroids* ordinarily lie either on the posterior surface of the thyroid gland near the junction of the upper and middle thirds, or along the branches of the superior thyroid artery. The *inferior parathyroids* usually lie on the posterior surface of the gland near the inferior margin of the lateral lobes. The relation of the parathyroids to the superior and inferior thyroid arteries and to their larger anastomotic branches is fairly constant.

Studies at the University of California Hospital based upon operative findings and cadaver dissections have shown that in 30 per cent of cases, one or more of the parathyroids is located on either the lateral or anterior part of the thyroid capsule. These parathyroids are removed in thyroidectomy unless care is taken to preserve part of the anterior and the lateral, as well as the posterior, part of the capsule (Millzner).

The connection between hyperplasia or tumor of the parathyroids and osteitis fibrosa cystica (von Recklinghausen's disease) has stimulated much recent investigation. So constant is this association, that parathyroid enlargement must be ruled out surgically in cases of osteitis fibrosa cystica. Hyperparathyroidism causes excessive mobilization of the skeletal calcium and results in hypercalcemia. Removal of the hyperplastic parathyroid or of the parathyroid tumor stops oversecretion and allows redeposition of calcium into the skeleton, a process which takes place within a very short time.

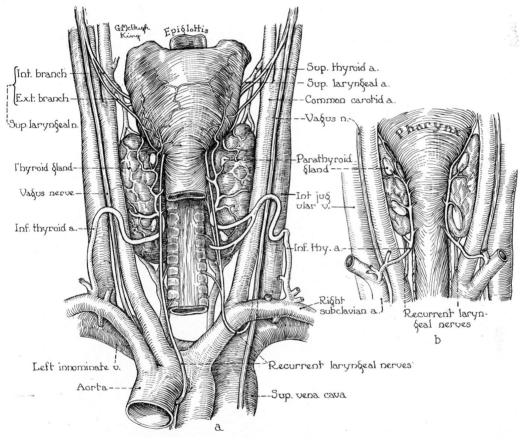

FIG. 178.—POSTERIOR VIEW OF THYROID, TRACHEA, AND ESOPHAGUS TO SHOW THE COURSE OF THE THYROID ARTERIES AND THEIR RELATIONS TO THE LARYNGEAL NERVES.

a, Accurate drawing from dissections; *b*, inaccurate representation. (Martin Nordland, Surg., Gynec. and Obst., Oct., 1930.)

5. Thyroid Vessels and Nerves.—Operative procedure on the thyroid gland requires an exact knowledge of its vessels and their relations to neighboring nerve trunks and to the parathyroid bodies. The thyroid gland is supplied by two paired arteries, the superior and inferior thyroid, and sometimes a single artery, the thyroidea ima.

The *superior thyroid artery* is the first branch of the external carotid. It arises opposite the thyrohyoid interval, a little above the thyroid cartilage, and is directed caudally and mesially, deep to the infrahyoid muscles. It lies on the outer surface of the inferior constrictor of the larynx with the superior laryngeal nerve situated only a little higher up (p. 173). This nerve may be included in ligation of the superior thyroid artery unless care is exercised. Its terminals anastomose within the gland with those of the inferior thyroid

and the superior thyroid arteries of the opposite side.   The superior thyroid artery may be
ligated near its origin by an incision similar to that employed for ligation of the exteranl
carotid (p. 204).   The *inferior thyroid artery*, the larger and more important, arises from the
subclavian artery by way of the thyrocervical trunk and turns mesially at a point about
2 cm. below the carotid tubercle (p. 156); at this point, it runs toward the gland in an arched
course with the convexity upward.   It may approach the gland directly by a downward

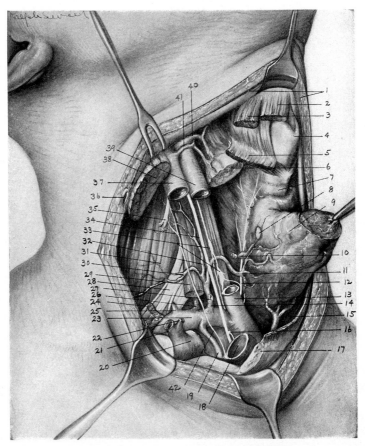

FIG. 179.—DEEP LATERAL VIEW OF THE THYROID REGION AND ITS RELATION WITH THE STRUCTURES
UNDER THE STERNOCLEIDOMASTOID MUSCLE.

The upper pole of the right lateral lobe of the thyroid has been sectioned to admit of drawing the lobe
toward the median line. (After Halsted.) 1, M. platysma; 2, M. sternohyoideus; 3, M. omohyoideus; 4,
cartilago thyreoidea; 5, M. sternothyreoideus; 6, glandula thyreoidea; 7, trachea; 8, glandula parathyre-
oidea; 9, glandula thyreoidea; 10, V. thyreoidea inferior; 11, A. thyreoidea inferior; 12, N. recurrens; 13,
A. carotis communis; 14, Truncus thyreocervicalis; 15, V. thyreoidea ima; 16, N. recurrens; 17, clavicula;
18, V. anonyma dextra; 19, A. mammaria interna; 20, V. subclavia; 21, V. jugularis externa; 22, V. jugularis
anterior; 23, A. subclavia; 24, M. omohyoideus; 25, A. transversa colli; 26, A. cervicalis profunda; 27, A.
transversa scapulae; 28, plexus brachialis; 29, M. scalenus anterior; 30, A. cervicalis superficialis; 31, M.
scalenus medius; 32, A. cervicalis ascendens; 33, ganglion cervicale medium; 34, N. vagus; 35, plexus cervicalis; 36, V. jugularis externa; 37, V. jugularis interna; 38, M. sternocleidomastoideus; 39, A. carotis
communis; 40, A. thyreoidea superior; 41, V. thyreoidea superior; 42, N. phrenicus.

curve.   The arch of the artery crosses anterior to the vertebral artery, the gangliated
sympathetic chain, and the middle cervical ganglion.   The segment of the artery proximal
to its division into terminal branches has important relations with the recurrent laryngeal
nerve, which runs upward in the tracheo-esophageal sulcus and enters the muscles of
the larynx.   The nerve lies either in front of the artery, among its branches, or behind
them.

The *thyroidea ima,* which branches from the innominate trunk or from the aortic arch, varies in size from a small arteriole to a vessel as large as the inferior thyroid. It runs upward over the anterior surface of the trachea to the inferior border of the thyroid gland. It may co-exist with the inferior thyroid artery or replace it. The possible presence of the vessel is to be borne in mind in low tracheotomy.

The thyroid arteries anastomose so thoroughly with those of the trachea and the esophagus that the trunks of all the thyroid arteries may be ligated without fear of necrosis of the gland.

The thyroid *veins* constitute a rich plexus mainly in front of the gland, and, as they leave, form the superior, middle, and inferior trunks. The upper trunk accompanies the superior thyroid artery and empties into the internal jugular vein by way of the common facial vein. The middle trunk empties inferiorly into the internal jugular vein. The inferior trunks are numerous and form an infrahyoid plexus which empties into the innominate vein. In some instances, these are greatly enlarged from the pressure of large goiters.

The thyroid *nerve supply* is derived from the sympathetic ganglia. The fibers from the middle and inferior cervical ganglia reach the gland as networks on the superior and inferior thyroid arteries. Excitation of these nerves may account for some of the symptoms and signs of exophthalmic goiter.

SURGICAL CONSIDERATIONS

1. **Goiter and Its Varieties.**—The term goiter signifies a pathologic enlargement of the thyroid gland. Under normal conditions, the volume of the gland varies within considerable limits in proportion to the engorgement of its vessels. In most females, the gland enlarges somewhat during each menstrual period. The right lobe frequently is larger than the left because of its greater blood supply.

The *simple parenchymatous goiter* is that in which the constituent parts of the thyroid apparently are increased in equal proportions, the consequence of a general tissue hyperplasia. In *cystic goiter* the glandular element distinctly predominates. In *fibrous goiter* the interglandular connective tissue stroma is increased out of proportion to other elements of the gland. Goiter may be *toxic* and be associated with exophthalmos, tachycardia, and tremor. This type of goiter is characterized by active hyperplasia of the gland with enlarged and newly formed follicles and an increase in the lymphoid tissue of the stroma. *Nodular* or *adenomatous goiter* may be toxic or nontoxic. Adenomata may develop in any or all parts of the gland; they exhibit a marked tendency to extend behind the trachea and sternum.

The gland presents a normal outline in uniform thyroid enlargement. Frequently, the enlargement is limited to one portion only and tends to compress and displace the structures with which it comes in contact. It may delve laterally beneath the sterno-cleidomastoid muscle, or inferiorly behind the sternum and clavicle. The trachea may be deviated or compressed by the enlargement, causing dyspnea; its lumen may be reduced to a mere slit. The pharynx and esophagus are subject to compression, causing difficult swallowing (dysphagia). Pressure upon the recurrent laryngeal nerve on either side is likely to be accompanied by paralysis of the laryngeal muscles it supplies, resulting in hoarseness (dysphonia) and even loss of voice (aphonia). With forward enlargement of the gland, the thyroid vessels, especially the veins, become enlarged and the infrahyoid muscles may be thinned out.

2. **Cretinism, Myxedema, and Cachexia Thyreopriva.**—Impaired function of the thyroid gland, known as hypothyroidism, presents a clinical picture characterized by peculiar conditions of the skin and subcutaneous tissue. Its clinical forms fall into three groups: cretinism, myxedema, and operative myxedema (cachexia thyreopriva). *Cretinism* may originate during fetal life or manifest itself any time before puberty. Thyroid secretion may be diminished or entirely lacking. The mental and physical development is stunted and the body activity is reduced. The skin is rough and scaly and the nostrils are

flaring. *Myxedema* occurs in adult life.   It carries with it a markedly lowered basal metabolism with tissue changes and slowed mentality.   When this clinical picture presents itself after extirpation of the gland, the condition is known as operative myxedema or *cachexia thyreopriva* (of Kocher).

3. **Thyrolingual or Thyroglossal Duct Cysts and Sinuses.**—The thyroglossal duct may persist between the foramen caecum and hyoid bone and develop into a *sublingual cyst* (p. 144).   That portion of the duct behind and below the hyoid bone sometimes develops into a *subhyoid cyst* which may rupture and become a *thyroglossal sinus*.   The duct may remain open from the mouth to the skin forming a *thyroglossal fistula*.   The presence of the duct frequently is made known by its involvement by infection.   Most of the cysts and fistulae are in the median line.   Effective treatment of either requires excision of all

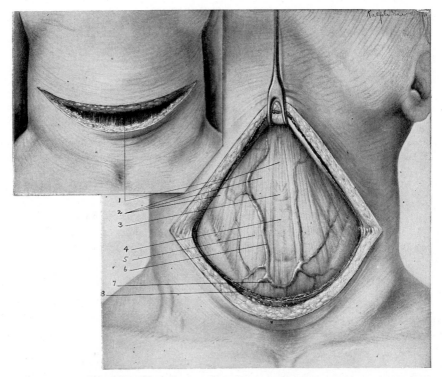

FIG. 180.—THE COLLAR INCISION FOR THYROIDECTOMY.

The inset indicates the incision developed to the platysmal muscle; the main drawing shows the incision developed through the platysma to the investing layer of deep cervical fascia; the flaps are dissected upward and downward (after Halsted). 1, M. platysma; 2, enveloping layer of deep cervical fascia; 3, cartilago thyreoidea; 4, glandula thyreoidea; 5, M. sternohyoideus; 6, V. jugularis anterior; 7, arcus venosus juguli; 8, M. platysma.

portions of the epithelium-lined walls, even to the point of curettement or division of the hyoid bone.

4. **Paths of Approach for Ligation of the Thyroid Vessels.**—The *superior thyroid artery* may be ligated through a small transverse incision located in a skin fold.   The incision should be directly over the point where the superior thyroid vessels enter the upper poles of the gland   This point can be determined only ·by palpating the gland against the thyroid cartilage.   The pole of the thyroid rests directly against the internal jugular vein and common carotid artery.   Adequate exposure, therefore, should be made.   The fibers of the omohyoid and the sternohyoid are separated longitudinally, and the fibers of the sternothyroid are cut across for the same distance as the skin incision.   The internal jugular vein and common carotid artery are retracted and the superior thyroid vessels are

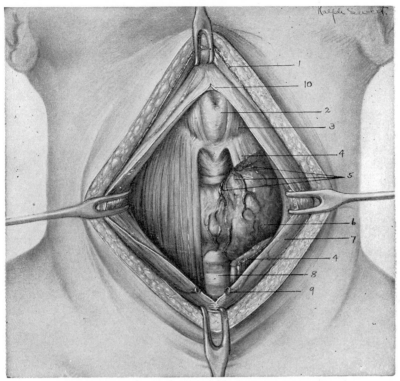

FIG 181.—VERTICAL INCISION DEVELOPED THROUGH THE INVESTING AND PRETRACHEAL LAYERS OF CERVICAL FASCIA BETWEEN THE INFRAHYOID MUSCLES.

A section has been removed from the left sternothyroid muscle to show the thyroid gland **covered with its** capsule (after Halsted). 1, M. platysma; 2, cartilago thyreoidea covered by its capsule; **3, M. thyreohyoideus;** 4, M. sternothyreoideus; 5, rami anteriores A. et V. thyreoideae superioris; 6, **glandula thyreoidea** covered with pretracheal fascia; 7, M. sternohyoideus; 8, trachea; 9, V. jugularis anterior; **10** enveloping and pretracheal layers of deep cervical fascia.

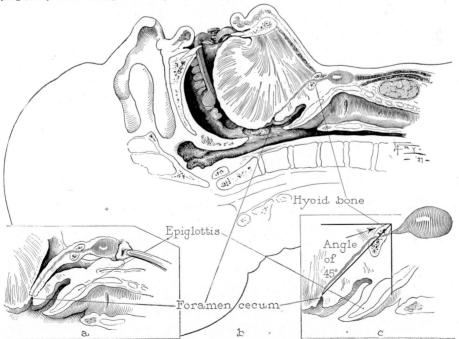

Hyoid bone

Epiglottis

Angle of 45°

Foramen cecum

FIG. 182.—EXCISION OF THYROGLOSSAL DUCT CYST.

a, Dissection of tract down to mucous membrane; *b*, direction of tract; tract runs through the **hyoid bone**; *c*, angulation of tract.   (W. E. Sistrunk, Surg., Gynec., and Obst. Jan., 1928.)

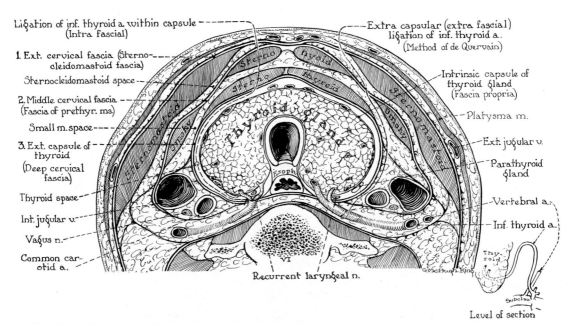

Ligation of inf. thyroid a. within capsule -------
(Intra fascial)

Extra capsular (extra fascial)
ligation of inf. thyroid a.
(Method of de Quervain)

1. Ext. cervical fascia (Sternocleidomastoid fascia)

Sternocleidomastoid space --

2. Middle cervical fascia --
(Fascia of prethyr. ms)

Small m. space ---

3. Ext. capsule of
thyroid
(Deep cervical
fascia)

Thyroid space --

Int. jugular v. --

Vagus n. --

Common car-
otid a. --

Intrinsic capsule of
thyroid gland
(Fascia propria)

Platysma m.

Ext. jugular v.

Parathyroid
gland

Vertebral a.

Inf. thyroid a.

Recurrent laryngeal n.

Level of section

FIG. 183.—TRANSVERSE SECTION THROUGH THE NECK TO ILLUSTRATE PATHS OF APPROACH TO THE INFERIOR THYROID ARTERY. (Martin Nordland, Surg., Gynec and Obst., Oct., 1930.)

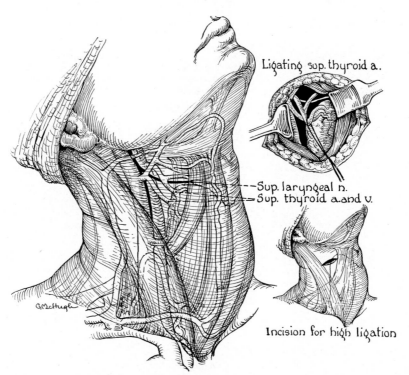

Ligating sup. thyroid a.

Sup. laryngeal n.
Sup. thyroid a. and v.

Incision for high ligation

FIG. 184.—LIGATION OF THE SUPERIOR THYROID VESSELS. THE SUPERIOR LARYNGEAL NERVE RELATIONS ARE INDICATED. (Martin Nordland, Surg., Gynec. and Obst., July, 1937.)

ligated.   Ligation just at the superior pole of the gland best insures avoidance of the superior laryngeal nerve.

Ligation of the *inferior thyroid artery*, which is more difficult, may be carried out mesial or lateral to the sternocleidomastoid.   The incision for mesial ligation is carried through the investing fascia along the anterior margin of the sternocleidomastoid.   The muscle is retracted laterally and the artery is sought by continuing the dissection deeply

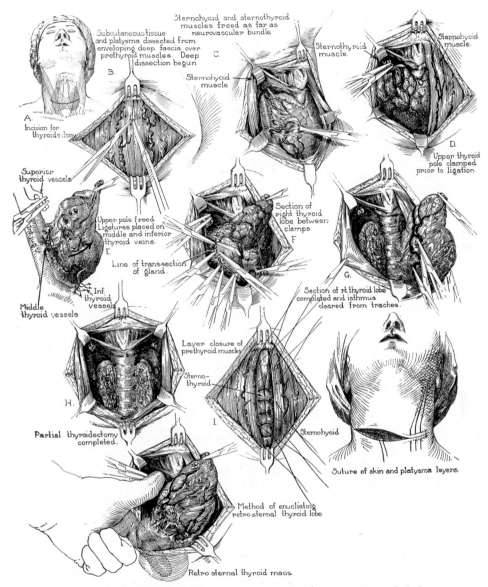

FIG. 185.—SUBTOTAL THYROIDECTOMY.   (Modified from Mont Reid.)

in the interval between the carotid sheath and the gland.   The gland is raised and displaced inward, and the artery is exposed where it arches mesially on the prevertebral fascia.   The ligature is applied over the main trunk of the artery in order that the recurrent nerve may be avoided (p. 182).

The inferior thyroid artery is more accessible by incision through the enveloping fascia along the posterior margin of the sternocleidomastoid.   The muscle is retracted forward and the artery is found on the prevertebral fascia, along the anterior margin of the anterior scalene muscle (p. 192), a little inferior to the carotid tubercle (p. 156). The artery can be felt as it arches mesially and its trunk, rather than its terminal branches, must be ligated in order to avoid the recurrent laryngeal nerve.

5. **Thyroidectomy.**—Satisfactory exposure of the thyroid gland is obtained by the collar incision of Kocher, which is directed transversely over the most prominent part of the goiter swelling. A natural fascial crease is followed to give the least possible scar, and the incision is deepened through the platysma to the enveloping fascia. The upper skin-platysma flap is dissected and retracted upward, and the lower flap is retracted downward to a lesser degree. The investing layer of the deep cervical fascia is divided vertically in the midline between the anterior jugular veins. The infrahyoid muscles then are identified and separated; in some cases, they are so thinned out by pressure from the underlying tumor that their edges are difficult to distinguish. Only rarely need they be cut transversely to afford adequate exposure of the gland. The loose tissue of the perithyroid sheath constitutes a cleavage plane which permits mobilization of the gland.

After the superior thyroid pedicle has been ligated, the lateral thyroid lobe may be displaced anteriorly. By rotating the lateral lobe mesially, the trunk of the inferior thyroid artery may be secured close to the gland. Resection of a portion of the gland may proceed between hemostats placed on the branches of the thyroid arteries as they ramify in the capsule.

In *intraglandular enucleation*, an incision is made into the gland and the offending mass is exposed and enucleated. Thus, an adenoma, or cyst of the gland, may be removed without disturbance of the surrounding glandular structure. Partial removal of the gland along with its corresponding portion of capsule may be performed in the same manner. Preservation of the posterior part of the capsule protects the recurrent nerves and preserves most of the parathyroid bodies.

A *subtotal excision* of the thyroid gland may be accomplished without preliminary ligation of the thyroid trunks by subcapsular resection between hemostats. This permits preservation of the lateral and posterior capsules, and part of the anterior capsule, obviating all danger of damage to the parathyroid bodies and the recurrent laryngeal nerves (Millzner, Searls, and Terry). The extensive operation of removing the entire thyroid gland obviously presents great risk of injuring the recurrent laryngeal nerves, more because of variability in their position than because of the vulnerability of the nerves themselves.

(IV) CERVICAL ESOPHAGUS

1. **Definition and Boundaries.**—The musculomembranous cervical esophagus is the direct continuation of the pharynx, the one merging with the other opposite the inferior margin of the cricoid cartilage at the level of the body of the sixth cervical vertebra. The carotid tubercle (p. 156) marks this level and is an important landmark in lateral esophagotomy (p. 206).

2. **Anatomic Summary.**—The esophagus, as well as the pharynx, is attached loosely to the prevertebral fascia by sagittal septa, which form retropharyngeal and retro-esophageal spaces. Abscesses occurring in these spaces are hindered from lateral extension by the septa, and fuse toward the mediastinum.

In the cervical region the trachea does not cover the esophagus completely, but leaves a portion of its left anterior margin exposed, affording natural surgical access. Despite its proximal fixation with the pharynx, the esophagus is capable of considerable upward and lateral displacement because of its intrinsic elasticity and loose connection with the trachea and prevertebral fascia.

The esophagus, when empty, is flattened anteroposteriorly, its lumen appearing as a transverse slit; when distended, it is irregularly cylindrical in form, presenting constrictions at certain points. The first and narrowest of these constrictions is at the beginning of the esophagus.

3. **Relations.**—The loose peri-esophageal tissue may be infected following injury to, or inflammation of, the walls of the esophagus, such as is caused by foreign bodies or by faulty instrumentation. Its chief lateral relation is with the carotid artery which lies 1 to 2 cm. from it. Deviation of the esophagus to the left relates it more intimately with the elements of the carotid sheath and the thyroid lobe on that side. The esophagus is related to the recurrent laryngeal nerves which lie in the tracheo-esophageal sulci, to the gangliated sympathetic chains, and to the inferior thyroid arteries.

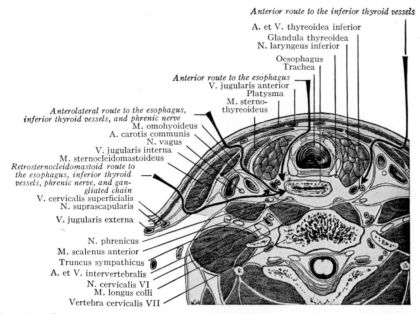

Anterior route to the inferior thyroid vessels

A. et V. thyreoidea inferior
Glandula thyreoidea
N. laryngeus inferior

Oesophagus
Trachea

Anterior route to the esophagus
V. jugularis anterior
Platysma
M. sterno-
thyreoideus

Anterolateral route to the esophagus,
inferior thyroid vessels, and phrenic nerve
M. omohyoideus
A. carotis communis
N. vagus
V. jugularis interna
M. sternocleidomastoideus
Retrosternocleidomastoid route to
the esophagus, inferior thyroid
vessels, phrenic nerve, and gan-
gliated chain
V. cervicalis superficialis
N. suprascapularis
V. jugularis externa

N. phrenicus
M. scalenus anterior
Truncus sympathicus
A. et V. intervertebralis
N. cervicalis VI
M. longus colli
Vertebra cervicalis VII

Fig. 186.—Diagrammatic Cross Section of the Neck at the Level of the Seventh Cervical Vertebra to Show the Cervical Approaches to the Esophagus, Inferior Thyroid Artery, Phrenic Nerve, and Sympathetic Gangliated Chain.

The posterior portions of the lateral thyroid lobe, when enlarged, may send out prolongations which insinuate themselves between the trachea and the anterior surface of the esophagus (retrotracheal and pre-esophageal). Prolongations may extend between the esophagus and prevertebral fascia and cause difficulty in swallowing.

Surgical Considerations

1. **Examination of the Esophagus.**—Use of the roentgen ray in examination of the esophagus has been of great value, not only in detecting foreign bodies lodged at the normal constrictions, but in demonstrating carcinoma, ulcers, diverticula, and strictures.

Esophagoscopy must be employed for the early diagnosis and treatment of esophageal lesions. Use of the esophagoscope requires accurate anatomical knowledge, dexterity, gentleness, and the cooperation of the patient. With the obturator in position, the esophagoscope is passed beyond the constriction at the esophageal inlet, whereupon the obturator is removed and the illuminated examining tube is passed downward under the direct vision of the operator. The closed cervical esophagus unrolls before the advancing instrument. Through the esophagoscope, local conditions may be treated, foreign bodies removed, strictures dilated, and biopsy tissue obtained.

2. **Obstruction of the Esophagus.**—A fibrous or cicatricial constriction of the esophagus may result from the healing of an ulcer, from traumatic or chronic inflammation (syphilitic or tuberculous), or from the swallowing of a corrosive or a hot liquid. The commonest cause of stricture in children is the swallowing of commercial lye, thoughtlessly left

about the kitchen. The first and chief symptom of obstruction is difficulty in swallowing (dysphagia) which becomes more pronounced until swallowing is impossible and regurgitation supervenes. With high stenosis, regurgitation is almost immediate; with low stenosis, and especially with proximal dilatation, it is delayed.

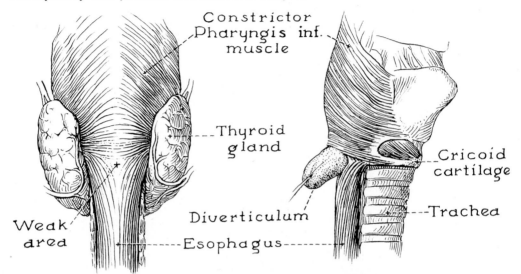

FIG. 187.—PULSION DIVERTICULUM OF THE ESPOHAGUS.

A, posterior view of pharyngoesophageal region showing the area at which the esophageal muscular wall gives way; B, right lateral view of protuding, mucosal sac.

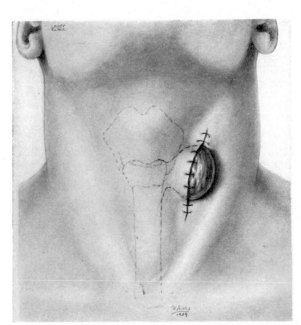

FIG. 188.—IMPLANTATION OF DIVERTICULUM INTO SKIN WOUND.

The sac is dissected completely from its bed, in the superior mediastinum when large, or from behind the esophagus when small.   (Frank Lahey, Surg., Gynec. and Obst., Aug., 1930.)

In adult life, carcinoma is the commonest cause of esophageal obstruction   The growth ulcerates the wall early and invades the deep cervical and posterior mediastinal lymph glands (mediastinitis).   It presents the same difficulty in swallowing as that accompanying ordinary cicatricial stenosis, and is followed quickly by regurgitation.

3. **Pharyngo-esophageal Diverticula.**—A diverticulum or outpocketing of the wall may occur in any part of the esophagus, but is most frequent in the upper part, because of the weakness in the longitudinal muscle layer at the level of the cricoid cartilage. The high diverticula of the posterior wall of the pharyngo-esophageal region are of the greatest interest as they are accessible surgically.

Esophageal diverticula may be congenital, the consequence of dilation proximal to a stricture, the result of pressure from within on a weak point of the wall, or of traction from without from the healing and subsequent cicatricial contraction of a peri-esophageal inflammatory process (diseased lymph glands).

Food, or any substance opaque to the x-ray, ordinarily goes to the stomach only after the diverticulum is filled, so that, under the fluoroscope, the pouch may be seen to fill and then to overflow into the esophagus. Diverticula in the neck may be extirpated and the esophagus sutured in a one-stage operation. Another method is to free the diverticulum and transplant it into the skin wound in the first stage of a two-stage operation. At the second operation, the paths of infection in the neck and toward the mediastinum, having been sealed off by adhesions, the diverticulum is removed. The procedure is endangered by the poor healing quality of the esophagus and the likelihood of infection following postoperative leakage into the mediastinum.

4. **Approach to the Cervical Esophagus.**—The esophagus is approached from the left side where it is more accessible (p. 188). A deepened presternocleidomastoid incision uncovers the left lateral lobe of the thyroid gland, which is drawn anteriorly and mesially, and the common carotid artery, which is displaced outward. The inferior thyroid artery is retracted or ligated to afford good exposure of the underlying esophagus. A vertical incision is made in the esophageal wall somewhat nearer its tracheal than its prevertebral aspect, carefully avoiding the recurrent laryngeal nerve in the tracheo-esophageal sulcus. Through this incision, foreign bodies may be removed, strictures dilated, and esophageal diverticula resected.

(V) PREVERTEBRAL REGION

1. **Definition and Boundaries.**—The prevertebral region includes only the thin and narrow musculo-aponeurotic layer which clothes the anterior surface of the vertebral column. Its surgical significance centers in the resistant prevertebral fascia and its relation to the inferior thyroid and vertebral arteries, the phrenic nerve, and the sympathetic gangliated chain. The region extends laterally to the apices of the cervical transverse processes.

2. **Sympathetic Gangliated Chain.**—The sympathetic gangliated chain in the neck is a prolongation of the thoracic sympathetic system, extending along the great vessels of the neck to the base of the skull. The cervical chain incorporates the superior, middle, and inferior ganglia, and plays an important rôle in pathologic changes when there is alteration of its powerful vasomotor action on the vessels to which it distributes plexuses. Section of the trunk and excision of the ganglia block the sympathetic impulses, both afferent and efferent; this is the theoretical basis for resection of the cervical sympathetic chain in exophthalmic goiter and angina pectoris.

The chain lies on the prevertebral fascia just mesial to the tuberosities of the cervical transverse processes, and is held in place by fibers derived from the underlying fascia. When the carotid sheath structures are retracted forward and mesially, the chain is not disturbed.

The broad, flat *superior cervical ganglion* is considered to be the coalescence of the sympathetic ganglia of the upper four cervical nerves. It lies in front of the transverse processes of the second and third cervical vertebrae, and is related anteriorly to the sheath of the internal carotid artery and internal jugular vein. Inferiorly, it is connected with the middle ganglion by the sympathetic trunk. Gray communicating branches connect the superior ganglion with the upper four cervical nerves The ganglion should not be excised unless its sympathetic communicating strand is shown leading to the middle cervical ganglion, to prevent its being mistaken for the ganglion of the vagus. From the lower part of the ganglion is given off the superior cardiac nerve, which contributes to the formation of the cardiac plexus.

The *middle cervical ganglion*, sometimes called the thyroid ganglion, is the smallest of the cervical ganglia, and occasionally is absent. It is located opposite the sixth cervical vertebra, usually in front of, or close to, the inferior thyroid artery. It sends gray communicating rami to the fifth and sixth cervical nerves, gives off the middle cardiac nerve, and communicates with the inferior ganglion by a well-developed strand.

The bean-sized *inferior cervical ganglion* is anterior to the first costovertebral joint in the angle made by the vertebral and subclavian arteries. It lies a very short distance from the first thoracic sympathetic ganglion, with which it sometimes unites to form the stellate ganglion. An inferior cardiac branch is given off deep to the deep cardiac plexus. Resection of the inferior cervical ganglion is a dangerous step in the removal of the gangliated chain because of its deep location and its relations to the vessels of the root of the neck.

3. Inferior Thyroid Artery.—The short, thick thyrocervical trunk arises from the subclavian artery, immediately above the origin of the internal mammary artery, and terminates about 0.5 cm. from its origin. Its three terminal branches are the transverse cervical and transverse scapular arteries, and the inferior thyroid trunk.

The *interior thyroid artery* ascends along the mesial margin of the anterior scalene muscle as far as the level of the cricoid cartilage. Just below the carotid tubercle, the artery changes direction abruptly to run horizontally, mesially, and then downward to ramify about the lower pole of the lateral thyroid lobe. It is bound down somewhat to the prevertebral fascia and must be freed to give exposure for ligation. In front, it is covered by the carotid sheath and middle cervical ganglion, and on the left by the thoracic duct. The vertebral vessels lie posterior to it and are separated from it by the prevertebral fascia. At the point where the inferior thyroid artery turns mesially, its ascending cervical branch is given off.

4. Vertebral Artery.—The vertebral artery is the first and largest branch given off by the subclavian artery. It arises from the posterior and upper part of the parent trunk opposite the interval between the anterior scalene and longus capitis muscles. The artery disappears from view at the apex of the triangular interval separating the anterior scalene and longus capitis muscles, to enter the foramen in the transverse process of the sixth cervical vertebra.

Its inferior and only surgically accessible portion is that between its origin and the point where it enters the vertebral foramen. It lies deep to the prevertebral fascia, is surrounded by a plexus of sympathetic fibers, and is overlain by the vertebral vein and the sympathetic trunk.

Surgical Considerations

1. Ligation of the Vertebral Artery.—True aneurysm of the vertebral artery is exceedingly rare; traumatic aneurysm, though rare on account of the depth of the vessel, is seen more frequently. The trunk of the artery may be compressed digitally below the carotid tubercle. The most accessible approach for ligation is through an incision low down along the posterior margin of the sternocleidomastoid muscle which permits forward displacement of this muscle and the internal jugular vein, and recognition of the carotid tubercle landmark. The artery is found in the triangular interval between the longus colli and anterior scalene muscles, and is identified by its pulsations.

The vessel can be reached by a presternocleidomastoid incision, identical with that used for ligation of the common carotid artery above the omohyoid muscle (p. 203). When well exposed, the carotid sheath and its contents are retracted laterally and the carotid tubercle is found at the level of the cricoid cartilage. The artery is felt in the depths between the longus colli and anterior scalene muscles. The point of election for ligation is 1.5 cm. below the carotid tubercle.

2. Approach for Cervical Sympathectomy and Ganglionectomy.—The incision for cervical ganglionectomy is made along the posterior margin of the sternocleidomastoid muscle as far down as the clavicle, and the muscle is retracted forward. The carotid sheath is drawn anteriorly and the sympathetic trunk is found on the prevertebral fascia. The trunk is delicate, appears to be a part of the fascia itself, and often is incorporated within it. The sympathetic chain must be differentiated from the phrenic nerve. The trunk of the chain is difficult to find until the *superior cervical ganglion* is located.

In the middle part of the neck, strands of the chain in front of the inferior thyroid artery sometimes enclose the vessel in their network. At this level lies the *middle cervical ganglion*. The *inferior cervical ganglion* is difficult to reach surgically. It always is connected intimately with, and usually is a part of, the first thoracic ganglion which is located deep at the entrance of the thorax, and lies against the neck of the first rib.

3. **The Phrenic Nerve and Its Section or Avulsion in the Neck.**—Division or avulsion of the phrenic nerve often is of great therapeutic value in pulmonary tuberculosis and other chest conditions. The diaphragm may temporarily be paralyzed almost completely by either procedure, but its paralysis does not render the muscle entirely immobile, as it re

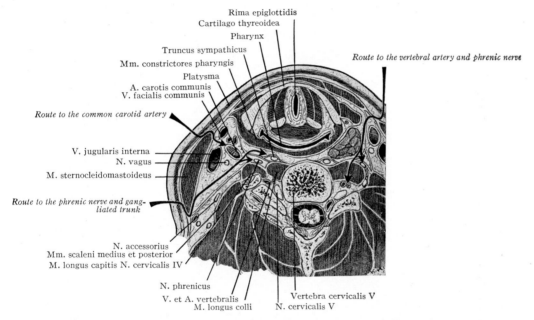

Rima epiglottidis
Cartilago thyreoidea
Pharynx
Truncus sympathicus
Mm. constrictores pharyngis
Platysma
A. carotis communis
V. facialis communis
Route to the common carotid artery
V. jugularis interna
N. vagus
M. sternocleidomastoideus
Route to the phrenic nerve and gang-liated trunk
N. accessorius
Mm. scaleni medius et posterior
M. longus capitis   N. cervicalis IV
N. phrenicus
V. et A. vertebralis
M. longus colli
Vertebra cervicalis V
N. cervicalis V
Route to the vertebral artery and phrenic nerve

FIG. 189.—DIAGRAMMATIC CROSS SECTION OF THE NECK AT THE LEVEL OF THE FIFTH CERVICAL VERTEBRA TO SHOW THE CERVICAL APPROACHES TO THE PHRENIC NERVE, SYMPATHETIC GANGLIATED CHAIN, AND TO THE COMMON CAROTID AND VERTEBRAL ARTERIES.

sponds to passive motion, being forced upward by abdominal pressure and downward by intrathoracic pressure. Regeneration of the nerve may occur after six months. In general, barring stiffening exudate or fibrotic changes in the muscle itself, there is a tendency for the paralyzed diaphragm to rise in the chest.

Incision for phrenic section is made at the posterior margin of the sternocleidomastoid muscle about 2.5 cm. above the clavicle. The posterior border of the muscle is exposed and the muscle and the carotid sheath are drawn forward. Dissection is carried deeper in the lower part of the wound until the posterior belly of the omohyoid muscle is recognized. Directly behind the great vessels and slightly oblique to their course lies the anterior scalene muscle, covered by the thin prevertebral fascia. The phrenic nerve descends vertically on this muscle, deep to the fascia, and can be followed upward to its origin in the cervical plexus. The nerve is smoother, larger, and more cylindrical than the sympathetic chain to which it lies lateral and from which it must be differentiated. Section of the nerve is safe and, in most instances, effects a satisfactory degree of diaphragmatic palsy.

13

An accessory phrenic nerve occurs in from 20 to 30 per cent of cases. Substitution of *avulsion* or *exeresis* for nerve section removes the accessory phrenic, as well as the phrenic, and increases the chances of securing complete paralysis of the corresponding half of the

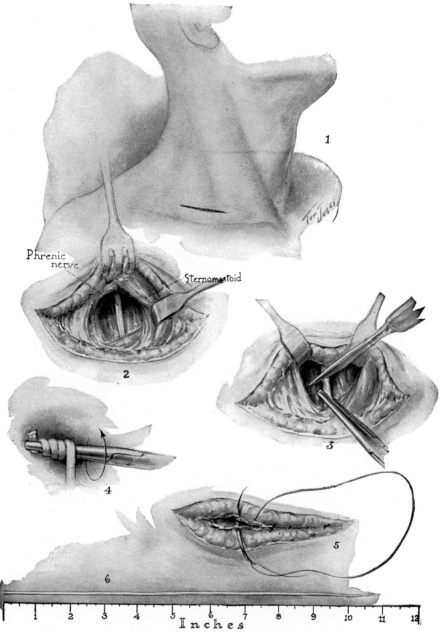

FIG. 190.—TECHNIC OF AVULSION OF THE PHRENIC NERVE. (From Carl A. Hedblom in Lewis' Surgery.) (Courtesy of W. F. Prior Company.)

diaphragm. The procedure is carried out by slowly winding the nerve upon a pair of forceps until the entire nerve and its branches are withdrawn. Avulsion should be abandoned if excessive pain accompanies traction on the phrenic nerve. Hemorrhage following avulsion probably comes from injury to the pericardiophrenic artery.

III. LATERAL REGIONS OF THE NECK

The lateral regions of the neck are the sternomastoid (carotid) and the supraclavicular.

A. STERNOMASTOID OR CAROTID REGION

1. **Definition and Boundaries.**—The broad sternocleidomastoid muscle covers a wide area of the lateral region of the neck. This area is known as the carotid region because the common, internal, and external carotid arteries run most of their courses within it. It is limited above by the mastoid process and below by the clavicle and upper sternum; it extends in depth to the prevertebral fascia.

2. **Landmarks.**—The *sternocleidomastoid muscle*, running from the mastoid process to the medial end of the clavicle, stands out in bold relief. The deep *sulcus* or *vascular groove* separating the muscle from the anterior neck regions leads superiorly to the retromandibular fossa. In thin individuals, the sulcus is much accentuated, particularly in the middle portion; in those with a strongly developed sternocleidomastoid, the sulcus is narrowed. In the depth of the groove, the great vessels of the neck may be palpated. The operative position of extension of the head puts the structures of the region on some tension, whereas flexion and rotation allow them to be palpated easily.

3. **Superficial Structures.**—Upon the surface of the sternocleidomastoid muscle, the superficial vessels and nerves run in duplications of the superficial cervical fascia. The *external jugular vein* is the only vessel of any surgical consequence. It is formed on the outer surface of the sternocleidomastoid muscle, inferior and posterior to the angle of the jaw, by the union of the posterior auricular vein and a branch from the posterior facial vein. Through the posterior facial vein, there is an anastomosis of the external and internal jugular veins. The external jugular emerges from the inferior part of the parotid compartment and penetrates the region at the angle of the jaw. From this point, it is directed downward and backward, and crosses the lateral surface of the sternocleidomastoid muscle obliquely to enter the supraclavicular fossa.

Four important superficial *branches* of the *cervical plexus* of nerves wind about the posterior margin of the sternocleidomastoid muscle. One of these, the great auricular, runs parallel to the external jugular vein to enter the nuchal region posterior to the ear. The cutaneous nerve of the neck crosses the muscle and supplies the region about the hyoid bone. Supraclavicular branches descend along the posterior margin of the sternocleidomastoid muscle and the lesser occipital nerve ascends to the scalp along the same margin. These structures are covered by the platysma muscle. The *superficial lymphatics* drain to the submaxillary lymph glands.

4. **Sternocleidomastoid Muscle and Its Enveloping Fascia.**—The sternocleidomastoid muscle is held securely in place by the duplication of the enveloping fascia of the neck (p. 158). The outer covering of deep fascia varies in structure. It is thick and fibrous above, where it passes over the inferior pole of the parotid gland in the retromandibular fossa, and is thin and transparent lower down.

The sternal and clavicular heads of the muscle are separated by a triangular interval, in the floor of which lies the inferior part of the carotid sheath. The sternal head may be severed and turned aside to obtain better exposure of the deeper structures. The *spinal accessory nerve* (eleventh cranial) enters the substance of the muscle about 4 cm. inferior to the tip of the mastoid process. The deep guides to the nerve are the posterior belly of the digastric muscle and the internal jugular vein, both of which the nerve crosses obliquely downward, laterally, and backward.

A thin deep fascial covering separates the muscle from the subjacent structures. Like the external layer, it is thicker and more resistant above than below. The sheath is sufficiently strong to hold fluid within it, as in a closed compartment. This fluid may be hemorrhage resulting from muscle rupture, or the contents of an abscess extending from a mastoiditis (*Bezold abscess*) (p. 110). Branchial cysts and sinuses present along the anterior border of the sternomastoid muscle (p. 206).

5. Cervical Lymph Glands and Their Relation to the Omohyoid Muscle and Pre-tracheal Fascia.—When the sternocleidomastoid muscle is retracted laterally, the internal jugular vein can be distinguished in the upper half or two thirds of the exposed area, lying in an abundant meshwork of areololymphatic tissue. The lymph glands disposed between the muscle and vein adhere more or less intimately to both structures. Adhesions caused by pathologic changes about the glands may be so dense as to require removal of the sterno-cleidomastoid muscle and internal jugular vein in gland dissection. After involving the lymph glands in the submaxillary region (p. 117), carcinoma of the lip and tongue metasta-

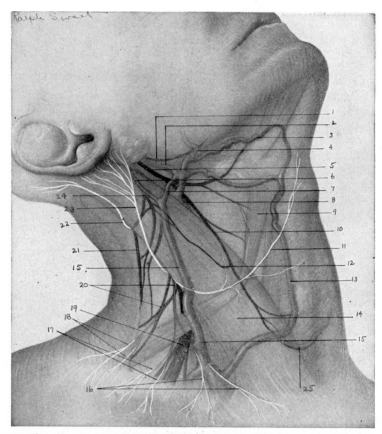

Fig. 191.—Surface Anatomy of the Lateral Region of the Neck, and the Distribution of the Superficial Veins and Nerves.

1, Ramus marginalis mandibulae n. facialis; 2, V. facialis posterior; 3, V. submentalis; 4, V. facialis anterior; 5, N. hypoglossus; 6, V. auricularis posterior; 7, V. facialis communis; 8, V. jugularis interna; 9, M. omohyoideus; 10, ramus descendens n. hypoglossi; 11, N. cutaneus colli; 12, ansa hypoglossi; 13, V. jugularis anterior; 14, M. sternocleidomastoideus; 15, V. jugularis externa; 16, Nn. supraclaviculares anteriores; 17, Nn. supraclaviculares medii; 18, Nn. supraclaviculares posteriores; 19, plexus brachialis; 20, trunks of supraclavicular nerves; 21, ramus externus nervi accessorii; 22, N. occipitalis minor; 23, N. auricularis magnus; 24, N. cervicalis III; 25, arcus venosus jugularis.

sizes to the *superior group* of *deep cervical lymph glands* which lie above the omohyoid muscle. The superior group communicates below with the *inferior set* of *deep cervical nodes* which lies inferior to the omohyoid muscle and deep to the pretracheal fascia; the nodes drain toward the supraclavicular region and mediastinum.

6. Carotid Sheath.—The carotid sheath is the tubular investment of deep cervical fascia which encloses the common and internal carotid arteries, internal jugular vein, and vagus nerve. Above the common carotid artery, its structure is somewhat attenuated. The posterior wall of the sheath is adherent to the prevertebral fascia. These adhesions however, do not prevent pus from passing from the carotid compartment to the adjoining supraclavicular region. The anterior wall of the sheath fuses with and, to some extent, is derived from, the pretracheal fascia (p. 159). It is thin over the internal jugular vein, but is thick and dense over the common carotid artery.

7. **Common Carotid Artery and Its Relations.**—The common carotid artery, the largest in the neck, arises from the innominate trunk on the right and from the arch of the aorta on the left. It emerges from behind the sternoclavicular joint, and ascends obliquely in the direction of the angle of the mandible. At the superior margin of the thyroid cartilage, each artery, after forming a swelling known as the carotid bulb, divides into two terminal branches, the internal and external carotid arteries. These continue upward and gently diverge; the internal carotid continues in the direction of the common trunk.

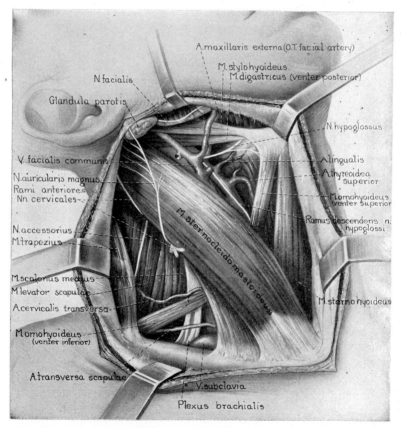

Fig. 192.—Structures of the Lateral Regions of the Neck with the Sternocleidomastoid Muscle in Situ.

The common carotid artery has posterior *relations* with the gangliated sympathetic chain, prevertebral fascia, underlying prevertebral muscles, and the anterior surface of the cervical transverse processes. The artery may be compressed easily against the bony transverse processes. The prominent carotid tubercle (p. 156) is an important landmark in the ligation of the common carotid artery.

Anteriorly, the common carotid is in relation with the cellular tissue of the neck in the upper two thirds of its course, and with the pretracheal fascia in the lower third. In its middle third, it is related to the omohyoid muscle, which crosses in front of the artery. That portion of the vessel below the omohyoid muscle is its surgically dangerous part, since there it has intimate relations with the great venous trunks at the base of the neck. Its course above the omohyoid, therefore, is the site of election for ligation.

8. **Internal Carotid Artery.**—The internal carotid artery begins at the termination of the common carotid opposite the superior margin of the thyroid cartilage, and terminates in the middle fossa of the skull by dividing into the anterior and middle cerebral arteries (p. 39). At its origin, it lies a little posterolateral to the external carotid, but as it ascends, it passes to the mesial side of the external carotid toward the lateral wall of the pharynx. When it reaches the pharynx, the artery runs vertically into the maxillopharyngeal space.

9. **External Carotid Artery and Its Branches within the Region.**—The external carotid artery arises from the common carotid opposite the upper border of the thyroid cartilage, somewhat mesial to, and in front of, the internal carotid artery. It then is directed upward and backward to the angle of the jaw. Here it changes direction and rises vertically to engage under the stylohyoid muscle and the posterior belly of the digastric; it pierces the

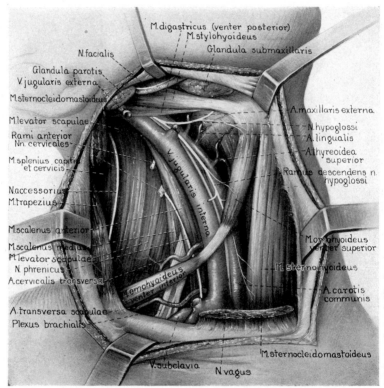

FIG. 193.—STRUCTURES EXPOSED IN THE LATERAL REGION OF THE NECK WHEN THE STERNOCLEIDOMASTOID MUSCLE IS REMOVED.

posteromesial surface of the parotid gland (p. 131). It continues upward through the gland just behind the neck of the mandible, where it ends by dividing into the internal maxillary and superficial temporal arteries. On either side, branches of the external carotid artery supply the upper neck and extracranial soft parts of the head. At its point of election for *ligation* it lies almost in contact with the great horn of the hyoid bone, which serves as an ideal surgical landmark. In front, it is overlain by areologlandular tissue and by the posterior belly of the digastric muscle.

The *superior thyroid artery* arises from the external carotid a little above the upper margin of the thyroid cartilage. It is overlapped by the anterior margin of the sternocleidomastoid muscle and runs downward and forward under cover of the omohyoid muscle to supply the thyroid gland. The *lingual artery* leaves the external carotid opposite the greater horn of the hyoid bone. It passes deep to the hyoglossal muscle to reach the sublingual compartment (p. 164). The greater horn of the hyoid bone is the surgical guide to the vessel, and the posterior belly of the digastric muscle is a guide to the depth to which the dissection has advanced. The *external maxillary (facial) artery* arises a little above the lingual artery, passes immediately upward under cover of the stylohyoid muscle and the posterior belly of the digastric, and enters the submaxillary region (p. 163). The *occipital artery* is given off at the same level as the external maxillary, but from the posterior aspect of the trunk deep to the posterior belly of the digastric, and disappears under the mastoid process and its attached muscles.

Collateral anastomoses between the internal and external carotid arteries are adequate to maintain circulation after ligation of either of these trunks. Many anastomotic rela-

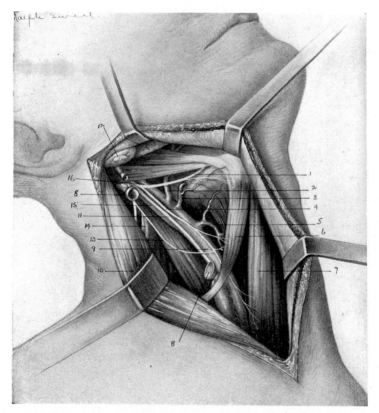

FIG. 194.—THE UPPER STERNOCLEIDOMASTOID REGION TO SHOW THE BRANCHES OF THE EXTERNAL CAROTID ARTERY.

1, N. hypoglossus; 2, A. maxillaris externa; 3, A. lingualis; 4, ramus descendens n. hypoglossi; 5, A. thyreoidea superior; 6, M. omohyoideus; 7, M. sternohyoideus; 8, V. jugularis interna (resected); 9, A. carotis communis; 10, M. sternocleidomastoideus; 11, N. vagus; 12, glandula parotis; 13, ansa hypoglossi; 14, Nn. cervicales III et IV; 15, A. carotis interna; 16, A. carotis externa.

tionships exist between the arteries of the ophthalmic territory of the internal carotid and the facial territory of the external carotid. An efficient anastomotic communication exists between the external carotid artery and the thyrocervical trunk through the superior thyroid branch of the former and the inferior thyroid branch of the latter. Free communication is present between the vertebral and internal carotid arteries by the posterior communicating artery of the circle of Willis. Numerous unions between the lingual, facial, occipital, posterior auricular, and ascending pharyngeal arteries, which make vast peribuccal and peripharyngeal circles, connect the external carotid arteries of the two sides. One internal carotid artery indirectly communicates with the other across the base of the brain by the anterior communicating artery and with the basilar trunk. Ordinarily, ligation of the common carotid artery does not stop the circulation, either anatomically or clinically, unless the anastomotic paths are disturbed.

10. **Internal Jugular Vein and Its Common Facial Branch.**—The *internal jugular vein* is the principal venous trunk of the neck and is the direct downward continuation of the transverse (lateral) sinus. The vessel rarely is seen surgically in its upper portion which lies deep to the styloid process and to the parotid compartment. It descends in the carotid sheath, and may be recognized easily by its bluish-gray color. The internal jugular vein runs to a point a little lateral to the sternoclavicular joint, where it unites with the subclavian to form the innominate vein. As it descends, it increases gradually in size upon receiving various tributaries.

The internal jugular is the largest of the relatively superficial veins of the body, and may be involved in piercing wounds. This vessel and the carotid artery usually escape

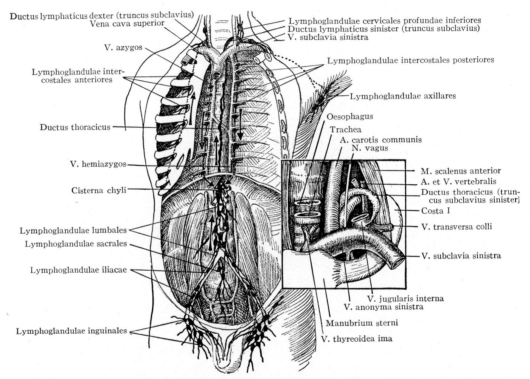

FIG. 195.—TRIBUTARIES AND TERMINATIONS OF THE LYMPHATIC CHANNELS OF THE THORAX AND ABDOMEN AND TOPOGRAPHY OF THE AZYGOS VENOUS SYSTEM.

injury in suicidal wounds, since the position assumed, with the chin tilted back and the sternocleidomastoid muscle made tense, protects them. The vein is influenced greatly by respiration, emptying during inspiration and filling during expiration, so that the thin-walled tube may be distended to 1.5 cm. in diameter, or be a flaccid ribbon-like structure with its walls in contact. During inspiration, air may be drawn into a rent in the vein and may embarrass respiration seriously by the formation of air emboli in the pulmonary veins, or cause death if sufficient air reaches the heart. The vein may be infected secondarily after intracranial sinus thrombosis, particularly that involving the transverse sinus. Infection is accompanied by pain and tenderness along the course of the vein.

The *common facial vein* (p. 164) is the most important contributing branch to the internal jugular. The trunk is formed about the submaxillary gland by the union of the anterior and posterior facial veins. It passes backward and downward to pierce the carotid sheath and enter the internal jugular vein opposite the great horn of the hyoid bone. It receives the thyroid and lingual veins and might be termed the "thyro-lingual-facial" trunk. The common facial vein, which often is joined by the anterior jugular vein, is a source of embarrassment in operations for lymph gland resection in the retromandibular area. The superior thyroid vein may enter the internal jugular directly, as do the middle thyroid veins.

11. **Vagus or Tenth Cranial Nerve.**—The vagus nerve lies between the internal jugular vein and the internal and common carotid arteries, and passes through the neck to its terminations in the thorax and abdomen. Injury to the nerve in ligation of the vessels is of serious consequence. The superior laryngeal branch is given off behind the carotid and traverses the thyrohyoid membrane with the superior laryngeal vessels. The inferior laryngeal nerve is the recurrent vagus branch from within the thorax.

12. **Thoracic Duct.**—As it leaves the thorax, the thoracic duct is applied closely to the left side of the esophagus. The duct ascends in the neck about 4 cm. above the clavicle and turns laterally behind the carotid sheath and in front of the inferior thyroid and vertebral arteries. At the medial margin of the anterior scalene muscle, it drops

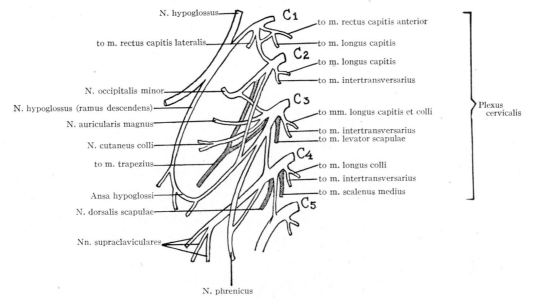

FIG. 196.—CERVICAL PLEXUS.

down to enter the angle of union of the internal jugular and subclavian veins. It drains the lymph from both lower extremities, the abdominal walls, most of the abdominal viscera, and the left half of the thorax. Near its opening, it usually is joined by the collecting lymphatic trunks from the left upper extremity and the left side of the head and neck.

13. **Retromandibular Fossa.**—The retromandibular fossa is a boundary region between the neck and head and, from the surgical viewpoint, is allied closely with the structures in the submaxillary compartment (p. 162). It is in vital connection with the structures of the sternomastoid region. The fossa is bounded in front by the posterior margin of the ramus of the mandible, and behind by the anterior border of the sternocleidomastoid muscle, and contains much of the posterior bellies of the digastric and stylohyoid muscles, deep to which lies the trunk of the external carotid artery. Into the region passes the facial nerve (seventh cranial), which emerges from the skull through the stylomastoid foramen and runs forward to and through the parotid gland (p. 132). An important content of the space is that portion of the parotid gland lying below the mandible.

14. **Hypoglossal Nerve.**—The hypoglossal (twelfth cranial) or motor nerve to the

tongue is an occupant of this region only in its proximal portion, where it lies deep to the parotid gland and descends between the internal carotid artery and the internal jugular vein. It appears beneath the lower margin of the posterior belly of the digastric muscle and turns forward almost at a right angle. After crossing the external and internal carotid arteries and continuing forward a little above the level of the hyoid bone, it disappears under the posterior belly of the digastric and reappears within the submaxillary compartment, lying on the hyoglossus muscle (p. 164). It enters the intermuscular cleft between the hyoglossus and mylohyoid muscles to reach the muscles of the tongue.

15. **Cervical Plexus.**—The cervical plexus is formed by the anterior rami of the first four cervical nerves, and each nerve receives a gray ramus communicans from the superior cervical sympathetic ganglion. These nerves are combined in an irregular series of loops under cover of the sternocleidomastoid muscle, deep to the longus capitis muscle, and on the scale nus medius. The roots of the plexus lie deep to the prevertebral fascia and are free from injury in radical removal of the glands of the neck. The terminal branches pierce the fascia to go to the muscles they supply and the nerves with which they communicate.

The *superficial cutaneous branches* radiate from the plexus and appear in the supraclavicular region by winding about the posterior margin of the sternocleidomastoid muscle. Of the *muscular* or *deep branches*, the phrenic nerve is the most important. It is derived mainly from the fourth cervical, reinforced by roots from the third and fifth cervical nerves, and passes downward in the neck deep to the prevertebral fascia. It runs on the anterior scalene muscle and enters the thorax at the root of the neck to be distributed to the diaphragm.

Surgical Considerations

1. **Excision of the Deep Cervical Lymph Glands.**—Lateral neck dissection of the deep cervical lymph glands is performed for metastatic carcinoma, primary endothelioma localized Hodgkin's disease, and intractable glandular tuberculosis. Deep cervical glandular dissection sometimes is carried out in combination with suprahyoid dissection (p. 164) for metastatic carcinoma of the buccal cavity, with or without metastases, for primary endothelioma arising in the lymph glands of the neck, and, with modifications, for glandular tuberculosis.

A T-shaped incision is used for lateral neck dissection. The horizontal portion of the incision is carried across the side of the neck, at the level of the hyoid bone, to the anterior margin of the trapezius. The vertical incision is dropped from the midpoint of the horizontal, striking the clavicle near the lateral edge of the sternocleidomastoid muscle. Two flaps are reflected, the posterior as far as the anterior edge of the trapezius, and the anterior to expose the ribbon muscles of the neck. The areologlandular tissue over the area is cleaned away down to the prevertebral fascia on the floor of the neck. The sternocleidomastoid muscle is cut transversely about 5 cm. above the clavicle at about the level of the crossing of the omohyoid muscle, and the subjacent internal jugular vein is ligated and divided. The clavicular stump of the muscle is turned down over the clavicle. The supraclavicular tissue is dissected to include the whole of the deep cervical lymph chain. The glands about the subclavian vein need not be removed save when the lowermost glands of the deep cervical chain are involved.

The dissection begins below and proceeds upward, following the floor of the neck (prevertebral fascia). The upward dissection can be completed without fear of mishap or danger to any important structures, since the vagus nerve and common carotid artery are visible. The roots of the cervical plexus and the phrenic nerve are protected by the prevertebral fascia, which is identified as a transparent tough covering, closely applied to the deep muscles of the neck. All of the important branches of the cervical plexus, save the phrenic nerve, pierce this fascia, and are divided at their points of emergence. In the upper portion of the incision, the superior thyroid artery is ligated and the tendinous part of the stylohyoid and digastric muscles at their insertion on the hyoid is exposed. Care is taken to isolate the hypoglossal nerve, which makes a loop below the level of the posterior belly of the digastric muscle.

The final procedure takes place at the upper lateral angle of the wound, and is concerned with cutting away the sternocleidomastoid muscle from the mastoid process, the removal of the lower pole of the parotid gland, and the ligation of the internal jugular vein at the base of the skull. The inferior 1 to 2 cm. of the parotid gland is resected because the uppermost glands of the deep cervical chain are embedded in it. Progress here is slow because of the necessity of division and ligation of numerous veins of the common facial trunk. The prevertebral fascia is cleared of all areolar tissue and the floor of the neck is left bare, save for a row of stumps remaining where the branches of the cervical plexus penetrate the fascia.

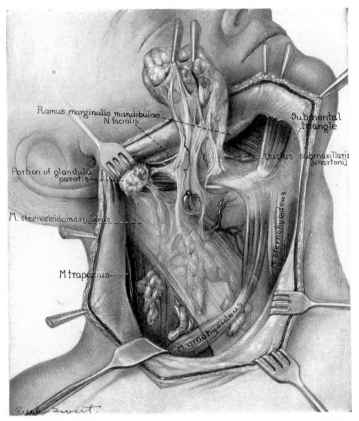

FIG. 197.—THE AREOLOGLANDULAR TISSUE TO BE REMOVED IN THE COMBINED SUPRAHYOID AND DEEP LATERAL NECK DISSECTION. (Bartlett and Callander.)

The contents of the suprahyoid area are suspended by clamps; the areologlandular tissue behind the sterno-mastoid muscle is shown in transparency.

2. **Ligation of Common Carotid Artery.**—The common carotid artery may require ligation to control profuse hemorrhage from deep wounds in the upper part of neck or from ulcerative lesions in the throat, or to interrupt circulation through an aneurysmal sac.

The vessel may be ligated above or below the omohyoid muscle, but the site of election is *above the omohyoid* crossing. The skin incision, about 7 to 8 cm. long, is made at the anterior margin of the sternocleidomastoid muscle, obliquely across the course of the vessel The center of the incision is at the level of the cricoid cartilage. After the superficial structures are divided, the enveloping fascia is incised along the anterior margin of the sternocleidomastoid muscle. When the muscle is retracted posteriorly, the omohyoid muscle is seen in the lower angle of the wound and is drawn downward and inward or is divided. The descending hypoglossal nerve is carried laterally, and the thyroid gland may

have to be drawn mesially.   The artery is located and ligatures are passed around it from
without inward to minimize the possibility of including the vagus nerve.

For ligation *below the omohyoid* crossing, the incision is anterior to the sternocleidomastoid muscle, but extends from the level of the cricoid cartilage to the sternoclavicular
joint.   The anterior jugular vein may require division.   The enveloping fascia is divided
and the sternocleidomastoid muscle is drawn backward.   The three flat infrahyoid muscles,
clothed in pretracheal fascia, are exposed, and the sternohyoid and sternothyroid muscles
are drawn mesially and inferiorly.   The omohyoid muscle is retracted laterally or is cut, as
occasion demands.   The lateral lobe of the thyroid gland conceals the carotid sheath and
must be retracted mesially.   On the left side, the internal jugular vein tends to overlie the

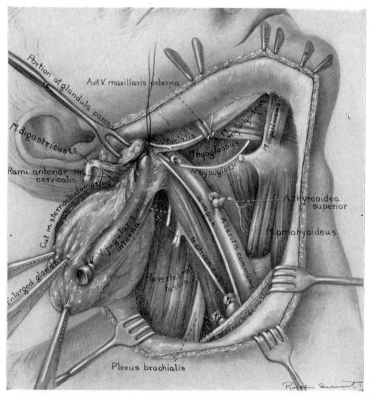

Fig. 198.—Final Steps in the Combined Suprahyoid and Deep Lateral Neck Dissection.   (Bartlett
and Callander.)

The sternomastoid and supraclavicular areas are cleared of all areologlandular content; the trunks of
the brachial plexus and the phrenic and vagus nerves are saved.   All of the lower branches of the external
carotid artery have been ligated or removed; the posterior half of the digastric muscle and the sternocleidomastoid muscle are removed along with the internal jugular vein.

artery, and, consequently, the common carotid lies deeper in the root of the neck, making
the operation more difficult.

3. **Ligation of External Carotid Artery.**—Ligation of the external carotid artery sometimes is indicated as a preliminary step in the more extensive operations on the face and
neck, as excision of the upper jaw for carcinoma or removal of a malignant growth from
the pharyngeal wall.

The site of election for ligation is between the emergence of the superior thyroid
and lingual trunks, but ligation may be performed proximal to the origin of the superior
thyroid vessel.   The incision is anterior to the sternocleidomastoid muscle, directed along
the course of the vessel, from a point opposite the angle of the mandible to the level of
the upper margin of the thyroid cartilage.   After dividing the superficial structures and

enveloping fascia, the anterior margin of the sternocleidomastoid muscle is freed and is retracted posteriorly. The inferior pole of the parotid gland may have to be retracted gently upward to expose the digastric tendon and the arching loop of the hypoglossal nerve, which cross the artery at this level. The ligature should be applied at about the level of the greater horn of the hyoid bone, which is the surgical landmark. The greatest embarrassment comes from the overlying thyroid, lingual, and facial branches of the common facial vein which require retraction or division. Care is taken to avoid the superior laryngeal nerve lying behind the artery

4. **Ligation of the Internal Carotid Artery.**—The internal carotid trunk contributes to the formation of the arterial circle at the base of the brain. Its middle cerebral branch has been emphasized (p. 39), and its main trunk has important pharyngeal and tonsillar relations (p. 146). Its relation to the cavernous sinus and ophthalmic artery is of prime importance (p. 32). The cervical part of the artery is accessible through the incision used for exposure of the external carotid artery.

5. **Exposure and Ligation of the Internal Jugular Vein.**—Ligation of the internal jugular vein occasionally is resorted to in transverse sinus thrombosis (p. 34) to prevent propagation of infection through the internal jugular to the general circulation. The vein may be found readily by a retrosternocleidomastoid incision through the deep fascia with forward retraction of the muscle, or by an incision directly over and through the sternocleidomastoid muscle. In its lower portion, the vein is isolated easily; in its upper part, it is ligated with difficulty, because of its tributaries. The ligation of one internal jugular vein can be made with impunity, and even bilateral ligation usually is tolerated well.

6. **Torticollis or Wryneck.**—The normal upright position of the head is maintained by the associated action of the muscles on both sides of the neck in such a manner that equilibrium is established. Any contraction, temporary or permanent, in one sternocleidomastoid muscle, with or without implication of the deeper muscles on the same side, particularly the scaleni, alters the attitude of the head and neck. The term "torticollis" or wryneck designates the altered position which the head and neck assume. The chronic contraction of one sternocleidomastoid muscle inclines the head and neck toward the affected side. At the same time, the head is tilted and rotated until the chin projects upward toward the unaffected side. The ear on the affected side approaches the corresponding shoulder. Because of the abnormal position of the cervical spine, a primary lateral curvature develops with its convexity toward the unaffected muscle. This cervical deviation is compensated by a thoracic curve.

There may be *transient contracture* from rheumatism, cold, acute myositis (myogenic), irritation of one or more inflamed deep cervical glands (reflex), or irritation of the spinal accessory nerve (neurogenic). Marked muscle spasm (spasmodic torticollis) may occur in the neurotic individual and is relieved with great difficulty.

In the group of *permanent contractures*, of which congenital torticollis is an example, the muscle cannot be lengthened to normal. Muscle retraction following a birth injury probably results from muscle rupture and subsequent scar formation. The muscle may feel hard and tendinous and stand out prominently, particularly at its sternal head, where a definite interval may be seen between the sternal and clavicular attachments. In aggravated cases, the deep muscles of the neck become rigid and contracted. For relief of permanent contractures, tenotomy is performed through an oblique incision across the lower part of the sternocleidomastoid muscle. The fascial sheath is divided with the muscle fibers. Occasionally, it may be necessary to open the underlying carotid sheath to get complete relaxation. The whole muscle may have to be excised or the spinal accessory nerve be sectioned.

7. **Aneurysm of the Common Carotid Artery.**—Aneurysm may develop in any part of the course of the common carotid artery. The usual locations are: at the origin from the innominate artery on the right; at the origin from the aortic arch on the left; and at the level of bifurcation into external and internal branches. A carotid aneurysm usually is small and the long axis lies parallel with that of the vessel.

On the medial side, the trachea, larynx, pharynx, and esophagus are compressed, obstructed, and displaced and afford locations for the rupture of aneurysm. The vagus, phrenic, sympathetic and recurrent laryngeal nerves and the internal jugular vein may become blended with the carotid sheath and eventually with the aneurysmal sac, a complication contributing to the difficulties of extirpation or even ligation.

8. **Branchial (Gr. gills) Cysts, Sinuses, and Fistulae.**—Early in embryonic life, entodermal pouches pocket out from the pharynx. Simultaneously, the cervical ectoderm becomes indented (branchial grooves or clefts) over the corresponding pharyngeal pouches. As the grooves approach the pouches, the intervening mesoderm is pushed aside so that for a time the ectoderm and the entoderm are in contact. The areas in contact are the closing membranes. The series of rounded bars of mesoderm, which have been pushed aside as the clefts and pouches are approximated, are the branchial arches. In gill-bearing animals, the closing membranes disappear, resulting in a series of gill-clefts, opening from the pharynx to the exterior. Figure 176 designates the branchial clefts, pouches, and arches and their ultimate derivatives.

Sinuses with external and internal openings, cysts with no internal or external or internal openings, and fistulous tracts with external and internal openings, and dermoids, are the vestigial branchial derivatives found in the sternomastoid area.

Clinically, a branchial cyst, unless secondarily infected, is a painless fluctuant tumor located characteristically at any level in the neck along the anterior margin of the sternomastoid muscle. The cyst extends under it to the deeper structures. Only complete surgical removal under general anesthesia will effect a cure. Injection of methylene blue helps greatly to locate the extent of the process.

9. **Presternomastoid Esophagotomy Approach.**—An incision anterior to the sternocleidomastoid muscle is made on the left side between the thyroid cartilage and the sternoclavicular joint. By retracting the sternocleidomastoid muscle laterally, the carotid sheath is exposed. The layer of infrahyoid muscles must be cut across to allow access to the cleft between the carotid sheath and the visceral mass of the trachea and thyroid At the depth of this cleft is the esophagus, which bulges to the left of the median line and lateral to the trachea. About a fingerbreadth below the cricoid cartilage, or at the level of the carotid tubercle, the inferior thyroid artery, flanked by its veins, crosses the esophagus. These, with the recurrent nerve and the overlying thyroid gland and trachea, must be retracted. The esophagus then can be drawn into the wound.

B. SUPRACLAVICULAR REGION OR FOSSA, OR POSTERIOR CERVICAL TRIANGLE

1. **Definition, Boundaries, and Superficial Structures.**—The supraclavicular fossa or posterior cervical triangle is a depressible space located above the middle third of the clavicle; its base rests upon the dome of the pleura. It corresponds to the area embraced by the posterior margin of the sternocleidomastoid muscle, the middle third of the clavicle, and the anterior edge of the trapezius. Its width and depth vary with the muscular development of the individual. The fossa is in broad communication with the sternomastoid, mediastinal, and axillary regions, which may be invaded by infections or tumors originating supraclavicularly. The upper part of the area is exposed in the removal of the superior group of deep cervical lymph glands. Its lower or deeper portion is of great surgical importance since it forms a communicating region between the root of the neck and the axillary and mediastinal areas. The supraclavicular region is exposed in operations upon the inferior group of deep cervical lymph nodes, in procedures directed toward lesions of the subclavian vessels, or of the brachial plexus, and in the removal of cervical ribs, which lie in intimate contact with the pleural dome. The nerve trunks are grouped about the lateral angle of the posterior triangle, while the vessels are deep and mesial.

The inferior portion of the region is covered by the platysma. Of the vessels piercing the platysma, only the external jugular vein is of surgical importance. It runs vertically over the sternocleidomastoid muscle to empty into the subclavian vein in the mesial angle of the base of the fossa (Fig. 191). The posterior belly of the omohyoid muscle swings across the fossa to the scapula, dividing it into a larger, superior, and lateral *omotrapezius area*, and a smaller, inferior, and medial *omoclavicular area*.

2. **Anterior and Posterior Walls of the Fossa.**—The investing layer of the deep cervical fascia divides to enclose the trapezius and sternocleidomastoid muscles. The intervening layer of enveloping fascia or the *anterior wall* of the fossa is a fairly loose aponeurosis which passes over, and is adherent to, the clavicle and extends into the thoracic region as the pectoral fascia. The pretracheal fascia sheathes the posterior belly of the omohyoid muscle and covers the lower part of the region deep to the enveloping fascia. The two fascial planes are separated by areolar tissue. The pretracheal layer can be traced downward behind the clavicle and the subclavius muscle, to both of which it adheres.

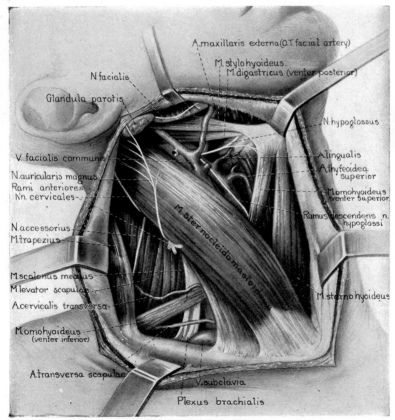

FIG. 199.—STRUCTURES OF THE LATERAL REGION OF THE NECK WITH THE STERNOCLEIDOMASTOID MUSCLE IN SITU.

It forms the outer fibrous investment for the subclavian vein. When the omohyoid muscle has close connections with the clavicle, the pretracheal fascia is limited in extent and the omoclavicular triangle is smaller.

The *posterior wall* or floor of the fossa is composed of groups of muscles which extend downward and outward from the cervical column. The scalenus medius and posterior muscles, although fused in their upper portions, form most of the anterior portion of the floor of the triangle, and are attached to the first and second ribs. The subclavian artery and the trunks of the brachial plexus, as they emerge from the cleft between the anterior and middle scalene muscles, lie on the floor of the triangle.

The anterior scalene muscle, normally completely covered by the sternocleidomastoid muscle, is exposed in operations within the supraclavicular region when the sternocleido-

mastoid is retracted mesially. The anterior scalene muscle arises from the transverse
processes of the third, fourth, fifth, and sixth cervical vertebrae and runs downward and
laterally to insert on the scalene tubercle and ridge, and on the medial margin of the first

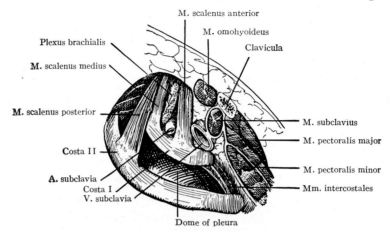

Fig. 200.—Apex of the Right Side of the Thorax Showing the Relations of the Subclavian
Artery and Vein to the Anterior Scalene Muscle and to the Apex of the Right Lung. (After
Corning.)

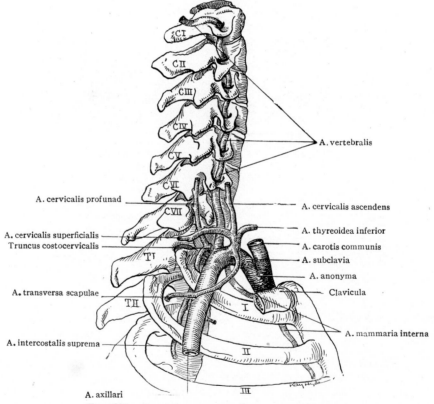

Fig. 201.—Branches of the Subclavian Artery.

rib. All of the muscles of the floor of the supraclavicular fossa are covered by prevertebral
fascia. The subclavian vein lies between the anterior scalene muscle and the clavicle, and
grooves the upper portion of the first rib. Behind this muscle lie the subclavian artery
and the large nerve trunks of the brachial plexus.

3. **Vessels of the Supraclavicular Fossa.**—The important structures within the supra-clavicular fossa are the vessels and nerves which cross the root of the neck, traverse the axilla, and supply the upper extremity. The lymph glands of the fossa establish communication between the axilla and the superficial and deep cervical glands.

The *right subclavian artery* branches from the innominate artery at a point deep to the right sternoclavicular joint, while the *left subclavian artery* branches directly from the aortic arch. From their points of cervical entry, both arteries arch laterally across the root of the neck from behind forward and from within outward, grooving the pleural dome. The height reached by the summit of the arch varies, the average being about 1 cm. above the sternal portion of the clavicle with the individual standing erect. The curve may be higher and more arched in those with slender necks and sloping shoulders,

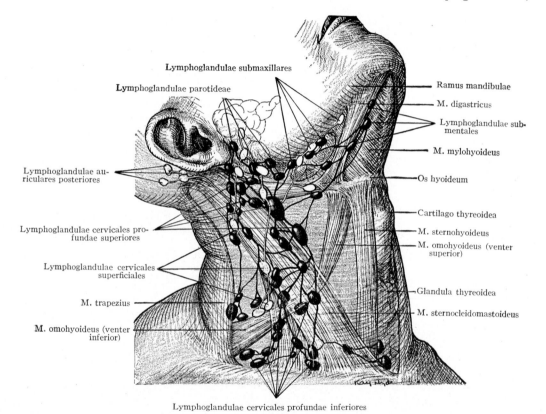

Lymphoglandulae submaxillares

Lymphoglandulae parotideae

Ramus mandibulae

M. digastricus

Lymphoglandulae sub-mentales

M. mylohyoideus

Lymphoglandulae au-riculares posteriores

Os hyoideum

Cartilago thyreoidea

Lymphoglandulae cervicales pro-fundae superiores

M. sternohyoideus

M. omohyoideus (venter superior)

Lymphoglandulae cervicales superficiales

Glandula thyreoidea

M. sternocleidomastoideus

M. trapezius

M. omohyoideus (venter inferior)

Lymphoglandulae cervicales profundae inferiores

FIG. 202.—SURFACE ANATOMY OF THE LATERAL REGION OF THE NECK SHOWING THE DISTRIBUTION OF THE SUPERFICIAL AND DEEP CERVICAL LYMPH GLANDS.

and scarcely exceed the upper margin of the clavicle in short-necked individuals. When a cervical rib is present, it is overlain by the artery, the expansile pulsations of which may be mistaken for a subclavian aneurysm.

Each artery, in its arched course, has three divisions, described with reference to its position, mesial, posterior, or lateral to the anterior scalene muscle. The third portion of the artery belongs definitely to the supraclavicular region and is relatively superficial. As the vessel descends behind the middle portion of the clavicle and lateral to the first rib, it becomes the axillary artery (p. 561).

Dorsally and laterally, the trunks of the brachial plexus are in relation to the sub-clavian artery, and accompany it to the apex of the axilla. Anteriorly, the artery is covered by the subclavian vein, which occupies the space between the anterior scalene muscle and the clavicle. Relations between the clavicle and artery vary considerably. When

14

the shoulder is elevated, the clavicle encroaches on the supraclavicular fossa and hides the artery in the deep recess formed behind the bone. When the shoulder is depressed, the fossa is largest and the artery is most superficial, so that pulsations sometimes are detected in the mesial angle.

Although well protected in the medial portion of its course by the overlying sterno-cleidomastoid muscle and the inner end of the clavicle, the subclavian artery is liable to injury by penetrating wounds in the lower neck region. The trunks of the brachial plexus, because of their proximity to the vessel, may be injured at the same time. The relationship of the pleura with the first and second portions of the artery must be borne in mind in ligating the artery. Circulation of the vessel may be controlled by firm pressure against the first rib. Tumors located deeply in the supraclavicular fossa so overlie the pleura that it may be torn easily in removing them.

The two branches of the subclavian artery in the supraclavicuar fossa are the transverse scapular and transverse cevrical, which, with the inferior thyroid artery, form the thyreocervical trunk (thyroid axis).

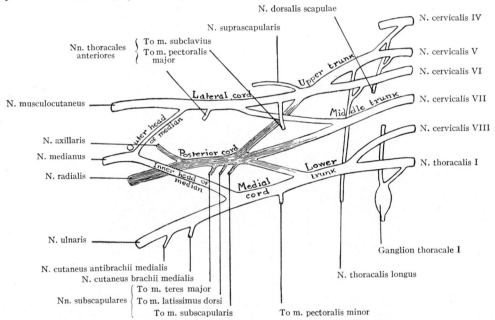

FIG. 203.—ANTERIOR PRIMARY DIVISIONS, TRUNKS, CORDS, AND TERMINALS OF THE BRACHIAL PLEXUS.
(After Tinel.)

The *subclavian vein* is the direct continuation of the axillary or main vein of the upper extremity, and is so named at the lateral margin of the first rib. Through its tributary, the external jugular, it collects blood from the head and neck. It runs mesially, a little below and in front of the corresponding artery, separated from it by the lower part of the anterior scalene muscle. More laterally, it is in relation with the subclavius muscle, which is applied to the inferior surface of the clavicle.

The *supra-omohyoid* and *infra-omohyoid groups* of *lymph glands* are continuous with the upper deep cervical glands of the sternomastoid region. These nodes drain the posterior scalp and the nuchal, pectoral, deltoid, and axillary regions. The relations of the nodes to the thoracic and right lymphatic ducts explain the gland involvement in visceral disease. The easily invaded, cellular tissue is in broad communication with the parotid, sternomastoid, and axillary regions, and with the mediastinum. The *right lymphatic duct*, not always present as a single trunk, drains the lymph from the right half of the supradiaphragmatic area of the body. The *thoracic duct* collects the lymph from the entire subdiaphragmatic portion of the body, as well as from the left half of the supradiaphragmatic area. From the mediastinum it runs forward and outward in an arched course to terminate in the confluence of the subclavian and left internal jugular veins. The arch of the duct lies above and crosses the subclavian artery. Injury to the duct in supraclavicular lymph gland dissection is accompanied by abundant lymphorrhea.

4. **Brachial Plexus.**—The individual nerves which make up the brachial plexus are the **anterior roots** or **primary divisions** of the fifth, sixth, seventh, and eighth cervical and first thoracic spinal nerves, with occasional twigs from the fourth cervical and second thoracic nerves. These roots emerge through the slitlike interval between the anterior and middle scalene muscles, and appear in the lower part of the posterior triangle of the neck.

On the middle scalene muscle, the anterior primary divisions unite to form **trunks.** Those of the fifth and sixth cervical nerves form the *upper trunk;* that of the seventh continues laterally alone as the *middle trunk;* and those of the eighth cervical and first thoracic nerves form the *lower trunk.* Each of the trunks continues undivided to a point just beyond the lateral margin of the anterior scalene muscle.

As these branches pass downward and laterally behind the clavicle, they are assembled in compact bundles or **cords,** which are named with reference to their location about the axillary artery. The anterior divisions of the upper and middle trunks constitute the *lateral*

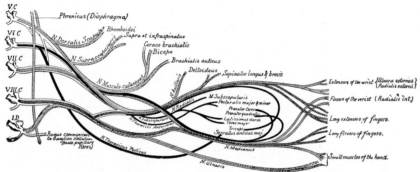

FIG. 204.—DIAGRAM OF THE BRACHIAL PLEXUS. (Kocher.)
Nerves to the muscles of the upper extremity are indicated.

cord; those of the lower trunk form the *medial cord.* The posterior divisions of the three trunks constitute the *posterior cord.* Before the cords divide to be distributed to the upper extremity, they form several important nerves. From the lateral cord, the lateral anterior thoracic nerve is given off to the pectorals; from the posterior cord are given off the subscapular nerves; and from the medial cord, the medial antibrachial, medial brachial cutaneous, and medial anterior thoracic (pectoral) nerves.

The cords then supply **terminals** to the extremity. The lateral cord divides into the *musculocutaneous* and the lateral head of the *median* nerve. The medial cord, after forming the medial head of the median nerve, continues as the *ulnar* nerve. The posterior cord, after giving off the subscapularis and axillary nerves, continues as the *radial* (musculospiral) nerve.

Trauma in the supraclavicular region may contuse, compress, or lacerate different portions of the plexus. The subclavian artery and vein, located distally and close to the clavicle, usually escape. Injuries in the region of the scaleni involve the roots of the plexus. Trauma within the confines of the supraclavicular fossa involves the trunks: injuries behind the clavicle and in the upper axilla involve the cords. Compression of the trunks and cords may be caused by tumors or aneurysm formation; they may be injured by a fractured clavicle.

5. **Skeletal Structures.**—The skeletal structures in the region are the clavicle and the first rib. The clavicle and scapula form the shoulder girdle, which suspends the upper

extremity and maintains it at a uniform functioning distance from the trunk. The *clavicle* has two curves, a medial with a convexity forward, and a lateral with a concavity forward. The longer medial curve presents important relations inferiorly and posteriorly with the subclavian vessels and with the cords and terminal nerves of the brachial plexus, being separated from them only by the subclavius muscle and its embracing sheath from the axilla. The lateral curve overlies the coracoid process, with which it is connected through the coracoclavicular ligaments.

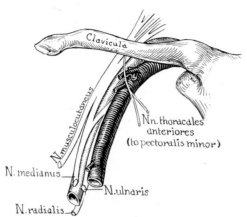

FIG. 205.—VASCULAR RELATIONS OF THE BRACHIAL PLEXUS BEHIND THE CLAVICLE AND IN THE AXILLA. (After Tinel.)

The sternal extremity of the clavicle has posterior relations with the innominate vein. On the right side, it is related to the bifurcation of the innominate artery, and on the left to the common carotid artery. On both sides, the sternohyoid and sternothyroid muscles separate the bone from these vessels. The sternal head of the sternocleidomastoid muscle overlies the clavicle in front. The shaft of the bone is superficial throughout.

The *body of the first rib* is placed so that its superior surface is almost flat. In its middle portion, it presents two transverse grooves, a posterior groove, through which courses the subclavian artery, and one just anterior to it, through which runs the corresponding vein. Between the two is the scalene tubercle for the attachment of the anterior scalene muscle.

SURGICAL CONSIDERATIONS

1. Cervical Rib and the Scalenus Anticus Syndrome.—The congenital anomaly of supernumerary ribs usually occurs in the cervical region, although occasionally in the lumbar. It seldom is discovered unless it causes symptoms, or unless attention is directed to the region in study or observation of other conditions. While supernumerary ribs are small and of little practical importance in the lumbar region, those in the cervical region may be of considerable importance.

A cervical rib attached to the transverse process and body of the seventh cervical vertebra may vary in size from a simple exostosis to a fully formed rib, and may be unilateral or bilateral. When very small, it may present a free ventral extremity or may be joined to the first thoracic rib by a fibrous attachment. When the rib is more than 5 cm. long, it displaces the subclavian artery and the brachial plexus upward. The anterior extremity of the rib, in a rare instance, may reach the sternum, but usually it articulates or fuses with the first (thoracic) rib. Since the chest is lengthened by one rib, there is a higher arch and a sharper curve in the subclavian artery. With the arch of the subclavian artery well up into the soft parts of the neck and above the clavicle, it runs greater risk of injury from trauma. The pulsation of an abnormally high subclavian artery may suggest the diagnosis of aneurysm; aneurysm of the axillary artery has been observed frequently in patients with cervical ribs.

Unless the rib is well developed, it is too short to support the artery, and may be crossed only by the lower trunk of the brachial plexus. The most frequent results of the anomaly are the nerve phenomena referable to the hand and arm, a consequency of pressure on roots of the brachial plexus. Neuritic symptoms of involvement of the lower trunk (C_8 and T_1) manifest themselves as pains running down the ulnar side of the arm and forearm, the areas supplied by the roots involved. Progressive paresis and wasting occur in the intrinsic hand muscles, and trophic changes in the arm accompany the atrophy and loss of power which correspond to the areas of anesthesia. Upward pressure on the

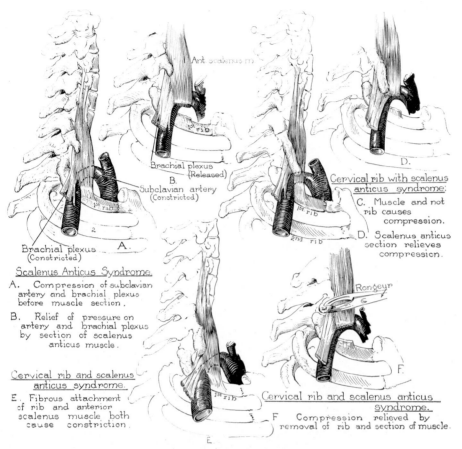

Ant. scalenus m

Brachial plexus
(Released)

B.

Subclavian artery
(Constricted)

Brachial plexus
(Constricted)   A.

D.

Cervical rib with scalenus
anticus syndrome.

C. Muscle and not
rib causes
compression.

D. Scalenus anticus
section relieves
compression.

Scalenus Anticus Syndrome.

A.   Compression of subclavian
artery and brachial plexus
before muscle section.

B.   Relief of pressure on
artery and brachial plexus
by section of scalenus
anticus muscle.

Rongeur

Cervical rib and scalenus
anticus syndrome.

E. Fibrous attachment
of rib and anterior
scalenus muscle both
cause constriction.

F.

Cervical rib and scalenus anticus
syndrome.

F   Compression relieved by
removal of rib and section of muscle.

Fig. 206.—Cervical Rib and the Scalenus Anticus Syndrome.   (Modified from Adson and Coffey.)

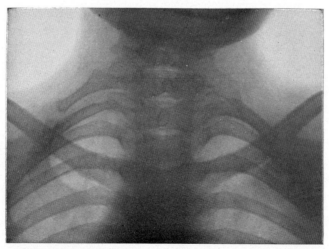

Fig. 207.—Cervical Rib on the Left Side.   (Andrews.)

artery may cause compression to the degree that pulsation at the wrist is absent and the limb becomes anemic.   If the collateral circulation proves inadequate, gangrene may occur in the fingers.

When the same symptoms are present and cervical ribs cannot be demonstrated, the clinical condition known as the *scalenus anticus syndrome* has been suggested. In this condition, the anterior scalene muscle compresses the subclavian artery and the brachial plexus against the first rib, or against the fibrous prolongation of a cervical rib when the rib itself causes no trouble. This muscle may produce an abnormal lift to the first rib and thereby cause upward compression of the subclavian artery and the brachial plexus. Excessive muscular development of the scalenus anticus in a young adult, or the sagging of the shoulder girdle in an older person, may cause this syndrome. High fixation of the sternum and ribs, low origin of the brachial plexus, or elevation of the first thoracic rib from spasm of the anterior scalene muscle may produce the same symptom-complex.

Cervical ribs causing pressure require removal. The whole area may be exposed widely by a curvilinear incision passing vertically down the posterior margin of the sternocleido-mastoid muscle and extending laterally along the clavicle. The brachial plexus and subclavian artery are displaced forward and the middle scalene muscle is separated from the under surface of the rib; care is taken to avoid injury to the pleura. The rib is divided as close as possible to its vertebral extremity. In the presence of a cervical rib without tendinous attachments, and without obvious pressure from behind, the condition may be alleviated by separating the tendon of the anterior scalene muscle from its attachment to the first rib or to the cervical rib or its anterior fibrous termination. In this way, the subclavian artery and whatever nerve elements of the brachial plexus are caught between the tendon and bony parts are able to free themselves by sliding downward and forward (Adson, Coffey).

2. **Lesions of the Brachial Plexus in General.**—The brachial plexus or any of its parts may be injured directly in penetrating wounds, by compression from a bony callus, foreign body, scarred fibrous mass, or simple hematoma in the supraclavicular or axillary fossa. The plexus may be injured extensively by upward or downward traction on the extremity or downward pressure on the shoulder, with or without dislocation. Injury may involve the roots, trunks, cords, or their branches, resulting in a great variety of clinical pictures. The cervical nerves divide almost immediately after their formation into anterior and posterior primary divisions. The posterior primary or dorsal division supplies not only the dorsal axial musculature but also the skin over the region of the back. Therefore, a lesion just outside the spinal canal shows, in addition to other signs of injury, an area of anesthesia to all forms of sensation over the region of the back supplied by the primary dorsal division affected. In an injury lateral to the primary division of the spinal nerve, the dorsal division escapes and anesthesia is not produced.

3. **Erb-Duchenne or Upper Arm Type of Paralysis.**—Paralysis from injury to the upper trunk of the brachial plexus is known as Erb-Duchenne or upper arm palsy. The fifth, and to a lesser extent, the sixth cervical nerves are involved. The injury commonly results from downward traction on the shoulder in complicated delivery. The pull tears the upper trunk proximal to the origin of the suprascapular nerve, but distal to the origins of the long thoracic nerve (of Bell) and dorsal scapular nerve (to the rhomboids). The deltoid, supraspinatus, infraspinatus, and teres minor, innervated by the suprascapular and axillary nerves, are paralyzed, and the arm is rotated mesially by the latissimus dorsi $(C_{6, 7, 8})$ and the sternal head of the pectoralis major, the latter because of its supply from the anterior primary branches of C_8 and T_1. The biceps and brachioradialis muscles are paralyzed and the forearm is pronated by the pronator quadratus $(C_{7, 8}, T_1)$, the pronator teres being supplied by C_6. Since the arm is fully pronated, the extensor digitorum communis and extensor carpi ulnaris muscles $(C_{6, 7, 8})$ may be able to produce slight flexion at the elbow.

When the lesion is confined to the anterior primary division of C_5, no sensory changes can be noted, since this nerve is not responsible for the exclusive supply of any definite area of skin. If C_6 also is involved, there usually is some loss of sensation on the outer aspect of the arm and forearm.

In treating such conditions, the paralyzed muscles must be relaxed, lest they become overstretched by the unopposed action of the unparalyzed antagonistic muscles. To accomplish relaxation and correct deformity, three postures of the arm must be maintained: abduction, lateral rotation, and flexion.

4. **Klumpke or Lower Arm Type of Paralysis.**—Klumpke or lower arm paralysis is the result of upward traction on the shoulder. It may be sustained in falling from a high place and seizing something to break the fall, or may occur in a breech presentation when the arms are carried over the head. The first thoracic spinal nerve is the one usually involved, but the whole lower trunk (C_8, T_1) may be torn across. Since the intrinsic muscles of the hand supplied by the ulnar nerve are paralyzed, a clawhand develops. In a clawhand, the fingers are hyperextended at the metacarpophalangeal joints and are flexed at the interphalangeal joints. Should all the lower trunk be affected, the flexor and extensor muscles of the fingers also are paralyzed. There is diminution of sensation over the mesial side of the arm, forearm, and hand.

5. **Injuries to Cords of the Plexus.**—The *medial cord* may be stretched or torn in subcoracoid dislocation of the head of the humerus or in rough methods of reduction of the dislocation. After such an injury, sensory changes are found in the domain of the cutaneous nerves of ulnar and median derivation. The muscles supplied by the medial cord are paralyzed. They are: the intrinsic muscles of the hand supplied by the ulnar nerve and the medial head of the median nerve, the flexor carpi ulnaris muscle, and the part of the flexor digitorum profundus muscle supplied by the ulnar nerve.

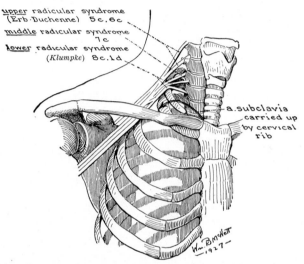

FIG. 208.—TYPES OF BRACHIAL PALSY. (Babcock.)

Upper radicular or Erb-Duchenne syndrome, middle radicular syndrome, and lower radicular or Klumpke syndrome. Effects of a cervical rib are shown.

When the *lateral cord* is injured, the muscles supplied by the musculocutaneous nerve, the biceps, coracobrachialis, and brachialis (anticus), are paralyzed partially. There is paralysis of the superficial and deep muscles of the anterior forearm, supplied by the lateral head of the median nerve. Partial loss of epicritic sensation exists in the areas supplied by the musculocutaneous and median nerves.

IV. THORACOCERVICAL REGION, "ROOT OF THE NECK"

1. **Definition and Boundaries.**—The thoracocervical region or the root of the neck forms a boundary between the neck and the thorax. The area adjoins the thoracic inlet and is occupied mainly by structures which enter and emerge from the thoracic cavity. It affords an approach in the operative treatment of innominate and subclavian aneurysms. To be considered here are: the inner extremity of the clavicle, the manubrium of the sternum, the sternoclavicular joint, and the subclavian vessels in their first and second portions.

2. **Suprasternal Fossa.**—A duplication of the enveloping fascia of the neck forms a triangular cavity above the manubrium (p. 167 and Fig. 296).

3. **Innominate and Subclavian Veins.**—When the sternothyroid and sternohyoid muscles, with their investing pretracheal fascia and the overlying enveloping fascia, are divided at their sternal attachments and reflected upward, the large vascular trunks at

the root of the neck are exposed. The terminal portions of the subclavian and internal jugular veins and their junction conceal most of the deeper structures. The innominate veins join opposite the first costal cartilage on the right to form the superior vena cava. To reach this point, the left vein passes behind the manubrium of the sternum; it is three times as long as the right vein.

The *right innominate vein* lies deep to the inner end of the right clavicle, from which it is separated by the attachments of the sternohyoid and sternothyroid muscles. It is in relation with the mesial surface of the right pleura and partly overlies the innominate artery. It runs downward almost vertically into the superior vena cava.

The *left innominate vein* passes from left to right and a little downward behind the upper part of the manubrium to the lower margin of the first right cartilage, where it terminates in the superior vena cava. It is covered in front by the left sternoclavicular joint, and on the right is overlapped slightly by the right pleura. The remains of the thymus lie between it and the sternum. It is on a level with, or slightly above, the upper margin of the manubrium. It may be endangered during a low thyroidectomy, a low tracheotomy, or in the removal of a tumor in the root of the neck.

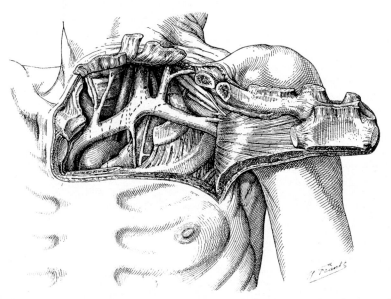

Fig. 209.—Thoracocervical Region After Retracting a Sternoclavicular Flap to Expose the Great Vessels in the Root of the Neck and in the Anterior Mediastinum. (Sencert.)

The *subclavian vein* on each side is a direct continuation of the axillary vein. At the junction of the clavicle and sternum, the subclavian unites with the internal jugular vein to form the innominate. Through its tributary, the external jugular vein, it receives blood from the head and neck. The subclavian vein begins at the outer border of the first rib and runs mesially, almost transversely, behind the clavicle. It lies in front of the subclavian artery, which it accompanies in its course, save where separated from the artery by the anterior scalene muscle. A penetrating wound may injure both vessels at any point along their course, and cause the formation of an arteriovenous fistula. The vein in its outer course has an anterior relation with the subclavian muscle, its anterior wall being united to the fascia which clothes that muscle.

Since the subclavian vein occupies the acute angle between the clavicle and the first rib and has slight resistance, it suffers compression from any outgrowth from these bones. In fracture, the interposed subclavian muscle protects the subclavian vein and artery and the brachial plexus. The connection of the vein with the fascia of the subclavian muscle and with the pretracheal fascia increases or maintains its caliber during inspiration. Elevation of the arm has a similar action, which fact should be remembered in the event of injury to the vein during operation, since elevation of the clavicle widens the rent. The internal jugular and subclavian veins unite in an acute angle which opens laterally. In the apex of the angle on the right, the external jugular vein and right lymphatic duct open into the subclavian vein. In the apex on the left, the external jugular vein and thoracic duct (p. 201) open into the subclavian vein.

4. First and Second Portions of the Subclavian Artery.—On the right side, the subclavian artery arises from the innominate artery posterior to the sternoclavicular joint; on the left, it arises from the aortic arch posterior to the upper half of the manubrium. It occupies not only the root of the neck, but also the superior mediastinum. As the subclavian artery turns laterally (*first portion*), it lies behind the beginning of the left innominate vein. The thoracic duct arches over it, and behind it lie the apex of the pleural sac and the lung. Ligation of the first portion is much more difficult on the left than on the right.

The *second* or *retroscalene portion* of the artery is located in the triangular space between the anterior and middle scalene muscles, the base or floor of the area corresponding to the first rib. Above and lateral to it are the trunks of the brachial plexus. To uncover the artery in this position, the anterior scalene muscle must be sectioned. On account of the presence of the phrenic nerve on its medial border, the section of the anterior scalene muscle cannot be complete; it can involve only the outer portion.

Aneurysm of the subclavian artery, as a rule, involves the *third* or *extrascalene portion* and appears as a swelling in the posterior triangle of the neck just above the clavicle. As it increases in size, it may fill the entire supraclavicular space and cause pressure phenomena of the brachial nerves, with motor and sensory disturbances over their respective areas of distribution. Edema of the upper extremity may occur as a consequence of pressure of the aneurysm against the subclavian vein, interfering with the venous return. The deep location and relations of the first portion of the subclavian artery and its numerous, closely grouped, large branches are sufficient to show that its ligation for subclavian aneurysm must be attended by considerable difficulty and some danger.

The large and important *vertebral artery* is the first branch from the subclavian and arises from the upper and posterior part of the first portion (p. 192). The *thyreocervical trunk* (p. 192) is the next large division arising from the first portion of the subclavian artery. The *internal mammary* is given off from the lower border of the first portion of the subclavian artery, inclines downward, forward, and inward behind the clavicle, and enters the thorax behind the first costal cartilage. The *costocervical trunk* (superior intercostal artery) branches from the posterior aspect of the second portion of the subclavian artery on the right and from the first part on the left. It courses upward and backward over the dome of the pleura to the neck of the first rib. This artery, which supplies the first and occasionally the second intercostal space, brings into the subclavian and axillary circulation an anastomosis with the whole intercostal (descending aorta) circulation.

To ligate the subclavian artery in its first or second portions, the inferior attachments of the sternocleidomastoid, sternothyroid, and sternohyoid muscles are severed and reflected superiorly. The common carotid artery is identified and followed downward until the subclavian artery is reached. As the vagus nerve is drawn mesially, a ligature is passed around the subclavian artery, mesial to the origin of the vertebral artery, carefully avoiding the pleura. To expose the artery properly, the inner extremity of the clavicle and its associated portion of the manubrium should be resected.

THE THORAX

THORAX IN GENERAL

THE bony thoracic cage is made up of the sternum, ribs, and vertebrae, covered in front and on the sides by a thin layer of soft parts. It houses and protects the main organs of circulation and respiration, and the esophageal portion of the digestive apparatus. External violence may cause injury through the intercostal spaces which are poorly protected areas, or may overcome the resistance of the shielding ribs which then become offending factors, wounding the structures within the costal cage. The entire cage is accessible to well-planned surgical approach.

1. **Shape.**—The thorax is a truncated cone, with its smaller base (superior) at the inlet and its larger (inferior) at the diaphragm. The narrow, restricted, and more rigid inlet

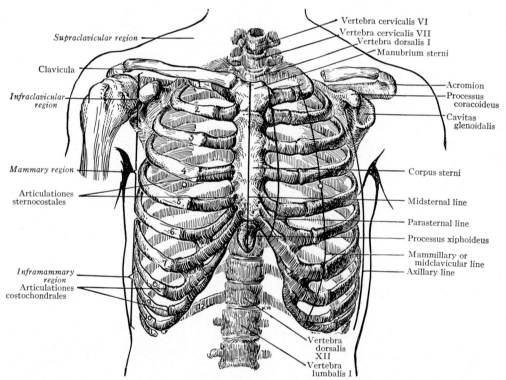

FIG. 210.—ANTERIOR VIEW OF THE BONY THORAX TO SHOW REGIONS, LANDMARKS, AND SURFACE MARKINGS.

affords ample protection to the important communicating structures between the thorax, neck, and upper extremities, but leaves little room for obstructive pathologic processes. From the inlet to the base, the thoracic cage assumes a gradually widening flare. The anterior bulge of the vertebral column makes the transverse section of the thoracic cavity kidney shaped.

Early in life, the anteroposterior and transverse diameters are about equal, making a rounded or barrel chest. In later life, the shape becomes oval owing to a widening of the transverse diameter. Any pathologic condition involving segments of the bony framework, especially if limiting its range of movement, tends to produce deformity with resulting changes in the shape and size of the cavity; to this deformity the visceral contents must

218

conform. The elasticity and freedom of movement of the ribs result from their cartilaginous attachment to the sternum and to the slight movement at the vertebral joints. Serious damage to the chest contents may occur with no injury to the bony framework.

2. **Surface Anatomy.**—The circulatory and respiratory organs are ever the object of clinical examination and surgical approach, and knowledge of their topographic relations to the chest wall is of equal importance to physician and surgeon. Over the entire thorax, the surface markings are conspicuous and readily palpable, making possible an easy comparative study of its two sides.

In examination, important muscle groups must be distinguished, and the degree of their range of motion, laxity, and rigidity must be noted with reference to disuse or par-

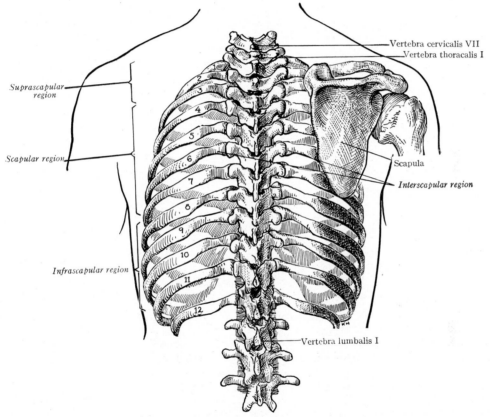

Suprascapular region

Scapular region

Infrascapular region

Vertebra cervicalis VII
Vertebra thoracalis I

Scapula

Interscapular region

Vertebra lumbalis I

FIG. 211.—POSTERIOR VIEW OF THE BONY THORAX TO SHOW THE REGIONS, LANDMARKS, AND SURFACE MARKINGS.

alysis. These groups include the spinal muscles lying in the trough between the vertebral column and the rib angles, and those to the shoulder girdle and upper arm. The crests of the angles of the ribs on either side are important markings in the study of curvatures of the spine.

Among the markings most useful for the thoracic projection of the enclosed viscera is a series of conventional *longitudinal lines* which parallel the long axis of the body. The midsternal line bisects the sternum and corresponds to the line of the midback; the midclavicular (mammary) line, dropped from the midpoint of the clavicle, usually passes somewhat mesial to the nipple; the parasternal line lies midway between the midclavicular and midsternal lines. The anterior, posterior, and midaxillary lines are dropped from the anterior and posterior axillary folds and from the middle of the axillary space, while the scapular line runs through the apex of the inferior angle of the scapula. The *sternal angle* (of Ludwig) is the anterior bulge made by the manubrium, or upper segment, with the body of the sternum.

3. Deformities.—*Rickets* sometimes presents characteristic chest markings. An anterior projection of the sternum and costal cartilages, with sinking in or depression of the costal wall at the costochondral junction, is known as *pigeon breast*. There also may be beadlike enlargements formed at the costochondral junctions, known in aggregate as *rachitic rosary*. In *funnel chest*, the inferior part of the sternum may be so sunken as almost to contact the vertebral column. The depressed sternum pulls down with it the inferior costal cartilages and rib ends.

Because of their firm vertebral attachments, the ribs are carried into deformity by functional and organic changes in the spine. Many chest deformities result from abnormal curvatures in the superior portions of the dorsal spinal column. In *kyphosis*, abnormal posterior curvature of the dorsal column, usually resulting from tuberculosis of the vertebral bodies, the superior spinal segment carries the corresponding ribs and sternum inferiorly, increasing the anteroposterior diameter of the thorax at the expense of the vertical and transverse measurements. In *scoliosis*, lateral curvature of the spine, the ribs, of necessity, follow the change in position and direction of the vertebral pedicles and laminae. Thus, the curvature is increased on the side of the spinal convexity and diminished on that of the concavity. In structural scoliosis, there is not only lateral deviation of the vertebrae, but also rotation or torsion about their longitudinal axes. The spinous processes incline toward the concavity of the curvature. On the side of the concavity, the intercostal spaces are diminished, the ribs even being approximated, while on the side of the convexity, the spaces are increased greatly. To these changes, the thoracic viscera must adapt themselves.

I. Thoracic Walls

A. Sternal Region

1. Definition, Division, and Boundaries.—The sternal region, occupying the median anterior thoracic wall, consists of the sternum with its three segments, named from above downward the *manubrium*, *body (gladiolus)*, and *xiphoid (ensiform) process*, and the clavicular and chondral attachments. The region extends superiorly to the jugular incisura (suprasternal notch), which forms the boundary between it and the infrahyoid region of the neck, and inferiorly to the epigastrium.

2. Surface Anatomy.—The superior margin of the sternum lies in the same horizontal plane as the inferior border of the body of the second thoracic vertebra, the distance separating them being about 5 cm. This is the inlet of the thorax. The junction of the manubrium and the body is a slight anterior prominence, the *angle of Ludwig*, which often can be seen and palpated, and which lies on the same plane as the body of the fifth thoracic vertebra. The *xiphisternal junction* corresponds to the level of the cartilage between the ninth and tenth thoracic vertebrae.

The sternal contour is modified by fracture, dislocation, and osteitis (tuberculous and syphilitic). The sternum is overlain by a thin musculotendinous layer derived from the decussating fibers of origin of both major pectoral muscles superiorly, and by certain mesial fibers of origin of the abdominal recti inferiorly.

3. Skeletal Layers.—The spongy and very vascular *sternum* is thickest at the upper extremity and gradually diminishes in thickness toward the xiphoid. It is developed in two lateral halves, which, in their failure to unite, leave openings or foramina in the midsternal line, through which extrasternal infection may extend into the mediastinum.

The *sternoclavicular joints* are strengthened greatly by the *interclavicular ligament* which stretches across the suprasternal space from one clavicle to the other. Free movement of the clavicle on the sternum is afforded by the double synovial joint, with its interposed articular disk. The shoulder girdles, which carry the upper extremities through their wide ranges of movement, are attached to the skeleton only through these joints, the unusual firmness and elasticity of which are shown by the infrequency of their dislocation and the exceedingly common occurrence of fracture of the clavicle. When the reinforcing ligaments are torn in exaggerated movements of the shoulder or by severe trauma, *dislocation* of the *inner end* of the *clavicle* occurs. The anterior variety of dislocation is the more usual, and does no harm to the great vessels which normally lie behind the joint.

The superior seven pairs of costal cartilages extend to the lateral margins of the sternum where they form *sternocostal joints*. Each joint is enclosed and reinforced by broad anterior and posterior sternocostal ligaments.

4. **Fractures and Infection.**—Fracture of the sternum is rare, but, when present, occurs most frequently at the manubriogladiolar joint. Here the bone is thinnest and the skeletal attachments are most rigid. Fortunately, however, the ligamentous coverings protect the fragments so that compound injury is rare and laceration of the mediastinal

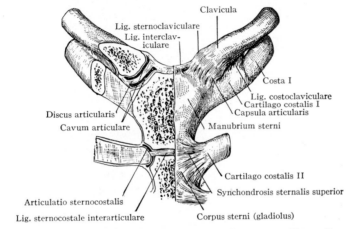

Fig. 212.—Sternoclavicular and Sternocostal Joints and Their Ligaments.

contents ordinarily is prevented. Advancing age, bringing complete ossification of the sternal pieces as well as of the costal cartilages, predisposes to fracture. The relatively superficial position and cancellous structure of the sternum expose it to trauma and infection. Syphilis and tuberculosis are relatively common.

B. COSTAL REGION

1. **Definition and Boundaries.**—The costal region comprises the chest wall between the sternum and the vertebral column, and extends in depth to the parietal pleura. Among the extrinsic structures, the breast is of sufficient importance to merit a description under its own heading (p. 227).

2. **Surface Anatomy.**—The rib cage is covered by much of the shoulder girdle and its connecting musculature. In the inferior and lateral portions of the region, the digitations of the serratus muscles can be palpated. Examination for fractured or diseased ribs begins with the second rib, because it lies opposite the sternal angle of Ludwig, which is easy to determine, whereas the first, being tucked behind the inner extremity of the clavicle, is difficult to make out.

The *intercostal spaces* are wider in the anterior and superior portions of the chest than elsewhere, and their breadth is modified considerably in the movements of flexion and extension. Posteriorly, the intercostal vessels occupy a protected position in front of the ribs; they lie protected in their respective grooves in the inferior rib borders. Anteriorly, these vessels lie exposed in the intercostal spaces.

3. **Extrinsic Musculature.**—The pectoralis major and minor and the serratus anterior

(magnus) form the extrinsic muscles on the anterior and lateral walls of the chest. The fan-shaped *pectoralis major*, of clavicular, sternocostal, and abdominal origin, converges toward the proximal extremity of the arm where it inserts mainly into the lateral lip of the

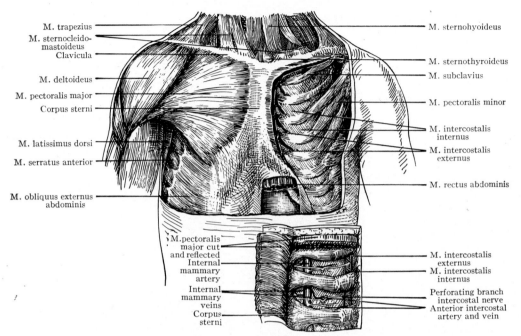

M. trapezius
M. sternocleido-mastoideus
Clavicula
M. deltoideus
M. pectoralis major
Corpus sterni
M. latissimus dorsi
M. serratus anterior
M. obliquus externus abdominis

M. sternohyoideus
M. sternothyroideus
M. subclavius
M. pectoralis minor
M. intercostalis internus
M. intercostalis externus
M. rectus abdominis

M. pectoralis major cut and reflected
Internal mammary artery
Internal mammary veins
Corpus sterni

M. intercostalis externus
M. intercostalis internus
Perforating branch intercostal nerve
Anterior intercostal artery and vein

FIG. 213.—MUSCLES OF THE ANTERIOR THORACIC WALL.
The inset shows the details of the structures in the intercostal spaces along the sternum.

intertubercular sulcus of the humerus. This muscle forms the anterior wall and fold of the axilla. The *pectoralis minor* is a thin, triangular muscle at the superior portion of the thorax under the pectoralis major. It arises from the third, fourth, and fifth ribs near

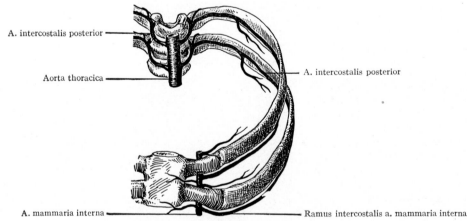

A. intercostalis posterior
Aorta thoracica
A. mammaria interna

A. intercostalis posterior
Ramus intercostalis a. mammaria interna

FIG. 214.—OBLIQUE CROSS SECTION SHOWING THE RELATIONS OF THE INTERCOSTAL ARTERIES TO THE RIBS AND INTERCOSTAL SPACES.
Posterior to the axilla the arteries are protected; anterior to the axilla, they are more exposed.

their cartilages and from their intercostal aponeuroses. The fibers insert into the coracoid process of the scapula. The nerve supply to both pectorals is from the anterior thoracic nerves ($C_{5, 6, 7, 8}, T_1$).

The *serratus anterior* (*magnus*) (long thoracic nerve, $C_{5, 6, 7}$) occupies the side of the chest and medial wall of the axilla. It is inserted mainly into the vertebral margin of the scapula. Contraction of this muscle draws the scapula forward on the chest wall. In beginning abduction of the humerus, it acts in association with the trapezius as a fixation muscle, and later is an active agent in the production of this movement. The movement of thrusting, as in fencing, is produced largely by the action of this muscle. It is the boxer's muscle, being the motive force in a forward punch. When the serratus is paralyzed or atrophied, the scapula no longer is held against the posterior chest wall and the deformity of "winged scapula" results.

The large, triangular *trapezius muscle* (spinal accessory nerve and $C_{3, 4}$) overlies the upper part of the back. From an extensive origin along the cervical and thoracic spine, its muscle fibers converge toward the clavicle, acromion, and spine of the scapula.

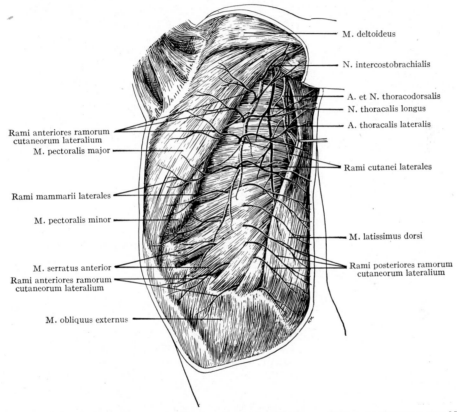

M. deltoideus

N. intercostobrachialis

A. et N. thoracodorsalis
N. thoracalis longus
A. thoracalis lateralis

Rami cutanei laterales

M. latissimus dorsi

Rami posteriores ramorum cutaneorum lateralium

Rami anteriores ramorum cutaneorum lateralium
M. pectoralis major

Rami mammarii laterales

M. pectoralis minor

M. serratus anterior
Rami anteriores ramorum cutaneorum lateralium

M. obliquus externus

FIG. 215.—LATERAL VIEW OF THE CHEST WALL TO SHOW THE EXTRINSIC MUSCLES, VESSELS, AND NERVES

The *latissimus dorsi* ($C_{6, 7, 8}$) is described in the Region of the Posterolateral Abdominal Wall (p. 312).

The *major* and *minor rhomboid muscles* (C_5) are described in the Posterior Scapular Region (p. 567).

4. **Intrinsic Musculo-osseous Structures.**—The upper seven ribs are *true* or *sternal ribs* in that they terminate directly at the sternum. The lower five are *false*, having no direct attachment to the sternum. The first three false ribs, the eighth, ninth, and tenth, are connected with the sternum through the intermedium of the cartilage of the seventh rib. The eleventh and twelfth ribs have neither direct nor indirect sternal attachment and are termed *floating ribs*.

The average width of the *intercostal spaces* is about 2 cm.; they are wider anteriorly than posteriorly and are broader between the upper ribs than between the lower ones. The

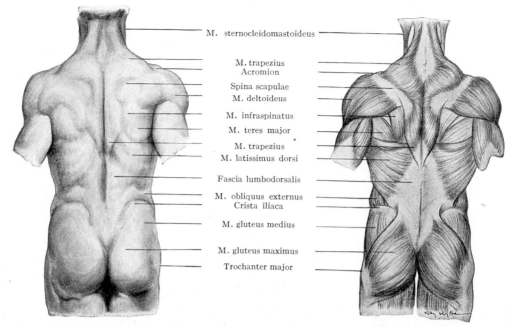

M. sternocleidomastoideus

M. trapezius
Acromion

Spina scapulae
M. deltoideus

M. infraspinatus

M. teres major

M. trapezius
M. latissimus dorsi

Fascia lumbodorsalis

M. obliquus externus
Crista iliaca

M. gluteus medius

M. gluteus maximus

Trochanter major

FIG. 216.—SURFACE ANATOMY AND MUSCULATURE OF THE BACK.   (After Richer.)

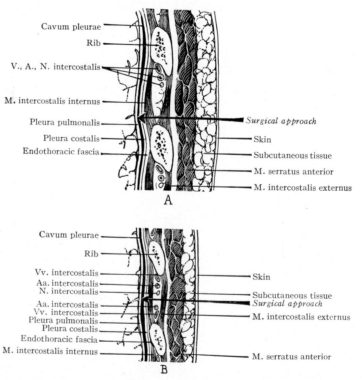

Cavum pleurae

Rib

V., A., N. intercostalis

M. intercostalis internus

Pleura pulmonalis

Pleura costalis

Endothoracic fascia

Surgical approach

Skin

Subcutaneous tissue

M. serratus anterior

M. intercostalis externus

A

Cavum pleurae

Rib

Vv. intercostalis
Aa. intercostalis
N. intercostalis

Aa. intercostalis
Vv. intercostalis
Pleura pulmonalis
Pleura costalis
Endothoracic fascia
M. intercostalis internus

Skin

Subcutaneous tissue
Surgical approach
M. intercostalis externus

M. serratus anterior

B

FIG 217.—VERTICAL SECTIONS THROUGH THE RIBS AND INTERSPACES; A, POSTERIOR TO AXILLA; B, ANTERIOR TO AXILLA.

To show the differences in the location of the intercostal vessels and nerves and the importance of these relations in intercostal thoracotomy.

spaces are occupied by the intercostal muscles, vessels, and nerves. The *intercostal muscles* are arranged in pairs, the internal and external, uniting the superior and inferior borders of adjacent ribs.

5. **Vessels and Nerves.**—Although there is an abundant vascular supply to the chest wall, there are no arteries of major size. The principal vessels are the intercostal and internal mammary arteries. The first two or three pairs of *intercostal arteries* arise from the superior intercostal branch of the costocervical trunk from the subclavian artery; the inferior nine pairs arise directly from the aorta. The location of the artery in the subcostal groove on the dorsal and dorsolateral chest wall explains the necessity of proceeding along the superior rib margin in aspiration of pleural exudates and in surgical approach through the interspaces. This bony bed and its vascular contents explain the danger of vessel injury in rib fracture.

The *internal mammary branch* of the subclavian artery passes inferiorly, anteriorly, and mesially, on the pleura. It lies behind the sternal extremity of the clavicle and descends into the chest along the lateral margin of the sternum, parallel to and about 1.25 cm. from it. At the level of the sixth intercostal space, the artery divides into a lateral branch, the *musculophrenic*, and a medial terminal branch, the *superior epigastric* (p. 280).

Injury to the internal mammary artery may result rapidly in a fatal hemorrhage. Although it can be ligated fairly readily in the first three or four intercostal spaces, it is difficult to ligate in the fourth or fifth space because of the narrowness of these intervals.

Although the cervical and brachial plexus partially supply the extrinsic musculature, the *intercostals* are the main *nerve supply* of the muscles of the chest wall. Irritation of the intercostal nerves produces symptoms of *intercostal neuralgia* which is difficult to differentiate from pleurisy.

SURGICAL CONSIDERATIONS

1. **Rib Fracture.**—Because of the curve, intrinsic elasticity, and extensive muscle attachment of the ribs, compression fracture is unusual, but may occur from severe anteroposterior compression of the chest. The break is likely to be directed outward at the apex of the main curve, and, for this reason, very rarely injures the pleura. Frequently, however, ribs are broken by direct violence, the site of fracture being at the point of injury. In such trauma, the fragments may injure the pleura and the intercostal vessels with resulting hemothorax, and, occasionally, subcutaneous emphysema.

The more exposed ribs, the fourth to the eighth, are most likely to be injured by direct violence. Fractures occur more often in adult life than in childhood, owing to the loss of elasticity incident to increasing calcification of the costal cartilages. Very little, if any, shortening or displacement occurs with fracture, because of the fixation of both extremities of the ribs and the attachment of the intercostal muscles. *Treatment* of rib fracture aims at immobilization of the injured part of the chest wall to alleviate pain and favor healing. Immobilization is effected by strapping in the general horizontal direction of the ribs.

2. **Intercostal Thoracotomy.**—Intercostal thoracotomy consists in exposure of the pleura through an intercostal space. It is a much simpler, but less satisfactory, operation than thoracotomy through the bed of one or more subperiosteally excised ribs. Closed drainage (Mazingo tube) through an intercostal thoracotomy incision is used in early cases of empyema with some success, but a more radical procedure usually is required later. The site of incision depends upon the findings of an exploratory puncture. The eighth or ninth space in the posterior scapular line is selected for incision, as it is sufficiently low to insure noninterference with the scapula and yet high enough to avoid the inadequate drainage which so frequently accompanies incision into the costophrenic sinus.

3. **Thoracotomy Through the Bed of One or More Subperiosteally Excised Ribs.**— The operation usually performed for evacuation of a purulent pleural effusion employs an incision in the bed of a rib, part of which has been excised subperiosteally. Simple rib resection contemplates the removal of part of one rib, but the unusual case demands partial excision of several. For a well-defined collection of pus, incision should be made directly

15

over the suspected area. Where fluid is free in the pleural cavity, the operative site generally chosen is the bed of the sixth and seventh ribs in the posterior or midaxillary line.

4· **Operations for Chronic Empyema in General.**—In chronic nontuberculous empyema, in which the lung is compressed and collapsed by the pressure of intrapleural fluid,

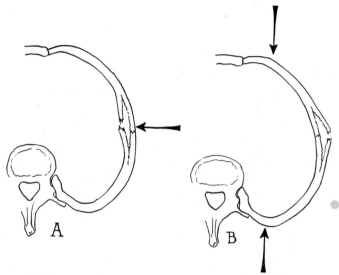

FIG. 218.—DIAGRAM OF RIB FRACTURE FOLLOWING COMPRESSION OF THE CHEST; A, LATERAL COMPRESSION; B, ANTEROPOSTERIOR COMPRESSION. (After Forgue.)

radical surgical intervention is necessary. The pleural infection causes the lung to be covered and bound down by an exudate of varying denseness and thickness. In the presence of an exudate of this kind, expansion of the lung is lost, even after evacuation of the effusion. In addition to a collapsed and restricted lung, a pleural dead space results, which is difficult to disinfect and obliterate.

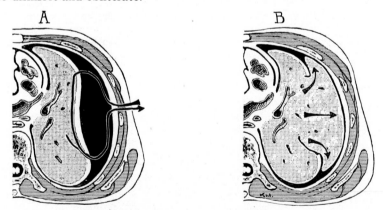

FIG. 219.—OPERATION OF PULMONARY DECORTICATION.
A, Visceral pleura being excised through an intercostal incision; B, released lung expanding to fill the chest cavity. (Modified after Testut and Jacob.)

There are two general surgical procedures which contemplate the approximation of the lung surface and the chest wall with elimination of the pus-secreting dead space. The more physiologic procedure for cases of nontuberculous empyema is *pulmonary decortication*, which endeavors to mobilize the lung, imprisoned against the mediastinum by dense plastic exudate. This operation is performed through a major thoracotomy exposure, and the layers of organized exudate gathered on the visceral pleura are freed by multiple incisions or are detached. When this layer has been freed sufficiently, the lungs gradually expand and fill the pleural cavity. The other procedure consists of subperiosteal removal of a sufficient number of ribs close enough to the vertebral column to permit the chest wall to fall in and meet the collapsed lung. This operation of *thoracoplasty* has a vogue at present in cases of advanced pulmonary tuberculosis in which all other attempts to immobilize the affected lung have failed, and intrapleural manipulation is contraindicated.

A   B

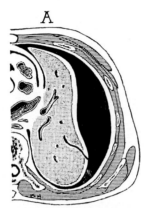 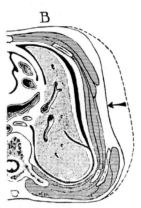

FIG. 220.—PRINCIPLES UNDERLYING THORACOPLASTY.

A, Large dead space exists between the thickened layers of visceral and parietal pleura; B, resection of a number of ribs allows the chest wall to fall in and obliterate the dead space. (Modified from Testut and Jacob.)

5. **Infection of the Ribs.**—Tuberculosis and typhoid fever sometimes cause osteitis in the ribs, and syphilis may cause periostitis. Localization here may be the result of repeated traumatism to which the ribs are exposed because of their subcutaneous position. Following rib resection for empyema, there may occur osteitis of the rib ends with infection traveling in the intercostal muscle planes.

C. BREAST OR MAMMARY REGION

The breast consists embryologically and morphologically of a group of exceedingly highly specialized cutaneous glands and, therefore, is a constituent element of the superficial layers of the costal region. Its function in the female, the frequency of breast lesions, and the importance of the lymphatic extension in the latter warrant special consideration.

1. **Definition and Boundaries.**—The mammary gland, with its fibrous and fatty tissue, occupies the interval between the third and seventh ribs, and extends in breadth from the parasternal to the midaxillary line. Surgically, the region extends in depth through the major and minor pectorals to the intercostal musculature, since lymphatic extension pervades these muscles. The glandular tissue rests in great part upon the pectoral fascia, and to a lesser degree upon the serratus anterior muscle. Very often breast tissue extends into the anterior axillary fold. This axillary prolongation may be visible as a definite mass simulating an axillary tumor or may be the seat of either benign or malignant tumors.

2. **Surface Anatomy.**—The shape and degree of development of the breast vary with the individual, the period of function, and age. The glandular portion in the male usually remains undeveloped and there is little surrounding adipose tissue, the result being that the male breast is flat and insignificant. The size of a breast is no true indication of its ability to secret, since fatty tissue makes up most of the bulk of the organ. The virginal breast is almost hemispherical, but is somewhat flattened above the nipple. In multiparae, the breasts become large and lax, and rarely regain their former shape and consistency. A shriveled breast indicates merely a disappearance of fat, as the gland still may be active functionally. After the menopause, much of the glandular tissue atrophies.

3. **Development and Congenital Abnormalities.**—The breast develops from invaginated ectoderm at the point where later the nipple is formed. In about the middle of fetal life, the mammary buds branch out into the superficial fascia, which condenses about the gland. By this enlargement, the mammary gland pushes aside the fatty tissue and comes to rest upon the fascia covering the underlying pectoral muscle.

In the young child, the breast structure consists almost entirely of a number of branching ducts with but little glandular tissue, the periglandular structures being connected with the skin by fibrous septa. As puberty is reached, the rudimentary gland buds grow rapidly and multiply, with resulting formation of acini and gland lobules. During pregnancy, there is a marked increase in gland development with corresponding diminution in the interglandular tissue, and the basal part of the breast comes into relationship with the subjacent pectoral muscles.

Imperfect development of the breast, evidenced by *absence of the nipple*, is an abnormality which may exist even with glands of normal development. In such instances, the

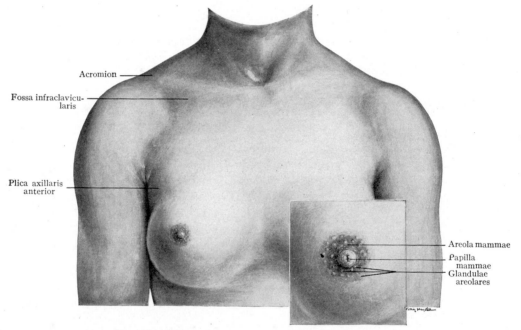

FIG. 221.—BREAST REGION IN A YOUNG ADULT FEMALE.

ducts open on a depression at the site of the nipple in the center of the areola. Defective development of the nipple commonly takes the form of excessive shortness or, though fairly well-formed, it may be surrounded by a deep fossa. Both of these defects tend to render nursing difficult.

Supernumerary breasts (*polymastia*) are of interest from the standpoint of excessive development. In certain mammalian embryos, there exists on each side of the ventral aspect of the median line a distinct ectodermic ridge which extends from the axillary region to the groin (inguino-axillary line). While there is some doubt as to whether similar epiblastic ridges are present in the human embryo, the occasional presence of supernumerary mammary glands or nipples makes their existence appear probable. Their position, when present in the human subject, appears as a rule to correspond to the direction of these lines, the most common location for a supernumerary gland being inferior and mesial to the gland, between it and the umbilicus. Four well-developed actively secreting breasts have been observed, the two extra ones being located in the axillae. Accessory breasts usually are imperfect, the nipple alone being present and in a rudimentary state, closely resembling a pigmentary spot or small nevus. A supernumerary gland rarely is present without a nipple and, when it occurs, can be explained most readily as a reversion to an ancestral type.

4. **Structure.**—The **skin** over the center of the breast is modified to form the areola and nipple. The circular *areola*, a cutaneous zone about 5 cm. in diameter, has many minute rounded elevations, indicating the presence of underlying cutaneous glands. These *areolar glands* (of Montgomery) are isolated sebaceous glands for lubrication of the nipple during lactation.

The color of the nipple and areola varies with the complexion of the individual, but in young subjects usually is rose pink. During pregnancy, the color becomes browner; the pigmentation never entirely disappears and increases slightly with each succeeding gestation. The areola may be the location of fissures, eczema, or abscess from infection in the areolar glands. The skin of the nipple is so delicate that trauma, to which it is subjected so frequently, often causes fissure-like abrasions. These openings are portals of entry for infection in the deeper glandular tissue. In nursing, pain accompanying nipple abrasion is so intense that it may be necessary to take the child from the breast.

The *nipple* or papilla mammae, a conical or wartlike elevation, is located in the middle of the areola on the approximate summit of each breast. In the young breast, the nipple usually lies opposite the fourth intercostal space, but after lactation the breast becomes

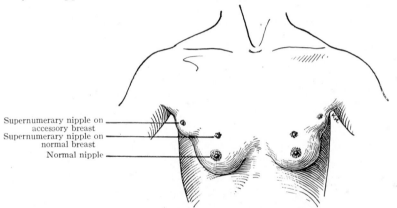

Supernumerary nipple on accessory breast
Supernumerary nipple on normal breast
Normal nipple

FIG. 222.—POLYMASTIA. (After Wiederscheim.)

pendant and the nipple no longer is a guide to intercostal spaces. By the action of the circular fibers at the base of the nipple and the longitudinal fibers attached to the lactiferous ducts, the nipple protrudes spontaneously upon touch. This phenomenon of erection, commonly attributed to the action of cavernous tissue within the nipple, probably is entirely muscular.

The nipple and the surrounding areola are supplied by a considerable network of lymphatic vessels, early involved in *Paget's disease*. This chronic, progressive lesion first appears as a keratosis of the nipple, soon followed by an itching, eczematous condition of the nipple and the surrounding skin. This extends in continuous concentric areas over most of the breast, producing a moist, indurated, partly eroded or scaling surface showing no tendency to heal. It is related to, and followed almost invariably by, carcinoma.

Beneath the skin is the areolo-fatty **subcutaneous tissue,** within which lie the glandular elements of the breast. The superficial fascia forms not only a general covering for the secreting apparatus, but sends into it partitions which aid materially in supporting the glandular as well as the fatty elements. Each duct is surrounded by an area of periductal connective tissue with attachments to the skin. When carcinoma invades any glandular area, the skin over that area is retracted, since the periductal strands of connective tissue fail to lengthen with the enlargement of the gland (peau d'orange). This connective tissue forms a network for the blood vessels as well as for the parenchyma, and gives firm-

ness and contour to the virgin breast.   During the periods of lactation, it undergoes a
varying degree of softening and atrophy which accommodates the increase in glandular
elements.   The laxity of the connective tissue with diminution in the breast fat results
in the pendulous breasts of multiparae.   Between the mammary gland and the pectoralis

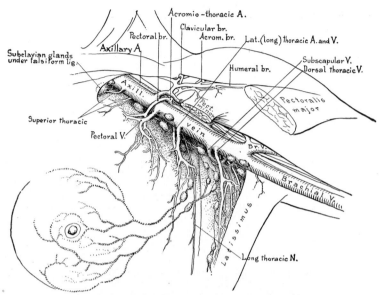

FIG. 223.—DISSECTION OF THE AXILLA SHOWING THE DISTRIBUTION OF THE VESSELS AND NERVES. (Finney
in "Keen's Surgery.")

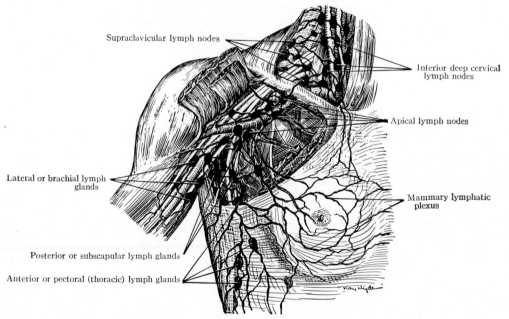

FIG. 224.—LYMPHATIC DISTRIBUTION IN THE BREAST REGION AND AXILLA.

major muscle is a thin retromammary layer of connective tissue, through which the pus
of a breast abscess may burrow readily.

The **secreting parenchyma** of the gland consists of a dozen or more separate irregular
lobes which radiate from the nipple.   Each lobe has its own excretory duct which converges

toward the nipple where it opens. Part of the secreting structure may lie deep to the pectoral fascia in the retromammary layers. To avoid the greatest number of breast radicles, radial incisions are made in drainage of *suppurative mastitis*, especially when abscesses are located near the base of the nipple. The subcutaneous connective tissue divides the lobes into lobules, and these into the ultimate secreting units, the alveoli. Each lactiferous duct, as it approaches the base of the nipple, presents a fusiform or ampullary enlargement, the lactiferous sinus, which acts as a temporary reservoir for the secretion of the gland. The duct narrows beyond the enlargement and passes into the nipple.

5. The **arterial supply** of the breast is derived from three sources: the lateral perforating branches of the anterior aortic intercostals; the perforating branches of the internal mammary; and branches of the pectoral division of the thoraco-acromial trunk of the axillary.

6. **Lymphatic Drainage of the Breast.**—A knowledge of the lymph drainage of the region is extremely important, because it is along lymph channels that breast cancer spreads.

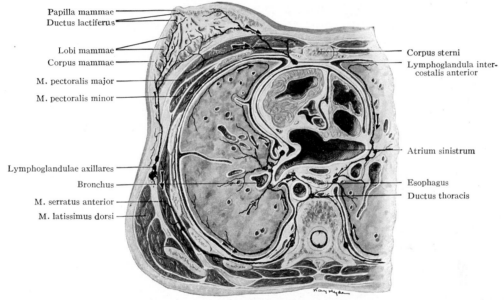

FIG. 225.—TRANSVERSE SECTION THROUGH THE THORAX SHOWING THE LYMPH DRAINAGE FROM THE BREAST REGION.

Practical application of the knowledge of paths of extension must be made if complete eradication of the growth is to be obtained.

Both the ducts and the acini of the gland are surrounded by a network of lymph vessels, the *periductal and periacinous* lymphatics. These communicate freely with *interlobar* lymphatics which ramify in the interglandular tissue, and with those lying in the subcutaneous and retromammary tissue, the latter traversing the pectoral fascia to form the chain along which the principal spread occurs. From the peripheral margin of the gland, efferent vessels run a classical path to the axilla. The major portion of the lymphatic drainage from the upper medial quadrant of the breast is along the perforating vessels directly into the chest rather than to the axillary lymph nodes.

In a very limited number of instances, there undoubtedly is lymph drainage by the mediastinal path into the anterior mediastinal nodes lying along the course of the internal mammary artery. These lymphatics pass from the mesial portion of the gland through openings for the perforating vessels at the medial extremities of the intercostal spaces to reach the mediastinal nodes. Their invasion by breast cancer, with dissemination into the lung, can be determined by *x*-ray examination; this invasion precludes the possibility of a cure by radical surgical methods. Lymph vessels sometimes pass from the deep surface of the gland through the whole thickness of the chest wall to join the intercostal lymphatics lying in the endothoracic fascia between the rib cage and pleura.

In cancer of the mesial side of the breast, there may be *cross involvement* of the lymph vessels with development of cancer in the opposite breast.

Stiles has shown that the inferior and mesial margin of the breast is only 2.5 cm. from the angular interspace between the xiphoid process and the costal arch. In this interval, the lymphatic plexus of the epigastric aponeurosis is separated from the extraperitoneal lymphatics only by the linea alba. Thus, when cancer cells extend mesially or inferiorly this distance beyond the breast, they have merely to pass through a single layer of fibrous tissue traversed by lymphatics to reach the peritoneum.

SURGICAL CONSIDERATIONS

1. Clinical Examination of the Breast.—The mobility of the normal breast is one of its most outstanding characteristics, but the ease with which its substance slips away from beneath the palpating fingers renders the detection of small tumors somewhat uncertain. For this reason, palpation of the gland is conducted most accurately with the patient in a supine position so that the palm of the hand may be applied flatly over the breast, and

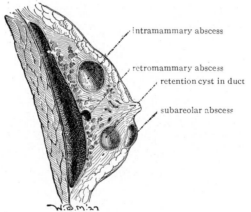

intramammary abscess

retromammary abscess

retention cyst in duct

subareolar abscess

FIG. 226.—VARIETIES OF MAMMARY ABSCESSES.
Development of a retromammary abscess from a deep-lying intramammary abscess is shown. (Babcock.

may compress the main part of the gland against the resistant chest wall. In this way, small cystic or solid tumors will be less likely to slip aside and escape detection. Tumors reveal their presence by their size and firm consistency.

2. Inflammation of the Breast.—Breast infection is observed with greatest frequency during the early stages of lactation when the gland tissue is highly vascular and functionally active. Abscesses occurring in the nonlactating breast follow infection of the glands of Montgomery and, therefore, are confined to the nipple zone.

Puerperal mastitis is the most frequent inflammatory lesion of the breast. The entrance of infection usually is at the nipple, and organisms rapidly invade the ducts and gland substance. This emphasizes the need for careful hygiene of the nipple. Infection spreads deeply from the superficial lesion, producing a suppurative lymphangitis (intramammary abscess). The abscess ramifies throughout the breast and gives rise to loculi traversed by fibrous septa. Inflammation, once started, has a tendency to spread from one lobule to another along the interglandular tissue, tunnelling the breast in various directions and leading to extensive destruction of the gland substance. Suppuration may take place outside the peripheral limits of the gland, either in the overlying tissue, *premammary abscess*, or in the loose areolar stratum upon which the gland lies, *retromammary abscess*.

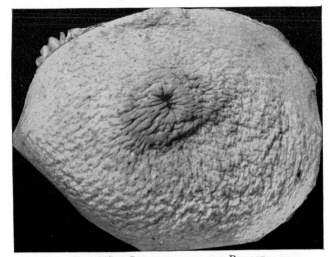

FIG. 227.—CARCINOMA OF THE BREAST.
Retraction of the nipple and orange peel or pigskin appearance of the skin.   (Boyd, "Surgical Pathology.")

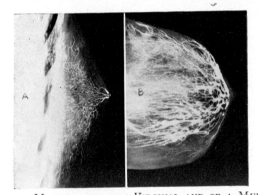

FIG. 228.—THOROTRAST MAMMOGRAMS OF A VIRGINAL AND OF A MULTIPAROUS BREAST.
A, Mammogram of a virginal breast during the resting phase of the menstrual cycle; B, Mammogram
of an early phase of lactation.
Mammography utilizes contrast fluids which are injected directly into the milk ducts, thus giving an
accurate roentgenographic pattern of the ducts and secretory system of the mammary gland.   (N. F.
Hicken, Surg., Gynec., and Obst., March, 1937.)

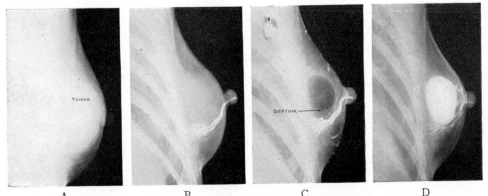

A   B   C   D
FIG. 229.—THOROTRAST MAMMOGRAMS OF A CYSTIC NEOPLASM OF THE BREAST.
A, Soft tissue x-ray outlines a single delimited breast tumor; B, Contrast medium injected into lactiferous duct does not enter the tumor but is displaced by the neoplastic mass; C, Cyst evacuated by aspiration, and content replaced by air.   Aeromammogram reveals a large bilocular cyst.   The tumor does not
communicate with the ducts; D, The air in the cyst is replaced by thorotrast.   Note how the cyst displaces
the injected duct.   (N. F. Hicken, Surg., Gynec., and Obst., March, 1937.)

The latter variety more commonly arises from a deeper cause, such as pleural empyema or tuberculous osteitis of a rib, and tends to push the breast and major pectoral muscle anteriorly.

Incisions for the intramammary and premammary abscesses are made to radiate from the nipple to avoid injury to the lactiferous ducts. If a retromammary abscess results from forward spread from deeper structures, the breast may be turned upward by a long incision in the inframammary groove.

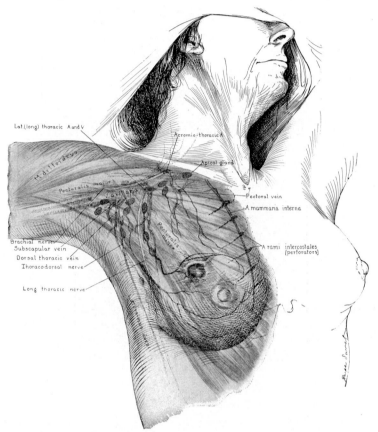

FIG. 230.—CARCINOMA OF THE BREAST.

Surface anatomy with transparency showing the position of the structures to be dealt with in the complete breast operation; the structures to be removed are the skin overlying the breast gland; the sub-cutaneous tissue over most of the area shown, the whole major pectoral muscle, and the axillary contents; the only axillary structures remaining at the completion of the dissection are the axillary artery and vein, and the brachial, long thoracic, and thoracodorsal nerves; note the perforating vessels; lymphatic vessels from the breast penetrate the chest wall alongside these vessels to communicate with the retrosternal lymph glands; note the apical lymph gland at the extreme apex of the axilla (Halsted's gland); note the glands on the outer surface of the minor pectoral muscle above the axillary vessels; these lie along the lymphatic vessels which communicate between the axillary and cervical glands. (After E. I. Bartlett; courtesy of Surgery, Gynecology, and Obstetrics.)

3. Benign Tumors of the Breast.—Benign tumors of the breast are either solid or cystic. The solid tumors are encapsulated and freely movable. They consist either of relatively dense connective tissue, enclosing islands of fairly normal acini—the *periductal fibroma* or *adenofibroma,* or of loose myxomatous connective tissue, through which are scattered compressed, greatly distorted duct structures—the *intracanalicular fibroma* or *myxofibroma.* These solid tumors tend to extrude themselves from the gland and to become superficial to the bulk of mammary tissue. They are removed by enucleation through a radial incision.

Mammary cysts result from the retention of duct secretion and may occur as single or multiple small, round tumors. They are found more frequently as one of the characteristic features of a diffuse process, *chronic cystic mastitis,* or abnormal involution. This lesion is very tender and painful, but usually requires no surgical treatment.

Papillomata are epithelial tumors arising from the walls of the breast ducts and are definitely precancerous lesions. Bleeding from the nipple is almost pathognomonic of the presence of a papilloma. These tumors may be intraductal, intracystic, or diffuse. The

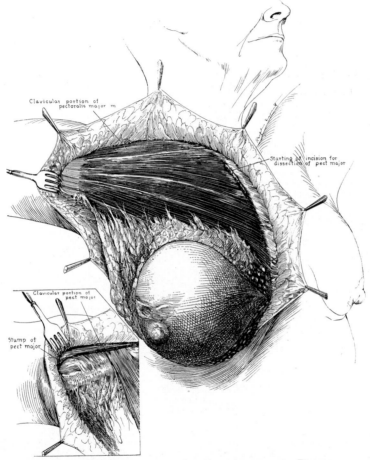

FIG. 231.—STAGE IN COMPLETE REMOVAL OF THE BREAST.

The upper and lateral limits of the subcutaneous dissection, the line of demarcation between the clavicular and sternal portions of the major pectoral muscle, and the beginning of the division of the major pectoral muscle fibers (vulnerable angle) at the border of the sternum; the whole sternal portion of this muscle will be removed; the outer end of the muscle is divided 2 cm. or less from the bone (humerus).

The inset shows the underlying structures in the outer axilla exposed by the removal of the sternal portion of the major pectoral muscle and the relationship of the pectoralis minor muscle and the clavicular portion of the pectoralis major to the axillary contents. (After E. I. Bartlett; courtesy of Surgery, Gynecology, and Obstetrics.)

last are called cystadenomata, and ramify throughout a varying portion of the duct system. The presence of a papilloma necessitates continued observation because of the possibility of its malignant degeneration. Occasionally, it is possible to localize the quadrant from which the bleeding arises and to remove the papilloma by exploring the major breast duct in this area. A cystadenoma simulates clinically an early carcinoma and always necessitates mastectomy.

4. **Carcinoma of the Breast.**—Carcinoma of the breast is so common that each palpable

tumor should be regarded as malignant until proved otherwise by surgical exploration. The progress of the lesion illustrates many points of interest in the structure of the mammary gland. The growth has its origin either in the columnar epithelium of the ducts, duct carcinoma, or in the glandular epithelium of the acini, acinous carcinoma, the latter being more common. It begins as a hard nodule which increases in size, the increase being characterized by progressive infiltration of the surrounding tissue.

Conspicuous in the pathologic changes of many breast carcinomata is the contractility of the fibrous connective tissue or stroma which surrounds the loculi where the cancer cells are lodged—*scirrhous variety.* In this type, which is chronic, fibrosis is developed to the highest degree, with hardness, marked puckering, and distortion of the surrounding tissues. In other types, which grow rapidly, the glandular element predominates—*medullary cancer*— and, because of the smaller amount of stroma present, there is less tendency for contraction.

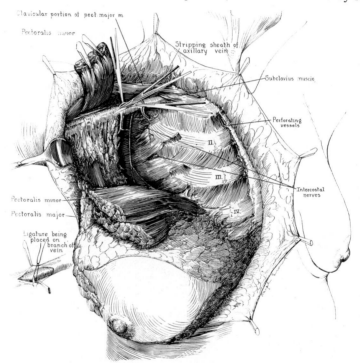

FIG. 232.—STAGE IN COMPLETE REMOVAL OF THE BREAST.
The early stage of axillary dissection; note the stump of the minor pectoral muscle used as a retractor, and the relationship of the subclavius muscle to the axillary vein; note the method of stripping the sheath of the axillary vein. (After E. I. Bartlett; courtesy of Surgery, Gynecology, and Obstetrics.)

Nipple retraction is caused by cicatricial changes in the tissues about the acini which are continuous superficially with those enveloping the large ducts traversing the nipple and opening on its summit.

Carcinomatous infiltrations of the fibrous bands (Cooper's ligaments) between the periglandular tissue, skin, and abundant pervading lymph channels explain the frequent involvement and final adherence of the overlying skin, which exhibits depressions making it appropriately comparable to the rough skin of an orange. Skin involvement effected in this way is in the form either of a number of small isolated nodules, or of a widespread growth which renders the skin hard and brawny. The rigid, unyielding character of this diffuse form of skin infiltration is known as "cancer en cuirasse."

The deep extension of the growth exceeds the limits of the gland and invades the retromammary tissue and the pectoral fascia, the progress being indicated by the loss of normal mobility of the breast. By continued extension in this direction, the disease eventually may work its way through the pectoral muscles to the chest wall and even to the pleura and lung. The lymph glands are involved usually at a comparatively early period by metastasis.

5. **Radical Removal of Breast Carcinoma.**—Any patient with a breast cancer can be cured if the primary growth and its extension are excised completely. This precept has led to the performance of very extensive operations upon the breast and axillary regions. Since there is no available clinical means of determining the limits of fascial, muscle, and lymphatic permeation, a wide circle of the deep fascia, the underlying musculature,

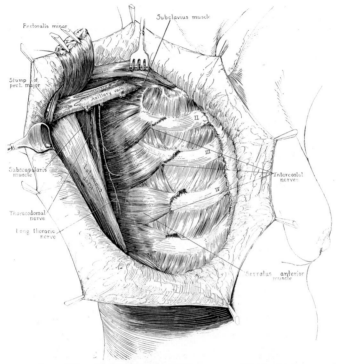

FIG. 233.—RADICAL BREAST OPERATION COMPLETED.

All of the structures shown should be as clearly identified as illustrated, and should be as clean of areolar tissue as shown in the sketch; note especially the relationship of the subclavius muscle to the under surface of the clavicular portion of the pectoralis major muscle and to the outer surface of the vein, artery, and nerves; note the long thoracic and thoracodorsal nerves lying free and undamaged; note the stump of the pectoralis minor muscle which is tucked into the dead space above the vessels and nerve plexus. (After E. I. Bartlett; courtesy of Surgery, Gynecology, and Obstetrics.)

and the tributary lymph glands must be removed, with a generous amount of the overlying skin. Malignancy extends less in the plane of the skin than in that of the underlying structures. The area included in the operation extends from the sternal margin to the center of the axilla.

D. DIAPHRAGM

1. **Definition.**—The diaphragm is a dome-shaped musculomembranous structure separating the thoracic and abdominal cavities. Its peripheral portion consists of muscle fibers which originate at the sternal, costal, and vertebral margins of the thoracic outlet and converge to an insertion in a central tendon. The diaphragm presents right and left vaults separated by a groove and depression upon which the heart and pericardium rest. The right vault mounts higher than the left; the highest point on each side is about 4 cm. mesial to the mammary line.

2. **Development of the Diaphragm.**—The diaphragm arises from five morphological elements—the central tendon, two ventrolateral, and two dorsal parts. The *central tendon*

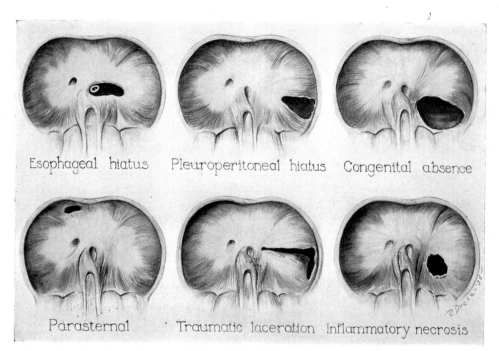

Esophageal hiatus   Pleuroperitoneal hiatus   Congenital absence

Parasternal   Traumatic laceration   Inflammatory necrosis

FIG. 234.—SITUATIONS OF CONGENITAL STRUCTURAL DEFECTS AND TRAUMATIC LACERATIONS OF THE DIAPHRAGM WHICH CAUSE THE MORE COMMON TYPES OF DIAPHRAGMATIC HERNIA. (S. W. Harrington, Western Jour. of Surg., Obst. and Gynec., May, 1936.)

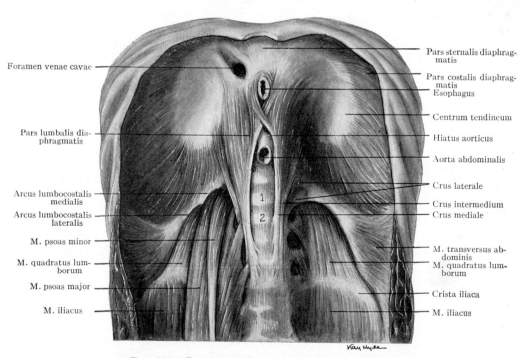

Foramen venae cavae

Pars lumbalis dia-phragmatis

Arcus lumbocostalis medialis

Arcus lumbocostalis lateralis

M. psoas minor

M. quadratus lum-borum

M. psoas major

M. iliacus

Pars sternalis diaphrag-matis

Pars costalis diaphrag-matis
Esophagus

Centrum tendineum

Hiatus aorticus

Aorta abdominalis

Crus laterale

Crus intermedium
Crus mediale

M. transversus ab-dominis
M. quadratus lum-borum

Crista iliaca

M. iliacus

FIG. 235.—DIAPHRAGM VIEWED ANTERO-INFERIORLY.

The thorax is bent backward; the fascia lumbodorsalis is removed to show the muscles of the posterior abdominal wall; the psoas muscles are removed on the left to show the M. quadratus lumborum and M. iliacus.

is formed from the transverse septum, an embryonic layer of tissue separating the heart from the liver. The *ventrolateral portions* of the diaphragm arise from the ventrolongitudinal muscle layer of the body. The *dorsal portions* are derived from the paravertebral musculature. These segments fuse and leave a pleuroperitoneal foramen on each side posteriorly between each dorsal and corresponding ventrolateral part. These apertures close early in fetal life by a fusion of their margins. The openings through which the congenital and acquired diaphragmatic herniae occur are the pleuroperitoneal openings behind, two small passages in front just behind the sternum, and the esophageal opening between the two dorsal divisions of the diaphragm. Of these openings, the esophageal presents the greatest weakness. The hiatuses for the aorta and vena cava are completely closed by the rigidity of the tendinous walls and the ability of the vessels to expand and completely fill their respective passageways.

Through the communications between the thorax and abdomen, there may be reciprocal spread of infection, permitting pleuritis to follow peritonitis and peritonitis to follow pleuritis.

3. **Relations.**—As a partition separating the thoracic and abdominal cavities, the diaphragm has important relations to the contents of both.

The *thoracic surface* of the diaphragm forms the floor of the chest cavity, contacts the diaphragmatic pleura and pericardium, and is in relation to the cellular tissue of the anterior and posterior mediastina and right and left pulmonary pleurae. Through the intermedium of the costodiaphragmatic (phrenic) sinus, the diaphragm has an important relation to the chest wall. The sinus contains a thin lappet of lung during inspiration, but is empty during expiration. Since the pleura does not reach the depth of the sinus, it is possible for a penetrating chest wound to enter the abdominal cavity without injury to either the lung or the pleura. Too low a thoracotomy for empyema may injure the diaphragm, and, because of the proximity of the diaphragm to the ribs, may inhibit free drainage of the thoracic cavity. It is well established that,

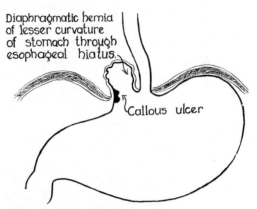

FIG. 236.—HERNIA OF LESSER CURVATURE OF STOMACH THROUGH THE ESOPHAGEAL HIATUS.

Callous gastric ulcer present at the neck of the hernial protrusion. (After Dewitt Stetten, Annals of Surgery, April, 1935, J. B. Lippincott Co., Publishers.)

subsequent to subdiaphragmatic or hepatic abscess, the pleural surfaces of the sinus may become adherent, an anatomic consideration which permits incision and drainage of such an abscess without invasion of the general peritoneal cavity.

The *abdominal surface* of the diaphragm is covered by peritoneum, save where it is attached to the posterior and superior surfaces of the liver and at the level of the pancreas, duodenum, and kidneys. It is related from right to left to the convex surface of the liver, the fundus of the stomach, the lateral surface of the spleen, and the left (splenic) flexure of the colon.

4. **Lymphatics and Nerves.**—The pleural *lymphatics* anastomose through the diaphragm with the peritoneal lymphatics, possibly accounting for reciprocal infection of the pleural and peritoneal cavities. The motor and sensory *nerve supply* is derived mainly from the cervical plexus through the two phrenic nerves ($C_{3, 4, 5}$), which descend in the thorax on the lateral surface of the pericardium and the mediastinal pleura, in front of the lung roots, to be distributed to the superior surface of the diaphragm. They terminate in branches which penetrate the muscle. The diaphragm also is innervated by the diaphragmatic plexus of the sympathetic and sometimes by fibers from the lower thoracic nerves.

SURGICAL CONSIDERATIONS

1. **Diaphragmatic Herniae.**—A diaphragmatic hernia is a protrusion of abdominal viscera through the diaphragm into the thoracic cavity. The reverse condition likewise could be defined, but does not occur because of the greater fixation of the thoracic structures. These herniae may be congenital or acquired.

Congenital herniae, those present at birth, usually have no sac. Two thirds of such herniae occur on the left side and most of these present through the left pleuroperitoneal foramen. Generally, those on the right pass through the right pleuroperitoneal passage. The majority of *acquired diaphragmatic herniae* occur through the esophageal hiatus, and a peritoneal sac is present almost invariably. The esophageal opening often is extensive because the stomach develops at this point and later descends, leaving a space between

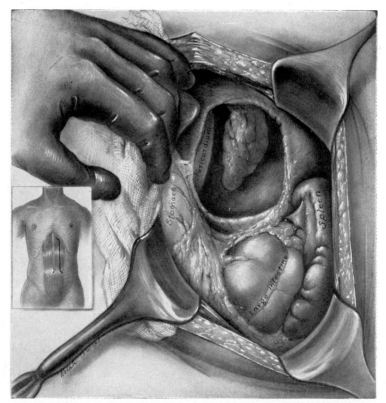

FIG. 237.—OPENING IN THE DIAPHRAGM IN A TRAUMATIC HERNIA. (J. H. Woolsey.)
Inset shows the operative incision.

the esophagus and the edge of the diaphragm. *Traumatic herniae* always are associated with a tear of the diaphragm, occurring usually on the left side in the central region, and are without a sac. This variety formerly was reported most frequently, but better clinical diagnoses and the use of the roentgen ray are bringing the congenital type into prominence. Localized pneumothorax sometimes is mistaken for diaphragmatic hernia. Hernia through the diaphragm must be distinguished from a condition in which one half of the diaphragm is greatly relaxed and elevated, usually from phrenic nerve paralysis. The latter condition is known as *eventration of the diaphragm*.

The routes of surgical approach for *diaphragmatic hernioplasty* are: abdominal, thoracic, and combined abdominal and thoracic. Some conditions cannot be dealt with from the abdomen alone, particularly those in which the contents of the rupture are adherent to chest structures. Closure of the diaphragmatic opening from below at times may be almost impossible.   Conversely, resection of the bowel and anastomosis can be done adequately only through an abdominal incision.   Since a thoracotomy incision permits easier approach for the repair of the diaphragm but does not allow sufficient room to explore the abdominal structures properly, the approach of choice is a combined one.   The single incision or two separate incisions employed permit the reduction of the abdominal organs, provide adequate exposure for dealing with injuries and strangulation as they present, and make possible the firm suturing of the defect in the diaphragm.

II. Thoracic Cavity and Its Contents

Unlike the abdomen, which contains but a single sac, the chest cavity presents three complete serous sacs.   These are the two pleurae and the pericardium.   The chest affords space for many important structures: the lungs and heart, and those structures whose function extends beyond the thorax, either to the abdomen or neck.   The more important of the latter are: the major portion of the great vessels from the heart and lungs, the esophagus, the trachea, the vagus and phrenic nerves, the thoracic duct, and the sympathetic nerve trunks.   For descriptive purposes, the thoracic cavity and its contents are considered in three sections: the pleurae and pleurothoracic topography, the lungs and pulmonothoracic topography, and the mediastinum.

A. PLEURAE AND PLEUROTHORACIC TOPOGRAPHY

The pleurae are two serous membranes which form independent closed sacs.   Into each sac at its mesial aspect is invaginated the respective lung.   Thus, two leaves or layers are present: one, applied over and adherent to the walls of the thorax, the parietal layer; and the other, intimately applied over the surface of the invaginated lung, the visceral or

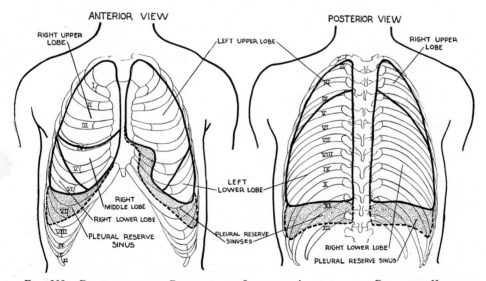

Fig. 238.—Borders of the Pleurae and Lungs in Anterior and Posterior Views.

pulmonary layer.   These layers are designed to effect excursion of the lungs over the walls of the thorax with a minimum of friction.   Between the layers is the pleural cavity, normally a potential space containing a minute amount of serous fluid, but, under certain pathologic conditions, constituting a true cavity.

1. **Pulmonary or Visceral Pleura.**—The very thin pulmonary pleura is bound down firmly to the lung surface and dips into the interlobar fissures, separating the lobes.   It cannot be detached without laceration of the lung substance.   It is continuous at the root of the lung with the pleura over the mediastinum.

16

2. **Divisions of the Parietal Pleura.**—The divisions of the parietal pleura are important from topographic and surgical points of view. The costal portion is in contact with the ribs, intercostal spaces, and endothoracic fascia, and the diaphragmatic portion with the superior surface of the diaphragm. The mediastinal division covers the lateral wall of the mediastinum.

The *costal pleura* is resistant, but, because of its loose attachment to the endothoracic fascia, is separated easily from the chest wall. It continues anteriorly into the mediastinal pleura and forms with it a vertical sinus or culdesac along the costomediastinal line of pleural reflection, known as the anterior costomediastinal sinus. In a similar fashion, the posterior costo(vertebro)mediastinal sinus is formed. The costal pleura dips inferiorly into the groove formed between the costal wall and the diaphragm to form, along the costodiaphragmatic line of pleural reflection, the inferior or costodiaphragmatic sinus.

The *diaphragmatic pleura* spreads over the diaphragm and is very adherent to the muscle, carpeting the area not covered by the diaphragmatic pericardium. It does not extend to the line of attachment of the diaphragm to the chest wall, but is separated from it by an interval containing fatty areolar connective tissue.

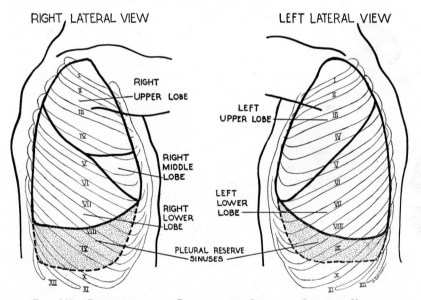

FIG. 239.—BORDERS OF THE PLEURAE AND LUNGS IN LATERAL VIEWS.

The *mediastinal pleura* is in loose contact with the structures against which it rests In the upper part of the cavity on each side, it extends without interruption from the sternum to the spine, but below is reflected from the pericardium over the root of the lung and becomes continuous with the pulmonary pleura.

3. **Lines of Pleural Reflection and the Pleural Reserve Sinuses.**—At certain levels the parietal pleura is folded upon itself as it is reflected from one wall of the chest cavity to the other. Two of these reflections, the anterior or costomediastinal, and the lower or costodiaphragmatic, possess a high degree of practical interest. Within these reflections are the pleural reserve sinuses, the costomediastinal and costodiaphragmatic spaces, which are invaded by the lung margins only in deep inspiration. During expiration, the pleural leaves of the recesses are approximated; during inspiration they allow the salient lung margins to expand to their capacity. These reflections and reserve sinuses are indicated graphically in Figures 238 and 239.

Knowledge of the exact levels of the *costomediastinal sinuses* permits transthoracic exploration of the pericardium, heart, and esophagus without opening the pleural sacs and incurring the complication of pneumothorax.

It reaches the column at the level of the twelfth thoracic spine about 1 cm. inferior to the head of the twelfth rib. The high level of the *inferior or costodiaphragmatic level of pleural reflection* permits of additional exposure through the inferior margin of the thoracic cage in difficult operations on the stomach and liver. The fatty areolar interval between the pleural reflection and the costal attachments of the diaphragm affords an extrapleural transthoracic approach to the diaphragm and to the underlying subdiaphragmatic space.

The pleural reflections are subject to some variation. Behind the sternum, one or the other costomediastinal reflection may advance farther anteriorly than usual or fall short of its normal limit and reach perhaps only to the anterior extremities of the costal cartilages. The practical significance of the variation is evident when considered with reference to the precordial region. With normal pleural reflections, the pericardium can be reached through the anterior extremities of the fifth and sixth interspaces without opening the pleura. If the left line of pleural reflection exceeds the normal limits and advances medially over the precordial area, it is injured in pericardial tap. There always is uncertainty as to how much of the pericardium is covered by pleura.

The *pleural dome* or *cervical pleura* is projected upward and forward into the neck. It is indicated on the surface by a curved line with an upward convexity, drawn from the center of the sternoclavicular joint to the junction of the sternal and middle thirds of the clavicle. The apices of the lung during both inspiration and expiration fill the domes completely. The anterior and middle scalene muscles lie upon the lateral surface of the cervical pleura before they attach to the upper surface of the first rib. The subclavian artery lies in a groove on the medial and ventral aspect of the pleural dome. The internal mammary vessels, the beginning of the vertebral and intercostal arteries, the inferior ganglion of the cervical chain, and the lower trunk of the brachial plexus also rest upon the cervical pleura.

SURGICAL CONSIDERATIONS

1. **Pressure Conditions within the Pleural Cavities.**—The pressure relations within the pleural cavities are of the utmost practical significance. The lungs normally fill the pleural cavities completely except for the pleural reserve sinuses (p. 242), these being, therefore, only potential spaces. The pleural surfaces are kept in contact by the negative intrapleural pressure and the cohesive property of the opposed serous membranes. The lungs, owing to their elasticity, tend to contract, but are prevented from doing so by the counteracting force of the negative intrapleural pressure. While the pleural cavities remain closed, the lung is unable to recede from the chest wall unless there is an alteration in the intrapleural pressure produced by fluid or air. As long as the parietal pleura is intact, the visceral layer lies in contact with it, but if the parietal pleura is opened, air enters, and the lung, greatly diminished in volume, falls away from the chest wall. The unopposed elasticity of the lung allows the viscus to collapse actively.

Collapse of the lung would not be of great moment were it not for the fact that the mediastinum is a very flexible composite and is capable of shifting rapidly (mediastinal flutter) with each respiration. Under altered pressure conditions, respiratory and circulatory embarrassment may be incompatible with life. This incompatibility is explained partly by the sudden pressure alterations, displacement of the heart and great vessels, and the diminished vital capacity of the good lung. Inability to cope with these alarming results for many years retarded the development of thoracic surgery. Clearer conceptions of respiratory mechanics and methods devised to maintain normal respiratory movements under positive pressure have furnished a marked impetus to surgery of the chest.

2. **Pneumothorax.**—Pneumothorax is the presence of air in the pleural cavity. Air may enter through a perforation in the lung, parietal pleura, or esophagus. Pneumothorax complicating pulmonary tuberculosis results from rupture of a tuberculous cavity in the periphery of the lung. This complication would be far more common were it not for the attendant adhesive pleuritis which often involves both layers of pleura and prevents air entering between them. Injuries of the chest may produce sucking wounds which produce progressively increasing pressure within the pleural cavity.

The production of pneumothorax in chest operations formerly caused serious symptoms and even death. Appreciation of the knowledge that lung collapse is much decreased when the pleural layers are adherent and the mediastinum is fixed by inflammatory deposits, together with the experience that mediastinal flutter may be stopped by grasping and holding the lung or limiting or closing the thoracic opening, have led to the adequate handling of these cases. Pneumothorax is induced artificially to put the lung at rest, to obliterate cavities within it, and to stop bleeding from the lung in hemothorax from lung injury. It is also of value in the differential diagnosis of intrathoracic tumors, whether in the lung, pleura, or mediastinum.

3. **Fibrinous Pleurisy** (Pleuritis).—The normal pleural surfaces are smooth and glistening, and are moistened by serous fluid which facilitates the movements between the opposed layers. When the pleura is inflamed, its surfaces are roughened from the deposition of fibrin, and a characteristic *friction sound* or *rub* may be heard on auscultation over the affected area. This is produced by the rubbing of the roughened surfaces against each other. The rub may be detected by applying the hand flat against the chest and, when perceived in this way, is called *friction fremitus*. Pleural inflammation may give rise to adhesions between the visceral and parietal layers.

The referred pain of fibrinous pleurisy varies according to the position of the pleura involved. The visceral pleura, which invests the lung, is not sensitive to painful stimuli, whereas the parietal pleura is supplied with sensory nerves through which stimuli are perceived acutely. Irritation of the costal pleura causes pain at the point of stimulation, but irritation of the diaphragmatic pleura causes pain referred to the neck, shoulder, scapula, back, or abdomen. Spasm of the muscles overlying a lung lesion (Pottenger's sign) may be of definite diagnostic value.

Irritation of the central portion of the diaphragm in *diaphragmatic pleurisy* causes neck, and sometimes shoulder, pain on the corresponding side. The pain is referred over the trapezius muscle and occasionally above the clavicle, where it is transmitted by the phrenic nerve. Irritation of the periphery of the diaphragm refers pain to the lower dorsal and lumbar regions, and to the flank and abdomen. There frequently is associated hyperesthesia of the skin areas innervated by the seventh to tenth spinal nerves. These symptoms are caused by the combined thoracic, abdominal, and diaphragmatic distribution of the lower intercostal nerves. Often the costal and diaphragmatic pleurae are inflamed at the same time.

The most severe pleural pain occurs in pleurisy secondary to basal pneumonia. In many instances, the pain is abdominal, and, on that account, frequently is misinterpreted as arising from an acute abdominal lesion, such as acute appendicitis, cholecystitis, or subdiaphragmatic infection. Differentiation between the conditions is aided by the knowledge that the common neck pain of diaphragmatic pleurisy does not occur in acute abdominal disease. Furthermore, the frequent relief of pain on deep pressure over the abdomen in pleurisy is in contrast to the accentuation of pain upon the same procedure in appendicitis and cholecystitis. The pleuritic pain is increased on deep inspiration. An acute inflammatory lesion just beneath the diaphragm offers the greatest difficulty in differential diagnosis, as the irritation of the peritoneal surface of the diaphragm refers pain after the same manner as does irritation of the pleural surface.

4. **Hydrothorax and Pleurisy with Effusion.**—*Hydrothorax* is noninflammatory and is produced by a transudate, commonly a part of a general dropsy, which results from cardiac decompensation. It is, as a rule, unilateral and on the right side. Unilateral hydrothorax also may occur in profound anemia or in compression of the venous trunks by an aneurysm of the aorta, tumor of the lung, or of the mediastinal structures. In renal disease, the hydrothorax almost always is bilateral. The symptoms produced by the fluid are the result of compression of the lung and displacement of the heart, and consist chiefly of dyspnea, cyanosis, and acceleration of the pulse.

The commonest cause of *pleurisy with effusion* is tuberculosis. The serous exudate may be the second stage of a dry pleurisy, but often the exudate is present from the onset.

When effusion occurs, the inflamed pleural surfaces are separated and the pain diminishes or disappears. At first, there is dyspnea from pain; later, unless the effusion has occurred very slowly, there is dyspnea from pressure of fluid upon the lung and mediastinal displacement. In severe cases, orthopnea and cyanosis are present. The fluid has the usual characteristics of an inflammatory exudate. In hydrothorax and pleurisy with effusion, the mediastinal structures are found displaced toward the unaffected side, and the diaphragm is depressed.

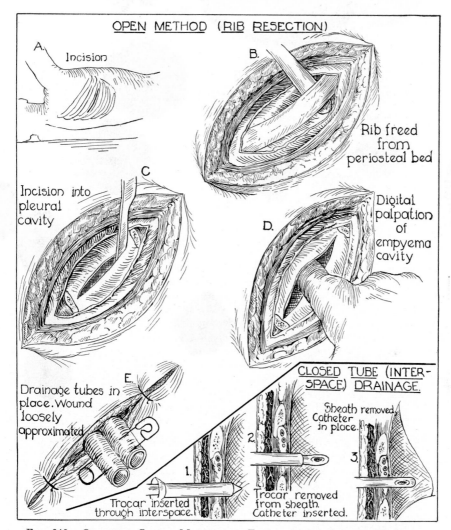

FIG. 240.—OPEN AND CLOSED METHODS IN TREATMENT OF EMPYEMA THORACIS.

5. Empyema.—Empyema is a pleuritis with a purulent exudate, and usually is secondary to a pulmonary lesion. Its presence is determined by clinical signs, roentgenologic examination, and aspiration.

Early empyema may occupy the entire pleural cavity (total), compressing the lung, displacing the heart and mediastinum, and even causing the interspaces of the affected side to bulge. More common than *total empyema* is that confined by adhesions to certain parts of the pleural cavity, *encapsulated or sacculated empyema*. The usual locations for encapsulated empyema are: between the base of the lung and the diaphragm, supradiaphragmatic; between the lung and the chest wall, parietal; in an interlobar fissure; or between the mesial lung surface and the mediastinum. Following rupture of a pulmonary lesion into the pleura, the empyema may be interlobar or loculated from the start. The presence of pus and air in the pleural cavity is called *pyopneumothorax*.

Diagnostic aspiration is of great importance as it largely determines the therapeutic procedure. The most common varieties of pus encountered are: the thin, stringy pus of

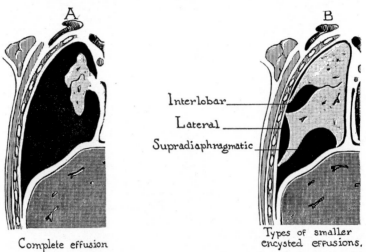

Fig. 241.—Frontal Sections Through the Thorax Showing Generalized and Encapsulated Effusions. (Modified from Testut and Jacob.)

streptococcus infection; the thick, yellowish or greenish pus of pneumococcus infection; and the seropurulent or serosanguineous exudate of tuberculous involvement.

Both the parietal and visceral pleurae change in empyema from thin, delicate membranes to markedly thickened, tough, fibrous, and sometimes almost cartilaginous layers,

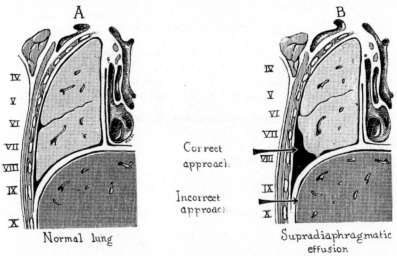

Fig. 242.—Frontal Sections Through the Thorax to Show the Relations of the Costodiaphragmatic Sinus to the Lungs, Diaphragm and Liver. (Modified from Testut and Jacob.)
Incision low in this sinus fails to evacuate the effusion.

with irregular surfaces covered by granulation tissue. These alterations, particularly in the visceral pleura, and the dense adhesions established are of serious consequence, as they limit, often to a marked degree, the expansile property of the lung, and prevent its reestablishing normal relationships within the pleural cavity.

Surgical drainage of empyema is employed to relieve respiratory and circulatory embarrassment, decrease toxic absorption, obviate rupture, and obliterate the pus cavity. In addition, it prevents thickening of the pleural membranes and the formation of adhesions. Respiratory and circulatory changes are relieved readily by aspiration during the toxic stages. In fact, frequent aspiration cures certain empyemas. Surgical drainage by rib resection is not attempted early as the sudden pressure change may result in shock from the sudden shifting of mediastinal structures. Subtotal evacuation by aspiration, with partial replacement by air, tides over the toxic phase, allows partial expansion of the lung, and, as the air is absorbed slowly, permits the mediastinal structures to return gradually to their normal position. Rib resection should not be performed in tuberculous empyema.

If aspiration and rib resection fail to obliterate the empyema cavity, the more radical procedures of pulmonary decortication (p. 226) and thoracoplasty (p. 227) can be employed.

An empyema, if left alone, may discharge its contents along any of a number of paths. Pus may break from the pleural cavity into a bronchus and be expectorated. It may ulcerate through and discharge into the esophagus, pericardium, diaphragm, or stomach, or may rupture externally through an intercostal space (empyema necessitatis), establishing a sinus. Large collections of pus have extended into the abdomen through the narrow intervals between the costal and vertebral attachments of the diaphragm and have continued along the spine, following the psoas muscle into the iliac fossa, there resembling lumbar and psoas abscesses.

B. LUNGS AND THEIR THORACIC TOPOGRAPHY

Each lung is roughly a half-cone with its base resting on the diaphragm and its apex occupying the cervical dome of the pleura. The mesial flat or concave surface lies against the mediastinum, and the outer convex wall against the rib-cage. The soft and spongy

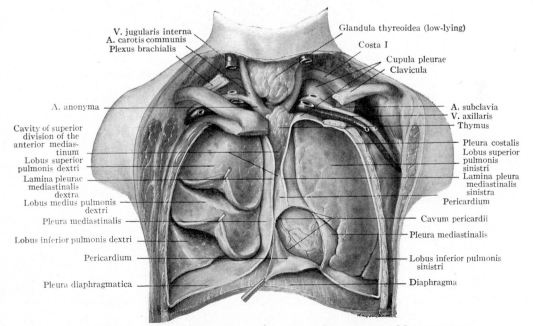

FIG. 243.—LUNGS AND THEIR RELATIONS TO THE PLEURAE AND MEDIASTINUM.

tissue is molded against the walls of the chest cavity and bears the impress of the various structures to which it is related. The lungs are separated by a complete interpulmonary septum, the mediastinum or central compartment of the thorax, which extends from the sternum to the spine. The lungs are somewhat asymmetrical because of the higher level of the diaphragm on the right side and the decided projection of the heart to the left of the median line.

   1. **Anatomic Summary.**—The lateral or *costal surface* of the lung is smooth and convex, is accurately adapted to the chest wall, and presents a series of oblique grooves and ridges which corresponds to the overlying ribs and rib spaces. It is traversed by a deep fissure which travels obliquely inferiorly and anteriorly and which terminates in the inferior free margin of the lung. This main fissure is very deep throughout, extending to the hilum. It is the only fissure of the left lung, dividing it into superior and inferior, or better termed, anterior and posterior lobes. A second or subsidiary fissure is present in the right lung, beginning behind at the main fissure and running anteriorly and slightly superiorly to the

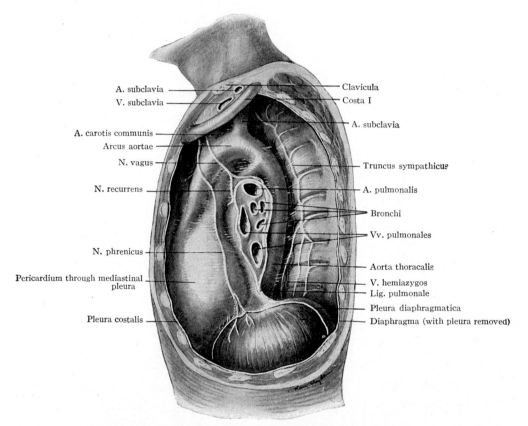

FIG.244.— STRUCTURES ON THE LEFT SURFACE OF THE MEDIASTINUM.

anterior free margin of the lung. Thus, three right lobes, a superior, middle, and inferior, are delimited. For diagrams of lung lobes and fissures, see Figures 238 and 239.

   The medial or *mediastinal surface* is irregularly concave, its principal relationship being with the heart and pericardium. The most important part of this surface corresponds to the pulmonary hilum, which, on section, presents an oval outline. The inferior extremity of the hilum is continued into a fold of the pleura, known as the pulmonary ligament. The structures grouped together at the hilum form the root of the lung. The hilum lies nearer the posterior than the anterior part of the lung, and somewhat nearer the apex than the base. The *apex* of the lung projects as a blunt cone above the plane of the thoracic inlet and fits accurately into the cervical dome of the pleura (p. 243), where it comes into close and surgically dangerous relationship with the thoracocervical (p. 215) and supra-clavicular (p. 206) areas of the neck.

2. **Thoracic Projection of the Borders and Lobes of the Lung.**—A knowledge of the surface projection of the lung borders and fissures affords the internist valuable aid in localizing pulmonary disease, and indicates to the surgeon the approach to the various types of encapsulated empyemas. The lung borders are indicated on the drawings which demonstrate the lines of pleural reflection (Figs. 238 and 239).

3. **Structures in the Lung Pedicle and Their Ramifications** (Fig. 254).—The structures in the root of the lung are: the bronchus, the pulmonary artery and veins, the bronchial arteries, veins, and lymphatics, the bronchial glands, the pulmonary nerve plexuses, and the pulmonary ligament. These structures are bound together with a small amount of connective tissue and pleura, which surrounds them as with a cuff

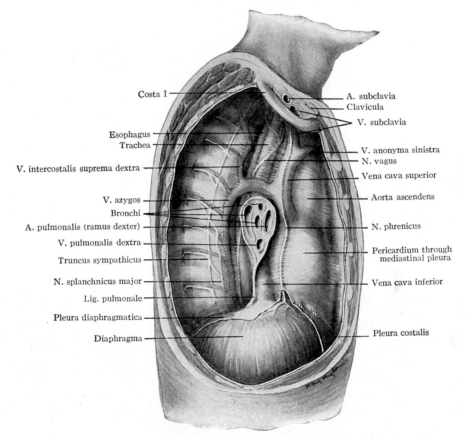

Fig. 245.—Structures on the Right Surface of the Mediastinum.

As the *bronchi* enter the lung, the tubes become smaller by repeated division, and their coats become correspondingly thinner. The lining mucosa, which plays an important defense rôle against invasion of the parenchyma, is exceptionally thin in the smaller bronchioles. When bronchial dilatation occurs, its site is the fibrocartilaginous portion of the bronchus, which, then devoid of support, is transformed into a fusiform cavity.

The *pulmonary artery*, after leaving the right ventricle. runs a superior course of about 4 cm. a little to the left of the ascending aorta. The right branch runs to the right lung behind the aorta, and the left branch runs to the left lung in the concavity of the aortic arch. In the lung pedicle, the right ramus divides into two branches and the left ramus is single. Their terminations spread out in a capillary network over the alveolar air cells, thus carrying impure venous blood from the right ventricle to the lung for aeration. A thrombus of the right side of the heart, of systemic venous origin, may release an embolus which blocks a branch of the pulmonary artery and causes a suppression of that part of the lung so supplied. A pulmonary infarct (p. 255) develops which may degenerate into a pulmonary abscess (p. 255).

The radicles of the *pulmonary veins* arise in, and carry the blood from, the pulmonary capillary plexuses about the alveoli. Their venules run in the interlobular spaces to enter,

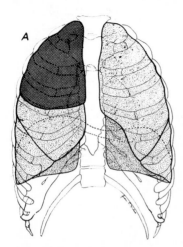 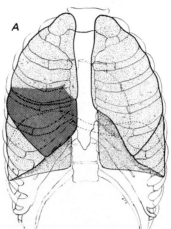 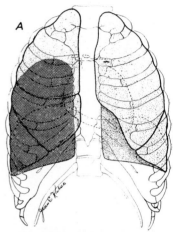

Figure I, A and B. Right upper lobe area and corresponding pneumonic consolidation.. Posterior — Anterior Views.

Figure II, A and B. Right middle lobe area and corresponding pneumonic consolidation...Posterior — Anterior Views.

Figure III, A and B. Right lower lobe area and corresponding pneumonic consolidation.. Posterior — Anterior Views.

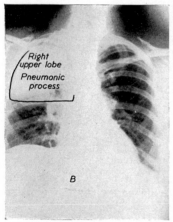 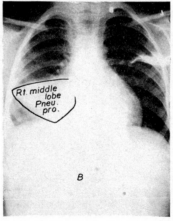 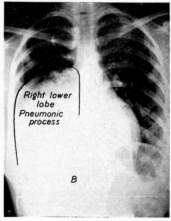

Fig. 246a.—x-Ray Appearance of Right Lobar Areas in Diagrams and in Corresponding Clinical Consolidations (Postero-anterior Views). (Modified from H. Brunn and J. Levitin in Radiology.)

and form the trunks of, the large pulmonary veins. Two main trunks from each lung open into the left atrium on its lateral borders.

The *bronchial arteries*, rather than the pulmonary arteries, nourish the lung. They are small branches from the aorta or the aortic intercostal vessels, and vary from 1 to 3 in number. They accompany the bronchioles to the lung lobules.

Below the root of the lung, the two layers of pleura investing it come into apposition and are prolonged inferiorly as a distinct fold, the *pulmonary ligament*. This fold stretches between the pericardium and the inferior part of the mediastinal surface of the pleura and ends below in a free border.

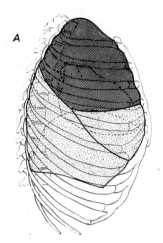
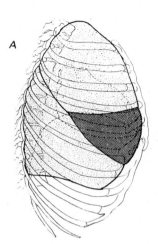
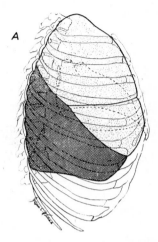

Figure I, A and B. Right upper lobe area and corresponding pneumonic consolidation..Lateral Views.

Figure II, A and B. Right middle lobe area and corresponding pneumonic consolidation...Lateral Views.

Figure III, A and B. Right lower lobe area and corresponding pneumonic consolidation...Lateral Views.

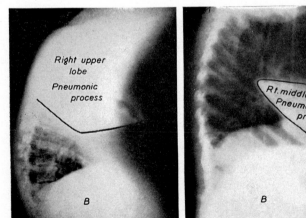
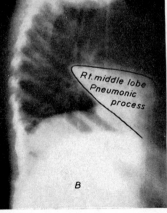
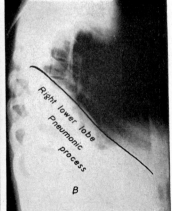

FIG. 246b.—x-RAY APPEARANCE OF RIGHT LOBAR AREAS IN DIAGRAMS AND IN CORRESPONDING CLINICAL CONSOLIDATIONS (LATERAL VIEWS). (Modified from H. Brunn and J. Levitin in Radiology.)

4. **x-Ray Appearance of Lobar Areas and Corresponding Clinical Consolidations.**—The most practical way to visualize and localize clinical pulmonary consolidations and interlobar effusions in x-rays is to study diagrams of lung areas and fissures which truly represent the normal x-ray findings. The diagrams in Figs. 246a to 250b were made from paraffin models of the lung lobes (Brunn and Levitin). These models, transparent to the x-ray, were fitted properly into the chest cage in order that the appearance and location

of the individual lobes could be studied. Lead foil was wrapped about the lobe under consideration and x-ray films were exposed in the postero-anterior and lateral positions. The accompanying illustrations are diagrams of these films. Each interlobar fissure was demonstrated by placing lead foil between the modelled lobes and exposing

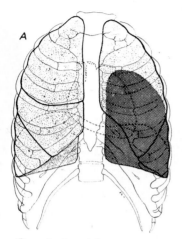 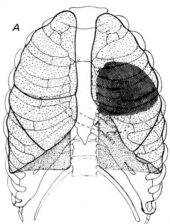 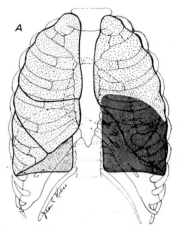

Figure I, A and B. Left lower lobe area and corresponding pneumonic consolidation... Posterior— Anterior Views.

Figure II, A and B. Superior division of left lower lobe and corresponding pneumonic consolidation... Posterior —Anterior Views.

Figure III, A and B Inferior division of left lower lobe area and corresponding pneumonic consolidation.... Posterior —Anter-ior Views.

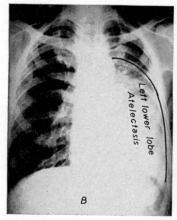 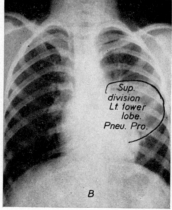 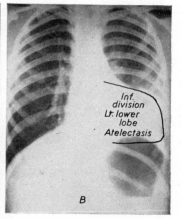

FIG. 247a.—x-RAY APPEARANCE OF LEFT LOBAR AREAS IN DIAGRAMS AND IN CORRESPONDING CLINICAL CONSOLIDATIONS (POSTERO-ANTERIOR VIEWS). (Modified from H. Brunn and J. Levitin in Radiology.)

films in the postero-anterior and lateral positions. The x-rays thus obtained were diagrammed.

In this series of figures, the x-ray shadows obtained experimentally are placed above the films of proved clinical cases of corresponding lobar consolidation and interlobar effusion. It is not implied that a pulmonary disease process occupies all of the corresponding lobar area designated in any one diagram. Previous disease in the lung may result in retraction, distortion, or the displacement of the whole lung or the lobe under consideration. Notwithstanding the factors which play a part in the distortion of lung shadows, the general configuration of the affected parts of the lung closely resemble the diagrams experimentally produced.

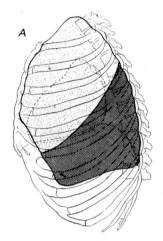
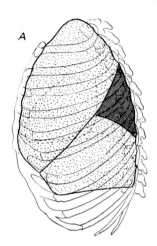
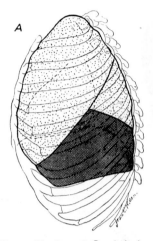

Figure I, A and B. Left lower lobe area and corresponding pneumonic consolidation.... Lateral Views.

Figure II, A and B. Superior division of left lower lobe area and corresponding pneumonic consolidation.... Lateral Views.

Figure III, A and B. Inferior division of left lower lobe area and corresponding pneumonic consolidation.... Lateral Views.

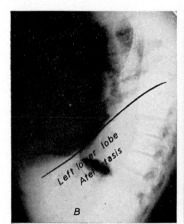
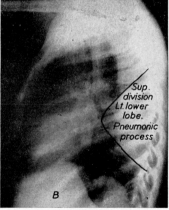
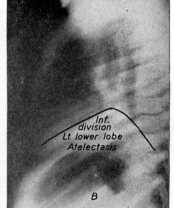

FIG. 247b.—x-RAY APPEARANCE OF LEFT LOBAR AREAS IN DIAGRAMS AND IN CORRESPONDING CLINICAL CONSOLIDATIONS (LATERAL VIEWS). (Modified from H. Brunn and J. Levitin in Radiology.)

Each lower lobe sometimes has two parts, a superior and an inferior division. The division of this lobe has an embryonic origin, for there is a distinct bronchial distribution to each of the divisions, and a fissure separating them may be present. Failure of fusion between the lung buds of the lower lobe accounts for an anomalous fissure.

The *superior division of the lower lobe* is the upper posterior part of the lobe (Fig. 247b), and shows well in the lateral view. It occupies a triangular area, with its apex at the hilus. This part of the lower lobe lies mainly behind the upper lobe. When the diaphragm is low, the upper division of the lower lobe appears to be in the central part of the chest in the postero-anterior x-ray view. Lung abscess is found most frequently in this part of the lung. Pneumonia of the lower lobe also develops commonly in this part of the lobe. Because of its central appearance on the roentgenogram, the disease often is called central pneumonia. The physical signs of the pneumonic process are found in a small, posterior, circumscribed area between the scapula and the vertebral column and between the fourth to the eighth ribs.

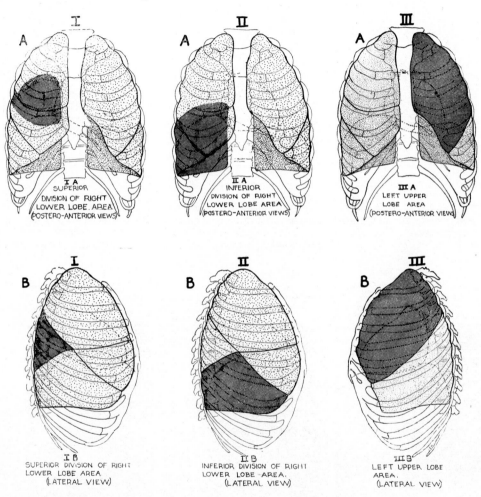

Fig. 248.—Diagrammatic x-Ray Appearance of Partial Right Lower Lobe and Left Upper Lobe
    Consolidations. (Postero-anterior and Lateral Views.) (Modified from H. Brunn and J.
    Levitin in Radiology.)

The *inferior division* is the larger part of the lower lobe. It extends posteriorly, anteriorly, and inferiorly to the diaphragm, and its shadow is continuous with that of the liver. In the postero-anterior view, the upper margin may be horizontal or oblique, depending on the nature of the disease process, *i. e.*, whether the lesion be consolidation or atelectasis. In the lateral view, the upper border usually is tented, although it, too, may be horizontal, depending on the nature of the disease process.

The *left lung* presents less complicating factors in its appearance on the roentgenogram than the right. The presence of only two lobes, with the one interlobar fissure, reduces the number of possible combinations of lobes involved and the variety of interlobar effusions

SURGICAL CONSIDERATIONS

1. **Pulmonary Embolism and Infarct.**—The pulmonary artery carries to the lungs all the blood from the caval system of veins. Any sudden stoppage of this most important carrier, as from a fragment of clot (*embolus*), will, according to the degree and point of obstruction, suppress the function of a part or all of the lung. No collateral circulation can be established because the pulmonary artery is a terminal artery. When the embolus is small, it may lodge in a minor branch of the pulmonary artery, eliminating but a small area of the lung from function. The consequence is the formation of an avascular segment of lung, known as an *infarct*.

2. **Lung Abscess.**—A nontuberculous lung abscess is the result of the destruction of pulmonary tissue by bacteria. The offending organisms are those found commonly in dental sepsis or in tonsil infection: streptococcus, fusiform bacillus, spirochete of Vincent, and the anaerobic bacillus, melaninogenicum. These bacteria may be aspirated with a foreign body, or with blood and tissue fragments following mouth or throat surgery, and may plug a small bronchus. By this mechanism, an abscess or gangrene may develop. It is probable that an infarct may become infected by the aspiration of organisms. The postpneumonic abscess doubtless is caused by invasion of devitalized tissue. A mixed hematogenous and aspiration origin is not uncommon.

Spontaneous cures of this condition occasionally occur. A cure may be effected by widening the opening of the cavity and evacuating its contents by aspiration through the bronchoscope. Sometimes an artificial pneumothorax will collapse an abscess and allow it to heal. Bronchoscopy is advisable whenever a foreign body or new growth is suspected, or when the etiology of the abscess is obscure. *Operative treatment* consists of thoracotomy and drainage.

3. **Bronchiectasis.**—Bronchiectasis is a more or less extensive dilatation of part of the bronchial tree associated with infection. The disease is chronic and is remarkable for its large amounts of exceedingly foul sputum. The epithelium lining the bronchi is destroyed and the muscularis of the bronchial walls atrophies. The organisms passing through the ulcerated walls penetrate the alveolar tissue, and give rise to multiple small abscesses. One lobe only may be affected, but both lungs may be involved uniformly. Bronchiectasis may follow the aspiration of a foreign body, or may be occasioned by a tumor within, or pressing upon, a bronchus. Bronchiectatic lesions may be demonstrated by x-ray by the injection of a radio-opaque oil (lipiodol) through the larynx into the bronchial tree.

Early bronchiectasis resulting from the presence of a foreign body often is cured by bronchoscopic removal of that body. Bronchoscopic treatment is no more than palliative if infection has become well established and pathologic changes are advanced. In late stages, the only curative treatment consists in the removal of the affected lobe or lobes, *lobectomy*. The diseased portion of the lung may be removed piecemeal by cauterization.

4. **Penetrating Wounds of the Lung.**—Wounds of the lung usually are accompanied by hemorrhage, the gravity of which depends upon the location of the lesion. The bleeding may be confined in the lung tissue and be spat up through a bronchus, or it may enter the pleural cavity, producing hemothorax. Wounds of the hilar zone are the most serious, as they may involve the large vascular trunks, while those of the outer zones are relatively harmless, the hemorrhage accompanying them being rapidly absorbed. Lung hemorrhage must be differentiated from that due to a torn intercostal vessel. Hemothorax may become infected, forming *pyohemothorax*.

5. **Pneumotomy.**—Pneumotomy denotes an incision into the lung substance with a view to reaching an intrapulmonary cavity. It is indicated mainly in pulmonary abscess. Hemorrhage is the principal danger attending the operation, and anticipation of it has led most surgeons to employ the cautery for penetrating the lung substance. The procedure is facilitated greatly if adhesions have formed between the visceral and parietal layers of the pleura, as extensive pneumothorax is obviated and the general pleural cavity is walled

off from infection. When adequate adhesions have not been formed, a two-stage operation is performed. In the first stage, adhesions are produced between the visceral and parietal pleurae by exposing the parietal pleura and packing against it. In the second stage, the abscess is opened. The presence of an abscess is determined best by *x*-ray examination after bronchoscopic injection of iodized oil. The multiplicity of abscesses resulting from

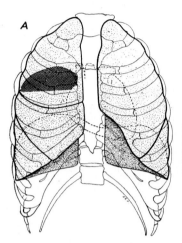 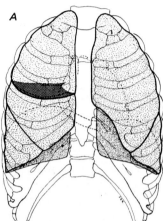 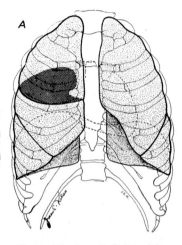

Figure I, A and B. Interlobar space and corresponding effusion between right upper and lower lobes... Posterior — Anterior Views.

Figure II, A and B. Interlobar space and corresponding effusion between right upper and middle lobes... Posterior — Anterior Views.

Figure III, A and B. Interlobar space and corresponding effusion between right upper and the lower and middle lobes... Posterior — Anterior Views.

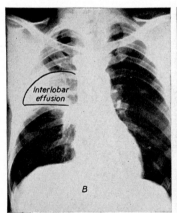 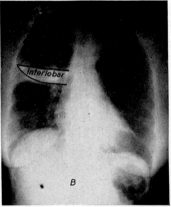 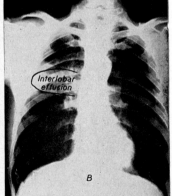

Fig. 249a.—*x*-Ray Appearance of Potential Right Interlobar Spaces in Diagrams and in Corresponding Clinical Effusions (Postero-anterior Views). (Modified from H. Brunn and J. Levitin in Radiology.)

the free branching of the bronchi greatly increases the danger of treating suppurative lesions in the lungs by surgical measures.

   6. *x*-Ray Appearance of Potential Interlobar Spaces and Corresponding Interlobar Effusions.—The method by which the *x*-ray opaque interlobar spaces were made experimentally and the manner of their appearance in postero-anterior and lateral roentgenograms has been explained (pp. 251 and 252).

It is apparent from Figs. 249 and 250 that a lateral *x*-ray view, taken in the same plane as the interlobar fissure, gives a totally different conception of the potential extent of the fissures than does a postero-anterior view. The same, of course, is true of the *x*-ray appearance of clinical effusions in the interlobar areas when lateral and postero-anterior roentgenograms are studied.

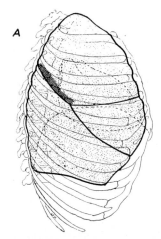

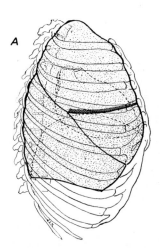

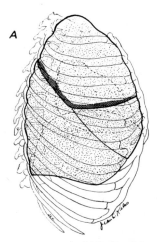

Figure I, A and B. Interlobar space and corresponding ef−fusion between right upper and lower lobes... Lateral Views.

Figure II, A and B. Interlobar space and corresponding ef−fusion between right upper and middle lobes... Lateral Views.

Figure III, A and B. Interlobar space and corresponding ef−fusion between right upper and the lower and middle lobes.

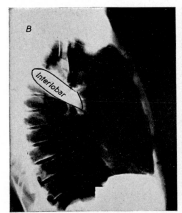

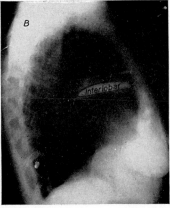

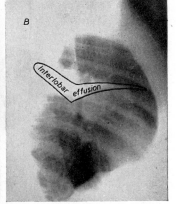

FIG. 249*b*.—*x*-RAY APPEARANCE OF POTENTIAL RIGHT INTERLOBAR SPACES IN DIAGRAMS AND IN COR-RESPONDING CLINICAL EFFUSIONS (LATERAL VIEWS). (Modified from H. Brunn and J. Levitin in Radiology.)

Two interlobar fissures divide the right lung into three lobes, the upper, middle, and lower. One fissure divides the left lung into two lobes, an upper and a lower.

The *interlobar fissure between the right upper and lower lobes* is the only area of contact between these lobes. This fissure extends obliquely upward and posteriorly from the lung hilus. In the postero-anterior view, it appears as a broad shadow which often is misin-

17

terpreted as lobar involvement.   The lateral view in the diagram and in the clinical effusion demonstrates clearly the oblique position of the fissure.

Physical signs of involvement of the fissure by an effusion may be absent.   This is easy to understand when we realize that this fissure only approaches the chest wall in the

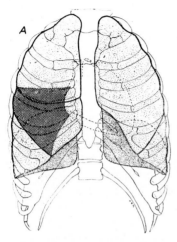 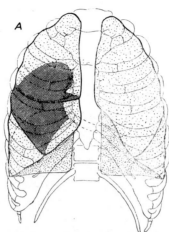 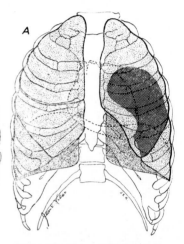

Figure I, A and B. Interlobar space and corresponding effusion between right middle and lower lobes....Posterior −Anterior Views.

Figure II, A and B. Interlobar spaces and corresponding effusion between right upper and the middle and lower lobes..... Posterior −Anterior Views.

Figure III, A and B. Interlobar space and corresponding effusion between left upper and lower lobes.... Posterior −Anterior Views.

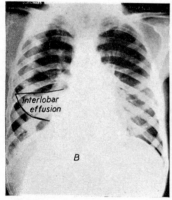 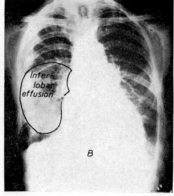 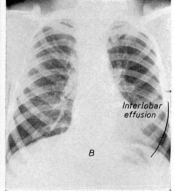

Fig. 250a.—x-Ray Appearance of Potential Interlobar Spaces in Diagrams and in Corresponding Clinical Effusions (Postero-anterior Views). (Modified from H. Brunn and J. Levitin in Radiology.)

axilla, its narrowest part.   In front of and behind this fissure is lung parenchyma, which if not involved, does not transmit the dulness of an interlobar effusion.

A study of the *interlobar fissure between the right upper and middle lobes* illustrates why physical signs of an effusion in this fissure are absent.   Here again the diseased process is overlapped both in front and behind by considerable lung tissue, which, if not involved, does not transmit the dulness of the effusion.

The shadow cast by an effusion in the *fissure which entirely surrounds the right upper lobe* is broad in the postero-anterior film. Since interlobar effusions most frequently follow pneumonia and cause subsequent temperature elevation, and since lung abscess is a frequent complication of pneumonia, the interpretation of the shadow caused by an effusion in this fissure is a pitfall which must be guarded against. The lateral view clearly

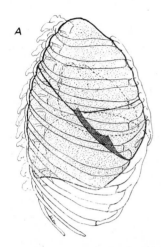

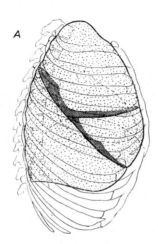

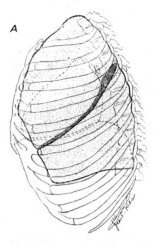

Figure I, A and B. Interlobar space and corresponding effusion between right middle and lower lobes.... Lateral Views.

Figure II, A and B. Interlobar spaces and corresponding effusion between right upper and the middle and lower lobes... Lateral Views.

Figure III, A and B. Interlobar space and corresponding effusion between left upper and lower lobes. . Lateral Views.

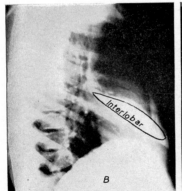

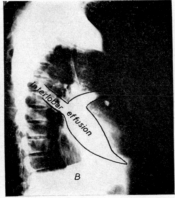

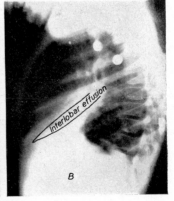

FIG. 250b.—x-RAY APPEARANCE OF POTENTIAL INTERLOBAR SPACES IN DIAGRAMS AND IN CORRESPONDING CLINICAL EFFUSIONS (LATERAL VIEWS). (Modified from H. Brunn and J. Levitin in Radiology.)

demonstrates the contour of this fissure. It is the posterior component of this fissure which casts the broad shadow.

Effusion in the *fissure between the right middle and lower lobes* is the most frequent of all fluid collections in the interlobar spaces and often is diagnosed incorrectly. The oblique course of this fissure, clearly demonstrated on the lateral view, explains the reason for the broad shadow seen on the roentgenogram in the postero-anterior view.

7. Partial Pneumectomy.—Excision of a portion of the lung is beset with great difficulties, and is a procedure to be used only in chronic cases when less radical measures have failed. In the absence of adhesions, one must pass through a large serous cavity to reach the involved lung. This step necessarily entails the development of pneumothorax and incurs the risk of infection. Total removal of a lobe is indicated when it contains many undrained bronchial dilatations or abscesses. A lobe may be resected for a lung tumor.

8. Postoperative Pulmonary Atelectasis (Collapse).—Atelectasis may be defined as the collapse of the whole, or any part of, a lung or of both lungs, resulting from disappearance of air from the alveoli. This deflation of the lung, with its group of variable symptoms and signs, is the predominant postoperative surgical complication. The major cause of this condition is any obstruction to free bronchial drainage, often a tenacious mucous plug.

The cardinal x-ray signs of a massive pulmonary collapse are: elevation of the diaphragm and narrowing of the rib spaces on the affected side, displacement of the mediastinum and trachea toward the affected side, and lung shadow. All of these signs result from the increased negative pressure which occurs with the disappearance of air in the involved lung distal to the obstruction.

Carbon dioxide induced hyperventilation, combined with frequent postural changes, should be employed as soon as this condition is recognized. A plug of tenacious sputum may require removal through the bronchoscope. The prognosis of uncomplicated postoperative atelectasis is excellent.

C. MEDIASTINUM (INTERPLEURAL SPACE)

The mediastinum or central compartment of the chest cavity is the space between the lungs bounded by the posterior aspect of the sternum, the anterior surface of the spine, the two pleuropulmonary areas ,and the diaphragm. It is not accurately median, but inclines somewhat to the left side. The mediastinum is shut off fairly securely from

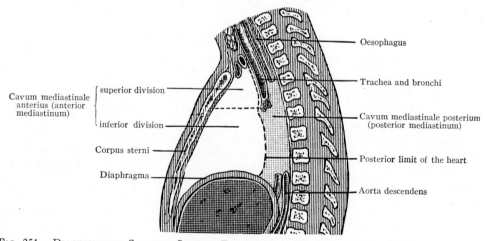

Oesophagus

Trachea and bronchi

Cavum mediastinale anterius (anterior mediastinum)

superior division

inferior division

Cavum mediastinale posterium (posterior mediastinum)

Corpus sterni

Posterior limit of the heart

Diaphragma

Aorta descendens

FIG. 251.—DIAGRAMMATIC SAGITTAL SECTION THROUGH THE THORAX TO SHOW THE ANTERIOR AND POSTERIOR DIVISIONS OF THE MEDIASTINUM. (Modified from Testut and Jacob.)
The anterior mediastinum is separated into superior and inferior divisions by the superior border of the heart.

the abdominal cavity save at three main points: a narrow interval anteriorly between the sternal and costal attachments of the diaphragm, filled with loose connective tissue; the aortic opening posteriorly; and the esophageal hiatus.

Many surgically important structures lie in the mediastinum: the heart with the great vessels and the pericardium, the trachea and bronchi, the esophagus, aorta, nerves, and lymph glands.   Until recently the region was considered inaccessible, but now it is explored extensively.   Arbitrary subdivisions are valuable for descriptive purposes.   The mediastinum is divided into anterior and posterior divisions by a frontal plane passing in front of the trachea and its bifurcation.   The **anterior mediastinum** is divided into superior and inferior divisions by a transverse plane passing through the union of the first and second portions of the sternum which marks the level of the superior border of the heart.

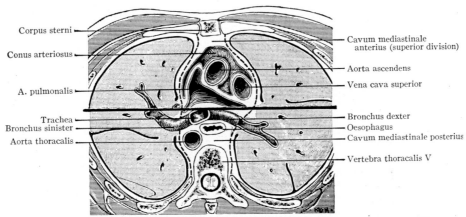

FIG. 252.—CROSS SECTION THROUGH THE THORAX AT THE LEVEL OF THE BIFURCATION OF THE TRACHEA TO SHOW THE ANTERIOR AND POSTERIOR DIVISIONS OF THE MEDIASTINUM.

The division line is marked by a horizontal plane anterior to the tracheal bifurcation; the structures of the anterior and posterior divisions are enclosed by broken lines.

The *superior division* includes the thymus and the great vessels passing to and from the heart.   The *inferior division* is occupied by the pericardium and heart.   In the **posterior mediastinum** are the trachea, bronchi, esophagus, descending aorta, thoracic duct, azygos veins, vagus, and sympathetic nerves.

(I) ANTERIOR MEDIASTINUM

(A) SUPERIOR DIVISION OF THE ANTERIOR MEDIASTINUM

Anteroposteriorly, the structures within the superior division of the anterior mediastinum are: the thymus, a venous layer composed of the innominate veins forming the superior vena cava, an arterial layer made up of the pulmonary arteries, the aorta, and the innominate and left common carotid arteries.   Between the vascular trunks of the area lie the vagus and phrenic nerves and the anterior mediastinal lymph glands.

1. **Thymus.**—The thymus is a transitory structure acquiring its greatest development in the first two years of life, after which time it normally regresses until, in the adult, it is replaced almost completely by adipose and connective tissue.   In the newborn, its two well-developed, elongated lobes, which rarely are symmetrical, lie in the anterosuperior part of the retromanubrial region in front of the great vessels and the trachea.   The lobes sometimes mold themselves over the upper circumference of the pericardial sac, and even may occupy a cervical position, reaching occasionally to the hyoid bone.   *Thymic enlargement* produces tracheal compression causing noisy, difficult inspiration and expiration, known as *thymic stridor*.   This is thought to progress to what commonly is called thymic asthma.   Attacks of thymic asthma are believed to be precipitated by very minor occurrences, and a few deaths on induction of anesthesia have been attributed to this cause. In patients suspected of having thymic asthma, an intralaryngeal or intrabronchial foreign body should be ruled out by bronchoscopy.

2. **Innominate Veins and Superior Vena Cava.**—The *innominate veins* (p. 216) unite at the inferior border of the first costal cartilage on the right to form the superior vena

cava.   The *superior vena cava* runs an inferior course of about 4 to 5 cm ,to the right atrium.   Its projection on the anterior chest wall corresponds to the first and second right intercostal spaces and the sternal extremities of the first two ribs.   It is extrapericardial in most of its course.

3. **Pulmonary Arteries.**—The trunk of the pulmonary artery, or the pulmonary aorta, directs the blood from the right ventricle to the lung.   Throughout most of its course, it lies within the pericardium at the base of the heart.   From the superior border of the artery, a short cord, the *ligamentum arteriosum*, runs to the inferior part of the aortic arch. This cord is the persisting portion of the *ductus arteriosus*, the fetal communication which

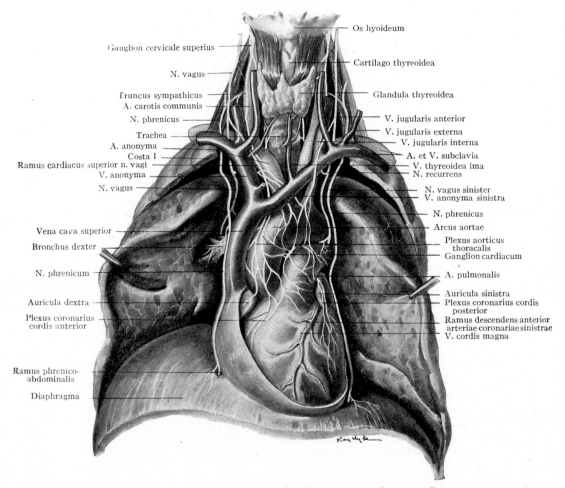

FIG. 253.—ANTERIOR VIEW OF THE STRUCTURES IN THE SUPERIOR AND INFERIOR DIVISIONS OF THE AN-
TERIOR MEDIASTINUM.

diverted blood from the pulmonary artery to the systemic aorta, sidetracking the then nonfunctioning lungs.   Incomplete occlusion of the duct occurs rather frequently, and generally is associated with a patent foramen ovale between the right and left auricles.   Both congenital defects make for insufficient aeration of the blood, and are common causes of death at birth and in early infancy.   The mixture of venous and arterial blood causes the cyanosis of the "blue baby."

4. **Ascending Aorta and Its Arch.**—The *ascending aorta* arises from the base of the left ventricle behind the left sternal margin opposite the third costal cartilage.   The aortic bulb, the dilated origin of the aorta, contains three secondary dilatations, the aortic

sinuses, which correspond to the three semilunar cusps of the aortic valve.   The right and left coronary arteries spring from the corresponding aortic sinuses.   At the second right costal interspace, the aorta is covered only by the thin anterior lappet of the right lung, so that, at this point, the aortic sound can be heard most readily.   The ascending aorta is enclosed completely by the pericardium.   The superior vena cava lies on its right, and the pulmonary artery on its left.

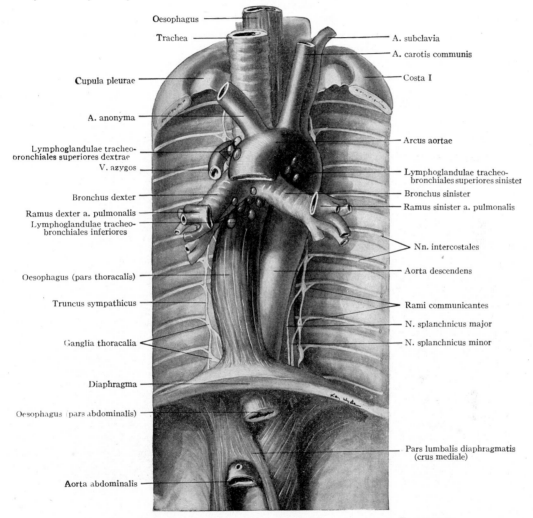

Oesophagus

Trachea

Cupula pleurae

A. anonyma

Lymphoglandulae tracheo-
bronchiales superiores dextrae

V. azygos

Bronchus dexter

Ramus dexter a. pulmonalis

Lymphoglandulae tracheo-
bronchiales inferiores

Oesophagus (pars thoracalis)

Truncus sympathicus

Ganglia thoracalia

Diaphragma

Oesophagus (pars abdominalis)

Aorta abdominalis

A. subclavia

A. carotis communis

Costa I

Arcus aortae

Lymphoglandulae tracheo-
bronchiales superiores sinister

Bronchus sinister

Ramus sinister a. pulmonalis

Nn. intercostales

Aorta descendens

Rami communicantes

N. splanchnicus major

N. splanchnicus minor

Pars lumbalis diaphragmatis
(crus mediale)

FIG. 254.—TOPOGRAPHY OF THE TRACHEA, AORTIC ARCH, AND ESOPHAGUS.

The *arch* of the aorta lies behind the lower part of the sternal manubrium.   It begins behind the right border of the sternum at the level of the second rib cartilage and extends dorsally to the left to reach the spine at the left of the body of the fourth thoracic vertebra.

5. **Innominate, Left Common Carotid, and Left Subclavian Arteries.**—From the arch of the aorta branch the innominate, left common carotid, and left subclavian arteries, in the order named.

(B) INFERIOR DIVISION OR PERICARDIUM AND HEART

1. **Pericardium, Its Layers, Cavity, and Relations.**—The *pericardium* is a closed fibroserous sac within which the heart and the proximal portions of its great vessels are enclosed.   It is cone-shaped and its base is directed inferiorly to a broad attachment at the diaphragm (p. 239).

Between its visceral and parietal layers is the *pericardial cavity*. Under normal conditions this is a potential space, with the serous walls in apposition. It becomes a true cavity when the walls are separated by fluid or air (hydropericardium, pneumopericardium). When the patient is in the erect position, pericardial fluid collects in the subcardiac reserve space or recess which lies anteriorly between the attachment of the pericardium to the diaphragm and the inferior margin of the heart.

The anterior portion of the pericardium lies against the anterior chest wall, and is divided into extrapleural and retropleural areas by the pleural reflections which lie upon it. When the anterior mediastinal pleural sinuses extend over the pericardium to the midsternal line, all of the front wall of the pericardium is retropleural, and there is no uncovered area. The extrapleural or uncovered area normally present is of extreme

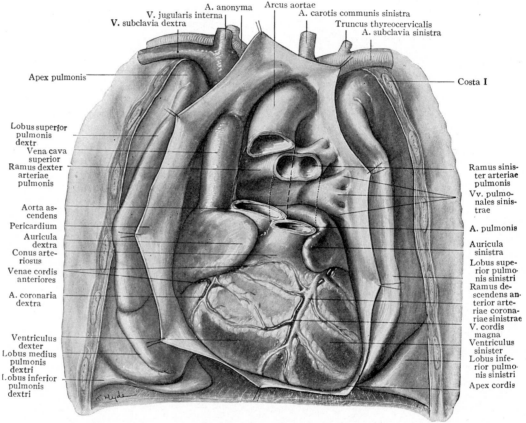

FIG. 255.—HEART AND THE GREAT VESSELS FROM THE FRONT, SHOWING THE REFLECTIONS OF THE PERICARDIUM.

importance from the surgical point of view, as it represents the only direct, accessible area of the pericardium where puncture can be made if pleural injury is to be avoided (p. 265). The intimate esophageal relations explain the difficulties in swallowing sometimes experienced in pericardial effusion and cardiac hypertrophy.

2. **Adhesive Pericarditis and Pericardial Effusion.**—Inflammatory lesions of the pericardium may modify the pericardial cavity by adhesions obliterating it, or by effusion enlarging it.

Obliteration of the cavity by *adhesive pericarditis* may not embarrass the heart action to any serious degree, but massive mediastinal adhesions, contracted by the pericardium as a whole, are a serious obstruction to competent heart action. This latter condition is the result of internal and external pericarditis in combination with hyperplastic mediastinitis, leaving a permanently adherent mass involving all the divisions of the pericardium and neighboring mediastinal structures. With each systolic contraction, the drawing in of the left chest taxes the heart severely. The operation of *cardiolysis* (of Brauer) has been devised to render heart action freer in such cases. This procedure consists of removal of sections of the ribs and the costal cartilages which overlie the pericardium, in order to substitute for the bony framework a more flexible musculocutaneous covering.

As the potential capacity of the pericardium is considerably greater than the volume of the heart and enclosed vessels, a large quantity of fluid may collect within the sac without causing untoward symptoms. If *pericardial effusion* develops slowly, the walls of the sac gradually stretch and the fluid content increases to an enormous amount, a liter or more, without causing serious disturbance. A sudden effusion, as of blood following a cardiac injury, collects rapidly and is not tolerated (cardiac tamponage).

As the pericardium becomes distended, its relations undergo important alterations. Generally, the anterior lung margins recede, and the lines of pleural reflection (costomediastinal) withdraw laterally until an abnormally wide area of the pericardium comes into immediate contact with the anterior chest wall. This is not invariable, for, in some cases,

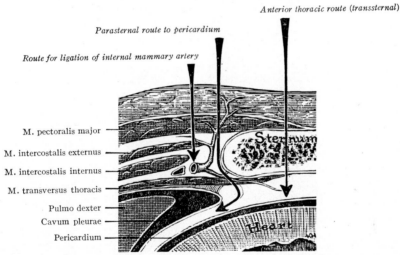

Anterior thoracic route (transsternal)

Parasternal route to pericardium

Route for ligation of internal mammary artery

M. pectoralis major

M. intercostalis externus

M. intercostalis internus

M. transversus thoracis

Pulmo dexter

Cavum pleurae

Pericardium

Sternum

Heart

FIG. 256.—SCHEMATIC CROSS SECTION THROUGH THE STERNAL REGION, PASSING THROUGH THE LEFT FIFTH INTERCOSTAL SPACE, TO SHOW THE RELATIONS OF THE INTERNAL MAMMARY ARTERY TO THE LEFT PLEURAL SINUS AND TO THE PERICARDIUM. (Modified from Testut and Jacob.)

the anterior pleural reflections remain in close apposition. Changed relationships between the pericardium and chest wall are recognized by percussion, which reveals an increased area of cardiac dulness roughly triangular in outline, broad inferiorly and narrowing superiorly. With a much distended pericardium, the dulness may extend from the first to the seventh ribs. Transversely, it may extend to the right as far as the mammary line.

The heart, suspended by the great vessels, is displaced posteriorly and superiorly in the fluid. As a result, its impulse becomes indistinct or imperceptible and its sounds inaudible. Fluid pressure exerted upon the heart, great vessels, and air passages causes progressive dyspnea. Difficulty in swallowing (dysphagia) sometimes is observed in consequence of compression of the esophagus. Repeated cardiac tapping (paracentesis) is indicated when exploratory puncture reveals no suppuration. If suppuration exists, rib resection with incision of the pericardium (pericardiotomy) is performed.

3. **Paracentesis of the Pericardium (Pericardiocentesis).**—Puncture or paracentesis of the pericardium is the piercing of the pericardium for the withdrawal of its content. This may be done as an exploratory or a therapeutic procedure. The selection of a site for the introduction of the needle must avoid the internal mammary vessels, pleura, and

heart. It should reach the largest collection of fluid in a favorable position for aspiration and, if deemed necessary, for incision.

Avoiding the internal mammary vessels is so important that all points of election for puncture lie lateral or mesial to them.

All the interspaces from the third to the seventh. either close to the sternum or lateral to the vessels, are satisfactory.

The danger incident to puncture of the pleura has been disregarded notably despite many reported cases of pleural infection following pericardial tap in septic cases. As one often is doubtful of the nature of the fluid in acute cases, it is safer to introduce the needle at a point where it is unlikely to injure either pleural sac. The diagrams of the pleural reflections (p. 242) show that the risk of injuring the pleura will be least if the needle is introduced through the anterior extremity of the fifth or sixth intercostal space, close to the sternum. The extreme narrowness of these spaces renders this a little difficult, especially as the interspace at this level often is reduced to a slit, and even that is blocked partially by cartilage. The sixth space is an excellent site for puncture as it overlies directly the large subcardiac pericardial recess, within which the bulk of the pericardial fluid is obtained; there is little risk of wounding the heart at this level. It rarely will be necessary to penetrate deeper than 2.5 cm., as the distended pericardium lies in close apposition to the sternochondral wall. The extreme thickness and toughness of the pericardium in some cases of purulent pericarditis make paracentesis difficult, as do adhesions of the serous layers and marked dilatation of the heart with only a limited effusion. The possibility of injuring the heart or a coronary vessel is a source of anxiety. The reasons for the election of puncture rather than open incision are its safety and simplicity.

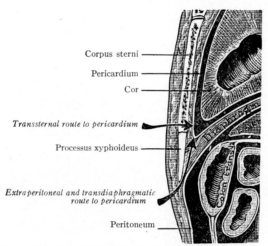

Corpus sterni

Pericardium

Cor

Transsternal route to pericardium

Processus xyphoideus

Extraperitoneal and transdiaphragmatic route to pericardium

Peritoneum

Fig. 257.—Schematic Sagittal Section Through the Sternal Region to Show the Anterior Relations of the Pericardium. (After Testut and Jacob.)

4. **Pericardiotomy.**—Pericardiotomy, or incision into the pericardium for the exposure and drainage of a purulent effusion, may be done after *subperichondrial excision* of the fifth left costal cartilage.

The internal mammary vessels are exposed, lying on the transversus thoracis (triangularis sterni) muscle. Incision is made through the perichondrium of the excised cartilage. More extensive exposure may require similar excision of the fourth and sixth cartilages. Greater access is obtained by chipping away the left border of the sternum. When the internal mammary vessels have been ligated, the transversus thoracis muscle is divided and the pericardium with its thin covering of mediastinal fat is exposed. The fat is wiped aside and the left pleural reflection is identified and displaced laterally with the fingers. The pericardium then is opened and drained.

The procedure may be carried out through a *transsternal approach*. A trephine opening is made in the sternum to avoid injuring the blood vessels and the margins of the pleura. By this route, the point of greatest and most dependent pericardial accumulation may be reached. By means of blunt dissection, the endothoracic fascia, the fibers of the triangularis sterni muscle (transversus thoracis), and the pleural margins may be pushed away. The pericardial sac can be seized, drawn into the opening, incised, and drained. The pericardium also may be exposed *inferior to the inferior end of the sternum*. This approach is simple, requires but little time, and drains freely the lowest available part of the cavity.

5. Heart in General.—The heart is a muscular organ so invaginated into the pericardium and so suspended by the great vessels at its base as to permit free movement. It has two separate receiving and pumping stations, a right venous unit and a left arterial unit. The right unit collects the blood from the systemic veins and drives it through the lungs. The left unit receives the purified blood from the lungs into its atrium; its ventricle drives the blood throughout the general arterial system.

The thin partition separating the two atria, the *atrial septum*, possesses near its middle an oval depression, the *fossa ovalis*. This depression marks the patent fossa ovalis of fetal life, by which blood from the right atrium was sidetracked from the lungs and transmitted directly into the left atrium to be emptied into the left ventricle; from this chamber it was forced into the systemic circuit. A small portion of the fossa may remain patent after birth as a consequence of insufficient development of the heart, and cause a mixture of non-oxygenated blood to enter the general circulation (cyanosis).

6. Means of Fixation of the Heart; Its Movements.—The heart is held in position mainly by its connection with the great vascular trunks at its base. It is further supported by the pericardium, which is in relation with the lungs and mediastinal pleurae and has actual attachment to the diaphragm. The right auricle is attached to the diaphragm by the inferior vena cava. Pathologic conditions arise in which the heart is displaced. For example, a large one-sided pleural effusion may displace the heart across the midsagittal plane to the uninvolved side, and pulmonary atelectasis may displace the heart to the side of the atelectasis.

The heart normally moves to the dependent side in the lateral recumbent posture and hangs more inferiorly in the standing position. In dorsal decubitus, the heart so recedes from the chest wall that the apex beat may become imperceptible. In forced inspiration, the heart descends perceptibly because of the attachment of the pericardium to the diaphragm.

7. Thoracic Projection of the Heart (Precordium) and Great Vessels.—The *projection* of the heart on the anterior chest wall (precordium) is outlined approximately as follows. The superior border of the heart is represented by a line drawn across the sternum at the level of the attachment of the third costal cartilage from points 2.5 cm. lateral to either sternal margin. This line is the clinical base of the heart, the line of demarcation from the great vessels. The normal extreme left margin of the heart is at a point a little inferior to the nipple in the left fifth intercostal space.

An anteroposterior *x*-ray film, with the tube 6 feet from the patient, shows a heart shadow accurate in outline. The location and shape of the heart can be seen to vary with the changes in position of the diaphragm. When the diaphragm is high, the heart lies in a more horizontal plane, the long axis through the base and apex forming a wider angle with the midsternal plane. In a long thorax with a low-placed diaphragm, the heart hangs in a more dependent position in the chest cavity, its axial or base-apex line forming a more acute angle with the midsternal line.

The thoracic projection of the right atrium reaches from the third to the sixth costal cartilage and is about 1 to 2 cm. lateral to the right sternal border. The right ventricle corresponds to the left half of the sternum and extends laterally to the left parasternal line from the third to the sixth left costal cartilage. The auricular appendix of the left atrium is the only part of that chamber that has a thoracic projection. This lies at the level of the sternal attachment of the left third costal cartilage. The dorsal projection of the left atrium lies at the level of the bodies of the seventh to ninth thoracic vertebrae. Only that small strip of the left ventricle, extending from the third to the sixth costal cartilage and forming the cardiac apex, can be seen from the front.

The *great vessel area* may be outlined by drawing a horizontal line across the sternum at the junction of the superior and middle thirds of the manubrium. This line should be a little less than 2.5 cm. inferior to the suprasternal notch and should extend to the right and left a sufficient distance to permit the drawing of vertical lines to the lateral limits of the superior margin of the cardiac area.

8. Thoracic Projection and Areas of Maximum Audibility of the Heart Valves.—In order to recognize the normal valve sounds and interpret properly pathologic findings by auscultation, it is necessary to locate the cardiac valves accurately. Consideration must be given to the depth of the valves from the chest surfaces and to the sound-transmitting quality of the intervening tissue, as well as to the direction of flow between the heart chambers. Of the four valves, the right auriculoventricular (tricuspid) and pulmonic lie nearer the surface than the left auriculoventricular (mitral) and aortic valves.

The *right auriculoventricular (tricuspid) valve* is located posterior and lateral to the lowermost quarter of the sternum behind the attachments of the right fourth, fifth, and sixth costal cartilages. Its area of greatest audibility is directly over its surface projection. The *pulmonary valve* lies mainly posterior to the third left costal cartilage, and the clearest sound of its closure is heard directly over its location in the second left interspace. The *left auriculoventricular (mitral) valve* lies at a much deeper level than the valves of the

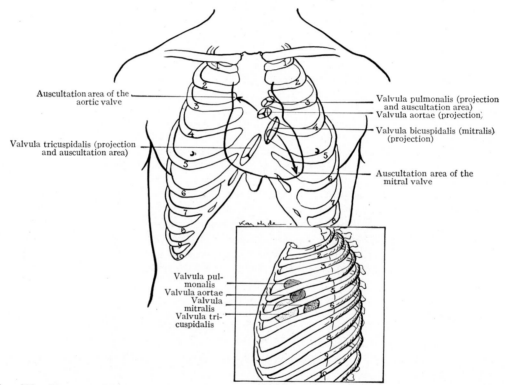

Fig. 258.—THORACIC PROJECTION OF THE HEART VALVES AND THEIR AREAS OF MAXIMUM AUDIBILITY

right side of the heart, and is located posterior to the left half of the sternum on a level with the fourth costal cartilage. Its auscultatory area is in the direction of the blood flow from the auricle to the ventricle, and is over the apex of the heart where the tip of the ventricle is in apposition with the chest wall. The *aortic valve* is overlain in part by the pulmonary valve, and is located posterior to the left sternal margin and the mesial part of the left third interspace. The sound of its closure is projected along the course of the blood stream and may be heard best in the second right interspace at the sternal margin.

9. Vessels and Nerves of the Heart.—The *arterial supply* of the heart muscle is derived from the right and left coronary arteries which spring from the aortic sinuses. Their origins are hidden anteriorly by the right auricular appendix and the pulmonary artery. The right coronary artery runs in the right portion of the coronary sulcus between the auricular appendix and the right ventricle. The left coronary artery is hidden at its origin by the pulmonary artery. Its short trunk divides into a descending ramus which runs down the anterior interventricular groove toward the apex, while the posterior circumflex branch is more horizontal and runs in the coronary sulcus to be distributed to the posterior portion of the heart. Coronary sclerosis or spasms, with obliteration of the arterial supply producing cardiac ischemia, may be the pathologic basis of angina pectoris.

Most of the *veins* of the heart enter the coronary sinus, a wide venous channel situated deep in the posterior part of the coronary sulcus. It opens into the right atrium between the auriculoventricular orifice and that for the inferior vena cava.

The *nerves* forming the cardiac plexus, which spreads over the aortic arch and heart, are derived from the vagus and from the cervical gangliated chain (p. 191).

10. **Exposure of the Heart.**—The heart may be exposed adequately by either of two methods, median sternotomy or intercostochondral thoracotomy. In *median sternotomy*, the skin is incised from the level of the second interspace to the midpoint between the

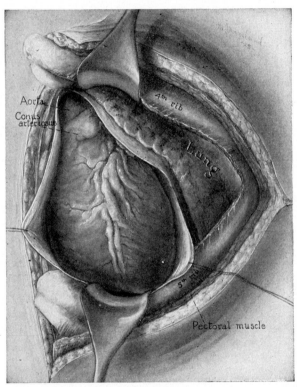

FIG. 259.—EXPOSURE OF THE HEART BY INTERCOSTOCHONDRAL THORACOTOMY. (After C. S. Beck; courtesy of Archives of Surgery.)

umbilicus and the xiphoid The overlying structures are freed from the sternum, which is split lengthwise to the upper level of the skin incision at which point the bone is cut across. The xiphoid is removed or is displaced laterally, and the internal mammary vessels are avoided carefully. The halves of the sternum are retracted and the pleura is pushed aside, after which the anterior portion of the diaphragm and peritoneum are incised. The pericardium is opened widely by an incision extending to the pericardial reflection over the diaphragm, and the heart is brought well into view.

In *intercostochondral thoracotomy*, an incision is made in the left fourth intercostal space from the anterior axillary line to the lateral border of the sternum. The third, fourth, fifth, and sixth costal cartilages then are sectioned, the internal mammary vessels are ligated, and the incision is carried into the pleura. The superior and inferior T flaps are retracted and the pericardium is opened. The left lung, left ventricle, and part of the right ventricle are exposed.

(II) Posterior Mediastinum

The posterior mediastinum lies behind the frontal plane, passing in front of the bifurcation of the trachea and the posterior surface of the heart. The most important structures contained in the abundant areolar tissue characteristic of the compartment are: the trachea, bronchi, thoracic esophagus, descending part of the thoracic aorta, thoracic duct, sympathetic gangliated trunk, and azygos vein with its tributaries. Abscesses from spontaneous or traumatic rupture of the esophagus, or from tuberculosis of the vertebral body, are fairly common here.

1. **Mediastinal Trachea and the Primary Bronchi.**—The thoracic part of the trachea runs from the superior margin of the sternum to the level of the junction of the first and second portions of the sternum where it bifurcates into two primary bronchi. The trachea occupies the median sagittal plane of the chest, and remains in front of the esophagus. The caliber and structure of the thoracic trachea are similar to those of the cervical part (p. 188). At the margins of the primary bronchi, a sagittal spur, the *carina*, which is seen clearly through the bronchoscope, runs upward into the lumen. The right bronchus continues nearly in the direction of the trachea, but the left is placed more horizontally. For this reason, foreign bodies are much more likely to drop into the right bronchus.

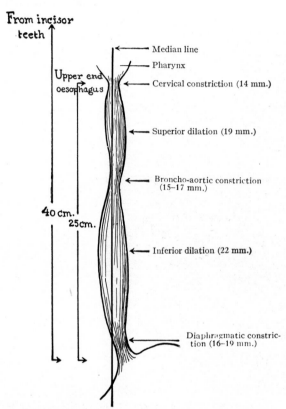

FIG. 260.—THE ESOPHAGUS FROM THE FRONT TO SHOW ITS DILATIONS, CONSTRICTIONS, AND MEASUREMENTS.

2. **Thoracic Esophagus.**—The thoracic esophagus is the continuation of the cervical esophagus and follows a somewhat curved course. It reaches the esophageal orifice of the diaphragm at the level of the tenth thoracic vertebra.

The *length* of the adult esophagus is 25 cm. An important measurement in esophageal manipulations is the distance from the teeth to the cardia. This is derived by adding the distance from the incisor teeth to the beginning of the esophagus at the cricoid cartilage, a distance of 15 cm., giving a total of 40 cm. All measurements are made carefully, since they may demonstrate accurately the site of tumors and strictures.

The esophagus presents three distinct *narrowings*. The first is at its beginning at the level of the cricoid cartilage. The second is behind the bifurcation of the trachea (broncho-aortic constriction) at the level of the fourth thoracic vertebra. The third constriction is at its point of passage through the esophageal hiatus into the abdominal cavity. These constrictions, particularly the second, have a tendency to stop foreign bodies, are subjected to maximum injury when chemicals are ingested, and are sites for carcinoma.

3. **Descending Part of the Thoracic Aorta.**—The descending part of the thoracic aorta extends from the termination of the arch at the inferior left side of the fourth thoracic vertebra to its diaphragmatic orifice. In the superior portion of its course, the aorta deviates a little to the left of the median line, but gradually regains the median plane to enter the abdomen through the aortic hiatus (p. 239). The intimate relation of the aorta with the pleura and the left lung explains the rupture of aortic aneurysm into the pleural sac

(Fig. 244). From the posterior surface of the aorta are given off nine or ten intercostal arteries.

4. **Thoracic Duct.**—The thoracic duct is the left main collecting vessel of the lymphatic system, and is far larger than the other terminal, the right lymphatic duct. The thoracic duct begins in the epigastric region at the height of the first and second lumbar vertebrae as an elongated dilation, the *cisterna chyli*, into which the right and left lumbar lymphatic trunks empty. From the cistern, the duct runs upward along the right side of the aorta, traversing the aortic hiatus. It crosses the median plane from right to left and ascends to the root of the neck, where it empties into the left innominate vein at the angle of union of the left internal jugular and subclavian veins (p. 200). The duct is provided with valves, the most perfect and important of which are at its termination to prevent the passing of blood into the duct.

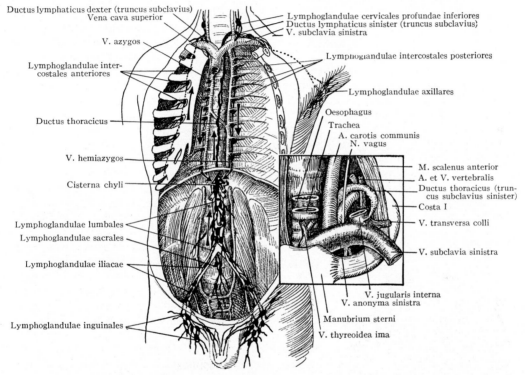

FIG. 261.—TRIBUTARIES AND TERMINATIONS OF THE LYMPHATIC CHANNELS OF THE THORAX AND ABDOMEN, AND TOPOGRAPHY OF THE AZYGOS VENOUS SYSTEM.

5. **Azygos System of Veins.**—The azygos vein and its main tributary, the hemiazygos, arise in the abdomen as continuations of the ascending lumbar veins and penetrate the chest, the azygos on the right and the hemiazygos on the left. They form a system of two parallel veins flanking the vertebral column, which on either side absorb the intercostal, esophageal, and bronchial venous flow. They anastomose at about the level of the seventh thoracic vertebra. The main trunk opens into the posterior surface of the superior vena cava at a point above the level at which the vessel is invested by pericardium (Fig. 245).

6 **Gangliated Sympathetic Chain.**—The gangliated sympathetic chain is the most laterally placed structure in the posterior mediastinum. It lies upon the heads of the ribs and is overlain by the costal pleura and the intercostal vessels. The thoracic portion of the chain contains ten or eleven ganglia, of which the first and largest lies on the neck of the first rib or may be fused with the inferior cervical ganglion (p. 192). A characteristic

of the thoracic ganglia is the almost unvarying connection each has with the thoracic spinal nerves through the rami communicantes.

Branches from the chain run to the subclavian vessels and the heart, contributing to the formation of the pulmonary and aortic sympathetic plexuses. From the lower part of the cord, the *splanchnic trunks* are given off and are distributed to the structures in the abdominal cavity. Between the fifth and ninth ganglia arises the *major splanchnic nerve,* which is of considerable size (Fig. 245). It descends through the posterior mediastinum, runs through the diaphragm, and joins the celiac ganglion. From the ninth and tenth ganglia, the *minor splanchnic nerve* descends to join the celiac ganglion plexus (aortico-renal ganglion).

SURGICAL CONSIDERATIONS

1. **Methods of Esophageal Examination.**—The most useful adjuncts to clinical examination of the esophagus are the esophagoscope and the *x*-ray. The esophagoscope is of the greatest value. By its use alone, early diagnosis may be made and local treatment, such as dilation, removal of foreign bodies, and excision of tissue specimens, may be performed. The examining tube is passed slowly and gently along the esophagus. The procedure requires knowledge of the region, dexterity, gentleness, and absolute control of the patient. Through the instrument, the esophagus is seen to unroll, and, if normal, the passage is visible down to the cardia. In trained hands, the procedure can be accomplished under local anesthesia in a very few minutes.

2. **Foreign Bodies in the Esophagus.**—A great variety of foreign bodies become impacted in the esophagus, usually above the broncho-aortic constriction (p. 270). Among the most common of these are false teeth, fish bones, pins, and pieces of food. The foreign body may burrow into the mucous membrane, form a diverticulum, and embed itself, setting up infection and possibly abscess which may rupture into the pleura, pericardial cavity, a neighboring vascular trunk, or even the aorta. A large bolus of food may engage behind the epiglottis, completely closing the laryngeal cavity. Cough or difficulty in breathing (dyspnea) suggests a foreign body in the air passages. A foreign body in the larynx or bronchi may be diagnosed as asthma. If the obstruction is in the inferior trachea, dyspnea will not be relieved by tracheotomy. The larynx should be examined first with a mirror and then with the laryngoscope; the trachea and bronchi should be viewed by means of the bronchoscope for further information. Difficulty in swallowing (dysphagia) may be caused by a foreign body in the esophagus. An esophageal foreign body occasionally produces marked dyspnea not relieved by tracheotomy. Accurate search demands esophagoscopy. A large body impossible of withdrawal through the esophagoscope requires esophagotomy.

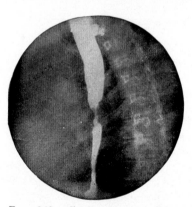

FIG. 262.—CARCINOMATOUS STRICTURE OF THE ESOPHAGUS. (Carman.)

3. **Esophageal Stricture.**—Stricture or stenosis, the commonest esophageal affection, results from a variety of causes. Corrosive stricture in children, caused by drinking chemicals such as lye, is appallingly frequent. Intrinsic stricture fairly often is caused by squamous-cell epithelioma, the type of neoplasm almost invariably found in the esophagus. Syphilis may cause a widespread stenosis.

Esophagoscopy must not be delayed, lest a tumor in the wall of the esophagus be overlooked until too late for resection. Obstructive extrinsic stenosis from the pressure of enlarged mediastinal glands, malignant disease in the mediastinum, aortic aneurysm, or spinal abscess is not uncommon.

When esophagoscopic examination has ruled out ulcerative conditions and the stricture is known to be benign, the treatment is mechanical dilation under direct vision through the esophagoscope. The blind use of bougies in the esophagus is obsolete, even in the hands of the most expert. Should the obstruction be so severe as to interfere with general nutrition, gastrostomy must be considered, and, if performed when the patient is in a fair state of nutrition, and under local anesthesia, the operation is neither dangerous nor difficult.

4. **Carcinoma of the Esophagus.**—Primary carcinoma of the esophagus is a squamous-cell growth arising from the epithelium of the mucous membrane. By annular invasion of the esophageal wall, the growth gradually obliterates the lumen, then ulcerates, and early invades the adjacent parts, involving the posterior mediastinal lymph glands. Accompanying the encroachment on the lumen is the development of dilation of the tube above the growth, into which the ingested food passes, to be vomited later or be aspirated and cause pneumonia. The earliest symptom of trouble is difficulty in swallowing. When the lumen becomes seriously encroached upon, there is intense dysphagia with the feeling of a foreign body in the throat, because of the arrest of food. Progressive emaciation is an early characteristic of the disease, succeeded by inanition and exhaustion. Early cases can be recognized only by esophagoscopy in conjunction with x-ray examination. In carcinoma of the esophagus, dilating instruments passed blindly are weapons rather than tools.

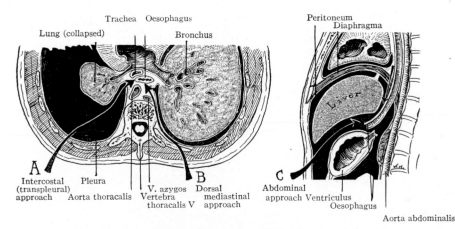

Fig. 263.—Routes to the Esophagus. (After Testut and Jacob.)

5. **Paths of Approach to the Esophagus.**—The posterior mediastinum may be approached by several incisions to give esophageal exposure: the dorsal mediastinal, the major intercostal or transpleural, and the abdominal transdiaphragmatic.

The *dorsal mediastinal* approach contemplates the removal of the posterior portion of several ribs, the resection being carried to the extremities of the transverse processes of the corresponding vertebrae. The pleura is retracted to expose the structures of the posterior mediastinum. On the left side, the main obstacle to exposure is the aorta, and on the right, the azygos vein.

The recent development of the *major intercostal (transpleural)* incision in chest exploration and in major procedures of lung surgery promises much for operations on structures of the posterior mediastinum. Several ribs may be resected or sectioned and the wound so spread as to give adequate exposure. The operation is made possible by positive pressure gas anesthesia.

The *abdominal route through the diaphragm* is applicable for operative procedures on that part of the esophagus just proximal to the stomach. It requires dilation of the esophageal orifice of the diaphragm and the dragging down of the esophagus through the orifice. It may be necessary to combine the abdominal and transpleural approaches.

18

ABDOMEN

I. Abdominal Walls

A. ANTEROLATERAL WALL IN GENERAL

1. Definition and Boundaries.—The anterolateral abdominal wall is bounded above by the flare of the costal margins and the xiphoid process of the sternum, and below by the iliac crests, inguinal ligaments, pubic crests, and pubic symphysis. Its lateral margins are conventional vertical lines dropped from the costal margins to the most elevated portions of the iliac crests.

2. Surface Anatomy.—The abdomen presents practical and reliable landmarks. The *linea alba* extends in the midline from the xiphoid to the symphysis. It is divided by the *umbilicus* into supra-umbilical and infra-umbilical segments of about equal length. The *rectus muscles* form bulging bands on each side of the linea alba. Across them stretch the

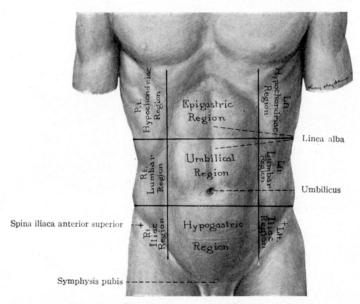

Fig. 264.—Regional Topography of the Anterolateral Abdominal Wall.

lineae transversae, tendinous intersections which, in more muscular individuals, produce palpable transverse depressions. These depressions are accentuated in active rectus contraction or in reflex muscle spasm associated with irritation of the peritoneum.

At the lateral margin of each rectus muscle is a depression, the *linea semilunaris*, which is directed toward the symphysis. In thin subjects, the *pubic spines* are palpable at the mesial attachments of the inguinal ligaments; in obese subjects, they are lost in the depth of the pubic fat. Their location is determined accurately as two fingerbreadths superior to the suspensory ligament of the penis, about 2.5 cm. lateral to the midline.

For clinical purposes, the anterolateral abdominal wall may be divided into nine regions by two vertical and two horizontal conventional lines. The *superior* of the *transverse lines* passes between the inferior margins of the costal flares (tips of the tenth ribs); the *inferior line* passes between the highest points of the iliac crests. The two *vertical* lines (mid-Poupart) bisect the two inguinal ligaments. Supero-inferiorly, the central regions are the *epigastric*, *umbilical*, and *pubic* or *hypogastric;* the lateral regions are the

274

hypochondriac, lumbar, and *iliac.* These regions facilitate the description of fixed viscera and of tumors.

The *contour* of the abdomen is subject to considerable variation. A greatly enlarged liver may cause undue prominence in the right hypochondriac and neighboring regions. Ovarian cysts or uterine tumors produce enlargement first in the lower abdomen above the pubes, which later extends superiorly. Common causes of generalized distention are ascites, paralytic ileus, mechanical bowel obstruction, and advanced peritonitis.

Retraction may be quite as striking as distention. The abdominal cavity may be reduced to very small dimensions and the anterior wall be depressed sufficiently to merit the description "scaphoid or boat-shaped" abdomen. The condition is seen in emaciated individuals, in certain forms of peritonitis, and, to a lesser degree, in some varieties of meningitis.

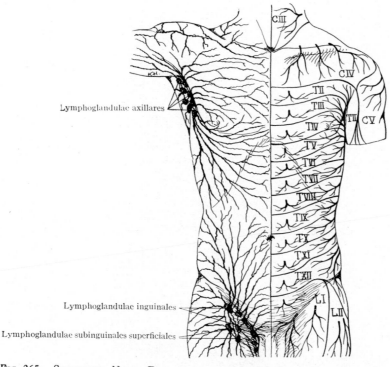

FIG. 265.—SEGMENTAL NERVE DISTRIBUTION AND LYMPH GLAND DRAINAGE OF THE ANTERIOR BODY WALL

A thick abdominal wall, whether from muscular development or abundance of fat, is an obstacle to palpation. A thin, flaccid abdominal wall greatly facilitates palpation. In certain cases, peristaltic movements along distended loops of intestine may be seen.

3. **Superficial Structures.**—The *skin* of the abdomen is attached loosely to the subjacent structures except at the umbilicus, where it adheres firmly.

The *superficial fascia* of the lower abdomen can be divided readily into two strata. In the superficial layer (Camper's fascia) lies the bulk of subcutaneous fat. The deep layer (Scarpa's fascia) is more dense, and is applied more closely to the abdominal muscles.

The subcutaneous tissue is supplied with *arteries* from various sources which contribute freely anastomosing branches. The area above the umbilicus receives branches from the superior epigastric, musculophrenic, and lower intercostal arteries. Below the umbilicus are three small branches from the femoral artery, the superficial epigastric, superficial circumflex iliac, and superficial external pudendal arteries.

The superficial epigastric, circumflex iliac, and pudendal *veins* converge toward the saphenous opening in the groin to enter the femoral vein and become tributary to the inferior caval system. The superficial veins above the umbilicus empty into the superior vena cava by way of the internal mammary, intercostal, and long thoracic veins. Both groups join freely with one another through the thoraco-epigastric vein which ascends from the groin to the region of the axilla. The two systemic groups of veins communicate indirectly at the umbilicus with the portal vein by means of potential anastomoses with the para-umbilical vein (of Sappey) which passes from the left branch of the portal vein along the round ligament of the liver to the umbilicus.

When the portal circulation is obstructed, as in hepatic cirrhosis, these anastomoses act as safety valves, and a large amount of blood, by reversal of flow, finds its way into

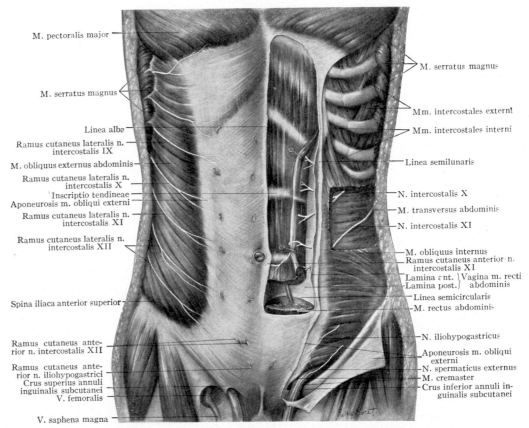

FIG. 266.—MUSCLES OF THE ANTEROLATERAL ABDOMINAL WALL.

The anterior layer of the sheath of the left rectus is removed to show the rectus compartment and the mode of entrance of vessels and nerves; a section of the left rectus is removed to show the inferior epigastric artery; all the external oblique muscle and a window from the internal oblique muscle are removed on the left side to show the intercostal musculature and transverse abdominal muscle.

the superficial veins about the umbilicus. In consequence, these veins assume a varicose appearance, fancifully termed "Caput Medusae."

Because of the ample anastomosis between the supra-umbilical and infra-umbilical veins of the caval system, a reversal of blood flow will be seen in superior or inferior caval obstruction, all the blood being borne toward the unobstructed cava.

The *lymphatics* are divided into two general groups: those arising in the supra-umbilical region draining to the thoracic group of axillary glands, and those arising in the infra-umbilical region draining toward the superficial glands of the thigh. Lymph vessels from the liver course along the ligamentum teres to the umbilicus to communicate with the lymphatics of the anterior abdominal wall. Cancer of the umbilicus occurs secondary to cancer of the liver, and metastases may spread to the lymph glands in the groin.

4. **Broad Abdominal Muscles, Transversalis Fascia, and Peritoneum.**—The flat muscles of the abdomen and the recti are arranged to form an elastic contractile layer about the abdominal cavity, protecting its contents. They function as a constricting mechanism, and the pressure they exert helps to maintain the abdominal viscera in their proper relative positions. The peristaltic contractions of the hollow viscera are supplemented by the uniform pressure of the abdominal muscles, as is well demonstrated in micturition and defecation.

The movements of the abdominal muscles alternate with those of the diaphragm, and are to be regarded as promoting the expiratory movements of the chest. Normal expiration is largely a result of the elastic recoil of the lungs and chest wall. When, as in emphysema, the lungs to a large extent lose their elasticity, the abdominal muscles partially compensate for the loss. Action of the abdominal muscles diminishes the intrathoracic space by contracting the thoracic outlet and pushing up the diaphragm.

By increasing the pressure brought to bear upon the abdominal contents, abdominal muscular contraction may be very forcible and lead to partial rupture of some of the muscle fibers, not an uncommon occurrence in the recti during parturition and other excessive muscular strains.

The muscles of the anterior abdominal wall help to approximate the lower thorax and the pelvis, acting in antagonism to the posterior spinal muscles. This is shown well in momentary loss of balance, where the tendency to fall backward is counteracted by the powerful effort the abdominal muscles exert in drawing the thoracic segment of the trunk anteriorly. This sometimes results in their partial rupture. The broad muscles cross each other, an arrangement designed to strengthen the abdominal wall and diminish the risk of hernial protrusions between separated muscle bundles. The external and internal oblique and transversus abdominis muscles form the encircling musculature, while the recti and pyramidales muscles are important in flexion and stabilization.

The most superficial of the **flat muscles,** the descending or *external oblique,* lies on the lateral (p. 312) and anterior parts of the abdomen. That portion of the aponeurosis which forms the inguinal ligament is rolled posteriorly and superiorly on itself and forms a groove to hold the spermatic cord. The mesial portion of the folded-back ligament is the *lacunar ligament* (of Gimbernat) which is attached to the pubic crest. It possesses a free lateral crescentic margin which is related intimately to the femoral (crural) canal (p. 703). Above the anterior extremity of the inguinal ligament, the spermatic cord emerges through the aponeurosis of the external oblique at the *subcutaneous inguinal ring.*

The *internal oblique muscle* is immediately deep to the external oblique. It arises from the lateral half of the inguinal ligament, from the anterior two thirds of the iliac crest, and from the lumbodorsal fascia, and runs superiorly, anteriorly, and mesially. It has no free posterior margin. The uppermost fibers are inserted into the lower ribs and their cartilages; the intermediate fibers form an aponeurosis which, above the semicircular line (of Douglas), divides into two lamellae at the linea semilunaris. The anterior lamella accompanies the external oblique aponeurosis to form the anterior rectus sheath. The posterior lamella is fused with the aponeurosis of the transversus abdominis to form the posterior rectus sheath. Below the semicircular line, the combined aponeuroses of the internal oblique, external oblique, and transversus abdominis muscles make up the anterior rectus sheath. The lowermost fibers of the internal oblique muscle arch over the spermatic cord, where they blend with the corresponding fibers of the transversus abdominis muscle to form the *inguinal falx* or *conjoined tendon.*

The *transversus abdominis* forms the most deeply placed muscle layer and is the most important constrictor. It arises from the lumbodorsal fascia, the iliac crest, the lateral third of the inguinal ligament, and the inner aspect of the lower six costal cartilages by slips which interdigitate with those of the diaphragm. The general direction of the fibers is toward the linea alba. Its aponeurosis runs posterior to the rectus abdominis muscle above the semicircular line, and anterior to it below. The lowermost fibers turn mesially downward and insert on the pubic crest as part of the inguinal falx.

The **transversalis fascia** covers the deep surface of the transversus abdominis muscle and lines the abdominal cavity, reinforcing unprotected areas. Below the semicircular line, where the posterior sheath of the rectus abdominis muscle is absent, the fascia is strong and is in immediate contact with the muscle. The fascia is attached below to the inner lip of the iliac crest, the outer half of the inguinal ligament, the lacunar ligament (of Gimbernat), and the pubic crest. Behind the mesial half of the ligament, it is continued over the femoral vessels into the thigh.

Against the transversalis fascia, the **peritoneum** is applied closely; the two are separated by a layer of areolar tissue, the *extraperitoneal fat*, which is developed to an unusual degree about the inguinal ligament and is prone to descend with hernial sacs in this area. The peritoneum may be separated from the transversalis fascia with great ease save at the

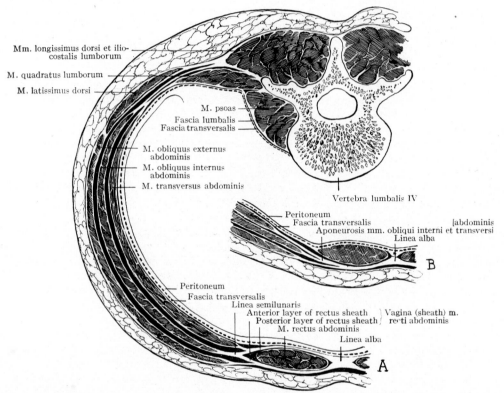

Fig. 267.—Transverse Section Through the Abdominal Wall with Particular Reference to the Formation of the Rectus Sheath.

A, Section at a level above the linea semicircularis (of Douglas); B, section taken at a level below the linea semicircularis (of Douglas).

abdominal inguinal ring where fusion has taken place. In the inguinal region, the peritoneum extends toward but does not reach the inguinal ligament, from which it is separated by an interval of fatty areolar tissue. In this tissue, the inferior epigastric artery, or even the termination of the external iliac artery, may be ligated without invading the peritoneal cavity. An incision parallel with and a little superior to the inguinal ligament affords exposure for ligation of these vessels, as well as exposes the neck of a femoral hernial sac (p. 704).

From the umbilicus, three folds of peritoneum diverge downward, marking obliterated structures of fetal life. The median fold sheathes the urachus, and the lateral folds contain the cordlike remnants of the obliterated umbilical arteries which continue the direction of the superior vesicular arteries. A description of the peritoneal fossae delimited by these folds and their practical significance in inguinal hernia is given more appropriately in the inguino-abdominal region.

5. **Linea Semilunaris.**—The lateral margin of each rectus abdominis muscle is indicated on the surface by a depression or vertically directed groove, the linea semilunaris This line begins at the pubic tubercle and passes upward midway between the umbilicus and the anterior superior spine, toward the tip of the ninth costal cartilage. Along this line, above the linea semicircularis, the aponeurosis of the internal oblique muscle splits to enclose the rectus muscle.

6. **Rectus Abdominis Muscle and the Rectus Sheath.**—Each *rectus abdominis* (Fig. 266) is a thick, flat band of muscle which arises from the anterior surface of the fifth, sixth, and seventh costal cartilages and from the xiphoid process, and extends downward in the interval between the linea alba and linea semilunaris to an insertion on the pubis between the crest and symphysis. Three to five irregular tendinous intersections, lineae transversae, cross the muscle, adhering to the anterior surface of the sheath only. To some extent, they limit fluid collections beneath the anterior sheath and prevent muscle rupture. Their attachment to the anterior sheath prevents retraction of the rectus in transverse incisions. A transverse rectus wound, in healing, forms essentially a new fibrous inter-

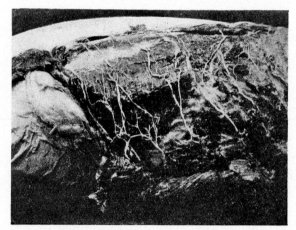

FIG. 268.—PHOTOGRAPH OF DISSECTION OF LEFT ANTEROLATERAL ABDOMINAL WALL TO SHOW PLEXUS FORMATION OF INTERCOSTAL NERVES.
All structures down to the transversus abdominis muscle have been removed. Note transverse direction of nerve trunk. (E. P. Stibbe.)

section. The muscle is not attached to the posterior sheath and is freely movable over this surface, so that it may be retracted mesially.

The *sheath* of the *rectus* is a strong, incomplete fibrous compartment formed by the aponeuroses of the three lateral abdominal muscles which criss-cross to make the linea alba. The composition of the sheath differs in its upper and lower portions. Above the midpoint between the umbilicus and the symphysis pubis, the rectus muscle has a well-defined investment, formed in front by the aponeurosis of the external oblique and the anterior lamina of the aponeurosis of the internal oblique, and behind by the aponeurosis of the transversus abdominis and the aponeurosis of the posterior lamina of the internal oblique. The posterior wall is not entirely aponeurotic, for the upper fleshy fibers of the transversus abdominis muscle lie behind the rectus abdominis and almost reach the linea alba.

Below the midpoint between the umbilicus and the symphysis, the aponeuroses of the three flat muscles pass entirely in front of the rectus, so that the inferior extent of the rectus muscle is devoid of a posterior fibrous covering. The posterior aponeurotic layer terminates in a free crescentic margin, the *linea semicircularis* (*semilunar fold*) (of Douglas), which is fused to the underlying transversalis fascia. The sheath contains, in addition to the rectus and pyramidalis muscles, the terminations of the lower six intercostal nerves and vessels, the last thoracic nerve, and the superior and inferior epigastric vessels.

7. **Linea Alba.**—The linear midline furrow, which can be seen in the anterior abdominal wall of muscular subjects, is the linea alba. It consists of a band of dense, crisscross fibers of the aponeuroses of the broad abdominal muscles, stretching from the xiphoid to the symphysis. Above the umbilicus, it widens out, but below that level, it is difficult to recognize. Increased intra-abdominal pressure widens the line and favors a spreading or *diastasis* of the *recti*. In the broad ribbon-like supra-umbilical portion of the line, the interlacing fibers of the aponeuroses leave small elliptical orifices through which the perforating vessels and nerves pass. Through these openings, extraperitoneal areolar tissue sometimes herniates into the subcutaneous tissue, producing an *epigastric* (linea alba) *hernia*. Extrusion of extraperitoneal fat may be accompanied by small sacs of the subjacent peritoneum. Whatever the volume and content of these herniae, they may give rise to subjective symptoms out of all proportion to the lesion, because of the direct pressure of the sac and contents against the nerves which sometimes emerge with them. In a person presenting an obscure upper abdominal disorder the possibility of such herniae should be investigated.

8. **Vessels and Nerves.**—The anterolateral abdominal wall receives its **arterial** supply from the last six intercostal and the four lumbar arteries, together with the superior and inferior epigastric and the deep circumflex iliac arteries. The trunks of the *intercostal* and *lumbar arteries* run with the intercostal, iliohypogastric, and ilio-inguinal nerves beween the transversus abdominis and internal oblique muscles. The arterial terminations

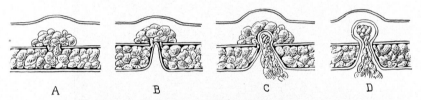

A   B   C   D

FIG. 269.—TYPES OF EPIGASTRIC LIPOMA AND EPIGASTRIC HERNIA.

A, Extraperitoneal lipoma broken through the linea alba; B, the peritoneum invaginates the lipoma; C, omental epigastric herniation into lipoma; D, omental epigastric herniation without a lipoma. (After DeQuervain.)

pierce the lateral margins of the rectus compartment at different levels and anastomose freely with the superior and inferior epigastric trunks.

The *superior epigastric artery*, one of the terminations of the internal mammary artery, reaches the posterior surface of the rectus muscle through the costoxiphoid interval in the diaphragm. It descends within the rectus sheath and anastomoses freely with the inferior epigastric artery. The *inferior epigastric artery* arises from the external iliac just proximal to the inguinal ligament, and at first lies in the midst of the extraperitoneal tissue at the medial side of the abdominal inguinal ring, in intimate relation with the posterior wall of the inguinal canal. The vas deferens, as it enters the abdomen, hooks around the lateral side of the artery. Accompanied by its satellite vein, the inferior epigastric artery ascends obliquely superiorly and medially toward the umbilicus, and, after piercing the transversalis fascia, enters the rectus compartment by passing in front of the linea semicircularis (semilunar fold) (of Douglas). It then pursues a vertical course and anastomoses freely with the superior epigastric artery. The inferior epigastric artery may be injured in a low right rectus incision, either in splitting muscle fibers or in retracting them mesially.

The *deep circumflex iliac artery* arises from the lateral aspect of the external iliac, opposite the origin of the inferior epigastric artery. A short distance above the iliac crest and near the anterior superior spine, the artery gives off an ascending branch of some size which is injured when the muscle-splitting incision of McBurney is prolonged laterally.

The anterior branches of the *lower six intercostal* **nerves** are continued forward into the abdominal wall and are accompanied by the *last thoracic nerve*. They run between the internal oblique and transversus abdominis muscles to the lateral margin of the rectus. There they enter the deep aspect of the sheath, and, after supplying the rectus, pass forward to pierce the anterior wall of the sheath and terminate in the subcutaneous tissue and skin. They give lateral cutaneous branches which supply the three broad muscles and the skin of the abdomen. The *iliohypogastric* and *ilio-inguinal nerves* are derived from the first lumbar nerve, and are distributed mainly to the inguino-abdominal region.

The position and course of the nerves should be borne in mind in planning abdominal incisions, for, although one or more may be severed without undesirable after-effect, the

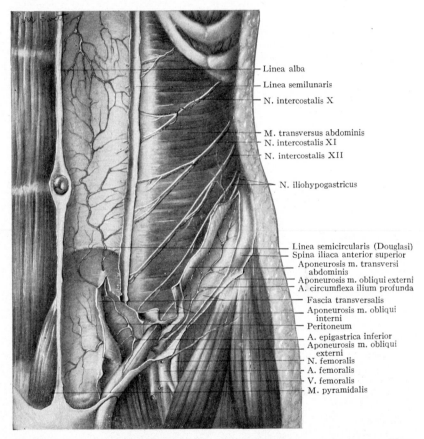

Linea alba
Linea semilunaris
N. intercostalis X

M. transversus abdominis
N. intercostalis XI
N. intercostalis XII

N. iliohypogastricus

Linea semicircularis (Douglasi)
Spina iliaca anterior superior
Aponeurosis m. transversi abdominis
Aponeurosis m. obliqui externi
A. circumflexa ilium profunda
Fascia transversalis
Aponeurosis m. obliqui interni
Peritoneum
A. epigastrica inferior
Aponeurosis m. obliqui externi
N. femoralis
A. femoralis
V. femoralis
M. pyramidalis

FIG. 270.—MUSCLES, APONEUROSES, ARTERIES AND NERVES OF THE ANTEROLATERAL ABDOMINAL WALL
The external and internal oblique muscles have been removed from the left side.

abdominal wall does not recover its muscle tone completely after section of the motor nerves.

The abdominal nerves supply not only the muscles, but also the overlying skin. This identity in nerve supply greatly favors reflex muscle action. Even a moderate stimulus applied to the surface of the abdomen, as for example, palpating with a cold hand, is sufficient to throw the abdominal wall into contraction.

Connections exist between the nerves of the abdominal wall and those of the viscera. When viscera are injured, or when peritonitis develops, the abdominal muscles contract through reflex action and exert a uniform pressure over the injured or inflamed parts. The muscles act more or less as splints to prevent movement as much as possible, thus keeping the injured or inflamed parts at rest. Their contraction places abdominal respiration in abeyance, fixes the lower ribs, and confines the respiratory movements chiefly to the upper region of the chest.

Pain referred to the front of the abdomen is not unusual in spinal tuberculosis, and is indicative of pressure on the main trunks of the intercostal nerves. Unless this be borne in mind, a serious mistake in diagnosis may be made, and the true nature of the case be overlooked.

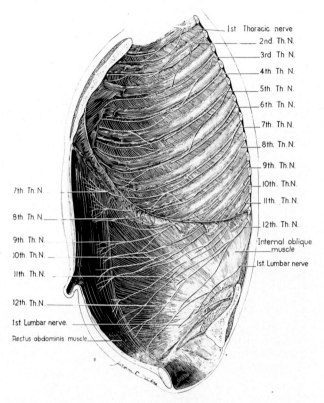

FIG. 271.—NERVE SUPPLY OF THE RIGHT THORACIC AND ABDOMINAL REGIONS.

The transversus abdominis muscle and the aponeuroses forming the posterior sheath of the rectus have been removed. Note the transverse direction of the intercostal nerves in the anterior abdominal wall. (Modified after Davies, Gladstone, and Stibbe.)

SURGICAL CONSIDERATIONS

Abdominal incisions are made through those parts of the abdominal wall which offer the freest access with the least sacrifice of vessels and nerves. Incisions in aponeurotic areas, such as the superior half of the linea alba and the linea semilunaris, are to be avoided because they predispose to postoperative hernia.

1. **Median Abdominal Section.**—Vertical section through the linea alba has the advantage of being almost bloodless, cutting no muscle fibers, injuring no nerves, and giving access to both sides of the abdomen. Above the umbilicus, the incision seldom is used since the single line of fascial sutures used in its repair cannot be relied upon to prevent weakness in the abdominal wall. Below the umbilicus, the median incision is employed almost universally in gynecologic operations. This incision invariably exposes the medial margin of one or the other muscle, because the recti are close together. Repair of this incision produces a strong abdominal wall. Median incision immediately above the symphysis pubis gives access to the bladder; this viscus should be emptied before operation except when it is to be operated upon.

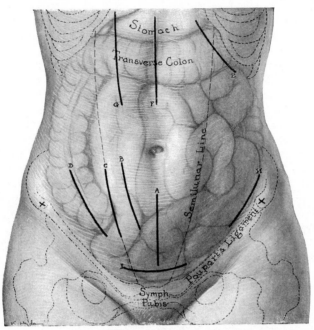

FIG. 272.—PRINCIPAL ABDOMINAL INCISIONS.

A, Median incision below the umbilicus; B, lateral rectus incision; C, semilunar line incision; D, Mc-Burney's incision; E, oblique subcostal incision; F, median incision above the umbilicus; G, right rectus incision; H, iliac incision; I, Pfannenstiel incision.

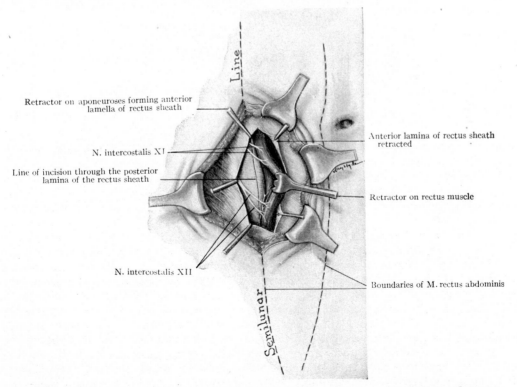

FIG. 273.—DIVISION OF THE STRUCTURES OF THE ABDOMINAL WALL IN A PARARECTUS INCISION.

2. Incision Through the Rectus Sheath and Muscle (Paramedian Section).

—The abdomen may be opened by vertical incision through the rectus sheath, an operation much less open to criticism than that through the linea semilunaris. Paramedian incisions are made over the rectus anywhere between the costal arch and the symphysis pubis. After the superficial parts are divided, the anterior sheath is incised. The sheath is closely adherent to the muscle at the tendinous intersections.

In the *muscle-splitting incision*, the fibers of the rectus are separated throughout the length of the wound and the posterior wall of the sheath is incised. If the epigastric vessels are seen, they are drawn aside. Incision of the subjacent and partially adherent transversalis fascia exposes the extraperitoneal fat and the peritoneum. In closure, the edges of the incision come together readily, and the wound heals with a strongly resistant scar which minimizes the risk of postoperative hernia. This approach is employed commonly for appendectomy. When the incision is carried through the rectus muscle below the semicircular fold (of Douglas), the transversalis fascia and peritoneum are encountered directly (p. 278). The inferior epigastric artery, lying on the transversalis fascia (p. 280), is exposed and may be retracted or divided.

A favorite paramedian (pararectus) incision contemplates opening the sheath of the rectus a little medial to its lateral border, freeing the muscle from its adhesions to the

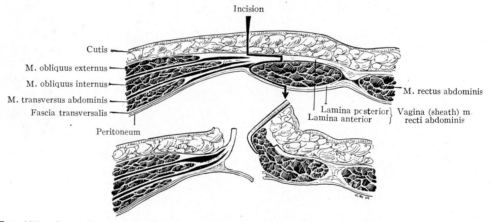

Fig. 274.—Cross Sections to Show the Division of the Strata of the Abdominal Wall in the Pararectus Incision.

compartment and the corresponding fibrous intersections, and *retracting the muscle mesially.* The intercostal vessels entering the compartment are ligated or retracted as exposure demands, and the posterior sheath and deeper structures are incised. The inferior epigastric artery should be ligated if it comes into the field. In closure, the posterior wall of the sheath is sutured and the retracted muscle is allowed to fall back over the deep-seated suture line.

Incision may be made over the medial aspect of the rectus sheath and the *muscle may be displaced laterally.* After the rectus is retracted laterally, the posterior layer of the sheath and the deeper structures are incised in the same plane as the incision in the anterior sheath. The chief advantage of this incision over that in the lateral rectus margin with mesial retraction of the muscle, is that the nerve supply of the rectus is not endangered, and that it affords good access to structures near the median line.

3. Incision in the Linea Semilunaris (Mediolateral Approach).

—Incision in the linea semilunaris occasionally is employed because of the excellent access it affords the underlying structures, notably the cecum and appendix. It has several disadvantages: the incision traverses the path of several intercostal nerves which supply the rectus muscle, and the partial paralysis which inevitably follows exerts a weakening tendency upon the anterior abdominal wall; reconstruction of the abdominal wall is unsatisfactory when dealing with aponeuroses alone. These circumstances favor the development of postoperative herniae. When the incision is made below the level of the umbilicus, it must be remembered that the inferior epigastric artery crosses the semilunar line.

4. Muscle-splitting Incision (of McBurney).—The muscle-splitting lateral abdominal incision (of McBurney) is planned to minimize postoperative weakness in the abdominal wall by dividing the three flat abdominal muscles in the direction of their fleshy and tendinous fibers. The incision begins a little above an imaginary line joining the anterior superior spine and the umbilicus, and is directed inferiorly and mesially, crossing this line about 4 cm. mesial to the anterior superior spine. It is from 5 to 8 cm. in length.

The incision is carried through the aponeurosis of the external oblique in the direction of its fibers. With the edges of the external oblique well retracted, the internal oblique and the transversus abdominis muscles are separated in the direction of their fibers, which, in this portion of their course, is almost horizontal. The incision then is carried through the underlying transversalis fascia and the peritoneum, carefully avoiding adherent bowel.

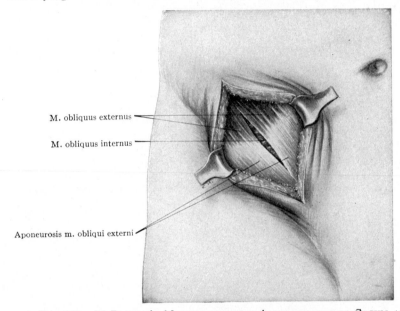

M. obliquus externus

M. obliquus internus

Aponeurosis m. obliqui externi

FIG. 275.—McBurney's Muscle-splitting Approach to the Cecum and the Appendix.

The incision is developed down to the external oblique muscle and aponeurosis; a slit is made in the direction of their fibers; the direction of the fibers of the underlying internal oblique and transversus abdominis muscles is seen to be almost transverse.

Before incision of the transversalis fascia and the peritoneum, much valuable information may be gained by palpating the underlying structures. A walled-off periappendiceal abscess may be located by palpation and be opened extraperitoneally, whereas blind incision in the mesial part of the wound may soil the general peritoneal cavity. If the intermuscular interval obtained does not afford sufficient access, the incision may be extended laterally toward the iliac crest or mesially through the anterior wall of the rectus sheath (Weir extension). The rectus then is retracted mesially and the posterior wall of the sheath is divided, care being taken to avoid or to ligate the inferior epigastric artery.

5. Iliac Incision.—Incisions parallel to, and in front of the anterior portion of, the iliac crest usually are employed to reach the extraperitoneal structures at and below the brim of the pelvis. The incision is carried directly through the musculature down to and through the transversalis fascia. The unopened peritoneum is loosened and is pressed mesially. The muscle guide to the major extraperitoneal structures is the medial border of the psoas major muscle. This incision is described in the section dealing with the approach to the ureter.

6. Oblique Subcostal Incision.—The oblique subcostal incision, carried from the xiphoid process laterally across the rectus sheath and across the lateral abdominal aponeuroses, affords excellent access to the bile passages and the inferior surface of the liver. The rectus muscle and the structures in the semilunar line are cut obliquely. Where further

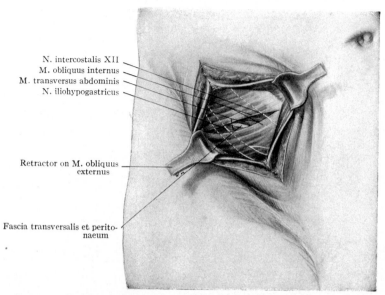

N. intercostalis XII
M. obliquus internus
M. transversus abdominis
N. iliohypogastricus

Retractor on M. obliquus externus

Fascia transversalis et peritonaeum

FIG. 276.—McBurney's Muscle-splitting Approach to the Appendix.

The external oblique muscle has been split in the direction of its fibers and its edges retracted; the transverse slit shows the slight difference in direction between the internal oblique and transversus abdominis muscles.

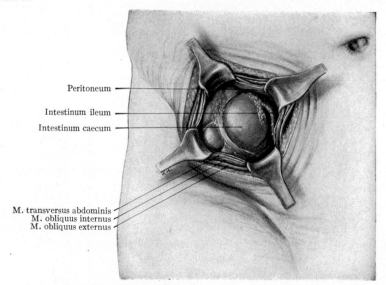

Peritoneum

Intestinum ileum
Intestinum caecum

M. transversus abdominis
M. obliquus internus
M. obliquus externus

FIG. 277.—McBurney's Muscle-splitting Approach to the Appendix.
The edges of the incision are retracted and the cecum and terminal ileum are exposed.

lateral exposure is required, the incision through the broad abdominal muscles is continued laterally in the same subcostal line. Since the broad rectus muscle is divided between its thoracic attachment and a fibrous intersection, it will not retract and can be reapproximated easily. The incision need divide no nerves which supply the rectus except the ninth thoracic, which lies almost directly in its course if the incision is extended. A supposed contraindication to this incision is the section of the rectus muscle, but it is accepted generally that a transverse rectus incision in healing leaves merely an added tendinous intersection which does not weaken the muscle.

A *bow-shaped* or *angular modification* of the oblique subcostal incision avoids the intercosto-abdominal nerves by passing first down the paramedian line and then laterally, parallel with the course of the nerves. The vertical limb of the incision begins in the median line at the xiphoid cartilage and descends 4 to 6 cm., a fingerbreadth to the right of the median plane. The anterior rectus sheath is divided in the line of the vertical part of the incision, and the medial border of the muscle is defined. The finger then can be inserted behind the rectus muscle in order to separate it from the posterior wall of the sheath. The anterior wall of the sheath and the rectus then are cut transversely. The posterior sheath is incised from the xiphoid to the lateral edge of the cut rectus in a gently curved line, and as much of the flat abdominal musculature is incised as adequate exposure

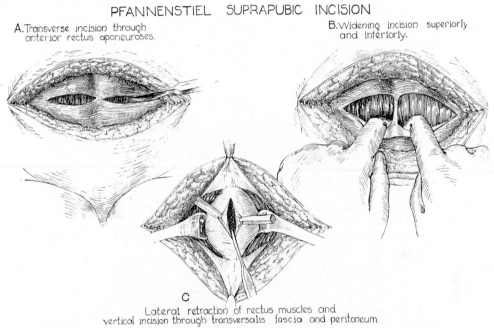

PFANNENSTIEL SUPRAPUBIC INCISION

A. Transverse incision through anterior rectus aponeuroses.

B. Widening incision superiorly and inferiorly.

C
Lateral retraction of rectus muscles and vertical incision through transversalis fascia and peritoneum.

Fig. 278.—Pfannenstiel Incision.
Transverse incision is carried through the skin and the anterior rectus aponeurosis.

demands. This approach produces little weakening of the abdominal wall since none of the motor nerves are destroyed.

7. Pfannenstiel Incision.—The Pfannenstiel incision is a suprapubic, transverse incision at the pubic hair line. The superficial structures and the anterior sheaths of the recti are incised transversely. The interval between the recti is developed superiorly and inferiorly by blunt and sharp dissection, thus mobilizing the rectus muscles. The recti are retracted laterally and the abdomen is opened by vertical incision through the transversalis fascia and the peritoneum. This approach has the advantage that no nerves are divided and that no visible scar remains. The wound is closed by vertical suturing of the posterior layer of the rectus sheath (transversalis fascia and peritoneum), and the uniting of the mesial margins of the recti. The cut edges of the transversely divided anterior sheaths are sutured and the skin wound is closed.

8. Transverse Incision for Appendectomy.—A useful transverse incision for appendectomy has its center over the linea semilunaris on or a little above the line joining the anterior superior iliac spines. The anterior sheath of the rectus is divided transversely and the muscle is displaced toward the median line. The abdomen is opened by transverse incision in the posterior sheath and semilunar line. The lateral continuation of the incision runs slightly oblique to the fibers of the external oblique and almost exactly in the direction of the fibers of the internal oblique and transversus abdominis muscles. The incision can be extended widely laterally and the rectus can be retracted mesially until excellent exposure is obtained.

9. **Abdominal Paracentesis.**—Abdominal paracentesis, or puncture of the peritoneal cavity, is done for diagnostic purposes or for the evacuation of peritoneal fluid. The site for the paracentesis generally is the linea alba, midway between the umbilicus and symphysis. Paracentesis may be done in the semilunar line or midway between the anterior superior iliac spine and the umbilicus. Before the trocar is introduced, the skin should be incised. If paracentesis is to be done in the linea alba, the patient should sit upright, since, in that position, fluid is caused to gravitate into the lower abdomen and pelvis.

(I) Inguino-abdominal Region (Inguinal Trigone)

1. **Definition and Boundaries.**—The inguino-abdominal region is the subsidiary area of the anterolateral abdominal wall which is limited by the inguinal ligament, the lateral margin of the rectus muscle, and a horizontal line from the anterior superior iliac spine to the lateral rectus margin. Its surgical importance is derived from the high incidence of

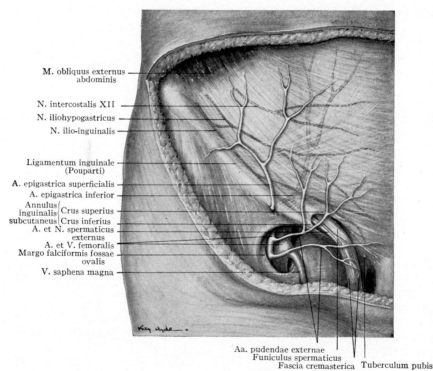

M. obliquus externus abdominis

N. intercostalis XII
N. iliohypogastricus
N. ilio-inguinalis

Ligamentum inguinale (Pouparti)

A. epigastrica superficialis
A. epigastrica inferior
Annulus inguinalis subcutaneus {Crus superius / Crus inferius
A. et N. spermaticus externus
A. et V. femoralis
Margo falciformis fossae ovalis
V. saphena magna

Aa. pudendae externae
Funiculus spermaticus
Fascia cremasterica   Tuberculum pubis

Fig. 279.—Superficial View of the Inguino-abdominal Region and the Inguinal Canal.

inguinal herniae. In the consideration of this area are reviewed the anatomic conditions which permit development of herniae, their classification, and the operative measures designed for their radical cure.

2. **Surface Anatomy.**—The landmarks of clinical and operative significance are the readily palpable *anterior superior iliac spine*, and the less easily palpable *pubic tubercle*. In obese individuals, the *pubic crest* is difficult to make out, but it may be determined

accurately enough in the male by measuring two fingerbreadths above the suspensory ligament of the penis. The *inguinal ligament*, especially under anesthesia, can be palpated readily. A swelling definitely located above the ligament is suggestive of inguino-abdominal origin, while one below is suggestive of origin in the thigh. The size and laxity of the *subcutaneous inguinal (external abdominal) ring* may be determined by invaginating the scrotum with the tip of the index finger, and carrying the finger over the tubercle against the opening. The ring, when normal in size, cannot be entered; but when dilated,

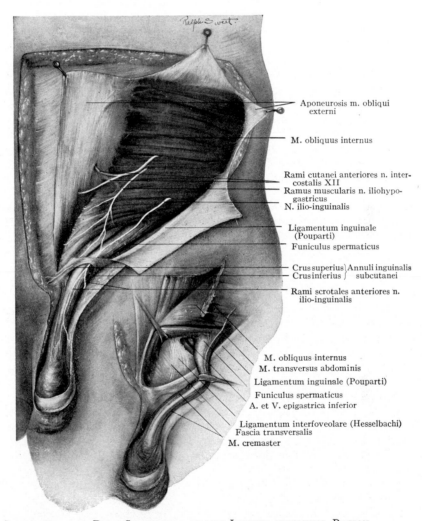

Aponeurosis m. obliqui externi

M. obliquus internus

Rami cutanei anteriores n. intercostalis XII
Ramus muscularis n. iliohypogastricus
N. ilio-inguinalis

Ligamentum inguinale (Pouparti)
Funiculus spermaticus

Crus superius ⎫ Annuli inguinalis
Crus inferius ⎭ subcutanei

Rami scrotales anteriores n. ilio-inguinalis

M. obliquus internus
M. transversus abdominis
Ligamentum inguinale (Pouparti)
Funiculus spermaticus
A. et V. epigastrica inferior
Ligamentum interfoveolare (Hesselbachi)
Fascia transversalis
M. cremaster

Fig. 280.—Superficial and Deep Structures of the Inguino-abdominal Region.

The inset shows the internal oblique muscle sectioned to indicate the underlying transversus abdominis; the cord is retracted inferiorly to show the floor of the inguinal canal; part of the transversalis fascia is removed to show the inferior epigastric vessels.

admits the finger readily. An impulse against the finger, produced by coughing, affords some appreciation of the resistance of the back wall of the canal and the presence of actual or potential hernia.

3. **Inguinal Musculature.**—The acknowledged weakness of the abdominal wall in the region of the inguinal trigone is accounted for in several ways: first, the substitution of an aponeurosis of no great strength for the thick muscular layer of the external oblique; second, the descent of the testis and the vaginal process of peritoneum in the male, and of the

round ligament and its vaginal process of peritoneum (canal of Nuck) in the female; and third, the fact that the inferior border of the internal oblique and transversus abdominis (conjoined muscle and tendon) falls short of the inguinal ligament over its medial two thirds. This disposition leaves a weak area between the inguinal ligament, the lower margin of these muscles, and the lateral border of the rectus; this weak area must bear the brunt of intra-abdominal pressure. The inguinal canal, by traversing the entire thickness of the abdominal wall, not only weakens it, but also provides an interstitial track along which hernial protrusions may travel. There is little doubt that the erect posture of man is a predisposing cause of inguinal hernia.

The **external oblique muscle** becomes tendinous over the confines of this region. Its lower fibers condense into the inguinal ligament and pubis, and a small mesial portion is reflected as the *lacunar ligament*. Immediately above the crest of the pubis, the aponeurosis presents a deficiency or gap, the *subcutaneous inguinal ring*, through which issues the spermatic cord in the male and the round ligament in the female. Arching *intercolumnar* (*intercrural*) *fibers* bind the borders of the ring together and form the outermost layer of the sheath of the cord. The fibers are designed to prevent the enlargement of the ring by further spreading of the external oblique aponeurosis. The margins of the ring can be made out distinctly only when the thin layer of fascia embracing the intercolumnar fibers, the *intercolumnar* (*intercrural*) *fascia*, is removed. The ring is triangular, and its long axis is directed obliquely inferiorly and mesially. The margins sometimes are called the medial and lateral *crura* (pillars) of the ring, but are described much more accurately as the superior and inferior crura. The inferior or lateral crus is formed mainly by the cordlike medial extremity of the inguinal ligament which is attached to the pubic spine. The superior or medial crus is thinner and flatter and attaches to the front of the symphysis. The shape and size of the ring vary widely in different individuals.

The anterior and inferior bulging of the external oblique muscle, before reflection posteriorly and superiorly as the inguinal l igament, forms a bed, the *inguinal groove*, for the spermatic cord, and a sharp free margin for the inguinal ligament.

Only the inferior fibers of the **internal oblique** and **transversus abdominis muscles**, those fibers which have a common origin over the lateral third or half of the inguinal ligament, properly belong in the inguinal region. Their superimposed muscle bundles become tendinous and fuse with one another at about the lateral margin of the rectus muscle. The resulting broad, frontally disposed *inguinal falx* or *conjoined tendon* inserts partly into the anterior sheath of the rectus muscle, but mainly into the crest of the pubis. When well developed, it forms a resistant arch behind the medial portion of the inguinal canal. The lateral margin of the inguinal falx sometimes can be palpated. The fibers of both muscles and their tendon arch inferiorly and medially, and cross the cord obliquely. They are first anterior to the cord, next superior to it, and then posterior to it.

From the muscular inferior border of the internal oblique, at the point where the testis emerged to descend into the scrotum, the *cremaster muscle* is given off. The lowermost fibers of the internal oblique muscle are impinged against by the testis in its descent, and form cremasteric loops over the cord, which maintain their lateral attachment at the inguinal ligament and their medial attachment at the pubis. Lateral, mesial, and anterior bundles of cremasteric fibers can be differentiated as contributing to the formation of the spermatic sheath.

4. **Transversalis Fascia.**—In the unprotected interval below the inferior margin of the internal oblique and transversus abdominis muscles, the transversalis fascia shows unusual development and reinforcement. It is inserted firmly into the iliac fascia above the line of fusion of the iliac fascia and inguinal ligament, is intimately fixed about the femoral vessels, and spreads out over the femoral ring like a diaphragm (*crural septum*). A vertical reinforcement for the fascia is afforded by the lateral expansion of the rectus tendon (*ligament of Henle*), which extends laterally to insert into the pubic crest and spine posterior to the insertion of the inguinal falx (conjoined tendon). The *interfoveolar ligament*, another strong, more or less vertical reinforcement, extends from the lowermost

margin of the transversus abdominis muscle to the superior ramus of the pubis. This ligament, hemmed by the inferior epigastric artery, holds the spermatic cord in the lateral angle of the weak inguinal region, and separates the abdominal inguinal ring from the *triangle of Hesselbach.* The base of the triangle is formed by the mesial portion of the inguinal ligament, the mesial side by the lateral border of the rectus abdominis muscle, and the lateral side by the inferior epigastric artery. Occasionally, hernia occurs through the transverslis fascia in the floor of Hesselbach's triangle (p. 298). The testicle, in its descent, evaginates the transversalis fascia, from which is derived the most intimate covering of the spermatic sheath, the *internal spermatic (infundibuliform) fascia.*

5. **Peritoneum, Extraperitoneal Areolar Tissue and Peritoneal Fossae.**—Before the parietal **peritoneum** covering the posterior surface of the inguino-abdominal region reaches the inguinal ligament, it is reflected posteriorly and superiorly to clothe the iliac fossa. The reflection of the peritoneal culdesac occurs at a higher level than the line of adhesion of the transversalis fascia to the iliac fascia. In consequence, there is a space between the

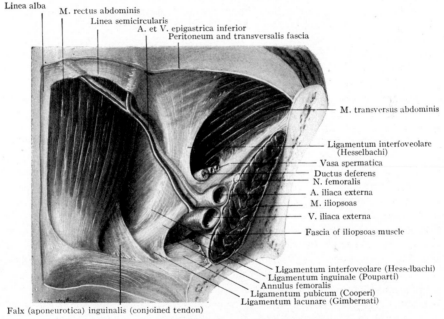

Linea alba — M. rectus abdominis — Linea semicircularis — A. et V. epigastrica inferior — Peritoneum and transversalis fascia

M. transversus abdominis

Ligamentum interfoveolare (Hesselbachi)
Vasa spermatica
Ductus deferens
N. femoralis
A. iliaca externa
M. iliopsoas
V. iliaca externa

Fascia of iliopsoas muscle

Ligamentum interfoveolare (Hesselbachi)
Ligamentum inguinale (Pouparti)
Annulus femoralis
Ligamentum pubicum (Cooperi)
Ligamentum lacunare (Gimbernati)

Falx (aponeurotica) inguinalis (conjoined tendon)

FIG. 281.—POSTERIOR VIEW OF THE INGUINO-ABDOMINAL AND INGUINOFEMORAL REGIONS AFTER THE PERITONEUM AND TRANSVERSALIS FASCIA HAVE BEEN REMOVED.

upward reflection of the serosa and the inguinal ligament which is filled with abundant **extraperitoneal areolar tissue.** The possibility of a part of the bladder occupying the space always must be considered in operating upon direct inguinal hernias (p. 299). An incision parallel to and 1 cm. above the ligament, with upward retraction of the contents of the inguinal canal, exposes the transversalis fascia over the inferior epigastric vessels. Here the inferior epigastric and external iliac arteries may be ligated extraperitoneally. The peritoneum is applied loosely to the transversails fascia except about the abdominal inguinal ring.

When the anterior abdominal wall is viewed from behind, certain peritoneal ridges, or cordlike structures, are seen converging from the pelvis and iliac fossa toward the umbilicus (Fig. 296). These are the urachus in the midline, and the obliterated umbilical and inferior epigastric arteries on each side. These folds delimit intervals or **peritoneal fossae** of surgical interest as they present important relations to various forms of herniae

The *external fossa* lies lateral to the inferior epigastric artery, and, when its peritoneal covering is removed, the internal abdominal ring is brought into view, with the vas deferens and spermatic vessels converging toward it.   When a hernia leaves the abdomen through the external inguinal fossa, it enters the inguinal canal at its inlet, and traverses its entire length before emerging through the subcutaneous inguinal ring.   For this reason, and because it lies outside the inferior epigastric artery, it is called an external or indirect inguinal hernia.

The *middle inguinal fossa* lies between the inferior epigastric artery laterally and the obliterated umbilical artery mesially.   At this level, the abdominal wall is weak, as the inferior margins of the internal oblique and transversus abdominis muscles fail to reach the inguinal ligament.   The result is that, over the lower part of the fossa, the transversalis fascia alone separates the sac of the hernia from the outlet of the canal at the external ring. A hernia originating within this fossa makes its way through the abdominal wall by pushing the transversalis fascia ahead of it and emerging through the subcutaneous inguinal ring.   It escapes to the lateral side of the conjoined tendon which normally overlies the main part of the fossa, but which in this variety of hernia is related closely to the neck of the sac on its superior and medial aspect.   This hernia, therefore, does not traverse the entire inguinal canal, but enters the canal near its outlet close behind the external abdominal ring.   It lies mesial to the inferior epigastric artery, and is designated an internal or direct inguinal hernia.   In direct hernia, the falx inguinalis occasionally may be pushed forward by the herniating mass.

The *internal inguinal fossa*, or *supravesical space*, is bounded laterally by the obliterated umbilical artery and mesially by the urachus.   At this level, the abdominal wall offers considerable resistance to intra-abdominal pressure because of the presence of the rectus muscle and the inguinal falx (conjoined tendon).   A hernia very rarely originates here because of these structures.

6. Vessels and Nerves.—The *inferior epigastric artery* arises from the anteromedial surface of the external iliac artery about 1 cm. superior to the inguinal ligament.   It runs mesially for a short distance, parallel to the inguinal ligament, and then obliquely upward and mesially in the extraperitoneal fat along the medial margin of the internal ring toward the linea semicircularis (of Douglas) (p. 280).

The principal nerves are the iliohypogastric and ilio-inguinal, both of which are branches of the first lumbar nerve.   The *iliohypogastric nerve* runs forward in the abdominal wall near the superior margin of the iliac crest, and there divides into hypogastric and iliac branches.

The *ilio-inguinal nerve* enters the region at a somewhat lower level than the iliohypogastric, and after crossing part of the iliac fossa, enters the inguinal canal.   It runs anteriorly beneath the aponeurosis of the internal oblique immediately above the inguinal ligament and emerges from the subcutaneous inguinal ring.

7. Descent of the Testicle and Its Relation to the Vaginal Process of Peritoneum.— The testicle develops between the transversalis fascia and peritoneum.   The gland is differentiated early in the lumbar region.   As growth and development proceed, the testicle occupies relatively lower levels, and toward the end of the third intra-uterine month has reached the vicinity of the anterior abdominal wall and lies in the iliac fossa close to the pelvic brim.   Passing upward from the gland is a fold of peritoneum, the *plica vascularis*, in which the spermatic vessels lie.   Passing downward from the testicle to the anterior abdominal wall is another fold, in which lies the *gubernaculum testis*.

A series of changes takes place preparatory to further movement of the testicle.   An outpocketing of peritoneum, the *processus vaginalis peritonei*, appears at the site of the future abdominal inguinal ring, and emerges through the anterior abdominal wall.   At this time there exists a rudiment of scrotum on each side of the rudimentary penis, made up of the coalescence of the two sides of the urogenital furrow.   The cordlike gubernaculum then extends into the bottom of the scrotal pouch.

The final stage of migration of the testicle occurs in the sixth or seventh month when the gland descends into the inguinal canal.   During the eighth intra-uterine month, the testicle, by vital growth along the gubernaculum, moves along the canal and, in the ninth

intra-uterine month, normally comes to rest in the scrotum.   The remnants of the gubernaculum form a short band which connects the inferior pole of the testicle with the depth
of the scrotum, and is designated the *scrotal ligament*.   Prior to the descent of the testicle

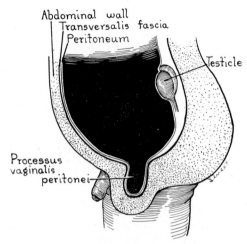

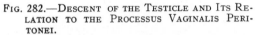

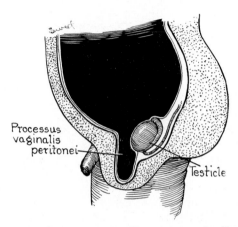

FIG. 282.—DESCENT OF THE TESTICLE AND ITS RE-
LATION TO THE PROCESSUS VAGINALIS PERI-
TONEI.

The testicle lies in the lumbar region between
the transversalis fascia and the peritoneum; the
vaginal process already is formed.

FIG. 283.—DESCENT OF THE TESTICLE AND ITS RE-
LATION TO THE PROCESSUS VAGINALIS PERI-
TONEI.

The testicle has reached the pelvic brim.

into the scrotal sac to the level it occupies at birth, the vaginal process of peritoneum
extends to the depth of the scrotum.   This saclike evagination of peritoneum applies itself
to the cord and testicle as an incomplete investment but at no point completely surrounds

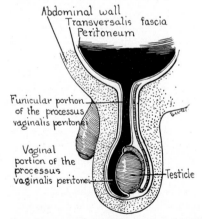

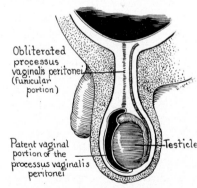

FIG. 284.—DESCENT OF THE TESTICLE AND ITS RE-
LATION TO THE PROCESSUS VAGINALIS PERI-
TONEI.

The testicle now has descended to the base of
the scrotum behind the vaginal process, the funicular part of which as yet is unobliterated.

FIG. 285.—DESCENT OF THE TESTICLE AND ITS RE-
LATION TO THE PROCESSUS VAGINALIS PERI-
TONEI.

The funicular portion of the vaginal process now
has become obliterated normally; the vaginal part of
the process normally remains unobliterated.

them.   As development advances, only the part of the process applied against the testicle,
the tunica vaginalis testis, remains patent.   That part of the vaginal process applied
to the spermatic cord between the tunica vaginalis testis and the abdominal inguinal
ring is the funicular portion, which, shortly after birth, loses its patency and becomes

a fibrous cord, the *vaginal ligament*. The vaginal process of peritoneum may remain patent throughout or in part, constituting developmental irregularities which have a most important bearing on certain forms of hernia and hydrocele.

Patency of the entire process affords a hernial sac of congenital origin, extending from the abdominal inguinal ring to the depth of the scrotum, and accounts for *vaginal hernia*. That part of the process opening into the abdomen may persist and supply the sac of a *funicular hernia*. There may be patency of the funicular part of the process, well into the inguinal canal and into the tunica vaginalis, making possible a *bilocular hydrocele* with an inguinal, as well as a scrotal, pouch. Isolated portions of the process may persist along the spermatic cord when both the superior and inferior parts have become obliterated, and allow formation of *hydroceles* or *cysts* of the *cord*. Longitudinal septa may form in an unobliterated part of the process and give rise to herniae with double or multiple sacs.

The condition of *undescended testicle* or *cryptorchidism* exists when the gland is retained in the abdomen or is arrested at some point along the inguinal canal.

8. **Walls of the Inguinal Canal.**—The inguinal canal is not a canal in the ordinary acceptance of the term. In the fetus, and for a varying period after birth, the abdominal wall in the male is traversed by the testicle and the spermatic cord and by the vaginal process of peritoneum. The last is a serous tube which is continuous with the peritoneal cavity above and extends to the depth of the scrotum. In the female, the abdominal wall is traversed by the round ligament and an outpocketing of peritoneum (canal of Nuck) which accompanies it.

The inguinal canal, then, is an oblique cleft in the inguino-abdominal wall above the mesial half of the inguinal ligament. Its length in the adult varies from 4 to 5 cm. The *inlet* of the canal, the *abdominal inguinal ring*, is located in the transversalis fascia a little above the center of the inguinal ligament. The *outlet*, the *subcutaneous inguinal ring*, through which the spermatic cord emerges from the abdominal wall, has been described (p. 290). The superior or deep end of the canal is lateral to the inferior or superficial end, an arrangement which compensates for the weakness in the wall caused by the passage of the spermatic cord. When, as in coughing, the viscera are pressed forcibly against the abdominal inguinal ring, they impinge against the posterior wall of the canal and force it into contact with its anterior wall, almost closing the canal.

The *anterior wall* is the aponeurosis of the external oblique, and in the lateral third, the fibers of the internal oblique muscle which arise from the middle third of the inguinal ligament help in the formation. The lowermost fibers of the internal oblique and, to a lesser degree, those of the transversus abdominis, as they pass mesially, arch over and form the *upper wall* or *roof* of the canal. They then descend mesially behind it and terminate in the inguinal falx (conjoined tendon). The inferior margin of the internal oblique is rendered rather indistinct by the muscle fibers which descend from it along the cord and make up the *cremaster muscle*. The *floor* of the canal presents a deep gutter, upon which the cord rests. This groove is formed by the fusion of the upper grooved surface of the inguinal ligament (of Poupart) with the lacunar ligament and the transversalis fascia. The *posterior wall* is formed by the transversalis fascia and is strengthened mesially by the inguinal falx, which lies in front of the transversalis fascia and behind the cord.

9. **Elements of the Spermatic Sheath.**—In their descent through the inguinal canal, the testicle and the spermatic cord push their way through the transversalis fascia at the abdominal inguinal ring and acquire therefrom an intimate investment, the *internal spermatic* or *infundibuliform fascia*. The testicle then encounters the lower border of the internal oblique muscle, from which it drags down fibers. This partial covering, lying outside the internal spermatic fascia, is the *cremaster muscle and fascia*. Stimulation of the cremasteric muscle fibers draws the testis up from the scrotum toward the subcutaneous inguinal ring (cremasteric reflex). Upon passing through the external oblique aponeurosis, the testicle gains its third and outermost covering, the *external spermatic* or *intercolumnar fascia*. Thus, the testicle and that part of the spermatic cord lying outside the inguinal canal acquire three coverings. The mesial part of the cord within the inguinal canal

acquires but two investments, while that part behind the internal oblique has only one, the internal spermatic fascia.

10. Spermatic Cord and the Round Ligament.—The **spermatic cord** may be examined in the inguinal canal, where it lies beneath the aponeurosis of the external oblique. The constituents of the cord are differentiated readily by splitting the sheath in which are bound together the deferent duct and the numerous blood vessels, lymphatics, and nerves.

The *ductus deferens (vas)*, or duct of the testicle, is a cylindrical, resistant, whitish structure lying posteriorly, surrounded by part of the pampiniform plexus of veins. It possesses a very thick muscular wall and a small lumen, and can be distinguished easily upon palpation of the cord. The *artery of the vas*, derived from the superior vesical artery, is applied closely to the vas and runs a visible, tortuous course upon it. A thickened vas in tuberculous epididymitis indicates extension of the disease to other parts of the genito-urinary tract.

The *pampiniform plexus of veins* ascends from the scrotum to the abdominal inguinal ring and there forms the spermatic veins. The varicosity of these veins may become very extensive (varicocele). The *internal spermatic artery*, a branch of the abdominal aorta, descends anteriorly in the cord in the midst of the pampiniform plexus. The *external spermatic (cremasteric) artery*, derived from the inferior epigastric, is distributed mainly to the elements of the spermatic sheath. It is the chief source of bleeding in manipulation of the spermatic sheath. The *lymphatics* ascend from the testicle to the lumbar and aortic glands.

Among the normal elements of the cord is a thin strand, the *vaginal ligament*, vestige of the vaginal process. A patent vaginal process constitutes the sac for a congenital inguinal hernia, into which class fall almost all indirect herniae. This process, when present, must be considered to be the prime abnormal element within the spermatic sheath.

The inguinal canal in the female is much smaller than that in the male, since it contains only the **round ligament** of the uterus. The subcutaneous inguinal ring is so small as to be difficult to palpate, unless it is enlarged by a hernial protrusion. The round ligament leaves the ring as a bundle of fanlike connective tissue strands which diverge to the tubercle and anterior surface of the pubis and are lost in the labium majus. Like the spermatic cord, the round ligament curves around the inferior epigastric vessels, accompanied by the ilio-inguinal nerve and surrounded by a sheathing layer of the transversalis fascia. During fetal life, the ligament is accompanied through the abdominal inguinal ring by a finger-like prolongation of peritoneum, the homologue of the vaginal process in the male, which occupies the entire length of the canal. Ordinarily, this diverticulum, the *canal of Nuck*, becomes obliterated by the end of the sixth intra-uterine month.

A persistent canal of Nuck explains the existence of cysts and herniae of congenital origin. As a hernia into the canal of Nuck increases in size, it may drag into the sac part of the suspensory ligament of the ovary, which, at its lateral extremity, is not far from the abdominal inguinal ring. This accounts for the fact that the ovary and the distal part of the uterine (fallopian) tube sometimes are found in the hernial sac.

Surgical Considerations

1. Varieties of Inguinal Hernia.—Inguinal herniae may be divided into two main groups: those which leave the abdomen lateral to the inferior epigastric artery and traverse part, if not all, of the extent of the inguinal canal (indirect, external, or oblique); and those which leave the abdomen through the middle inguinal fossa (p. 292) mesial to the inferior epigastric artery and enter the inguinal canal near its outlet (internal or direct). Another classification divides them into congenital and acquired varieties.

2. Congenital Indirect Inguinal Hernia; Congenital Hydrocele.—All of the congenital varieties of hernia and hydrocele result from developmental defects which occur in connection with failure of obliteration of the vaginal process (p. 292). The term "congenital" does not imply that a hernia exists at birth, but that there exists a patent process which will allow the descent of abdominal elements. The process is patent in 50 per cent of infants up to a month after birth. The entrance of abdominal elements into the process, constituting hernia, may not occur for months or even years. The failure of abdominal elements to enter the sac, even though a congenital sac exists, perhaps is accounted for by the obliquity of the inguinal canal.

When the vaginal process remains patent throughout, as in the fetal condition, and the opening of the neck of the sac is sufficiently wide, bowel or omentum may enter the vaginal process and pass down to the depth of the scrotum. This constitutes the **vaginal indirect inguinal hernia.** The contents of the sac are in contact with the testicle, separated from it only by the visceral layer of the patent tunica vaginalis. The normal elements of the spermatic cord usually lie posterior to and to the medial side of the sac, but, in exceptional instances, they are invaginated into the sac, at times appearing as though suspended within it by a serosal duplication.

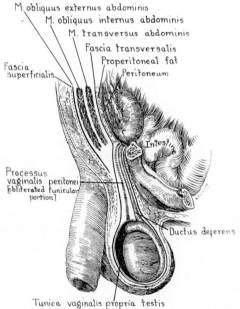

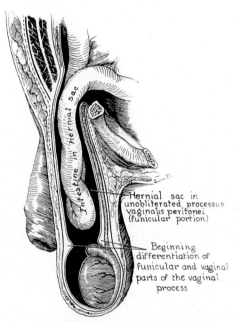

FIG. 286.—PARAMEDIAN SAGITTAL SECTION THROUGH THE LEFT INGUINAL HERNIAL REGION.

The funicular part of the vaginal process of peritoneum is obliterated normally from the origin at the abdominal inguinal ring to the superior border of the testicle; the tunica vaginalis testis is that portion of the vaginal process that normally remains patent.

FIG. 287.—CONGENITAL INGUINAL HERNIA.

The intestine has invaded the patent funicular part of the vaginal process almost down to the testicle; if and when the intestine extends to the base of the scrotum, the hernia becomes complete; the funicular and vaginal portions are beginning to be differentiated just above the testicle.

When the opening at the neck is too small to admit the passage of abdominal contents, serous peritoneal fluid may find its way into the sac and cause an *intermittent vaginal hydrocele.* When the individual lies down, the fluid passes back into the general peritoneal cavity. This type of hydrocele may be mistaken for hernia.

In most congenital herniae, only the proximal or funicular portion of the vaginal process maintains its fetal connection with the general abdominal cavity. This condition gives rise to the **funicular indirect inguinal hernia.** If the neck of the sac is not large enough to admit abdominal contents, an *intermittent funicular hydrocele* may occur.

In **encysted herniae,** almost all of the vaginal process remains patent, but there is a thin septum of closure at the abdominal inguinal ring. The hernial contents, in making their way into the canal, must invaginate the septum before them, stretching it in some cases to the degree that it bulges downward into the cavity of the tunica vaginalis testis.

Interparietal herniae are of congenital origin and occur commonly in connection with an incompletely descended testicle, but the testicle may be in the normal position in the scrotum. When the gland is retained within the inguinal canal, the vaginal process almost always is patent, and the hernia occurring within it occupies any of a variety of interparietal positions. The sacs often are bilocular. In the bilocular variety of *properitoneal hernia,* the proximal loculus lies between the peritoneum and the transversalis fascia, and the distal loculus usually lies in the inguinal canal. However, the distal loculus may lie between the other layers of the abdominal wall. In *inguinosuperficial hernia* the proximal division of the sac lies between the external oblique muscle and the skin, sometimes extending nearly to the anterior superior spine. Great care is necessary in making the herniotomy incision, as the sac is very superficial. In certain cases, the proximal loculus of the sac lies beneath the aponeurosis of the external oblique muscles. It may push the inferior margins of the internal oblique and transversus abdomini muscles superiorly.

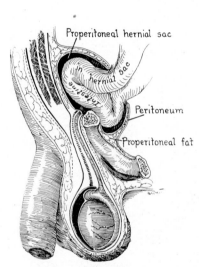

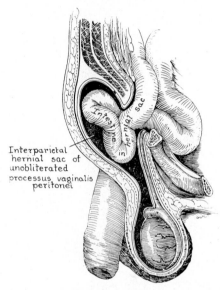

FIG. 288.—CONGENITAL INTERPARIETAL PROPERIT-
ONEAL HERNIA.

The hernial contents lie in a sac formed by the unobliterated uppermost part of the funicular portion of the vaginal process.

FIG. 289.—CONGENITAL INTERPARIETAL INGUINAL
HERNIA.

The intestine has invaded the patent vaginal process, and has extended anteriorly and superiorly between the external and internal oblique muscles.

The funicular division of the vaginal process may be shut off from the tunica vaginalis testis and from the general peritoneal cavity, and yet remain patent in its intermediate part (along the spermatic cord). Should this sac become distended with fluid, an **encysted hydrocele of the cord** results. The vaginal process may be obliterated at different levels, so that the patent parts permit the combination of a funicular hernia, an encysted hydrocele of the cord, and a hydrocele of the tunica vaginalis testis. Not infrequently, the vaginal process is obliterated only at the abdominal ring, and a large monolocular or bilocular hydrocele of almost the entire vaginal process results.

Congenital inguinal hernia in the **female** rarely is seen in adult life, but is fairly common in infants and young girls. The canal of Nuck remains pervious, and forms the sac of a hernial protrusion. The ovary and uterine tube frequently occupy the sac of the hernia. An imperfect closure at any point in the canal of Nuck may lead to an *encysted hydrocele* of the *round ligament.*

3. **So-called "Acquired Indirect Inguinal Hernia."**—In exceedingly rare instances, after extraordinary trauma, a hernia, whose sac is not formed at the expense of the funicular part of the vaginal process (which remains tightly obliterated), enters the inguinal

canal at the abdominal inguinal ring through the peritoneal dimple or depression which marks the upper limit of obliteration of the funicular process. The sac and its contents make their way down the spermatic cord parallel to the fused funicular process, covered by the spermatic sheath. The sac of this hernia, as opposed to that which occupies the funicular process, is overlain loosely by the elements of the cord and can be dissected from them easily.

A rare variety of acquired inguinal hernia occurs when there is obliteration of the vaginal process only at the abdominal inguinal ring, below which it remains patent and passes without interruption into the tunica vaginalis testis. An acquired hernial pouch appears behind this and traverses the inguinal canal. This rupture may lead to some confusion at herniotomy, especially when the hernial sac is emptied of its contents at the time of operation. The cavity within the vaginal process, which lies in front of that which contained the hernial contents, passes freely upward into the inguinal canal and, when

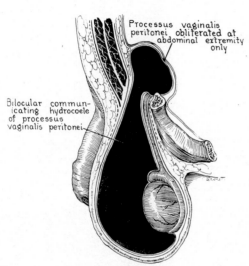

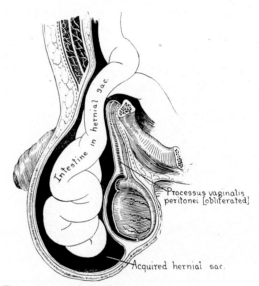

FIG. 290.—CONGENITAL BILOCULAR COMMUNICAT-
ING HYDROCELE.

The vaginal process of peritoneum is obliterated only
at the abdominal extremity.

FIG. 291.—ACQUIRED COMPLETE INDIRECT IN-
GUINAL HERNIA.

In this very unusual type of inguinal hernia, the hernial sac is not derived from the vaginal process of peritoneum, but springs from parietal peritoneum about the abdominal ring; the obliterated vaginal process can be found among the elements of the spermatic cord as a fibrous ligamentous structure.

opened, may be mistaken for the true hernial sac which lies behind, if the observation is not made that the cavity of the vaginal process is closed above at the abdominal ring. The real or acquired hernial sac is found to communicate freely with the abdominal cavity.

4. Direct Inguinal Hernia.—A direct or internal inguinal hernia enters the inguinal canal through Hesselbach's triangle, a little lateral to or opposite the subcutaneous inguinal ring. It passes directly through or lateral to the inguinal falx (conjoined tendon), and its subsequent course in the inguinal canal is the same as that of an indirect hernia. An important difference between direct and indirect herniae lies in their relationship to the inferior epigastric artery. The neck of the sac of an indirect hernia lies lateral to the artery, while that of a direct hernia is mesial to it. Direct hernia is observed most frequently in adult life when, from various causes, a heavy strain is thrown upon the abdominal wall, especially when there is a diminution of muscle tone. The lax muscles yield easily and the inguino-abdominal region bulges forward characteristically. Certain diseases predispose to rupture because of the frequent sudden increase in intra-abdominal pressure which they entail. Among these may be mentioned chronic bronchitis, prostatic enlargement, and urethral stricture. Direct hernia is of slow development, and its beginning is indicated by an exaggeration of the internal or the middle inguinal fossa, usually the middle (p. 292). After increasing sufficiently in size to occupy the inguinal canal, the hernia emerges through the external ring and forms a protrusion above the pubic spine, a *bubonocele*. The volume increases by degrees until it occupies and distends the scrotum on the same side, constituting a *complete direct inguinal (scrotal) hernia*.

If the hernia has existed for some time, it will have altered profoundly the length and direction of the inguinal canal. Because of the traction which it exercises, it may become so large as to contain the greater part of the small intestine and a part of the large bowel. The inguinal rings approximate each other more and more until the canal is reduced to a short, wide passage leading the exploring finger directly backward through the abdominal wall.

In long-standing inguinal herniae, some difficulty may be experienced in deciding which variety is present. The inferior epigastric artery in an old indirect rupture is deflected medial to its normal course, and may be found curving upward and medially close to the lateral edge of the rectus muscle. If a long-standing hernia becomes strangulated, it is advisable to incise the constricting neck in an upward and medial direction from the neck of the sac to avoid injuring the inferior epigastric vessels. If a direct hernia is mistaken for an indirect hernia, and the neck of the sac is incised in a lateral direction, these vessels will be injured. If an old indirect hernia is mistaken for a direct hernia, and the constricting neck is cut in a mesial direction, the same accident will occur.

In a *primary direct hernia of the bladder*, a part of the viscus, usually that not covered by peritoneum, or a bladder diverticulum, may be extruded, and with it a large quantity of prevesical fat, constituting practically a "lipoma," so that the true condition of affairs may be quite unsuspected. As more of the bladder becomes involved, the part covered by peritoneum will be included, and with it an extension of peritoneum from behind that part of the bladder which first became extruded. Part of the bladder covered by peritoneum, therefore, will lie within the sac, while the extraperitoneal portion will be devoid of a sac.

Herniation of the bladder may be *secondary* when an inguinal rupture, usually of the direct type, already exists. As the hernial sac increases at the expense of the parietal peritoneum about the abdominal aperture, the bladder gradually is included. In young children, much of the bladder lies in the abdomen above the level of the symphysis and may extend laterally almost to the abdominal inguinal ring, so that it is possible in the course of herniotomy to injure the viscus. Traction upon the hernial sac in an attempt to ligate its neck high up may draw a part of the bladder wall into close proximity of the abdominal ring, or even into the ring itself, where it may be injured in the placing of the sutures transfixing the sac. This awkward accident has led to urinary infiltration in the deeper parts of the wound, and to fistulae discharging into the hernial region.

5. **Inguinal Herniotomy.**—The two main reasons for subjecting herniae to operative treatment are the need for radical cure and the relief of strangulation. The two essential procedures in operative treatment are: removal of the sac after carefully reducing its contents and ligating it at its neck, and reconstruction of the inguinal canal.

The operation which seems most suitable to these requirements is that devised by Bassini, or one of its numerous modifications. The features of the **Bassini operation** are briefly as follows. An incision is developed along the line bisecting the angle formed by the inguinal ligament and the lateral margin of the rectus muscle, beginning a little above the abdominal ring and extending to the pubic spine. The aponeurosis of the external oblique is exposed after division of the superficial fasciae of Camper and Scarpa (p. 275), and of the superficial epigastric and external pudic arteries lying between them. At the mesial portion of the wound, the spermatic cord is exposed and the subcutaneous inguinal ring is defined. Beginning at the apex of the ring, the aponeurosis of the external oblique is incised as far as the abdominal ring.

If the hernia is *indirect*, the sac must be sought in combination with the cord and within its sheath. Forceps are applied to the margins of the sheath, which consists of the cremasteric and the internal spermatic (infundibuliform) fascia, and it is separated longitudinally, exposing the elements of the cord. The sac is separated from the deferent duct and the pampiniform plexus, and its neck is isolated carefully, ligated, and divided at the point of exit from the abdominal inguinal ring. The distal portion of the sac then is excised. Excessive traction upon the sac is to be avoided, lest the bladder be drawn into the canal. The stump of the sac is allowed to retract flush with the abdominal peritoneum, or it may be drawn superiorly beneath the musculature of the roof of the canal and sutured there. If the sac is of the complete (vaginal) type, the inferior part is ligated by purse-string suture to form a closed tunica vaginalis testis.

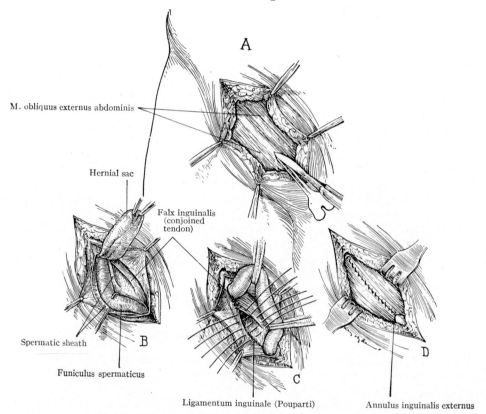

FIG. 292.—BASSINI OPERATION FOR INGUINAL HERNIA.

Reconstruction of the inguinal canal strengthens the hernial region and minimizes recurrence. The procedure contemplates closure of the gap between the inferior border of the internal oblique and transversus abdominis muscles superiorly, and the inguinal ligament inferiorly. After the cord is freed from its sheath and retracted superiorly or inferiorly out of the wound, the inferior border of these muscles is brought down and sutured to the shelving margin of the inguinal ligament. The close relations of the femoral vessels deep to the inguinal ligament must be borne in mind when these sutures are inserted. Care is taken not to constrict the spermatic cord where it emerges from the abdominal ring. The cord is laid upon the sutured muscles (transplanted), the incision in the aponeurosis of the external oblique muscle is sutured, and the external abdominal ring, if unduly large, is reduced to dimensions which will not constrict the emerging cord.

The incision for *direct inguinal hernia* is the same as that employed for the indirect variety, but the coverings of the sac are different. The spermatic sheath, with its cremasteric and infundibuliform coverings and the cord, are found lying to the lateral side of the hernial bulge. The rupture, bearing outward through Hesselbach's triangle, is covered by a thin expansion from the inguinal falx, and a sheath, which, though derived from the transversalis fascia, is quite free and distinct from the internal spermatic (infundibuliform) fascia of the cord. The sac usually has a broader neck, and is much more difficult to resect than that of the indirect variety. The Bassini technic in the reconstruction of the new posterior wall for the cord is similar to that devised for indirect hernia. An additional strengthening layer for Hesselbach's triangle may be added by turning down a flap of the anterior sheath of the rectus muscle, or even fibers from the lateral margin

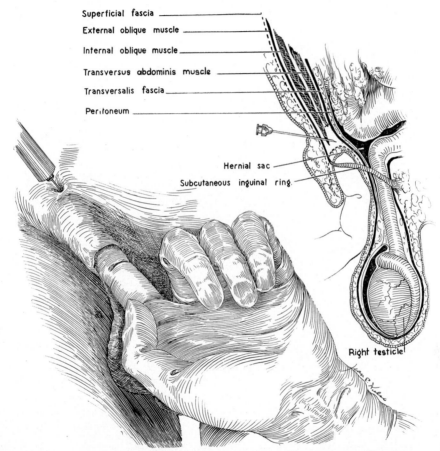

Superficial fascia

External oblique muscle

Internal oblique muscle

Transversus abdominis muscle

Transversalis fascia

Peritoneum

Hernial sac

Subcutaneous inguinal ring

Right testicle

FIG. 293.—METHOD OF INJECTING RIGHT INGUINAL CANAL IN NONOPERATIVE TREATMENT OF HERNIA

The scrotum is invaginated through the subcutaneous inguinal ring to act as a guide for the injection of a fibrosing solution through the external oblique aponeurosis into the inguinal canal.

The sagittal section indicates how the invaginating finger orients the injection needle. (Harris and White, Surg., Gynec. and Obst., Aug., 1936.)

of the rectus muscle itself, and suturing them to the shelving edge of the inguinal ligament.

A favorite **modification of the Bassini technic** (*Ferguson operation*), more applicable in indirect than in direct hernia, allows the cord to remain *in situ* against the original back wall of the canal after the sac is excised. A new anterior wall is made for the cord by suturing the inferior margin of the internal oblique and transversus abdominis muscles and their inguinal falx to the inguinal ligament anterior to the nontransplanted cord. In this procedure, the elements of the cord are not disturbed, and therefore are less traumatized. For a direct hernia or a large indirect hernia, it has the disadvantage of not allowing complete closure of the new wall at the pubic spine, where space must be left for the cord to emerge.

Another procedure contemplates **transplantation of the cord entirely out of the inguinal canal** (*original Halsted operation*) into a position between the skin and the aponeurosis of the external oblique. A stronger wall is formed posterior to the cord by the approximation to the inguinal ligament of not only the internal oblique and transversus abdominis muscles, but also the aponeurosis of the external oblique.

6. **Injection Treatment of Inguinal Hernia.**—Much interest has been aroused recently in the nonoperative injection treatment of inguinal hernia. The principles underlying this type of therapy and the mechanics of the cure will be outlined.

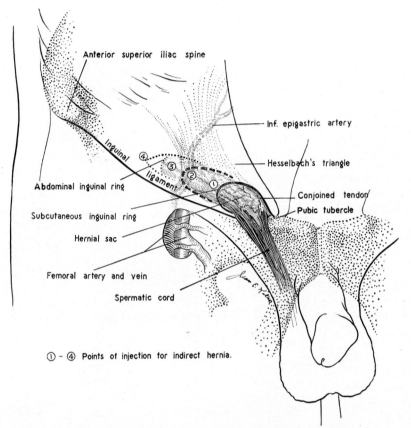

Fig. 294.—Points of Injection of Sclerosing Solution in Nonoperative Treatment of Indirect Inguinal Hernia.

In direct hernia, all of the injection points are within Hesselbach's triangle.

When the hernia is a combined direct and indirect hernia, the entire inguinal canal and Hesselbach's triangle are injected. (Harris and White, Surg., Gynec. and Obst., Aug., 1936.)

If an indirect or direct inguinal hernia is to occur, the walls of the inguinal canal must be relaxed sufficiently to allow abdominal contents to enter and travel down the hernial sac. Only when contents occupy a sac does hernia really occur. The presence of a sac alone, therefore, does not constitute rupture. Any mechanical agent which prevents the separation of the structures forming the inguinal canal stops the descent of abdominal contents into the hernial sac, and thereby prevents hernia. Wearing a well-fitted truss accomplishes this by exerting pressure directly on the walls of the canal. The external oblique aponeurosis is pressed tightly against the underlying musculature, cord, and transversalis fascia and the potential space in the inguinal canal is obliterated. The sac of course, remains patent.

The injection of a fibrosing solution into the inguinal canal acts in a fashion similar to a truss. The fibrosis caused by the injected material obliterates the inguinal canal, and thereby keeps abdominal contents out of any variety of hernial sac which may exist.

Truss pressure must be maintained over the injected area during the period of injection treatment and for a considerable time thereafter in order to prevent the destruction of the newly-formed connective tissue, which would occur if abdominal contents were allowed to descend the hernial sac, and to allow this tissue to become organized uniformly and firmly.

(II) UMBILICAL REGION

1. Definition and Boundaries.—The umbilical region occupies the central portion of the anterolateral abdominal wall. It derives its surgical interest from the occurrence of a special form of hernia (umbilical) and a number of congenital anomalies related to the fetal circulation, the vitello-intestinal duct and the urachus.

2. Development of the Umbilical Region.—The surgical anatomy of the region is incomplete without brief reference to its development, which is given with a view toward rendering intelligible the abnormal conditions found at the umbilicus and associated conditions within the abdominal cavity, the result of arrested or imperfect development in fetal life.

In the early human embryo, the alimentary canal communicates freely with the yolk sac by the *vitello-intestinal duct*. Caudal to this communication, the alimentary tube throws out a diverticulum, the *allantois*. The cavity of the allantois is continuous with that of the *urachus*, which grows out anteriorly into the *umbilical pedicle*. This pedicle is the means of attachment of the embryo to the chorion, and contains the vessels which supply the fetus. At this period, the lining of the true body cavity, or *coelom*, is directly continuous with the lining of the outside body cavity or *exocoelom*. These cavities communicate broadly with one another. As the embryo enlarges, its ventral enclosed area, bounded by the edge of the amnion, becomes relatively smaller. The tubular structure contained within the ventral enclosed area is the *umbilical cord*. The cord encloses the yolk stalk,

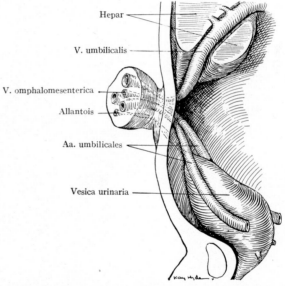

FIG. 295.—SAGITTAL VIEW OF A RECONSTRUCTION OF THE UMBILICAL REGION OF A HUMAN EMBRYO 5.5 CM. IN LENGTH. (After Cullen.)

allantois, and the fetal blood vessels which pass to and from the placenta. Thenceforth, the umbilical cord connects the embryo to that part of the outer fetal membrane which constitutes the fetal surface of the placenta, the *chorion*.

By the end of the third month, the body walls have closed in except at the umbilical ring, to the periphery of which the cord is adherent. The amnion invests the cord externally and is continuous with the skin of the abdomen. The amniotic cavity, during the same interval, has increased greatly in size and is filled with amniotic fluid in which the fetus is suspended.

Since the abdominal portion of the alimentary canal increases in length much more rapidly than does the coelomic or body cavity, much of the gut extrudes itself through the large patent defect in the abdominal wall and lies in the umbilical cord. As the body cavity becomes large enough to contain the abdominal viscera, the intestinal loop to which the vitello-intestinal duct is attached returns to the body cavity. Later, when the body walls are formed, this narrow duct runs along the cord and connects the intestine with its shriveled yolk sac. The abdominal walls, in their ventral growth, gradually close off the body cavity until, at birth, no trace of the yolk stalk remains. Should all of the bowel contents of the umbilical cord fail to return to the abdomen, or should a part of the cord remain open, maintaining a communication with the abdominal cavity, a *hernia into the cord* results.

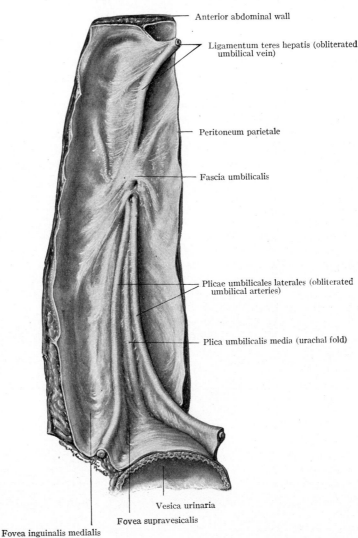

FIG. 296.—UMBILICAL AND SUPRAVESICAL REGIONS FROM WITHIN.

Attention is directed to the medial inguinal and supravesical peritoneal fossae and the median and lateral umbilical folds. (After Cullen.)

Under normal conditions, the vitello-intestinal duct, omphalomesenteric vessels, and urachus atrophy into fibrous cords. In consequence of this process, the umbilical ring, which is traversed by these structures, is reduced to a very small orifice. After birth, blood no longer circulates in the vessels of the cord, and a small umbilical crust remains where the cord has been ligated and cut. This heals rapidly and epithelializes without suppuration. As healing progresses, fibrous changes take place within the vessels and urachus and draw the scar against the circumference of the umbilical ring. The force of the retraction of the umbilical vein draws the scar against the uppermost circumference of the ring, but the adhesion thus formed is less dense than that resulting from the adhesion of the scar to the inferior contour of the ring, caused by the inferior pull of the two obliterated umbilical arteries and the urachus. Thus it occurs that, in the superior part of the ring, there is an area of lesser fusion where the subcutaneous tissue is almost in contact with the extraperitoneal fat. This area is the site of election for the development of umbilical hernia. In the infant, the umbilicus bulges slightly forward; in the adult it usually is retracted. Retraction is explained by the fact that the urachus and obliterated umbilical arteries form unyielding cords which are incapable of elongating as the abdominal walls and pelvis continue to grow.

Slight herniae commonly bulge through the umbilicus in the newborn, but prompt reduction, followed by suitable and persistent padding, assures such healing as will insure a resistant abdominal wall.

3. Surface Anatomy.—Between the umbilical papilla and the contour of the ring is a circular or elliptical depression, about which is a superficial bulge caused by the presence of fat in the subcutaneous tissues. The papilla usually is a little elevated, very irregular, and surmounted by the scar. At the ring, the fat is absent, so that the very thin skin is fused directly to the ring margins, the adhesion being particularly dense over the inferior contour of the ring (see above). Upon reducing an umbilical hernia, the finger invaginates the abdominal cavity, readily palpating the fibrous contour of the ring. After multiple pregnancies, or with ascites, the ring may be dilated and enlarged.

4. Fibro-aponeurotic Umbilical Ring.—The fibrous contour of the ring, formed within the linea alba by the abdominal aponeuroses, constitutes the framework for the region and contains the umbilical débris overlain by skin. When the ring is examined on its deep aspect after the peritoneal layer has been stripped away, two sets of semicircular fibers with their opposed concavities are exposed. The fusion of the umbilical remains to the ring contour at first is soft and unresistant; toward the end of the first year, the papilla presents a definite resistance, closing the orifice firmly.

Surgical Considerations

It is customary to describe three distinct forms of umbilical hernia: hernia into the umbilical cord, infantile, and acquired.

1. Hernia into the Umbilical Cord.—Hernia into the cord may be explained on the basis of the failure of the abdominal muscles on the two sides to approximate and unite properly at the midline, because of the intervention of viscera which should have receded into the abdominal cavity during the later period of intra-uterine life. The hernia which results is present at birth. In other words, instead of an umbilical cord emerging from a small opening, there is no proper umbilicus, only a broad funnel-shaped defect in the central part of the abdominal wall, through which the viscera protrude into the umbilical cord.

A segment of intestine may be found lying in the cord, the umbilical vessels either spreading over it or being pushed to one side. The protruding part may be a loop of normally developed intestine, which may be replaced with little difficulty. In large herniae, the liver and spleen may lie within the cord together with the major part of the bowel. Sometimes the rupture contains the remains of the vitello-intestinal duct which is connected by its proximal or basal end with the small intestine within the abdomen, a Meckel's diverticulum. Occasionally, the original umbilical loop of intestine may fail to withdraw itself into the abdomen and may remain within the cord, perhaps connected at its apex with the narrowed stalk of the yolk sac.

The covering of these large herniae consists of the amnion externally, and, deep to it, a delicate layer prolonged from the parietal peritoneum. In many instances, unfortunately, these herniae have not been recognized, and the protruding parts have been included in ligating the cord. Care should be taken to examine the cord in every case before applying a ligature, lest this disastrous accident occur. Inclusion of a patent vitello-intestinal duct is followed, after separation of the ligature, by an umbilical fecal fistula. Should the intestine be included, an absolute and probably fatal obstruction is the inevitable conse-

20

quence. The only evidence of hernia may be an abnormal thickening of the cord near the base. When this thickening presents, the cord must be ligated some distance from the abdominal wall. Congenital umbilical hernia often is accompanied by other congenital deformities, such as harelip and imperforate anus.

2. **Infantile Umbilical Hernia.**—Infantile umbilical hernia, as distinguished from hernia into the umbilical cord, appears within a few days or weeks after the stump of the

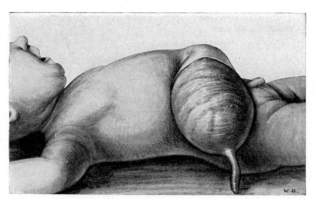

FIG. 297.—HERNIA INTO THE UMBILICAL CORD.

cord has dropped off. Infantile hernia is covered with true skin and not with gelatinous cord tissue as is a hernia into the cord. As a rule, a hernia in an infant remains a small rounded protrusion, rarely larger than a walnut, appearing in the superior rather than in the inferior margin of the umbilical ring. It is easily reducible, and becomes prominent when the child cries or coughs; it is symptomless, its strangulation is rare, and increase in size is uncommon.

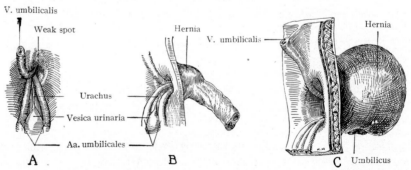

FIG. 298.—DIAGRAM OF THE UMBILICAL RING TO SHOW ITS SIGNIFICANCE IN THE DEVELOPMENT OF UM-
BILICAL HERNIA.

A, A dissection of the umbilical ring in an eight months' human embryo, viewed from within; the peritoneum and extraperitoneal connective tissue have been removed and there is exposed a funnel-shaped opening above and to the right of the umbilical arteries. The umbilical vein lies to the left of this weak spot. The umbilical arteries are the strongest structures within the ring and a hernial protrusion usually occurs above or to one side of them. B is a side view of the umbilical ring, showing the usual position of the small hernial protrusion often seen in the newborn. C is a larger hernia which represents a later stage of the same type. Note how the umbilicus is lodged at the inferior part of the hernial protrusion.

The cause of the protrusion is a weakness in the adhesion between the scarred remains in the cord and the umbilical ring (p. 305). When the abdomen is large and distended, the overstretched linea alba has a tendency to widen, and the gap may be so extensive that a median bulge appears between the recti when the child cries. In such cases, infantile umbilical hernia not uncommonly exists. These herniae tend to undergo spontaneous cure, especially if firm, constant pressure is maintained over the ring for some time.

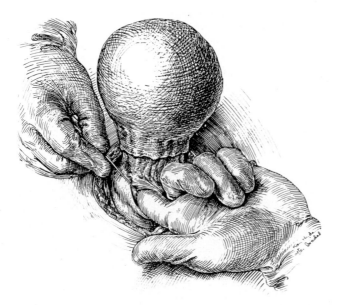

FIG. 299.—MAYO OPERATION FOR REPAIR OF UMBILICAL HERNIA.

After wide exposure of the neck of the protrusion, the abdomen is entered at a point sufficiently remote from the sac to avoid structures adherent to the neck of the sac. (After Cullen.)

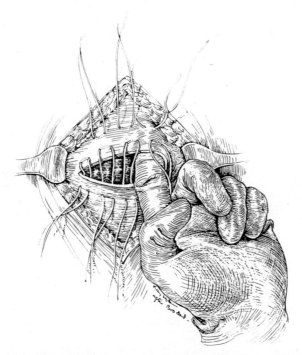

FIG. 300.—MAYO OPERATION FOR REPAIR OF UMBILICAL HERNIA.

The sac has been removed by excision at the margins of the umbilical ring; after closure of the peritoneum, the flaps of the widened linea alba are overlapped and held in place by mattress sutures, the second row of mattress sutures is laid in such a fashion as to avoid injury to underlying structures. (After Cullen.)

3. Acquired Umbilical Hernia.

3. **Acquired Umbilical Hernia.**—The hernial protrusion of an acquired umbilical hernia makes its appearance at some period remote from the closure of the umbilical ring. In order for the condition to supervene, it is obvious that the cicatricial tissue closing the ring must yield gradually. This is most likely to take place at the upper margin of the ring, because the scar between the débris of the cord and the ring is not as strong there as at the inferior margin. As predisposing factors, there may be mentioned the excessive

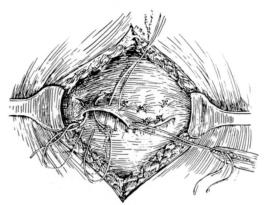

FIG. 301.—MAYO OPERATION FOR REPAIR OF UMBILICAL HERNIA.
The final steps in closure illustrate the overlapping of the flaps of aponeurotic tissue.   (After Cullen.)

stretching of the abdominal wall which occurs with pregnancy, hard labor, ascites, and obesity. Deposition of fat in the superior part of the ring also may weaken it.

Adult hernia, as contrasted with the infantile variety, does not tend to spontaneous recession, but rather tends to steady increase in size. In adult hernia, the sac always is thin and its coverings may be so stretched and attenuated as to make it appear that the hernial contents are just under the skin. If the contents be intestine, peristaltic move-

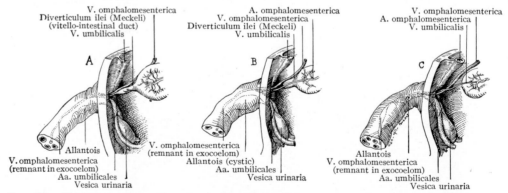

FIG. 302.—DIAGRAM TO SHOW FAILURE OF EMBRYONIC STRUCTURES IN THE UMBILICAL REGION TO RE-
GRESS NORMALLY.

A shows a persistent omphalomesenteric vein and a patent vitello-intestinal duct; B indicates persistent omphalomesenteric vessels and a diverticulum of the ileum (Meckel), as well as a cystic allantois in the umbilical cord; C illustrates persistent omphalomesenteric vessels.

ment may be visible. The contents often consist of a mass of omentum with perhaps part of the transverse colon or small intestine. These herniae often are lobulated in outline, the lobulation apparently being caused by the irregular manner in which the hernial sac expands. By following the lines of least resistance, the sac insinuates itself between the resisting bands of fascia which connect the skin to the subjacent aponeurosis. The loculi or sacculations may be seen by opening the sac and turning aside the contents which may be adherent to it. As the hernia usually makes its exit immediately below the superior border of the ring and not at its center, the umbilical scar usually is found at some distance to one side or inferior to the bulk of the protruding mass. Contrasted with infrequent strangulation in the infantile hernia is the frequent strangulation in the adult hernia.

4. **Radical Cure of Acquired Umbilical Hernia.**—With no sharp differentiation, umbilical herniae are grouped as small and large. The small are those in which the protrusion is a rounded mass not over 2 cm. in diameter, with a sac neck much smaller. The large are those above this size, some of them enormous, in which the broad sac neck forms an ovoid opening with its long diameter transverse to the body axis.

In the repair of *small herniae*, a vertical oval incision is made around the umbilicus down to the sheath of the rectus. The sac is opened, its contents are reduced, and the sac with the skin over the umbilicus is excised. The neck of the sac is closed and the rectus sheaths are united across the defect, after which the skin is sutured.

A *large hernia* with a wide transverse neck, accompanied by a diastasis of the recti, is a far more difficult surgical problem than a small hernia. In the Mayo repair, a transverse elliptical incision is made outside the hernial mass and carried down to the abdominal aponeurosis. The abdomen is opened by incising the linea alba a short distance from the umbilical ring, or through the peritoneum of the sac at the margin of the ring where adhesions are not likely to be present. The sac is opened, the contents are reduced, and

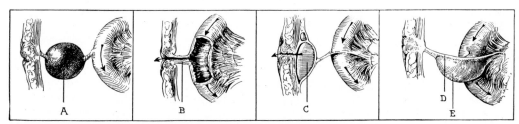

FIG. 303.—VARIETIES OF OMPHALOMESENTERIC PATHOLOGY.

A, Cyst resulting from torsion of omphalomesenteric duct; B, patent omphalomesenteric duct; C, cyst of the umbilicus, the result of a remnant of the omphalomesenteric duct; D, fibrous cord formed from the omphalomesenteric vessels; E, Meckel's diverticulum. (After Cullen.)

the sac with the overlying skin is removed. The superior margin of the cleft in the linea alba is drawn down as a flap in front of the inferior margin. This results in a double flap or overlay effect across the former position of the umbilical ring. These flaps are maintained in superapposition by a double row of mattress sutures.

5. **Abnormal Conditions Resulting from Partial or Complete Persistence of the Omphalo-(Vitello-)Intestinal Duct.**—In early fetal life, the midgut has a wide communication with the yolk sac. As the abdominal walls approximate one another, the vitello-intestinal duct becomes narrower and lies within the umbilical cord. Under normal conditions, the intestine finally is set free from all connection with the yolk sac and retires within the abdominal cavity, leaving no trace of the former connection with this structure. The vitello-intestinal duct may fail to undergo complete obliteration, and parts sometimes are found to persist up to adult life.

The incompletely-obliterated duct may be found with its *proximal* or *intestinal end attached* to some portion of the ileum near the ileocecal valve and its distal end free. This abnormality is known as *Meckel's diverticulum*. It springs from the antimesenteric border of the intestine and resembles in structure the intestine with which it is connected. The distal extremity terminates in a culdesac in the manner of a glove finger. It varies in length, but 5 to 8 cm. may be regarded as the average. The diverticulum may be so small as to appear as a mere budlike process from the intestinal wall.

A diverticulum is a source of danger in the abdomen because of its tendency to create an intestinal obstruction. This may be done by twisting itself around an adjacent coil of intestine, or by becoming adherent to some neighboring part, the abdominal wall, intestine, or mesentery, thus forming a cord about which a coil of intestine may fold and become constricted.   The *distal end of the diverticulum may be continued into a fibrous cord* and may maintain its connection with the intestine and umbilicus.   This is likely to bring about an intestinal strangulation and obstruction.   The duct may *remain open throughout its length* and constitute one of the varieties of umbilical fistula in which the constant escape of feces and mucus constitutes a great source of annoyance.   Occasionally, certain forms of cystic adenoma are found which apparently have risen from *vestiges of the duct* in the *umbilical region.*

6. **Congenital Defects in the Allantois.**—In the fetus, the allantois consists of an abdominal and an extra-abdominal portion.   After birth, the abdominal portion, between the urinary bladder and the umbilicus, shrinks and is converted into a fibrous cord, the *urachus.*   The extra-abdominal portion lies among the contents of the umbilical cord.   The urachus may be patent throughout, with a consequent fistulous opening at the umbilicus through which urine escapes.   Closure of the urachus at the two ends sometimes occurs with the intervening portion remaining patent, a condition which may cause a cystic tumor of considerable size.   The cyst is extraperitoneal.

B. POSTEROLATERAL ABDOMINAL WALL (LUMBAR OR ILIOCOSTAL REGION)

Surgical interest in the lumbar or iliocostal region arises from the fact that surgical access to the kidneys and the proximal portion of the ureters is offered therein.

1. **Definition, Boundaries, and Landmarks.**—Superficially, the posterolateral abdominal wall comprises the quadrilateral area between the lowermost ribs, the iliac crest, the vertebral column, and a vertical line erected at the anterior superior iliac spine.   Deeply, the region takes in the parietal peritoneum and the retroperitoneal space, which includes the lumbar and iliac fossae.   The lumbar and iliac fossae are described in the section devoted to the retroperitoneal structures of the abdomen.   The *landmarks* are: the lumbar vertebral column, the iliac crest, the eleventh and twelfth (floating) ribs, and the depression lateral to the bulky mass of the erector spinae muscle.

2. **Superficial Structures.**—The superficial fascia is disposed in two layers, between which an excessive quantity of loculated fatty tissue is deposited.   This loose tissue frequently is the seat of extensive suppuration which gravitates down to, but does not extend into, the corresponding tissue of the anterolateral wall.   The arteries, veins, and nerves are small and of no surgical import.

3. **Lumbodorsal (Lumbar) Fascia.**—It is convenient to consider the three divisions of the lumbodorsal fascia as fusing lateral to the erector spinae and quadratus lumborum muscles into a broad aponeurosis which extends anteriorly as the transversus abdominis muscle (p. 277).   The *posterior,* and by far the thickest, *layer* of this fascia originates over the lumbar spinous processes and the supraspinous ligaments and gives a stout dorsal investment to the erector spinae muscle.   This lamella is covered by the latissimus dorsi and the serratus posterior inferior muscles, to which it partly gives origin.

The *middle layer* of fascia is attached to the posterior surfaces and tips of the lumbar transverse processes, and lies in front of the erector spinae muscle and behind the quadratus lumborum.   At the lateral margin of the erector spinae muscle, the middle and posterior layers fuse to enclose this powerful muscle mass in a dense aponeurotic compartment.   In its upper portion, the middle layer is strengthened by the *posterior lumbocostal ligament,* which connects the transverse processes of the first and second lumbar vertebrae to the outer margin of the lowest rib.   The medial attachment of the upper portion of the ligament to the transverse process of the first and second lumbar vertebrae is constant in all cases.   The lateral termination of both portions of the ligament is attached to the twelfth rib if it be present and of normal length; otherwise, it is attached to the eleventh rib.   The sharp edge of the ligament is an extremely important landmark for the inferior line of pleural reflection (p. 243), and should be avoided in operating.

The *anterior layer* of the lumbodorsal fascia is the least resistant, arises from the anterior surfaces of the lumbar transverse processes and their bases, and forms an anterior investment for the quadratus lumborum muscle. In its upper portion the layer is strengthened by the *lateral lumbocostal (external arcuate) ligament*, which is anterior and lateral to the posterior lumbocostal ligament, and serves as origin for some of the posterior fibers

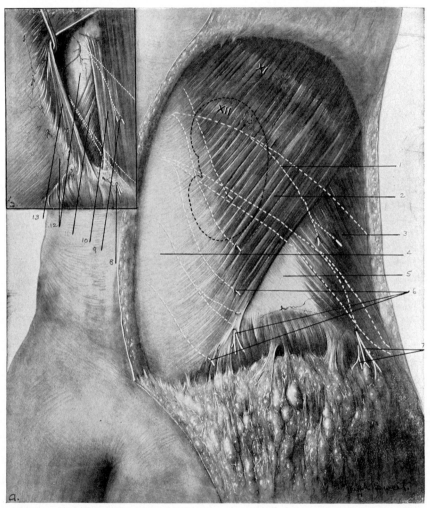

Fig. 304.—Superficial Muscular Layer of the Posterolateral Abdominal Wall.

The main drawing shows the excessive fatty tissue of the loin, and an unusually wide lumbar trigone (of Petit); the inset shows a narrow lumbar trigone, with the internal oblique muscle cleared of fatty tissue; the outline of the kidney is shown in projection. 1, Ramus cutaneus posterior n. thoracalis XII; 2, M. latissimus dorsi; 3, M. obliquus externus; 4, fascia lumbodorsalis; 5, trigonum lumbale (Petit's triangle); 6, Nn. clunia superiores (rami cutanei dorsales a. rami posterioribus n. lumbalium I, II, III); 7, ramus cutaneus lateralis n. iliohypogastrici; 8, ramus cutaneus lateralis n. iliohypogastrici; 9, ramus cutaneus posterior n. thoracalis XII; 10, M. obliquus externus; 11, M. obliquus internus; 12, fascia lumbodorsalis; 13, M. latissimus dorsi. (After Kelly, Burnam.)

of the diaphragm (Fig. 235). The ligament serves to protect the pleura in surgical exposure of the kidney and sometimes may be a considerable obstruction, particularly if the kidney lies high in the lumbar fossa. The anterior layer meets the fusion aponeurosis of the posterior and middle fascial layers at the lateral margin of the quadratus lumborum muscle, whence the broad lumbar aponeurosis runs laterally to merge into the fleshy band of the transversus abdominis muscle (p. 277). Through this broad aponeurosis lateral to the quadratus lumborum muscle, access is gained to the retrorenal spaces.

4. **Posterior Abdominal Musculature.**—Superficial, middle, and deep muscle groups may be considered in the musculature of the region.

The **superficial musculature** consists of the latissimus dorsi posteriorly and the external oblique laterally. Within the region, the *latissimus dorsi muscle* arises from the posterior third of the outer ridge of the iliac crest, from the lumbar and sacral spinous processes, and from the dorsal leaf of the lumbodorsal fascia. Its fibers converge superiorly and laterally to attach by a flat tendon into the intertubercular (bicipital) groove of the humerus. In kidney incisions, it may be cut or retracted posteriorly without serious damage to vessels or nerves deep to it. The anterior border of the latissimus dorsi, as it crosses the external oblique, may be separated below from the posterior margin of that muscle by a small triangular interval, the *inferior lumbar triangle* (of Petit). The base of the triangle is a portion of the iliac crest, and the floor is the internal oblique muscle.

The *superior* or *surgical lumbar triangle* lies under cover of the latissimus dorsi muscle and above and mesial to the lumbar triangle of Petit. Above, it is bounded by the twelfth rib; mesially, by the depression along the lateral margin of the sacrospinalis muscle; and below, by the superior border of the internal oblique near its origin from the lumbodorsal fascia. The floor of the space is the transversus abdominis aponeurosis, made up of the union of the three leaves of the lumbodorsal fascia. The triangle affords ready access to the retroperitoneal structures, and all kidney incisions, whatever their outside configuration, pass through it.

The fibers of the *external oblique muscle* which arise from the ninth, tenth, and eleventh ribs, descend obliquely downward and forward, and form a free posterior margin for that muscle within the region. In the kidney approach, the posterior fibers may be drawn ventrally, save where the external oblique reaches very far back. If the muscle must be sacrificed in the incision, it should be cut parallel to the lower ribs to avoid cutting nerves.

In the **middle muscle group** are the sacrospinalis, internal oblique, and serratus posterior inferior muscles. The *sacrospinalis (erector spinae) muscle* occupies the aponeurotic compartment formed by the dorsal and middle layers of the lumbodorsal fascia. It lies in the groove along the spinous processes from the sacrum to the neck, and is about a palm-breadth wide. In kidney incisions, only the lateral bundles of the sacrospinalis muscle require consideration. When they must be cut, which rarely is the case, the incision should be made transverse to the fibers, 3 or 4 cm. below and parallel to the twelfth rib to avoid the larger vessels, the lateral and ventral branches of the last thoracic and first lumbar nerves, and the dorsal branches of the tenth and eleventh thoracic nerves.

The *internal oblique muscle*, which arises from the iliac crest and inferior portion of the lumbodorsal fascia, sends fibers upward and forward which are encountered in operations in this region. Its superior margin is the lateral boundary of the superior lumbar triangle. Any incision in the superior lumbar triangle which is enlarged anterolaterally will cut the muscle. The incision should parallel the lower rib to avoid cutting vessels and nerves.

The *serratus posterior inferior* is a thin, flat, quadrangular muscle which lies in the upper confines of the region, covered by the latissimus dorsi muscle and partly by the trapezius muscle. It arises from the dorsal layer of the lumbodorsal fascia and runs horizontally laterally to insert by digitations on the lowest four ribs. Its lowermost fibers are the upper boundary of the superior lumbar triangle. The lowermost bundle of the muscle lies superficial to the posterior lumbocostal ligament in almost the same relative position. As the pleura is on a level with the lumbocostal ligament (p. 310) or only a little above it, incisions should avoid injuring the muscle or the ligament deep to it. If it is necessary for the sake of good exposure to remove the lateral portion of the twelfth rib, the rib periosteum should be preserved carefully to avoid injury to the pleura.

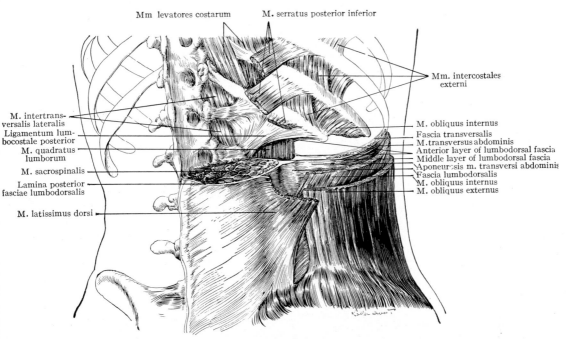

Mm levatores costarum   M. serratus posterior inferior

Mm. intercostales externi

M. intertransversalis lateralis
Ligamentum lumbocostale posterior
M. quadratus lumborum
M. sacrospinalis
Lamina posterior fasciae lumbodorsalis
M. latissimus dorsi

M. obliquus internus
Fascia transversalis
M. transversus abdominis
Anterior layer of lumbodorsal fascia
Middle layer of lumbodorsal fascia
Aponeurosis m. transversi abdominis
Fascia lumbodorsalis
M. obliquus internus
M. obliquus externus

FIG. 305.—TRANSVERSE SECTION THROUGH THE MUSCLES OF THE POSTEROLATERAL ABDOMINAL WALL.

Attention is called to the three layers of lumbodorsal fascia which fuse at the lateral margin of the quadratus lumborum muscle to form the aponeurosis of the transversus abdominis muscle.   (After Kelly, Burnam.)

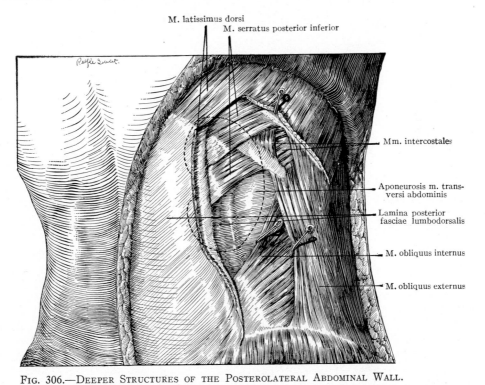

M. latissimus dorsi
M. serratus posterior inferior

Mm. intercostales

Aponeurosis m. transversi abdominis

Lamina posterior fasciae lumbodorsalis

M. obliquus internus

M. obliquus externus

FIG. 306.—DEEPER STRUCTURES OF THE POSTEROLATERAL ABDOMINAL WALL.

Part of the latissimus dorsi muscle has been removed to show the aponeurosis of the transversus abdominis, which all posterolateral kidney incisions must traverse.   (After Kelly, Burnam.)

The **deep** or **anterior muscle group** includes the quadratus lumborum, the psoas major, and the origin of the transversus abdominis. The *quadratus lumborum muscle* arises below from the iliac crest and from the iliolumbar ligament which runs between the crest and the fifth lumbar transverse process. It narrows as it passes upward to an insertion into the twelfth rib. The quadratus lumborum is contained within the fibrous compartment formed by the middle and anterior lamellae of the lumbodorsal fascia, and is separated from the transversalis fascia by the anterior lamella. In the upper portion, it is strengthened anteriorly by the lateral lumbocostal ligament. The kidney, in normal position, **extends from 1 to 3 cm.** lateral to the lateral margin of the quadratus lumborum. Since this muscle can be drawn medialward, it is necessary only in an extraordinary case to sacrifice its lateral bundles.

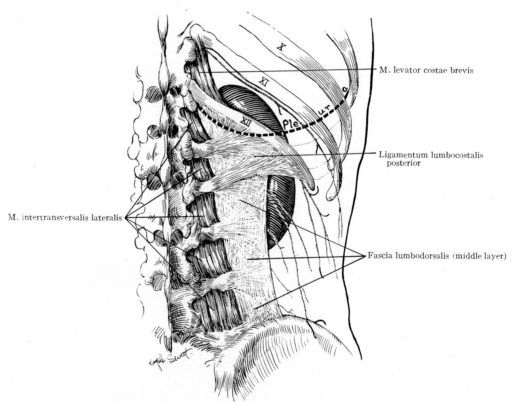

Fig. 307.—The Relations of the Kidney with the Deep Structures of the Posterolateral Abdominal Wall.

The posterior lumbocostal ligament and its relations to the inferior pleural reflection are emphasized.

The *psoas major muscle* occupies the gutter between the bodies and transverse processes of the lumbar vertebrae. It arises from the twelfth thoracic vertebra and all the lumbar vertebrae, and passes downward and laterally along the margin of the pelvic brim. As it passes beneath the inguinal ligament, it enters the thigh and inserts into the lesser trochanter of the femur. It forms a buffer between the kidney and the vertebral column. Because of its depth and medial position, the psoas does not come directly into consideration in renal operations. This muscle is enclosed in a stout membranous sheath. Pus tracking downward from tuberculous spondylitis of the thoracic vertebrae enters this muscular compartment and is directed into the thigh.

The part of the *transversus abdominis muscle* which figures in this region arises from the fusion aponeurosis of the three leaves of the lumbodorsal fascia. This broad aponeurosis, in the lateral part of the region, assumes fleshy characteristics as it extends over the anterolateral abdominal wall toward the linea alba. The upper part of the transversus aponeurosis is strengthened considerably by the posterior lumbocostal ligament. The peritoneum is applied against the transversus abdominis muscle, from which it is separated by the transversalis fascia and the extraperitoneal fat.

5. **Vessels and Nerves.**—The vessels of this area are the lowest or twelfth intercostal arteries and veins and the lumbar arteries and veins. The main trunks lie at a higher level than the terminal trunks which supply the region. The superior lumbar triangle is a relatively avascular space, the *twelfth intercostal artery* lying well in the upper part of the region. This artery has a larger area of distribution than have the other intercostals, or the lumbar vessels. The ventral branch runs anterior to the quadratus lumborum muscle, while the dorsal branch runs behind it and the sacrospinalis muscle and supplies both of them. The main ventral branch passes laterally and downward to the broad abdominal muscles. It frequently is cut in superior lumbar trigone incisions.

The superior lumbar trigone lies between the twelfth intercostal and first lumbar nerves. The *twelfth intercostal nerve* runs along the upper margin of the trigone, and the *first lumbar nerve* along its medial and lower border. The ventral division of the first lumbar nerve has a larger iliohypogastric and a smaller ilio-inguinal branch. These emerge between the psoas major and quadratus lumborum muscles and pass downward and laterally at a variable distance from the iliac crest. The higher-placed of the two, the *iliohypogastric nerve*, pierces the transversus abdominis aponeurosis and runs forward for a short distance between it and the internal oblique muscle (p. 281). The lower or *ilio-inguinal nerve* continues along the inner surface of the transversus aponeurosis until it perforates the transversus abdominis muscle near the anterior part of the iliac crest. It then pierces the internal oblique muscle and enters the inguinal canal (p. 292).

SURGICAL CONSIDERATIONS

1. **Lumbar Approach to the Kidney.**—No single incision admits of kidney exposure appropriate to, or adequate for, all surgical procedures on that organ. The incision must be sufficiently large to admit free manipulation of the kidney with the hands, but must sacrifice a minimum of nerves, muscles, and vessels. The severing of nerves is followed by long-standing disagreeable paresthesias. Individual variations in the distance between the twelfth rib and the iliac crest are many, and the deep and occasionally high location of the kidney often is a cause of despair to the surgeon. Although exposing the kidney as much as possible, the incision must not injure the pleura (p. 243).

The minor or major nature of the operation determines to some extent the length and direction of the incision, the exposure for simple fixation of the kidney varying greatly from that which permits careful handling of a large infected kidney. Resection of the twelfth and even the eleventh rib may be required. In all lumbar kidney procedures, the patient is placed with the sound side upon a lumbar support which rounds out the involved region prominently, increasing the costo-iliac space to the maximum.

In simple operations upon the kidney, such as nephropexy or the draining of a perinephric abscess, the *intermuscular approach* suffices. An incision through the superior lumbar triangle, beginning just above the twelfth rib, is carried antero-inferiorly in a direction about midway between the lumbar transverse processes and the anterior superior spine and a little lateral to the bulge of the sacrospinalis muscle. After division of the skin and fascia, the fibers of the latissimus dorsi muscle present in the wound. Below and lateral is the free edge of the external oblique muscle. The lumbar trigone is exposed by drawing the lateral border of the latissimus dorsi mesially and the mesial margin of the external oblique laterally. The upper part of the trigone is denser in consistency because of the reinforcement given it by the anterior and posterior lumbocostal ligaments. The lumbar aponeurosis of the transversus abdominis muscle, which floors the trigone, is incised at a point about 2 cm. below the last rib, which is about midway between the last thoracic and first lumbar nerves.

The wound is enlarged by blunt dissection to admit the hand. The rounded lateral border of the quadratus lumborum muscle is seen and felt, and, in the lower portion of the wound, the iliohypogastric and ilio-inguinal branches of the first lumbar nerve may be seen. The subcostal or twelfth thoracic nerve skirts the upper margin of the wound.

An extensive layer of retrorenal fat may or may not be found between the lumbar aponeurosis and the retrorenal leaf of the perinephric fascia. The retrorenal leaf is incised

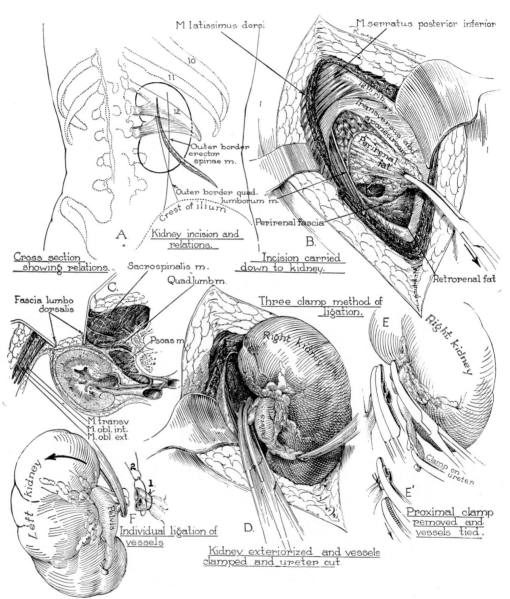

FIG. 308.—LUMBAR NEPHRECTOMY.

and access is gained to the perirenal fat, which surrounds the kidney as a fatty capsule and continues around the pelvis, great vessels, and ureter. The perirenal fat is stripped away from the surface of the kidney until the freeing of both poles admits the delivery of the kidney into the wound; the kidney is attached only by its vessels and the ureter. If exposure is difficult, the incision is extended.

The opening in the lumbar aponeurosis may be enlarged by cutting downward and forward through the oblique muscles of the abdomen. For additional exposure, the

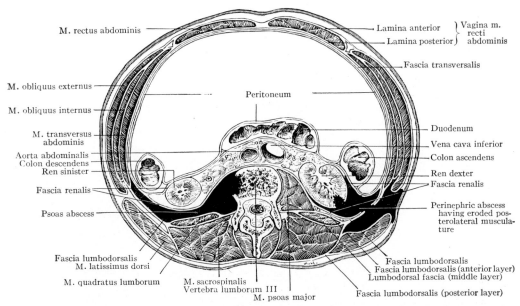

M. rectus abdominis

Lamina anterior } Vagina m.
Lamina posterior } recti
abdominis

Fascia transversalis

M. obliquus externus

Peritoneum

M. obliquus internus

M. transversus abdominis

Duodenum

Vena cava inferior

Aorta abdominalis
Colon descendens
Ren sinister

Colon ascendens

Ren dexter
Fascia renalis

Fascia renalis

Psoas abscess

Perinephric abscess having eroded posterolateral musculature

Fascia lumbodorsalis
M. latissimus dorsi

M. quadratus lumborum

M. sacrospinalis
Vertebra lumborum III
M. psoas major

Fascia lumbodorsalis
Fascia lumbodorsalis (anterior layer)
Lumbodorsal fascia (middle layer)

Fascia lumbodorsalis (posterior layer)

FIG. 309.—CROSS SECTION TO SHOW EXTENSION OF PERINEPHRIC AND PSOAS ABSCESSES.

incision is carried forward through the transversus abdominis parallel to the iliac crest. To supplement mesial exposure, the latissimus dorsi may be cut in the line of the incision and the lateral fibers of the quadratus may be incised.

II. ABDOMINAL CAVITY AND CONTENTS

A. INTRAPERITONEAL VISCERA

The intraperitoneal viscera include the subdivisions of the gastro-intestinal tube and the glands associated with them, the liver, spleen, and pancreas.

In the primitive stages, the tube and adnexed glands are enveloped by peritoneum. Therefore, although rotation and posterior peritoneal fixation carry certain of the intestinal segments and the glands from their primitive intraperitoneal sagittal position to positions which are secondarily retroperitoneal, all of the elements of the tube must be considered developmentally as intraperitoneal structures.

Topographically, these structures may be classified with reference to the transverse colon and mesocolon, which form a definite transverse barrier across the abdomen. Above this barrier are the supramesocolic viscera, the stomach, spleen, liver, and bile passages, with portions of the duodenum and pancreas. Below the barrier are the inframesocolic viscera, which include a part of the duodenum, the subdivisions of the large bowel, and the jejunum and ileum.

(I) SUPRAMESOCOLIC VISCERA

(A) STOMACH

The stomach is a local expansion of the alimentary tube interposed between the termination of the esophagus and the beginning of the small intestine. It is shaped like a cornucopia which, when filled with barium and viewed under the fluoroscope, appears as a reversed cone with its lower extremity curved mesially to the right. Its shape is modified by various factors, among which are: functional activity, volume of contents, disease, and changes in the surrounding viscera. The stomach varies greatly in size, being enlarged enormously in postoperative atony or in pyloric obstruction, and so shrunken in esophageal cancer that it may be no larger than the transverse colon. In this event, the arterial networks on its curvatures lie in close apposition.

1. **Gastric Orifices.**—The *cardiac orifice* (*cardia*) is the point of junction of the esophagus and stomach and marks the level at which the curvatures begin. The *pylorus* is more mobile than the cardia, and is more likely to vary in position. The junction of the stomach with the duodenum is marked externally by a circular narrowing, the duodenopyloric constriction, and internally by the pyloric valve. The pylorus occupies a plane anteroinferior to the cardia.

2. **Subdivisions of the Stomach and Their Relations.**—The *fundus* is that expanded upper extremity of the stomach lying to the left of the cardia and surmounting the body

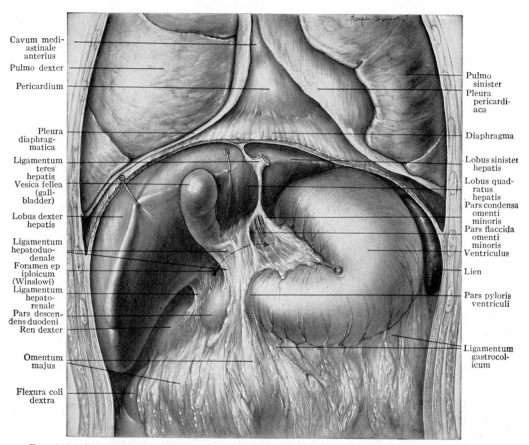

Fig. 310.—Supramesocolic Viscera and Their Relations with the Thoracic Contents.

like a dome. In the supine position, it bulges markedly upward into the left cupola of the diaphragm until its superior limit extends behind the apex of the heart and the pericardium at the level of the fifth rib posteriorly. Distention of the fundus may produce cardiac discomfort mechanically by direct pressure. In the erect position, the volume of the fundus is diminished, and its outline tends to become absorbed into the greater curvature. The *body* of the stomach lies between the fundus and the pylorus, and its general direction is oblique.

The *pyloric portion* of the stomach is the attenuated right extremity, limited externally by the *duodenopyloric constriction*, and internally by the pyloric orifice. This portion, when distended, has a sacculated outline, divided into lesser sacculi by an intermediate sulcus. The larger sacculus, lying to the left, is the *pyloric vestibule*, and the much narrowed part to the right is the *pyloric antrum*. The tube-shaped *pyloric canal* is about 2.5 cm. long and communicates with the duodenum through the pylorus.

Part of the anterior surface of the stomach comes forward into the epigastrium and lies behind the anterior abdominal wall. The lower boundary of the stomach, when the

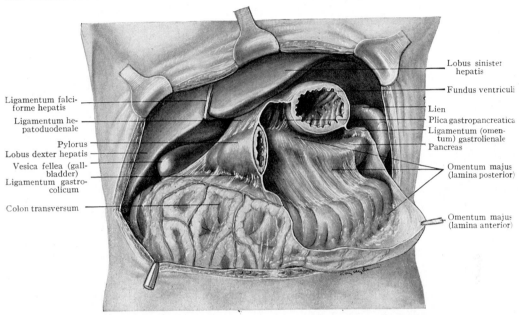

Fig. 311.—Section of the Stomach Removed to Show the Gastric Orifices and the Relations of the Viscus to the Lesser Peritoneal Cavity.

viscus is distended moderately, corresponds to a horizontal surface line connecting the tenth costal cartilages. By resection of a portion of the left costal margin, it is possible to gain wider access to the stomach without risk of opening the pleural cavity.

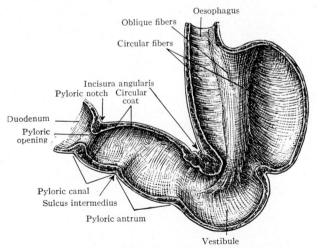

Fig. 312.—Muscular Coats and Divisions of the Stomach. The anterior half of the stomach has been removed. (After Cunningham.)

Posteriorly to the left, the stomach rests upon the spleen, which is hollowed to receive it. In the narrow interval between the spleen and pancreas, only the peritoneum of the lesser sac lies between the stomach and the anterior surface of the left kidney. The anterior surface of the body and tail of the pancreas is molded to the stomach. Because of these relations, adhesions of the posterior wall of the stomach to the peritoneum of the lesser sac over the pancreas, celiac axis, and aorta commonly occur following penetrating and perforated gastric ulcer, and are very troublesome in operative procedures on the stomach.

3. **Curvatures and Their Relations.**—The convex *greater curvature*, on the left side of the stomach, begins at the cardia in the depth of the sharp angle between the esophagus and the fundus. It is directed posterosuperiorly over the fundus and then anteriorly from left to right with an inferior inclination. It assumes an upward bend as it approaches the pylorus. Below the level of the fundus, the curvature is related to the arterial arch formed from the right and left gastro-epiploic arteries lying within the layers of the gastrocolic ligament

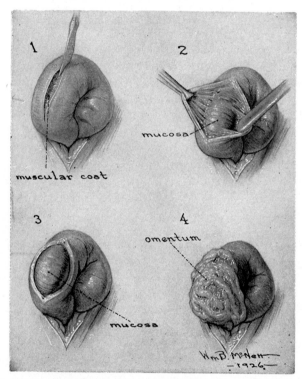

Fig. 313.—Rammstedt's Pyloroplasty for Congenital Pyloric Stenosis.

1, Incision through the serosa; 2, spreading of muscle fibers until the mucosa is reached; 3, mucosa allowed to bulge through the incision; 4, omentum applied to defect in the muscle. (Babcock, "Textbook of Surgery.")

The concave *lesser curvature* defines the right margin of the stomach and possesses vertical and horizontal segments which join at the angular incisura. It is continuous without any line of demarcation into the right margin of the esophagus. The curvature affords attachment for the gastrohepatic or lesser omentum, and is related to the arterial circle contained therein, which consists of the right and left gastric (coronary) arteries.

4. **Position of the Stomach.**—By far the greater part of the stomach lies in the left hypochondrium, and the remainder in the epigastrium where it is supported, to a considerable degree, by the sloping transverse mesocolon upon which it rests. The organ is maintained in position mainly by its continuity with the abdominal esophagus which is fixed solidly to the esophageal hiatus in the diaphragm. Below, it is held firmly in position by continuity with the duodenum, which is anchored securely over most of its extent to the posterior parietal peritoneum. The arteries from the celiac trunk and the various

peritoneal ligaments and omenta contribute to the stability of its position. The small intestine pressing upward prevents any marked degree of inferior displacement

The position of the stomach is subject to wide variation. In erect posture, the postero-inferior surface of the stomach slides downward and forward on the sloping ledge of the transverse mesocolon which supports it. Further change in position is rendered possible by the slight descent of the diaphragm and the elasticity and loose attachment of the peritoneum. At the same time, the pylorus undergoes a considerable change in position, permitted by the two factors enumerated and by the normal mobility of the first portion of the duodenum. Because of the uniformity with which this downward displacement is observed in roentgenograms in erect posture, the presence of an immobile, high-placed pylorus suggests the possibility of its immobilization by adhesions to the gallbladder and neighboring structures.

5. **Structure of the Stomach.**—An investment of peritoneum gives the stomach a complete *serous* coat, save at the reflections of the omenta at the curvatures, and a small area at the left of the cardia which is in direct contact with the diaphragm. The *musculature* consists of three layers of involuntary muscle, an outer longitudinal, a middle

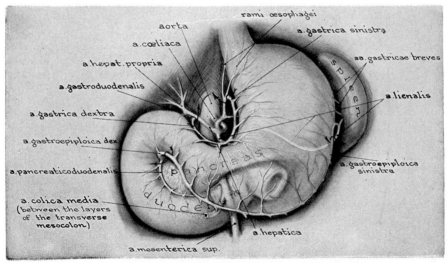

Fig. 314.—Arteries of the Stomach, Indicating Their Points of Ligation in Partial Gastrectomy. (Babcock, "Textbook of Surgery.")

circular, and an inner oblique. At the pylorus, the circular middle layer thickens to form the pyloric sphincter. In infants, excessive thickening of the circular layer at the pylorus from continued spasm or actual hypertrophy may give rise to *congenital pyloric stenosis*. Operative relief of this condition contemplates longitudinal division of all the layers of the pylorus save the mucosa, which is allowed to bulge into the wound (Rammstedt). This division sufficiently reestablishes the pyloric lumen to relieve the obstructive symptoms.

The *mucosa* is thick, highly vascular, and has such ready play over its submucosal base that in incisions into the stomach, as into the esophagus, it may be pushed easily ahead of the knife. In small puncture wounds, the mucosa may plug the opening so effectively that there is no escape of gastric contents. The toughness of the loose *submucosa* explains its ability to hold gastric sutures.

6. **Arteries and Veins of the Stomach.**—The stomach receives a rich arterial supply from the celiac (axis) artery which arises from the aorta just above the neck of the pancreas and at once trifurcates into the left gastric (coronary), splenic, and hepatic arteries. These trunks and their branches form two arterial arches related respectively to the greater

21

and lesser curvatures.   The arch of the lesser curvature consists of the right gastric branch of the hepatic artery running from right to left, and the left gastric (coronary) artery running from left to right.   The arch of the greater curvature is contained within the layers of the great omentum, and is made up of the gastro-epiploic artery from the gastro-duodenal and the left gastro-epiploic artery from the splenic artery.   The relations of these arches to the stomach vary.   When the stomach is empty, each arch is very tortuous and is from 1 to 2 cm. distant from the corresponding curvature.   With distention of the stomach, both arches come into close contact with the wall, but are not stretched to any marked degree.

The **hepatic artery** runs to the right along the upper border of the pancreas, turns forward just below the epiploic foramen, and reaches the first part of the duodenum. Together with the common bile duct and portal vein, it turns upward and ascends to the liver (p. 341) in front of the epiploic foramen between the two layers of the lesser omentum. In passing around the epiploic foramen, it gives off the *right gastric (pyloric) artery* and, at the upper border of the first part of the duodenum, it gives off the *gastroduodenal artery*, which descends behind the duodenum to its lower margin where it divides into the *superior pancreaticoduodenal* and *right gastro-epiploic arteries.*

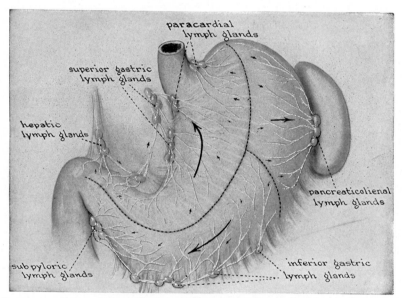

FIG. 315.—LYMPHATIC DRAINAGE OF THE STOMACH IN RELATION TO PARTIAL GASTRECTOMY FOR CAR-
CINOMA.   (Babcock, "Textbook of Surgery.")

The **left gastric (coronary) artery** runs upward to the left to the beginning of the lesser curvature at the cardia, and divides into two parallel branches which anastomose with the right gastric (pyloric) artery.

The **splenic artery** runs to the left under the peritoneal floor of the lesser peritoneal sac (omental bursa) along the upper margin of the body and tail of the pancreas, until it reaches the hilus of the spleen.   The *short gastric* and *left gastro-epiploic arteries* arise from the splenic artery near its termination and run forward in the gastrosplenic omentum to the greater curvature of the stomach.   The short gastric arteries are distributed to the fundus, and the left gastro-epiploic artery anastomoses with the right gastro-epiploic artery.

In brief, the celiac artery supplies the stomach directly by the left gastric (coronary) artery) and indirectly by the right gastric and right gastro-epiploic arteries from the hepatic artery and the short gastric and left gastro-epiploic arteries from the splenic artery.   The branches given off by these vessels supply adjoining areas of both surfaces of the stomach and run at right angles to its long axis.

The **gastric veins** correspond to the arteries and empty into the large splenic and superior mesenteric trunks of the portal vein or into the portal vein itself. The *left gastric (coronary) vein*, tributary to the portal system, anastomoses freely with the lower esophageal veins. The lower esophageal veins anastomose with the upper esophageal veins which are tributary through the azygos veins with the caval venous system. This forms a very important anastomosis between the portal and systemic venous systems. The veins at the inferior end of the esophagus become varicose in portal obstruction (p. 342), and their rupture, with resulting hematemesis, may be the first sign of the condition.

7. **Lymphatics of the Stomach.**—The abundant lymph vessels of the stomach originate in the mucosa and ramify in plexuses in the submucosa and muscularis. As the networks are invaded rapidly in gastric carcinoma, the connections and paths of extension are of prime importance. The lymph vessels drain to regional lymph nodes along the gastric curvatures.

SURGICAL CONSIDERATIONS

1. **Roentgenologic Examination of the Stomach.**—In the erect position, the normal stomach appears horn-shaped or J-shaped in roentgenograms taken after an opaque meal (barium). The longer limb of the J is vertical, and is to the left of the median line. The barium is well supported in the vertical segment by the muscle of the healthy stomach wall, and fills the shorter limb which corresponds to the pyloric portion. The usual roentgenogram of a normal stomach shows a small, caplike shadow immediately above the

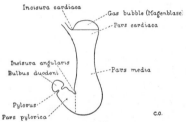

FIG. 316.—FISHHOOK STOMACH.

This is the usual vertical type, indicating the parts shown in the roentgenogram. (Carman.)

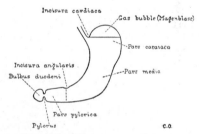

FIG. 317.—STEER-HORN STOMACH.

A transversely placed stomach, seen occasionally by roentgenogram. (Carman.)

barium in the pyloric antrum, separated from it by a clear area. The cap is the barium contained in the first part of the duodenum, and the clear area corresponds to the pyloric canal which is closed by the contraction of the pyloric sphincter.

2. **Examination of the Stomach at Operation.**—When the abdomen is opened above the umbilicus, the greater omentum is exposed with the transverse colon visible through it. The omentum is traced readily to the greater curvature of the stomach; the stomach can be brought down to permit a view of the pylorus and the first part of the duodenum. The muscular thickening of the pyloroduodenal junction renders its recognition easy. The walls of the normal stomach are firm, while those of a dilated atonic stomach are thinner and flaccid and the pylorus is somewhat difficult to identify. The pyloric vein, which runs across the anterior surface of the bowel, is a guide to the pyloroduodenal junction. The cardiac end and the fundus of the stomach are difficult to examine because of their fixation and their shielded position in the left hypochondrium.

In searching for a perforated ulcer, all of the anterosuperior surface of the stomach and the accessible surface of the first part of the duodenum must be examined carefully first. If there are no gastric contents in the supramesocolic compartment when the abdomen is opened, the postero-inferior surface of the stomach must be exposed and explored. The epiploic foramen (of Winslow) is examined first, and if it is closed by adhesions, a perforated ulcer leaking into the omental bursa should be suspected. To gain access to the postero-inferior surface of the stomach, the omental bursa must be opened.

This is done easily by incising carefully through the gastrocolic ligament at some distance to the left of the pylorus and immediately below the gastro-epiploic vessels. The greater curvature then is turned superiorly, affording exposure of much of the postero-inferior

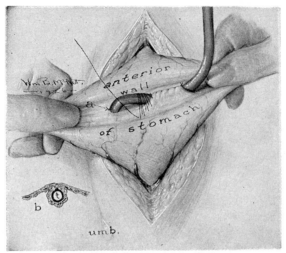

FIG. 318.—WITZEL GASTROSTOMY.

In this method, a soft rubber tube is placed into the stomach and held there by a suture; about 5 cm. of the tube then is buried by sutures in a groove formed on the outer wall of the stomach; the tube is brought out through the anterior abdominal wall. (Babcock, "Textbook of Surgery.")

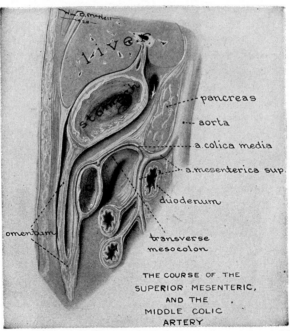

FIG. 319.—SHOWING THE PROXIMITY OF THE MIDDLE COLIC ARTERY TO THE VESSELS OF THE GREAT OMENTUM.

Accidental ligation of this artery in partial gastrectomy may be followed by gangrene of the transverse colon. (Babcock, "Textbook of Surgery.")

surface of the stomach. Part of the cardia can be examined through a rent in the thinnest part of the lesser omentum by everting the stomach through the aperture.

3. **Gastrostomy.**—Gastrostomy is the establishment of an artificial stoma in the

stomach wall for administering nourishment, and is resorted to in fibrous or malignant stricture of the esophagus. In such conditions, the stomach is contracted (p. 317). It is likely to recede deep into the gastric compartment, and, not infrequently, the transverse colon is found to have risen so as to intervene between the stomach and the anterior abdominal wall. The main feature of all the technics described for this operation is the provision of a valvular opening, leading from the skin surface into the stomach cavity, which will prevent the escape of gastric contents and admit food. The stomach is sutured to the anterior abdominal wall after the fixation of the gastrostomy tube into the stomach wall. The operation may be performed through an oblique subcostal or upper left rectus incision.

4. **Pyloroplasty.**—Pyloroplasty is an operation designed to enlarge the lumen at the pylorus or the pyloroduodenal junction in simple hypertrophic stenosis or in cicatricial stricture from ulcer. In the latter condition, the stomach is opened close to the pylorus

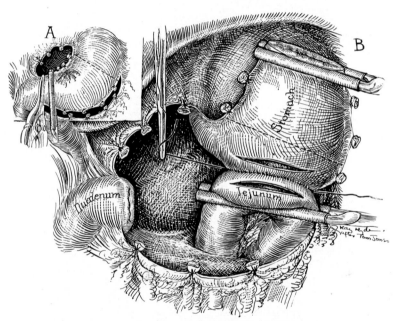

Fig. 320.—Second Billroth Partial Gastrectomy.

In A, the duodenum is clamped prior to section after ligation of the arteries of the stomach in the lesser and greater omenta; in B, the duodenum is closed and a transmesocolic gastrojejunostomy is performed before the partial gastrectomy is completed.

by an incision directed in the long axis of the pyloric canal. The stenosed pyloric orifice is examined and the section continued through it into the duodenum. The edges of the incision are separated as widely as possible, so that the midpoints in the edges of the wound become the ends of the opening. The wound thus assumes a direction at right angles to the original section in the long axis of the tube. Suturing the wound edges in this position materially widens the lumen of the canal.

5. **Pylorectomy or Partial Gastrectomy.**—In partial gastrectomy, the condition of the part to be removed and its immediate surroundings should be noted very carefully. Adhesions causing fixity of the stomach are a contraindication to resection. An incision in the gastrocolic ligament sufficiently large to permit examination of the posterior wall of the stomach enables one to judge of the presence or absence of adhesions in that locality. After the feasibility of the operation has been determined, the gastrohepatic and gastrocolic ligaments and their enclosed vessels are ligated as close to the stomach as possible. The vessels divided are: the gastroduodenal, right gastric (pyloric), right gastro-epiploic,

left gastric, and left gastro-epiploic arteries.   The diseased part is removed with a margin
of healthy duodenal and gastric tissue.

   Kocher's pylorectomy consists of a partial gastrectomy and a side-to-end gastroduodenostomy.   The involved area of stomach is removed and the gastric wound closed com-

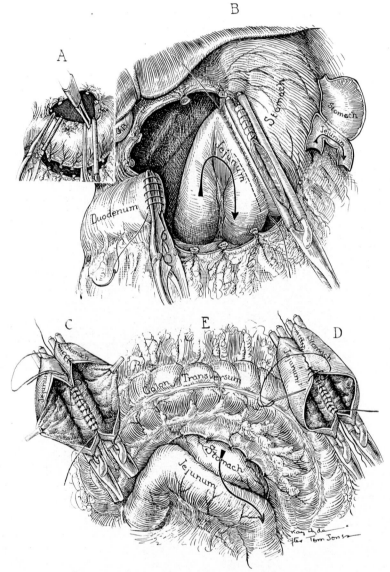

Fig. 321.—Mayo-Polya Partial Gastrectomy.

   In A, the segment of stomach to be removed is isolated preparatory to section by the cautery; in B,
the duodenum is closed and anastomosis is made between the jejunum and part of the distal end of the
stomach; in C and D, the sutures of the gastrojejunal anastomosis are placed; E shows the stomach brought
down through the rent in the transverse mesocolon and sutured; the anastomosis is well out of the peritoneal
sac and the stomach contents gravitate down the distal limb of the jejunal loop.

pletely, after which the open end of the duodenum is implanted in the posterior wall of the
stomach a little behind the line of gastric suture.

   In the *first Billroth operation*, after partial gastric resection, the open end of the
stomach is closed partially by a suture running from the lesser curvature to the greater

until the stomach opening at the greater curvature corresponds in size to the cut end of the duodenum. The gastric and duodenal openings are united by end-to-end anastomosis. The procedure is essentially an end-to-end gastroduodenostomy.

The *second Billroth operation* is a partial gastric resection, in which the open ends of both the duodenum and stomach are closed by suture. Alimentary continuity is obtained by performing a posterior gastrojejunostomy.

Intestinal continuity in the *Mayo-Polya pylorectomy* is gained by closure of the duodenum and anastomosis of a loop of jejunum to the partially sutured or entirely open end of the stomach. A loop of jejunum selected about 18 inches from the duodenojejunal angle is drawn through a rent either in the avascular part of the transverse mesocolon or anterior to the transverse colon. The operation is a partial gastrectomy with closure of the duodenum and a gastrojejunostomy by the end-to-loop method.

6. **Gastrojejunostomy.**—The object of gastrojejunostomy is to establish a permanent communication between the stomach and the upper part of the small intestine without

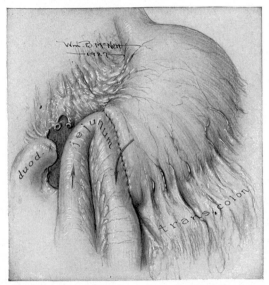

FIG. 322.—ANTECOLIC PARTIAL GASTRECTOMY BY THE POLYA METHOD

This is an antecolic anastomosis between the end of the stomach and the side of the jejunum; this avoids the tension and difficulties of the retrocolic union, especially when the residual part of the stomach is small, high, and fixed; entero-enterostomy should be added to avoid reflux distention of the proximal loop. (Babcock, "Textbook of Surgery.")

removing a segment of the stomach. Generally, it is required in cases where the stomach fails to empty itself efficiently because of pyloric obstruction. In the presence of gastric or duodenal ulceration, the operation is performed to provide a new outlet for the stomach, thus giving the ulcer the necessary rest from irritation.

A coil of jejunum may be anastomosed to the stomach by one or another of the following methods. In the *anterior* or *precolic gastrojejunal anastomosis*, the greater omentum and the transverse colon are turned upward and search is made to the left of the spine for the duodenojejunal flexure in the angle between the root of the mesentery and the transverse mesocolon. A loop is selected from 30 to 40 inches from the duodenojejunal flexure and is brought up over the greater omentum in front of the colon. It is anastomosed to the anterior surface of the stomach close to the greater curvature. This operation is performed only when a posterior gastrojejunostomy is contraindicated by inability to mobilize the posterior wall of the stomach, because of adhesions within the lesser sac or excessive shortness of the transverse mesocolon.

The method of choice is the *posterior* or *retrocolic no-loop gastrojejunostomy*. When the abdomen is opened, the duodenojejunal flexure and the first few inches of the jejunum are identified. An avascular area in the transverse mesocolon is selected and an opening made in it through which the stomach wall is exposed and with which a communication is

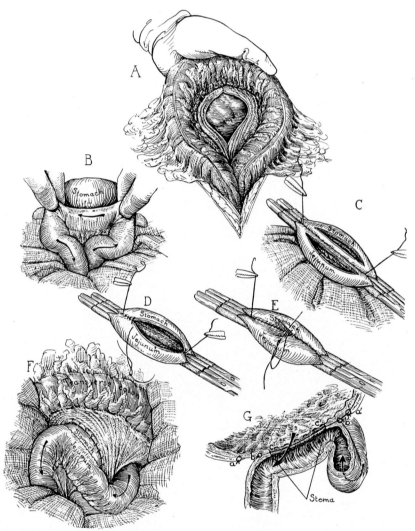

FIG. 323.—POSTERIOR GASTROJEJUNOSTOMY.

A, An opening is made in the avascular area of the transverse mesocolon, exposing the posterior surface of the stomach; B, an isoperistaltic alignment is made between the jejunum and stomach, a short loop of jejunum being used; C, the posterior layer of the continuous serous suture has been placed; incisions have been made into the stomach and duodenum; D, the posterior and part of the anterior through-and-through sutures have been placed; E, the continuous serous suture is being completed in front; F, the edges of the opening in the transverse mesocolon are united to the posterior wall of the stomach with fine sutures about the anastomosis; G, frontal section shows the dependent large stoma, absence of angulation, lines of continuous serous sutures, *bb'*; *cc'*, through-and-through suture around the stoma and closure of the lesser peritoneal cavity, *aa'*.

established between the stomach and jejunum. The gastric site for anastomosis is at the most available dependent part of the greater curvature. The margins of the rent in the transverse mesocolon are stitched to the posterior wall of the stomach. This procedure hinders retraction of the anastomosis through the opening and prevents herniation of the small bowel into the lesser sac.

The posterior or transmesocolic operation has distinct advantages over the anterior precolic procedure. In the anterior operation, the transverse colon incurs considerable risk of being compressed, especially if the length of jejunum intervening between the

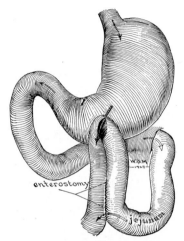

FIG. 324.—ANTERIOR GASTROJEJUNOSTOMY.

This operation is used when a posterior gastro-enterostomy is not feasible; a long loop of jejunum is required to pass without tension under the omentum and in front of the transverse colon. An antero-entero-anastomosis also is performed to prevent regurgitation. (Babcock, "Textbook of Surgery.")

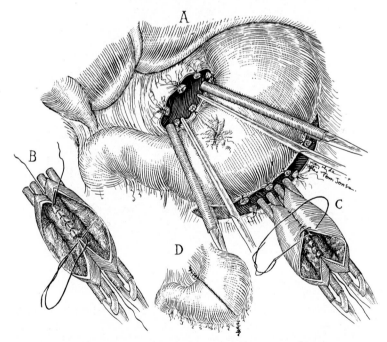

FIG. 325.—SLEEVE RESECTION OF PART OF THE STOMACH.

In A, the segment of the stomach to be resected is isolated; B and C show the steps in the end-to-end anastomosis; D shows the shortened stomach after the operation is completed.

duodenojejunal flexure and the site of the anastomosis is inadequate. In the posterior operation, the stomach is reached by the shortest route, the stoma is in a fully dependent position which facilitates the outflow of gastric contents, and the danger of intestinal obstruction is lessened by not drawing the jejunal loop over the transverse colon.

(B) DUODENUM

1. Definition and Boundaries.—The duodenum begins opposite the right side of the spine at the level of the first lumbar vertebra.   It extends from the pylorus to the duodeno-jejunal flexure, a total length of about 25 cm., and forms a C-shaped bend, the area of which is occupied roughly by the head of the pancreas.   This segment is differentiated clearly from the rest of the bowel by its deep position, marked fixation, and connection with the secretory ducts of the liver and pancreas.   Its lumen is larger than that of the jejunum.

2. Divisions and Relations.—With the body in the recumbent position, the *superior* or *first part* of the duodenum (duodenal cap) passes backward and slightly upward from the pylorus to the neck of the gallbladder.   With the body in the erect position this part of the duodenum passes vertically upward, and the level of the first flexure of the duodenum drops to the level of the second lumbar vertebra.   The proximal 2.5 cm. is freely movable, and is invested by a continuation of the same two layers of peritoneum as enclose the

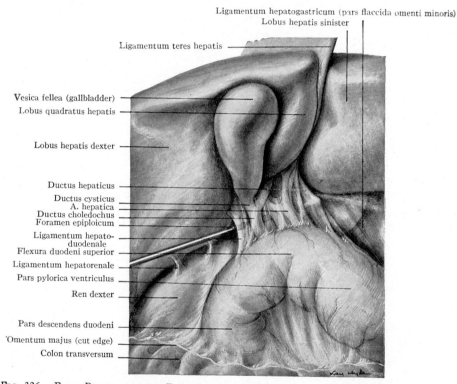

Ligamentum hepatogastricum (pars flaccida omenti minoris)
Lobus hepatis sinister

Ligamentum teres hepatis

Vesica fellea (gallbladder)
Lobus quadratus hepatis

Lobus hepatis dexter

Ductus hepaticus
Ductus cysticus
A. hepatica
Ductus choledochus
Foramen epiploicum
Ligamentum hepato-
    duodenale
Flexura duodeni superior
Ligamentum hepatorenale
Pars pylorica ventriculi
Ren dexter

Pars descendens duodeni
Omentum majus (cut edge)
Colon transversum

FIG. 326.—FIRST PORTION OF THE DUODENUM AND ITS RELATIONS TO THE EXTRAHEPATIC BILE PASSAGES
A probe is placed in the epiploic foramen.

stomach.   The intimate relations with the gallbladder explain the adhesions between these structures and the frequency of spontaneous passage of gallstones into the duodenum (p. 349).   The distal 2.5 cm. or more is covered only in front by peritoneum, so that the range of movement permitted depends upon the elasticity of the peritoneal coat.   The posteromesial surface is in immediate relation with the common bile duct, portal vein, and gastroduodenal artery.   The inferior vena cava is separated from the segment only by a layer of areolar fusion fascia.

All of this portion of the duodenum lies in the supramesocolic subdivision of the peritoneal cavity.   The most common site of duodenal ulcer is on the anterolateral surface, and the perforation affects the supracolic area primarily.   A posteromesial perforation close to the pylorus involves the omental bursa.   More distal perforation results in extra-peritoneal infection which may pass upward along the vena cava to the subdiaphragmatic area and cause subdiaphragmatic abscess (p. 344).

The *descending (vertical) second division* forms an acute angle with the first division and descends from the neck of the gallbladder, anterior to the hilum of the kidney and the beginning of the ureter, to the inferior duodenal flexure by which it passes into the third division.   The second division is crossed by the transverse colon, which, at this point, may or may not possess a mesentery.   Above the attachment of the transverse colon, the descending duodenum lies in the supramesocolic compartment; below, it lies in the infra-colic area and is related to the ascending colon.   Posteriorly, it is related to the right

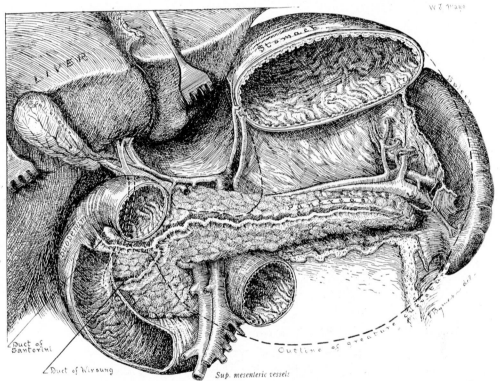

FIG. 327.—NORMAL RELATIONS OF THE PANCREAS TO THE STOMACH, DUODENUM, LIVER, AND EXTRA-HEPATIC BILE PASSAGES.   (William J. Mayo, Surg., Gynec. and Obst.)

kidney, renal vessels, and inferior vena cava.   Its left border is related to the head of the pancreas and to the common bile duct for a short distance before its termination.   The common opening of the bile and pancreatic ducts is upon the summit of a papilla about half-way down the posteromesial aspect of the division.   In the anterior groove between the head of the pancreas and the descending duodenum runs the superior pancreaticoduodenal branch of the gastroduodenal artery.

This division of the duodenum is fixed definitely in position by its peritoneal relations. By dividing the peritoneum at the right lateral edge of the upper portion of the segment (Kocher's maneuver), the descending duodenum can be mobilized so as to render surgically accessible the retroduodenal part of the common duct (Figs. 348, 349).   The bowel then may be turned forward, downward, and to the left.

The *third* or *transverse division* of the duodenum runs horizontally to the left in front of the ureter, inferior vena cava, lumbar column, and aorta, and ends at the left of the third lumbar vertebra.   It lies behind the peritoneum in the right inframesocolic compart-ment, and near its termination is crossed by the root of the mesentery of the jejuno-ileum.

The superior mesenteric artery runs downward over the anterior surface of the transverse division to enter the root of the mesentery. Tight stretching of the artery over the segment may be responsible for certain duodenal obstructions. Duodenojejunal anastomosis furnishes free alimentary continuity. The pancreas is applied closely to the upper border of the segment, and is separated from it by a groove in which lies the inferior pancreatico-duodenal artery. Most of the anterior surface of the segment is overlain by small intestine.

The *fourth* or *ascending part* of the duodenum runs upward and slightly to the left along the left side of the spine to the duodenojejunal flexure at the root of the transverse mesocolon. At the left of the second lumbar vertebra, the terminal part of the duodenum bends sharply downward, forward, and to the left to form the *duodenojejunal flexure* which is a readily recognized landmark to guide the search for obstruction in the small bowel, and to locate a loop of upper jejunum for gastrojejunostomy (p. 327). It is found by passing the hand backward to the posterior abdominal wall behind the greater omentum and palpating upward along the left of the spine until the flexure is encountered. The

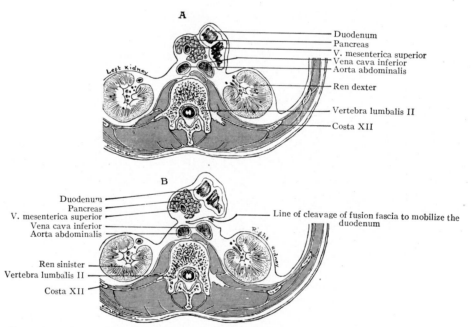

FIG. 328.—CROSS SECTIONS TO SHOW SURGICAL MOBILIZATION OF THE DUODENUM.
A shows the duodenum and head of the pancreas after fusion; B shows the surgical cleaving of the fusion fascia to mobilize duodenum.

bend is in contact with the inferior margin of the pancreas through the root of the transverse mesocolon.

3. **Fixation of the Duodenum.**—A relatively short duodenum in a fixed, secondarily retroperitoneal position occurs first among the primates. In lower vertebrates, the duodenal loop is relatively longer, has a well-developed mesoduodenum, and enjoys great mobility, as there is no secondary posterior fusion fixation. In man, all the duodenum, save the first portion, ultimately is anchored in position by the fusion between its peritoneum and that of the head of the pancreas to the posterior parietal peritoneum. Variations in its fusion to the posterior abdominal wall account for variations in mobility.

The duodenum is held in place to a slight degree by connections with the common bile and pancreatic ducts, as well as by the vessels and nerves running to and from it. The duodenojejunal angle is stabilized by the *suspensory muscle of the duodenum* (*Treitz*), a bundle of involuntary muscle fibers described as running from the left pillar of the diaphragm to the angle. The right colic flexure and the fixed portion of the transverse mesocolon

and mesocolon anchor the duodenum still more securely, and render it doubly retroperitoneal. It acquires additional fixation through the adhesion of the greater omentum to
the transverse colon, mesocolon, and lateral margins of the diaphragm. In its deep position, the duodenum would appear to be well protected from injury, yet it sometimes
is crushed and even torn against the spine in severe abdominal contusions, partly because
of the rigid peritoneal fixation. A rupture of the posterior surface is difficult to recognize
and to repair. The escaping contents may make their way downward beneath the peritoneum toward the right iliac fossa and lead to peritonitis.

The cap or first portion of the duodenum is covered entirely by peritoneum and has
considerable mobility, which is advantageous in that it offers facility for the performance
of plastic operations upon the pylorus and the duodenum. Pyloroplasty and pylorectomy
manipulations are performed with greater ease and safety when the pylorus and adjoining
duodenum can be drawn forward into the abdominal wound. Mobility of the duodenum
simplifies cholecystoduodenostomy (p. 357).

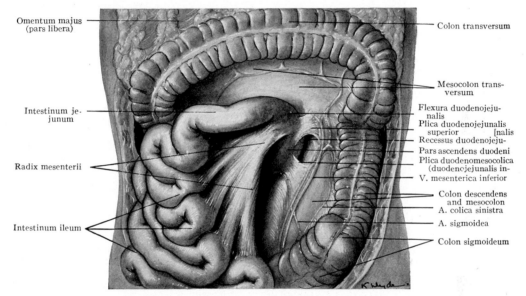

Omentum majus
(pars libera)

Colon transversum

Mesocolon trans-
versum

Flexura duodenojeju-
nalis
Plica duodenojejunalis
superior   [nalis
Recessus duodenojeju-
Pars ascendens duodeni
Plica duodenomesocolica
(duodenojejunalis in-
V. mesenterica inferior

Intestinum je-
junum

Radix mesenterii

Colon descendens
and mesocolon
A. colica sinistra

A. sigmoidea

Colon sigmoideum

Intestinum ileum

FIG. 329.—DUODENOJEJUNAL FOLDS AND FOSSAE.
Attention is called to the relation between the inferior mesenteric vessels and the superior duodenojejuna
fold.

4. Peritoneal Duodenal Fossae.—Several inconstant peritoneal recesses are found
about the duodenojejunal flexure, and sometimes are responsible for strangulated intraperitoneal herniae. The pockets and peritoneal folds which form the fossae are developed
to a greater or less extent depending upon the fixation of the terminal duodenum.

The *superior duodenal fossa* lies behind the superior duodenojejunal fold, the concave
free border of which is directed inferiorly. This fold extends to the left from the flexure
for about 2.5 cm. The upper segment of the inferior mesenteric artery may run in the
free margin of the fold. The mouth of the fossa looks downward, while its cavity passes
upward toward the pancreas. The *inferior duodenal fossa* (of Jonnesco) has its apex or
blind extremity directed downward to the right, its depth being about 2.5 cm. The inferior
duodenojejunal fold, forming the anterior wall, stretches from the left side of the duodenum
to the left of the aorta and spine. The upper or free edge of the fold contains no vessels
of consequence. The *paraduodenal fossa* (of Landzert), when present, is the longest of the
peritoneal culdesac, and lies to the left of the terminal stage of the duodenum. Its existence appears to depend upon the peritoneal fold raised by the ascending branches of the
left colic artery and the inferior mesenteric vein. Its mouth looks mesially, and its free

crescentic margin, which may be 5 cm. long, may unite the superior and inferior duodenal fossae when they are present.

When a herniating loop of small intestine enters one of these fossae, it makes a deep sac at the expense of the posterior parietal peritoneum (intraperitoneal hernia) lying anterior to the left ureter and kidney. When strangulation occurs, care must be taken in dividing the neck of the sac lest the inferior mesenteric vein or left colic artery be injured.

5. **Vessels of the Duodenum.**—The arterial supply of the duodenum is derived from the pancreaticoduodenal arteries. The superior pancreaticoduodenal artery is a branch of the gastroduodenal artery from the hepatic artery, and the inferior pancreaticoduodenal

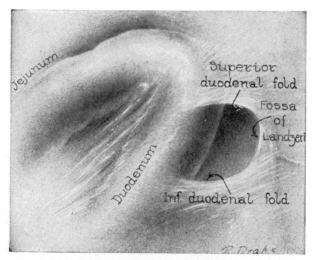

FIG. 330.—DUODENOJEJUNAL FOLDS AND FOSSAE.

Arrows indicate how intraperitoneal herniae are formed at this level. (G. W. Nagel; courtesy, Jour. Amer. Med. Assoc.)

artery is the first branch of the superior mesenteric artery. These arteries run in the groove between the descending and transverse divisions of the duodenum and the head of the pancreas. The anastomotic circle they form is overlain by the transverse colon, transverse mesocolon, and greater omentum, and rarely comes into surgical prominence.

SURGICAL CONSIDERATIONS

1. **Roentgenologic Examination of the Duodenum.**—Roentgenologic examination of the duodenum is made after an opaque meal. The first segment, the cap or bulb, is the most expanded part of the duodenum and is of special diagnostic interest. Viewed from the front, it appears as a smoothly outlined conical chamber with its base at the pyloric ring. The conical peak of the cap suggests a marked narrowing of the duodenum at that point. This apparent change in caliber results from the course of the duodenum backward, laterally, and downward from the cap. The shadow of the barium-filled bulb under normal conditions is more dense than the remainder of the duodenal shadow because of the more anterior position of the bulb, its greater size, and the tendency of the barium to remain in it for a short time. By reason of the rapid transit of the duodenal contents through the second, or descending, portion of the duodenum, that part often is not well visualized. The duodenal cap can be shifted about to some extent by manipulation through the abdominal wall, but the other divisions are fixed and respond but slightly to passive movement.

2. **Duodenal Ulcer.**—Ulcers of the duodenum, in the majority of instances, are located within 5 cm. of the pylorus, and, therefore, are in the mobile part of the bowel. They

occur most frequently on the anterior wall toward the right. Perforation of an ulcer so situated produces a generalized peritonitis. Fluid from a perforated ulcer has a tendency to localize in the right renal pouch, whence it is guided downward and to the right by the obliquity of the mesenteric attachment as well as by the shape of the posterior abdominal wall, often reaching the ileocecal region. The usual location of an ulcer explains perforation into the gallbladder, liver, and colon, since the first attempt to localize infection is the formation of an adhesive barrier uniting the duodenum to these structures. Perforation sometimes causes a subdiaphragmatic abscess. Duodenal, as well as gastric, ulcers tend to extend deeply, and the floor of the ulcer may be formed by the liver, gallbladder, or pancreas, adhesions having been formed previously between the apposed serous surfaces. The proximity of the duodenum to the gallbladder explains the frequency with which adhesions are found in patients having had attacks of cholecystitis, and also explains the

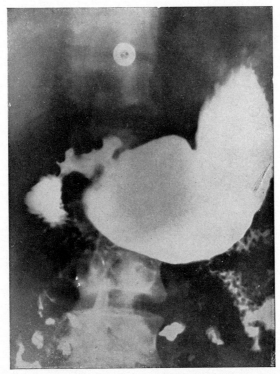

Fig. 331.—Duodenal Ulcer with Marked Deformity of the First Part of the Duodenum.
(Boyd, "Surgical Pathology.")

ulceration of gallstones into the duodenum. Cicatrization of an extensive duodenal ulcer may cause stenosis of the bowel with subsequent dilation of the stomach.

When the perforation is easy of access, as is usual, two technical operative possibilities present: suture of the perforation with or without resection of the ulcer, and suture or resection of the ulcer with some method of gastrojejunal anastomosis. When surgical closure of a perforation markedly constricts the lumen, gastro-enterostomy should be done lest complete obstruction supervene. If the perforation be difficult of access so that no suturing can be done, the only possible procedure is to attempt to wall off the area and afford adequate drainage through the anterior abdominal wall.

3. **Duodenitis.**—The understanding of the pathologic changes of duodenal ulcer has been advanced in recent years by the study of tissues removed at operation. The study demonstrates the occurrence of an inflammatory lesion which might be called duodenitis. Duodenal ulcer is seen in two forms: the indurated, calloused ulcer capable of being seen

and felt from the serosal surface; and the nonindurated ulcer which neither can be seen nor felt, and is recognized with difficulty when the intestine is laid open. The first, recognized by the congestion of the serosal surface, is the true ulcer, having more or less scar formation with duodenal adhesion and deformity. The wall is indurated and tumor formation results from the defense reaction of the surrounding tissues when the ulcer slowly perforates the bowel. The mucosal surface reveals a crater ulcer. The second type of lesion, called by Judd and Nagel "duodenitis" or "submucous ulcer," is characterized by congestion and stippling of the serosa with little or no induration. Its site may be marked only by a slight abrasion of the mucosa. The submucosa and sometimes the muscle layers are infiltrated with lymphocytes. Clinically, there is little to differentiate the two lesions.

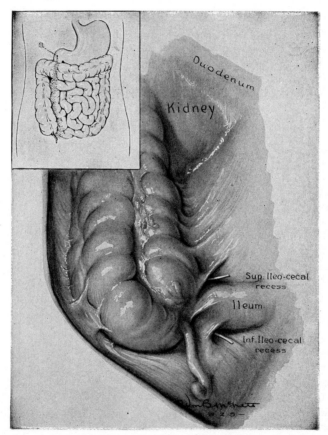

Fig. 332.—Fossae about the Kidney and the Ileocecal Angle Which May Catch Fluid Escaping from a Perforated Duodenal Ulcer.
Inset shows leakage to these fossae from perforated duodenal ulcer, *a*. (Babcock, "Textbook of Surgery.")

The roentgenogram shows spasmodic deformity of the duodenum in both lesions. Duodenitis does not develop of necessity into true ulcer, although in most cases of chronic ulcer more or less duodenitis is present. The therapeutic procedure found most suitable in duodenitis is excision of the diseased area together with the anterior half of the pyloric sphincter, and approximation and transverse stitching of the cut ends of the stomach and duodenum over the remaining posterior half of the sphincter.

4. Herniae about the Duodenojejunal Flexure.—When the peritoneal fixation of the duodenojejunal flexure is less than normal, fossae are present which permit enlargement by peritoneal cleavage. The practical significance of these fossae lies in the fact that they furnish sites for the development of intraperitoneal herniae. The proximal part of the jejunum may press into any one or several of the fossae about the flexure and enlarge the cavity into a hernial sac, allowing the contents to burrow in all directions, but mainly to the right and upward behind the duodenum. More and more of the bowel passes into the enlarging pouch until the greater part of the small intestine may lie within it. Recurrence has been reported, but may be prevented if all the incarcerated intestine can be withdrawn and the entrance to the sac sutured.

5. **Duodenal Diverticula.**—Duodenal diverticula, both congenital and acquired, have been recognized as occasional and inconsequential findings on *x*-ray examination or at autopsy. Most of the *developmental diverticula*, usually multiple, are located within 3 cm. of the duodenal papilla (of Vater) and are united closely with the pancreas, many being buried completely in its substance. Infection apparently plays no rôle in their production. Most of them include only the mucosa and submucosa in their walls.

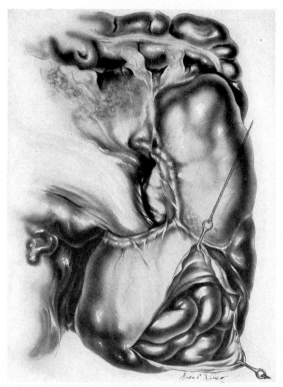

Fig. 333.—Intraperitoneal Hernia into the Duodenojejunal Fossae. (Callander, Rusk, and Nemir Surg., Gynec. and Obst., June, 1935.)

The *acquired diverticula* form a more important group and are located usually in the first part of the duodenum. Some may be associated with the pull of adhesions from gall-bladder disease, but the majority are definitely the result of duodenal ulceration. Any process producing adhesions and scar tissue in the wall of the duodenum may distort the wall so as to predispose to diverticulum formation. All the coats of the bowel are included in this type of diverticulum. As the upper margin of the duodenum just distal to the pylorus is the most frequent site of ulcer, most of the shortening occurs there, leaving the lower border redundant and favorable to diverticulum formation. The diverticula apparently are not involved directly in inflammatory processes, as their peritoneal surface is smooth and free from adhesions in nearly all instances and they cause no symptoms. At operation, noninflammatory pouches can be ignored or be invaginated into the lumen of the bowel.

22

(C) LIVER

1. **Definition and Boundaries.**—The liver, by far the largest glandular organ in the body, is located mainly in the upper abdomen on the right side. It occupies the right hypochondriac and epigastric regions and extends into the left hypochondrium and downward into the right lumbar region. It lies immediately beneath the diaphragm, and is

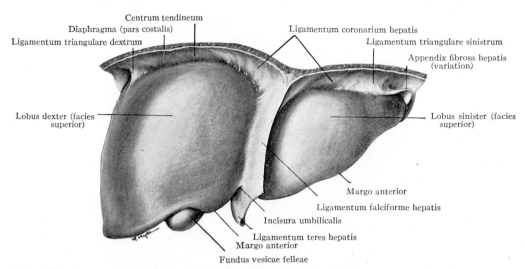

Fig. 334.—ANTEROSUPERIOR SURFACE OF THE LIVER AND ITS CONNECTION WITH THE DIAPHRAGM.

covered by the ribs over the greater part of its lateral surface, there being but a small part of its anterior surface in contact with the anterior abdominal wall.

2. **Surfaces and Relations.**—The *convex* or *anterosuperior surface* of the liver is molded to both halves of the diaphragm. It is almost hidden at the costal margin, save in the

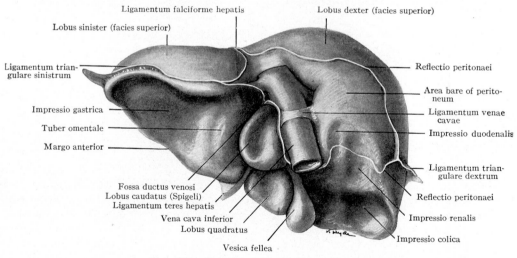

Fig. 335.—POSTERIOR VIEW OF THE LIVER.

This shows how the bare area and the peritoneal reflections suspend the liver from the diaphragm.

subcostal angle where it contacts the anterior abdominal wall and can be examined by palpation and percussion.

The convex surface of the right lobe is in relation with the right lung and pleura. This explains the erosion of hepatic cysts and abscesses through the diaphragm into the pleural cavity and right lung, and the evacuation of their contents into the bronchi. To reach a liver abscess high on the convex surface, the pleura, diaphragm, and peritoneum must be traversed. When tumors and abscesses occur in the anterior part of the convex surface, they usually distend the surface sufficiently to bring it into contact with the abdominal wall over a considerable area, thus making themselves surgically asiblocese without extra-

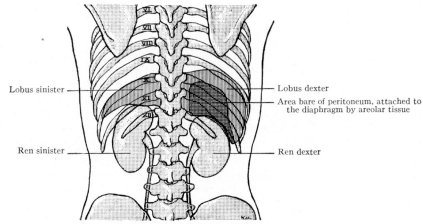

Lobus sinister

Lobus dexter

Area bare of peritoneum, attached to the diaphragm by areolar tissue

Ren sinister

Ren dexter

FIG. 336.—PROJECTION OF THE LIVER ON THE POSTERIOR SURFACE OF THE TRUNK.

pleural resection of the costal margin. Violin-string adhesions between the parietal surface of the liver and the adjacent anterior abdominal wall and the diaphragm not infrequently occur in patients with coincident residual gonococcal tubal disease (Curtis).

The convex surface of the left lobe is small, and has very little relationship to the anterior abdominal wall.

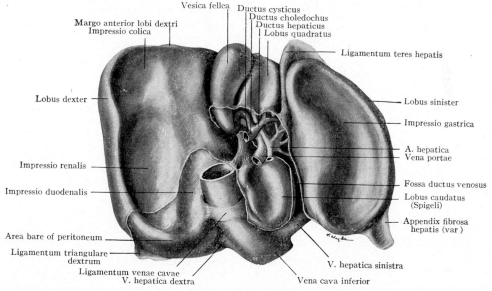

Vesica fellea Ductus cysticus

Margo anterior lobi dextri
Impressio colica

Ductus choledochus
Ductus hepaticus
Lobus quadratus

Ligamentum teres hepatis

Lobus dexter

Lobus sinister

Impressio gastrica

A. hepatica
Vena portae

Impressio renalis

Impressio duodenalis

Fossa ductus venosus

Lobus caudatus
(Spigeli)

Appendix fibrosa
hepatis (var.)

Area bare of peritoneum

Ligamentum triangulare
dextrum
Ligamentum venae cavae
V. hepatica dextra

V. hepatica sinistra

Vena cava inferior

FIG. 337.—INFERIOR SURFACE OF THE LIVER.

The *right lateral surface* lies just beneath the costal margin in the midaxillary line. It rests against the diaphragm and is related indirectly to the thin edge of the base of the right lung, to the costodiaphragmatic pleural recess, and to the thoracic wall from the seventh to the eleventh rib and is covered entirely by peritoneum.

The peritoneum of the superior surface is not continued over the *posterior surface*, but is reflected to the diaphragm to form the coronary ligament. The peritoneum of the inferior surface of the right lobe is reflected to the kidney (posterior layer of the coronary ligament), so that the right half of the posterior surface of the liver is devoid of peritoneal covering, and is in direct contact with the diaphragm. It is known as the "bare area," and is contained within the reflections of the coronary ligament whose lateral edges form the triangular ligaments. This is the site of extraperitoneal subdiaphragmatic abscesses which occur from the upward spread of retroperitoneal abscesses on the right side of the abdomen.

3. **Surface Anatomy of the Liver.**—Owing to the deep location of the liver under the arching vault of the diaphragm, its surface projection is indicated by an outline confined mainly to the thorax, but including a small portion of the epigastrium. It is important to know accurately the upper and lower limits of the normal liver in order to determine an increase or decrease in size, or a change in level. The limits are determined by the physical diagnostic methods of palpation and percussion. It is difficult to determine the upper and lower boundaries with precision because the lower edge of the lung overlaps the liver above, and the lower thin edge of the liver overlaps the stomach and intestine below.

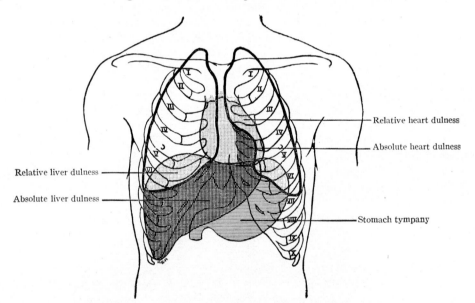

FIG. 338.—PERCUSSION OUTLINES OF THE HEART, LIVER, AND STOMACH.

The area within the epigastrium where the liver is accessible to palpation is important, especially when the organ is enlarged. The lower margin rises and falls during respiration and affords a useful diagnostic sign in the differentiation of obscure abdominal tumors which may or may not be attached to it. When the gallbladder is enlarged, the outline of its fundus sometimes can be made out distinctly, especially in thin-walled persons.

When the liver enlarges upward, the base of the lung rises with the diaphragm, but the depth of the pleural recess is essentially unchanged. This disposition is important in surgery of the liver, since it happens frequently that the most direct route to a hepatic abscess or cyst in the right lobe is by way of the thorax. In such cases, the lung is displaced upward out of the pleural recess, and the diaphragm lies in contact with the thoracic wall to an abnormal extent. To reach the liver through the diaphragm, the pleural recess usually is opened. This constitutes the transpleural route for hepatotomy (p. 343).

4. **Blood Vessels of the Liver.**—The liver is supplied with blood from both the hepatic artery and the portal vein. After circulating through the liver, the blood is returned to the inferior vena cava by the hepatic veins.

The *common hepatic artery* is one of the trunks of trifurcation of the celiac artery. It is directed at first almost horizontally from left to right behind the peritoneal floor of the lesser sac.   Destruction of the right or left terminal branches of the hepatic artery does not cause necrosis of the corresponding liver area supplied, since an accessory system of hepatic arteries supplements these vessels.

The *portal vein* carries to the liver blood which has passed through the capillaries of the whole abdominal alimentary tube, the pancreas, spleen, and gallbladder.   It is a thick trunk about 7.5 cm. long, formed behind the head of the pancreas by the union of the splenic and superior mesenteric veins.   It ascends at first behind the first division of the duodenum, but emerges between the two layers of the gastrohepatic omentum as far as the hepatic porta.   It is accompanied closely by the bile ducts (p. 353) and the hepatic artery.

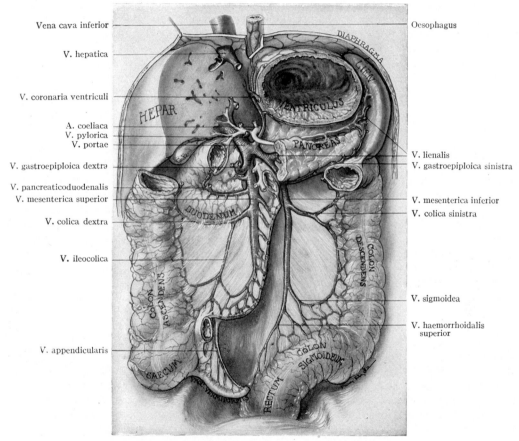

FIG. 339.—VEINS OF THE PORTAL SYSTEM.

Infections which localize in the wall of the portal vein cause *portal phlebitis* or *pylephlebitis*.   If this lesion progresses to an occlusive thrombosis, embarrassment of the portal circulation supervenes, with consequent ascites and the development of an accessory portal circulation.

The *hepatic veins* carry the blood away from the liver by draining into the inferior vena cava in its groove on the posterior aspect of the organ.

5. **Accessory Portal System.**—Definite natural channels of anastomosis exist between the portal and caval systems of veins, but they do not function unless obstruction to the portal vein, either in its intraperitoneal or intrahepatic course, so demands.   These communications constitute a portal system accessory to the main trunk.   Essentially, they

are anastomoses between the portal radicles of the gastro-intestinal and hepatic territories and the caval radicles of the surrounding structures.

Chief among the anastomosing channels between the portal and hepatic systems are the para-umbilical veins, which run in the falciform ligament of the liver and unite the left branch of the portal vein with the epigastric venous network of the abdominal wall (caval system). These veins, when enlarged, form a varicose network under the skin of the anterior abdominal wall known clinically as the "caput medusae." Occasionally, a single vein may attain the size of the small finger and run directly between the liver hilum and the epigastric vein at the umbilicus. Veins about the gallbladder, lesser omentum, and lesser curvature (portal system veins) sometimes connect with the para-umbilical veins and thereby with the caval system of the anterior abdominal wall. These same portal radicles sometimes anastomose with the diaphragmatic and intercostal tributaries of the azygos veins (caval system).

At the distal end of the esophagus, the left gastric veins (portal system) communicate in the submucous layer with the esophageal veins (caval system). In portal obstruction, the esophageal veins may become dilated and produce large varices which project into the esophageal mucosa. These veins, being almost unsupported, may rupture when the patient apparently is in excellent health, and result in a rapidly exsanguinating hemorrhage. Passage of a stomach tube, or any other form of esophagogastric instrumentation is an exceedingly dangerous practice in any patient who may have esophageal varices.

Anastomoses exist about the lower rectum between the superior hemorrhoidal veins (portal system) and the middle and inferior hemorrhoidal veins (caval system). The degree of communication is variable, since, in many cases of portal obstruction, hemorrhoidal varices are not evident. In the region of the bare area of the liver, collateral paths exist between the veins of the liver (portal system) and the veins of the diaphragm (caval system). The veins of Retzius unite the radicles of the splenic and mesenteric trunks of the portal with the branches of the inferior vena cava. To this group belong whole collections of retroperitoneal veins lying about the abdominal viscera which are fixed to the abdominal wall and diaphragm. These viscera are the liver, suprarenal bodies, duodenum, pancreas, and the ascending and descending portions of the colon. These veins divert blood from the portal circulation into the following caval tributaries: lower intercostal, diaphragmatic, lumbar, iliolumbar, epigastric, and circumflex iliac veins.

These anatomical connections between the two venous systems seldom suffice to effect compensation in portal obstruction. Since venous connections arise when inflamed abdominal viscera become adherent to the abdominal walls, it has been proposed, in an uncompensated portal block, to establish an artificial connection between the omentum or other abdominal structure and the abdominal wall. The apposed peritoneal surfaces of the liver and spleen (portal circulation) and those of the diaphragm and anterior abdominal wall (caval system) are irritated to encourage the formation of adhesions and thus facilitate an artificial anastomosis (Talma-Morison operation). In addition, the greater omentum (tributary to the portal system) may be sutured to the peritoneum of the anterior abdominal wall (tributary to the caval system).

SURGICAL CONSIDERATIONS

1. **Hepatic Abscess.**—In the absence of an open wound, pus-forming organisms may reach the liver along various channels, most frequently by the portal and hepatic vessels. In the majority of instances, infection is conveyed to the liver by emboli, or by a thrombophlebitis spreading along the portal vein from any part of the area drained by the tributaries of this vessel. Usually, the infection begins in the intestinal canal in the ulcerations of dysentery, in appendicitis, or in the wounds of rectal operations. If there is a general pyemia, infective emboli, after traveling through the lungs, find their way to the hepatic artery. A not uncommon infective focus is the lateral sinus, which may become inflamed and thrombosed as a complication of middle ear disease. Long before the pathologic connection between remote foci of suppuration was understood clearly, attention was drawn to the frequent association of intracranial suppuration and liver abscesses.

Liver abscesses are multiple or solitary. *Multiple abscesses* generally are of pyemic origin; they are small, diffusely scattered through the liver, and quite beyond the scope of surgical treatment. The *solitary* or *tropical abscess*, however, is of surgical interest because of the complications to which it may give rise and the form of treatment it demands. The tropical abscess is a manifestation of amebiasis and is associated with acute or chronic dysentery. Abscesses may occur anywhere in the liver structure, but four fifths of them appear in the right lobe. The favorite locations for abscess are the dome and the under surface of the liver. The abscess at first is deep but, as it increases in size and causes progressive liver destruction and localized or uniform liver enlargement, it tends to make its way to the surface. Upon reaching the surface, an abscess may rupture into a neighboring cavity or viscus. It may burst into the general peritoneal cavity, or, if adhesions have been formed, into the stomach, colon, or duodenum.

When an abscess erodes through the diaphragm and reaches the pleural cavity, it sets up a diffuse pleurisy. This complication usually is prevented by pleural adhesions between the lung and diaphragm, in which case the abscess may invade the lung, empty into a bronchus, and be evacuated by expectoration. The pus, if copious in amount, may cause suffocation. If the abscess is located posteriorly, it may penetrate the loose tissue behind the liver and diaphragm and extend along the perinephric tissue toward the lumbar region. It has been known to erode between the ribs, and to make its way forward through the anterior abdominal wall.

2. **Surgical Routes to the Liver.**—The evacuation of a large hepatic abscess by surgical measures (hepatotomy) is indicated as soon as the presence of pus has been ascertained. The location of the abscess and the direction in which it enlarges most freely determine the route by which it must be evacuated, whether subcostally through the abdominal wall, or through the chest wall either subpleurally or extrapleurally.

Admirable exposure of the anterior aspect of the liver is obtained by an oblique, subcostal incision immediately below the costal arch, that is, by the *abdominal transperitoneal route.* Continuation of the incision allows exposure of the left lobe. Where adhesions have formed between the parietal peritoneum and the hepatic serosa, incision may be made directly into the liver substance

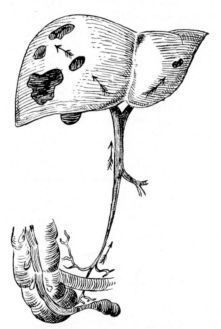

Fig. 340.—Portal Pyemia.

Abscess of the liver secondary to suppuration in the appendix. (After Rutherford Morison.)

and the operation be completed in one stage. Where no adhesions have formed between the liver and the abdominal wall and the patient's condition brooks no delay, the suspected area of liver may be walled off carefully and the abscess evacuated through the abdominal incision without contaminating the abdomen. The edges of the abscess cavity then are sutured to the abdominal opening. If the patient's condition permits, the parietal peritoneum may be sutured to the liver about the suspected area and the suture line be protected by a ring of gauze packing. The incision may be made directly into the liver or be deferred until the general cavity has been walled off from the suspected abscess area.

In the *thoracic transpleural route*, the site of the abscess is exposed by partial excision of one or two ribs. Where the pleural walls are united by adhesion and the liver is adherent to the diaphragm, the abscess is entered boldly. If the pleural walls are not adherent, they must be sutured at the periphery of the site within which the deeper incision is to be made, and the wound packed with gauze for several days to promote adhesions. If urgency demands, the incision may be made as soon as the several layers have been sutured. Should the diaphragm be found not adherent to the liver, it is sutured to the liver and the incision is developed through the sutured area.

An approach to the diaphragm by the *thoracic subpleural route* contemplates subperiosteal excision of one or more of the lower ribs in the midaxillary line, at a level above the diaphragm but below the line of pleural reflection (p. 242). If the pleural reflection is encountered after excision of the posterior layer of periosteum and the endothoracic fascia, it is detached by blunt dissection and reflected upward out of the way. The diaphragm is divided preferably in the direction of its fibers. When adhesions exist between the diaphragmatic and hepatic peritoneum, the abscess may be opened at once and drainage established. When no adhesions are present, the margins of the diaphragmatic opening may be sutured to the liver and the suture line protected by gauze packing so that the abscess may be opened.

3. **Echinococcus (Hydatid) Cysts.**—Hydatid cysts develop from the ovum of the taenia echinococcus (dog tapeworm), and are found more frequently in the liver than in any other part of the body. Generally, a single cyst occurs. The ovum is carried to the stomach with the food, and its outer envelope is dissolved, setting the embryo free in the intestinal tract. The embryo makes its way through the intestinal mucous membrane into one of the portal radicles. On reaching the liver, it develops into a hydatid cyst which may attain large dimensions, causing the liver to increase greatly in size. When the enlarging cyst invades the subdiaphragmatic region, it compresses the lungs and heart, impeding respiration and causing cardiac distress. During a coughing spell it may rupture into the pleural cavity, but more commonly it ruptures into one of the bronchi, where the sudden gush of its contents may cause suffocation.

The treatment consists of incision of the cyst and evacuation of its contents. This may be done either by the abdominal or transpleural route, and in one or two stages, depending on the presence or absence of serosal adhesions. Care must be taken to prevent the contents of the cyst from entering the peritoneal or the pleural cavity, lest the disease be spread.

4. **Contusions and Lacerations of the Liver.**—The overlying ribs protect the liver from direct violence, but sometimes it is contused and even lacerated seriously. Some injury is attributable no doubt to its solidity and fixation, and to the somewhat yielding nature of the lower ribs. The friability of the organ renders it liable to rupture, an accident which is even more likely to occur when the liver size is increased by disease. Sometimes, Glisson's capsule and the peritoneum surrounding the liver may remain untorn, and the liver substance suffer severe damage. The more serious injuries cause deep fissures, especially upon the visceral aspect, complicated by free hemorrhage and extravasation of bile into the peritoneal cavity. The blood in the liver is under very slight pressure, and careful packing generally is efficient both in checking the hemorrhage and furnishing the necessary drainage. A penetrating wound of the chest wall below the horizontal level of the fifth rib in the mammary line, if deep enough, may traverse the pleural cavity and diaphragm, and penetrate the liver. Such a wound usually implicates the lower thin edge of the lung in the costodiaphragmatic pleural recess. Sharp ends of fractured ribs may be driven through the diaphragm into the liver.

5. **Suprahepatic and Infrahepatic Divisions of the Subdiaphragmatic Space and Their Relation to Subdiaphragmatic Abscess.**—In general, the subdiaphragmatic (subphrenic) space is an extensive one. It is closed or hooded above by the diaphragm, and is partially barred from the rest of the abdominal cavity below by the transverse mesocolon and transverse colon. In the presence of infection, these structures and the great omentum adhere firmly to the anterior abdominal wall, and limit the downward extension of inflammatory products. On the right, the large right lobe of the liver is interposed between these two natural boundaries. The falciform ligament, sagittally placed, divides the area into right and left segments. On the left side are the small left lobe of the liver above

and the frontally disposed gastrohepatic (lesser) omentum and stomach below. Because the liver occupies the bulk of this space, and because its peritoneal connections are the key to a correct understanding of the area beneath the diaphragm in which residual abscesses may form, we propose to orient our discussion with reference to the liver rather than to the diaphragm itself, which surmounts the whole area as does a cupola.

The abdominal surface of the liver is covered everywhere by peritoneum, except over that portion which lies in direct contact with the diaphragm. It is important to visualize this "bare area," bare of peritoneum, lying almost directly posteriorly—placed against the posterior part of the diaphragm (Fig. 335). The superior and inferior reflections of peritoneum

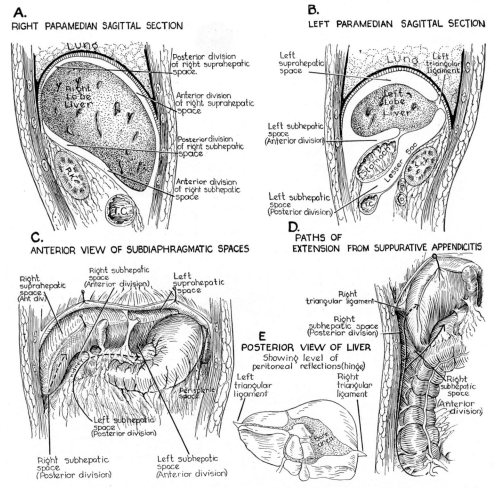

FIG. 341.—LOCATIONS OF SUBDIAPHRAGMATIC (SUPRAHEPATIC AND INFRAHEPATIC) ABSCESSES. (Callander.)

from the liver to the diaphragm which outline the bare area are continued directly laterally as the triangular (lateral) ligaments of the liver. The bulk of the liver is located superior to this composite line of peritoneal reflection; at this line, the superior or convex surface of the right and left liver lobes practically begins. The concave surface of the liver lies inferior to this line of reflection. Intraperitoneal subdiaphragmatic collections of fluid, as we interpret them, lie superior to this posteriorly placed hinge of peritoneal reflection, or inferior to it.

On the **right side,** a *suprahepatic* collection of fluid may be located posteriorly near the peritoneal reflection, or it may form more anteriorly near the costal margin. These areas we consider as the anterior and posterior divisions of the suprahepatic space. An abscess occasionally overlies all the suprahepatic space. A *right subhepatic abscess* may occupy all the area between the concave surface of the right lobe of the liver and the barrier formed by the kidney and the transverse colon and mesocolon. A subhepatic collection may be limited to a posteriorly and superiorly placed abscess. It then lies between the inferior peritoneal reflection and the upper pole of the right kidney (Fig. 341), and is designated as an abscess in the posterior division of the subhepatic space. By far the majority of subdiaphragmatic abscesses are subhepatic and lie in this posteriorly located space. The reason for the frequency of abscess formation here is that the exudate from suppurative appendicitis naturally gravitates superiorly along the paracolic gutter, impinges against

POSTERIOR EXTRAPERITONEAL APPROACH TO SUBDIAPHRAGMATIC ABSCESS

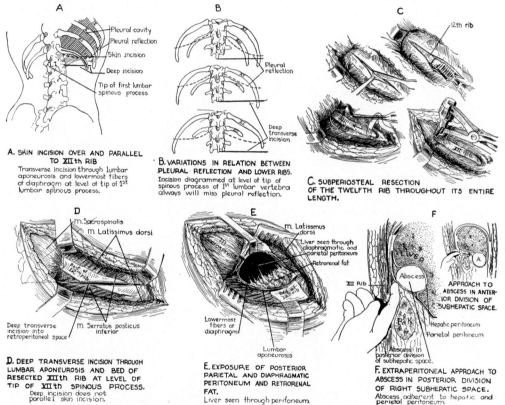

A. SKIN INCISION OVER AND PARALLEL TO XIIth RIB
Transverse incision through lumbar aponeurosis and lowermost fibers of diaphragm at level of tip of 1st lumbar spinous process.

B. VARIATIONS IN RELATION BETWEEN PLEURAL REFLECTION AND LOWER RIBS.
Incision diagrammed at level of tip of spinous process of 1st lumbar vertebra always will miss pleural reflection.

C. SUBPERIOSTEAL RESECTION OF THE TWELFTH RIB THROUGHOUT ITS ENTIRE LENGTH.

D. DEEP TRANSVERSE INCISION THROUGH LUMBAR APONEUROSIS AND BED OF RESECTED XIIth RIB AT LEVEL OF TIP OF XIIth SPINOUS PROCESS.
Deep incision does not parallel skin incision.

E. EXPOSURE OF POSTERIOR PARIETAL AND DIAPHRAGMATIC PERITONEUM AND RETRORENAL FAT.
Liver seen through peritoneum.

F. EXTRAPERITONEAL APPROACH TO ABSCESS IN POSTERIOR DIVISION OF RIGHT SUBHEPATIC SPACE.
Abscess adherent to hepatic and parietal peritoneum.

Fig. 342.—Posterior Extraperitoneal Approach to Subdiaphragmatic (Infrahepatic) Abscess. (Modified after Nather and Ochsner.)

the right triangular lateral ligament of the liver, and is guided to a posteriorly placed subhepatic position. Residual infection from a ruptured gallbladder or duodenal ulcer more readily gravitates into the more anterior area of the subhepatic space.

An intrahepatic infection, posteriorly located, may erode the liver substance in the area devoid of peritoneum and form an abscess there between the liver and the diaphragm in the *right extraperitoneal space*.

On the **left** of the falciform ligament lies the small left lobe of the liver with its superior convex and inferior concave surfaces. The left triangular ligament along the posterior margin of the lobe hinges the two areas. An abscess located superior to this line of peritoneal reflection is a *left suprahepatic abscess*. Because of the small size of the left lobe of the liver, an abscess here is rare and, of necessity, small. The frontally disposed stomach and gastrohepatic (lesser) omentum naturally subdivide the *left subhepatic area* into anterior and posterior divisions. The posterior of these areas is the lesser peritoneal sac. Residual abscess in the lesser sac may occur after rupture of a posteriorly located gastric ulcer. The anterior area of the left subhepatic space lies between the lesser omentum and the stomach and the anterior abdominal wall. It is limited inferiorly by the ready adhesion of the transverse colon and great omentum against the anterior abdominal wall, which occurs with contiguous infection. Rupture of an anteriorly situated gastric ulcer, or rupture of the gallbladder in which infected contacts spread to the left, locate a subhepatic abscess in this location.

A *left extraperitoneal subdiaphragmatic abscess* may form about the upper pole of the left kidney, extend upward and strip the peritoneum off the diaphragm. The cause of this may be a high perinephric and, therefore, extraperitoneal abscess, or perforation of a carcinoma of the abdominal esophagus in its posterior and, therefore, extraperitoneal area.

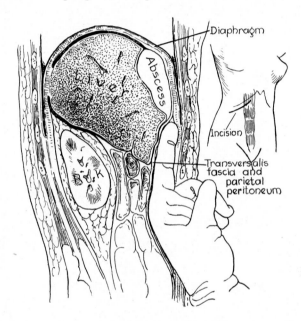

FIG. 343.—ANTERIOR EXTRAPERITONEAL APPROACH TO SUBDIAPHRAGMATIC (SUPRAHEPATIC) ABSCESS
(Clairmont after Nather and Ochsner.)

The abscess in the anterior division of the subdiaphragmatic space is drained by blunt dissection extraperitoneally.

6. **Paths of Approach to Subdiaphragmatic Abscess.**—The treatment of subdiaphragmatic abscess is incision and drainage performed so that uninvolved portions of pleural and peritoneal cavities are not contaminated. This basic surgical principle often is disregarded. The paths of approach are transdiaphragmatic and transabdominal, and each variety of approach may be transserous or extraserous.

The **transdiaphragmatic** *extrapleural* approach is accomplished through rib resection below the costodiaphragmatic pleural reflection, or through rib resection and upward mobilization of the unopened pleural reflection. Upward mobilization of the pleura on the diaphragm is difficult. Transdiaphragmatic *transpleural* drainage through rib resection and suture of the opposed costal and diaphragmatic layers of pleura in one or two stages is a procedure used much too frequently. The walling-off practice often does not protect the rest of the pleural cavity.

Transabdominal *transperitoneal* drainage which permits of contamination of uninvolved areas of peritoneum is disastrous. Transabdominal *extraperitoneal* drainage is the method best adapted to the evacuation of all varieties of subdiaphragmatic abscess, and the approach is anterior or posterior according to the location of the infected area.

Abscesses located in the right and left suprahepatic spaces and those situated in the anterior division of the left subhepatic area can be drained extraperitoneally through the anterior abdominal wall (Clairmont) (Fig. 343).   An incision just below, and parallel to, either costal margin is developed through the abdominal musculature and transversalis fascia down to the anterior parietal peritoneum.   The peritoneum is separated from the under surface of the diaphragm by blunt dissection until the abscess cavity is reached. The cavity is opened extraperitoneally through the abscess wall, which is intimately adherent to the mobilized diaphragmatic peritoneum.

The posterior extraperitoneal approach devised by Nather and Ochsner (Fig. 342) should be employed in dealing with abscesses in the anterior or posterior division of the right subhepatic area or with abscess in the right or left extraperitoneal spaces.   The posterior part of the suprahepatic space can be reached through this incision.   The principle of this, as well as that of the anterior approach, is that the peritoneum on the diaphragm can be dissected bluntly toward the dome until the abscess cavity is reached. The abscess can be opened directly, since its wall is adherent to the mobilized diaphragmatic peritoneum.

(D) EXTRAHEPATIC BILIARY PASSAGES

The extrahepatic bile tract consists of the hepatic or excretory duct of the liver, the gallbladder, a reservoir in which bile accumulates, the cystic duct which is the continuation of the gallbladder, and the common duct, which is the union of the hepatic and cystic ducts.   With these structures in the hepatic pedicle, or hepatoduodenal ligament, are the portal vein and branches of the hepatic artery.   These elements are disposed in two layers, the ventral, containing the bile ducts and the hepatic artery, and the dorsal containing the portal vein.

The anatomy of the bile passages and the vessels so intimately related to them clarifies the rationale of operations performed for the removal of gallstones, and for the treatment of the various inflammatory complications which they incur.

1. **Hepatic Duct.**—The hepatic duct is formed in the depth of the transverse fissure of the liver by the union of the right and left hepatic ducts.   The resulting trunk runs downward, backward, and mesially in the gastrohepatic ligament (lesser omentum).   The length of the duct averages about 4 cm., but may vary considerably, depending upon the level at which it is joined by the cystic duct.

At the liver hilus, the duct crosses the portal vein and the branches of the hepatic artery.   As it leaves the hilus, it lies over the anterolateral aspect of the portal vein and maintains that position to its termination.   The hepatic duct is related to the hepatic artery proper which sometimes runs closely along its left margin, but which usually lies some distance from it, especially when the finger introduced into the epiploic foramen draws the lesser omentum forward.   From the right branch of the hepatic artery, the cystic artery runs dorsal to the hepatic duct to ramify over the anterior surface of the neck of the gallbladder.

2. **Gallbladder.**—The gallbladder, a thin-walled, pear-shaped sac about 8 to 10 cm. long with a capacity of about 50 cc., lies in a fossa of the inferior surface of the liver which separates the right lobe from the quadrate lobe.   Loose connective tissue and the peritoneum reflected from its sides attach the gallbladder to the liver.

The large bulbous extremity, or *fundus*, is covered partly with peritoneum, and is directed downward, forward, and to the left.   It occupies the cystic notch in the margin of the liver and exceeds it for a distance of 1 cm. or more.   When the gallbladder is full, the fundus comes into contact with the anterior abdominal wall opposite the ninth costal cartilage, where it can be marked out in the angle between the right rectus muscle and the costal margin.

The *body* of the gallbladder is united to the inferior surface of the liver.   While normally there is no peritoneum between the body of the gallbladder and the liver fossa, occasionally the gallbladder is attached so loosely as to be freely mobile and is suspended from the liver as by a mesentery. The degree of difficulty experienced in isolating the gallbladder and separating it from its bed depends somewhat upon the degree to which the peritoneum binds it to the liver. Small vessels and even small biliary channels may connect the two. Hemorrhage from these vessels usually is slight.

The body is continued into the tapering extremity or *neck* of the gallbladder, which presents a sinuous or S-shaped curve downward to reach a termination in the cystic duct. It occupies the deepest part of the cystic fossa, and lies in the uppermost free portion of the lesser omentum. It contains the remainder of the embryonic spiral valve (of Heister) which makes catheterization from above difficult. Between the body and the cystic duct is a forward bulging which is the *ampulla*.

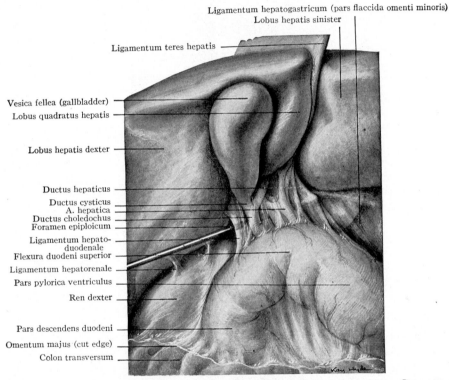

Ligamentum hepatogastricum (pars flaccida omenti minoris)
Lobus hepatis sinister

Ligamentum teres hepatis

Vesica fellea (gallbladder)
Lobus quadratus hepatis

Lobus hepatis dexter

Ductus hepaticus
Ductus cysticus
A. hepatica
Ductus choledochus
Foramen epiploicum
Ligamentum hepato-
duodenale
Flexura duodeni superior
Ligamentum hepatorenale
Pars pylorica ventriculus
Ren dexter

Pars descendens duodeni
Omentum majus (cut edge)
Colon transversum

Fig. 344.—Extrahepatic Biliary Passages and Their Relations with the Stomach, Duodenum and Liver.
A probe is placed in the epiploic foramen.

The *mucosa* is so rich in mucus-secreting glands that when the ampulla or cystic duct is obstructed by an impacted calculus, the gallbladder may dilate and form a *mucocele*. As this obstruction offers no obstacle to the free passage of bile from the liver into the duodenum, the inflammation of the gallbladder sometimes associated with it need not cause jaundice.

The *relations* of the gallbladder to the duodenum and transverse colon explain their not infrequent adhesion and the passage of gallstones from the one to the other. They also explain the rationale of surgical anastomosis between the gallbladder and duodenum or stomach for an irremovable calculus in the terminal common duct or for carcinoma in the head of the pancreas.

The gallbladder undergoes great changes in size under normal conditions, but in the pathologic state its size varies from enormous distention to contraction into a fibrous mass. When it becomes distended, it enlarges in a downward and medial direction, forming a readily palpable, movable tumor which may be mistaken for a floating kidney. Obstruction in the terminal portion of the biliary apparatus from a noninflammatory lesion, such as cancer of the head of the pancreas or of the termination of the common duct, causes the gallbladder to dilate. Obstruction caused by a calculus usually carries with it

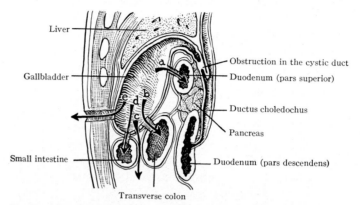

FIG. 345.—PARAMEDIAN SAGITTAL DIAGRAM SHOWING PATHS OF SPONTANEOUS RUPTURE OF AN EMPYEMA OF THE GALLBLADDER.

a, Rupture into the duodenum; *b*, erosion into transverse colon; *c*, rupture into the general peritoneal cavity; *d*, rupture into the small intestine; *e*, erosion through the abdominal wall.

inflammation of the bile passages (cholangitis), and the gallbladder generally is contracted as a result of the accompanying infection (*Courvoisier's law*). The gallbladder may acquire such adhesions with the surrounding tissues as to render its resection and even its recognition difficult.

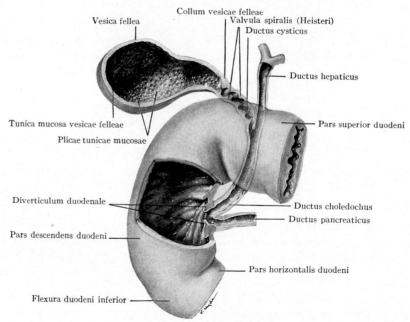

FIG. 346.—GALLBLADDER AND BILE DUCTS AND THEIR RELATIONS WITH THE DUODENUM.

3. **Cystic Duct.**—The cystic duct, continuing the neck of the gallbladder, is about 4 cm. long, but is folded upon itself so that its union with the hepatic duct occurs close to the neck of the gallbladder. It usually runs some distance beside the hepatic duct before opening into it. The redundant lining is arranged into a series of folds which produce the

spiral *valve of Heister*. This valve obstructs the passage of an instrument, save when the duct is dilated greatly by the passage of stones or by obstruction of the common duct. The folds may offer sufficient obstruction to cause calculi to become impacted. The cystic artery accompanies the duct, usually running on the left side.

4. **Common Bile Duct.**—The common bile duct, although conveniently regarded as the union of the cystic and hepatic ducts, really is the direct continuation of the hepatic duct. It is about 9 cm. long, and passes downward in the lesser omentum (supraduodenal portion), behind the duodenum (retroduodenal portion) in a groove of, or behind, the pancreas (pancreatic portion), and obliquely into the descending duodenum (intraduodenal portion).

The *supraduodenal*, or *first, part of the duct* is about 3.5 cm. long, but may be shortened by the opening of the cystic duct into the hepatic duct very close to the superior margin of the duodenum. It descends along the right margin of the lesser omentum to the right of the hepatic artery, anterior to the portal vein. The lymph glands related to the common duct at its beginning and termination may become enlarged in infections of the bile passages and in malignancy of the stomach and pancreas, and be mistaken for impacted gallstones. Downward pressure on the duodenum and division of the hepatocolic ligament, if present, expose the supraduodenal and retroduodenal parts of the duct. The index finger of the left hand is passed into the epiploic foramen and the supraduodena

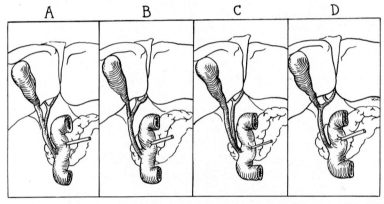

FIG. 347.—VARIATIONS IN THE UNION BETWEEN THE CYSTIC AND HEPATIC DUCTS. (Modified after Ruge.)

part of the duct is palpated between the left forefinger and thumb. A stone may be milked from more distal locations in the duct. If a calculus is present in the termination of the common duct, the proximal parts of the duct including the supraduodenal portion are dilated, a condition which admits of surgical exploration upward into the hepatic ducts and downward into the duodenum through an incision in the supraduodenal portion.

The *retroduodenal*, or *second, part of the duct* descends behind the first part of the duodenum anterior to the vena cava and to the right of the portal vein. There are 1 or 2 cm. of the upper duodenal wall to which the duct does not adhere, and which may be exposed by incising the anterior layer of the lesser omentum at the upper margin of the duodenum and drawing the duodenum downward. To examine the second part of the duct, the forefinger is placed in the epiploic foramen and the thumb on the anterolateral aspect of the first part of the duodenum. Between the two fingers, the presence of impacted stones can be recognized. It sometimes is necessary to mobilize the descending duodenum to expose the second part of the bile duct, but usually stones can be manipulated upward into the supraduodenal part or downward into the duodenum.

The *pancreatic*, or *third, part of the duct* begins at the upper margin of the head of the pancreas, the posterior surface of which it either grooves or tunnels. This part passes downward and terminates by piercing the posteromesial aspect of the descending duodenum at about its middle. It is separated from the inferior vena cava by connective tissue alone or by a thin layer of pancreas. It has no direct relationship with the portal vein which approaches it obliquely from below and from the left. On its left side, the duct is accompanied by the gastroduodenal artery, which, a variable distance down its course,

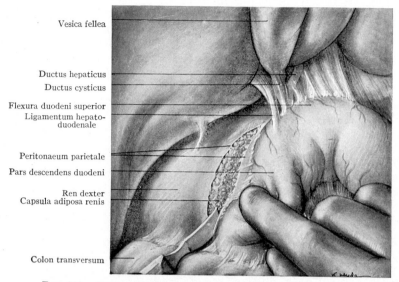

Vesica fellea

Ductus hepaticus
Ductus cysticus

Flexura duodeni superior
Ligamentum hepato-
duodenale

Peritonaeum parietale

Pars descendens duodeni

Ren dexter
Capsula adiposa renis

Colon transversum

FIG. 348.—SURGICAL MOBILIZATION OF THE DESCENDING PART OF THE DUODENUM.
Mobilizing this part of the duodenum offers a direct approach to the retroduodenal and pancreatic divisions of the common duct; this is accomplished by incising the parietal peritoneum along the descending duodenum, allowing medial retraction. This maneuver also facilitates pyloroplasty.

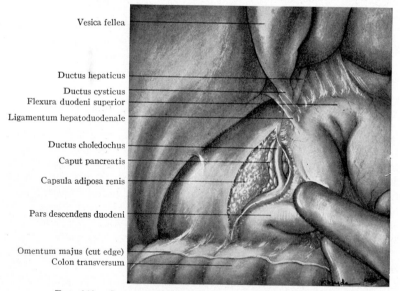

Vesica fellea

Ductus hepaticus
Ductus cysticus
Flexura duodeni superior
Ligamentum hepatoduodenale

Ductus choledochus
Caput pancreatis

Capsula adiposa renis

Pars descendens duodeni

Omentum majus (cut edge)
Colon transversum

FIG. 349.—SURGICAL MOBILIZATION OF THE DESCENDING DUODENUM COMPLETED.
The common duct is exposed where it grooves the head of the pancreas; this maneuver renders the intrapancreatic portion of the common duct accessible for removal of calculus. It also facilitates pyloroplasty.

gives off the superior pancreaticoduodenal trunk (p. 322). This trunk crosses the common duct either anteriorly or posteriorly. Its presence and its interlacing branches to the duct explain the hemorrhage which occurs in exposure of the third portion of the duct. Hemorrhage also may be caused by injury to a vein issuing from the posterior aspect of the head of the pancreas and running upward along the mesial aspect of the bile duct to join the portal vein (p. 360)

The common duct begins its *intraduodenal portion* where it enters the wall of the duodenum obliquely and is joined on the left by the pancreatic duct. The short common reservoir formed by the two ducts partly within the duodenal wall is the *ampulla of Vater*. The ampulla becomes constricted and opens into the duodenum on the summit of the *duodenal papilla*. The opening is so small that gallstones, having passed the cystic and common ducts, often become impacted. When this occurs, pancreatic as well as bile secretion may be prevented from entering the duodenum unless a communication exists between the main and accessory pancreatic ducts (p. 359). This condition and spasm of the sphincter (of Oddi) about the duodenal opening favor reflux of bile into the pancreatic duct with consequent pancreatitis. The common bile duct sometimes narrows a little before opening into the ampulla of Vater and causes impaction of stones. In this case, the pancreas is not so likely to be affected. Direct access to a stone impacted in the ampulla of Vater is gained by the transduodenal route (p. 357).

5. **Modes of Termination of the Bile and Pancreatic Ducts.**—Considerable variation exists in the modes of termination of the pancreatic and bile ducts. Normally there is an ampulla, common to both ducts, opening on the duodenal mucosa on the summit of the

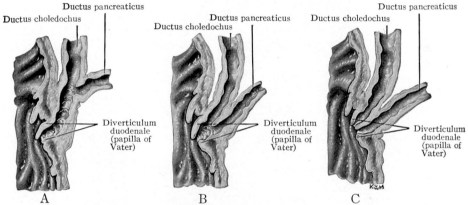

FIG. 350.—COMMONER VARIATIONS IN THE UNION OF THE PANCREATIC AND COMMON BILE DUCTS. A, The communication takes place outside the wall of the duodenum; B, the union is within the duodenal diverticulum; C, each duct opens by a separate orifice on the duodenal papilla.

duodenal papilla. The two ducts may open independently into the duodenum, each on the summit of a small papilla or in the depth of a slight depression, in which case a stone impacted in the terminal common duct will not cause pancreatic obstruction. The common duct may open at the papilla and the pancreatic duct unite with the common duct at a higher level.

6. **Vessels.**—The arteries surgically related to the extrahepatic bile passages are derived from the common hepatic trunk of the celiac axis. The hepatic artery divides early in its course behind the pylorus into two diverging trunks, the hepatic artery proper and the gastroduodenal artery.

The *hepatic artery proper* runs superiorly to the right in the lesser omentum (hepatoduodenal ligament), during which course it gives off the right gastric artery to the pyloric side of the lesser curvature. Near the liver, the hepatic artery divides into right and left branches for the corresponding liver lobes. The cystic artery usually arises from the right hepatic branch and runs to the cystic duct and the neck of the gallbladder. In the majority of cases, the right branch of the hepatic artery lies to the right of the hepatic duct so that the cystic artery does not cross it. At the left margin of the cystic duct, the cystic artery divides into inferior and superior branches which anastomose about the gallbladder.

23

The *gastroduodenal artery* runs downward and backward along the mesial voncace margin of the descending duodenum to the left of the common duct. The interlacing branches given to the common duct must be kept in mind in operations on its supra-duodenal and retroduodenal portions. Its terminal branches are the right gastro-epiploic and the superior pancreaticoduodenal arteries.

The *portal vein* and its relations have been considered (p. 341).

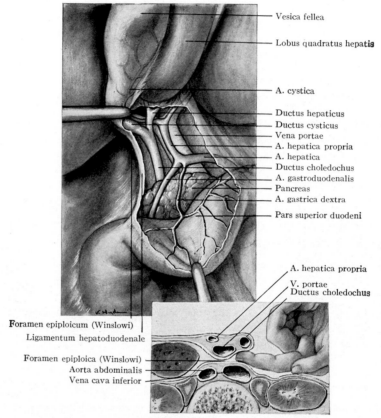

Vesica fellea

Lobus quadratus hepatis

A. cystica

Ductus hepaticus
Ductus cysticus
Vena portae
A. hepatica propria
A. hepatica
Ductus choledochus
A. gastroduodenalis
Pancreas
A. gastrica dextra

Pars superior duodeni

A. hepatica propria
V. portae
Ductus choledochus

Foramen epiploicum (Winslowi)
Ligamentum hepatoduodenale

Foramen epiploica (Winslowi)
Aorta abdominalis
Vena cava inferior

FIG. 351.—TOPOGRAPHY OF THE VESSELS AND DUCTS IN THE HEPATIC PEDICLE.
The inset is a cross section through the structures of the pedicle; it is evident that the portal vein lies considerably to the left of the common duct and at a deeper level. Right gastric artery usually branches from the proper hepatic artery.

The *lymphatics* of the gallbladder and cystic duct drain not only to the lymph glands at the hilus of the liver. but also along lymph channels into the liver substance. By the latter efferent vessels, the liver may be infected from a diseased gallbladder. The lymph vessels along the hepatic and common ducts drain into nodes along the common duct, which, when hypertrophied, feel like calculi in the common duct.

SURGICAL CONSIDERATIONS

The gallbladder lies in the supramesocolic compartment of the abdominal cavity, in the forward part of a deep recess, directed from before obliquely backward and upward under the inferior surface of the liver. The exploring hand, upon passing deeply into the subhepatic recess, comes into contact with the kidney, and is arrested by the reflection of the peritoneum between the kidney and the posterior surface of the liver.

Inferior to the neck of the gallbladder, the finger may be passed into the epiploic for-amen, in the layers of the front wall of which lie the supraduodenal part of the common duct, the portal vein, and the hepatic artery. Beneath the liver, the pyloric end of the stomach passes posteriorly into the first portion of the duodenum, which in turn can be traced farther to its union with the descending duodenum. A lateral counterdrainage, opening at the posterior extremity of the hepatorenal recess to the right of the hepatic flexure of the colon, conducts an extravasation of fluid from the space without soiling the contents of the abdomen below the transverse colon and mesocolon. This opening drains well because of its dependent position in recumbency.

When a calculus becomes impacted in the cystic duct, or the duct is occluded by a cicatricial contraction, the gallbladder becomes distended by the clear mucinous fluid secreted by its mucous membrane (*hydrops of the gallbladder*). If suppurative cholecystitis is superimposed, the gallbladder will contain pus to the extent of forming an abscess sac (*empyema*).

1. **Cholecystostomy.**—To perform a cholecystostomy, a small abdominal incision is made. and, after palpation of the ducts and examination of the gallbladder, the fundus is drawn into the wound as far as possible and protected carefully by gauze packs. If there are stones in the cystic duct or in the neck of the gallbladder, effort is made to milk them into the gallbladder before opening it. The gallbladder is evacuated with an aspirating trocar, the puncture wound in the fundus is enlarged, and the cavity is searched for calculi. A rubber drainage tube is introduced 5 to 8 cm. into the gallbladder and held in place by a purse-string suture, with the serosa inverted. The viscus may or may not be sutured to the peritoneum at the upper margin of the incision.

When a stone is removed from the common duct, cholecystostomy often is advisable so that the gallbladder may remain as a guide to the deep ducts, in which subsequent infection may occur. The gallbladder also is of great value for cholecystenterostomy, if stricture of the common duct should occur.

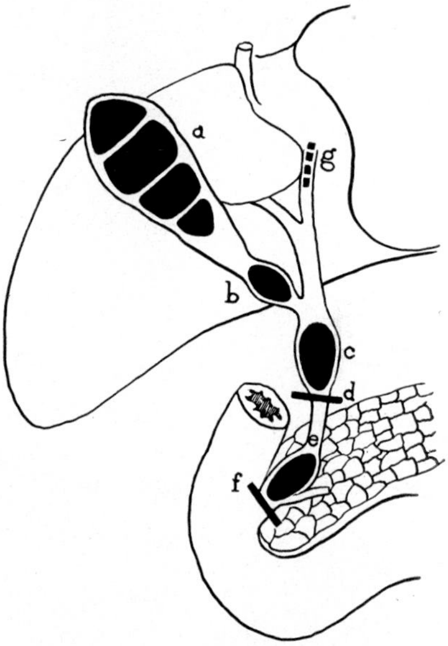

2. **Cholecystectomy.**—Cholecystectomy consists of resection of the gallbladder, the usual indications for which are calculi and diseased gallbladder walls which might resist cure by drainage. Excision may be performed from the fundus downward or from the cystic duct upward.

FIG. 352.—SCHEMA OF THE LOCATION OF CALCULUS AND TUMORS IN THE EXTRAHEPATIC BILE PASSAGES.

a, Facetted gallstones in the gallbladder; b, solitary stone in cystic duct; c, stone in supraduodenal part of the common duct; d, tumor obstruction of common duct; e, stone in pancreatic portion of common duct; f, tumor of intraduodenal part of common duct; g, small calculi in left primary hepatic duct. (After De Quervain.)

Removal from the fundus downward affords free anatomical dissection, and is indicated when the neck of the gallbladder is more or less hidden by dense adhesions. Incision is made through the serous and subserous layers along each side of the gallbladder and over the fundus at a sufficient distance from the liver attachment to afford peritoneal covering for the cystic fossa after the viscus has been removed. The fundus is drawn downward from the liver and separated from it by blunt dissection. As the dissection is carried toward the neck of the bladder, the cystic artery is seen beside the cystic duct. The artery and duct are exposed and followed into the hepatic pedicle where the artery is ligated and divided proximal to its division into terminal branches. The peritoneal flaps are sutured across the raw surface of the liver bed.

The more usual approach is to carry the *dissection from the cystic duct upward*, so that the most difficult steps in the operation are completed at once. Isolation. ligation, and

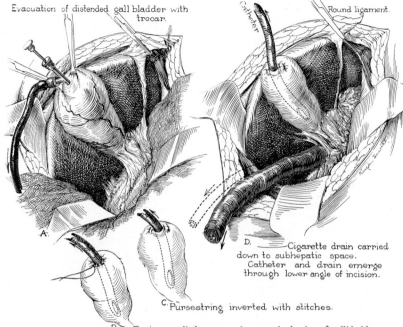

Evacuation of distended gall bladder with trocar.

Catheter

Round ligament.

D. — Cigarette drain carried down to subhepatic space.
Catheter and drain emerge through lower angle of incision.

C. Pursestring inverted with stitches.

B. — Drainage catheter pursestrung into fundus of gallbladder

FIG. 353.—CHOLECYSTOSTOMY.

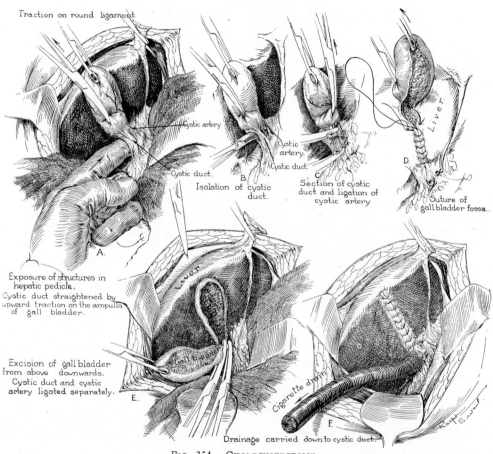

Traction on round ligament

Cystic artery.

Cystic duct.

Cystic artery.

Cystic duct.

B. Isolation of cystic duct.

C. Section of cystic duct and ligation of cystic artery

Liver.

D. Suture of gall bladder fossa.

A.

Exposure of structures in hepatic pedicle.
Cystic duct straightened by upward traction on the ampulla of gall bladder.

Excision of gall bladder from above downwards.
Cystic duct and cystic artery ligated separately.

Liver.

Gall bladder

E.

Cigarette drain

F.

Drainage carried down to cystic duct.

FIG. 354.—CHOLECYSTECTOMY.

division of the cystic duct and artery create a bloodless field for removal of the gallbladder. In the event of hemorrhage in the depth of the wound, compression of the hepatic pedicle between the thumb and forefinger will arrest the hemorrhage by occluding the hepatic artery. The bleeding vessel, generally the cystic artery, then can be looked for in a dry field.

3. Operations on the Common Duct (Choledochotomy).—Choledochotomy is an operation designed for the removal of a calculus from the common bile duct, most frequently from its uppermost (supraduodenal) segment.

In *supraduodenal choledochotomy*, the common duct is incised in its free portion between the origin at the junction of the cystic and hepatic ducts and the upper margin of the duodenum. The object is the extraction of a calculus from the site of the incision or of calculi lying above or below, within reach of the incision. The common duct, together with the other structures contained within the hepatoduodenal ligament, is drawn forward and the incision is made in the long axis of the duct. Usually, the incision in the duct is sutured about a drain. If complete suture of the duct is performed, a cholecystostomy

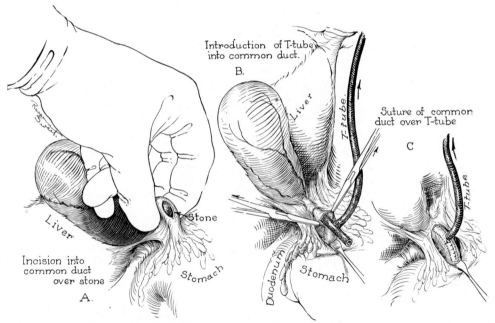

FIG. 355.—CHOLEDOCHOTOMY WITH COMMON DUCT DRAINAGE.

may be performed to act as a drain to the biliary system and to relieve tension on the sutures in the common duct.

Transduodenal choledochotomy is employed for the removal of stones impacted in the ampulla (of Vater). The operation contemplates incision through the anterior wall of the duodenum and a search for the stone behind the mucous membrane at the posterior wall of the duodenum just above the duodenal papilla. The mucous membrane is incised and the stone is extracted. Other stones in the intrapancreatic portion may be pressed downward and removed.

4. Cholecystenterostomy.—An anastomosis between the gallbladder and some available segment of the gastro-intestinal tract must be made in irremovable obstruction of the common duct, such as is encountered in tumors of the head of the pancreas or of the common duct, in inaccessible stone in the common duct, or in fibrotic stenosis. The operation furnishes a new pathway for the ingress of bile into the gastro-intestinal system, and is performed usually by the suture method. Union may be accomplished by some such mechanical contrivance as the Murphy button. Connections with the stomach or duodenum are preferable, as the bile then is emptied into the tract near its normal point of entry.   A fistula with the jejunum or colon is an undesirable alternative because of the possibility of infection ascending to the liver.

(E) PANCREAS

1. **Definition and Location.**—The pancreas is an elongated, hammer-shaped gland, resembling very closely in outward appearance one of the larger salivary glands (Fig. 327). It lies in the epigastrium and left hypochondrium in an ultimately retroperitoneal position behind the serosal floor of the omental bursa (lesser sac), at the level of the first and second lumbar vertebrae.   Its deep location explains the difficulty in clinical diagnosis between inflammatory and tumor involvement of the gland, and lesions of the overlying stomach, transverse colon, and omentum.   Adding to the confusion with lesions of other supra-mesocolic viscera is the fact that lesions of the pancreas are prevented from posterior extension by the resistant posterior abdominal wall, and extend forward into the lesser sac.   Furthermore, since the anterior surface of the organ is covered by peritoneum form-ing the floor of the lesser peritoneal sac, an acute inflammation of the pancreas may cause

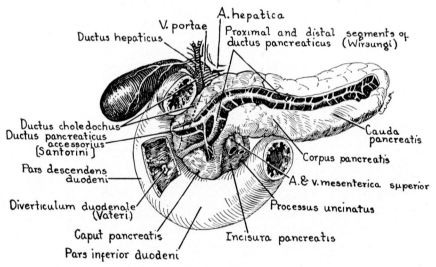

FIG. 356.—NORMAL RELATIONS BETWEEN THE DUODENUM, BILE PASSAGES, AND PANCREAS, WITH SPECIAL REFERENCE TO THE PANCREATIC DUCTS.

a peritonitis with effusion, which, at first, is limited to the lesser sac.   If the epiploic for-amen is blocked simultaneously by inflammatory adhesions, the exudate will be confined to this region and will give the physical signs of a tumor.

2. **Division and Relations.**—The pancreas is divided into a head, neck, body, and tail. The *head* or right extremity is embraced by the duodenum and bends downward over the duodenum for some distance below the general level of the gland.   This intimate relation to the duodenal loop, particularly to its descending portion, explains how lesions of the head of the gland, notably carcinoma, may encroach upon the lumen of the duodenum and cause obstructive symptoms necessitating gastrojejunostomy.   A rare anatomic anomaly has been observed in which the head of the pancreas surrounds the duodenum like a ring.   By the swelling of chronic pancreatic inflammation, this arrangement may lead to actual stenosis of the duodenum.   Anteriorly, the head is covered by the pylorus above and the transverse colon below.   The root of the transverse mesocolon divides the head into supramesocolic and inframesocolic areas.   Posteriorly, the head is related to the inferior vena cava, left renal vein, and aorta.   Tumors of the gland may compress the inferior vena cava and the portal tributaries, causing edema of the extremities and ascites. The common bile duct, near its termination, lies in a groove at the right extremity of the

gland and may be embedded in it. This explains the jaundice from biliary retention found in chronic pancreatitis and in carcinoma of the head of the gland. In obstruction caused by carcinoma of the head of the pancreas, the gallbladder is dilated by the gradual accumulation of bile, whereas, in obstruction resulting from gallstones, the gallbladder is contracted (Courvoisier's law). The uncinate process of the head of the pancreas hooks behind the superior mesenteric vessels.

The *neck* is a comparatively short, narrow portion directed upward and to the left to join the body. It supports the pyloric end of the stomach. At its upper border, the common duct, portal vein, and hepatic artery enter the gastrohepatic (lesser) omentum, behind the neck, the superior mesenteric and splenic veins unite to form the portal vein.

The *body* of the pancreas forms a well-marked anterior convexity where it lies in front of the vertebral column at, or a little below, the transpyloric plane. It is somewhat triangular in cross section and presents three surfaces. The anterior surface is covered by the peritoneal floor of the omental bursa. An ulcer on the posterior wall of the stomach may adhere to this surface of the gland and penetrate its substance (p. 320). A solid or cystic pancreatic tumor will bulge forward through the overlying peritoneum and present through the gastrohepatic (lesser) omentum, gastrocolic ligament, or transverse mesocolon. These modes of presentation are the rationale for the surgical approaches to the organ.

The inferior surface is separated from the anterior surface by the anterior border of the gland, along which lies the attachment of the root of the transverse mesocolon. The

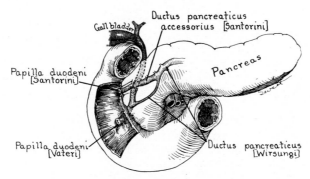

FIG. 357.—PANCREATIC DUCT SYSTEM IN WHICH THE ACCESSORY DUCT (OF SANTORINI) CARRIES MOST OF THE SECRETION OF THE PANCREAS.

underlying splenic vein and left renal vessels indicate the danger of attempting to reach the pancreas by a posterior lumbar approach. The upper margin of the body of the pancreas has a close relation with the celiac trunk, and is grooved or tunnelled by the splenic artery.

Without demarcation, the body merges into the *tail*, which usually lies within the peritoneal duplication of the lienorenal ligament and is related below to the left colic flexure. When the tail is short, it does not reach the hilus of the spleen; when long, it lies at the hilus, surrounded by the splenic vessels. These intimate relations of the pancreas and spleen always should be considered in splenectomy (p. 367), since a ligature placed en masse on the splenic vessels easily may include the tail of the pancreas.

3. **Duct System of the Pancreas.**—The *main pancreatic duct* (of Wirsung) begins in the tail and traverses the whole gland near its posterior surface, receiving branches from all sides. It emerges from the right border of the head and, together with the common bile duct, opens into the ampulla of Vater. An *accessory pancreatic duct* (of Santorini) drains the upper part of the head of the gland, opening by one extremity into the main pancreatic duct and by the other into the duodenum, cephalad to the opening of the main duct. When the communication with the main pancreatic duct is free, the accessory duct may convey all of the pancreatic secretion to the duodenum in the event of obstruction to the terminal part of the main duct.

The chief point of surgical interest lies in the relation of the common bile duct to the main pancreatic duct. The common duct traverses the wall of the duodenum obliquely and ends in an ampulla and sphincter (of Oddi). The sphincter guards the outlet of the common duct into the duodenum and controls the bile outflow. In three quarters of cases, the pancreatic duct empties into the common bile duct just above, or at the site of, the ampulla, affording a common channel for bile and pancreatic juice. An impaction of a calculus at the ampulla of Vater converts the two ducts into a continuous passage. It is demonstrated fairly well that this mechanism accounts for the passage of bile into the pancreatic duct, causing pancreatitis.

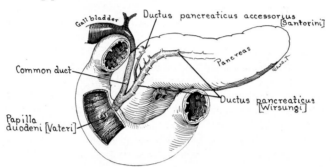

FIG. 358.—DUCT SYSTEM OF THE PANCREAS IN WHICH THE ACCESSORY DUCT IS RUDIMENTARY AND HAS NO CONNECTION WITH THE DUODENUM.

The pancreas elaborates two *secretions*, an internal and an external. The external secretion, containing three ferments, is discharged through the pancreatic duct system and promotes protein, carbohydrate, and fat metabolism. The internal secretion, elaborated by the islands of Langerhans, is absorbed directly into the blood, and largely controls sugar metabolism.

4. **Vessels of the Pancreas.**—The body and tail of the pancreas derive most of their rich arterial circulation from the *splenic artery*. The head is supplied largely by the anastomosing superior and inferior pancreaticoduodenal trunks from the gastroduodenal and superior mesenteric arteries respectively.

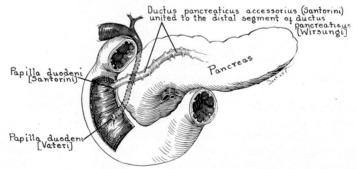

FIG. 359.—PANCREATIC DUCT SYSTEM IN WHICH THE ACCESSORY DUCT IS UNITED TO THE DISTAL SEGMENT OF THE MAIN PANCREATIC DUCT. THERE IS NO PROXIMAL SEGMENT OF THE MAIN PANCREATIC DUCT.

The *veins* of the pancreas join the splenic vein, but a large trunk issues from the dorsal aspect of the gland and runs upward along the left of the common bile duct to join the portal vein. This vessel may be injured in exposure of the pancreatic part of the common duct (p. 353).

Scarcely an organ in the abdomen possesses as extensive a *lymphatic distribution* as does the pancreas. The glands drain into the pancreaticosplenic nodes at the hilus of the spleen, and into the pancreaticoduodenal and preaortic nodes near the origin of the superior mesenteric artery.

Surgical Considerations

The deep location of the pancreas and the important structures surrounding it emphasize the difficulties and the dangers which attend surgical procedures involving the organ. The only part of the gland permitting practical resection is that lying to the left of the spine, although partial excision of the head of the pancreas has been performed successfully.

1. Paths of Surgical Approach.—There are three anterior transperitoneal approaches, in addition to the lumbar approach to the pancreas for the dependent drainage of pancreatic fluid. Access to the pancreas, and especially to its superior margin, is afforded *through the gastrohepatic ligament* (lesser omentum). The liver is raised and the stomach drawn down as far as possible to permit an opening in the lesser omentum, exposing the lesser peritoneal sac. Easy access to the body and tail of the gland is not afforded by this route unless the pathologic condition is localized in their uppermost margins superior to the lesser curvature. Because of the confines of the space, very little room is available for operative manipulation by this route.

By far the best exposure of the pancreas is gained *through the gastrocolic ligament*. After making an incision between the stomach and transverse colon, the gastrocolic ligament may be incised throughout its entire breadth, sparing the gastro-epiploic arteries.

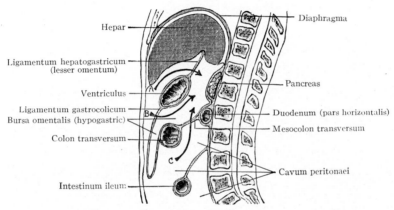

Hepar — Diaphragma

Ligamentum hepatogastricum (lesser omentum)

Pancreas

Ventriculus

Ligamentum gastrocolicum

Duodenum (pars horizontalis)

Bursa omentalis (hypogastric)

Mesocolon transversum

Colon transversum

Cavum peritonaei

Intestinum ileum

Fig. 360.—Sagittal Section to Show Surgical Approaches to the Body of the Pancreas. A is the approach through the gastrohepatic ligament; B is the approach through the gastrocolic ligament; C is the transmesocolic approach.

The edges of the incision are drawn apart and the greater curvature of the stomach is retracted upward and forward, opening the lesser sac widely. The anterior surface of the pancreas can be explored from its enclosure in the duodenal loop to its termination at the hilus of the spleen. The gland is recognized by its lobulated appearance, which is quite distinct through its thin peritoneal covering. This approach is the most direct route to the posterior aspect of the stomach (p. 323), the upper or supramesocolic area of the left kidney, and the splenic vessels. The structures are brought into view much more prominently with the patient in dorsal decubitus with a support under the midback.

Access to the lesser sac and the pancreas lying on its floor is afforded by incision *through the transverse mesocolon* in an avascular area. This route exposes satisfactorily only the middle portion of the gland.

2. Wounds of the Pancreas.—Because of the deep location of the pancreas in the floor of the lesser sac and the protection afforded it by the costal arch, injury to it is exceedingly rare. The hemorrhage consequent upon serious damage to the gland forms a large fluctuant tumor of blood and pancreatic fluid in the lesser sac, especially when adhesive peritonitis has blocked the epiploic foramen. In pancreatic wounds, torn vessels may be ligated without endangering the viability of the gland as there is an extensive vascular supply. In penetrating wounds involving both surfaces of the stomach, careful investigation of

the pancreas always should be made, lest a laceration be overlooked and the patient suc-
cumb from pancreatic necrosis and peritonitis.   The most important procedure is to secure
the general peritoneal cavity from the outflowing pancreatic juice.   For this purpose,
careful drainage to the exterior is necessary.   A pancreatic fistula is prone to occur in any
operative intervention on the pancreas; therefore, the gland should be drained by the
gastrohepatic or gastrocolic routes, depending upon where the effusion points.

   3. **Pancreatitis.**—In the last three decades, pancreatitis has received considerable
attention from both surgeon and pathologist.   At present, the etiology is thought to
be the admission of bile, or possibly duodenal contents, into the pancreatic duct.   The
disease is characterized by primary necrosis and secondary reactional inflammation, accompanied by symptoms of violent epigastric pain, often with shock, by toxemia from the
absorption of necrotic tissue products, by peritonitis, and by paralytic ileus.   Because of
the close relationship of the pancreatic and common bile ducts in the duodenal ampulla, a

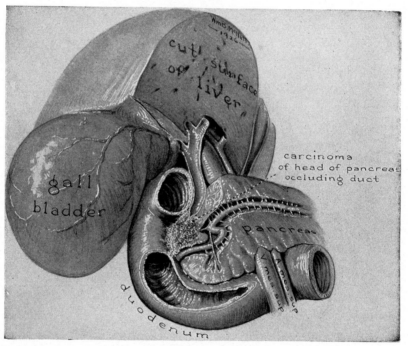

FIG. 361.—DISTENTION OF THE GALLBLADDER AND BILIARY DUCTS FROM CARCINOMA OF THE HEAD OF
THE PANCREAS OBSTRUCTING THE COMMON DUCT.   (Babcock, "Textbook of Surgery.")

stone of biliary origin impacted within the ampulla is a very likely source of pancreatic
disorder, but spasm of the sphincter (of Oddi) at the termination of the common duct likewise allows reflux of bile into the pancreatic duct.   A large stone may occupy the ampulla,
and actually occlude the orifices of the common bile and pancreatic ducts, producing disturbances in the liver and pancreas associated with retained secretion.   Simple inflammatory invasion of the pancreatic duct from the duodenum is a factor in some cases of
pancreatitis.   Blood stream infection sometimes causes pancreatitis.

   The development of peritonitis in pancreatitis usually is late, since the reaction at
first is confined to the lesser sac.   The chief aim in treatment should be direct drainage of
the pancreas, which probably is obtained best by the gastrocolic ligament approach.

   In patients who are not too acutely ill, an effort should be made to prevent further
entrance of bile into the pancreatic duct.   This is accomplished by inserting a safety valve
into the biliary system in the form of a drainage tube into the gallbladder, thus preventing
the possibility of any appreciable rise in bile pressure.

4. **Carcinoma of the Head of the Pancreas.**—Carcinoma is the tumor most commonly encountered in the pancreas, and its usual occurrence in the head of the gland almost invariably involves the common bile and pancreatic ducts by pressure. The gradually increasing jaundice which results from biliary obstruction without infection of the bile passages is a constant sign. The gallbladder gradually distends with bile until it presents as an ill-defined or a well-defined tumor against the anterior abdominal wall. The growth may encroach upon the descending duodenum to the degree of absolute obstruction. When the tumor presses upon the portal vein and the inferior vena cava, there may be evidences of venous congestion, ascites, and edema of the lower limbs. The only justified treatment is palliative, the standard operation being the union of the distended gallbladder with either the stomach or the duodenum (cholecystogastrostomy or cholecystoduodenostomy) (p. 357).

5. **Cysts of the Pancreas.**—Pancreatic cysts sometimes attain considerable size. While some originate behind obstruction of the main pancreatic duct by calculus or by pressure from without by a gallstone, the majority represent cystic transformations of destroyed pancreatic tissue, the result of acute pancreatic necrosis. Pseudocysts lie outside the pancreas, usually in the lesser sac. Generally, they are initiated by an attack of pancreatic necrosis.

A pancreatic cyst or pseudocyst usually presents an elastic swelling nearly always in the midepigastrium, but extending farther to the left than to the right. With increase in size, the cyst presses forward, but the projection appears at different levels. The progress of cyst growth may be upward and may appear above the lesser curvature of the stomach. In most instances, it presses straight forward, flattening out the stomach, and pressing the transverse colon downward until the cyst presents below the greater curvature at the gastrocolic ligament. It may burrow downward between the leaves of the transverse mesocolon, or present below the transverse mesocolon.

Cysts are exposed ordinarily by an incision in the median line above the umbilicus, through which they may be extirpated or their edges be sutured to the deeper layers of the abdominal wound (marsupialization), thereby establishing drainage.

(F) SPLEEN

1. **Definition and Location.**—The spleen, the vascular lymphoid organ located in the left hypochondrium under cover of the ninth, tenth, and eleventh ribs, is the largest of the ductless glands. Deeply concealed beneath the diaphragm and costal arch, it is hidden in great measure by the stomach.

2. **Thoracic Projection of the Spleen.**—The surface projection of the spleen is indicated by an oval area confined entirely to the thoracic region. Because of its concealed position, the normal spleen cannot be palpated. The enlarged spleen extends ventrally and lies close beneath the costal arch. With decided enlargement, the organ emerges from beneath the rib cage so that it is possible, especially if the abdominal wall is thin, to palpate the splenic notches of the anterior margin. The direction taken by an enlarging spleen is obliquely downward and mesial, since the phrenicocolic ligament and splenic flexure hinder its enlargement directly downward. This has a certain diagnostic value in differentiating an enlarged spleen from abdominal tumors. It is difficult to outline the spleen by percussion, because the lower border of the left lung intervenes between its upper half and the chest wall, and the stomach is applied against its visceral aspect.

3. **Peritoneal Connections.**—The layers of the *gastrolienal (splenic) omentum* separate at the hilus of the spleen. The outer layer invests the gland and then is reflected to the peritoneum over the anterior surface of the left kidney. The deep layer covers the splenic vessels and is continuous with the peritoneum of the floor of the lesser peritoneal sac. Behind and mesial to the spleen, these two layers contain the splenic vessels and form the *pancreaticolienal* or *lienorenal ligament* which passes between the hilum of the spleen and the ventral aspect of the kidney. The inferior extremity of the spleen lies upon, and sometimes is connected with, the *phrenicocolic ligament*, a fold of peritoneum connecting the splenic flexure of the colon with the diaphragm.

4. Displacements of the Spleen.—In addition to the support the spleen receives from its peritoneal connections, it is maintained in position by the pressure of the surrounding viscera, particularly the left kidney, the splenic flexure of the colon, and the stomach.

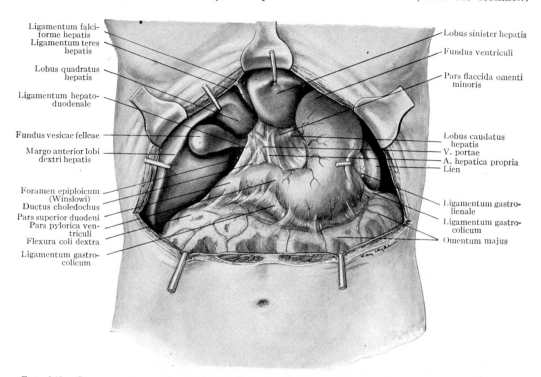

FIG. 362.—SUPRAMESOCOLIC VISCERA WITH SPECIAL REFERENCE TO THE LOCATION OF THE SPLEEN.

Abnormal mobility of the spleen occasionally is encountered as a congenital, but more frequently as an acquired, defect. Mobility is facilitated by stretching or tearing of the splenic ligaments by trauma or by the downward traction of the organ when enlarged.

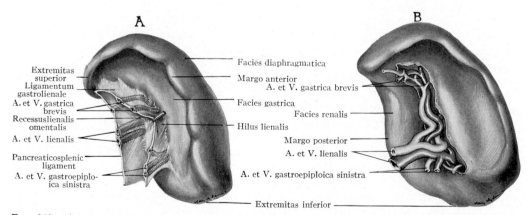

FIG. 363.—ANTERO-INTERNAL SURFACE OF THE SPLEEN WITH AND WITHOUT THE PERITONEAL CONNECTION AT THE HILUS.

The supporting ligaments may be elongated to a remarkable degree and the spleen may come to rest in the abdomen or pelvis, in which case it is known as a *prolapsed, ectopic,* or *wandering spleen.*

When the pedicle is elongated greatly and permits the spleen to float about the abdominal cavity upon the coils of intestine, it may rotate on its horizontal axis, resulting in torsion of the pedicle. The organ may become fixed in an abnormal position by adhesions forming between it and the parietal peritoneum or the viscera.

5. Vessels of the Spleen.—The arterial supply of the spleen comes from the large **lienal (splenic) artery** which runs a generally transverse course from right to left along the superior margin of the pancreas. Near the hilus, and within the lienorenal ligament, the artery divides into numerous branches, chief of which are: the superior polar, left gastro-epiploic, superior terminal, and inferior terminal arteries. The well-developed *superior polar artery* arises some distance from the hilus, and, before entering the spleen

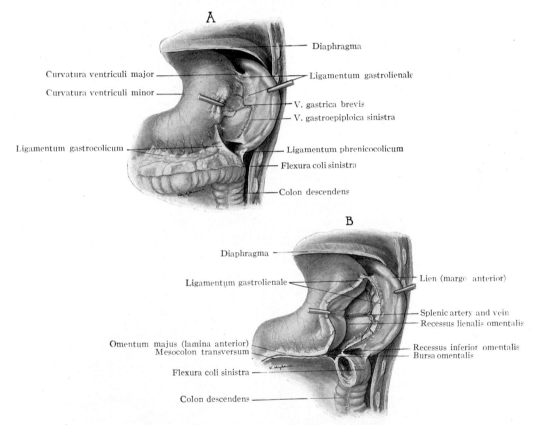

Fig. 364.—Anterior Views of the Splenic Recess to Show the Routes to the Splenic Vessels after the Lesser Sac Has Been Opened Through the Gastrosplenic Omentum.

A shows the enlarged spleen drawn laterally and the gastrosplenic ligament made tense; B shows the splenic vessels on the floor of the lesser sac after the gastrosplenic ligament has been divided.

gives off the short gastric arteries to the stomach. The *left gastro-epiploic artery* passes along the inferior pole of the spleen to supply part of the greater curvature of the stomach and the great omentum.

The *superior* and *inferior terminal arteries* resolve into secondary branches which penetrate the splenic parenchyma at the hilus along an irregularly disposed line drawn from one splenic pole to the other. The ultimate branches are end-vessels, each of which supplies a wedge-shaped area, the base of which is directed toward the periphery of the spleen. If one of these vessels is plugged, no blood passes directly into the area it supplies, and an *infarct* results. The central portion of the infarcted area is pale in color, but its outlying parts are stained deeply with blood which has diffused into it from the surrounding ascular zones. Infarction is common in heart disease in which emboli may be detached from the valves of the left side of the heart and carried into the aortic branches.

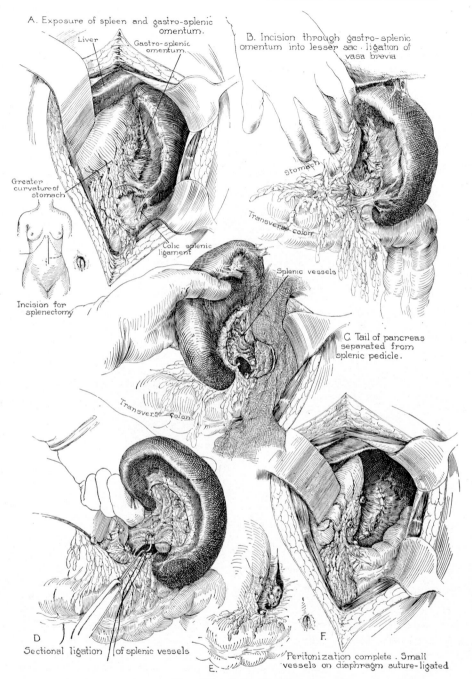

A. Exposure of spleen and gastro-splenic omentum.

Liver

Gastro-splenic omentum.

B. Incision through gastro-splenic omentum into lesser sac. ligation of vasa brevia

Stomach

Transverse colon

Greater curvature of stomach

Incision for splenectomy

Colic splenic ligament

Splenic vessels

C. Tail of pancreas separated from splenic pedicle.

Transverse colon

D
Sectional ligation of splenic vessels

F.

E.

Peritonization complete. Small vessels on diaphragm suture-ligated

FIG. 365.—SPLENECTOMY.

The **splenic vein** begins in several large branches leaving the hilum of the spleen. It pursues a much straighter course than the artery, and runs dorsal to the pancreas from left to right, joining with the superior mesenteric vein to form the portal vein (p. 341). The junction occurs behind the head of the pancreas and ventral to the inferior vena cava.

The **lymphatics** of the splenic capsule enter the lymph glands of the hilus, which, in turn, drain to the nodes along the splenic artery and into the celiac glands.

SURGICAL CONSIDERATIONS

1. **Injuries of the Spleen.**—The normal spleen is protected from injury better than are the other parenchymatous organs in the abdomen because of the overlying thoracic wall and its position against the resilient diaphragm. A blow of slight force may suffice to rupture a spleen that is enlarged, softened, or adherent. The contusion may leave no external sign indicating the severity of the internal trauma.

Injuries of the spleen are attended by very serious consequences because of the profuse hemorrhage which occurs. Splenic injury is complicated very frequently by wounds of the diaphragm, pleura, lungs, stomach, colon, and kidney. The spleen has been found partially or completely herniated through extensive wounds of the thoracic and abdominal walls. The generally accepted procedure in injuries to the spleen is splenectomy, as it is the surest way to control bleeding and is effective in all degrees of injury.

2. **Splenectomy.**—Access to the spleen is obtained by an oblique subcostal incision, by an angular or bow-shaped incision, or by a vertical incision similar to, but on the side opposite to that described for operation on the bile passages. There are two methods available for the removal of the organ. The splenic vessels may be exposed for ligation by incising the gastrocolic and gastrosplenic ligaments just above the transverse colon and opening the omental bursa (lesser sac). The stomach is retracted upward and the transverse colon and mesocolon are retracted downward. The peritoneum of the floor of the lesser sac is divided cautiously at the upper border of the pancreas at, or beyond, the tail, and beneath it the splenic vessels are located readily, the vein lying just caudal to the artery. Both vessels are ligated in this situation, and hemorrhage is controlled immediately. First the gastrosplenic, then the lienorenal ligament, is ligated and divided segment by segment, freeing the spleen.

If the spleen can be drawn forward into the abdominal wound, and there are no serious adhesions to the diaphragm and kidney, the left side of the lienorenal ligament may be exposed and ligature of the pedicle be undertaken from the general peritoneal cavity. The ligament is ligated and divided segment by segment, and the spleen drawn over to the left so that the same process may be instituted on the gastrosplenic ligament, thus freeing the spleen completely.

(II) INFRAMESOCOLIC VISCERA

The inframesocolic viscera include the bulk of the small intestine (jejuno-ileum), the ileocecal segment, and the ascending, transverse, and descending portions of the colon.

(A) JEJUNUM AND ILEUM (JEJUNO-ILEUM)

1. **Definition and Boundaries.**—The small bowel, extending from the duodenojejunal flexure to the cecum, is freely movable. The upper two fifths is *jejunum* and the lower three fifths *ileum*, but there is no morphologic demarcation between the two segments. The small bowel in the adult averages 22 feet in length. Its caliber is not uniform but diminishes from above downward, being narrowest at the termination.

2. **Position and Arrangement.**—The jejuno-ileum, contained within a limited space, of necessity is coiled in a complicated fashion. It is connected to the posterior abdominal wall by a fold of peritoneum, the mesentery proper, which allows great range of mobility. For the most part, the jejuno-ileum is contained in that part of the abdomen which lies below the subcostal plane and in the pelvis. The coils are related anteriorly to the anterior abdominal wall and the greater omentum, which, as a rule, is spread over them. They are hemmed in by the large bowel and related posteriorly to the posterior abdominal wall and retroperitoneal structures.

The position of the intestinal coils in the abdomen cannot be predetermined accurately. Several anatomic facts suggest that the largest part of the adult small intestine occupies the left half of the abdomen. These facts are: the natural position with reference to the mesenteric insertion, the elevated position of the left colic flexure, and the direct communication between the left half of the abdominal cavity and the pelvis.

Like its mesenteric attachment, the small intestine is disposed in an irregularly curved line from the upper left to the lower right quadrant. The uppermost portion lies in the left hypochondrium, reaching the left colic flexure, and is covered, to a degree, by the transverse colon and mesocolon. The succeeding loops lie in the right abdominal cavity, whence they extend into the left iliac fossa and then again to the right to fill the pelvis. From the pelvis, a terminal loop passes upward into the right iliac fossa to join the large bowel. In pelvic peritonitis of tubal, ovarian, or appendiceal origin, the pelvic loops become involved and adherent. Pelvic coils are most liable to strangulation by obstructive bands from an adhesive peritonitis.

3. **Mesentery of the Jejuno-ileum.**—A mesentery suspends the jejuno-ileum from the posterior abdominal wall and contains the neurovascular system of the intestines. Its

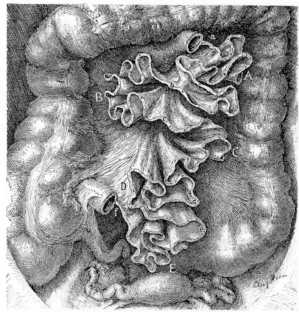

Fig. 366.—Mesenteric Ruffle Showing the Groups and Disposition of the Coils of the Jejuno-ileum.

A attaches to the proximal coils of jejunum; B attaches to a more terminal group of jejunal coils; C marks the attachment of coils which are part jejunum and part ileum; D attaches to the proximal coils of ileum and E attaches to the terminal coils of ileum. (Kelly, Hurdon, "Vermiform Appendix.")

parietal or root attachment extends from the left side of the second lumbar vertebra downward to the right across the aorta and inferior vena cava to the right sacro-iliac joint, a distance of about 15 cm. It crosses the ventral surface of the transverse stage of the duodenum where it contains between its layers the superior mesenteric vessels, the lymphatics, and the nerves. Removal of a cyst or solid tumor of the mesentery endangers the terminal blood supply of the intestines and exposes them to gangrene. The mesentery in traversing the inframesocolic compartment converts it into two spaces, that to the right being much the smaller and terminating in the right iliac fossa, and that to the left being much the larger and passing uninterruptedly into the true pelvis.

The distance between the intestinal and parietal mesenteric attachments is insignificant at the upper and lower extremities, and is greatest where the attachment crosses the spine. The depth of the mesentery, as a rule, does not exceed 20 to 25 cm. The length, in many instances, permits the descent of the small bowel into the sac of an inguinal

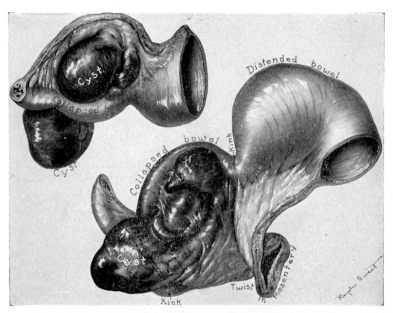

FIG. 367.—MESENTERIC CYST. (Roller, Surg., Gynec. and Obst., June, 1935.)

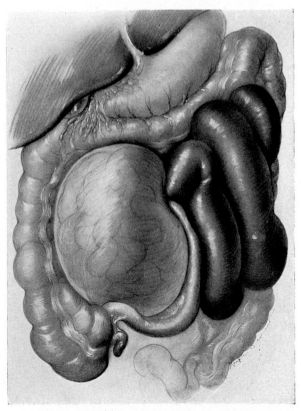

FIG. 368.—MESENTERICOPARIETAL HERNIA OF WALDEYER. (F. Foote, Calif. and West. Med.)

or femoral hernia.   When the mesentery seems unusually long, it probably is not actually lengthened, but is able to slide downward on a loose extraperitoneal attachment.

Fat deposition is marked along the mesenteric root and diminishes toward the intestinal attachment.   The amount of fat is greater in the distal end of the mesentery than in the proximal.   A group of infected lymph nodes in the mesentery may become adherent to an adjoining loop of small bowel and cause a mechanical intestinal obstruction.   An acute terminal *mesenteric lymphadenitis* frequently is indistinguishable from acute appendicitis.   Near the duodenojejunal flexure can be seen semitranslucent areas of peritoneum, separated from one another by branches of the superior mesenteric vessels.   These areas or "windows" become more obscure as the jejunum is traced distally, until, in the distal part of the ileum, they scarcely can be distinguished because of the deposition of fat near and about the bowel.   An examination of the mesentery, therefore, may determine whether a loop of small intestine drawn through an abdominal wound belongs to a proximal or a distal segment.

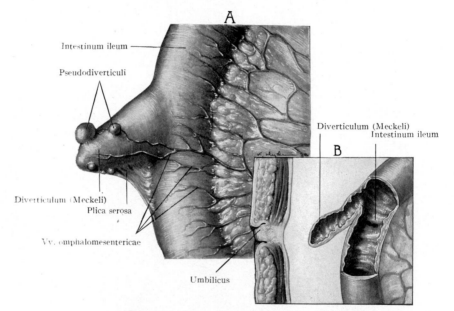

FIG. 369.—ILEAL DIVERTICULUM (OF MECKEL).

A shows the diverticulum along which lie the omphalo(vitello)-intestinal vessels; B shows a section removed from the ileum and from the diverticulum.   (After Cullen.)

Failure of the root of the mesentery to fuse over its entire extent with the posterior parietal peritoneum allows a pocket to be formed between it and the peritoneum which may form the sac of an intraperitoneal hernia (*mesentericoparietal hernia of Waldeyer*).

4. **Structure.**—Beneath the serosa, the small bowel possesses a strong muscle coat, which consists of an outer longitudinal and an inner circular layer.   Plicae circulares (valvulae conniventes), ridges of the thick mucosa which begin in the descending duodenum, are numerous in the proximal jejunum.   By grasping the jejunum between the thumb and finger, these folds can be felt through the wall of the gut; their absence in the distal ileum serves to distinguish the proximal from the distal segment.   In the ileum, but not in the jejunum, are numerous aggregated lymph nodules which vary in length from 2 to 10 cm.   They form granular patches (Peyer's patches) in the mucosa along the antimesenteric border.

5. **Abnormalities of the Omphalo(Vitello)-intestinal Duct.**—In the early human embryo, the convexity of the umbilical loop of the primitive gut communicates freely with the yolk sac by the *omphalo(vitello)-intestinal* duct.   As development proceeds, the

duct normally becomes occluded and later disappears entirely. All or any part of the duct may persist. With the *duct completely permeable*, a *congenital fecal fistula* at the umbilicus results. The duct may be several inches in length or so short that the ileum itself appears to open on the surface.

In the latter instance, the mesenteric wall of the bowel may prolapse through the opening and produce intestinal obstruction. Persistence of the intra-embryonic duct is to be differentiated from *persistence* of a *small part* of the *extra-embryonic duct* which causes a mucous discharge. Probing of the duct indicates which condition is present.

With the *duct partially persistent*, only that part of the duct immediately deep to the umbilicus may remain patent, and a *cyst opening on the umbilicus* occur, or only the middle portion may persist and a *cyst of the duct* occur. A free *blind diverticulum attached to the ileum* (*Meckel's diverticulum*) is the commonest anomaly. It usually occurs within a meter of the terminal ileum, and may or may not possess a mesentery. When the opening into the cavity is larger than the caliber of the tube in general, there is little danger of infection (*Meckel's diverticulitis*) from fecal impaction or from a foreign body. The free diverticulum may be attached to the umbilicus by a fibrous cord, around which intestinal loops may become obstructed. Occasionally, the *vitello-intestinal vessels may persist* with no trace of the diverticulum. In inflammation, the free diverticulum may acquire adhesions to any neighboring structure and cause intestinal obstruction.

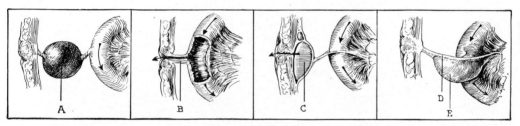

FIG. 370.—VARIETIES OF OMPHALO(VITELLO)-INTESTINAL PATHOLOGY.

A, Cyst caused by torsion of the omphalomesenteric duct; B, patent omphalomesenteric duct; C, cyst of the umbilicus, the result of a remnant of the omphalomesenteric duct; D, fibrous cord from omphalomesenteric vessels; E, Meckel's diverticulum. (After Cullen.)

6. Vessels and Nerves.—The arteries supplying the jejuno-ileum spring from the left aspect of the *superior mesenteric artery* which arises from the aorta about 2 cm. below the origin of the celiac trunk, behind the head of the pancreas. This artery leaves the deep surface of the gland at the incisura and enters the root of the mesentery. As it descends toward the right iliac fossa, it describes a curve with a convexity directed to the left. It terminates at the mesial aspect of the cecum by anastomosing with one of its own branches, the ileocolic artery.

Close to the origin of the trunk, the inferior pancreaticoduodenal artery is given off. It runs to the right between the head of the pancreas and the duodenum, supplying both these structures and anastomosing with the superior pancreaticoduodenal artery (p. 360). The intestinal arteries break up into a series of arcades which are more complex in the ileum than in the jejunum. From the convexities of the terminal arcades, small parallel vessels (vasa recti) pass to the mesenteric border of the bowel and bifurcate. In the intestinal wall, the vessels run parallel to the circular muscle coat, traversing successively the serous, muscle, and submucous layers. Injury to the mesentery containing these vessels is likely to cause gangrene in the part of the bowel they supply, because the anastomoses of the superior mesenteric artery with the celiac and inferior mesenteric arteries are not adequate to reestablish circulation if a large trunk or one of its main branches is destroyed. In sectioning the bowel for anastomosis, it is advisable to remove less of the mesenteric than of the antimesenteric border in order that the cut margin may have a good blood supply.

The middle colic, right colic and ileocolic arteries are described in the civic and ileo-cecal regions.

The *superior mesenteric vein* returns blood from the small intestine, and from the ascending and transverse colon.   Behind the neck of the pancreas, it unites with the splenic vein to form the portal vein (p. 341).   The superior mesenteric vein may be the site of a thrombosing phlebitis, terminating in intestinal venous engorgement, gangrene, intestinal obstruction, and peritonitis.

The *lymphatics* originate in the central lacteals of the mucosal villi and are directed to rich plexuses in the submucous coats.   The plexuses join the superior mesenteric lymph glands within the mesentery where they lie in close relation to the arterial arches.   This intramesenteric group of glands may be infected with tuberculosis directly from the ali-

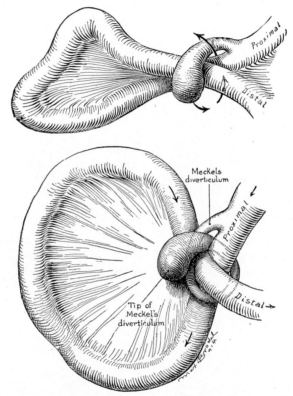

FIG. 371.—A DIVERTICULUM TYING OFF A LOOP OF SMALL BOWEL.
This indicates the manner in which the obstruction occurred; a Meckel's diverticulum has dropped over a loop of bowel which has been twisted; after passing under the loop, the diverticulum curves upward and passes through the space between the base of the diverticulum and the adjacent small bowel; there is consequent distention of the constricted bowel and complete obstruction has resulted.   (Cullen.)

mentary tract.   Tuberculous infection, spreading along the lymphatics from an ulcerated aggregated lymph nodule (Peyer's patch) may cause a stricture of the bowel.   Acute miliary tuberculosis commonly arises in this way in consequence of the large numbers of bacilli passing from the lymphatics into the lymphatic duct and thence into the general circulation.   Aggregated lymph nodules are most numerous in the terminal ileum which is consequently the most common site for tuberculous stricture.

The *nerve supply* of the small intestine is derived from the celiac plexus of the sympathetic system and from the vagus.   Referred pain in connection with a lesion of the small bowel is experienced in areas supplied by the ninth, tenth, and eleventh thoracic nerves. Clinically, the pain usually is about the umbilical region, and only occasionally spreads to the lumbar region and back.

SURGICAL CONSIDERATIONS

1. Intestinal Injuries.—Of all the abdominal viscera, the small bowel is exposed most to injury, but the elasticity and ease with which the coils glide over one another and elude pressure serve to protect it.

A minute puncture wound of the bowel may not lead to extravasation of intestinal contents as the muscle coats may contract so as to close the opening. If the rent is large and mucosa is everted into the wound, spontaneous closure becomes difficult. The bowel may be injured to the point of severance by traumatic compression against the spinal column or sacral promontory. Intestinal perforation should be closed surgically at the earliest possible moment.

2. Enterostomy.—An enterostomy is the formation of an artificial fistulous communication between the lumen of some part of the small bowel and the surface of the skin, to serve, temporarily at least, as an intestinal outlet. The procedure is usually

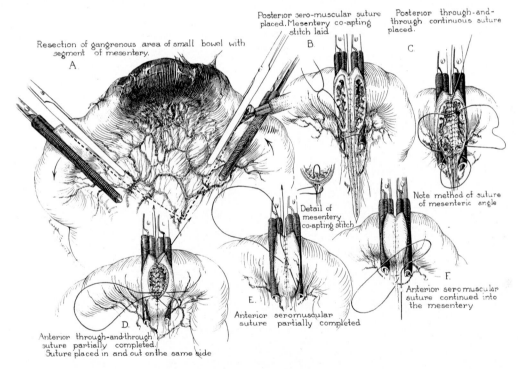

FIG. 372.—OPEN METHOD OF SMALL BOWEL ANASTOMOSIS.

resorted to as a means of emptying the bowel in intestinal obstruction, or as an inlet to furnish nourishment.

An *ileostomy* is an enterostomy generally performed in the right inguinal region for obstruction about the ileocecal segment. The opening is made proximal to the obstruction and often is intended to be temporary. The first distended loop proximal to the cecum is withdrawn through the abdominal wound and attached to its edges on a level with or a little above its surface. If the bowel must be opened at once, a tube may be purse strung into the antimesenteric border of the ileum and the liquid and gaseous contents of the loops be evacuated. Adhesions form to seal off the peritoneal cavity before the suture holding the tube in position becomes loose. If the bowel need not be opened at once, and time is allowed for the peritoneal union of the bowel to the margins of the wound, the presenting antimesenteric border of the small intestine may be cauterized or incised axially and the contents be allowed to escape on the dressings in and about the wound.

An ileostomy which is to establish a **permanent** artificial anus for the small intestine differs from the temporary fecal fistula in that the operation is performed to relieve an irremovable obstruction. It contemplates attaching a knuckle of bowel rather than a flat surface of bowel into the abdominal wound. A sufficient length of intestinal loop is brought out and anchored into the wound to insure a spur formation of the mesenteric border.

A *jejunostomy* is that form of enterostomy in which a fistulous communication is made between the upper jejunum and the skin surface. It is regarded as a standard operation for the formation of a nourishment-giving fistula in cases in which the stomach no longer is pervious or cannot be rendered so by operation, as in advanced gastric malignancy where neither gastro-enterostomy nor gastrostomy is possible. Often, it is a life-saving procedure in relieving the obstruction of postoperative paralytic ileus.

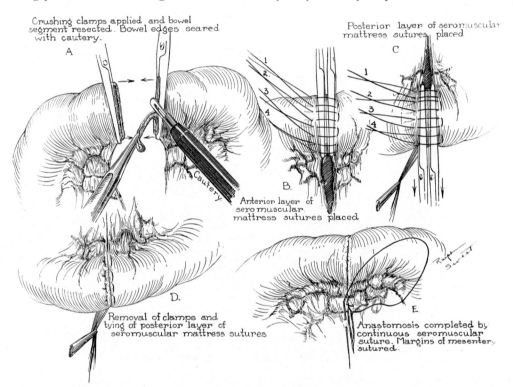

FIG. 373.—CLOSED (ASEPTIC) METHOD OF SMALL BOWEL ANASTOMOSIS.

3. Enterectomy or Intestinal Resection.—The intestinal segment to be resected is drawn outside the abdomen. Pairs of clamps are placed transversely on the bowel above and below the selected part, and the bowel is divided with a cautery between each pair of clamps. Section of the mesentery is made as close as possible to the intestinal attachment. Resection of a wedge-shaped segment of mesentery with the intestine has been advocated. It is recommended that the intestine be divided, not at right angles to its long axis, but somewhat obliquely, with removal of more of the antimesenteric than the mesenteric margin. This spares the transverse vessels which run toward the convexity of the bowel and assures a better blood supply to the sutured ends, with avoidance of a zone of necrosis.

The divided ends may be united by end-to-end or by lateral anastomosis. In *end-to-end union*, the mode of attachment of the mesentery to the bowel is important. The layers of the mesentery diverge slightly as they approach the intestine, and the intervening space is occupied by lymphatics, blood vessels, and fatty areolar tissue. When the divided ends of the intestine are brought together for suture. it is necessary that the junction be effected in such a way that the outer or serous surfaces of the two ends come into accurate apposition along the suture line.   It long has been recognized that the two peritoneal surfaces connected in this way adhere very quickly and securely.   At the mesenteric attachment, the ends of the intestine come together over a narrow area devoid of peritoneum. Union of the apposing surfaces is not effected as rapidly at this point and may result in subsequent leakage of bowel contents.

In *lateral intestinal anastomosis* after partial enterectomy, the free ends of intestine are closed by suture and the lateral aspect of the closed upper segment is approximated to and united with the lateral aspect of the closed lower segment.   The technic for the lateral anastomosis is similar to that for gastrojejunostomy (p. 327).

(B) ILEOCECAL-APPENDICEAL REGION

The few terminal centimeters of the ileum, the cecum, and the appendix may be grouped into an important surgical anatomic composite.

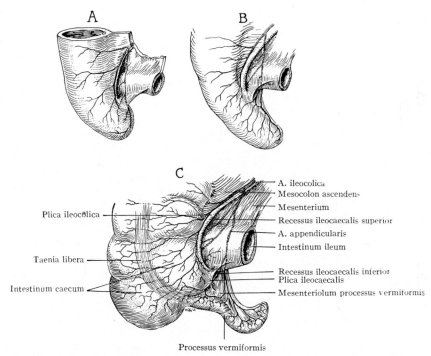

FIG. 374.—DEVELOPMENT OF THE CECUM AND APPENDIX AND THEIR BLOOD SUPPLY.   (After Kelly, Hurdon)

During early development, the large intestine is a tube of uniform dimensions and its cecal segment presents no distinguishing features.   The lower part of the cecal segment lags in growth, while the upper part keeps pace with the growth of the colon.   As the difference in size becomes greater, the lower tapering extremity becomes the vermiform appendix, and the roomy part above it, the cecum.   At birth, the cecum has a conical shape, a smooth external appearance, and a well-marked curve in its long axis with its concavity directed upward and inward, so that the tip of the appendix comes into close proximity with the end of the ileum.   By the third year, longitudinal bands, or taeniae, with sacculi between them, are developed.   The sacculus between the anterior and lateral bands develops out of proportion to the others and causes the cecum to assume a globoid form.   This large sacculus forms the most dependent part, or fundus, and the greater part of the anterior wall of the cecum.   The appendix is attached, then, to the medial and posterior aspect of the cecal segment

The large intestine differs from the small intestine in several particulars. It is not surrounded entirely by its longitudinal muscle coat, but derives from it three narrow bands, the taeniae coli, which are clearly visible through the serosa. Its wall is thinner, chiefly because of the deficiency in the longitudinal coat. It has epiploic appendices, small peritoneal sacs filled with fat, which are attached mainly to the transverse and sigmoid portions of the colon.

1. Anatomic Summary of the Cecum.—The cecum comprises that part of the large bowel located below a transverse line passing just above the ileocecal valve. It is about 6 cm. long and 7 cm. wide, and lies normally upon the iliopsoas muscle in the right iliac fossa in the angle formed by the flare of the ilium and the anterior abdominal wall. When filled with gas and fluid, the cecum reaches the mesial border of the psoas muscle and may form a palpable, and sometimes visible, tumor mass. Manipulation of this tumor often produces gurgling. In certain cases of obstruction in the large bowel, *perforation of the uninvolved cecum* sometimes occurs. Certain factors cause the cecum, rather than other parts of the colon, to give away. The cecum is the thinnest walled part of the colon. Second, carcinoma at the splenic flexure, for example, produces partial obstruction for some time. Chronic distention and hypertrophy of the proximal large bowel occur. The bowel wall hypertrophy gradually diminishes toward the cecum, which is thinner and relatively weaker. For cecal perforation to occur, the ileocecal valve must be closed to localize distention at the cecum. Incompetence of the ileocecal valve makes diastasic perforation of the cecum as rare as it is (Saeltzer and Rhodes). As a rule, the cecum is covered by peritoneum and is freely dependent in the general cavity. Coils of small intestine usually conceal the empty cecum. The anterior cecal band is a guide to the appendix, as it is continued, with the two other bands, into the outer longitudinal muscle of that structure.

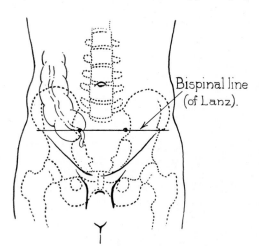

FIG. 375.—LOCATION OF BASE OF APPENDIX ALONG LANZ' LINE.
Point located at junction of right and middle thirds of Lanz' line.

As a consequence of incomplete development of the colon, the cecum may occupy a high position and lie on the right kidney below the liver. In its low position, it may lie in the depth of the pelvis. In the fetus and infant, it lies high in the iliac fossa. In adults, and especially in old people, it lies lower down. Its elongation and descent with advancing age favor the presence of the cecum and appendix in the sac of an inguinal hernia. Because of the proximity of the cecum and appendix to the right abdominal inguinal ring, they occasionally present in a right inguinal hernia, even in children. As a result of faulty development, rotation, and fixation of the intestine, the ileocecal-appendiceal segment may occupy almost any portion of the abdomen.

Abnormal positions of the cecum possess a high degree of practical surgical interest because of the difficulty in diagnosis and the complications they introduce should appendicitis supervene. Occasionally, the cecum and colon retain their fetal peritoneal connections and are suspended from the posterior abdominal wall by a mesentery, allowing an abnormal range of mobility. This condition makes it possible for the ileocecal segment to become twisted upon its own mesenteric axis or about an adjacent coil (volvulus), and greatly enhances the occurrence of an intussusception (p. 380).

2. Appendix.—The vermiform process, or appendix, attaches to the posteromesial border of the cecum about 2.5 cm. below the ileocecal junction and always can be located by tracing the anterior longitudinal band distally. The excessive growth of the right wall of the cecum causes the appendix to lie to its medial side. It is uniformly cylindrical and usually is from 6 to 12 cm. long and about 0.8 cm. wide, but the length is extremely variable. It possesses the same layers as does the large bowel. The muscular coat in areas, however, may be so deficient that the peritoneum and mucous membrane are separated only by a thin layer of connective tissue, through which infection can spread easily. Divertication of the mucosa, with or without infection, is not uncommon. Its orifice into the cecum is guarded by a crescentic mucosal fold, absence or incompetence of which may account for the presence of fecal material within the process. The mesoappendix is a triangular peritoneal fold attached to the left, or lower aspect of the mesentery of the ileum, or, if shortened, to the posterior abdominal wall near the pelvic brim.

Although the relation of the base of the appendix to the cecum is constant, the appendix possesses a wide range of movement and may occupy a great variety of positions.

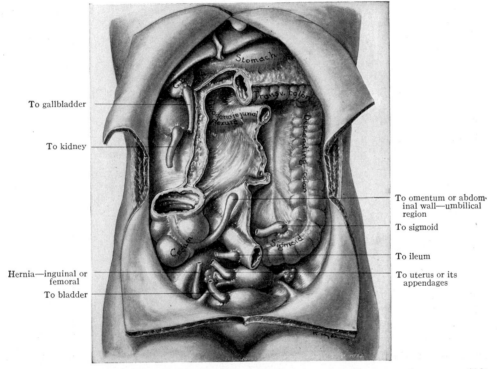

To gallbladder

To kidney

To omentum or abdominal wall—umbilical region

To sigmoid

To ileum

To uterus or its appendages

Hernia—inguinal or femoral

To bladder

Fig. 376.—Diagram to Show the Various Points of Attachment of an Inflamed Appendix. (After Kelly, Hurdon.)

It sometimes crosses the psoas muscle, and its apex hangs over the pelvic brim. When the appendix becomes inflamed and fixed to the psoas muscle, stretching of the muscle by extension or hyperextension of the thigh causes pain. This finding is a valuable diagnostic sign. If the appendix hangs over the pelvic brim, it will rest on the pelvic fascia overlying the obturator internus muscle. If the organ becomes inflamed in this situation, the underlying peritoneum and fascia also may become inflamed. Stretching the obturator internus muscle by flexing and rotating the thigh medially causes the patient pain by irritating the overlying fascia and peritoneum (*obturator internus test*). An inflamed appendix in a pelvic position (*pelvic appendicitis*) may result in adhesions connecting it with the rectum and bladder which may produce painful defecation and micturition. An inflamed appendix in a pelvic position in the female is difficult to differentiate from infection of the tube and ovary because of the close relationship of the structures. Pelvic appendicitis or culdesac abscess in the female causes less bladder irritation than in the male because the pelvic partition in the female protects the bladder. Differential diagnosis is aided by the relation of the pain to the menstrual period and by rectal or vaginal examination.

The appendix may ascend behind the cecum, where its relationship with the peritoneum varies. It may possess a mesentery and be free in the retrocecal fossa, be plastered against the posterior aspect of the cecum, lie on the anterior wall of the fossa, or lie against the iliac fascia on the posterior wall of the fossa. An inflamed retrocecal appendix may be attached secondarily to the parietal peritoneum of the false pelvis. An abscess from a retrocecal appendix becomes walled off, overhung by the cecum and, at times, by the inferior part of the ascending mesocolon.

3. **Colic (Ileocecal) Valve.**—The colic valve is located at the entrance of the ileum into the large intestine opposite the junction of the cecum and ascending colon. *In situ*, it appears as a buttonhole slit. The soft, rounded edges of the valve project prominently

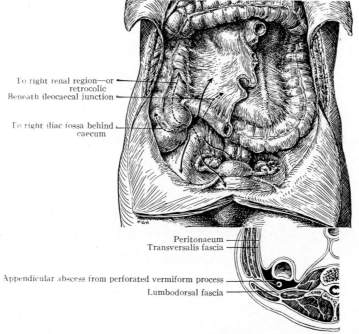

To right renal region—or retrocolic
Beneath ileocaecal junction
To right iliac fossa behind caecum

Peritonaeum
Transversalis fascia

Appendicular abscess from perforated vermiform process
Lumbodorsal fascia

FIG 377.—MORE COMMON PATHS OF INFECTION FROM THE APPENDIX AND THE USUAL LOCATIONS OF APPENDICEAL ABSCESSES.

Inset is a cross section showing location of a retrocecal abscess.

into the lumen of the large bowel. The valve consists of an upper and lower segment which are formed by a duplication of the wall of the small and large bowels. The circular muscle of the terminal ileum is the ileocolic sphincter; it regulates the flow of chyme into the cecum, preventing regurgitation into the ileum.

4. **Peritoneal Folds and Recesses about the Cecum and Terminal Ileum.**—The cecum and appendix usually have a complete investment of peritoneum, so that all of the cecum, or only its caput, hangs free in the iliac fossa much as the heart does in the pericardium. The usual line of peritoneal connection and fixation is at the beginning of the ascending colon. Sometimes, part or all of the posterior surface of the cecum, and even the appendix, is fused to the primitive parietal peritoneum of the iliac fossa. Even though the cecum is fixed in this way, a cellular fascial layer lies between it and the actual extraperitoneal tissue. This retrocecal fusion fascia is derived from embryonic fusion between the dorsal peritoneum of the cecum and the primitive parietal peritoneum of the iliac fossa. By inci-

sion of the iliac peritoneum just lateral to the cecum, the cecum can be pulled mesially, making the appendicocecal segment more accessible surgically. A fixed cecum, by sliding downward and laterally, may engage in the abdominal inguinal ring and present in the inguinal canal as a hernia with a partial sac or no sac (sliding hernia) (p. 382).

The appendicocecal peritoneum is lifted into folds by vessels which run to the different segments. These folds bound fairly constant peritoneal recesses.

The *ileocolic fold* is attached over a variable extent to the anterior surface of the mesentery of the terminal ileum and to the anterior aspect of the ascending colon. The free border of the fold, looking downward and to the left, contains the anterior cecal branch of the ileocolic artery. This fold is the anterior boundary of the *superior ileocecal (ileocolic) recess* which lies in the angle between the ileum and the ascending colon.

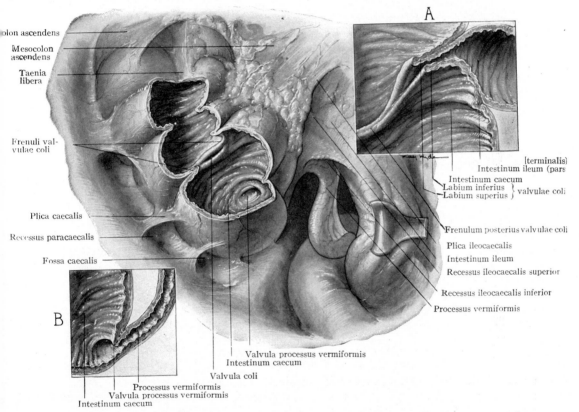

Colon ascendens

Mesocolon ascendens

Taenia libera

Frenuli valvulae coli

Plica caecalis

Recessus paracaecalis

Fossa caecalis

A

B

[terminalis]
Intestinum ileum (pars
Intestinum caecum
Labium inferius }
Labium superius } valvulae coli

Frenulum posterius valvulae coli

Plica ileocaecalis

Intestinum ileum

Recessus ileocaecalis superior

Recessus ileocaecalis inferior

Processus vermiformis

Valvula processus vermiformis
Intestinum caecum

Valvula coli

Processus vermiformis
Valvula processus vermiformis
Intestinum caecum

FIG. 378.—ILEOCECAL REGION WITH PART OF THE ANTERIOR WALL REMOVED TO DEMONSTRATE THE ILEOCECAL VALVE AND THE ORIGIN OF THE APPENDIX.
A, a detailed drawing of the ileocecal valve; B, a frontal section through the proximal end of the cecum and appendix.

The *ileocecal fold* is avascular, occupies the ileocecal angle, and forms the forward wall of the *ileocecal (appendicular) recess*. The posterior wall of the fossa is formed by the mesoappendix.

An avascular *retrocecal fold* sometimes extends from the ascending colon and cecum across the lower part of the right paracolic gutter to the peritoneum of the iliac fossa. This fold helps to limit the retrocecal fossa and the beginning of the ascending colon. The depth of the fold depends upon the height at which the peritoneal reflection from the intestine to the iliac fossa or lumbar region occurs. The fossa may be very large and its blind extremity reach to the level of the kidney. The appendix, twisted on itself, often is found here. While these recesses very rarely contain small bowel or form intraperitoneal herniae, they have real significance in connection with encysted appendiceal abscesses.

5. Vessels and Nerves.—The cecum, the inferior part of the ascending colon, the appendix, and the terminal ileum are supplied by the *ileocolic artery*. This vascular distribution is one indication of the anatomic individuality of the ileocecal segment. The artery arises from the superior mesenteric trunk below the transverse portion of the duodenum and runs downward and to the right across the ureter and psoas major muscle toward the ileocolic angle. It divides into four terminal branches. The anterior and posterior cecal arteries supply corresponding surfaces of the cecum. The appendiceal artery runs behind the terminal ileum to the tip of the appendix and sends out en route a series of straight branches. It is a terminal vessel and, if kinked or obstructed entirely, the blood supply of the appendix is cut off so that gangrene ensues. The ileal artery supplies the terminal ileum.

The *veins* of the ileocecal segment are tributary to the superior mesenteric trunk of the portal, and phlebitis involving them may result in liver abscesses (p. 342).

The *lymphatics* of the cecum and appendix terminate in a group of glands lying about the origin of the terminals of the ileocolic artery. Excessive enlargement of these nodes may encroach upon the lumen of the terminal ileum sufficiently to cause intestinal obstruction. These lymphatics anastomose with the lumbo-iliac chain. This connection accounts for infection of the retroperitoneal tissues of the posterior wall of the pelvis following appendicitis.

Surgical Considerations

1. Appendicitis.—Certain anatomic conditions predispose the appendix to inflammation. Among the principal of these are: the relatively large amount of lymphoid tissue within its walls, the long, narrow lumen ending in a culdesac, the dependent position, and the open communication with the cecum where fecal material collects.

Attention is directed to the limited anastomosis of the artery of the appendix with the vessels of the cecum. In the event of obstruction of the appendiceal artery from any cause, gangrene of the appendix may supervene. A stricture of the appendix, or varying degrees of obliteration of its cavity. predisposes to recurrent attacks of appendicitis by obstructing the escape of contained fluids into the cecum.

2. Surgical Access to the Appendix.—Save in collapse from severe peritonitis, appendectomy is indicated in any stage of appendicitis or in the interval between attacks. An appendiceal abscess may require drainage independently of appendectomy to prevent the spread of infection consequent upon the trauma of removal of an organ exceedingly difficult of access.

The surgical approach is determined by the duration of the infection. Operations early in the disease require the smallest incisions and the simplest technic. The intermuscular approach (of McBurney) (p. 285) and the pararectus incision (p. 284) are used most commonly. Operation in advanced chronic infection may require wide incision and careful manipulation because of attendant adhesions. In appendiceal abscesses, the McBurney approach best protects the general cavity.

3. Intussusception.—An intussusception is a prolapse or invagination of a portion of the intestine into the lumen of an immediately adjoining segment. Many cases of acute intestinal obstruction, especially in infants and young children, originate in intussusception. The high incidence in infants is accounted for by the fact that there exists during the first year the greatest relative disproportion between the large and small intestine. The most frequent site for an invagination is the ileocecal region, since incipient intussusception always is present because of the normal invagination of the circular muscle coat into the segments of the ileocecal valve. The condition can occur only when the terminal ileum or ascending colon possesses a mesentery of considerable length. The existence of a mobile ascending mesocolon makes it possible for a considerable invagination of the cecum into the ascending colon to occur without interfering with the blood supply of either viscus. Whereas the existence of a mesentery predisposes to intussusception, it protects the blood supply of the bowel, at least for a time, against strangulation and gangrene.

Certain terms are applied to the parts of a completely developed intussusception. The entering or invaginating tube is the *intussusceptum;* the sheath or receiving tube is the *intussuscipiens.* The apex of the entering or invaginating tube is the *head* of the intussusception and the junction of the ensheathing and entering layers of the intussuscipiens is the *neck.* Once the process of invagination has begun, the entering tube acts as a foreign body and stimulates the receiving tube to advance the prolapsed part. The growth of the intussusception occurs at the expense of the receiving tube.

In the ileocecal form of intussusception, the ileocecal junction is the head of the intussusception and the wall of the ascending colon the intussuscipiens. The wall of the colon turns in more and more until the head of the intussusceptum finally may reach the rectum and protrude through the anal aperture. For an intussusception as extensive as this to occur, the large intestine must have a free range of mobility, such as it possesses when it retains its original mesentery.

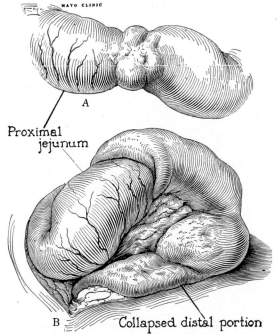

FIG. 379.—TUMOR OF JEJUNUM CAUSING INTUSSUSCEPTION
A, Tumor of jejunum after reduction of intussusception; B, intussusception in the jejunum. (Dixon and Stewart, Surg., Gynec. and Obst., April, 1933.)

Infolding of the intussusception is arrested if the mesentery of the intussuscipiens is too short to permit further invagination. This mechanism is illustrated in the ileocecal segment where the ascending colon acquires varying adhesions with the primitive parietal peritoneum.

Complications which may supervene in an unreduced intussusception are gangrene of the whole or part of the entering tube and obstruction to the passage of the intestinal contents. When the mesentery is constricted at the neck of an intussusception, the venous return is obstructed. Swelling of the intussusceptum and oozing of blood into the bowel lumen result. The arterial flow finally is obstructed and the intussusceptum undergoes partial or complete necrosis and may be cast off into the bowel as a slough. If adhesions have formed at the neck of the intussusception before the necrosis occurs, a spontaneous cure may result.

An intussusception is recognized by its sudden onset, the presence of a tumor mass localized resistance, the colic pain of obstruction, and the discharge of blood-stained mucus.

4. Cecal Herniae.—A prolapsed low-lying cecum may present in a variety of ways in a right inguinal hernia. The degree of peritoneal fixation of the prolapsed bowel influences materially the results of operation to restore the hernial contents to the abdominal cavity and remake the abdominal wall.

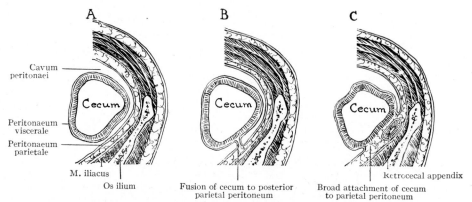

FIG. 380.—CROSS SECTIONS AT THE LEVEL OF THE CECUM AND THE ILIAC FOSSA TO SHOW VARIATIONS IN THE DEGREE OF FUSION OF THE CECUM TO THE PERITONEUM OF THE ILIAC FOSSA.

In A, the cecum is unattached and free; in B, the cecum is bound down by a narrow fold; in C, the cecum with a retrocecal appendix is bound down to the iliac peritoneum over an extensive area. (After Testut and Jacob.)

A mobile cecum, entirely covered by peritoneum, sometimes is found *free in a hernial sac* and presents no operative difficulties as it can be replaced easily in the abdomen, allowing ligation and excision of the sac.

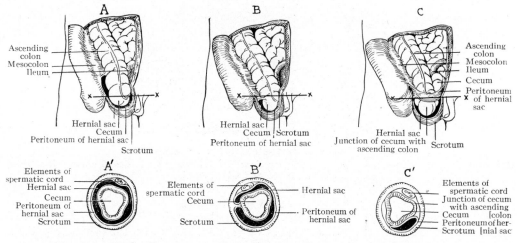

FIG. 381.—THREE VARIETIES OF HERNIA OF THE CECUM AND ASCENDING COLON.

A is a hernia of a mobile or unfixed cecum and the sac is complete (see A′); in B, the cecum in the hernia has a narrow mesentery and therefore the hernial sac is incomplete (see B′); C is a hernia of the junction of the cecum and ascending colon and is almost without a sac; most of the bowel is directly in contact with the hernial coverings, no sac intervening; there is a vestige of sac at the upper portion of the hernia (see C′).

A′, B′, and C′ are horizontal sections through the ruptures taken along the lines *xx*. (After Testut and Jacob.)

When the cecum is fixed partially to the parietal peritoneum by a mesentery-like attachment and presents in a hernial sac, the *sac is incomplete* over the attached area of the bowel behind. In this instance, the prolapsed cecum cannot be reduced until the cecum is mobilized by blunt or sharp dissection.

When the cecal hernia presents *no sac*, as may occur late in life, the cecum or junction of the cecum and ascending colon is fixed over all its posterior surface to the parietal peritoneum, and this area of attachment overlies or slides downward until it covers the abdominal inguinal ring. When a hernia occurs under these conditions, the bowel itself may be mistaken for the hernial sac and be incised unwittingly.

The existence of a mesentery on the ascending colon, in whole or in the lower part, renders the cecum and lower ascending colon mobile. Under these circumstances, the cecum may become twisted on its long axis (*volvulus*). The lower ascending colon and cecum frequently are involved together, and are a fairly common cause of acute mechanical intestinal obstruction. Reduction of the volvulus and cecostomy relieve the condition and safeguard against recurrence.

(C) DIVISIONS OF THE COLON AND MESOCOLON

1. **Anatomic Summary.**—The colon begins in the right iliac fossa distal to the cecum and terminates opposite the body of the third sacral vertebra where it becomes continuous with the rectum. With the exception of its terminal portion, its general outline resembles an M or an inverted U. Beneath the arch which it forms lie the coils of the jejuno-ileum and a part of the duodenum.

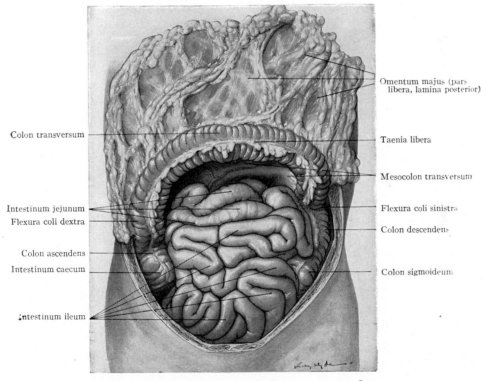

FIG. 382.—RELATIONS BETWEEN THE LARGE BOWEL AND THE JEJUNO-ILEUM.

The colon is not more than one fourth of the length of the small intestine, and is fixed much more securely. Because of its fixation, its position is much more constant. Two of the subdivisions, the transverse colon and sigmoid colon, however, are suspended by a mesocolon and have a great range of mobility.

In external appearance, the large bowel differs very decidedly from the small. It possesses three longitudinal muscle bands or *taeniae* which are plainly discernible. Because of the manner in which the taeniae shorten the bowel, it presents a series of pouches or *haustra* separated by transverse furrows. Numerous pedunculated bodies, the *appendices epiploicae*, are attached to the outer serous layer of the colon.   They sometimes attain considerable size from the amount of fat deposited within them.

The size of the colon diminishes gradually from a diameter of 6 cm. at its cecal extremity to 2.5 cm. at the termination of the sigmoid colon, which usually is narrowest.   The diameter of the colon in an empty and contracted state may not exceed that of the thumb, but it is capable of great increase, especially proximal to malignant stricture of the distal extremity of the sigmoid or of the rectum.

The *relations* of the ascending and descending colon to the right and left kidneys explain the resonant note obtained by percussion over renal tumors.   The colon may

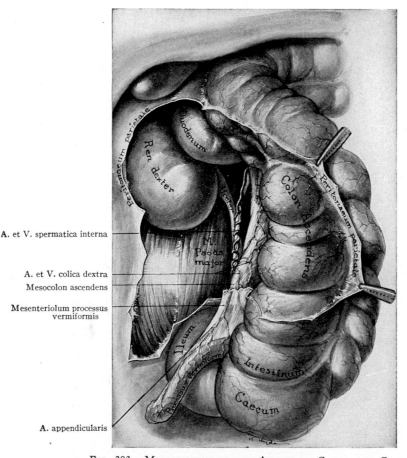

A. et V. spermatica interna

A. et V. colica dextra
Mesocolon ascendens

Mesenteriolum processus
vermiformis

A. appendicularis

FIG. 383.—MOBILIZATION OF THE ASCENDING COLON AND CECUM.

The ascending colon and mesocolon are mobilized by incising along the lateral margin of the bowel and cleaving the fusion fascia which results from the coalescence of the posterior layer of the ascending mesocolon and the right primitive parietal peritoneum.

acquire adhesions from an enlarged or inflamed kidney and be in danger of injury in nephrectomy.   Nephric and perinephric abscesses have been known to discharge their contents into the colon.   The proximity of the hepatic flexure to the inferior surface of the right lobe of the liver explains the adhesions between the liver or gallbladder and the colon, and the possibility of gallstones ulcerating into the colon when such adhesions have formed.   Liver abscesses may rupture into this part of the large bowel.

2. **Ascending Colon.**—The ascending colon lies between the cecum and the right colic (hepatic) flexure, and varies in length as the cecum occupies a high, middle, or low position.   The inferior margin usually is tangent to the iliac crest and the upper margin

is on a horizontal plane where the right tenth rib crosses the midaxillary line.   It is from 12.5 to 20 cm. long.

Posteriorly, the ascending colon is related to the iliac fascia over the iliacus muscle, to the fascia covering the quadratus lumborum, and to the lower part of the right kidney. It is separated from the kidney by the extraperitoneal and perirenal fat, and the anterior layer of perirenal fascia (p. 401).   Its medial aspect is related to the psoas muscle and the descending duodenum.   The ascending colon separates the right paracolic gutter from the right inframesocolic compartment, and is bound to the posterior abdominal wall by the peritoneum clothing its posterior surface.   At times, the right margin of the great omentum

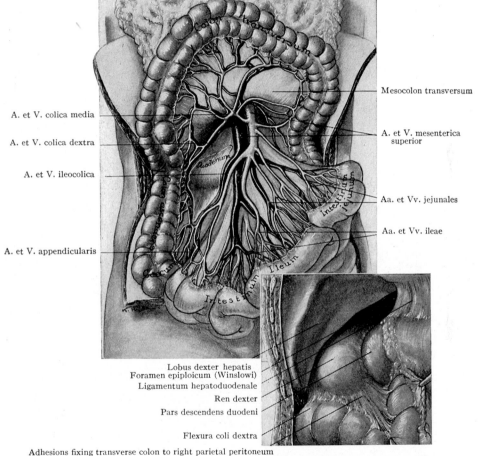

A. et V. colica media

A. et V. colica dextra

A. et V. ileocolica

A. et V. appendicularis

Mesocolon transversum

A. et V. mesenterica superior

Aa. et Vv. jejunales

Aa. et Vv. ileae

Lobus dexter hepatis
Foramen epiploicum (Winslowi)
Ligamentum hepatoduodenale
Ren dexter
Pars descendens duodeni

Flexura coli dextra
Adhesions fixing transverse colon to right parietal peritoneum

FIG. 384.—ASCENDING AND TRANSVERSE COLON AND MESOCOLON WITH THE VASCULAR CONNECTIONS
The inset shows the method of fixation of the right colic angle and the right portion of the transverse colon.

is fused with the peritoneum of the ascending colon, in which instance, the right half of the transverse colon often comes into approximation with the ascending colon, forming a "double-barreled" arrangement.

The ascending colon and mesocolon, primitively suspended by a dorsal common mesentery, after rotation lie intimately against the right primitive parietal peritoneum. The serous surfaces in apposition coalesce into a fusion fascia, which, in the kidney region, is known as Toldt's fascia (p. 401).   In resection of the ascending colon, the peritoneum along the lateral margin of the bowel is incised and the colon is drawn medialward by blunt cleavage of the fusion fascia   In this manipulation, neither the vessels in the ascend-

25

ing colon and in its mesocolon, nor the ureter and vessels to the kidney, lying deep to the fusion fascia, are injured.

When the ascending colon is supplied (as primitively) with a mesocolon, the ascending colon falls away from the loin and drags the hepatic flexure and the cecum with it. While this condition of mobile ascending colon may be symptomless, it may play an important part in cecal stasis, cecal volvulus (p. 383), and ileocecal intussusception (p. 381), and perhaps in mobility of the right kidney. The drag which a mobile ascending colon makes on the superior mesenteric artery may cause that artery to compress the transverse portion of the duodenum against the lumbar column sufficiently to cause symptoms of duodenal obstruction requiring duodenojejunostomy. The ascending colon throughout its entire length may be sutured to the posterior parietal peritoneum.

3. **Right Colic (Hepatic) Flexure.**—The right colic flexure, formed by the junction of the ascending colon and the transverse colon, lies under the ninth and tenth costal car-

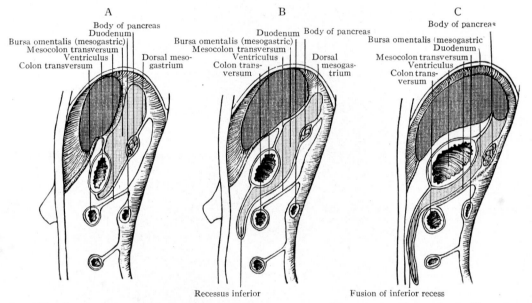

FIG. 385.—SAGITTAL SECTION TO SHOW THE DEVELOPMENT OF THE MESOGASTRIC BURSA AND ITS INFERIOR RECESS, THE GREATER OMENTUM.

In A, rotation of the gastro-intestinal tube has occurred, but no peritoneal fixation has taken place; in B, the mesogastric bursa is growing redundantly downward toward the pelvis, no peritoneal fusion as yet having taken place; in C, posterior peritoneal fixation has occurred between the left primitive parietal peritoneum and the dorsal mesogastrium containing the pancreas; the inferior recess of the mesogastric (omental) bursa in the greater omentum has reached the pelvis and its cavity has become obliterated by the fusion between the apposed serous surfaces; the peritoneal layer of dorsal mesogastrium has fused to the primitive transverse mesocolon and to the colon.

tilages in the interval between the inferior surface of the right lobe of the liver and the anterior surface of the lower pole of the right kidney. It is related by its medial surface to the fundus of the gallbladder anteriorly, and to the descending duodenum posteriorly. A peritoneal band from the gastrohepatic (lesser) omentum, or hepatoduodenal ligament, sometimes passes downward from the right extremity to the flexure, and is known as the *hepatocolic ligament*. Not infrequently, a peritoneal fold leaves the peritoneal surface of the right lobe of the liver to spread out over the colic flexure. The right flexure occasionally has an adhesion, the *cysticocolic ligament*, between itself and the gallbladder. By cleaving the embryological fusion fascia behind the flexure, the colic angle may be mobilized sufficiently to render its excision possible.

4. **Transverse Colon.**—The transverse colon crosses the abdominal cavity from the right to the left colic flexure with a downward curve. In recumbency, it reaches its lowest

position in the midline at, or a little below, the umbilicus. In many patients, it lies at a much lower level because of its excessive length, as obtains in cases of undescended cecum, and in excessive length of the transverse mesocolon. In the erect position, the transverse colon descends and often may be seen lying behind the symphysis; both flexures become very acute and the proximal part of the transverse colon descends in front of, or just mesial to, the ascending colon. Should these adjacent portions of large bowel become attached to each other by peritoneal adhesive bands, the kinking becomes permanent and may give rise to obstructive phenomena.

The right and more fixed portion of the transverse colon is related to the gallbladder, with which it sometimes establishes a fistulous communication through which gallstones

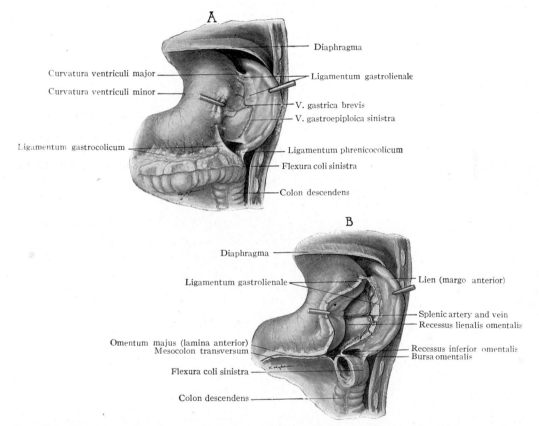

FIG. 386.—PERITONEAL CONNECTIONS BETWEEN THE STOMACH, SPLEEN, TRANSVERSE COLON, AND LEFT COLIC FLEXURE.
In A, the gastrosplenic ligament (omentum) is intact; in B, it is incised to show the splenic recess of the lesser sac.

may be extruded into the large bowel (p. 349). The left segment is related closely to the greater curvature of the stomach and ascends slightly as it approaches the splenic flexure. Between the flexures, the transverse colon is connected to the posterior abdominal wall by the transverse mesocolon.

5. **Transverse Mesocolon.**—The transverse mesocolon forms a horizontal partition across the abdominal cavity, suspending the transverse colon from the posterior abdominal wall and separating the cavity of the omental bursa and the supramesocolic structures from the inframesocolic compartment. It is the natural barrier to reciprocal infections between these areas. The posterior parietal attachment of the transverse mesocolon is to the anterior surface of the head, neck, and body of the pancreas, but it may extend farther to the right and cross the anterior surface of the descending duodenum.

6. **Greater Omentum.**—The greater omentum develops from the primitive peritoneal duplication, the dorsal mesogastrium, which extends from the greater curvature of the stomach to the posterior abdominal wall, independently of the colon and transverse meso-colon. As the stomach assumes its ultimate position in the abdomen, this fold bulges to the left and develops in a forward and downward direction until it forms a baglike structure, the mesogastric (omental) bursa. The epiploic foramen or open end of this pouch is directed to the right, and the closed lower end enlarges downward until it hangs over the transverse colon and mesocolon and the small intestine and becomes the greater omentum.

Toward the middle of intra-uterine life, the posterior layer of the greater omentum fuses with the serosal layer of the transverse colon and mesocolon with which it is in con-

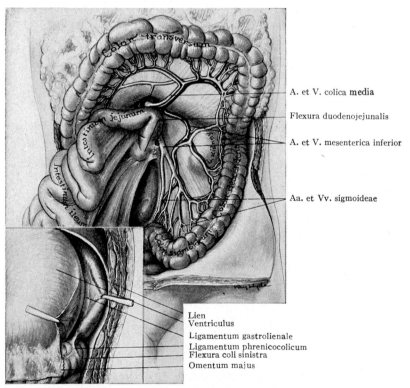

A. et V. colica **media**

Flexura duodenojejunalis

A. et V. mesenterica inferior

Aa. et Vv. sigmoideae

Lien
Ventriculus
Ligamentum gastrolienale
Ligamentum phrenicocolicum
Flexura coli sinistra
Omentum majus

FIG. 387.—TRANSVERSE, DESCENDING, AND SIGMOID PORTIONS OF THE COLON AND ITS MESOCOLON, WITH THEIR VASCULAR CONNECTIONS.

The inset shows the peritoneal connections at the left colic angle and their relations to the spleen.

tact. Often in the infant, and occasionally in the adult, the cavity of the greater omen-tum remains open below the level of the transverse colon. Generally, however, the cavity of the greater omentum is obliterated to within a short distance of the greater curvature of the stomach by adhesion between the apposed serous surfaces, so that the omentum appears to arise from the convexity of the transverse colon. Obliteration on the left is not as complete as that on the right, so that the unobliterated interval on the left between the stomach and transverse colon offers readier access to the cavity of the lesser sac. That part of the greater omentum connecting the greater curvature of the stomach with the transverse colon is the *gastrocolic ligament*. The greater omentum spreads over the large and small bowel and helps to anchor the colic angles by fusing to the diaphragm.

7. **Left Colic (Splenic) Flexure.**—Because of the small left lobe of the liver, the left colic flexure is placed higher than the right and its angle is more acute than that of the

hepatic flexure.   The splenic flexure may overlie the left kidney anywhere from its upper to its lower pole; it is located deeply under cover of the costal margin and is overlain partly by the stomach.   Examination of the flexure is difficult, and tumors escape early recognition.   The upper and forward aspects of the flexure receive an attachment from the left margin of the greater omentum, and the posterior aspect is attached to the pancreas by the left extremity of the transverse mesocolon.   From the lateral aspect of the flexure, the peritoneum passes to the diaphragm as the *left phrenicocolic ligament*.   The inferior pole of the spleen rests upon the ligament, which, in consequence, also is known as the supporting ligament of the spleen.

8. **Descending Colon.**—The descending colon varies from 8 to 12 cm. in length, and extends from the left colic flexure to the iliac crest.   In its descent, it inclines mesially, curving around the lower extremity of the left kidney.   Its posteromesial aspect lies directly upon the fascia covering the quadratus lumborum muscle; the remainder of the descending colon is covered by peritoneum.   The descending colon is more deeply placed than the ascending colon and rarely possesses a mesentery.

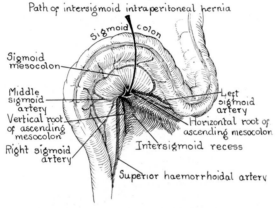

FIG. 388.—SIGMOID COLON, ITS MESENTERY AND ARTERIAL SUPPLY, AND THE INTERSIGMOID RECESS.

The sigmoid colon and mesocolon are raised forward and upward to show the vertical and horizontal attachments of its two roots; the arrow indicates the apex of the intersigmoid recess into which a loop of small bowel may insinuate, and travel up behind a partially unfused descending mesocolon to form an intraperitoneal hernia; the superior hemorrhoidal artery, which is the main arterial supply to the rectum, lies between the leaves of the vertical root of the sigmoid mesocolon and is accessible there for ligation in removal of the rectosigmoid area for carcinoma.

9. **Sigmoid Colon and Mesocolon.**—The sigmoid colon or flexure begins at the iliac crest and terminates at the third sacral vertebra.   It is divisible into a fixed (iliac) and a mobile (pelvic) segment.

The *iliac segment* is that part of the sigmoid flexure which lies in the iliac fossa and has no mesentery.   It descends on the iliacus muscle to the level of the anterior superior iliac spine and turns mesially just above and parallel to the inguinal ligament.   It extends to the pelvic brim where it becomes continuous with the pelvic colon.   A tumor of the iliac colon is recognized readily as it can be palpated by rolling the gut against the ilium.

The *pelvic segment*, or mobile division of the sigmoid, is a long, omega-shaped coil of bowel which is continuous above with the iliac colon and below with the rectum.   It is suspended from the posterior wall of the pelvis by a mesentery, the *pelvic mesocolon*.   The line of mesenteric attachment resembles an inverted V.   It begins at the mesial border of the psoas major muscle and passes upward and medially along the medial aspect of the external iliac vessels.   After crossing the hypogastric (internal iliac) vessels, it turns sharply downward and ends in front of the third sacral vertebra.   The terms "ascending" and "descending" limbs are used to indicate the segments of gut which this arrangement of the mesentery encloses.   The length, location, and degree of mobility of the loop and the length of its mesentery are subject to wide variation. Usually, the pelvic colon is situated partly in the pelvis and partly in the abdomen. When it possesses a long meso-

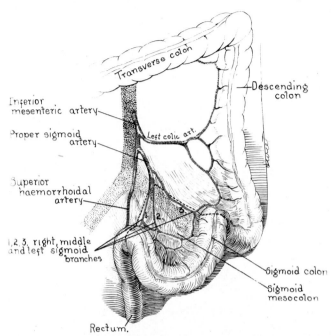

FIG. 389.—SIGMOID COLON AND MESOCOLON WITH SPECIAL REFERENCE TO THE ARTERIAL SUPPLY.

The arteries to the sigmoid are the left (3), middle (2), and right (1) sigmoid arteries which are branches from the inferior mesenteric artery; the large single branch of the inferior mesenteric artery is the superior hemorrhoidal artery which supplies the upper rectum; the area within the dotted lines is to be removed from its attachments to show the sigmoid relations to the posterior parietal and pelvic peritoneum and intersigmoid recess.

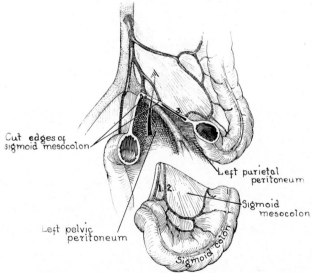

FIG. 390.—DIAGRAM OF THE SIGMOID REGION TO SHOW THE LOOP OF THE SIGMOID COLON AND PART OF ITS MESENTERY REMOVED TO SHOW THE LEFT PARIETAL AND PELVIC PERITONEUM.

The arrow shows the path of an intersigmoid intraperitoneal hernia behind the descending mesocolon.

colon, it may cross the median line, where, not infrequently, it comes into view in the course of an appendectomy. In certain instances, the pelvic colon is short, presents no loop, has little mesentery, and passes directly from the iliac colon into the rectum. This disposition of the colon is unsuitable for permanent colostomy.

The *intersigmoid recess* is a small, funnel-shaped pouch quite commonly present at the junction of the two roads of the sigmoid mesocolon. In this recess may lodge a loop of small bowel, which, by a process of cleavage, may insinuate itself between the meso-colon and the primitive parietal peritoneum and form a not uncommon variety of internal or intraperitoneal hernia.

10. **Vessels of the Colon.**—The arterial supply to the ascending colon, right colic (hepatic) flexure, and transverse colon is derived from the right and middle colic branches of the **superior mesenteric artery.** The left colic branch and the sigmoid arteries from the inferior mesenteric artery supply the descending and sigmoid portions of the colon.

The *right colic artery* arises just above, or in common with, the ileocolic artery and runs behind the peritoneum of the right inframesocolic space. Near the bowel, it divides into a descending branch which anastomoses with the colic branch of the ileocolic artery

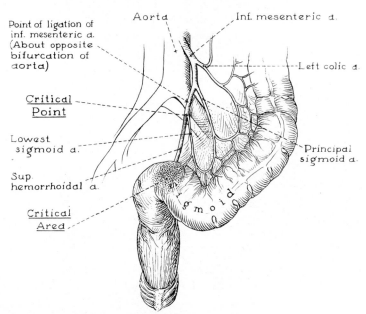

FIG. 391.—"CRITICAL POINT" IN THE ARTERIAL SUPPLY OF THE SIGMOID AND RECTUM, AND THE "CRITICAL AREA" OF THE SIGMOID AND RECTUM.

A, Point for ligation of the inferior mesenteric artery; B, junction of sigmoid and rectum poorly supplied with arterial blood.

and an ascending branch which anastomoses with the right branch of the middle colic artery. Both of these branches supply the ascending colon.

The *middle colic artery* arises from the superior mesenteric at the lower margin of the pancreas and runs in the transverse mesocolon where it divides into right and left branches which anastomose with the right and left colic arteries. The right branch supplies the right third of the transverse colon, and the left, the left two thirds. Since the main trunk lies to the right of the midline, an operative opening through the transverse mesocolon is made on the left side.

The **inferior mesenteric artery** through its left colic, sigmoid, and superior hemorrhoidal branches, supplies the descending and sigmoid colon and the proximal part of the rectum. The inferior mesenteric artery arises from the aorta about 10 cm. above the bifurcation. As it runs downward and slightly to the left, it gives off the *left colic artery* to the descending colon and part of the transverse colon, and the *sigmoid arteries* to the iliac and pelvic segments of the sigmoid colon.

The several sigmoid arteries anastomose freely with one another to form arterial arches and a marginal artery in the pelvic mesocolon. The uppermost of these arteries anastomoses with the descending branch of the left colic artery. The lowermost sigmoid artery has no marginal artery connection with the superior hemorrhoidal artery. In abdominoperineal removal of the rectum, or in resection of the pelvic colon, the inferior mesenteric artery must be ligated proximal to the origin of the lowest sigmoid branch if the lower part of the pelvic colon is to maintain a blood supply. The inferior mesenteric artery, beyond the origin of the lowest sigmoid artery, continues downward into the pelvis on the dorsal surface of the rectum as the *superior hemorrhoidal artery* (p. 436).

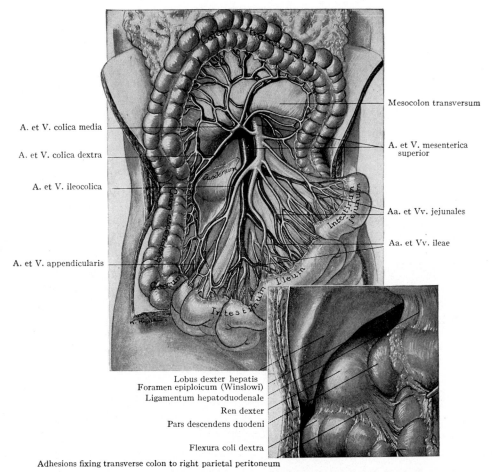

A. et V. colica media

A. et V. colica dextra

A. et V. ileocolica

A. et V. appendicularis

Mesocolon transversum

A. et V. mesenterica superior

Aa. et Vv. jejunales

Aa. et Vv. ileae

Lobus dexter hepatis
Foramen epiploicum (Winslowi)
Ligamentum hepatoduodenale
Ren dexter
Pars descendens duodeni

Flexura coli dextra

Adhesions fixing transverse colon to right parietal peritoneum

FIG. 392.—VESSELS OF THE ASCENDING AND TRANSVERSE COLON AND MESOCOLON.
The inset shows the peritoneal connections at the right colic angle.

The point of junction between the superior hemorrhoidal artery and lowest sigmoid artery, therefore, is the "critical," or, better, the "indispensable point" in the vascularization of the terminal sigmoid and the upper rectum. Ligation of the inferior mesenteric artery just proximal to the critical point will maintain circulation between the lowest sigmoid artery and the superior hemorrhoidal artery. Ligation of either of these trunks (distal to the critical point) may result in gangrene of the distal area of the sigmoid, or of the proximal part of the rectum. These two adjoining areas of large bowel well might be called the "critical areas" of the sigmoid and rectum.

The **veins** correspond largely to the arteries and join the superior and inferior mesenteric trunks which send their blood to the portal vein.

The **lymph vessels** of the large bowel follow mainly the course of the chief blood vessels. They may be considered to form four groups: epicolic, paracolic, intermediate, and main or central. The *epicolic glands* lie on the wall of the bowel in the epiploic appendices. The *paracolic glands* lie behind the peritoneum along the mesial borders of the ascending, descending, and iliac colon on the upper border of the transverse colon and the mesenteric margin of the pelvic colon. The *intermediate glands* lie along the branches of the colic arteries and *central* or *main groups* lie about the vascular trunks, from which the colic arteries rise. Most of the lymph drainage is to the group of glands about the upper part of the superior mesenteric artery and thence by the efferents of these glands to the common intestinal lymphatic trunk.

SURGICAL CONSIDERATIONS

1. Resection of the Cecum and the Ascending Colon.—Most of the ascending colon and mesocolon, and frequently part of the cecum, with their blood and lymph vessels lie behind the ultimate posterior parietal peritoneum. For this reason, resection of these parts presents more difficulty than the removal of a segment of small intestine and its mesentery which are freely movable. Irrespective of the degree of tuberculous or malignant involvement of the ascending colon and cecum, it is advisable to remove the hepatic flexure in addition to the cecum, ascending colon, and a small portion of the terminal ileum in order to allow anastomosis of the ileum with the mobile transverse colon and to eradicate the immediately tributary lymphatic drainage.

The abdomen is opened by an appropriate incision. To free the bowel, a vertical incision is made through the peritoneum of the right paracolic gutter along its whole extent and is continued below the cecum and terminal ileum. Both the cecum and ascending colon then are freed by blunt dissection with the fingers and carried with their blood supply toward the median line. The ileocolic and right colic arteries may be ligated before or after the bowel is freed. Care must be exercised not to injure the right spermatic vessels, the second part of the duodenum, or the ureter.

After the mobilized segments are drawn out of the abdomen and turned toward the left, the ileocolic and right colic vessels are secured on the deep surface of the mobilized ascending mesocolon. The ileum and the transverse colon beyond the hepatic flexure are clamped and divided with a cautery. The intervening portion of bowel along with the adjoining area of mobilized mesocolon up to the point where the vessels have been divided then is removed. Since the ileocolic artery has been ligated, the terminal portion of the ileum must depend for its arterial supply on the anastomosis between the termination of the superior mesenteric and the ileocolic arteries. This small segment therefore is rendered unsuitable for anastomosis with the large bowel, and must be removed in order that the part of the ileum utilized may possess an ample blood supply.

2. Resection of the Left (Splenic) Colic Flexure and Part or All of the Descending Colon.—Resection of the left colic flexure and part or all of the descending colon involves the removal of the left third of the transverse colon and the upper part or all of the descending colon. Mobilization of these parts requires division of the peritoneum in the left paracolic gutter, and of the left phrenicocolic ligament and the left part of the transverse mesocolon. When the flexure is mobilized, it can be stripped downward and mesially by the fingers. Care must be taken not to injure the kidney and ureter. The ascending branch of the left colic artery is ligated on the posterior surface of the mobilized mesocolon and the left branch of the middle colic artery is ligated before the bowel is divided. The remainder of the transverse colon or the terminal ileum then may be anastomosed to the sigmoid.

The frequency of obstruction in the clinical course of cancer in the left side of the colon makes cecostomy (p. 395) advisable as the initial operation in many cases.

3. Excision of the Pelvic Colon.—Removal of the pelvic colon presents little difficulty when the bowel is long and has a long mesentery. In the event of a short pelvic colon and mesocolon, the distal part of the iliac segment must be mobilized by stripping the peritoneum along the left paracolic gutter and bluntly dissecting the bowel mesially on a hinge of mobilized mesocolon. The deferent duct, internal spermatic vessels, ureter, and inferior mesenteric artery may be injured unless care is taken in this dissection, for they are crossed by one or other of the limbs of the root of the pelvic mesocolon. The mode of restoration of intestinal continuity depends upon the length of bowel available.

4. **Volvulus.**—Volvulus is a term employed to denote certain forms of twisting of the intestine. In one, and much the commonest, form, the bowel is twisted around its mesenteric axis. In other forms, the bowel is wound about some neighboring coil, a postoperative adhesive band, or certain of the remains of the vitello-intestinal duct.

The sigmoid colon is concerned in by far the majority of the recorded instances of volvulus as it affords the most favorable predisposing conditions. The loop of the sigmoid

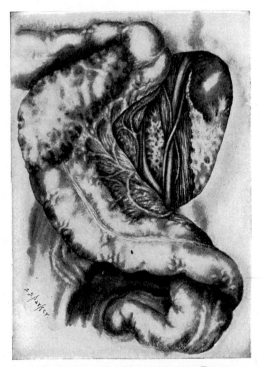

Fig. 393.—Mobilization of the Left Colic Flexure and the Descending Colon and Mesocolon

By incising the peritoneum immediately lateral to the attachment of these segments of the bowel to the posterior parietal peritoneum, the bowel is mobilized by cleaving the fusion fascia which has resulted from the coalescence between the posterior layer of the descending mesocolon and colon and the left primitive parietal peritoneum; no vessel in the mesocolon or behind the primitive parietal peritoneum need be injured. (Bickham, "Operative Surgery.")

colon varies considerably in length and its extremities are comparatively close to one another. The gap between the two may be diminished further as a result of the traction exercised upon the mesentery by the loaded condition of the bowel, so common in chronic constipation. Under traction, the pelvic mesocolon elongates considerably. A twist of the loop occurs readily, and the bowel becomes distended and the vessels constricted by the mutual pressure of the two ends of the loop. The obstruction to the venous return causes the twisted loop to become greatly swollen and edematous so that it assumes a livid hue. The arterial flow subsequently is arrested, and, if the vascular constriction remains unrelieved, gangrene of the loop ensues. While these changes are occurring, the bowel distends and rises gradually until it may fill the greater part of the abdominal cavity and come into contact with the liver or compress the diaphragm.

In volvulus of the sigmoid, signs of obstruction come on slowly, and vomiting is a late manifestation. In volvulus of the small bowel, vomiting is an early and persistent occurrence. This follows the general rule that in intestinal obstruction the higher the seat of obstruction the more likely vomiting is to occur early, because of the greater fluidity of the contents higher in the intestinal canal.

5. **Colostomy.**—By colostomy is meant the establishment of an artificial opening either temporary (fecal fistula), or more or less permanent (artificial anus), between some part of the colon and the skin. Colostomy in the large bowel corresponds to enterostomy in the small bowel (p. 373).

When a *temporary colostomy* is designed, only the convexity of the intestinal loop is anchored into the wound, but when a *permanent colostomy* is performed, the loop is drawn well out of the wound and anchored so as to prevent retraction. A tube, fastened by a purse-string suture, may be used to convey the intestinal content to the outside without endangering the abdominal cavity during the period of formation of adhesions between the colostomized loop and the wound margins.

A colostomy is designed to form an artificial anus proximal to a bowel obstruction, usually in the rectum or rectosigmoid junction, with or independent of removal of the obstruction. The operation may be performed to furnish a temporary fecal outlet for relief of colitis or proctitis and to provide an avenue for local bowel treatment.

The location of the colostomy depends upon the segment of colon chosen. Usually, a left iliac colostomy of the sigmoid loop is selected. Not infrequently, the transverse colon is the loop utilized; in which case, the colostomy is situated above the umbilicus. On the right side, cecostomy is the operation of choice.

6. **Intestinal Exclusion.**—By intestinal exclusion is meant the diverting of the intestinal contents from some limited part of the intestinal tract by means of a short-circuiting operation which does not interfere with the intestinal flow in the remainder of the bowel. When a lesion, which cannot or should not be removed, obstructs the colon or requires rest, this procedure is adopted. The lesion must be located at some point below which sufficient uninvolved bowel is available for an anastomosis. Exclusion is accomplished by uniting two portions of the bowel so that the content of the upper or proximal part empties into the lower or distal portion without traversing the interposed loop.

The intermediate or short-circuited portion is said to be partially excluded when some part of the intestinal flow occurs through one or the other end of the short-circuited part into the remainder of the bowel. A *partial exclusion* of the large bowel is obtained by ileocolostomy. In this procedure, the ileum just proximal to the cecum is anastomosed with either the sigmoid or the transverse colon to allow the major part of the bowel contents to pass directly from the ileum into the terminal colon, thus short-circuiting to a degree the interval of large bowel proximal to the anastomosis. When, as so frequently happens, the large bowel becomes blocked by the disease for which the ileocolostomy was done so that satisfactory fecal elimination from the excluded part is interfered with, it becomes necessary to provide a colostomy in the short-circuited area.

If it is desired to prevent the fecal current from passing upward through the ileocecal-ascending colon segment, the ileum may be divided near the cecum and its distal extremity closed or brought out through the abdominal wall as an ileostomy to function for drainage purposes. The proximal ileum then is anastomosed laterally to the transverse colon or sigmoid.

Complete exclusion of a segment of bowel requires more than a simple short-circuiting anastomosis, for, unless there is an organic or spastic constriction distal to the stoma, a part of the feces continues to pass into the short-circuited loop. Complete exclusion demands that anastomosis be combined with the division of the bowel proximal and distal to the lesion and that both ends be brought out on the abdominal wall as mucous fistulae, or, at least, that the bowel be closed proximal to the lesion and the distal free end be brought out to the skin. In either of these procedures, the segment actually is excluded from the fecal current.

7. Diverticula of the Colon (Diverticulosis) and Diverticulitis.—Diverticula of the large bowel (*diverticulosis*), present mainly in the sigmoid, are herniations of areas of mucosa and submucosa through interstices in the muscle coats, "blowouts of the inner tube (of mucosa)." They probably develop along the course of the blood vessels penetrating the intestinal wall, and usually are innocuous. Diverticula perforating the wall through a narrow opening and ballooning out the peritoneal covering are those most likely to become inflamed. The muscularis is thin or disappears except at the neck of the diverticulum. Intestinal contents entering the diverticulum set up inflammatory changes and ulceration.

Although walling off by adhesions is more active in *diverticulitis* than in appendicitis, internal fistulae may occur from ulceration into neighboring viscera. The urinary bladder is the organ involved ordinarily in this unusual anastomosis. The mesosigmoid may become infiltrated and thickened by inflammation or even become the seat of an acute abscess which may open through the abdominal wall or into the vagina or rectum.

An acute diverticulitis may require surgical treatment because of the effects of perforation into the general abdominal cavity, but recession of the inflammatory process is usual, and a large tender mass may disappear entirely. When symptoms of obstruction present, colostomy proximal to the obstructing mass should be performed in preference to resection. Infection of the mesentery, so common in diverticulitis, makes intestinal resection a dangerous procedure.

B. RETROPERITONEAL SPACE AND CONTENTS

(I) LUMBO-ILIAC REGION

1. Lumbar and Iliac Fossae.—In the lumbar and iliac regions, between the peritoneum and the posterior parietal wall of the abdominal cavity, lie the contents of the retroperitoneal space.

On each side, the *lumbar fossa* extends from the twelfth dorsal vertebra and twelfth rib to the base of the sacrum and the iliac crest. The lateral boundary is indicated by a vertical groove directed between the sacrospinalis and the flat abdominal muscles. Viewed from the abdominal aspect, after the contents of the space have been removed, the lateral margin of the region corresponds to the lateral border of the quadratus lumborum muscle. The floor of the space is formed by the quadratus lumborum and psoas major muscles, and extends from the lateral lumbocostal arch above to the iliolumbar ligament below. Both muscles of the floor have a definite fascial covering, that for the quadratus being derived from the lumbodorsal fascia as its anterior layer, and that for the psoas being directly continuous below with the fascia covering the iliacus muscle. These fascial layers are overlain by a varying amount of areolofatty tissue which fills the interstices between the muscles and furnishes a pliable bed for the superjacent viscera: the kidney, ascending colon, and duodenum on the right, and the kidney and descending colon on the left.

The retroperitoneal tissue is traversed by the ureter, renal vessels, spermatic vessels in the male, and ovarian vessels in the female. The tissue abuts against the inferior vena cava on the right and the aorta on the left.

The *iliac fossa* is overlain by peritoneum, beneath which is a layer of retroperitoneal tissue directly continuous with that of the adjoining regions, the anterior and lateral aspects of the abdominal wall, the lumbar region above, and the pelvis below. Within the subperitoneal tissue of the iliac fossa are found the iliac vessels, ureter, genitofemoral nerve, spermatic or ovarian vessels, and the iliac lymph glands. The iliacus muscle lies deep to the retroperitoneal tissue, separated from it by the iliac fascia. This fascia is continued upward over the psoas major muscle, is attached mesially to the linea terminalis or to the brim of the pelvis, and anteriorly to the proximal margin of the deep aspect of the inguinal ligament in its lateral half where it fuses with the transversalis fascia (p. 278).

Surgical Considerations

1. Iliolumbar Abscesses.—The lumbar and iliac regions are of special interest in connection with certain forms of abscesses and their manner of extension. It is evident that there are two available sites for abscesses: within the extraperitoneal tissue, and beneath the iliac fascia and its extension over the quadratus lumborum and psoas major muscles.

The commoner sources of abscesses *within the extraperitoneal tissue* are: appendiceal abscess, perinephric abscess, infected lymph glands, and the lateral extension of a pelvic abscess which has originated in the areolar tissue of the broad ligament (parametritis). The looseness of the areolar tissue and the laxity of the surrounding structures permit widespread diffusion of the infection.

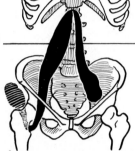

Follows sheath of psoas to head of femur and around it to gluteal region   Follows sheath of psoas and ends at Poupart's ligament

Fig. 394.—Psoas Abscess.

Subfascial abscesses develop mainly from tuberculosis (caries) of the spine (Pott's disease). Pus from the diseased vertebral bodies is limited in its forward extension by the anterior longitudinal ligament of the spine. Its usual egress is directly into the body of the psoas muscle or between that muscle and its anterior sheath, but if the abscess is in the thoracic region or even higher, the purulent collection may gravitate down the posterior mediastinum and pass into the abdomen behind the lateral lumbocostal arch and enter the psoas compartment behind its sheath. The purulent collection within the psoas sheath may destroy the muscle completely and occupy the entire compartment. Usually,

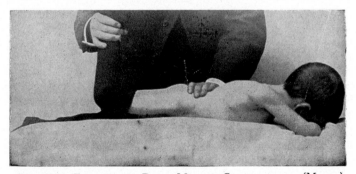

Fig. 395.—Testing for Psoas Muscle Contraction. (Moore.)

with increasing amounts of pus, the subfascial space distends and the abscess descends to the iliac fossa. Further distention causes pus to pass beneath the inguinal ligament at the lateral margin of the femoral vessels into the thigh, where it may follow one of a number of courses. Most frequently, it passes down to the apex of the femoral triangle (of Scarpa), and points lateral to the femoral vessels at a point superficial to the attachment of the psoas tendon into the lesser trochanter. Sometimes the abscess appears to follow the femoral sheath to the origin of the femoral profunda artery and then to follow the course of this vessel beneath the adductor longus muscle and subsequently to become superficial, forming a fluctuant swelling at the medial side of the thigh. Occasionally, the abscess travels backward and points in the lumbar region (p. 543), or it may seek an exit through the suprapyriformic and infrapyriformic foramina of the pelvis, pointing in the gluteal region along the course of the sciatic nerve. Pus may spread laterally, burst the psoas sheath, and fuse laterally on the iliacus muscle between it and its sheath, simulating an appendiceal abscess. If the iliac fascia is not strong enough to limit the abscess, pus may point on the skin near the anterior superior spine where it may be evacuated extraperitoneally through a muscle-splitting incision. Very infrequently, the pus may make its way backward along the course of the last dorsal or upper lumbar nerves, and point over the superior lumbar triangle or against the floor of the inferior lumbar triangle (of Petit). Usually, an extension is debarred from the pelvis by the firm attachment of the iliac fascia to the pelvic brim.

A well-developed psoas abscess may consist of a sinuous channel in the psoas muscle, an expanded area beneath the iliac fascia, a narrow neck beneath the inguinal ligament and a lower expanded portion on the medial aspect of the thigh. The thigh is likely to be flexed because of irritation of the psoas muscle and the attempt to relieve muscle tension to prevent pressure on the lumbar nerves within the psoas sheath.

(II) Kidney Region

1. **Suprarenal Glands.**—The adrenal or suprarenal bodies are two small flattened glands of internal secretion comprised of a thin, but resistant, fibrous capsule and a cortical and medullary parenchyma. They are located in the upper median portion of each kidney fossa between the upper pole of the kidney and the great vascular trunks of the abdomen. The concave base of the gland rests upon the upper pole of the kidney like a cap; its posterior surface lies against the diaphragm and its anterior margin extends toward the kidney hilum. On the anteromedian surface of the gland, vessels enter and leave.

Between the capsule of the suprarenal body and the kidney is a layer of loose connective tissue admitting of easy separation of the kidney from the adrenal in nephrectomy. Both the kidney and adrenal lie within the perirenal fibrous capsule.

The *arterial supply* consists of the superior suprarenal artery from the inferior phrenic artery, a small direct branch from the aorta, and an inferior suprarenal branch from the renal artery.

2. **Kidneys.**—The kidneys are solid, glandular organs, one on each side of the spine opposite the twelfth dorsal and first three lumbar vertebrae. Because of the great size of the right lobe of the liver, the right kidney usually lies at a somewhat lower level than the left. Each organ is about 12 cm. long and 7 cm. broad. The middle of the mesial border of the kidney is hollowed out and constitutes the hilum where the renal arteries and nerves enter and the renal vein, the principal lymphatics of the organ and the ureter emerge. This hilar aggregate forms the *renal pedicle*. Because of the gradual increase in bulk of the psoas muscles as they descend, the inferior poles of the kidneys are directed forward and are wider apart than the upper poles.

The kidney is covered completely by a thin, but resistant, fibro-elastic membranous *capsule*. Expansions of the capsule extend over the pelvis of the kidney and its excretory duct, the ureter. It is because of the solidity and tenacity of its investing membrane that the otherwise friable kidney bears suturing. Even when the parenchyma is destroyed by infection, the capsule usually resists destruction. Inversely, it may constrict and strangulate the organ in an acute nephritis; hence the procedure of capsular decortication to relieve parenchymal congestion. Normally, the capsule is connected loosely to the kidney parenchyma by delicate vascular connective tissue and can be stripped away readily.

The kidney hilum expands into a central cavity, the *renal sinus*, which contains the uppermost and expanded part of the kidney pelvis and calices. The kidney parenchyma consists of an inner medullary and an outer cortical substance. The *medulla* is composed largely of a number of conical pyramids. These are arranged with their bases directed toward the surface and their apices toward the renal sinus where they form prominent papillae which project into the interior of the calices.   The bases of the pyramids do not reach the surface of the kidney, but are separated from it by a thin layer of kidney substance, the *cortex*.   The cortical substance not only covers the bases of the pyramids, but sends prolongations, called renal columns, between the pyramids toward the sinus.   The

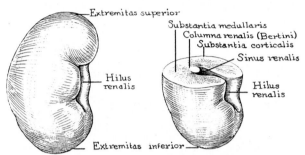

Extremitas superior

Substantia medullaris
Columna renalis (Bertini)
Substantia corticalis
Sinus renalis

Hilus
renalis

Hilus
renalis

Extremitas inferior

FIG. 396.—HILUS AND SINUS OF THE KIDNEY.

medullary part of the kidney in section is striated in appearance, while the cortical part is granular and usually different in color   The larger blood vessels lie between the pyramids.

At its proximal extremity, the ureter widens into the funnel-shaped sac, the *renal pelvis*, which is contained, for the most part, within the renal sinus behind the vessels.

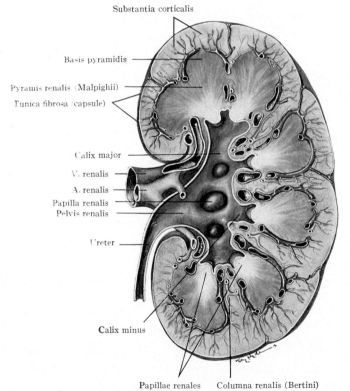

Substantia corticalis

Basis pyramidis

Pyramis renalis (Malpighii)

Tunica fibrosa (capsule)

Calix major

V. renalis

A. renalis

Papilla renalis
Pelvis renalis

Ureter

Calix minus

Papillae renales   Columna renalis (Bertini)

FIG. 397.—FRONTAL SECTION THROUGH THE KIDNEY.

As a rule, the extrarenal portion of the pelvis, that projecting beyond the kidney sinus, is larger than the intrarenal part.   However, the whole pelvis may lie within the renal sinus and be invisible at the kidney hilum.   The renal vessels lie anterior to the pelvis on each side, but, occasionally, branches of the vein and artery lie on the dorsal aspect.

The renal pelvis lies among the larger renal vessels and is formed usually by the junc-tion of three thin-walled tubes, the superior, middle, and inferior *major calices;* occasionally, there may be only two major calices. Into each major calix open a number of smaller or *minor calices.* Their wide, somewhat funnel-like ends enclose the renal papillae and receive the urine. When the kidney pelvis is very small and consists only of the major calices, there is no extrarenal pelvis and a stone can be removed only by incising through the kidney substance.

3. **Vessels.**—The **renal arteries** are derived from the abdominal aorta at about the level of the second lumbar vertebra, the left at a somewhat higher level than the right. The right artery is 1 to 2 cm. longer than the left, since it must extend from the aorta across the median line behind the vena cava. Either at or before reaching the kidney hilum, each renal artery divides into *prepelvic* and *retropelvic branches* or groups of branches. Within the sinus, these ventral and dorsal branches divide into rich prepelvic and post-pelvic arterial networks. The branches of the anterior network are the more numerous. The terminations of the peripelvic networks penetrate the renal parenchyma around the papillae and ramify over the medullary pyramids from the apex to the base.

These vessels are end-arteries and do not anastomose. As a consequence, each is responsible for its own portion of parenchyma and a lesion in any one vessel results in an

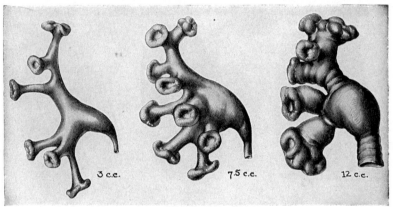

FIG. 398.—CASTS OF TYPES OF THE HUMAN RENAL PELVIS SHOWING MAJOR AND MINOR CALICES.
Actual size and capacity.

infarct of the area it normally supplies. The lack of anastomosis between the prepelvic and retropelvic arteries and their medullary terminals produces an *avascular frontal plane* in the kidney, noted by Brödel to lie at the junction of the posterior with the middle third of the gland. By incising the kidney in this plane, the hemorrhage encountered can be controlled by pressure on the vascular pedicle.

Supplementary or *supernumerary renal arteries* may be present on either side, arising from the abdominal aorta and entering the different portions of the kidney cortex. These arteries more frequently enter the kidney over its anterior surface and lower pole. In excision of the kidney, their occurrence always must be borne in mind before the main vessels at the hilum are encountered. A supernumerary artery at the lower pole may kink the ureter and cause urinary obstruction, pelvic retention, and hydronephrosis. These accessory arteries probably persist from the embryonic period when the kidney is more or less lobulated, and each vessel supplies a limited area of the lobulated mass.

The **renal veins** have much the same disposition as the arteries. They descend from the surface of the kidney through the cortex to the bases of the pyramids to become the *interlobular veins.* In the renal sinus, these are grouped into prepelvic and postpelvic trunks which converge to form the renal vein. As the renal vein leaves the hilum, it lies anterior and somewhat inferior to the level of the artery. Because the inferior vena cava lies on the right of the median plane, the left renal vein is longer than the right.

There are superficial and deep **lymphatic systems** in the kidney. The superficial system drains the fat capsule about the kidney and the true renal capsule. The deep system drains the parenchyma. The vessels of both systems are afferent to lymph nodes located for the most part behind the pelvis at the hilum. These nodes are involved in renal carcinoma. Spread of carcinoma into the left renal vein may involve the left spermatic vein, with resulting varicocele (p. 521). Efferent vessels from the renal lymph nodes drain to the lumbar lymph glands along the aorta and inferior vena cava.

4. **Fixation of the Kidney; Perirenal Fascia; Retrorenal and Perirenal Fat.**—The kidneys in their niches in the hypochondria are *maintained in position* against the posterior abdominal wall by a variety of mechanisms; they are held in place chiefly by the fascial and fatty structures lying about them, partly by the attachment of the renal pedicles, and partly by intra-abdominal pressure. The left kidney position is reinforced by the pancreas which is applied over it.

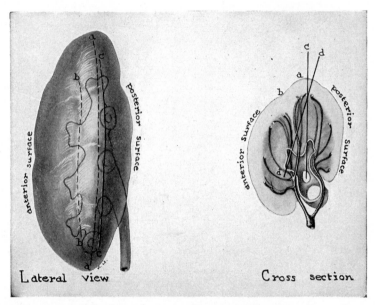

F I G. 399.—SIDE VIEW AND CROSS SECTION OF THE KIDNEY TO SHOW THE POPER PLANE FOR INCISION

Line *a-a* represents the periphery of the convex border; an incision along the line *b-b* would sever many vascular trunks and should be avoided; line *c-c* is along a relatively avascular plane between the anterior and posterior vessels and is the proper location for an incision through the kidney; line *d-d* indicates an incision not in the frontal plane and one which, if continued, will cut through the large vessels in the depth of the kidney. (After Kelly, Burnam.)

The transversalis fascia splits into prerenal and retrorenal fascial layers at the lateral border of the kidney and forms a fascial compartment known as the *perirenal fascial space* (of Gerota) which incloses both the kidney and the suprarenal gland. A loose layer of connective tissue separates the two organs in such a manner that the kidney may be dislocated dorsally, while the suprarenal gland remains in place. The compartment is open mesially where the anterior (prerenal) and the posterior (retrorenal) layers are continued across the median line. The compartment is in broad communication below with the extraperitoneal tissue of the lumbo-iliac region. Superior and lateral to the kidney, the layers are approximated. Below the lower pole of the kidney, the layers remain spread apart for quite a distance, affording an anatomical cleavage area predisposing to movable kidney. Where the primitive ascending and descending portions of the mesocolon have fused with the primitive parietal peritoneum a fusion fascia (of Toldt) is formed; it reinforces the subjacent prerenal leaf of fascia. The retrorenal fascia overlies the quadratus lumborum and psoas muscles and is very resistant.

26

Between the posterior layer of the perinephric fascia and the transversus abdominus aponeurosis lies the *retrorenal (pararenal) fat*, which is a portion of the extraperitoneal fat

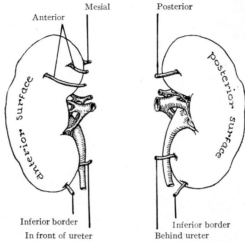

FIGS. 400 AND 401.—COMPOSITE VIEWS OF THE ANTERIOR AND POSTERIOR SURFACES OF THE KIDNEYS TO SHOW THE USUAL POINTS OF ENTRANCE OF ACCESSORY ARTERIES.

The arteries entering the upper pole are particularly dangerous in nephrectomy; the branches near the ureter may be factors in producing ureteral kinks and hydronephrosis. (After Kelly, Burnam.)

pad lying behind all the abdominal contents. It is continuous with the extraperitoneal fat of the anterolateral and posterior abdominal walls and with the extrapleural areolo-adipose tissue above the edges of the diaphragm. The amount of pararenal fat varies

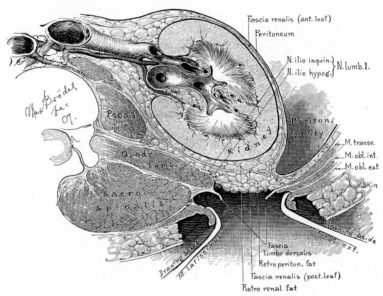

FIG. 402.—CROSS SECTION THROUGH THE KIDNEY AND THE SUPERIOR LUMBAR TRGIONE TO SHOW THE STRUCTURES ENCOUNTERED IN THE LUMBAR APPROACH TO THE KIDNEY.

The perirenal fasciae and areas of fat about the kidney are emphasized. (After Kelly, Burnam.)

from a layer 5 mm. thick to a cushion of enormous dimensions, upon which the perirenal fascial space and the fatty tunic rest.

Within the fibrous envelope of the kidney is the *perirenal fat capsule* or *tunic*, a special-ized fatty tissue designed to hold the kidney and its pedicle *in situ*. The fat is more abundant along the borders of the kidney and behind it than in front. Its almost fluid consistency allows the kidney to execute the normal movements transmitted to it by the diaphragm. The fat passes into the hilum and insinuates itself between the renal blood vessels, affording them protection; it fuses with the outer coat of the calices. Delicate fibrous septa pass from the perirenal fascia to the true kidney capsule and loculate the fatty tissue. The more fat present, the more rigidly the kidney is held in position. Lesions of the perirenal tunic occur in perinephritis.

5. **Relations of the Kidney to the Vertebrae, Diaphragm, and Pleura.**—The upper pole of the kidney lies almost at the level of the middle or lower portion of the eleventh or twelfth thoracic vertebra, while the inferior pole extends as low as the body of the second or third lumbar vertebra. Extension beyond these points is abnormal. The right kidney usually is placed 1 to 2 cm. lower than the left, because the large right lobe of the liver arrests its ascent. The kidneys generally lie about half the thickness of a vertebra lower in females than in males. In early childhood, the kidneys lie at a definitely lower level than at any subsequent time, because of their relatively greater size and the relatively shorter

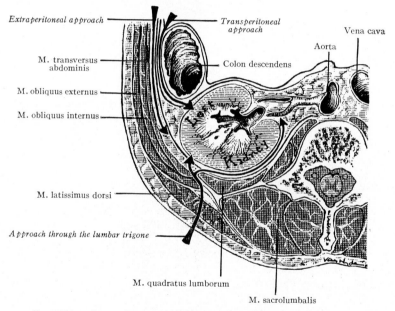

FIG. 403.—CROSS SECTION TO SHOW THE PATHS OF APPROACH TO THE LEFT KIDNEY.

lumbar region. A line connecting the tips of the lumbar transverse processes marks the median border of the kidney.

About one fourth of the right kidney and one third of the left lie in contact with the diaphragm. If there are weak portions in the opposing areas of diaphragm (p. 239), the posterior surface of the kidneys may come into close relationship with the pleura Weak areas in the right diaphragm are protected, in a large measure, by the right lobe of the liver, which may explain the small number of right perinephric abscesses pervading the diaphragm and causing pleural empyema.

The posterior costodiaphragmatic pleural reflections divide the kidneys into covered and uncovered areas. The reflection of the posterior costal pleura to the diaphragm occurs along a horizontal line beginning at the lateral surface of the twelfth thoracic vertebra on the same level as, or a little below, the origin of the twelfth rib, and passes obliquely downward and laterally. The twelfth rib crosses the reflection about three fingerbreadths lateral to the median line, so that the proximal 4 cm. of the rib lie above the level of the pleura while the distal portion extends below it. Irrespective of the length of the rib or its absence, the lower line of pleural reflection remains the same; for this reason, it is important to know whether the last palpable rib is the eleventh or twelfth. This is determined by counting from above downward. About half of the left kidney and one third of the right lie above the pleural line, the left kidney being the higher placed. In renal

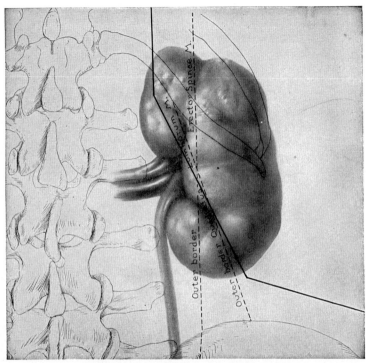

FIG. 404.—DIAGRAM OF THE POSTERIOR PROJECTION OF THE KIDNEY.
The heavy black line indicates one lumbar approach to the kidney. (W. J. Mayo, Annals of Surgery.)

surgery, production of an artificial pneumothorax may be prevented by observance of the natural protection afforded the pleural reflection by the lumbocostal ligaments externally and the lumbocostal arches intra-abdominally.

SURGICAL CONSIDERATIONS

1. Movable Kidney.—Being closely applied to the arch of the diaphragm, the normal kidneys move downward in respiration through an excursion of about 2 cm. An excessive range of mobility is encountered rather frequently, especially in women. Because of the displacing effect of the liver, the right kidney is mobile much more frequently than is the left.

Several problems present themselves in the consideration of a movable kidney: first, demonstration of the mobility; second, evaluation of the symptoms arising from the condition, and third, treatment. The displaced kidney often can be detected by abdominal examination, one hand being placed in the costo-iliac space posterior and lateral to the sacrospinalis muscle, and the other laid flat upon the subcostal abdominal wall lateral to the semilunar line. On deep inspiration, a movable kidney may be felt as a smooth rounded body well below the costal arch where it may be held between the thumb and forefinger. If an effort be made to compress its lower extremity, it usually slips upward out of reach and reappears when the patient stands or inspires deeply.

A movable right kidney must not be confused with a large gallbladder. On either side, an ovarian cyst with a long pedicle may simulate a movable kidney, as the tumor may be manipulated into the position normally occupied by the kidney.   The discomfort in movable kidney probably results from tension on the peritoneum and on the renal nerve plexuses passing to and emerging from the kidney pedicle.   The pain is referred to the abdominal wall along the sensory nerves derived from the tenth thoracic to the first lumbar segment.

Correction of this condition requires fixing the kidney in its normal position and maintaining it by nonoperative or operative measures.   Nonoperative treatment consists of application to the abdomen of variously devised supports and belts.   Operative fixation

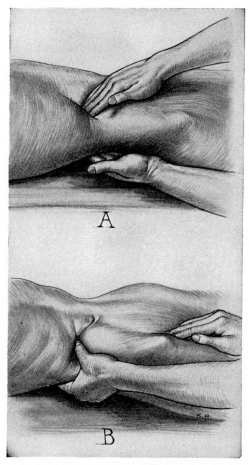

FIG. 405.—BIMANUAL PALPATION OF THE RIGHT KIDNEY.

In A, the patient is in the dorsal posture; after a deep inspiration, the right hand presses down sharply below the costal margin, thus catching a movable kidney after it has descended with the deep breath; in B, the displaced kidney is held with the left hand to prevent ascent during expiration. (After Kelly, Burnam.)

consists in suturing the kidney in its normal fossa (*nephrorrhaphy* or *nephropexy*).   The kidney is approached by the lumbar incision (p. 315), and its posterior aspect is denuded of its fatty tunic.   The ureter is freed for a considerable distance to prevent kinking.   In freeing the kidney and ureter, the renal and ureteral sympathetic plexuses are stripped away.   Sutures are passed from the substance of the kidney into the muscles at about the level of the twelfth rib.

2. **Injuries of the Kidneys.**—Severe contusions and penetrating wounds of the kidney are minimized by the deep position of the organ and its protection by the lower costal margin and the viscera applied against its abdominal aspect.   Since the eleventh and

twelfth ribs rarely are fractured, kidney laceration from dircet impact of broken ribs seldom occurs. Rupture may occur from hydrostatic pressure from impact of the twelfth rib. Contusions sufficiently serious to injure the kidney usually are received in the ilio-costal space and are likely to cause more serious injury if the abdominal walls are relaxed at the moment of impact. The kidney is pushed back and is wedged tightly into the costo-vertebral angle, and may be crushed against the last rib and the upper two lumbar vertebrae.

Kidney rupture may be incomplete, the cortex and parenchyma only being lacerated, or it may be complete, and extend from the exterior to the interior of the organ, from the capsule into the pelvis. The tear may involve the overlying peritoneum and result in serious intra-abdominal hemorrhage. In complete rupture, an extravasation of blood and urine may spread diffusely into the perirenal tissue and give rise to a large extraper-itoneal extension which may bulge the flank and pass downward into the iliac fossa.

3. **Hydronephrosis.**—Hydronephrosis, or perhaps better, uronephrosis, designates urinary retention in a distended kidney pelvis and its calices, resulting from some impedi-ment to urinary outflow. Whether the urine so backed up is or is not infected determines the conditions of infected hydronephrosis or simple hydronephrosis. When marked infection occurs in the hydronephrotic sac, the condition becomes one of *pyonephrosis*.

Blockage to the urinary outflow may occur anywhere in the ureter or urethra, and distention may occur in the calices or pelvis alone, or in both these portions of the excre-tory system. Retentive phenomena may be caused by an abnormal position of the kidney or by an aberrant vessel which kinks the ureter.

4. **Perinephric Abscess.**—Perinephric abscess or abscess in the lumbarextraperit oneal fatty-areolar tissue rarely occurs secondary to primary pathologic change in the kidney substance, pelvis, or ureter. A large group of perinephric infections is secondary to pyogenic skin conditions, the usual organism being the staphylococcus. Urinary findings in perinephric abscess secondary to skin lesions usually are within normal limits Pain, if present, radiates along the course of the twelfth intercostal nerve and the iliohypogastric and ilio-inguinal branches of the first lumbar nerve. Roentgenological examinations of the lumbar and lower dorsal regions almost uniformly show certain diagnostic signs: ob-literation of the psoas muscle shadow, or marked dulness of its ordinarily sharp contour; obscuring of the kidney outline on the affected side; and a scoliosis of the lumbar spine with the concavity toward the lesion. The scoliosis may be the result of splinting action through muscle spasm or of the instinctive effort to increase the loin space. x-Ray find-ings often are the sole criteria by which an early diagnosis may be made. There may be local tenderness, overlying edema, and flexion and adduction of the thigh, since the upper lumbar nerves control those movements.

The abscess, if untreated, may extend posteriorly and point in the lumbar region, usually becoming superficial in the lumbar triangle of Petit (p. 312). It may burrow upward through the diaphragm into the pleural cavity and lung, or travel downward and form a large collection in the iliac fossa. Abscesses involving the perirenal tissue secon-darily may spread upward in the extraperitoneal tissue following appendicitis or pelvic cellulitis, or pass downward from the pleura by eroding the diaphragm in the interval behind its vertebral and costal attachments.

5. **Anomalies of the Kidney.**—Kidney anomalies assume a practical clinical impor-tance in connection with the diagnosis of intra-abdominal swellings and in the operative relief of renal conditions. During early life, the primitive kidney occupies a position in the region of the future pelvic cavity. In the course of development, it usually ascends to the ultimate lumbar position. As a consequence of incomplete migration, the kidney may assume permanently an abnormal position. This condition is known as *renal ectopia*. The kidney may lie within the corresponding iliac fossa upon the pelvic brim or within the pelvic cavity between the bladder and rectum. In developmental ascent from the pelvis, the kidney may pursue an unusual course and take a position in front of the spine or it may cross to the opposite side and lie beneath the normal kidney. The ectopically placed kidney sometimes is misshapen, or retains a greater or less degree of embryonic lobulation.

In contrast to the movable kidney, the ectopic kidney is firmly fixed. Both kidneys may be ectopic and, in such instances, they not infrequently fuse at their lower extremities forming a *horseshoe kidney*.

One kidney may be absent or exist in rudimentary form. When only one is present, it attains considerably greater dimensions than those of the normal organ.

6. **Lumbar Nephrectomy.**—The approach for lumbar nephrectomy is discussed in the region of the posterolateral abdominal wall (p. 315).

7. **Pyelotomy.**—The principal indication for incision into the kidney pelvis is the removal of renal calculi. This incision sometimes is employed as a substitute for approach through the kidney parenchyma. Incising a greatly distended kidney pelvis is a simple and entirely bloodless procedure. The kidney should be delivered into the loin incision whenever possible. Pyelotomy is not feasible when there are very many or very large stones or when the stones are high in the kidney parenchyma. Many kidneys have major calices so small that it is impossible to extract even a small stone through them. The minor calices may have such a configuration that any attempt to locate a small stone through the pelvic incision fails.

When a kidney has a large, well-defined extrarenal pelvis, it is well to begin all explorations for moderately large stones through the pelvic incision. If necessary, the incision may be extended obliquely through the posterior parenchyma in a caudad direction. If the pelvic incision is too small for the removal of the calculus, it cannot be extended in an upward direction because of the posterior branch of the renal artery which is a large vessel skirting the pelvis. The incision may be enlarged safely in an oblique downward direction over the posterior surface of the kidney. This incision combines pyelotomy and nephrotomy. It often is convenient to remove a part of the stone through the pelvic incision and the remainder through the nephrotomy opening. Incisions in the pelvis heal well if there is not too much infection of the kidney and drainage down the ureter is free. The incisions should be closed by suture in layers when possible.

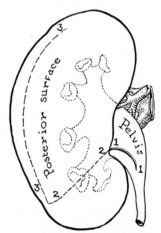

FIG. 406.—MOST BLOODLESS INCISION FOR OPENING THE KIDNEY PELVIS AND KIDNEY SUBSTANCE.

1-1 indicates pyelotomy incision; this can be carried obliquely through renal parenchyma as shown in 2-2, thus opening the lower calices; continued incision along 3-3 opens the entire pelvis. (After Kelly, Burnam.)

8. **Nephrotomy.**—Nephrotomy, or incision into the kidney, is designed to evacuate an abscess or remove calculi. The kidney is exposed as for lumbar nephrectomy and an incision is made into it, avoiding injury to the vessels and parenchyma as much as possible. A knowledge of the projection of the avascular plane on the periphery of the kidney is the key to the operation. The branches of the renal arterial supply resemble the stems and branches of a bush, in that they may be separated readily by division from within outward. Incision is made from within the kidney outward, usually with a wire or thread. The kidney first is palpated carefully to ascertain the presence of calculi, their usual sites being the calices or pelvis. In this operation, the entire kidney occasionally is slit open along the avascular plane in order to expose these cavities thoroughly. Hemorrhage is controlled by compressing the vessels in the pedicle.

(III) Ureter, Great Vessels, and Nerves

1. **Ureter.**—Toward the level of the inferior end of the kidney, the part of the pelvis lying outside the renal sinus diminishes in caliber to form a musculomucous tube, the ureter, which conveys the urine to the bladder.

In its *abdominal portion*, the ureter pursues an almost vertical course downward and medially on the anterior surface of the psoas major muscle which separates it from the tips of the transverse processes of the lumbar vertebrae. The abdominal segment is divided by the iliac crest into lumbar and iliac portions, each of which measures about 8 cm. On the right side, the abdominal ureter lies deep to the peritoneum of the right infracolic compartment. Just before it enters the pelvis, the ureter is crossed by the root of the mesentery and the terminal ileum. In its proximal portion, it lies behind the descending and transverse parts of the duodenum. Between the duodenum and the root of the mesentery of the jejuno-ileum, the spermatic, right colic, and ileocolic vessels cross the anterior surface of the ureter and separate it from the peritoneum. Because of these vascular relations, the extraperitoneal lumbo-inguinal approach (p. 415) to the ureter is preferable to the transperitoneal approach (p. 284). The ureter is attached so closely to the peritoneum that the two are not dissociated when the peritoneum is stripped forward.

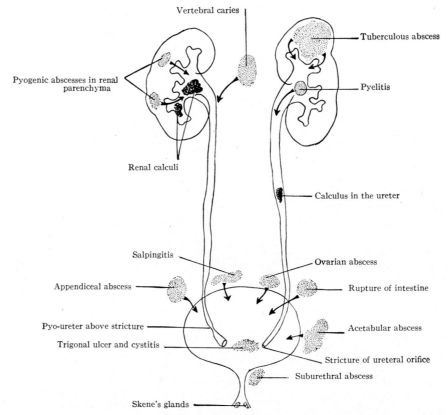

FIG. 407.—DIAGRAM TO SHOW THE VARIOUS SOURCES OF PUS IN THE URINE.

On the left side, the ureter lies deep to the peritoneum covering the left infracolic space. As it enters the pelvis, it is crossed by the pelvic mesocolon. The spermatic, left colic, and sigmoid vessels cross its anterior surface.

The *pelvic portion* of the ureter consists of parietal and intravesical divisions and makes up half of the length of the entire tube, about 15 cm. The parietal division, closely related to the peritoneum, crosses the brim of the pelvis in front of, or a little lateral to, the bifurcation of the common iliac artery. It descends abruptly between the peritoneum and the hypogastric (internal iliac) artery which separates it from the posterior wall of the pelvis and the great nerve trunks. As it approaches the base of the bladder, it is related to the superior vesical artery lying above it. Just before entering the bladder in the male, it is crossed lateromesially and on its upper aspect by the deferent duct which intervenes between it and the peritoneum.

In the female, the ureter passes to the posterior peritoneal layer of the broad ligament and enters the parametrium, through which it passes forward toward the cervix, inclining downward and medially to reach the wall of the bladder. As the ureter traverses the parametrium, it is separated from the supravaginal part of the cervix by a distance of 2 cm. At this level, it is situated a little more than 1 cm. above the lateral vaginal fornix and is enveloped closely by the veins of the vesical and vaginal plexuses. It is crossed above by the uterine artery which passes medially to the uterus from the pelvic wall. From the cervix forward, the ureter converges toward its fellow and, as it runs forward and medially, lies first beside the lateral fornix of the vagina and subsequently between the anterior vaginal wall and the base of the bladder, still within the parametrium.

The intravesical course of the ureter measures about 0.5 to 1 cm. and is the most contracted part of the duct, being but 3 to 4 mm. in diameter. Calculi naturally lodge at this point.

The *caliber* of the normal ureter is not uniform, but is constricted in certain locations and has long spindle-shaped dilations between the constrictions. The uppermost of these constrictions lies about 5.5 cm. from the kidney pelvis, the next at the brim of the pelvis where the ureter crosses the common iliac artery, and the lowermost just outside the ureteral orifice. The constricted segments are the points of arrest of ureteral calculi. Blockage of the ureter by a calculus often produces an acute hydronephrosis, the symptoms of which may overshadow symptoms directly referable to the seat of impaction of the offending stone. The subjective symptoms of a calculus are explained by the interrelation of the ureteral, vesical, and genital nerve supply through the great sympathetic plexuses.

The renal, spermatic, and superior and inferior vesicular arteries constitute the *arterial supply* of the ureter. The branches anastomose freely with one another to form the ureteric plexus. Because of its vascularity, the ureter withstands a considerable amount of surgical trauma, large segments of it may be mobilized without subsequent sloughing, and injuries to it heal quickly.

2. Abdominal Aorta.—The abdominal aorta extends from the aortic hiatus of the diaphragm to the body of the fourth lumbar vertebra, where it divides into three terminal branches, a small median branch, the middle sacral artery, and two lateral branches, the common iliacs. The projection of the termination of the aorta to the anterior abdominal wall corresponds to the midpoint of a line joining the summits of the iliac crests. The aorta gives off visceral and parietal branches.

The **visceral branches** comprise the celiac, superior and inferior mesenteric, renal, spermatic, and ovarian arteries. The *celiac artery* arises from the anterior surface of the aorta just below the aortic opening into the diaphragm. It is a short trunk projecting forward above the upper margin of the pancreas. The *superior mesenteric artery* springs from the anterior surface of the aorta at the level of the first lumbar vertebra about 12 mm. distal to the origin of the celiac artery, usually between the points of origin of the third and fourth paired lumbar parietal branches. The *inferior mesenteric artery* arises from the aorta 3 or 4 cm. above the bifurcation into the two common iliac arteries.

The **parietal branches** are the paired *inferior phrenic arteries*, arising near the aortic hiatus and supplying the lumbar part of the diaphragm. From them, superior branches to the suprarenal glands frequently arise. The *lumbar arteries* correspond to the intercostal arteries from the thoracic aorta and are arranged in four pairs. At the mesial border of the psoas muscle, each artery divides into dorsal branches which supply the muscles of the spine, and ventral branches which supply the muscles of the abdominal wall.

3. Common and External Iliac Arteries.—The two *common iliac arteries* pass obliquely laterally, downward, and forward to about the level of the sacro-iliac synchondroses where each bifurcates into an internal iliac (hypogastric) and an external iliac trunk. Save for their terminals, neither common iliac has collaterals. The terminal ileum on the right and the pelvic colon on the left rest upon them. The left common iliac artery is crossed by the superior hemorrhoidal branch of the inferior mesenteric artery.

Of the two main trunks of the common iliac, the *external iliac artery* alone remains in the abdominal cavity. It runs from the sacro-iliac synchondrosis to the lateral side of the lacunar ligament beneath the inguinal ligament where it becomes the femoral artery. The two branches of the external iliac, the inferior epigastric, and the deep circumflex iliac arteries are derivations of the terminal part of the trunk. The external iliac artery is most accessible by the extraperitoneal approach (p. 415).

4. Inferior Vena Cava.—The inferior vena cava caval system includes the veins of the body wall below the diaphragm, those of the lower extremities, and those from the abdominal and pelvic cavities, save the veins of the portal system.

From its origin in the two *common iliac veins*, the inferior vena cava increases in size from below upward with the accession of the various tributaries, and becomes the largest of the body veins. It maintains a close relationship with the abdominal aorta throughout the major part of its course, and its paired branches correspond mainly with those of the aorta. Laterally, it lies in contact with the right psoas major muscle, and is related closely to the descending duodenum, the head of the pancreas, and the medial margin of the right kidney.

A *thrombosis of the inferior vena cava*, or any part thereof, demands an accessory path to the superior cava for the tributary blood. The collateral burden borne by the anastomosing veins of the abdominal wall and the azygos and hemiazygos systems aids materially in shunting the flow from the inferior to the superior cava. In *portal obstruction*, portal blood passes into the caval system along well-defined collateral pathways (p. 341).

5. Retroperitoneal Lymphatics.—The retroperitoneal space is very rich in lymphatic structures, which form a chain extending from the inguinal ligament to the diaphragm. The many nodes and vessels are grouped about the great vascular trunks of the region and unite the lymphatic drainage from the extremities, pelvis, and abdomen with that of the mediastinum.

The more differentiated groups of lymph nodes are the iliac and lumbo-aortic glands. The *iliac lymph glands*, grouped about the external and common iliac vessels, receive afferent vessels from nodes in many different areas, including those draining almost the whole of the pelvic contents and also the inguinal and subinguinal nodes draining the lower extremity. The *lumbo-aortic nodes* are remarkable for their large number. They lie in superficial and deep groups about the aorta and inferior vena cava and receive the efferents of the intestines and their mesenteries. The vessels leading from the lumbo-aortic glands open into the *cisterna chyli*, which is scarcely more than a dilated ampulla of the *thoracic duct*.

6. Abdominal and Pelvic Divisions of the Sympathetic Gangliated Chain and Their Plexuses.—The *abdominal* or *lumbar division* of the gangliated chain consists of ganglia and connecting association cords lying in the retroperitoneal space, anterior to the lumbar vertebrae and mesial to the psoas major muscles. The left cord is concealed partially by the aorta, and the right cord by the vena cava. Association cords connect the abdominal with the thoracic and pelvic divisions. Central branches or communicating rami pass in an irregular fashion from the gangliated trunk to the anterior rami of the lumbar nerves. They run beneath the origins of the psoas major muscle over the vertebral bodies. Occasionally, they pierce the fibers of the muscle. Peripheral branches supply the aortic subdivision of the celiac plexus.

The *pelvic* or *sacral division* of the gangliated chain lies on the pelvic surface of the sacrum mesial to the anterior sacral foramina. Irregular central or communicating rami connect the sacral ganglia with the anterior rami of the sacral and coccygeal nerves.

The peripheral branches of the gangliated chain are characterized as in the neck and thorax, by the formation of, or association with, plexuses in their neighborhood. These plexuses lie on a plane anterior to that of the gangliated cords. The celiac, hypogastric, and pelvic plexuses serve to distribute nerves to the viscera and vessels of the abdominal and pelvic cavities. They are elaborated by peripheral branches from the lower thoracic, abdominal, and upper pelvic divisions of the gangliated chain, and are related to the central nervous system by communicating rami to the lower thoracic, upper lumbar, and sacral nerves. The hypogastric plexus is a connection between the celiac and pelvic plexuses.

7. **Lumbar Sympathetic Ganglionectomy and Trunk Resection.**—The removal of these structures can be performed through a midline transperitoneal incision, or it can be done extraperitoneally through a large, lateral, muscle-splitting incision. The transperitoneal approach has the advantage that both lumbar chains can be removed through the one incision.

After the lower midline incision is made, the patient is placed in the Trendelenburg position and the intestines are packed off superiorly, thus insuring exposure of the struc-

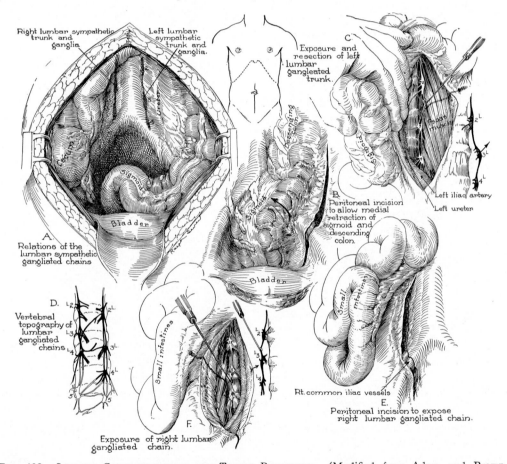

FIG. 408.—LUMBAR GANGLIONECTOMY AND TRUNK RESECTION. (Modified from Adson and Brown.)

tures overlying the lumbar ganglia. To expose the *left lumbar sympathetic chain*, it is necessary to loosen and elevate the attachment of the mesosigmoid and of the lower descending colon. When the line of cleavage is established, the large bowel is elevated readily and retracted medially. The retroperitoneum is exposed, and the left lumbar gangliated chain, which lies on the lumbar vertebrae, is found just medial to the psoas muscle. The aorta overlies it. The second, third, and fourth lumbar ganglia, the trunk, and rami are dissected free and removed. The fourth ganglion lies at the brim of the pelvis.

The *approach to the right lumbar gangliated chain* is similar to that on the left, except that the peritoneal incision is made just lateral to the inferior vena cava and is continued inferiorly over the right common iliac vein into the true pelvis. It is carried superiorly and medially along the root of the mesentery of the small bowel and partially across the vena cava. The cecum, small intestine, and ureter are retracted superiorly and to the right. Retraction of the vena cava medially and of the right common iliac vein inferiorly exposes the location of the lumbar ganglia, chain, and rami. These structures are excised Closure consists in apposition of both retroperitoneal incisions and suture of the abdominal wall.

Left lumbar ganglionectomy removes the inhibitory fibers to the lower left colon. This operation often has allowed the motor parasympathetic fibers to this bowel to preponderate, and has enabled the distended bowel in Hirschsprung's disease (megacolon) to empty itself. The operation may be of value in removing the vasospastic nerve elements, thought by some to be responsible for Raynaud's disease.

8. **Resection of the Presacral (Superior Hypogastric) Plexus.**—This operation has restored normal bladder functions in certain cases of chronic urinary retention from cord lesions, and has lessened the symptoms of dysmenorrhea and pelvic pain.

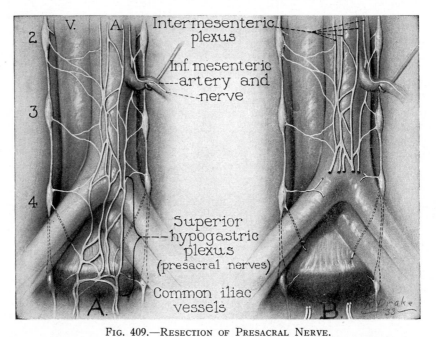

Fig. 409.—Resection of Presacral Nerve.

A, Presacral nerves and their connections; B, presacral nerves (superior hypogastric plexus) removed. (Adson and Masson, Mayo Clinic.)

The explanation of these results lies in the double sympathetic innervation of the pelvic contents. The bladder obtains its motor (emptying) impulses through the sacral gangliated chain and gets its inhibitory fibers from the thoracicolumbar outflow, which passes through and contributes to the presacral plexus. Removal of the presacral plexus removes the brake mechanism to these structures and allows the motor fibers from the sacral outflow to function more efficiently. Excision of these nerve fibers interrupts the pathway of the sensory (afferent) sympathetic fibers from the bladder and pelvic genitalia and sometimes alleviates the pain of dysmenorrhea. Fibers which contribute to the presacral (hypogastric) plexus reach it from the preaortic collateral ganglia. The plexus occupies a varying extent between the two common iliac arteries. Occasionally, the nerve elements are gathered into a single nerve, the presacral nerve, and not into a plexus. The nerve or plexus is easy of access in front of the fifth lumbar vertebra and lies in the median line immediately under the peritoneum. Posteriorly, it is separated from the great vessels by loose connective tissue. Lower down on the sacrum, it becomes more intimately

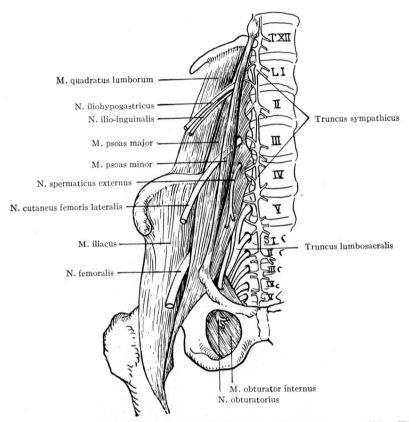

M. quadratus lumborum

N. iliohypogastricus

N. ilio-inguinalis

M. psoas major

M. psoas minor

N. spermaticus externus

N. cutaneus femoris lateralis

M. iliacus

N. femoralis

Truncus sympathicus

Truncus lumbosacralis

M. obturator internus
N. obturatorius

FIG. 410.—RELATIONS OF THE LUMBOSACRAL PLEXUS AND ITS BRANCHES. (After Tinel.)

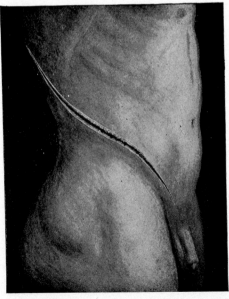

FIG. 411.—INCISION FOR THE LUMBAR EXTRAPERITONEAL EXPOSURE OF THE KIDNEY, AND FOR THE EX-
TRAPERITONEAL LUMBO-ILIO-INGUINAL EXPOSURE OF THE ENTIRE URETER.

The incision begins about the middle of the twelfth rib, and runs downward and forward in the direction of a midpoint between the center of the iliac crest and the anterior superior spine; thence it skirts the
anterior superior iliac spine, and passes downward and forward, parallel with the inguinal ligament. (Bickham, "Operative Surgery.")

related to the underlying bone. The attachment of the mesentery of the small bowel is cephalad to the presacral plexus, and the root of the mesosigmoid lies to its left.

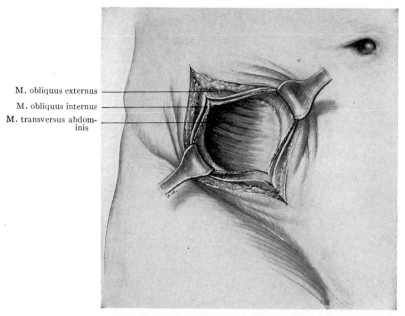

M. obliquus externus
M. obliquus internus
M. transversus abdom-
inis

FIG. 412.—ILIAC EXTRAPERITONEAL APPROACH TO THE PELVIC URETER AND GREAT VESSELS.
The external and internal oblique muscles are incised in the direction of the skin incision.

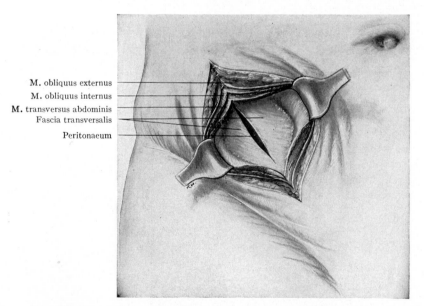

M. obliquus externus
M. obliquus internus
M. transversus abdominis
Fascia transversalis

Peritonaeum

FIG. 413.—ILIAC EXTRAPERITONEAL APPROACH TO THE PELVIC URETER AND GREAT VESSELS.
The external and internal oblique and transversus abdominis muscles are incised in the line of the skin incision; incision is made in the transversalis fascia preliminary to extraperitoneal exposure of the ureter and pelvic vessels.

9. **Lumbar Plexus.**—The lumbar plexus is formed by the anterior rami of the first three lumbar nerves and a part of the fourth lumbar nerve. The plexus lies in the substance of the psoas muscle anterior to the transverse processes.

10. **Surgical Approach to the Ureter.**—For purposes of repair, removal of stones, or excision, the ureter can be reached most readily by the retroperitoneal approach. The approach permits of wide examination, and is chosen when the nature or exact location of the lesion is not known. With the patient in lateral decubitus and well-arched over a sand bag, a lumbo-iliac incision is made, beginning below the last rib, as in lumbar nephrectomy (p. 315). The wound is extended downward and forward 2.5 cm. mesial to the

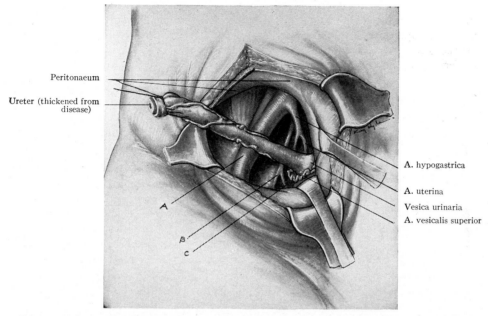

Peritonaeum

Ureter (thickened from disease)

A. hypogastrica

A. uterina

Vesica urinaria

A. vesicalis superior

FIG. 414.—ILIAC EXTRAPERITONEAL APPROACH TO THE PELVIC URETER AND GREAT VESSELS.
The peritoneum has been dissected bluntly medianward and downward and a greatly thickened ureter and the pelvic vessels are exposed; A, A. iliaca externa; B, ligamentum umbilicale laterale; C, A. vesicalis inferior.

anterior superior spine, and may be continued just above and parallel to the inguinal ligament, to the lateral margin of the rectus. The adherence of the ureter to the peritoneum must be borne in mind when that membrane is reflected toward the median line. Its presence under the membrane may be detected readily by running the tip of the finger lightly across its course. It can be detached easily from the peritoneum to permit surgical exploration and removal of a calculus.

PELVIS

THE pelvis is the skeletal base of the trunk and transmits the weight of the super-jacent torso to the lower limbs.   The bones which enter into its formation, the sacrum and coccyx behind and the innominate bones laterally and anteriorly, articulate with each other to form a complete ring and are maintained in position by large and powerful ligaments.   Topographically, the pelvis consists of a bony and ligamentous framework and includes the soft parts clothing its inner and outer aspects and the pelvic contents.   It is closed inferiorly by layers of muscle and fascia which constitute the pelvic diaphragm.

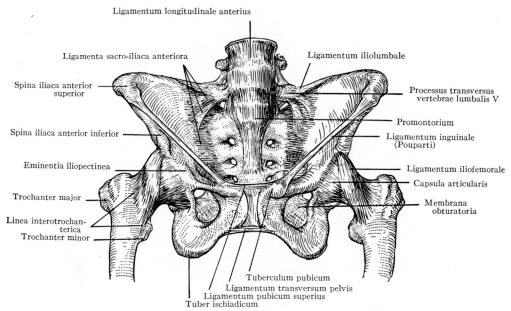

Ligamentum longitudinale anterius

Ligamenta sacro-iliaca anteriora

Ligamentum iliolumbale

Spina iliaca anterior superior

Processus transversus vertebrae lumbalis V

Spina iliaca anterior inferior

Promontorium

Ligamentum inguinale (Pouparti)

Eminentia iliopectinea

Ligamentum iliofemorale

Capsula articularis

Trochanter major

Membrana obturatoria

Linea interotrochan-terica
Trochanter minor

Tuberculum pubicum
Ligamentum transversum pelvis
Ligamentum pubicum superius
Tuber ischiadicum

FIG. 415.—ANTERIOR VIEW OF THE PELVIS.

From the surgical viewpoint, certain parts of the pelvic composite are discussed best in other regions.   The pelvic diaphragm serves as the floor of the perineum.   The structures lying on the iliac floor of the false pelvis are considered in that region.   The soft parts related to the outer wall of the pelvic framework are discussed in the gluteal region, the adductor region of the hip, and the anterior region of the thigh.

I. BONY AND LIGAMENTOUS PELVIS

The bony and ligamentous pelvis is divided into: the bony pelvis as a whole and the sacro-iliac and sacrococcygeal regions.

A. BONY PELVIS AS A WHOLE

1. **Definition and Boundaries.**—The bony pelvis is formed anteriorly and laterally by the innominate bones, and posteriorly by the sacrum and coccyx.   These bones are united by a number of strong and resistant ligaments.   In contrast to the shoulder girdle, designed for freedom of motion, the pelvic girdle is adapted for strength, support, and locomotion. In the erect position, the pelvic girdle is inclined forward so that the plane of the inlet subtends an angle of about 60 degrees with the horizontal, and the axis of the sacrum forms an angle of about 110 degrees with the lumbar spine.

416

The plane of the *pelvic inlet* (*superior strait*) is regular in outline and connects the promontory of the sacrum with the superior margin of the pubis. It forms the boundary between the true and false pelves.

The circumference of the *pelvic outlet* (*inferior strait*) is very irregular and presents median and lateral notches. The median subpubic notch is formed by the union of the pubic rami at the pubic symphysis, and is traversed by the urogenital apparatus. Each lateral sciatic (sacrosciatic) notch lies between the lateral margin of the sacrum and coccyx and the body and tuberosity of the ischium. The sciatic notch is transformed into greater and lesser sciatic foramina by the sacrospinous and sacrotuberous ligaments. These foramina offer anatomic and pathologic communication between the intrapelvic and gluteal areas. On each side of the median line anteriorly is the obturator foramen, which is closed by the obturator membrane and clothed without and within by the obturator muscles.

2. **Surface Anatomy.**—The pubic symphysis and the pubic tubercle, about 2.5 cm. lateral to it, usually can be palpated. The anterior superior spine is made out readily, but the anterior inferior iliac spine is too deep to be felt. The outer lip of the iliac crest can be followed to the posterior superior iliac spine which lies on a level with the middle of the sacro-iliac joint. In the erect position, a line drawn from the posterior superior iliac spine to the anterior superior spine inclines forward and downward, making an angle of about 15 degrees with the horizontal. The angle is increased in the heavy anatomical type and decreased in the slender type. The gluteal musculature masks the lateral flare of the ilium. The dorsal surface of the sacrum and its spinous processes, the ischial tuberosity, and the inferior ramus of the pubis can be palpated. By vaginal and rectal examination, the framework of the pelvic canal can be felt.

3. **Development and Structure.**—At birth, the pelvis is small and poorly developed. It is cone shaped and the sacrum is almost vertical. The characteristics of the adult pelvis are determined gradually during the process of growth. Abnormal weight distribution, such as that caused by deviation of the vertebral column or infection in the innominate bones, sacrum, or pelvic joints, tends to produce deformity of the pelvis. Recognition of deformed pelves is of the greatest importance in obstetrics.

The innominate bone presents two groups of ossifying centers, acetabular and marginal. Of the *acetabular centers*, that for the development of the ilium appears during the second fetal month and grows rapidly toward the upper part of the bone. A center for the ischium appears below the acetabulum at the fourth month, but the pubic center is later in development (fifth to sixth month). The union of these ossifying centers, as a rule, occurs near puberty. The pubic and ischial rami unite at about the tenth year.

The *marginal centers* include those for the crest of the ilium, anterior superior spine, tuberosity of the ischium, angle of the pubis, and the spine of the ischium. The site of predilection for osteitis is the bone about actively growing centers. Osteitis of the regions about the acetabulum occurs early during the active growth of the acetabular centers, but marginal osteitis is a postpuberty disease occurring between the fifteenth and thirtieth years.

4. **Function.**—The bony and ligamentous pelvic mechanism is designed to subserve three functions: to protect the pelvic viscera, support the vertebral column, and facilitate locomotion.

The pelvic girdle *protects the viscera* contained within its canal from all ordinary trauma, so that only through the abdominal wall above or the perineum below are they likely to be injured, although they may be damaged in penetrating wounds through the obturator foramina and the sciatic notches. If the resistance of the bony pelvis is overcome, resulting in fracture, the bony fragments may become damaging factors and produce bladder laceration or perforation (p. 447), or rupture of the urethra (p. 498). For this reason, all fractured pelves require scrupulous clinical observation.

In *supporting the weight* transmitted through the spine, the sacrum is forced downward so that the sacral promontory faces forward and downward in the pelvis. In sitting, the weight is transmitted to the ischial tuberosities; in standing, it is transmitted down the thighs.   The acetabulum, in order to act efficiently as a supporting mechanism, must be of sufficient strength to resist the heavy pressure from the head of the femur in the erect posture   Its only weak feature (p. 692) is the thinness of its floor, the result of the union of the three acetabular centers of ossification.

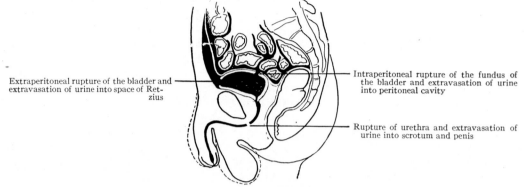

Extraperitoneal rupture of the bladder and extravasation of urine into space of Retzius

Intraperitoneal rupture of the fundus of the bladder and extravasation of urine into peritoneal cavity

Rupture of urethra and extravasation of urine into scrotum and penis

FIG. 416.—MOST FREQUENT COMPLICATIONS OF FRACTURE OF THE PELVIS.

Ignoring the flares of the ilia, the bony pelvic ring or girdle may be regarded as a *stabilizing mechanism adapted to locomotion*.   It is comprised of a main posterior arch and a complementary anterior or counterarch for the support and distribution of the body weight in standing and the additional thrust in locomotion.   The posterior arch consists of the three upper sacral vertebrae contributing to the sacro-iliac joint, the sacro-iliac

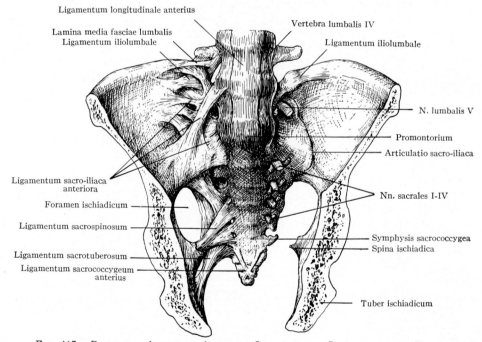

Ligamentum longitudinale anterius

Lamina media fasciae lumbalis
Ligamentum iliolumbale

Vertebra lumbalis IV

Ligamentum iliolumbale

N. lumbalis V

Promontorium

Articulatio sacro-iliaca

Ligamentum sacro-iliaca anteriora

Foramen ischiadicum

Ligamentum sacrospinosum

Ligamentum sacrotuberosum

Ligamentum sacrococcygeum anterius

Nn. sacrales I-IV

Symphysis sacrococcygea
Spina ischiadica

Tuber ischiadicum

FIG. 417.—POSTERIOR ARCH AND ANTERIOR LIGAMENTOUS SUPPORT OF THE PELVIS.

articulations, and the exceedingly strong pillars of the hip bone running from the sacro-iliac joint into the acetabular cavities.   The anterior or counterarch consists of the bony masses which run forward from the bodies of the ilium and ischium to form the pubis at the summit of the arch.   The line of union of the two arches lies in a frontal plane through the acetabular cavities.

The segments of the arches are tied together by three joints, an interpubic and two sacro-iliac. The slight elasticity in the pelvic girdle, afforded by the presence of these joints, materially lessens shock. Their comparative freedom from movement affords stability indispensable in efficient locomotion. Laxity in these joints causes pain and interferes materially with locomotion.

5. **Sexual Differences in the Pelvis.**—The female pelvis differs in form and dimensions from that of the male. The pelvic inlet in the female is oval; that in the male is heart shaped. In general, the female pelvis is more regular in outline. In the male pelvis, the sacral promontory is more prominent and the sacrum is longer and more curved. Although the extreme width of the pelvis does not differ materially in the sexes, the flares of the ilia are flatter, the pelvic cavity is broader and shallower, the acetabula and the ischial tuberosities are set farther apart, the bony walls of the pelvic canal are more vertical, and the subpubic angle is broader in the female than in the male.

6. **Obstetrical Measurements.**—The diameters of the superior strait (pelvic inlet), middle strait (pelvic canal), and inferior strait (pelvic outlet) are of practical importance in obstetrics.

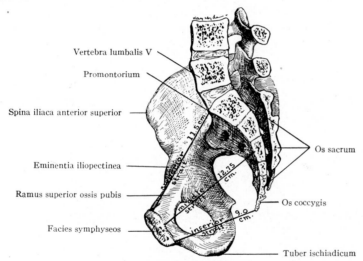

Fig. 418.—Lateral View of the Female Pelvis, Indicating the Planes and Measurements of the Anteroposterior Diameters.

The transverse diameter of the *superior strait* is the greatest distance between the linea arcuata on either side, and measures from 13 to 14 cm. The anteroposterior diameter measures 11 cm. from the sacral promontory to the superior margin of the symphysis. The oblique diameter, measured from the sacro-iliac joint to the opposite pectineal eminence, is about 12.5 cm. If the superior strait is contracted, the fetal head cannot engage in the pelvis.

The greatest diameter of the *middle strait* of the pelvis, the anteroposterior, is 12 cm., measured from the third sacral vertebra to the middle of the pubic symphysis. The fetal head, after traversing the inlet by way of the greatest available diameter, accommodates itself by rotation to the greatest available diameter of the middle strait. The diameters of the superior and middle straits are bony and incapable of distention.

The anteroposterior diameter of the *inferior strait*, which extends from the tip of the coccyx to the inferior margin of the symphysis, is 9 cm., but it may be increased 2 or 3 cm. because of the movability of the coccyx. The transverse diameter of the outlet, between the two ischial tuberosities, is from 10 to 12 cm.

7. **Fractures of the Pelvis.**—The bony pelvis has great power of resistance to trauma and gives way and fractures in its weak areas only when the limits of its elasticity are reached. Its strongest portions are the lateral parts of the innominate bones; its weak-

est, the sacro-iliac region, the alae of the ilia, and the pubo-obturator areas. Pubo-obturator fractures are very frequent and, because of their proximity to the bladder, are exceedingly dangerous.

When the pelvis is compressed anteroposteriorly by *indirect violence*, as in a squeezing accident, the brunt of the acting force is borne by the weak anterior counterarch, with resulting fracture of the pubic rami. The strong ligaments uniting the pubes tend to maintain the integrity of the symphysis. If the force continues to act, the strong posterior arch is spread forcibly, throwing a strain upon the sacro-iliac joints. The joints are bound so firmly by ligaments that they seldom tear; fracture of the adjacent bones is much more frequent.

When the squeezing force is applied transversely, the acetabula are pressed forcibly toward one another. Since the anterior arch is weaker than the posterior, the former often gives way and continuing violence forces the two ilia together. Continued strain falls upon the sacro-iliac joints, and their posterior ligaments may tear away a portion of adjacent bone.

In falls upon the feet or upon the ischial tuberosities, the main arch may escape injury because of its strength, but the anterior arch sometimes is fractured, or the acetabulum may be injured and the femur be driven through the thinnest part of the acetabular

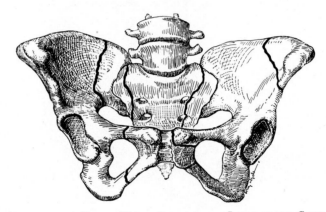

FIG. 419.—WEAK AREAS OF THE PELVIS WHICH INDICATE THE LINES OF THE COMMONER FRACTURES.

fossa into the pelvis (p. 692). In young individuals, the acetabulum may be broken into its three anatomical segments or its rim may be torn away. When a double vertical fracture occurs through both ischiopubic rami anteriorly and the ilium near the sacro-iliac joint posteriorly, there is a large pelvic fragment, more or less movable with the femur, which sometimes presents the picture of fracture of the neck of the femur (p. 688).

Any part of the pelvis, even the sacrum, may be broken by well-localized *direct trauma*. The crest or any of the spines of the ilium may be knocked off or torn away, or the epiphyses of the iliac crest and spines be separated. In spite of the tremendous pull on the ischial tuberosities by the hamstring muscles, injury of the tuberosities is comparatively rare.

Much of the gravity of pelvic fractures depends upon the occurrence of *visceral complications*. Large pelvic vessels frequently have been born in fractures running to the brim of the pelvis. Rupture of the bladder (p. 448) or urethra (p. 498) may result from the penetration of a splinter or fragment of bone.

B. SACRO-ILIAC REGION

1. **Definition and Boundaries.**—The sacro-iliac joints embrace the expanded portion, or three upper segments, of the sacrum and the articular surfaces of the ilia. The two joints are important elastic buffers between the spinal column and the lower extremities and contribute to the posterior arch of the pelvic girdle (p. 418).

2. Surface Anatomy.—Mesial to the easily palpable, blunt, posterior superior iliac spine is a depression corresponding to the sacro-iliac joint line. The underlying, tense soft parts offer great resistance to deep palpation in examination for tenderness following strain. On the sacrum near the joint line, a row of dorsal projections, corresponding to the rudimentary, fused transverse processes of the sacral vertebrae, may be palpated. Mesial to the transverse processes are the posterior sacral foramina.

3. Sacro-iliac Joint.—The articulating surface of the sacrum is directed posteriorly and laterally, while that of the ilium is directed forward and mesially. The plane of the joint looking from the pelvis is directed posteriorly and mesially, and the joint space is an unevenly curved slit. The articular surfaces, in the main, are smooth, but they have several irregular projections and depressions which help to lock and stabilize the joint.

Posterior to the articulating areas, the bony surfaces of the sacrum and ilium are rough, for the attachment of the strong reinforcing *ligaments*. The short, posterior inter-osseus ligament crosses the longitudinal depression behind the joint. The long and short

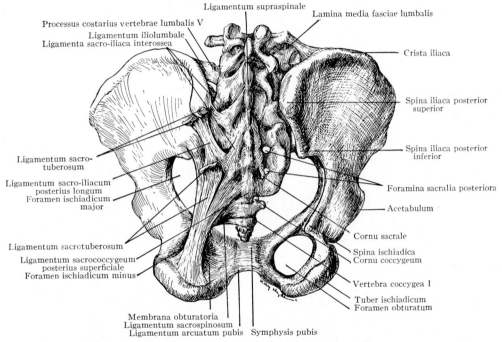

FIG. 420.—POSTERIOR LIGAMENTOUS SUPPORT OF THE PELVIS

posterior sacro-iliac ligaments constitute a strong expansive mass of fibrous bands, extending obliquely outward to the ilium from the lateral sacral crest, and also reinforce the posterior joint line. The sacrotuberous and sacrospinous ligaments, which arise over the whole area of the posterior sacro-iliac ligaments and are anchored into the ischial tuberosity and spine, further stabilize the joint. The anterior sacro-iliac ligament consists of broad, thin, fibrous plates extending from the sacrum to the medial surface of the ilium. The iliolumbar ligament is a strong, expansive, fibrous band extending from the posterior part of each iliac crest and the adjacent sacrum to the transverse process of the fifth lumbar vertebra. As the transverse processes of the fifth lumbar vertebra lie at a lower level than the crests of the ilia, the iliolumbar ligaments act as a hammock for this vertebra. In this way, they oppose the shearing force of the superimposed body weight. The short thin capsule which connects the margins of the articular surfaces of the sacro-iliac joint is reinforced anteriorly by the iliolumbar and anterior sacro-iliac ligaments.

Weight-bearing in unfavorable conditions of posture and muscle balance may strain one or the other joint and weaken it so that recurrence of injury is common, even to the point of producing a chronically relaxed or strained joint. A strained joint requires fixation or stabilization sufficient to restrain the movements of the lower segments of the spine, particularly those at the lumbosacral connection. A subluxated joint may require manipulative reduction in addition to fixation and stabilization.

The ordinary tests to demonstrate a lesion in the sacro-iliac joint are straight leg-raising (Kernig's sign), hyperextension of the extremity on the trunk, and prone knee flexion. *Straight leg-raising* takes advantage of the insertion of the sacrotuberous ligament on the ischium, where the great hamstring muscles from the hip to the leg originate. When the hamstrings are stretched in this maneuver, they pull on the ischium and strain the sacro-iliac joint because they tend to rotate the ilium posteriorly. *Forced hyperextension* of the

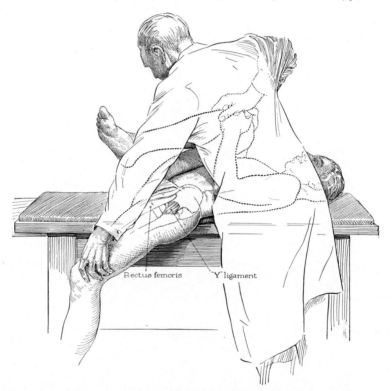

Rectus femoris   "Y" ligament

Fig. 421.—Test for Differentiation Between Lumbosacral and Sacro-iliac Lesions.

The sketch shows forcible hyperextension of the left hip, with the pelvis and lumbar spine fixed by means of extreme flexion of the right hip. Pain generally is present in sacro-iliac lesions and absent in umbosacral lesions. (Gaenslen.)

extremity puts strain on the anterior ligaments of the hip joint and on the corresponding sacro-iliac joint, tending to rotate the ilium forward.

Knee flexion with the body in the prone position also rotates the ilium forward by tensing the quadriceps muscle and making traction upon the anterior iliac spines (Pitkin).

In lesions of the sacro-iliac joint, there is radiation of pain to any or all of the following locations: buttocks, posterior and lateral portions of the thigh, posterior and lateral leg, lateral side of the foot, and occasionally the groin. A characteristic list of the trunk to one side or the other for relief from pain, and induced spasm in the spinal muscles cause scoliosis and are common manifestations of sacro-iliac strain.

Chronic osteo-arthritis with spur formation is potential of disability upon slight injury. In old age, the sacro-iliac articulation may undergo bony changes resulting in an immovable joint (synarthrosis).

Hyperextension of the hip with fixation of the pelvis and lumbar spine is a valuable diagnostic procedure in the differentiation between sacro-iliac and lumbosacral lesions, and between right and left sided lesions. The patient, lying supine, flexes the knee and hip on the same side acutely, the thigh being crowded against the abdomen with the aid of both the patient's hands clasped about the flexed knee. This brings the lumbar spine firmly in contact with the table, and fixes both the pelvis and the lumbar spine. The patient then is brought well to the side of the table, and the opposite thigh is hyperextended slowly by the examiner with gradually increasing force by pressure of the examiner's hand on the top of the knee. With the opposite hand, the examiner assists the patient in fixing the lumbar spine by pressure over the patient's clasped hands. The hyperextension of the hip exerts a rotating force on the corresponding half of the pelvis in the sagittal plane

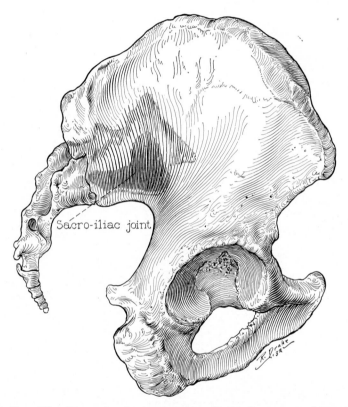

FIG. 422.—PROJECTED SURFACE OF THE RIGHT SACRO-ILIAC JOINT.
The level of the inferior margin of the sacro-iliac joint runs parallel to the superior margin of the sacro sciatic notch. (Ghormley, Jour. Amer. Med. Assoc., Dec. 2, 1933.)

through the transverse axis of the sacro-iliac joint. The pull is made on the ilium through the Y ligament and the muscles attached to the anterior superior and anterior inferior spines. As a result of the impaired ligamentous support on the diseased side, this rotating force causes abnormal mobility accompanied by pain, either local or referred on the side of the lesion. Confirmation of the observations thus made by carrying out this test on the opposite side generally is possible (Gaenslen).

Inordinate and disadvantageous stress and strain may occur also at the union between the fifth lumbar vertebra and the sacrum. The fifth lumbar vertebra shows many irregularities and developmental anomalies which play a rôle in low-back injuries. Remedy of strain in the lumbosacral joint, as in the sacro-iliac joint, requires restraint of movements by fixation.

4. Sacro-iliac Tuberculosis.—The masses of cancellous bone contiguous to the sacro-iliac articulation are sites for tuberculous infection. The pus may course deep to the ilio-lumbar ligament and reach the psoas muscle which it follows into the thigh (p. 397). The products of the infection may escape from the pelvis through the greater sciatic foramen and elevate the gluteus maximus muscle (p. 398), follow the pyriformis muscle, and point at the posterior thigh near the great trochanter or follow the sheath of the sciatic nerve. Infectious products may run along the curve of the sacrum and rupture into the rectum or invade the ischiorectal fossae (p. 501).

5. Approaches to the Sacro-iliac Joint.—The sacro-iliac joint is exposed for the curettement of diseased tissue in tuberculosis, for the removal of débris and drainage in osteomyelitis, and for joint fusion in posttraumatic disabling conditions which have resisted conservative methods of treatment.

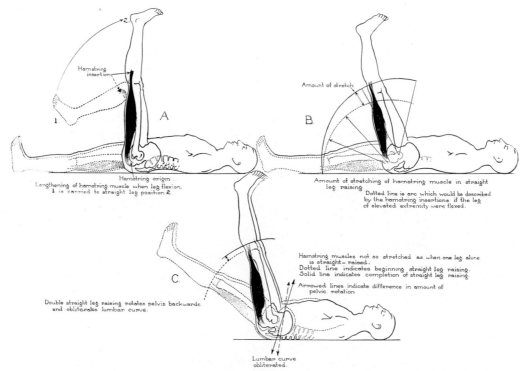

Fig. 423.—The Effect of Straight Leg Raising upon the Hamstring Muscles, Pelvis, and Lumbar Spine. (Modified from M. Brahdy.)

In the *Smith-Petersen approach,* an incision is made along the posterior two thirds of the iliac crest, curving around the posterior superior spine and then running parallel to the fibers of the gluteal muscles for a distance of from 8 to 10 cm. The soft tissues are reflected subperiosteally until the posterior portion of the lateral surface of the ilium is exposed. The center of the surface overlying the joint is 2.5 cm. superior to the upper border of the sciatic notch and 2.5 cm. anterior to the posterior superior spine. With this point as a center, a block or window of ilium, 2.5 by 4 cm., is removed, the longer side being parallel to the upper margin of the notch. This exposure is adequate for curettement and drainage of the joint. In an arthrodesis, the cartilage is removed from the sacral joint surface, exposing cancellous bone, and from the joint surface of the block of ilium. The bone block is replaced and countersunk so that its cancellous portion comes into contact with the cancellous bone of the sacrum.

In *Picque's approach,* an incision is made along the posterior surface of the iliac crest and continued downward to the border of the sacrum at a point midway between the posterior superior and inferior spines of the ilium. The soft parts are reflected downward subperiosteally from the crest of the ilium. The bone of the crest is divided from the forward confines of the incision to the posterior inferior spine, exposing the sacroiliac joint.

Campbell has devised an entirely *extra-articular fusion operation* to avoid contamination of the joint. A subperiosteal incision over the posterior half of the iliac crest exposes the posterior surface of the dorsum of the ilium, and a downward vertical continuation of the incision exposes the lateral half of the posterior surface of the sacrum. A portion of the crest is removed and the mesial surface of the overhanging part of the crest and the adjacent posterior surface of the ilium are denuded. This makes a raw gutter parallel to the sacro-iliac joint, formed by the posterior surface of the sacrum and the medial surface of the ilium behind the sacro-iliac joint. Into this space, the graft from the crest is placed, as well as grafts or "shavings" from the dorsum of the ilium, until the interval is filled.

Occasionally, the lumbosacral joint also must be fused. A graft from the crest of the ilium or one from the tibia can be employed. It is inserted into the spinous processes of the lower lumbar vertebrae and sacrum.

C. SACROCOCCYGEAL REGION

1. **Surface Anatomy.**—The spinous processes of the sacrum, of which the second and third are the most prominent, may be palpated in the median line. Following the median crest toward the base of the coccyx, two lateral bony prominences are palpated, the sacral

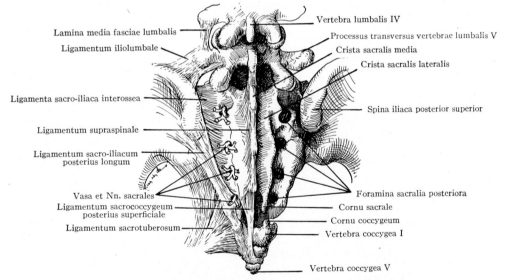

FIG. 424.—POSTERIOR VIEW OF THE SACROCOCCYGEAL REGION.
On the right side, the vessels, nerves, and ligaments have been removed to indicate the topography of the sacral foramina.

and coccygeal cornua, which bound the sacral hiatus or external opening of the sacrococcygeal canal. The prominent posterior superior iliac spines may be palpated at the sides of the region. A line joining the posterior superior spines passes between the first and second sacral foramina and indicates the level of the termination of the subarachnoid space (p. 548).

The lateral crest of the sacrum, made up of the fused transverse processes of the sacral vertebrae, is one thumbbreadth lateral to the median sacral crest. The lateral crest, lying just to the outer side of the sacral foramina, serves as a landmark for injection through the foramina in extradural sacral anesthesia.

The pelvic surface of the sacrum and coccyx may be palpated through the rectum or vagina, a fact of considerable importance in determining the form and dimensions of the pelvis or the existence of irregularities which may be obstructive to parturition. Pelvic examination may reveal soreness along the sacral nerves emerging from the anterior foramina. The sciatic notch, through which the important pelvic nerves and vessels emerge to the thigh, also is palpable, and the presence of tumors or abscesses causing pressure on pelvic structures may be determined. Ordinarily, the sacral promontory is not reached by the examining finger.

2. **Soft Parts.**—The *skin* of the sacrococcygeal region is thick and resistant. It is bound down closely in the region of the anal crease, but generally is loose over the convexity of the sacrum. In emaciated or thin subjects, the bony prominences, otherwise well covered and protected, are brought into relief, and the overlying skin is subject to pressure ulceration (decubitus ulcer). The *musculo-aponeurotic layer* over the sacrum is the inferior portion of the dorsal layer of the lumbodorsal fascia (p. 310), which covers and fuses with the expansive tendinous origin of the spinal musculature. It is attached to the median crest of the spinous processes and the lateral sacral crests. At the base of the sacrum, overlying the lumbosacral articulation, the musculotendinous mass is thick and strong, affording much strength to the stabilizing mechanism of the lower back.

3. **Skeletal Structure.**—The *sacrum* is a single bone representing the developmental fusion of its five vertebral components. It is triangularly wedge shaped, with its broad thick proximal base, from which the thick lateral parts gradually diminish in size and taper to the distal apex. The transversely flattened, posteriorly placed sacral canal runs throughout the length of the mass, and opens on the dorsal surface of the sacrum, somewhat proximal to its apex, at the sacrococcygeal hiatus. A series of openings lead directly anteriorly and somewhat laterally from the sacral canal. These are the anterior sacral foramina through which the sacral nerves emerging from the cord may be reached in sacral anesthesia (p. 549). Posteriorly, at the entrance and exit of the canal are the lumbosacral and sacrococcygeal spaces through which subarachnoid and extradural anesthesia respectively are induced.

The lumbosacral space is 1 cm. high and 2 cm. wide. The sacrococcygeal space, which is of an inverted V shape, is 2 cm. high and 1 cm. wide; it arises from the incomplete closure of the arch of the fifth sacral vertebra because of the absence of its laminae and spinous process. Both spaces are closed by resistant fibrous membranes. Sacral decubitus ulceration and infected abrasions of the skin in this region expose the sacral canal and its contents, and may result in neuritis, meningitis, or myelitis. In embryonic development, there may be incomplete closure of the canal posteriorly, exposing the canal contents as a hernia which is known as spina bifida.

The base of the sacrum presents the ordinary markings of a vertebra. In the mid-anterior portion of the base is a flat, slightly depressed, oval articular surface for the fifth lumbar vertebra. Posterior to the articular surface is the opening into the sacral canal. The thick, massive, lateral part of the sacrum represents the fusion of the transverse processes of the five sacral vertebrae. Through that part of the sacrum which represents the fusion of the first, second, and third sacral vertebrae, there is articulation with the ilium. Fusion processes at the base of the sacrum present a variety of anomalies, such as a fused sixth lumbar vertebra or one fused on one side only. The lateral margins of the sacrum distal to the sacro-iliac joint are thin and narrow, affording an expansive attachment to the stabilizing sacrotuberous and sacrospinous ligaments.

Each sacral vertebra develops from three primary centers, one for the body, and one for each half of the neural arch. These centers appear between the third and eighth months. In addition to the primary centers, there are secondary nuclei fusing to form the massive lateral parts of the sacrum. These nuclei form the spinous processes and the two epiphyseal plates of each sacral segment. The development of the sacrum is essentially the development of the separate segments which fuse into the adult bone by the twenty-fifth year.

The *coccyx*, the small, triangular, terminal segment of the spine, is made up of the distal four or five incompletely developed vertebrae joined to, and continuing in the direction of the sacrum. The whole coccyx may be ossified to the apex of the sacrum. The lateral margins of the coccyx and its tip continue the expansive origin of the sacrotuberous ligament and afford attachment to the muscles of the pelvic floor.

4. **Contents of the Sacral Canal.**—The roots of the lumbar, sacral, and coccygeal nerves leave the cord in the lower dorsal and upper lumbar regions. The lowermost roots pass downward through the sacral canal, which contains the last five sacral nerves and the coccygeal nerves of each side, together with the terminal filament of the cord. The culdesac formed by the dural and arachnoid membranes of the spinal cord occupies only the upper part of the canal and usually does not descend below the level of the second sacral segment, so that neither the dural tube nor its contained subarachnoid space is opened by a section traversing the bone below this level. An anesthetic for infiltration of the sacral and coccygeal nerves must be injected into the sacral canal distal to the blind ending of the dural culdesac. Within the sacral canal lies also some loose fatty tissue traversed by numerous veins and by branches of the lateral sacral arteries.

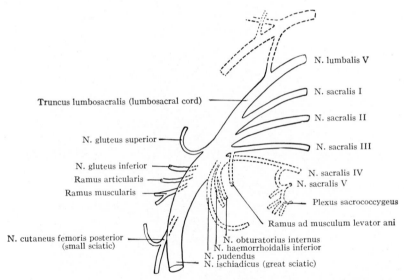

FIG. 425.—SACROCOCCYGEAL NERVE PLEXUS. (After Tinel.)

The sacral nerves, after dividing into anterior and posterior branches, leave the canal through their respective foramina. Several of the sacral nerves are concerned directly in resection of the sacrum. The serious consequences attending destruction of the third and fourth sacral nerves are dependent upon the fact that they innervate both the anorectal region and the external anal sphincter through the inferior hemorrhoidal branch of the internal pudendal nerve. The nerve supply of the levator ani muscle is derived chiefly from the third, but partly from the second and fourth sacral nerves, and the external sphincter receives an independent filament from the fourth sacral nerve through its perineal branch. The second, third, and fourth sacral nerves are the principal sources of visceral branches to the bladder, prostate, and urethra in the male, and to the bladder, urethra, and vagina in the female.

5. **Sacral Anesthesia.**—The details of sacral anesthesia are outlined in the discussion of the vertebral canal (p. 549).

6. **Sacralization of the Fifth Lumbar Vertebra.**—The formula for the elements of the vertebral column is not fixed, and the process of shortening the lumbar spine is continuing. This is shown by the frequency with which the fifth lumbar vertebra takes on sacral characteristics. Lumbar sacralization implies fusion of the transverse processes of the fifth

lumbar vertebra to the subjacent alae of the sacrum. Sometimes the lumbar transverse processes articulate with, or are fused to, the iliac crest through ossification of the ilio-lumbar ligament. Any of these conditions may cause persistent low back pain.

II. Soft Parts Lining the Pelvis

The soft parts lining the pelvis include the muscles lining its walls, those forming the pelvic diaphragm, the fascia and peritoneum covering them, and the vessels and nerves.

1. Intraparietal Musculature, Intermuscular Foramina, and Parietal Fascia.—The obturator internus and piriformis muscles smooth out the contour of the true pelvis before entering the gluteal region through the greater and lesser sciatic foramina to insert on the femur.

The *obturator internus muscle* ($L_{4, 5}$ S_1) springs from the circumference of the obturator foramen and the medial surface of the obturator membrane, from which broad area of

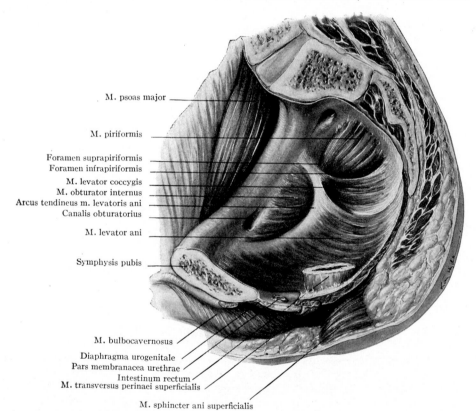

M. psoas major

M. piriformis

Foramen suprapiriformis
Foramen infrapiriformis

M. levator coccygis
M. obturator internus
Arcus tendineus m. levatoris ani
Canalis obturatorius

M. levator ani

Symphysis pubis

M. bulbocavernosus

Diaphragma urogenitale
Pars membranacea urethrae
Intestinum rectum
M. transversus perinaei superficialis

M. sphincter ani superficialis

Fig. 426.—Muscles of the Lateral Wall and Floor of the Male Pelvis.

attachment the muscle bundles converge toward and almost fill the lesser sciatic foramen. The converging tendon is flanked by the gemelli muscles arising outside the pelvic cavity on the ischial spine and tuberosity. The composite muscle tendon bends about the margin of the foramen to insert on the medial surface of the great trochanter just above the trochanteric (digital) fossa (p. 680). With this posteromedial insertion, the obturator internus acts as an external rotator of the thigh.

Like the obturator internus muscle, the *piriformis muscle* ($S_{1, 2}$) arises on the osseo-ligamentous framework of the interior of the pelvis. It springs mainly from the anterior surfaces of the second, third, and fourth sacral vertebrae lateral to the anterior sacral foramina, and, to a lesser degree, from the sacrotuberous ligament. Its fibers run outward and converge inferiorly into a musculo-aponeurotic tendon which leaves the pelvis by the greater sciatic foramen (p. 417). The piriformis does not occupy all of the cavity of the greater foramen, but leaves two areas comparatively open, one above and one below the muscle. These openings are the suprapiriformic and infrapiriformic spaces or foramina.

The *suprapiriformic foramen* is bounded above by the greater sciatic notch and below by the upper margin of the piriformis muscle, furnishing a passage for the superior gluteal vessels and nerves from the pelvis to the gluteal region (p. 675). The *infrapiriformic foramen*, bounded by the lower border of the piriformis muscle above and by the ischial spine and sacrospinous ligament below, is traversed by pelvic vessels, the sciatic nerve, and the nerves running to the perineal region. These openings and the obturator canal (p. 711) are areas of lessened resistance, through which intrapelvic structures may herniate.

The *parietal pelvic fascia* clothing the obturator internus and piriformis muscles is fused densely with the sheaths of the vessels and nerves which emerge through the foramina. A reinforced area termed the tendinous arch or linea terminalis extends backward from the posterior surface of the pubis to the spine of each ischium and serves as the line of origin for the levator ani muscles.

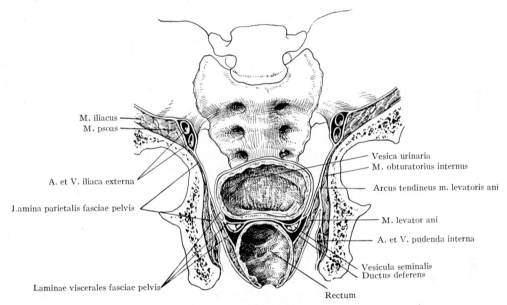

FIG. 427.—OBLIQUE FRONTAL SECTION THROUGH THE MALE PELVIS SHOWING THE FASCIAE OF THE PELVIS AND PERINEUM.

2. **Structure of the Pelvic Diaphragm.**—The outlet of the pelvis is closed by a concave musculo-aponeurotic hammock, the pelvic diaphragm. The main pelvic or muscular diaphragm, consisting of the paired levator ani and coccygeus muscles, is incomplete anteriorly. The levators are separated by a definite interval, the interlevator cleft, which is closed on the perineal side by the accessory pelvic or *urogenital diaphragm;* this diaphragm is stretched across the subpubic arch and is densely adherent to the under surface of the mesial borders of the separated levators (p. 494).

Each *levator ani muscle* (N. pudendal S_3, $_4$) is composed of a lateral and a mesial portion. The lateral portion arises from the posterolateral aspect of the body of the pubis and from the linea terminalis of the parietal pelvic fascia. Its fibers run obliquely downward and backward, without adhering to the prostate, vagina, or lateral surface of the rectum, to form the anococcygeal raphe. The mesial or pubococcygeal portion arises from the pubic body nearer to the median line than to the lateral segment. It is directed posteriorly along the lateral surface of the prostate or vagina and, after entering into the composition of the central tendinous area of the perineum, blends with the longitudinal muscle of the rectum near the anal margin (p. 499).   The *coccygeus muscle* (S₃, ₄), which completes the main pelvic diaphragm behind, overlies the sacrospinous ligament and extends fanwise from the spine of the ischium to the coccyx.   It lies immediately inferior to the piriformis muscle.   The *visceral layer* of the *pelvic fascia* is that which overlies the pelvic surface of the muscular diaphragm.

The pelvic diaphragm has the unique and important function of supporting much of the weight of the superimposed viscera when the body is erect.   Hernias through the diaphragm, such as prolapse of the bladder and rectum and descensus of the uterus, are frequent.

3. **Extraperitoneal Space of the Pelvis; Pelvic Peritoneum.**—A commodious *extraperitoneal space* separates the pelvic diaphragm from the pelvic peritoneum.   It contains areolar tissue which is in communication with the gluteal and obturator regions.   Extraperitoneal pelvic abscesses may progress upward into the iliac fossae and anterior abdominal wall.   In the extraperitoneal space, lateral rectal, retrorectal, and retrovesical compartments are differentiated.

The *pelvic peritoneum* is lifted into folds and depressed into culdesacs by the bladder, rectum, and pelvic genitalia.   The peritoneum is depressed into lateral recesses about the rectum and into a deep culdesac (of Douglas), which separates the rectum from the uro-

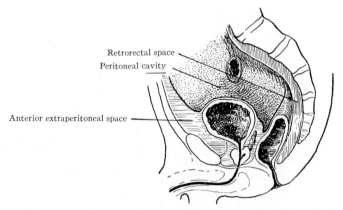

Retrorectal space
Peritoneal cavity

Anterior extraperitoneal space

Fɪɢ. 428.—Sᴄʜᴇᴍᴀᴛɪᴄ Sᴀɢɪᴛᴛᴀʟ Sᴇᴄᴛɪᴏɴ Tʜʀᴏᴜɢʜ ᴛʜᴇ Pᴇʟᴠɪs ᴛᴏ Iɴᴅɪᴄᴀᴛᴇ ᴛʜᴇ Dɪᴠɪsɪᴏɴs ᴏғ ᴛʜᴇ Ex-
ᴛʀᴀᴘᴇʀɪᴛᴏɴᴇᴀʟ Sᴘᴀᴄᴇ ᴏғ ᴛʜᴇ Pᴇʟᴠɪs.

genital organs and descends to within 6 or 7 cm of the perineum.   In the male, the culdesac descends just below the level of the seminal vesicles.   In the female, the recto-uterine pouch (p. 434) is bounded laterally by the uterosacral ligaments which divide it into two parts.   The upper and broader division is in relation to the posterior surface of the uterus, and the inferior and narrower division, to the posterior fornix of the vagina.

4. **Vessels and Nerves.**—The pelvic vessels and nerves, all of which run in the extraperitoneal cellular spaces, are known as parietal or visceral, according to whether they supply the soft parts of the pelvic walls, or are distributed to the pelvic viscera.

The **hypogastric (internal iliac) artery,** a branch of the common iliac, is the main artery of both the interior and exterior of the pelvis.   It runs mesial to the psoas muscle along the sacro-iliac joint line and descends almost vertically into the pelvis.   After the iliolumbar and lateral sacral arteries are given off, the hypogastric artery divides, at the upper margin of the greater sciatic foramen, into a posterior trunk and a smaller anterior trunk.

Of the *parietal branches*, the superior gluteal artery is the continuation of the posterior division of the hypogastric artery, and is distributed to the gluteal region of the hip through the suprapiriformic space (p. 675).   The anterior division of the hypogastric artery, in addition to giving off the obturator, inferior gluteal, and internal pudendal branches, is the main arterial supply of the pelvic viscera.   The inferior gluteal and internal pudendal branches leave the pelvis through the infrapiriformic space (p. 429), and the obturator artery leaves the pelvis through the obturator foramen (p. 711). Not infrequently, the obturator artery arises from the inferior epigastric artery, crosses the femoral canal, and becomes of surgical interest in the operation for femoral hernia (p. 704).

All of the *visceral branches* to the pelvic contents are derived from the anterior trunk of the hypogastric artery. They have a certain degree of mobility necessitated by the changing conditions in the uterus, bladder, and rectum. This mobility is facilitated by the investment of these vessels in a large amount of lax extraperitoneal connective tissue. Groups of branches supply the bladder, genitalia, and rectum, and are described with the viscera to which they are distributed.

The visceral and parietal **veins** form rich anastomotic plexuses, the efferent trunks of which are directed to the hypogastric vein.

The anterior divisions of the sacral and coccygeal **nerves** form the sacral and pudendal plexuses. The *sacral plexus* is formed by the anterior divisions of the fourth and fifth lumbar and the first, second, and third sacral nerves. These nerves lie largely on the mesial surface of the piriformis muscles and form a marked thickening on the pelvic wall which is overlain by the pelvic vessels. The nerves converge toward the lower part of the greater sciatic foramen (infrapiriformic space), and unite to form a flattened band which is con-

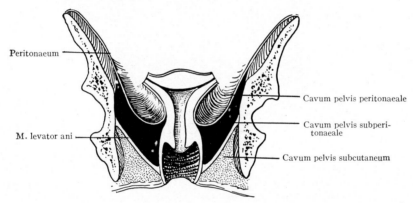

Peritonaeum

M. levator ani

Cavum pelvis peritonaeale

Cavum pelvis subperi-
tonaeale

Cavum pelvis subcutaneum

FIG. 429.—SCHEMATIC FRONTAL SECTION THROUGH THE FEMALE PELVIS TO EMPHASIZE THE SIZE OF THE
EXTRAPERITONEAL SPACES. (After Corning.)

tinued as the sciatic nerve (p. 676) into the gluteal region. The inferior gluteal nerve leaves the pelvis through the infrapiriformic space of the greater sciatic foramen to supply the gluteal musculature (p. 675).

The *pudendal plexus* is not marked off sharply from the sacral plexus. It is formed usually by branches from the anterior division of the second and third sacral nerves, all of the anterior division of the fourth and fifth sacral nerves, and the coccygeal nerve; it lies on the posterior wall of the pelvis. Its main branch, the pudendal (internal pudic) nerve (p. 502), leaves the infrapiriformic space, enters the gluteal region, and terminates by supplying the external genitalia and much of the perineum.

The obturator nerve from the lumbar plexus runs along the mesial margin of the psoas muscle, the sacro-iliac joint, and the linea terminalis and enters the obturator foramen en route to the adductor region of the thigh (p. 711).

5. **Ligation of the Common Iliac Artery.**—By the *transperitoneal method*, the common iliac artery is approached through a median incision from the umbilicus to the symphysis. On the right side, the vessel is not overlain by any structures of importance, and may be reached by direct division of the peritoneum over it. The vena cava and both common iliac veins are in close relation to the artery on this side. The common iliac vein passes deep to the artery. On the left side, the sigmoid mesocolon, containing the sigmoid and the superior hemorrhoidal branches of the inferior mesenteric artery, covers almost all of

the common iliac artery. To avoid injury to the vessels of the mesocolon, the mesentery must be incised carefully. The common iliac vein usually lies somewhat behind and mesial to the artery.

The approach in the *extraperitoneal exposure* is through a high iliac incision (p. 414). The abdominal muscles and transversalis fascia are divided and the peritoneum is lifted

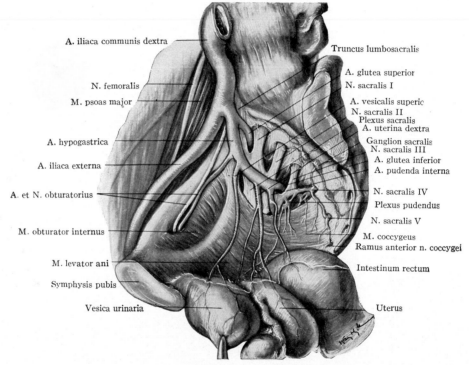

A. iliaca communis dextra
N. femoralis
M. psoas major
A. hypogastrica
A. iliaca externa
A. et N. obturatorius
M. obturator internus
M. levator ani
Symphysis pubis
Vesica urinaria

Truncus lumbosacralis
A. glutea superior
N. sacralis I
A. vesicalis superic
N. sacralis II
Plexus sacralis
A. uterina dextra
Ganglion sacralis
N. sacralis III
A. glutea inferior
A. pudenda interna
N. sacralis IV
Plexus pudendus
N. sacralis V
M. coccygeus
Ramus anterior n. coccygei
Intestinum rectum
Uterus

FIG. 430.—LATERAL VIEW OF THE FEMALE PELVIS TO SHOW THE MAIN ARTERIES AND NERVES. The bladder, rectum, and the pelvic genitalia are drawn downward to show their arterial supply.

away from the iliac fascia along the line of the direction of the iliac crest. The peritoneum must be pressed forward away from the psoas muscle and the iliac vessels lying along the mesial margin of that muscle. The ureter remains attached to the peritoneum and with it is lifted out of danger.

III. PELVIC VISCERA IN THE MALE

The viscera which occupy, and are fixed to, the floor and walls of the male pelvis are the rectum, bladder, prostate, pelvic ureters, seminal vesicles, and deferent ducts. Loops of ileum, the sigmoid colon, and occasionally the appendix are distinguished from the intrinsic contents of the true pelvis on the basis of their fixation to the walls of the abdomen and the false pelvis.

A. RECTUM

1. **Definition, Boundaries, and Divisions.**—The rectum, or terminal portion of the large intestine, begins anterior to the body of the third sacral vertebra, and, after traversing the pelvic floor, terminates at the anus. It is customary to divide the rectum into the pelvic rectum and the perineal or anal rectum (p. 503).

The pelvic rectum lies within the pelvic cavity and is from 12 to 14 cm. in length. At its beginning it usually lies in the median line, and, in its downward course, describes a curve corresponding closely to that of the sacrum and coccyx. At its lower level, the puborectal portion of the levators (p. 429) comes into contact with its lateral surfaces. This level lies at the apex of the prostate in the male and opposite the lower fourth of the posterior vaginal wall in the female. Description of the anal rectum properly belongs in the perineum (p. 503). The pelvic rectum, especially when distended, presents a series of lateral foldings or inflections which produce horizontal shelflike projections within the bowel. These projections, the rectal valves (of Houston), partially divide the rectum into a series of compartments. The lumen of the rectum is not uniform, but is narrow at its upper and lower extremities. Toward the lower portion of the bowel, the lumen expands to form the rectal ampulla. The anterior wall of the ampulla bulges and angulates forward and downward immediately proximal to the anal canal. This bulging is particularly marked in females who have borne children and in subjects with a relaxed pelvic floor. In the male, the ampulla projects forward almost to the apex of the prostate and to the membranous urethra. The attachment of the recto-urethralis muscle to the ampulla of the rectum and to the superior fascia of the urogenital diaphragm (p. 497) causes this

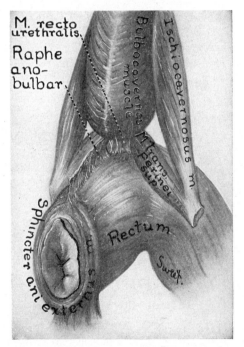

FIG. 431.—RELATIONS BETWEEN THE AMPULLA OF THE RECTUM AND THE BULB OF THE URETHRA.
The anterior angulation of the ampulla of the rectum brings the rectum into contact with the urethral bulb; connection is maintained by the recto-urethralis muscle. (After Hinman.)

anterior angulation of the bowel. The bowel must be avoided when the muscle is divided in perineal prostatectomy. The varied pathologic changes of the pelvic rectum and the numerous surgical interventions designed to cope with them give this division unusual clinical and topographic interest.

2. **Location and Attachments.**—The rectum lies in the midst of the areolar tissue of the pelvic extraperitoneal space. Extraperitoneal tissue separates the anterior surface of the rectum from the posterior surface of the seminal vesicles and prostate. Cellulitis may develop in the prerectal tissue as a result of lesions in the prostate, seminal vesicles, or bladder, but it arises more frequently from lesions of the rectum. Inflammatory processes in the region may burrow into the rectum or may perforate the levator ani muscle and point in the ischiorectal fossa.

The rectum is maintained in position by the peritoneum which incompletely surrounds its upper part, by sheaths from the visceral division of the pelvic fascia, and by lateral fibrous prolongations carrying the middle hemorrhoidal vessels. The firm adhesion

28

of the rectum to the levator ani muscles forms a fixed point of attachment. Each rectal support must be freed in extirpation of the viscus. When the elements holding the rectum in position become lax, rectal prolapse tends to occur (p. 508).

3. **Relations.**—The rectum rests upon the sacrum, coccyx, and middle sacral artery, and is separated from them by the visceral layer of pelvic fascia and by extraperitoneal connective tissue. The extraperitoneal relationships form the rationale for the sacro-coccygeal approach to the rectum. The close relationship of the rectum to the lumbosacral plexus explains the sciatic and perineal distribution of pain noted at times as an early symptom of carcinoma of the rectum.

The peritoneum covering the apposed surfaces of the rectum and bladder forms the rectovesical culdesac (of Douglas), which extends to the uppermost margin of the recto-vesical fascia bridging the extraperitoneal portions of the rectum and bladder. Not all of the posterior aspect of the bladder has a peritoneal covering, for the peritoneum usually descends only to within 1 cm. of the base of the prostate. Only the anterior and lateral surfaces of the upper two thirds of the rectal ampulla receive a peritoneal investment. In the newborn, this peritoneal pouch descends until it clothes all of the posterior surface of the bladder, seminal vesicles, and a part of the posterior surface of the prostate. It some-times reaches the pelvic diaphragm. Adults may manifest the persistence of fetal con-

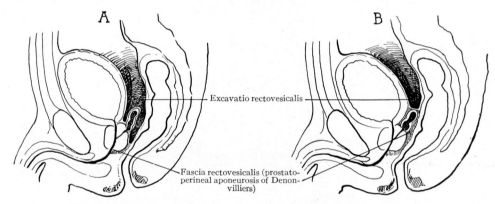

FIG. 432.—VARIATIONS IN THE DEPTH OF THE RECTOVESICAL CULDESAC.
In A, the rectovesical culdesac extends below the level of the superior surface of the prostate; in B, the culdesac does not reach the seminal vesicles, and the rectum is in direct relation with the bladder, seminal vesicles and prostate.

ditions as a consequence of the lack of fusion of the two embryonic layers of the pouch which lie in contact. In pronounced nonfusion, there may be an intestinal hernia into the perineum. A deep rectovaginal pouch may allow an intestinal loop to evaginate into the vagina as a vaginal enterocele, or cause a perineal hernia.

When the rectum is filled, two peritoneal folds pass from the lateral walls of the bladder to the ampullary portion of the rectum, and bound the entrance to the lowermost cavity of the pelvic peritoneal pouch. These vesicorectal folds or ligaments (of Douglas) contain smooth muscle fibers which give them a supporting rôle in the fixation of the blad-der. Morphologically, these folds are analogous to those which unite the uterus to the rectum and sacrum (uterosacral ligaments) (p. 470).

The extraperitoneal portion of the rectum is in relation to that part of the base of the bladder lying between the deferent ducts (interdeferent triangle or rectovesical trigone) through the intermedium of the rectovesical fascia of Denonvilliers. This frontally placed aponeurosis or septum offers no obstacle to digital examination of the prostate and seminal vesicles through the rectum, but explains the fact that carcinoma of the rectum invades anterior structures only in the late stages of the disease.

4. **Development and Congenital Malformations.**—In early embryonic life, the terminal segment of the intestine and the bud which forms the primitive bladder and urethra con-

stitute a single cavity, the *cloaca*, which is separated from the exterior by the *cloacal membrane*. The cloaca is transformed gradually into two cavities by the downgrowth of a frontally placed partition, the *urorectal septum*. The ventral space represents the urogenital sinus, and the dorsal space forms the rectum. The cloacal membrane is not broken through to the outside until the urorectal septum has divided the cloaca. The anal por-

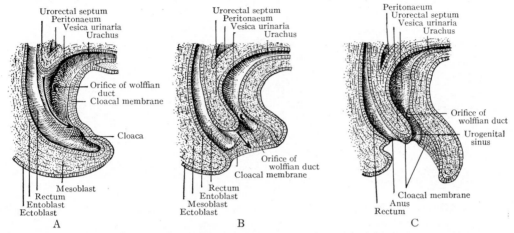

FIG. 433.—DIAGRAM OF THE DEVELOPMENT OF THE RECTUM, ANUS, AND BLADDER.
In A, the arrow indicates the direction of growth of the uro(ano)rectal septum toward the cloacal membrane; in B, the urorectal septum almost has partitioned the cloaca into vesical and rectal compartments; in C, the urorectal septum has reached the cloacal membrane; the membrane has given way at the caudal termination of the bladder and rectum; separate exits are formed for these structures.

tion of the cloacal membrane, which separates the rectum from the surface, breaks through first, forming the anal orifice. The urogenital sinus opens through the urogenital part of the membrane into the urethral orifice in the male and the urethrovaginal orifice in the female.

Various *congenital malformations* occur as a result of failure of these parts to develop properly. The most frequent anomaly is anal atresia, which results from failure of the

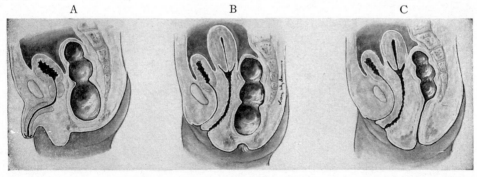

FIG. 434.—ANOMALIES IN THE DEVELOPMENT OF THE PELVIC AND ANAL PORTIONS OF THE RECTUM.
A, Complete absence of the anus; B, failure of the pelvic rectum to connect with the anal depression; in C, the terminal part of the pelvic rectum and the anal canal are narrowed greatly.

anal portion of the cloaca to open to the exterior through the cloacal membrane. Abnormal union may occur between the rectum and the urogenital sinus, and the rectum may open into the anterior urogenital structures. The rectum may be absent or may open externally by a narrow fistula. The terminal rectum and the vagina may be connected by a fistula. The prognosis in these malformations depends upon the variety. Imperforations are fatal in a few days unless a permanent outlet is established.

5. **Vessels.**—The *arteries* forming the rich anastomoses in the rectum are the superior, middle, and inferior hemorrhoidals and the middle sacral. The middle and inferior hemorrhoidal arteries are bilateral vessels with a symmetrical arrangement. The superior hemorrhoidal and middle sacral arteries are single.

The superior hemorrhoidal artery is the direct continuation of the inferior mesenteric artery into the pelvis. After crossing the left common iliac artery, it runs downward

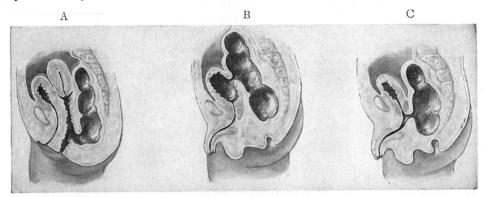

FIG. 435.—ANOMALIES IN THE DEVELOPMENT OF THE RECTUM AND THE UROGENITAL APPARATUS.

In A, the pelvic rectum opens into the vagina; there is complete absence of the anal canal; in B, the pelvic rectum opens into the bladder; parts of the anal canal and terminal pelvic rectum are absent; in C, the pelvic rectum opens into the male urethra; parts of the anal canal and terminal pelvic rectum are absent; these conditions are known as atresia ani vaginalis, atresia ani vesicalis, and atresia ani urethralis.

between the layers of the pelvic mesocolon near their parietal attachment. Upon reaching the rectum, the artery usually bifurcates into right and left divisions, both of which are surrounded by a layer of areolo-adipose tissue lying between the rectal fascia and the bowel wall. Its branches spread over the rectum posteriorly, laterally, and anteriorly.

The middle hemorrhoidal artery usually is represented by two or more branches which originate either in the trunk of the hypogastric artery or in one of its larger branches, the internal pudendal or the inferior vesicular.

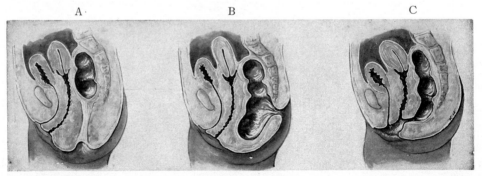

FIG. 436.—ANOMALIES IN THE DEVELOPMENT OF THE RECTUM AND UROGENITAL APPARATUS.

In A, the anorectal tract is impervious and fibrous; in B, the pelvic rectum opens just below the coccyx; in C, there is a cloaca formation in which the bladder, vagina, and rectum open into a common cavity.

The inferior hemorrhoidal artery is distributed to the perineal rectum. It arises on each side from the internal pudendal artery in Alcock's canal (p. 502) in the ischiorectal fossa. The middle sacral artery arises from the abdominal aorta near its termination and runs downward in the median plane on the posterior surface of the rectum, to which it supplies a few twigs.

The *rectal veins* differ from those of the other divisions of the large bowel in that they form a rich hemorrhoidal plexus within the thickness of the bowel. This plexus is developed best in the anal region (p. 504). The superior hemorrhoidal vein is tributary to the portal system, but the middle and inferior hemorrhoidal veins drain to the inferior vena cava.

Most of the *lymphatics* of the pelvic rectum drain to rectal lymph nodes lying along the course of the superior hemorrhoidal veins and thence to the nodes in the mesentery of the pelvic colon. Some of the rectal lymphatics follow the middle hemorrhoidal vessels and empty into the hypogastric lymph nodes. The majority of the inferior hemorrhoidal lymphatics traverse the perineal region and medial aspect of the thigh and join the medial group of subinguinal glands. Carcinoma of the rectum metastasizes by way of the lymphatics along three courses of spread (Miles). Downward extension involves the ischio-

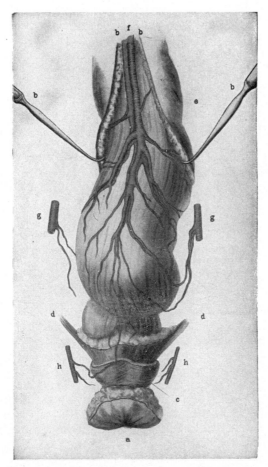

Fig. 437.—Posterior View of the Anorectum.

a Anus; *b, b,* posterior reflection of the peritoneum; *c,* external sphincter ani; *d, d,* levator ani; *e,* nonperitoneal aspect of the posterior aspect of the rectum; *f,* superior hemorrhoidal artery and vein; *g,* middle hemorrhoidal artery; *h,* inferior hemorrhoidal artery. (Bickham, "Operative Surgery.")

rectal fat, the external anal sphincter, and the perianal skin. The lateral extension involves the levator ani muscles, the sacral and internal iliac glands, the base of the bladder, and the seminal vesicles. In women, the posterior vaginal wall, cervix, and base of the broad ligament are involved also. Upward extension attacks the pelvic peritoneum, the whole of the pelvic mesocolon, and the glands at the bifurcation of the left common iliac artery.

Rectal carcinoma may be disseminated by vascular distribution along the route of the portal circulation. Rectal carcinoma, although locally operable, often is inoperable because of metastases to the peritoneal cavity and to the liver. When vascular extension occurs by way of the middle and inferior hemorrhoidal veins, the caval venous system is involved by the propagation of metastases into the internal pudendal and iliac veins. Without visceral metastasis, rectal carcinoma runs a long course before lymphatic dissemination contraindicates operation, and early excision of the growth in these cases offers a fair chance of cure.

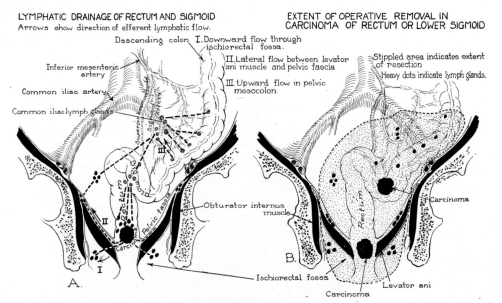

LYMPHATIC DRAINAGE OF RECTUM AND SIGMOID
Arrows show direction of efferent lymphatic flow.

EXTENT OF OPERATIVE REMOVAL IN
CARCINOMA OF RECTUM OR LOWER SIGMOID

FIG. 438.—LYMPHATIC DRAINAGE FROM THE SIGMOID AND RECTUM TO SHOW THE EXTENT OF RESECTION FOR CARCINOMA. (Modified after Miles.)

SURGICAL CONSIDERATIONS

1. **Rectal Examination.**—Rectal examination may be made instrumentally or digitally. The patient may be examined in the knee-chest, exaggerated lithotomy, lateral prone, or squatting position, or hinged almost at right angles over a specially constructed table. Any position with the body dependent causes the intestines to gravitate toward the diaphragm, empties the rectovesical and rectovaginal pouches, relieves downward pressure upon the sigmoid, and permits the rectum to dilate upon the admission of air. A dependent position facilitates the introduction of an examining instrument such as the rectoscope or sigmoidoscope. Stout people should be placed either in the knee-chest or in the exaggerated lithotomy position, as the anal canal cannot be examined easily in the lateral prone position.

Valuable information about the interior of the rectum and the structures adjacent to it is obtained by digital examination. On passing the well-lubricated index finger through the anal orifice, the grasp of the external sphincter is felt. The finger may be advanced upward and forward about 4 cm., where it slips past the internal sphincter and enters the rectal ampulla. The definite constriction at the upper level of the anal canal is caused by the attachment of the rectum to the levator muscles. If the anal orifice is constricted tightly, anal fissure (p. 506) should be suspected, and further examination should be conducted under anesthesia. If the patient is made to strain, that part of the bowel lying just out of reach of the examining finger can be "threaded" on the finger. A squatting position facilitates digital examination in rectal prolapse and hemorrhoids.

Within the ampulla, the examining finger should be directed backward to the hollow of the sacrum. At this stage, the middle rectal valve may be felt as an inwardly projecting fold. This valve very commonly is the cause of difficulty in passing a rectal tube. The finger, on palpating from side to side, readily explores the anterior aspect of the coccyx and the lower part of the sacrum, upon which the rectum moves with great freedom. The mesial wall of the pelvis may be examined, and, posterolaterally, enlarged hypogastric lymph nodes can be made out. Anteriorly, through the lowest part of the wall of the rectal ampulla, enlarged bulbo-urethral glands (of Cowper) (p. 499) can be felt. About 4 cm. from the anus, the apex of the prostate is palpated; above it, the posterior surface of the gland is outlined readily because of its firm consistency and regular contour. Above the prostate, enlarged seminal vesicles are felt as nodular projections. Between the seminal vesicles, the finger is in contact with the interampullary area of the base of the bladder (p. 444).

In rectal examination in the female, the finger contacts the vagina, and above it, the cervix. The cervix, because of its proximity to the rectum and its firm consistency, has been mistaken for a rectal tumor. Bimanual examination, which is examination with one or two fingers in the rectum and the other hand applied to the abdomen, is a valuable adjunct to the diagnosis of the position and condition of the uterus, ovaries, and tubes (p. 474).

2. **Combined Abdominal-perineal Operation for High Rectal and Rectosigmoid Carcinoma.**—Excision of the rectum by the combined abdominal and perineal approach

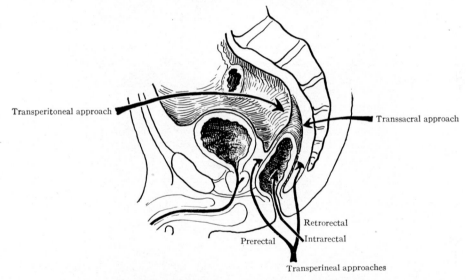

FIG. 439.—SURGICAL APPROACHES TO THE RECTUM.

contemplates the surgical exposure and exploration of the tumor mass through median abdominal section, proximal division of the intestinal canal, and the establishment of a permanent iliac anus. Through the perineal approach, the segment of bowel containing the growth is removed. The special indication for the removal of a growth by the combined approach is its location in the upper rectum, lower sigmoid, or rectosigmoid junction. The approach affords an opportunity for exploring the mass, determining the presence of vascular metastases to the liver, and for ascertaining the local and contiguous lymphatic involvement.

In the *abdominal part* of the operation, the abdomen is opened through an incision just to the left of the midline from the symphysis to a point above the umbilicus. With the patient in Trendelenburg position, the lowest loop of sigmoid is drawn to the right, exposing the peritoneum reflected from the pelvis to the mesosigmoid and mesorectum. An incision divides the pelvic peritoneum at this point of reflection, and is continued through the peritoneum around the anterior portion of the rectum at the most dependent accessible level of the culdesac. The lower sigmoid and upper rectum are drawn toward the median line, carrying with them the blood supply in the mesosigmoid. The superior hemorrhoidal artery, which is the downward continuation of the inferior mesenteric artery, is ligated about a fingerbreadth proximal to the promontory of the sacrum to the left of the median line. The point of ligation is proximal to the origin of the sigmoid arteries from the inferior mesenteric artery. The sigmoid arteries must be preserved because they supply the lower loop of the sigmoid which is used as a permanent colostomy.

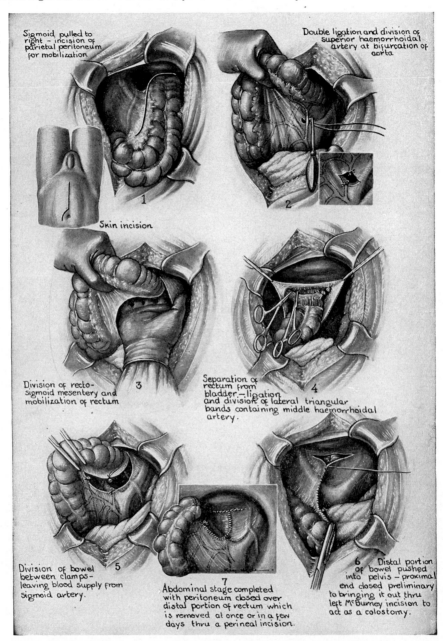

Sigmoid pulled to right – incision of parietal peritoneum for mobilization

Double ligation and division of superior haemorrhoidal artery at bifurcation of aorta

Skin incision

1

2

Division of rectosigmoid mesentery and mobilization of rectum

3

Separation of rectum from bladder – ligation and division of lateral triangular bands containing middle haemorrhoidal artery.

4

Division of bowel between clamps – leaving blood supply from sigmoid artery.

5

Abdominal stage completed with peritoneum closed over distal portion of rectum which is removed at once or in a few days thru a perineal incision.

7

6 Distal portion of bowel pushed into pelvis – proximal end closed preliminary to bringing it out thru left McBurney incision to act as a colostomy.

FIG. 440.—STEPS IN THE ABDOMINAL PORTION OF THE COMBINED ABDOMINAL-PERINEAL RESECTION OF THE RECTUM FOR CARCINOMA. (Modified from Lewis' Surgery.)

After ligation and division of the inferior mesenteric artery proximal to the origin of the lowest sigmoid branch, the mesial layer of the mesosigmoid is incised alongside the bowel. The incision connects with that in the left leaf of the mesosigmoid, making a complete line of separation between the bladder and rectum. The right hand is slipped into the hollow of the sacrum beneath the bowel, and is carried down to the sacrococcygeal junction, developing a cleavage line between the rectum and bladder anteriorly at the depth of the culdesac. The bowel is freed bluntly to the level of the seminal vesicles and prostate in the male and to the vagina in the female. The bands of fascia containing the middle hemorrhoidal arteries reach the rectum from the side at this level and are ligated and divided.

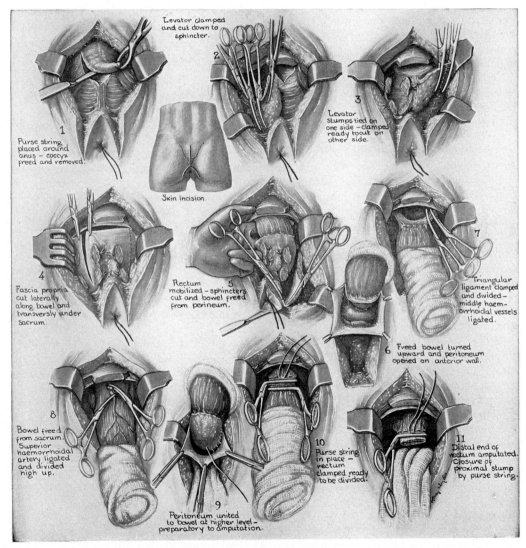

FIG. 441.—PERINEAL REMOVAL OF THE LOWER SIGMOID AND RECTUM FOR CARCINOMA. (Modified from Lewis' Surgery.)

An area low in the sigmoid loop is selected for the point of division of the bowel. The bowel is divided and the ends are closed by suture. The completely mobilized rectum is depressed into the hollow of the sacrum, and the pelvic peritoneum is closed over it tightly. The proximal closed end of the sigmoid is brought out on the abdomen through a muscle-splitting incision, and is opened later into an artificial anus.

For the *perineal part* of the operation, the patient is placed on his face in a reversed Trendelenburg position, or on his back in the lithotomy position. A median incision is made over the sacrum and coccyx to the anus, which then is circumscribed. Lateral incisions extend to the levator ani muscles on either side. With the finger inserted under the levator from above, the muscle is cut, first on one side and then on the other, at a considerable distance from the rectum. A transverse incision is made in the pelvic fascia between the sacrum and rectum, and is carried forward on one side of the rectum, opening the cleavage space between the rectum and the prostate. After dividing the levator ani muscle and the pelvic fascia, access is obtained to the hollow of the sacrum, and the extra-peritoneal mobilized bowel lying there is pulled out. The sphincter region finally is separated from the perineum anteriorly.

A *two-stage abdominal-perineal operation* is used for patients whose condition will not permit a one-stage procedure. The first stage consists of abdominal section and exploration of the abdomen, complete or partial mobilization of the bowel to be removed, and the establishment of a colostomy. The second stage is the perineal removal of the partially mobilized bowel; it is performed several days later. Interference with the blood supply in the carcinoma-bearing segment of the bowel in the process of its mobilization may occur in the two-stage operation; gangrene of this segment may cause peritonitis before the perineal stage of the operation.

3. Two-stage Abdominal and Perineal Operation for Carcinoma Low in the Rectum.— In carcinoma of the rectum below the peritoneum or at the peritoneal reflection, a two-stage operation is the more satisfactory. The first stage consists in an abdominal exploration and the formation of an inguinal colostomy, and the second stage, following in from ten days to two weeks, consists in the perineal removal of that part of the rectum which contains the tumor.

In the *abdominal stage*, a low, right paramedian rectus incision is made which amply exposes the rectovesical or recto-uterine culdesac. The local relations of the tumor are examined and the liver is palpated for the possible presence of metastases. If necessary, the sigmoid is mobilized to the extent that it can be lifted easily through an accessory small muscle-splitting incision. The second or perineal stage of the operation is performed two weeks after the first or abdominal stage when the patient is having normal bowel movements through the colostomy.

The *perineal removal* of that part of the rectum which contains the tumor is performed through an incision similar to that described for the perineal portion of the combined abdominoperineal operation (p. 441). After the rectum has been separated from the prostate or vagina anteriorly, the lower rectum is mobilized by sharp dissection. The hollow of the sacrum is entered through the opening in the pelvic fascia, and the fascial bands containing the middle hemorrhoidal vessels are divided, freeing the upper rectum. With the mobilized bowel retracted over the sacrum, the peritoneum is incised close to the anterior bowel wall. After the mobilized bowel has been allowed to fall back into the wound, the superior hemorrhoidal vessels can be felt as a firm strand on the posterior wall of the rectum. These vessels are ligated high and divided so that the bowel comes down still further and can be divided a considerable distance proximal to the upper limit of the growth. Before dividing the bowel, the peritoneum is sutured to it proximal to the point of proposed division.

4. Rectal Prolapse and Intussusception.—Rectal prolapse and intussusception are described under the anal part of the rectum (p. 508).

B. BLADDER

1. Location and Shape.—The urinary bladder is located anteriorly in the pelvis, immediately posterior to the pubes. When the bladder is empty and contracted, it is wedged in the forward part of the pelvis; its walls lie in contact and its cavity is reduced to a mere slit. Looking toward the pelvic cavity, the upper or posterosuperior surface of the bladder is rounded and is covered by the peritoneum of the anterior wall of the pelvis. This surface is triangular in shape; its apex, which is directed forward, lies behind the symphysis and is connected with the urachus; the lateral or basal angles correspond to the points at which the ureters reach the bladder. The interval between these angles indicated by a ridge, is the posterior or basal margin of the bladder.

When the bladder is distended, it undergoes marked alterations. The posterior and lateral boundaries become rounded and the viscus assumes an oval outline. The upper or posterosuperior wall of the bladder rises and gradually encroaches upon the pelvic cavity. The lateral surfaces are increased and consequently more of the bladder comes into relation with the pelvic organs. The line of peritoneal reflection rises to a much higher level, and the bladder floor bulges downward. As the bladder expands, it mounts gradually over the pubes. The pubovesical reflection of peritoneum rises a variable extent, so that the bladder wall lies directly against the abdominal wall except for some intervening fatty tissue. Even when the viscus is distended greatly, the peritoneal reflection anteriorly may rise but slightly. Occasionally, the peritoneum is more than usually adherent behind the symphysis, and elevation of the pubovesical reflection is prevented. Advantage is taken of the rising of the pubovesical peritoneum is aspirating the overdistended bladder suprapubically, and in the operation of suprapubic cystotomy. The same relationship may be obtained by distending the viscus artificially.

The bladder occupies a higher position in the very young child than in the adult because of the smaller relative size of the pelvis and the greater relative size of the bladder.

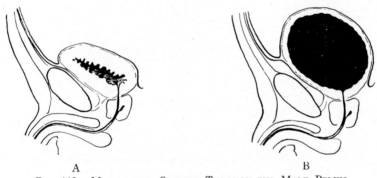

A   B

FIG. 442.—MIDSAGITTAL SECTION THROUGH THE MALE PELVIS.

In A, the bladder is empty; in B, the bladder is distended; distention of the bladder usually elevates the prevesical fold of peritoneum.

The neck of the bladder lies almost on a level with the upper margin of the symphysis, and most of the bladder lies in the abdomen. For this reason the bladder should be evacuated before making any incision in the lower part of the anterior abdominal wall, especially in inguinal hernioplasty (p. 299).

2. **Perivesical Spaces.**—The bladder, like the rectum, is encompassed partly by extraperitoneal, areolar, connective tissue spaces, an arrangement which accommodates the distention demanded of the viscus. Of the tissue spaces, the prevesical area is clinically important because of the infections set up in it or propagated to it.

The *prevesical space* (of Retzius) lies partly in the pelvis and partly in the abdomen, and is a division of the extraperitoneal space which extends from the pelvic floor to the umbilicus. The space is bounded anteriorly by the posterior sheath of the rectus muscle and the posterior surface of the pubes. An effusion here may extend rapidly into the extraperitoneal tissue of the abdominal wall and pelvis. The continuity of the extraperitoneal areas about the inguinal and femoral hernial regions explains the presence of a segment of bladder in herniae. Inflammatory involvement of the space follows vesical infection, urinary extravasation in extraperitoneal rupture of the bladder, and infection which gravitates into the pelvic part of the space from urinary extravasation after suprapubic cystotomy. The guiding principle in treatment of these infections is free evacuation and adequate drainage.

3. **Fixation of the Bladder.**—The bladder is anchored securely only at its base where it is fixed by continuity with the prostate and urethra, which, in turn, are bound to the urogenital diaphragm (triangular ligament) (p. 497). The neck of the bladder is fixed also by the pubovesical and puboprostatic ligaments which bind it to the symphysis. These ligaments are bundles of fibers derived from the visceral layer of pelvic fascia. The median umbilical ligament, containing the urachus, maintains the bladder in position anteriorly and superiorly. The lateral umbilical ligaments, containing the atrophied supravesical portions of the fetal umbilical arteries, stabilize the bladder. The lateral and median umbilical ligaments are bladder supports only in the sense that they act as guides in maintaining the bladder against the anterior abdominal wall when the bladder fills and rises out of the pelvis. Posteriorly, the bladder is reinforced by the rectovesical fascia (of Denonvilliers) (p. 445). The viscus lies within the visceral layer of pelvic fascia. After

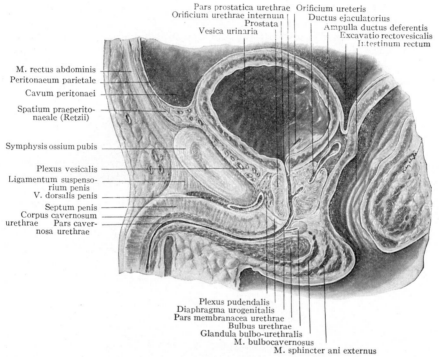

Fig. 443.—Midsagittal Section Through the Pelvis and Perineum with the Bladder Distended. The structures in relation to the bladder are shown in detail.

difficult deliveries, the bladder may be loosened from its attachment to the pelvic floor and may prolapse into the perineum, appearing at the vulva as a cystocele.

4. **Relations of the Bladder.**—Anteriorly and inferiorly, the bladder is related to the pubic bones, symphysis, retropubic fat, anterior vesical veins, and the vesical portion of the pelvic fascia. Fragments from a pubic fracture may penetrate the prevesical space and lacerate the bladder. Traumatic separation of the symphysis may cause bladder rupture from the sudden pull exerted on the pubovesical ligaments. The lateral aspect of the bladder is related to the levator ani and obturator internus muscles, the parietal layer of pelvic fascia, and the vesicoprostatic venous plexus.

In the male, the postero-inferior (basal) aspect of the bladder is related to the rectum, but is separated from it by the seminal vesicles, the deferent ducts and their ampullae, and the rectovesical fascia (of Denonvilliers). A small interval exists between the deferent ducts and the inferior reflection of the bladder serosa. This area, the interdeferent triangle (p. 450), increases slightly in size as the bladder becomes distended. For puncture of the bladder by the old-fashioned rectal route, a trocar was passed through this extraperitoneal area. The terminal parts of the ureters lie between the upper rounded extremities of the seminal vesicles and the bladder wall. In the female, the bladder is related posteriorly to the shallow uterovesical pouch of peritoneum separating it from the body of the uterus. Below this peritoneal pouch, the bladder is in direct relation with the cervix and the

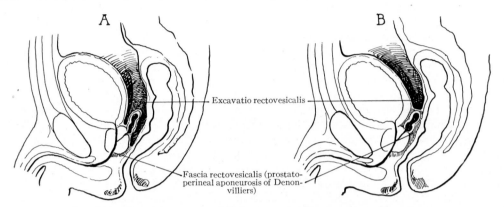

Fig. 444.—Variations in the Depth of the Rectovesical Culdesac.

In A, the rectovesical culdesac extends below the level of the superior surface of the prostate; in B, the culdesac does not reach the seminal vesicles; in this instance, the rectum is in direct relation with the bladder, seminal vesicles, and prostate.

anterior vaginal wall. Lateral to the ureter, the bladder is related to the anterior layer of the broad ligament (p. 462). The bladder has posterosuperior relations with the pelvic colon and loops of small bowel. It is overlain by the fundus and body of the uterus. The erosion of adhesions between the bladder and small bowel may form an intestinovesical fistula.

5. **Rectovesical (Prostatoperitoneal) Fascia (of Denonvilliers).**—The extent to which the prostate and seminal vesicles are covered by peritoneum depends upon the depth of

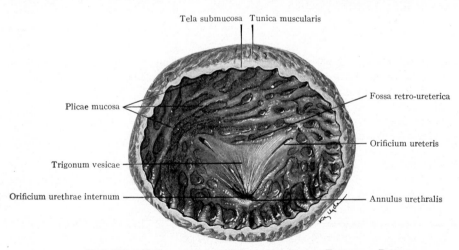

Fig. 445.—Fundus of the Bladder and the Trigonal Region.

the rectovesical pouch. As a developmental anomaly, this pouch occasionally may reach to within 1 or 2 cm. of the anus or even lower, and may contain intestinal loops which have herniated into the perineum. At about the fourth or fifth intra-uterine month, the culdesac extends to the pelvic floor; in the newborn, it reaches to the base of the prostate. The peritoneum of the anterior and posterior walls of the embryonic pouch approximates and fuses from below upward so that there is formed a frontally disposed fascia, the recto-vesical or prostatoperitoneal fascia (of Denonvilliers).

6. Interior of the Bladder.—The appearance of the bladder varies according to the degree of tension on the lining mucosa which is loosely adherent to the muscle layer through a relatively loose submucosa. In the contracted organ, the mucosa is thrown into folds and presents a wrinkled appearance. In the distended organ, the mucosa has fewer folds, but even with the fullest distention there remains a corrugated appearance caused by the interlacing subjacent muscle columns.

In the region of the urethral orifice, the mucosa undergoes a striking modification. It is comparatively smooth over a triangular area known as the *trigone*. The apex of the trigone lies at the *urethral orifice;* the base corresponds to an imaginary line, indicated usually by a well-defined elevation, the *interureteric ridge,* which connects the orifices of the ureters. The prominence of the ridge depends upon the elevation of the mucosa over the muscle elements which are raised by the oblique passage of the ureters through the bladder wall. The distance between the orifices measures from 2 to 3 cm. and varies with the size and degree of distention of the viscus. The center of the trigone is depressed toward the urethral orifice and is the most frequent area of localization of disease of the bladder (pathologic zone). The urethral orifice is not circular because of a median elevation, the *vesical crest* or *uvula,* in its posterior circumference. The crest consists of a thickening of mucous membrane over a framework of muscle tissue, and is continued through the ure-

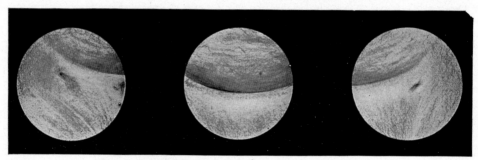

Fig. 446.—Cystoscopic Views of an Hypertrophied Trigone with a Moderately Deep Pouch Behind It. Ureteral Orifices Are Normal. (Young, "Practice of Urology.")

thral orifice to the floor of the prostatic urethra. Inflammatory lesions about the urethral orifice are characterized by painful and frequent urination, often accompanied by muscle spasm and urinary retention.

The obliquely placed *ureteral orifices* open upon the mesial extremities of a well-defined ureteric fold. They usually are slitlike, but may be oval or round, and their direction is obliquely transverse. The lateral margin of each orifice is guarded by a valvelike projection, while the mesial margin lies embedded in the fold.

The interior of the fundus of the bladder or *retrotrigonal fossa* is depressed. When the fossa is rendered large and deep by increased intravesical pressure from prostatic hypertrophy, urinary residues accumulate within it and stagnation occurs. Foreign bodies gravitate to the fossa and bladder ruptures occur through it.

7. Mucosa of the Bladder.—The mucosa of the bladder is located midway in the genito-urinary tract, and is prone to pathologic changes, of which cystitis is the most common. Cystitis nearly always is transmitted from the kidneys. From the urethra, there easily develops a trigonitis, but scarcely ever a cystitis. The generous nerve supply of the region explains the exquisite pain and sensitiveness coincident with infection and edema. Spasmodic contraction of the muscle elements in the vesical and upper urethral walls causes the colicky type of pain (tenesmus) of cystitis.

8. Vessels and Nerves.—The *arterial* supply of the bladder reaches it laterally, anteriorly, and posteriorly from the visceral branches of the hypogastric artery or from the hypogastric artery itself. Small branches from the internal pudendal and obturator arteries supply the anterior portion of the bladder. The superior vesicular arteries, which are the unobliterated portion of the umbilical arteries, supply the superolateral walls. They reach the bladder under the lateral reflection of the pelvic peritoneum. The inferior vesicular arteries from the hypogastric artery share their distribution between the floor of the bladder, the prostate, and the prostatic urethra. A vesicular branch from the middle hemorrhoidal artery partially supplies the posterior surface of the bladder and the seminal vesicles These vessels form a perivesical network and their rami penetrate the mucosa. Erosion of these vessels explains the hematuria so common in bladder disease.

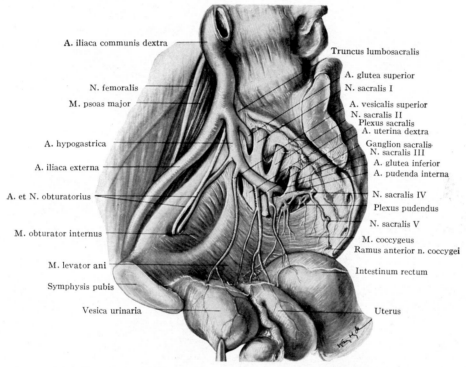

FIG. 447.—LATERAL VIEW OF THE FEMALE PELVIS TO SHOW THE MAIN ARTERIES AND NERVES. The bladder, rectum, and pelvic genitalia are drawn downward to show their arterial supply.

The vesical *veins* are arranged in a plexiform manner throughout the walls. The larger stems are directed to the plexuses in the basal region, which, in the male, lie in the groove between the bladder and prostate (vesicoprostatic plexus). Phlebitis of these veins is a grave condition because they propagate infection to the large hypogastric vein.

The *lymphatics* draining the bladder are connected with glands arranged along the external iliac and hypogastric vessels.

SURGICAL CONSIDERATIONS

1. **Injuries of the Bladder.**—The infrequency of bladder wounds may be accounted for largely by the well-protected position of the viscus within the pelvic cavity. Bladder injury may occur in various ways: the viscus may be lacerated by sharp bony fragments in fractures of the pubes; if the bladder is distended considerably, it may rupture from a direct blow over the hypogastrium; it may be injured by penetrating wounds through the hypogastrium; or it may be torn by violence exerted through the rectum and vagina or by trauma to the perineum. Penetrating wounds directed through the greater sciatic or the obturator foramina may penetrate the bladder.

Bladder rupture rarely follows distention alone if the bladder walls are healthy, but it may occur spontaneously through an ulcerated area or through a wall long subjected to pressure from urinary obstruction. In neglected cases of urethral stricture, the bladder

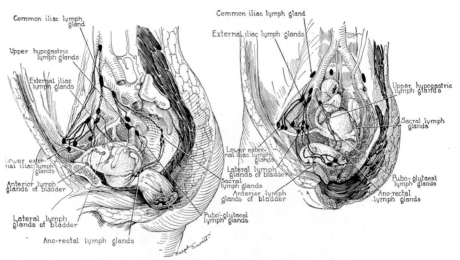

FIG. 448.—LYMPHATIC DRAINAGE OF THE MALE AND FEMALE BLADDER. (Hinman.)

usually maintains its integrity and the urethra proximal to the stricture gives way (p 498). In a bladder rendered immobile by pericystitis or pelvic cellulitis, less force is required to produce rupture. The likelihood of injury from trauma is proportionate to the degree of distention of the bladder and the consequent elevation of the viscus from the

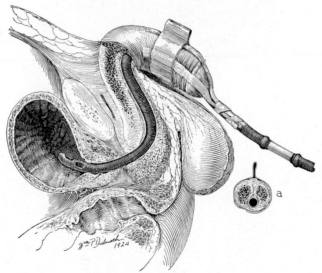

FIG. 449.—DIAGRAM OF A RETENTION CATHETER IN PLACE.

An additional fenestra is cut at the tip of the catheter; the catheter is fastened closely to the glans with adhesive plaster strips which are retained on the penis by a circular band. The expansion "pleat" on the band, shown in the main drawing and in the inset a, allows for erections, thus preventing constriction. (Young, "Practice of Urology.")

protection of the pelvis. Drunkenness predisposes to bladder distention, and a blow, scarcely appreciated by the patient in his stuporous condition, may rupture it. The walls of a distended bladder lose their elasticity, and force applied to its contained fluid produces a rupture at the weakest point.

Intraperitoneal rupture occurs in that part of the bladder covered by peritoneum, and *extraperitoneal rupture* in that not covered by peritoneum; when the tear involves only the mucomuscular coats, the lesion is *subperitoneal* and the urine extravasates beneath the peritoneal covering. The commonest location for rupture is the posterosuperior aspect of the bladder Rupture involving the anterior surface alone is unusual.

The symptoms of bladder rupture are dependent largely upon the escape of urine into the surrounding regions and vary with the location of the lesion. Urine in the abdominal cavity produces the most evident symptoms. If the patient is unable to void, the diagnosis

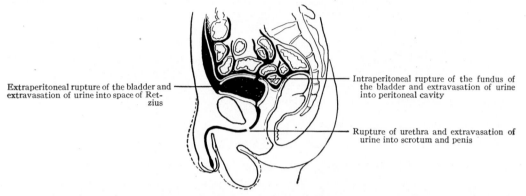

Extraperitoneal rupture of the bladder and extravasation of urine into space of Retzius

Intraperitoneal rupture of the fundus of the bladder and extravasation of urine into peritoneal cavity

Rupture of urethra and extravasation of urine into scrotum and penis

FIG. 450.—MOST FREQUENT COMPLICATIONS OF FRACTURE OF THE PELVIS.

of rupture of the bladder may be made by immediate catheterization. If catheterization withdraws only a little bloody urine or cannot withdraw all of a measured quantity of fluid instilled, rupture of the bladder is certain. Whether the rupture be intraperitoneal or extraperitoneal, immediate closure must be done and egress be given the urine by a suprapubic cystotomy or by the placement of an indwelling urethral catheter, or both. Roentgenograms of the bladder after intravenous injection of a radio-opaque dye which is secreted by the kidney reveal the outlines of the bladder and may reveal a defect in its walls

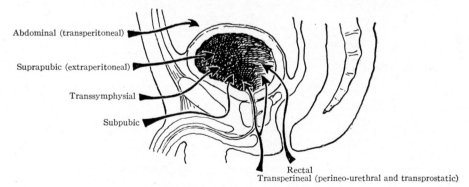

Abdominal (transperitoneal)

Suprapubic (extraperitoneal)

Transsymphysial

Subpubic

Rectal
Transperineal (perineo-urethral and transprostatic)

FIG. 451.—SURGICAL APPROACHES TO THE BLADDER.

2. **Routes to the Bladder.**—The *urethral* or *cystoscopic route* to the bladder is employed for diagnostic purposes. The use of the cystoscope has proved an invaluable aid in the diagnosis and treatment of bladder conditions. It makes possible examination of the mucosa, catheterization of the ureters, and removal of small bladder growths, foreign bodies, and calculi. Because of the comparative shortness and dilatability of the urethra in the female, cystoscopy in the female is much simpler than it is in the male.

The *perineal approach* is discussed in the section on the Perineum (p. 504).

The median hypogastric or *suprapubic route* usually is selected for surgery of the bladder, since it affords excellent access for the removal of calculi and new growths, and for

29

prostatectomy (p. 459). Suprapubic cystotomy frequently is performed for the purpose of draining the bladder. It is the aim of the operation to expose the bladder below the line of reflection of the peritoneum from the abdominal wall so that the peritoneal cavity is not opened. As a preliminary step, it is necessary that the viscus be distended fully.

A vertical median incision is made through the anterior abdominal wall in the suprapubic region. It reaches to a point just above the symphysis and is carried deeply into the interval between the pyramidalis and rectus abdominis muscles. Behind these muscles, but separated from them at the upper border of the symphysis by a definite interval containing fatty tissue, lies the transversalis fascia. The prevesical space is exposed by division of this fascia. The bladder, if distended, is palpated readily by a finger introduced into the lower angle of the wound. The peritoneal reflection is drawn upward out of the way without difficulty, because the connection of the peritoneum to the bladder is loose. The prevesical fat and the visceral layer of pelvic fascia are incised, avoiding the anterior vesical veins, if possible. The bladder wall is drawn forward and incised vertically. The urethral orifice, because of its proximity to the symphysis, may be reached by introducing the finger into the suprapubic wound.

C. INTRAPELVIC PORTION OF THE DEFERENT DUCTS; SEMINAL VESICLES; PROSTATE; PROSTATIC URETHRA

1. **Intrapelvic Portion of the Deferent Ducts.**—The intrapelvic portion of each deferent duct extends from the abdominal inguinal ring to the base of the prostate. On leaving the inguinal canal, it descends into the pelvic cavity by crossing the lateral and posterior aspect of the inferior epigastric artery. It then runs downward, backward, and

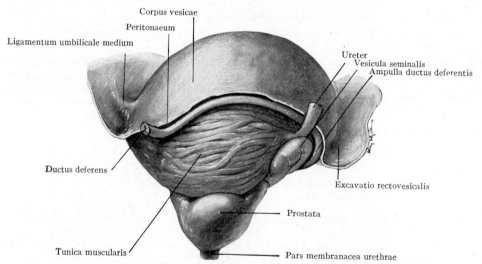

Corpus vesicae

Peritonaeum

Ligamentum umbilicale medium

Ureter
Vesicula seminalis
Ampulla ductus deferentis

Ductus deferens

Excavatio rectovesicalis

Prostata

Tunica muscularis

Pars membranacea urethrae

FIG. 452.—LATERAL VIEW OF THE BLADDER AND MALE PELVIC GENITALIA.

mesially, and crosses over the external iliac vessels to reach the lateral walls of the true pelvis. After crossing the ureter, it runs beneath the peritoneum to the angle formed by the seminal vesicles. In this angle, the two ducts contribute to the formation of the interdeferent triangle. In its terminal part, each duct is enclosed within the thickness of the frontally disposed rectovesical fascia (of Denonvilliers), and widens into an *ampulla*. The ampullae converge and unite with the excretory ducts of the seminal vesicles to form the ejaculatory ducts which traverse the prostate and open on the prostatic urethra.

2. **Seminal Vesicles.**—The seminal vesiclesare sacculated membranous reservoirs which are off-shoots from the deferent ducts. They are invested partially by the peritoneum of the rectovesical pouch, and the terminal parts of the ureters separate them from

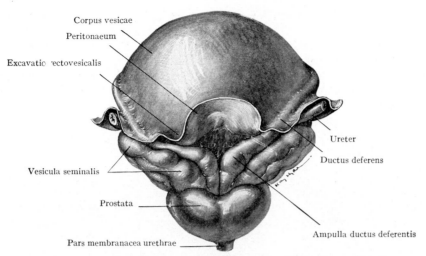

Corpus vesicae

Peritonaeum

Excavatio rectovesicalis

Ureter

Ductus deferens

Vesicula seminalis

Prostata

Ampulla ductus deferentis

Pars membranacea urethrae

FIG. 453.—POSTERIOR VIEW OF THE BLADDER AND MALE PELVIC GENITALIA.

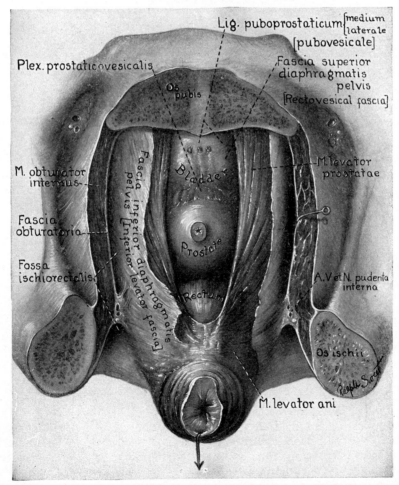

Lig. puboprostaticum {medium / laterale [pubovesicale]

Plex. prostaticovesicalis

Fascia superior diaphragmatis pelvis [Rectovesical fascia]

Os pubis

Bladder

M. levator prostatae

M. obturator internus

Fascia obturatoria

Fascia inferior diaphragmatis pelvis [Inferior levator fascia]

Prostate

Fossa ischiorectalis

Rectum

A. V et N. pudenta interna

Os ischii

M. levator ani

FIG. 454.—PERINEAL ASPECT OF THE LEVATOR ANI PORTION OF THE PELVIC DIAPHRAGM.

The ischium or inferior part of the bony pelvis has been cut away; the urogenital diaphragm has been removed to show the interlevator cleft and the intrapelvic structures.

contact with the bladder wall. The lower pointed extremity of the vesicle narrows to form the excretory duct and is received into the fissure of the base of the prostate, where it joins the lateral aspect of the ampulla of the corresponding vas. From their communication at the base of the prostate, the ejaculatory ducts run forward and downward between its median and lateral lobes and in front of the posterior lobe of the prostate to converge and empty into the prostatic urethra close to the orifice of the prostatic utricle (p. 457).

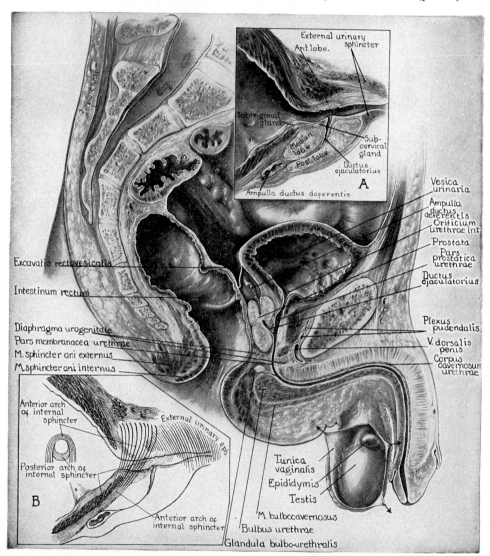

Fig. 455.—Sagittal Section Through the Male Pelvis, Perineum, and External Genitalia. A is a sagittal section through the neck of the bladder and the prostate; B is a diagram of the musculature at the vesical orifice. (After Wesson.)

Seminal vesiculitis usually is secondary to infection elsewhere in the genito-urinary tract. Gonococcal vesiculitis sometimes succeeds prostatitis and may terminate in abscess formation. The abscess may discharge its contents into the rectum or bladder, or even into the pelvic peritoneal cavity, although this usually is prevented by the adhesions resulting from a localized peritonitis. The infection may extend downward through the pelvic diaphragm to the perineal region by a mechanism similar to that for the spread of prostatic abscess (p 458).

Tuberculosis of the epididymis (p. 519) is thought to be secondary to tuberculous vesiculitis, extension being along the vas. The infection may originate in the kidney. Rectal examination reveals the extent of the swelling of the seminal vesicles. The seminal vesicles are approached through an incision anterior to the anus, similar to incision for perineal prostatectomy (p. 461).

3. **Prostate.**—The prostate is a solid musculoglandular body of firm consistency, comparable in size and shape to a chestnut. Its apex is directed downward and rests upon the superior fascia of the urogenital diaphragm (p. 497). The posterior surface of the organ

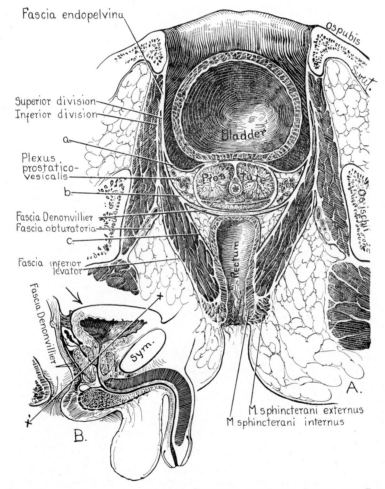

FIG. 456.—OBLIQUE TRANSVERSE SECTION THROUGH THE MALE PELVIS AND PERINEUM.

The inset, B, is a sagittal section through the male pelvis and perineum; the line x–x′ is the level at which the main drawing was made; a, b, c represent the superior, middle, and inferior divisions of the superior or rectovesical division of the pelvic fascia.

is in contact with the rectum through the intermedium of the rectovesical fascia and can be palpated readily on rectal examination. The lateral surfaces lie against the mesial borders of the levators and also can be examined through the rectum. The prostate is traversed from its base to its apex by the first or prostatic part of the urethra. A groove separates the lateral margins of the prostate from the base of the bladder. The ejaculatory ducts traverse the gland downward and forward and empty into the posterior wall of the prostatic urethra.

There is scant periprostatic tissue at the sides of the gland, but abundant tissue anteriorly, consisting largely of the periprostatic venous plexus. This tissue is the seat of periprostatic abscess. Pus from such an abscess, or the extravasated urine following prostatic rupture, tends to invade the extraperitoneal space of the pelvis (p. 430) rather than the perineum.

4. **Capsule and Sheath of the Prostate.**—For the prostate, as for the thyroid (p. 179), there is an intrinsic capsule incorporated with the fibrous elements, and an extrinsic sheath. The *prostatic capsule* consists of parallel layers of fibromuscular tissue continuous with, and forming part of, the stroma of the organ. The prostatic capsule is of such strength that adenomata of the prostate grow superiorly into the bladder along the line of least resistance. The *prostatic sheath* or *false capsule* is formed anteriorly and laterally by

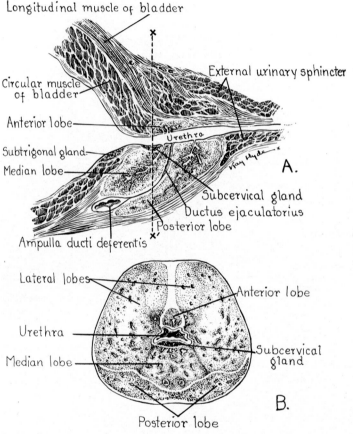

Fig. 457.—A, Midsagittal Section Through an Embryo to Show the Structures at the Neck of the Bladder. B, Cross Section at the Neck of the Bladder at the Level of x–x′ in Drawing A. These drawings illustrate the development of the lobes of the prostate. (After Lowsley.)

periprostatic connective tissue derived from the pelvic fascia in which the prostatovesical plexus of veins lies. A few veins lie in the loose tissue between the sheath and capsule. Posteriorly, the sheath is formed by the avascular rectovesical fascia of Denonvillier's. This fascia is of fair thickness and acts as an efficient barrier to the reciprocal spread of prostatic or rectal malignant disease. In the enucleation of hypertrophied glandular elements of the prostrate, injury to the periprostatic venous plexuses must be avoided. The capsule and sheath must not be damaged lest there be urinary extravasation into the extraperitoneal tissues of the pelvis.

5. **Development of the Prostate; Mechanism of Urinary Obstruction.**—For a proper appreciation of the mechanism of urinary obstruction from glandular hypertrophy, a knowledge of the development of the prostate is essential. In intra-uterine life, longitudinal

depressions appear on the walls of the urethra just inferior to the bladder. By a process of budding, these depressions are elaborated into a number of glandular masses or lobes which penetrate the surrounding muscle and connective tissue to form the ultimate prostate gland.

The lobules forming the *anterior lobe* bud from the anterior wall of the urethra. The glandular elements are few and gradually disappear until, at birth, the lobe of the prostate gland thus formed has no surgical significance, since its few glandular elements do not encroach upon the lumen of the urethra.

The glands forming the *median* or *prespermatic lobe* originate on the posterior surface of the floor of the urethra just superior to the urethral openings of the ejaculatory ducts. The lobe, therefore, is posturethral and prespermatic. The glands grow backward and upward toward the bladder in such a fashion that median lobe hypertrophy causes urinary obstruction by pushing the urethra forward at the apex of the trigone. When this lobe hypertrophies upward, it lifts the bladder mucosa which is behind the urinary orifice and dilates and destroys the internal sphincter; sometimes it gives rise to a large irregular mass which seriously deforms the bladder orifice, hinders spontaneous urinary evacuation, and makes urethral catheterization difficult. In median lobe enlargement, the normally straight prostatic urethra becomes definitely, and sometimes abruptly, curved.

The two *lateral lobes* arise as tubular outgrowths from the prostatic furrows on the lateral walls of the urethra. They expand laterally, anteriorly, posteriorly, and upward. until they occupy most of the base or upper portion of the prostate. During development, they are separated from the median lobe by fibrous partitions which do not exist in the adult gland. As they grow, they nearly approximate one another anterior to the urethra, especially in the inferior part of the gland near its apex. Hypertrophy of the lateral lobes causes urinary obstruction by lateral encroachment on the prostatic urethra. If one lobe greatly exceeds the other in size, the urethra is deviated laterally and is increased in length.

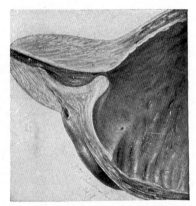

FIG. 458.—LONGITUDINAL SECTION THROUGH THE NECK OF THE BLADDER AND THE PROSTATE.

A typical median bar is elevated above the trigone; there is no enlargement of the prostate. (Young, "Practice of Urology.")

The tubules of origin of the *posterior lobe* arise in the posterior wall of the urethra inferior to the orifices of the ejaculatory ducts, and grow superiorly to occupy a plane behind the ducts. As they grow upward toward the base of the bladder, they are both posturethral and postspermatic. This lobe in the ultimate gland is separated definitely from the lateral and median lobes and the ejaculatory ducts by fibrous interlobar partitions. It forms all the posterior surface of the gland and, therefore, is the lobe encountered in rectal examination. The lobe thins out toward the superior surface of the gland, and presents a median longitudinal furrow. Enlargement of this lobe rarely occurs.

In perineal prostatectomy (p. 461) it is necessary to incise the posterior surface of the prostate deeply enough to penetrate the posterior lobe completely and divide the fibrous septum anterior to it. The lateral lobes and median lobe, the true offenders in prostatic hypertrophy, are enucleated through the incision or incisions in the posterior lobe. Attempt at enucleation of these lobes through the posterior lobe is difficult if the incision is too shallow and extends only into and not through the substance of the posterior lobe. With an adequate incision, both the lateral and median lobes may be removed in such a way as to leave a median bridge of tissue which contains the thickness of the posterior lobe as well as the ejaculatory ducts.

The *subcervical glands* develop beneath the mucosa of the urethra just outside the bladder, but within the confines of the internal urinary sphincter. As they are proximal to the internal sphincter, their position is most important, since even a slight increase in their size may cause marked interference with the passage of urine from the bladder.

The small nodules of *subtrigonal gland tissue* lie beneath the mucosa of the middle of the bladder trigone and near its apex. Although their size is comparatively insignificant, those near the apex of the trigone occupy a strategic intravesical position. A very

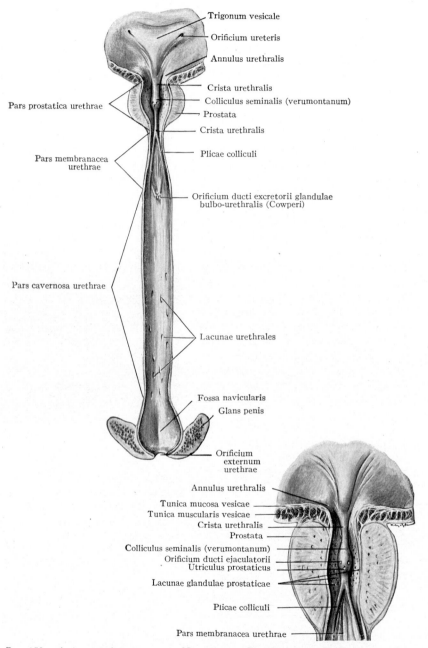

FIG. 459.—ANTERIOR ASPECT OF THE NECK OF THE BLADDER AND THE POSTERIOR ASPECT OF THE URETHRA. The inset shows the details of the prostatic urethra.

slight hypertrophy may encroach on the lumen of the vesical orifice and form a marked obstruction to urinary outflow. The tubules, in some instances, become so pedunculated as to lie almost free about the vesical orifice, and are in a position to block it in a ball-valve fashion as effectively as a much hypertrophied prostate.

6. **Prostatic Urethra.**—The prostatic urethra, normally about 3 cm. long, traverses the gland from base to apex, that is, from the internal urethral orifice to the superior layer of the urogenital diaphragm (triangular ligament) (p. 497). It does not follow the axis of the prostate, but lies much nearer the anterior than the posterior surface. The lumen of the urethra, although admitting of considerable dilation, normally is obliterated by the approximation of its anterior and posterior walls. It appears in cross section as a horizontal slit, save where the seminal colliculus (verumontanum) bulges forward from the posterior urethral wall. In lateral lobe hypertrophy, pressure of the lobes transforms the slit into an anteroposterior fissure.

The *urethral crest* extends along the posterior wall or floor of the urethra from its origin on the vesical trigone (p. 446) to its termination at the membranous urethra. On each side of the crest is a depressed fossa, the *prostatic sinus*, the floor of which is perforated by numerous apertures, the *orifices of the prostatic ducts*. The *seminal colliculus* (*verumontanum*), the greatest prominence of the urethral crest, lies over the middle of the prostatic urethra where the lumen of the channel, because of the forward projection of the colliculus, appears crescentic in outline. It is surmounted by the slitlike opening of the *prostatic utricle*. The culdesac of the prostatic utricle is directed backward and upward a variable distance (10 to 12 mm.) into the prostate. Upon the seminal colliculus, and lateral to the edges of the lips of the 'utricle, open the *orifices of the ejaculatory ducts*. Seminal colliculitis (verumontanitis) may cause constriction or obliteration of the ejaculatory ducts.

Much clinical interest attaches to the relations of the urethra with the prostate, for chronic urethral infection involves the prostatic ducts opening at different levels into the canal. When the inflammation is propagated to the openings of the ejaculatory ducts, a deferentitis or an epididymitis may result. It is from infection localized in the prostatic urethra that prostatic abscesses arise.

7. **Internal and External Urinary Sphincter.**—The *vesical (internal urinary) sphincter* (Fig. 455) is derived from the outer longitudinal and middle circular muscle layers of the bladder. Certain of the longitudinal muscle

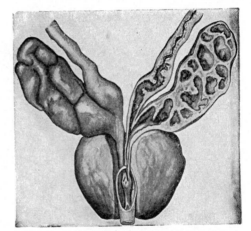

FIG. 460.—RELATIONS OF THE EJACULATORY DUCTS TO THE PROSTATE AND PROSTATIC URETHRA. (Bickham after Spalteholz.)

bundles, after winding about the convexity of the bladder, do not end at the vesical orifice, but sweep downward inferior to and behind it. They then arch forward and mesially about the origin of the urethra in such a way as to form an arch over it. To assist in forming a sphincter about the initial part of the urethra, a few of the circular fibers of the bladder continue a short distance down the posterior and lateral walls of the urethra and form a contractile posterior arch (Wesson).

The *urethral (external urinary) sphincter* consists of concentrically placed striated muscle fibers which invest the prostatic and beginning membranous parts of the urethra distal to the anterior arch of the internal sphincter. Only toward the apex of the prostate do the fibers entirely surround the urethra, enabling them to exert a sphincter action. It is unlikely that this voluntary sphincter is the sole agent in urinary retention distal to the involuntary internal sphincter. The intrinsic involuntary muscle supply of the prostatic urethra probably plays an important role in urinary retention. The rare instances of urinary incontinence following suprapubic prostatectomy no doubt are a result of the destruction of much of the prostatic urethra and its intrinsic involuntary musculature.

Part of the explanation of the incontinence which occasionally follows the perineal removal of the obstructing masses in the prostate may be injury of the vesical sphincter from long-standing distention by the hypertrophied prostatic lobes or from operative trauma. Incontinence after this operation may be caused by external membranous urethrotomy and removal of much of the prostatic urethra and its involuntary musculature.

SURGICAL CONSIDERATIONS

1. **Prostatitis and Prostatic Abscess.**—*Prostatitis* usually is preceded by urethritis, especially the gonococcal form. The inflammation tends both to acute suppuration and chronicity of infection because of the imperfect drainage from the prostatic tubules. When the infecting organisms have entered a prostatic duct, edema of the walls of the duct occurs, which blocks the egress of pus formed in the deeper structures. The increased vascularity of the tissue of the gland causes swelling. The symptoms of bladder tenesmus and painful urination are caused partly by mechanical obstruction but probably more by the spread of inflammation to the trigonal region (p. 446). The acute infection soon passes into a chronic stage. Infection persists in the glands of the prostate and in the crypts of the prostatic urethra.

Eventually, *prostatic abscess* may make its appearance, either in the form of a single large cavity or of several discrete foci. The abscess usually points in the direction of

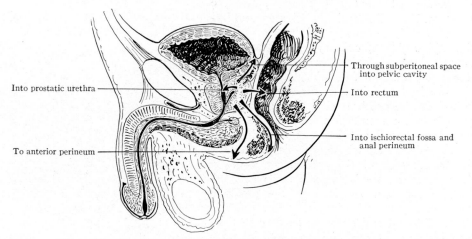

Into prostatic urethra —

To anterior perineum —

Through subperitoneal space into pelvic cavity

Into rectum

Into ischiorectal fossa and anal perineum

FIG. 461.—PATHS OF EXTENSION FROM A PROSTATIC ABSCESS.
The arrows indicate rupture through the subperitoneal space into the pelvic cavity, into the rectum, into the ischiorectal fossa and anal perineum, and into the prostatic urethra.

least resistance and ruptures into the urethra. An abscess not opening into the urethra may form a periprostatic suppuration which can extend in many directions. The dense investment of pelvic fascia resists its progress through the peritoneum into the pelvic cavity, but the collection of pus may lie above the prostate and tend to localize about the seminal vesicles. It scarcely can reach the most anterior part of the perineum because of the strong urogenital diaphragm. To reach the perineum, it points toward the rectum, from which it is separated by the less resistant rectovesical fascia. It may erode this fascia and invade the rectum, or be guided by the fascia into the perineum through the interval between the urogenital diaphragm and the anus. The abscess sometimes fuses forward and breaks through the pubovesical ligaments into the prevesical space (of Retzius). The periprostatic diffusion from the abscess may lie lateral to the gland and reach the ischiorectal fossa by invading the levator ani muscle.

The investment of the prostate in an unyielding capsule serves, in part, to explain the severe pain occasioned by abscess. Since the prostatic nerve supply is derived from the lower dorsal and upper lumbar segments, referred pain may occur over a large area. It is common in the back about the twelfth rib and the sacrum, and may be referred to the foot through the third sacral nerve.

To minimize the amount of prostatic tissue destroyed and the danger of extension of infection, the abscess should be evacuated immediately upon its discovery. A spreading thrombophlebitis in the veins of the periprostatic plexus is a serious complication.

Deliberate evacuation of a prostatic abscess can be performed through the *perineal incision* (devised for prostatectomy) (p. 461). Should the abscess be intraprostatic, the posterior surface of the gland is reached without encountering pus. Lateral incision through the posterior lobe allows exploration of the abscess cavity, and blunt dissection serves to explore its wall and break down intervening septa. If the abscess has become periprostatic, pus is encountered before the prostrate is reached. Lateral and retroprostatic

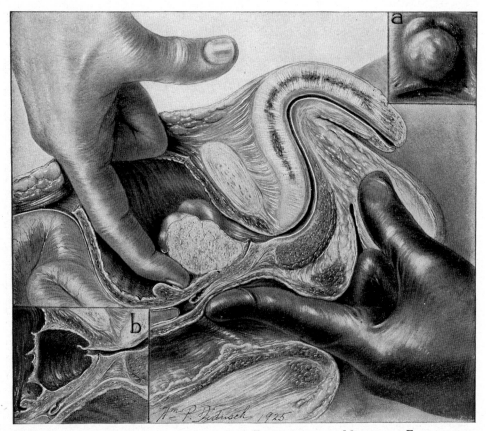

FIG. 462.—SUPRAPUBIC PROSTATECTOMY BY THE EXTRA-URETHRAL METHOD OF ENUCLEATION.
Enucleation is begun after breaking through or incising the mucous membrane at the peripheral edge of the intravesical projecting prostatic lobes (see inset *a*); through this opening, the finger is inserted and the enucleation is carried out laterally and posteriorly as shown in the main drawing; lateral, median, and sometimes anterior hypertrophied tissue is removed in one mass; the final procedure is to break through the urethra near the apex of the prostate; inset *b* shows the urethra ruptured just proximal to the ejaculatory ducts and the torn edge of the vesical mucosa adjacent to the cavity. (Young, "Practice of Urology.")

collections are evacuated easily, but supraprostatic suppuration requires freeing of the posterosuperior aspect of the gland.

The abscess may be evacuated into the urethra through a *median perineal urethrotomy* incision. The finger is introduced into the membranous urethra and carried into the prostatic urethra. A knife is directed along the palpating finger and an incision is made through the wall of the prostatic urethra and the intervening normal prostatic tissue into the abscess cavity. The abscess may be made to open into the urethra by fulguration of the posterior wall of the prostatic urethra through the cysto-urethroscope.

2. **Prostatectomy.**—The object of prostatectomy for nonmalignant enlargement of the gland is to remove permanently the cause of obstruction to urinary outflow, allow satis-

factory emptying of the bladder, and, at the same time, preserve vesical control. Preservation of the ejaculatory ducts is desirable, but should not jeopardize the object of the operation. The obstacle to urination usually is hypertrophy of the prostatic glandular elements. Prostatectomy for malignancy of the prostate entails radical removal of the gland. Either partial or complete enucleation can be accomplished through the suprapubic or the perineal route.

Suprapubic intracapsular adenectomy is performed by opening the bladder through the suprapubic incision (p. 449), with the patient in the Trendelenburg position. The mucous membrane which covers the upwardly projecting lobes of the prostate is incised, the index finger is introduced into the rent thus made, and enucleation of the median and lateral lobes is performed (extra-urethral method). The same object may be accomplished by plunging the finger into the prostatic urethra to the apex of the gland and enucleating the

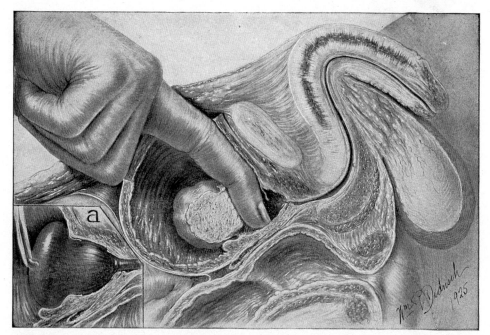

FIG. 463.—SUPRAPUBIC PROSTATECTOMY BY THE INTRA-URETHRAL METHOD OF ENUCLEATION.

The finger is introduced into the prostatic urethra as far as the apex and tears through the mucous membrane in front of the lateral lobes on each side; the finger is shown pushing the median lobe of the prostate backward into the bladder along with the lateral lobes; enucleation may be in one piece or separately, depending on how closely attached the lobes are to each other; inset *a* shows the Hagner bag drawn into the cavity to stop hemorrhage. (Young, "Practice of Urology.")

offending lobes from that position (intra-urethral method). While the prostatic masses are being removed, the bladder floor may be steadied with two fingers in the rectum pressing the prostate forward in the direction of the suprapubic wound. When the enlargement is caused by an adenoma, the true prostatic tissue is thinned out and compressed against the capsule. Enucleation is comparatively easy and the periprostatic venous plexus is not in danger.

When enlargement results from hypertrophy of the fibrous tissue components, the whole gland, including its capsule, must be enucleated from the sheath which contains the prostaticovesical venous plexus (*suprapubic extracapsular enucleation*). In extracapsular enucleation, the finger is insinuated into the interval between the capsule and the sheath. The sheath may be likened to the peel of an orange, and the capsule to the covering of the individual segments. To define the cleavage interval further, the finger is swept around one side of the prostate and then the other, the pad of the finger hugging the capsule to avoid injury to the sheath. In this procedure, some prostatic veins are torn through as they pass outward to joint the prostaticovesical plexus. The prostate remains fixed only by the distal end of the prostatic urethra which, at this stage, is torn across where it pierces the urogenital diaphragm. If the interval between the sheath and the capsule is not defined and the sheath is broken through, severe hemorrhage from the veins of the prostaticovesical plexus results.

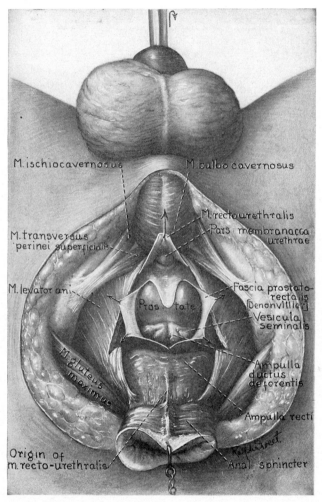

FIG. 464.—PROSTATE AND SEMINAL VESICLES EXPOSED THROUGH THE PERINEAL APPROACH.

The anobulbar raphe and the recto-urethralis muscle are divided; the interlevator space is widened by transverse incisions into the levator ani muscles; pressure exerted on the intravesical tractor exposes the structures at the neck of the bladder which are seen through the anterior layer of the prostatorectal fascia (of Denonvilliers); attention is called to the sharp anterior angulation of the ampulla of the rectum.

In partial or complete removal of the prostate, the prostatic urethra is replaced by a fibrous sac, the prostatic capsule, in adenectomy, and the prostatic sheath in extracapsular enucleation. The neck of the bladder opens into the sac above, and the urethra descends from it below. The cavity, filled at first with blood and urine, soon collapses and the walls gradually become lined by mucous membrane which grows downward from the bladder and upward from the urethra.

For *perineal prostatectomy*, the patient is placed in the exaggerated lithotomy position and a sound is passed into the bladder. A curved or inverted V-shaped incision is made anterior to the anus and deepened to the central tendinous point of the perineum, the lateral limits of which are defined by blunt dissection. The central tendon is divided in the line of the skin incision, exposing the interval between the rectum and the corpus cavernosum of the urethra (bulb). After the recto-urethral muscle is divided, the bulb can be drawn forward and the rectum backward. The prostate then is exposed in the depth of the wound. The urethra is incised at the apex of the prostate by cutting down on the sound. The incision must not injure the urethral sphincter. The sound is withdrawn and a prostatic tractor is passed into the bladder through the incision in the urethra. By use of the tractor, the prostate is levered downward and backward into the perineal wound and the offending prostatic tissue, usually the median and lateral lobes, is removed intracapsularly through one or two vertical incisions through the posterior lobe of the gland.

A central wedge, containing the prostatic urethra and the ejaculatory ducts, is preserved if possible. The perineal approach avoids an extensive wound in the base of the bladder, and dependent drainage is obtained through the urethrotomy incision. Dependent drainage is important where chronic cystitis is a complication.

IV. PELVIC VISCERA IN THE FEMALE

The female pelvis is differentiated abruptly from the male pelvis by its intrapelvic genitalia; the ovaries, uterine (fallopian) tubes, the uterus and its ligaments, the vagina, and rectum. As the uterus in its development rises upward and forward from the extraperitoneal space, it lifts the serosa into a peritoneal covering for the uterine fundus and the contents of the two broad ligaments. The broad ligaments, with the uterus, form a transverse partition dividing the pelvis into two separate cavities, the vesico-uterine and recto-uterine culdesacs.

A. BROAD LIGAMENT

1. **Definition and Anatomic Summary.**—Each broad ligament is a tentlike reflection of peritoneum, irregularly quadrilateral in outline; it contains between its layers the uterine tube, the ovary and its ligaments, the round ligament, the uterine and ovarian blood vessels, nerves, lymphatics, a variable amount of fibromuscular and fatty areolar tissue, and a part of the ureter. Each ligament has a free, mobile upper margin and a broad base. The free upper margin forms a ridge extending from the cornu of the uterus to the lateral pelvic wall, and contains the uterine tube, the suspensory ligament of the ovary, and the round ligament. The broad base brings the contents of the broad ligament into continuity with the extraperitoneal spaces of the pelvis, so that inflammatory conditions from the uterus and upper vagina can extend readily into the paravesical and prevesical extraperitoneal spaces anteriorly and into the pararectal and prerectal extraperitoneal spaces posteriorly.

That part of the ligament enclosing the uterine tube, its blood vessels, and the epoophoron (parovarium) is the *mesosalpinx*, and the area attaching itself to the ovary is the *mesovarium*. Between the ovary and uterus, a fold of broad ligament is modified into the *utero-ovarian ligament*. The *infundibulopelvic ligament* (*suspensory ligament of the ovary*) extends from the ovary to the lateral pelvic wall. The *round ligament* extends from the cornu of the uterus to the labium majus. The lower extent of the broad ligament is thickened progressively toward the pelvic floor, forming the *mesometrium*. Within the lowermost portion of the mesometrium lie the uterine vessels, the ureter, and a musculoconnective tissue band, the *transverse ligament of the cervix*. Anteriorly, the peritoneum of the droab ligament is reflected over the bladder and the adjoining areas of the lateral pelvic wall; the posterior layer of the broad ligament has much greater expanse than the anterior layer and sweeps downward and backward to the lateral and posterior pelvic walls and the rectum so that it is in contact with the intrapelvic loops of intestine. At the level of the upper part of the cervix behind, the peritoneum of the broad ligament helps to form the uterosacral folds (p. 470).

When the uterus presents its usual anterior position (p. 472), each broad ligament presents a corresponding forward inclination at its medial or uterine attachment, but is directed almost vertically at its lateral or pelvic attachment.

2. **Vessels.**—There are three **arteries** in the broad ligament—the uterine and the ovarian arteries and the artery of the round ligament. The *uterine artery* branches from the anterior division of the hypogastric (internal iliac) artery and descends in its parietal portion in contact with the lateral pelvic wall. In its parametrial portion, it turns mesially and traverses the base of the broad ligament. After crossing the ureter, it reaches the lateral surface of the uterus at a level just below the internal os. After giving off a branch which descends to supply the cervix and upper vagina, it ascends in its juxta-uterine portion along the lateral border of the uterus to which it supplies numerous branches. Just before anastomosing with the ovarian artery at the cornu of the uterus, it gives off an important branch which ascends to supply the fundus of the uterus. Its termination

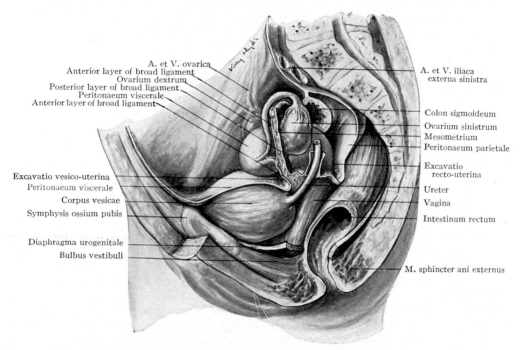

FIG. 465.—LEFT PARAMEDIAN SAGITTAL SECTION THROUGH THE FEMALE PELVIS TO SHOW THE REFLECTIONS OF THE BROAD LIGAMENT AND THE PELVIC PERITONEUM.

supplies the isthmus of the uterine tube and anastomoses with the uterine end of the ovarian artery.

The location of the artery is important surgically, especially where it crosses the ureter ("water runs under a bridge") near the level of the internal os, 1 or 2 cm. from the lateral border of the cervix. At this crossing, the ureter may be caught in ligation of the artery. In a conservative panhysterectomy, the artery is tied close to the uterus in order to avoid the ureter, but when a parametrial dissection is performed, the ureter must be isolated to avoid danger. When the more usual supravaginal hysterectomy is performed, the artery may be ligated on the lateral surface of the uterus at or above the level of the internal os without danger to the ureter.

The *ovarian artery* arises from the abdominal aorta both on the right and left sides and passes downward and laterally on the psoas major muscle to reach the brim of the pelvis. At the attached lateral portion of the broad ligament, it enters the suspensory ligament of the ovary. The ovarian artery supplies branches to the uterine tube and to the ovary, continues mesially, and anastomoses with the uterine artery within the broad ligament.   In the terminal portion of its course, the artery is tortuous and is surrounded by the pampiniform plexus of veins which forms the ovarian vein.   Because of the free anastomosis of the ovarian and uterine arteries and the danger of vessel retraction in the broad ligament, ligation of the ovarian vessels should be done by transfixing the broad ligament.

The *artery to the round ligament* arises from the inferior epigastric artery where the round ligament crosses that vessel.

The **veins** form plexuses mainly about the uterine and ovarian arteries.   Deep in the broad ligament, the network of veins which surrounds the base of the bladder, vagina, and rectum anastomoses with the uterine and ovarian plexuses.   Therefore, infection in the broad ligament veins soon may become generalized throughout the pelvis (puerperal sepsis) and may involve the lymphatics.   The *uterine veins* arise in the cavernous venous spaces in the uterine wall and leave the lateral aspect of the organ mainly at the level of the cervix where they form a plexus of thin-walled vessels surrounding the ureter.   The uterine veins anastomose with those of the vagina and form the *uterovaginal plexus*.   The trunks from this plexus converge into the internal iliac vein or into one of its large tributaries.   The

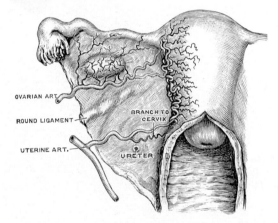

OVARIAN ART.

ROUND LIGAMENT

UTERINE ART.

BRANCH TO CERVIX

URETER

FIG. 466.—BLOOD SUPPLY OF THE UTERUS AND VAGINA.   (Sutton and Giles.)

ovarian (pampiniform) venous plexus empties into the inferior vena cava on the right and into the renal vein on the left.   The ovarian veins frequently are varicose (*pelvic varicocele*).

The **lymphatics** of the broad ligaments form rich plexuses for the uterus, tubes, and ovaries and anastomose with the lymphatics of the neighboring structures.   The *uterine lymphatics* are both superficial and deep.   The superficial lymphatics run transversely to the external iliac glands, posterolaterally to the hypogastric glands, and posteriorly to the nodes on the common iliac vessels.   Most of the deep lymphatics from the fundus and body of the uterus run laterally in the broad ligaments and are continued upward with the ovarian vessels to the lateral and pre-aortic lymph glands.   A few channels run to the external iliac glands and the superficial subinguinal nodes.   The *ovarian lymphatics* accompany the ovarian vessels in the suspensory (infundibulopelvic) ligament and terminate in the lumbar lymphatics.

The *pelvic lymphatics* play an important part in the spread and localization of pelvic infection.   Most of the lymphatic vessels arise in the layers of the uterus, particularly in the musculosa.   An upper group drains the body of the uterus, the tubes and ovaries.   These lymphatics follow the ovarian vessels and enter the lumbar lymph nodes.   The middle group receives the lymphatics of the round ligament which traverse the inguinal canal to empty into the lymph glands of the groin.   The inferior group is by far the most important surgically as it drains most of the body of the uterus, the cervix, and the vaginal vault. The vessels of the inferior group course with the uterine vessels in the base of the broad ligament in the midst of the extraperitoneal cellular tissue, and terminate in the uppermost group of the external iliac nodes. These lymphatics are involved early in carcinoma of the cervix.

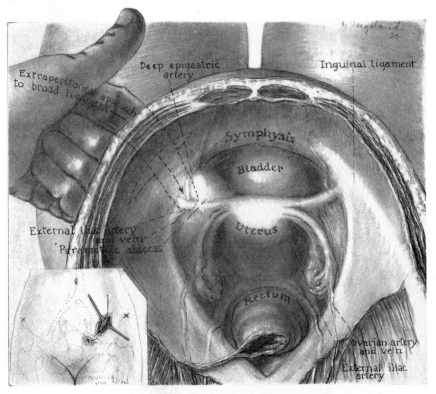

FIG. 467.—EXTRAPERITONEAL INGUINAL APPROACH TO BROAD LIGAMENT CELLULITIS. (M. Douglas after Cullen.)

SURGICAL CONSIDERATIONS

1 Broad Ligament Cellulitis.—The normal broad ligament is too soft to be felt in vaginal and rectal examination. When the broad ligament is infected, it becomes brawny and indurated. Circumscribed abscesses may be located and differentiated from generalized thickness in the ligament resulting from diffuse cellulitis. The cellular tissue within the ligament is exposed both to trauma and to infection which may bring about a localized or diffuse cellulitis.

In the presence of infection, *traumatic cellulitis* may occur from pressure or tears during labor, or from use of a badly fitting pessary which injures the cellular tissue about the vaginal fornices (paracolpium). Thrombosis of the veins sometimes occurs, and the cellular tissue becomes edematous and swollen.

Septic cellulitis usually is caused by infection complicating labor or abortion, and sometimes is produced by intra-uterine instrumentation or operation. Infected wounds following vaginal operations may give rise to septic cellulitis. In labor or abortion, there often are lacerations extending more or less deeply into the cervix or through it into the parametrium. These lacerations afford an entrance for infective organisms which gain access to the cellular tissue directly or by way of the lymphatics or veins.

An exudate in the parametrial tissue either undergoes resolution and gradually becomes absorbed, or localizes, softens, and forms an abscess. The more virulent infections may exhibit no local manifestations but may pass through the intermediate lymphatics of the broad ligament and enter the general circulation. Pus from an abscess, if not released by

30

incision, may burrow along the wall of the vagina, bulge into the vaginal fornices, and rupture into the vagina or rectum.   The abscess may be discharged into the bladder, into an adherent loop of intestine, or into the pelvic cavity.   A large para-uterine abscess may elevate the peritoneum, extend forward, and present behind the symphysis.   It may burrow laterally and be accessible to evacuation by extraperitoneal inguinal incision.   This method of evacuation may be employed before a broad ligament abscess points in the inguinal region.   Rarely, infection may diffuse outside the lateral pelvic peritoneum to present externally in the loin.   Pus has been known to burrow through the pelvic floor and localize in the ischiorectal fossa.

Extraperitoneal pelvic cellulitis must be differentiated from intraperitoneal pelvic peritonitis.   The palpable mass in extraperitoneal pelvic cellulitis is continuous with, and fixed to, the pelvic wall.   In intraperitoneal pelvic peritonitis, the mass usually occupies a position in the recto-uterine culdesac.

B. UTERUS

The uterus is the pivotal organ of the female genitalia.   It occupies an intermediate position between the bladder, rectum, and broad ligaments.   The uterus and vagina represent those parts of the müllerian ducts which fuse at an early period in fetal life.   The uterine tubes represent the upper portions of the müllerian ducts which do not fuse.   The

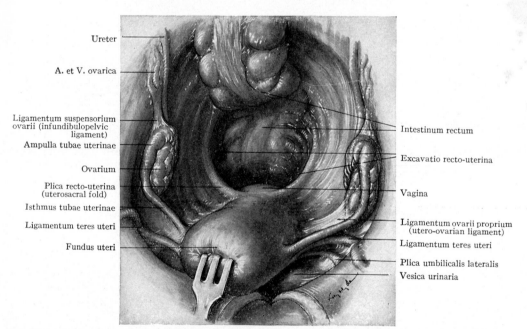

Fig. 468.—Contents of the Female Pelvis with the Bladder Empty and the Uterus Drawn Anteriorly.

wall of the uterus is very thick and muscular and that of the vagina is comparatively thin. The small cavity of the uterus communicates through the external os with the cavity of the vagina.

1. **Shape, Division, and Size.**—The uterus is a pear-shaped organ, flattened anteroposteriorly.   Its truncated inferior extremity, just below its middle portion, presents a circular constriction, the *isthmus*, which divides the organ into a larger, rounded upper part, the *body*, and a smaller, almost cylindrical lower part, the *cervix*.   Internally, the boundary line of the isthmus is defined by a constriction of the upper part of the cervical canal which is known as the *internal os*.   In nulliparae, the neck of the uterus is about

equidistant from the *fundus*, or upper portion of the body, and the orifice of the cervix; in multiparae, the body is longer and more globoid. The opening of the cervical canal into the vagina is circular in the virgin, but in multiparae it is flattened into a transverse opening with somewhat everted anteroposterior lips.

The cervix, like a cylindrical plug, is invaginated into the vaginal vault. The inferior extremity of the cervix presents itself free within the vaginal canal and rests in contact with

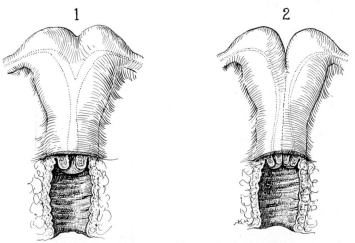

Fig. 469.—Malformations of the Uterus.
1, Arched bicornuate uterus; 2, bicornuate bicervical uterus.

its posterior wall. The area of the cervix above the attachment of the vagina is the *supro-vaginal segment;* that below it is the *vaginal segment.*

The uterus is about 7.5 cm. long and 5 cm. broad in its widest portion. The total length of the uterine cavity from the external orifice to the fundus is about 6.25 cm. The length of the cervical portion is 2.5 cm.

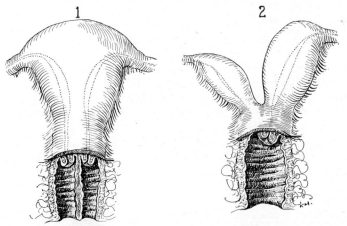

Fig. 470.—Malformations of the Uterus.
1, Biseptate uterus with duplex vagina; 2, double uterus; one side is rudimentary and the other functions.

2. **Development and Malformations.**—Malformations of the uterus result from anomalies in the development of the müllerian ducts. In the embryo, each of the two ducts is a thick-walled tube possessing an independent cavity. In the course of development, each duct is divided into a uterine tube, uterus, and vagina; later, the inferior extremities of the ducts become apposed and fuse in the median line. Fusion takes place over the parts

which form the uterus and vagina.   The upper or tubal parts retain their independence indefinitely as the two uterine tubes.   The fused uterus and vagina at first are partitioned by a midsagittal septum which later disappears and the double uterine and vaginal canals become a single cavity.

The absorption of the median partition occurs from the vulva upward to the fundus of the uterus.   According to the degree of septum absorption, there may be found: a partitioned vagina with a partitioned uterus; a completely developed single-cavity vagina and a partitioned uterus; or a single vagina and a single uterus.   An arrest in the development of the müllerian ducts explains the actual *absence of the uterus and vagina*.   Rarely, the ducts remain separate throughout their length and form two entirely *separate uteri and vaginae*.   Each of these cavities has the function of the normal organ.   The body of the uterus may be cleft completely, the *bicornuate uterus*, and the cervix be single or divided. The duplexity of the uterus may be partial and be limited to a branching fundus with a well-formed partition in the body and cervix.   The only evidence of duplexity may lie within the uterus where a more or less definite septum divides the uterine cavity (*uterus septus*).   If one component of a müllerian duct fails to keep pace with the other in development, all varieties of asymmetry result, from suppression of a tube in a bicornuate uterus to simple unilateral deviation of the fundus.   A localized stenosis or imperforation at any point in the uterine or vaginal canal is a serious developmental accident caused by incomplete resorption or defective cavity formation in the primitive müllerian duct.   Stenosis may cause retention of menses proximal to the obstruction and form a tumor of very considerable size, known as a *hematocolpos*, *hematocolpometra*, or *hematometra*, according to whether the tumor occupies the vagina, the vagina and uterus, or the uterus alone.

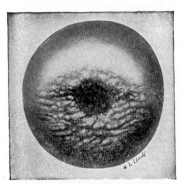

FIG. 471.—EROSION OF THE EXTERNAL ORIFICE OF THE UTERUS WITH PAPILLARY HYPERTROPHY. (Montgomery in "Keen's Surgery.")

3. **Cervix.**—The cervix is divided into supravaginal and vaginal portions.   The *supravaginal division* is covered by peritoneum on its posterior aspect only.   Anteriorly, the supravaginal portion is related to the bladder, from which it is separated by cellular tissue.   The *vaginal division* normally projects downward and backward into the posterosuperior part of the vaginal vault, and receives a squamous epithelial covering similar to that lining the vagina.

The cervix is traversed by the *cervical canal*, which communicates with the cavity of the uterus by the internal orifice and with the vagina by the external orifice.   The external orifice in nulliparae is a circular depression which is directed against the posterior vaginal wall.   In multiparae, the orifice is an irregularly transverse slit which usually will admit the tip of the finger.

4. **Supports of the Uterus.**—The mobility of the uterus has definite physiologic limits imposed upon it by various means of fixation: the peritoneum covering it, the ligaments holding it to the walls of the pelvis, the vessels reaching and leaving it, and the pelvic floor.

The *peritoneum* is reflected from the bladder over the anterior surface of the uterus at the level of the isthmus.   It covers the anterior and posterior surfaces of the uterus, the fundus, the supravaginal portion of the cervix posteriorly, and a little of the posterior culdesac of the vagina before it is reflected over the anterior surface of the rectum.   The peritoneum is attached loosely to the cervix and fundus.   The fixation rôle of the peritoneum under normal conditions is not as important as that in pathologic conditions where adhesions are formed between the serosa covering the uterus and the adjoining peritoneum. Adhesions between the posterior surface of the uterus and the recto-uterine pouch may be such as to fix the fundus of the organ deep in the pelvis.   When pregnancy occurs in a uterus fixed in this manner, abortion may take place early in gestation.

The tendency of serous surfaces to adhere is utilized to fix and maintain the organ in a correct position. To correct retroversion and descensus of the uterus, the anterior surface of the fundus may be sutured into the anterior abdominal wall by the procedure termed "abdominal hysteropexy." This abdominal fixation should not be done without assurance that no further pregnancy can occur.

The broad, round, and uterosacral ligaments are powerful suspensory mechanisms for the uterus. The *broad ligaments* (p. 462) form a frontal partition across the true pelvis and are the most efficient uterine supports. The broad ligaments allow anteroposterior movement of the uterus, but oppose lateral movement. One broad ligament may be longer than the other and permit the uterus to deviate laterally.

The *round ligaments* are two fibromuscular cords situated between the layers of the broad ligaments. Each round ligament begins at the lateral angle of the uterus, anterior

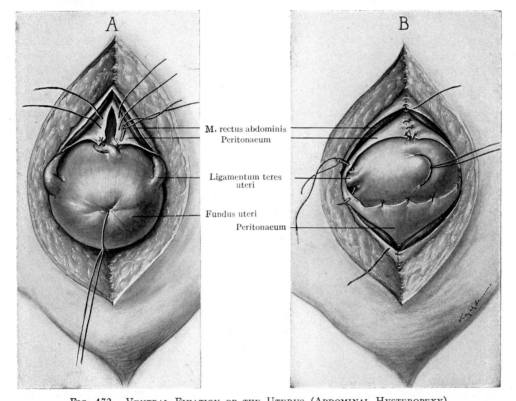

M. rectus abdominis
Peritonaeum

Ligamentum teres
uteri

Fundus uteri
Peritonaeum

FIG. 472.—VENTRAL FIXATION OF THE UTERUS (ABDOMINAL HYSTEROPEXY).

In A, the parietal peritoneum is sutured into the fundus of the uterus; in B, the round ligaments are sutured to the parietal peritoneum: the anterior wall is sutured in layers across the embedded uterine fundus.

to the attachment of the uterine tubes. From this point, the ligament passes forward, upward, and laterally, within a peritoneal duplication of the broad ligament, to the abdominal inguinal ring. It passes through the inguinal canal and inserts into the labium majus. In the fetus, a tubular process of peritoneum, the *canal of Nuck*, accompanies the round ligament in its course to the labium majus. The canal generally is obliterated in the adult, but sometimes remains pervious. The canal of Nuck is analogous to the vaginal process of peritoneum in the male (p. 292), and furnishes the serosal sac of a congenital indirect hernia in the female. The round ligaments aid in maintaining the uterus in its anterior position. Shortening of the ligaments brings the fundus of the uterus nearer the anterior abdominal wall (uterine suspension).

The reflection of peritoneum from the posterior vaginal fornix to the rectum forms the depth of the recto-uterine pouch. Part of the lateral boundaries of the pouch are crescentic folds of peritoneum (*uterosacral ligaments*), which pass backward from the cervix at the level of the isthmus around the rectum to the first sacral vertebra. These ligaments contain fibrous tissue and nonstriped muscle fibers. They partially divide the recto-uterine culdesac into upper and lower divisions, are stationary supports to the uterus, and oppose displacement of the cervix toward the symphysis. The uterine attachment of these ligaments marks the most fixed part of the uterus, about which torsion, flexion, and version take place.

The *fibrous expansions surrounding the uterine vessels* in the extraperitoneal space of the pelvis and the *transverse ligament of the cervix* (p. 462) aid in the support of the uterus. The connection between the uterus and bladder contributes support to the uterus, but

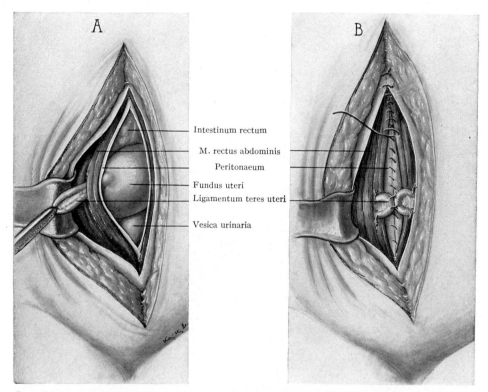

Intestinum rectum

M. rectus abdominis

Peritonaeum

Fundus uteri

Ligamentum teres uteri

Vesica urinaria

FIG. 473.—SUSPENSION OF THE UTERUS BY ANTERIOR FIXATION OF THE ROUND LIGAMENTS.
In A, the right round ligament is drawn through the peritoneum and rectus muscle; in B, both round ligaments are sutured in front of the rectus muscle; the anterior rectus sheath is closed over the round ligaments.

the *pelvic floor*, although it is not adherent to the uterus at any point, is its most powerful supporting mechanism. Through the intermedium of the vagina, the neck of the uterus lies on the pelvic floor. Weakening of the floor by the perineal tears of parturition contributes to prolapse of the uterus. Uterine prolapse is treated by tightening the suspending structures (uterine suspension) and supporting the pelvic floor (perineorrhaphy).

5. **Relations of the Uterus.**—The *anterior* or *vesical surface* of the uterus lies posterior to the bladder but is separated from it by the uterovesical pouch of peritoneum. The depth of the culdesac depends partly upon the fulness of the bladder. In nulliparae, the reflection of peritoneum scarcely reaches to the isthmus, but in multiparae it may extend to the anterior fornix of the vagina. Below the level of the peritoneal reflection, a layer of connective tissue separates the uterus from the bladder for a vertical distance of about 2 cm. This layer is of a fairly loose texture in the median line, but increases in density

as it approaches the sides of the cervix where it is continuous with the tissue of the broad
ligament surrounding the ureter and the uterine blood vessels (p. 463).   It is unusual to
find a pathologic effusion or serious adhesions in this pouch.   When the bladder is empty
and the uterus is retroverted, loops of intestine lie between the bladder and the uterus.   In
marked anteversion and anteflexion, the uterus rests upon the bladder.

The *posterior* or *intestinal aspect* of the body of the uterus and the supravaginal portion
of the cervix are overlain by the sigmoid colon and coils of small intestine.   In uterine
retroversion and retroflexion, the relations between the uterus and rectum are extensive.

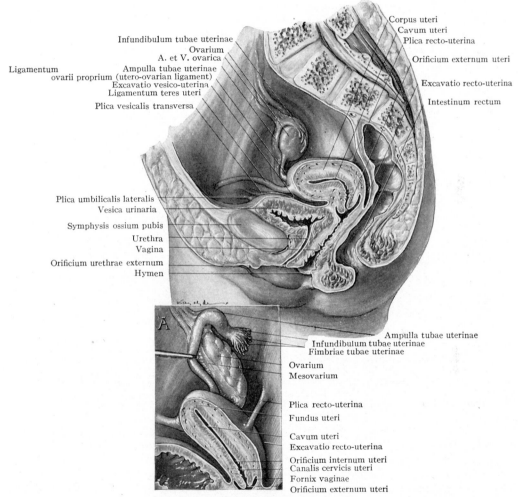

FIG. 474.—MIDSAGITTAL SECTION THROUGH THE FEMALE PELVIS TO SHOW THE MECHANISM OF THE SUP-
PORT OF THE UTERUS.
The inset, A, shows the suspending mechanism furnished by the round ligament and the recto-uterine fold
(uterosacral ligament).

The relations of the *supravaginal segment of the cervix* are important in operations for
the removal of the uterus (hysterectomy).   Anteriorly this segment is in contact with
the base of the bladder through a thin and readily separable layer of connective tissue.
Injury to this septum in childbirth may result in vesicocervical fistula, which is difficult
to repair.   Posteriorly, the segment is in relation to the rectum through the recto-uterine
culdesac.   Its lateral margins are related to the uterine arteries, the venous plexuses
accompanying them, and the terminal portion of the ureter.

6. Positions of the Uterus.—The uterus has no fixed position and its axis has no fixed direction. It is a movable pelvic organ in equilibrium between the rectum and bladder and suspended between the lateral pelvic walls by its broad ligaments. Being interposed between these elastic structures, the uterus responds to impulses communicated to it from any direction. Pressure by a finger in the vagina displaces the uterus upward in the direction of the abdominal cavity. Distention of the intestines or manual pressure from above pushes it toward the perineum. The uterus is susceptible at all times to the varying distention of the bladder. A full rectum or a mass of small bowel in the uterine culdesac may push the uterus forward into anteversion. The simultaneous filling of the rectum and bladder pushes the uterus upward. The organ can be moved considerably in bimanual vaginal examination without causing any distress. The entire uterus may be raised until its fundus contacts the anterior abdominal wall. It may be drawn downward until the external os lies just within the vaginal introitus, and may be moved freely from side to side or backward into the hollow of the sacrum. Inclination of the uterus to the side is known as *right* or *left lateral deviation*.

Right and left displacements may be caused by traction or pressure applied to the uterus by a tumor lying lateral to it. An ovarian cyst in the pelvis may push the body

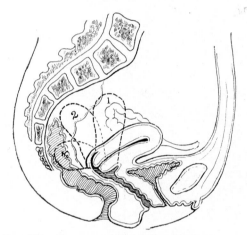 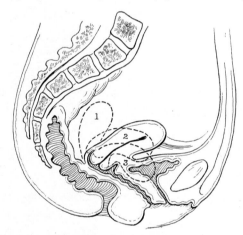

Fig. 475.—Diagram of Uterine Displacements.
The uterus in the solid black outline is in the normal position of anteversion; 1, retroversion; 2, moderate retroflexion; 3, marked retroflexion. (Moorhead, "Traumatic Surgery.")

Fig. 476.—Diagram of Uterine Displacements.
The uterus in the solid black outline is in the normal position of anteversion; 1, retroversion; 2, moderate anteflexion; 3, marked anteflexion. (Moorhead, "Traumatic Surgery.")

of the uterus to the opposite side, while one which has extended into the abdomen may pull the uterus over to the side on which the growth originated.

The uterus, considered as a whole, may be inclined forward (*anteversion*) or backward (*retroversion*). Any fixed displacement which disturbs the function of the uterus is pathologic. A common cause of fixation is inflammation of the tubes and ovaries (pelvic inflammatory disease).

The difference in direction between the axes of the body and cervix of the uterus is such that angulation (flexion) is present between these two segments. The uterus is in *anteflexion, retroflexion,* or *lateral flexion* respectively as the angle between the body and cervix opens forward, backward, or laterally. Slight anteflexion is the usual position assumed by the uterus.

Too great freedom of movement of the uterus is as abnormal a condition as is marked limitation of movement. The supporting structures may be so lax that the uterus lies upon the pelvic floor instead of maintaining a position of equilibrium within the pelvic cavity. This displacement is known as *descensus*. It may be a stage in descent which progresses to the appearance of the cervix at the vaginal outlet, a condition known as *partial*

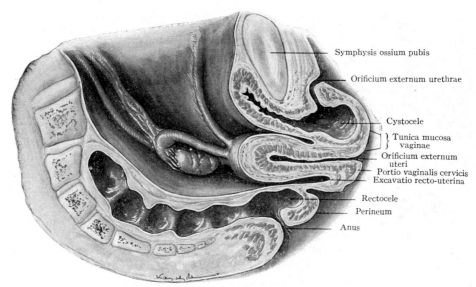

FIG. 477.—PARTIAL PROLAPSE OF THE UTERUS.
A cystocele and a rectocele accompany the prolapse; the cervix projects through the vulva.

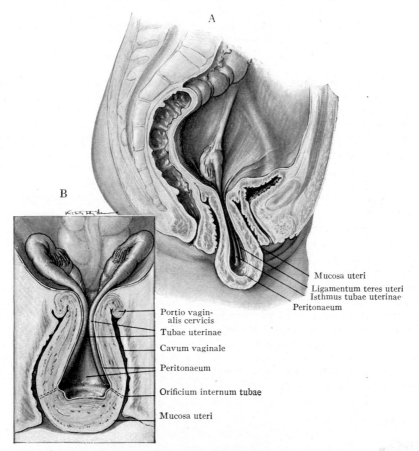

FIG. 478.—INVERSION OF THE UTERUS.
A, Partial extravaginal inversion; B, intravaginal inversion.

prolapse; or progresses to complete extrusion of the uterus, a condition known as *complete prolapse.* In the latter condition, the protrusion forms a large mass between the thighs, the apex of which is formed by the external os and the outer investment of which is formed by the everted lining of the vagina. Descensus and the varying degrees of uterine pro- lapse usually are found in parous women who have suffered injury to the pelvic floor. The uterus, in the course of its descent, draws the bladder with it and causes the anterior vaginal wall to protrude at or through the vulva (*cystocele*). As this is taking place, the posterior vaginal wall descends, but because of its lax connection with the rectum, it does not as readily draw the rectum down with it (*rectocele*).

7. Inversion of the Uterus.—Inversion of the uterus is an abnormal condition in which the organ is turned partially or completely inside out. The uterine mucosa becomes the covering of the inverted organ. In partial or *intra-uterine inversion*, part of the uterus is invaginated into the uterine cavity without presenting through the cervix. In *intra- vaginal inversion*, part or all of the body of the uterus is evaginated through the external os into the vaginal canal. In *extravaginal inversion*, the evaginated uterus is partially or com- pletely outside the vagina, and requires an evagination of the vagina.

The displacement usually results from a relaxed condition of the uterine walls and may be produced by traction on the cord in ill-advised attempts at delivery of the placenta. In the nonpuerperal variety of inversion, a submucous fibroid of the sessile type fills the cavity of the uterus until the cervix is distended partially. Contractile efforts to expel the growth as a foreign body lead to further dilatation of the cervix and dragging downward of the fundus by the weight and attachment of the tumor. The expulsive efforts and downward traction continue until the inversion or evagination becomes complete.

SURGICAL CONSIDERATIONS

1. Vaginal Examination of the Uterus and Adnexa.—*Examination* of the *external genitalia* consists in noting the orifices of Bartholin's glands and examining any swellings or other evidences of infection. The condition of the hymen is noted, whether intact, dilated, or torn. A puffy, red condition about the urethral orifice is an evidence of inflam- mation (p. 528), and an attempt is made to express pus from Skene's gland by milking down the urethra through the anterior vaginal wall against the pubic arch. *Simple vaginal examination* may be done preliminary to bimanual examination. The labia majora are separated to expose the labia minora. The strength of the muscles surrounding the vaginal outlet is determined by making pressure against the posterior vaginal wall in the presence of voluntary contraction of the muscles of the perineum. The cervix is felt as a knoblike prominence in the vault of the vagina. Its axis points backward toward the sacrum or forward toward the symphysis, according to the position of the uterus. A lacerated cervix, or one studded and infiltrated with follicles, or indurated with carcinoma, can be distin- guished readily from the normal smooth cervix. If the uterus is in slight anteposition, the body cannot be felt with one hand alone; if acutely flexed, it can be felt as a resisting mass by tapping the anterior vaginal wall anterior to the cervix.

Bimanual examination consists in palpating the abdominal wall above the symphysis with one hand and palpating through the vagina with the other. The bladder should be empty at the time of examination. Pressure is made upon the abdomen to prevent upward displacement of the uterus and adnexa by the fingers in the vagina.

Despite the assistance given by the external hand, bimanual examination often would afford insufficient information if the vaginal examination were limited to the length of the index and middle fingers. A considerable additional range of exploration may be gained by forced invagination of the pelvic floor.

Bimanual palpation anterior and posterior to the cervix determines whether the body of the uterus lies in anteposition or retroposition. When the fundus lies markedly anterior to the cervix, the vaginal finger palpates the body of the uterus through the anterior vaginal wall and transmits each movement to the abdominal hand. The ovary usually may be held and palpated by carrying the vaginal fingers far up into the lateral fornix of the vagina while deep pressure is made by the abdominal hand over the corresponding semilunar line. The ovary is manipulated between the fingers until its surfaces and free border are ex-

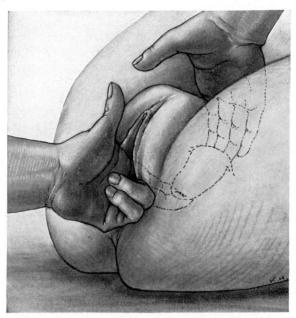

FIG. 479.—METHOD OF BIMANUAL PALPATION OF THE UTERUS AND ADNEXA.

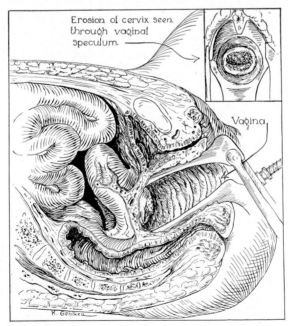

FIG. 480.—SPECULUM EXAMINATION OF THE CERVIX.

amined thoroughly. The ovary normally is a freely movable firm body about the size of a large almond. Normally, the tubes cannot be felt, but when they are thickened by disease, their uterine ends can be rolled between the fingers and can be traced laterally toward the pelvic walls.

When there is obscure or deep-seated pelvic disease, bimanual vaginal examination combined with rectal examination (*abdominovaginorectal examination*) frequently is of great diagnostic value.

Examination under general anesthesia is of the utmost importance n obscure intrapelvic disease. Ether or spinal anesthesia eliminates voluntary muscle resistance, completely relaxes the abdominal musculature, and prevents muscle resistance when tender areas are palpated. The examination can be conducted with a thoroughness impossible otherwise; the uterus may be pressed down, adhesions pulled upon, the perineum invaginated deeply, and the inflamed ovaries and tubes examined satisfactorily. In indefinite pelvic conditions, this examination should precede exploratory laparotomy.

2. **Hysterectomy.**—Hysterectomy or removal of the uterus may be partial or complete. Partial hysterectomy may be done at any level above the vagina and is either

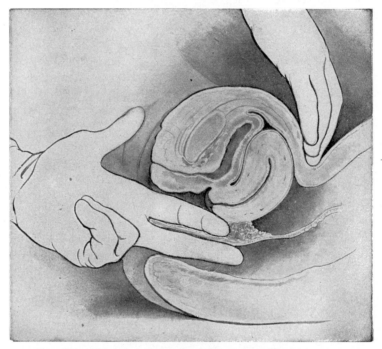

FIG. 481.—BIMANUAL ABDOMINOVAGINORECTAL EXAMINATION.

This method of examination is a useful diagnostic procedure in the identification of deep-seated pelvic disease. (Curtis, "Textbook of Gynecology.")

supravaginal or supracervical. Removal of the fundus alone is defundation of the uterus. Complete removal of the uterus is panhysterectomy.

In *partial* or *supravaginal abdominal hysterectomy*, the segment removed includes the body of the organ and that part of the cervix above the line of vaginal attachment. After the abdomen is opened by a midline incision between the umbilicus and symphysis, the uterus is pulled upward. Both round ligaments are ligated doubly at their uterine extremities and are cut across. This procedure allows the layers of the broad ligament to be separated. A clamp is passed readily through the posterior layer of the broad ligament just below the ovarian vessels. That portion of the broad ligament containing the ovarian vessels is ligated doubly and divided. The ligation controls the uterine anastomoses with the ovarian artery. The dissection of the broad ligament from the lateral surface of the uterus may be carried down to the level of the internal os without danger from hemorrhage. If the tubes and ovaries are to be removed, the ovarian vessels are ligated and divided by ligating the suspensory ligament of the ovary (infundibulopelvic ligament).

The reflection of peritoneum from the bladder to the anterior surface of the uterus then is cut transversely as far up on the uterus as possible and the bladder is separated

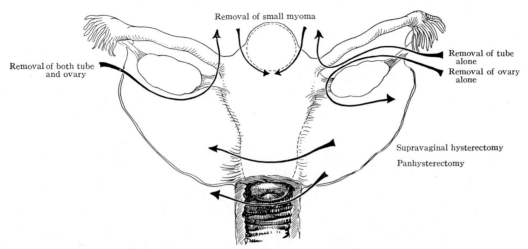

Removal of small myoma

Removal of both tube and ovary

Removal of tube alone

Removal of ovary alone

Supravaginal hysterectomy

Panhysterectomy

FIG. 482.—DIAGRAM OF THE COMMONER OPERATIONS ON THE UTERUS AND ADNEXA.

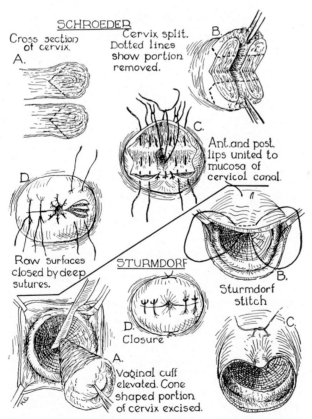

SCHROEDER

Cross section of cervix. A.

Cervix split. Dotted lines show portion removed.

B.

C.

Ant. and post. lips united to mucosa of cervical canal.

D.

Raw surfaces closed by deep sutures.

STURMDORF

D. Closure

B. Sturmdorf stitch

C.

A. Vaginal cuff elevated. Cone shaped portion of cervix excised.

FIG. 483.—TYPES OF CERVICAL REPAIR.

The sketches of the Curtis-Schroeder and Sturmdorf technics are taken from p. 51 of "Operative Procedure," published by Johnson and Johnson.

from the anterior surface of the cervix by blunt dissection. The uterine artery and vein are caught in suture ligatures which transfix a small portion of cervical tissue   Ligation of the uterine vessels at the cervix eliminates the danger of including the ureter. The cervix is divided by two incisions sloping from the anterior and posterior aspects downward to the cervical canal. The two remaining flaps of the cervix are sutured to close the cervical canal. With a purse-string suture, the round ligament, the anterior and posterior layers of the broad ligament, and the proximal extremity of the tube, if it remains, are sutured on each side to the cervical stump. These structures support the cervix and the vaginal vault. The peritoneum detached from the anterior surface of the uterus is drawn back over the uterine stump and sutured to the peritoneum of the recto-uterine pouch. If the tube and ovary are removed, the stump of the suspensory ligament of the ovary is inverted and the peritoneal edges of the broad ligament are sutured.

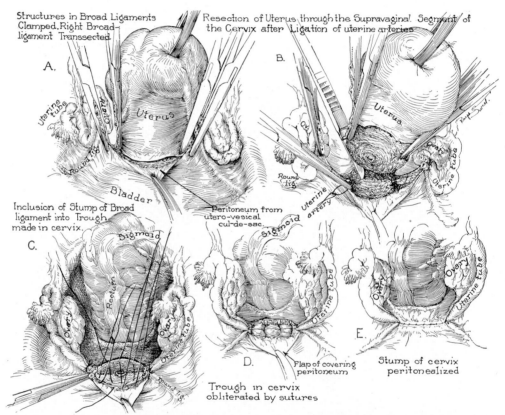

FIG. 484.—SUPRAVAGINAL HYSTERECTOMY.

Uterine tumors which extend into the broad ligament (intraligamentary) may prevent ready dissection downward through the broad ligament. It is advisable to dissect downward on the less involved side, cut across the cervix, and approach the intraligamentary tumor from beneath. Usually, the tumor can be removed without difficulty when this approach is possible. If downward dissection is not possible through either broad ligament, the body and part of the cervix of the uterus are bisected by a sagittal incision. The incision is carried laterally to either side beneath the tmors and dissection is continued from below upward.

Partial hysterectomy has several advantages. The cervix which remains leaves a normal vaginal tract and supports the vaginal vault. The operation may be done even though the cervical glands are infected, as they may be cauterized in the preliminary stage of the abdominal operation. Subsequent infection in them also may be controlled by cauterization. In young women, a high amputation of the body of the uterus, which leaves a small amount of endometrium, is desirable from the endocrine aspect.

Complete abdominal hysterectomy (panhysterectomy) is the removal of the entire uterus The operation, as far as the ligation of the uterine vessels, is the same as that outlined for supravaginal hysterectomy. In conservative panhysterectomy, the uterine vessels are ligated independently of the cervix. The downward dissection along the cervix is continued until the fornices of the vagina are opened laterally, posteriorly, and anteriorly and the entire uterus is removed. There is no danger to the ureter. The bleeding from the small vaginal vessels is controlled by suture. In a radical panhysterectomy, the uterus first must be freed from its bed in order that dissection of the glands in the base of the broad ligament can be performed without danger to the ureter. The vault of the vagina then is closed and peritonealized.

Vaginal hysterectomy, or removal of the uterus through the vaginal canal, may be performed when the vaginal outlet is relaxed sufficiently to afford an approach by the vaginal route. Dense adhesions or large tumors do not allow this approach. The operation permits rapid repair of the vaginal outlet, and the chief indication for its use is uterine prolapse in elderly women.

With the patient in the lithotomy position, a speculum is introduced into the vagina to retract the posterior vaginal wall. The cervix is grasped and brought down to the vulva and the vaginal mucous membrane surrounding the cervix is divided. The incision is continued forward on the anterior vaginal wall to the urethra; the connections between the bladder and uterus are separated by blunt dissection to the point where the peritoneum is reflected from the bladder to the uterus. The peritoneum of the vesico-uterine cul-desac is divided as far as the broad ligaments. An incision is made through the posterior vaginal wall into the recto-uterine pouch, and extended laterally to the posterior layer of the broad ligament.

Either the ovarian or the uterine vessels may be divided next. If the anterior vaginal wall is relaxed, the fundus of the uterus can be drawn downward easily, affording ready access to the ovarian vessels. The vessels, round ligament, uterine tube, and upper margin of the broad ligament are clamped, divided, and transfixed. The broad ligament is dissected from the lateral margin of the uterus. The uterine vessels then are clamped, divided, and transfixed close to the uterus in the base of the broad ligament and the uterus is removed. The uterine and ovarian vessels of one side may be ligated before ligating those of the opposite side.

If the uterine vessels are to be divided first, two clamps are placed on the base of each broad ligament close to the uterus. The tissue between the clamps is transfixed and ligated, and the upward dissection between clamps is continued until the upper border of the broad ligament, the round ligament, uterine tube, and ovarian vessels are transfixed and ligated.

C. UTERINE TUBES

1. **Definition and Divisions.**—The uterine tube is a duct about 12 cm. long. It opens into the lateral and uppermost part of the uterine cavity by a minute orifice, the *uterine ostium*, and extends laterally in the free upper margin of the broad ligament toward the pelvic wall where it is related closely to the medial surface of the ovary (p. 484). By its lateral or free extremity, it communicates with the general peritoneal cavity through the *abdominal ostium.*

That part of the tube embedded in the uterine wall is the *pars uterina.* Lateral to it, in the portion termed the *isthmus*, the tube has well-differentiated longitudinal and circular muscle coats and a very small lumen. Beyond the isthmus, the tube widens somewhat and, for the remainder of its extent, is known as the *ampulla*. In this segment, the muscle coat is less developed but the mucosa is very much thicker. The outer extremity of the ampulla widens into the *intundibulum*, which is a funnel-like expansion of the tube, the walls of which are formed by numerous narrow processes, the *fimbriae*. In the pit of the infundibulum, the uterine tube communicates with the peritoneal cavity by the abdominal ostium, and the peritoneal endothelium merges into the ciliated epithelium which lines the tube.

The tube normally courses laterally from the lateral angle of the uterus almost horizontally for a short distance, and, at the level of the junction between the isthmus and ampulla, turns abruptly upward opposite the lower or uterine pole of the ovary. It ascends almost vertically along the medial edge of the ovary in close relationship to its anterior attached border and the mesovarium. After reaching the upper pole of the ovary, it arches backward over it. The tube descends along the upper part of the posterior margin of the ovary and the adjoining portion of its medial surface with which the fimbriae are in contact. One fimbria, longer than the others, usually is attached to the upper pole of the ovary and serves to direct the contents of the ruptured follicle into the lumen of the tube. The curves characterizing the ampullary portion are an obstacle to free evacuation of inflammatory collections in the tube and favor the development of a cystic condition, *hydrosalpinx*, or an encysted purulent collection, *pyosalpinx*. The lining of the tube has longitudinal folds which render drainage of a tubal infection difficult and explain partly the recurrences which so frequently follow the initial attack of salpingitis.

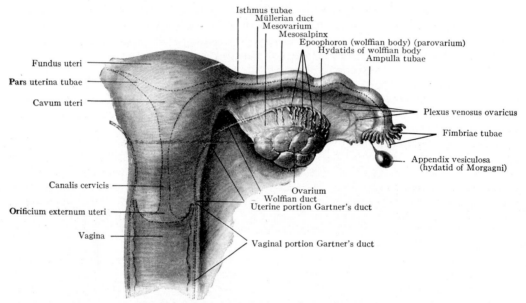

FIG. 485.—RELATIONS OF THE MÜLLERIAN, WOLFFIAN, AND GARTNER'S DUCTS TO THE UTERUS AND ADNEXA
Gartner's duct is the inferior continuation of the wolffian duct. (After Cullen.)

2. Structure.—In addition to an outer or serous investment from the broad ligament, the uterine tube is surrounded by a stratum of subserous connective tissue. Beneath the connective tissue layer is the muscle coat, continuous with that of the uterus. The mucosa lining the tube is peculiar in that it is arranged in folds directed longitudinally. Each of the longer folds is provided with duplications of mucosa, especially in the ampulla where they encroach on the lumen of the tube, causing an arborescent appearance. At the lateral extremity of the tube, the mucosa lines the inner surface of the fimbriae and ends abruptly at the free margins where it meets with and merges into the peritoneum.

The muscle layers of the tube are sufficiently resistant to withstand considerable dilation from contained fluids. Tubal rupture, which may complicate tubal pregnancy, is not caused alone by pressure necrosis in the tube, but also by alterations in its wall caused by placental attachment. In salpingitis, the inflammatory lesion may remain localized in the mucosa as an endosalpingitis. If infection extends to the outer layer of the tube, the tube atrophies.

The arteries supplying the tube are the tubal branches of the uterine and ovarian trunks (p. 463).

3. **Attachments and Relations of the Tube.**—The tube, from its uterine attachment to its fimbriated extremity, is enveloped by the *mesosalpinx*, a superior fold of the broad ligament. The isthmus of the tube has a short mesosalpinx and moves with the uterus, while the ampulla and infundibulum, with a comparatively long mesosalpinx, are nearly as mobile as the ovary. The inflammatory process in salpingitis causes the tube to become adherent to the adjoining structures.

The tube is related to the intestinal coils in the pelvis and to the bladder and rectum. The relation of an inflamed tube to the bladder explains the painful urination (dysuria) and urinary frequency so often occurring in pelvic inflammatory disease. The dense adhesions of the tube to surrounding structures explain the spontaneous evacuation of tubal abscesses into the intestinal loops, bladder, and vagina, and particularly into the rectum. At operation, adhesions are separated carefully by finger dissection.

4. **Vestigial Structures.**—Pelvic disease may arise from vestigial elements of the embryonic wolffian duct. When the wolffian duct persists, it is represented by a tube beginning close to the lateral extremity of the uterine tube. This tube runs medially between the layers of the broad ligament and downward in the superficial tissue of the cervix and lateral aspect of the vagina to an opening at the vulva close to the orifice of Bartholin's gland. Usually no trace remains of Gartner's duct which is the lower or uterovaginal segment of the wolffian duct. A vestige of the upper or mesosalpingial portion of the wolffian duct, the epoophoron, usually is found between the layers of the mesosalpinx or in the broad ligament. These fetal remnants may give rise to cystic tumors which are termed *parovarian cysts*. They vary in size, though usually they are not large, and generally are unilocular; sometimes, they contain clear fluid. They may be mistaken for ovarian cysts, but they always lie within the broad ligament. A parovarian cyst sometimes may be recognized by the greatly elongated uterine tube stretching over its upper surface. The cysts may burrow downward in the broad ligament and come into contact with and adhere to the ureter. In removal of these tumors, the greatest danger is that of injuring the ureter. The tumors are approached best by downward dissection through the broad ligament.

SURGICAL CONSIDERATIONS

1. **Salpingitis.**—Salpingitis is infection of the uterine tube. The continuity of the mucosal lining of the uterus with that of the tube explains the readiness with which ascending infection, chiefly gonococcal, occurs. Blood stream infection is responsible for tuberculous salpingitis, and lymphatic involvement for streptococcal salpingitis associated with pregnancy. The commonest result of tubal infection is the sealing up of the abdominal ostium by adhesions which tend to prevent the products of infection from entering the pelvic cavity. The secretions which collect in the infected tube, having insufficient drainage into the uterus, cause the tube to distend so that it may be palpated easily (*pus tube*, *pyosalpinx*). Absorption of the purulent exudate in the tube and its replacement by clear fluid results in *hydrosalpinx*, which resembles a retention cyst. The tube may be distended by blood (*hematosalpinx*).

Leakage of infective material into the pelvic cavity may produce a pelvic peritonitis which may extend upward and result in a *generalized peritonitis*, or remain localized and produce *adhesive pelvic peritonitis*. In the latter condition, it is not uncommon to find the ovary, tube, the adjoining part of the broad ligament, one or more coils of small intestine and the sigmoid glued together firmly and adherent to the pelvic wall. This constitutes *adnexal disease*. When an infection occurs in both the tube and ovary, adhesions form between them and wall off a single pus cavity known as a *tubo-ovarian abscess*. There often is so much inflammation in the surrounding tissues that it is difficult to attribute to each structure its proper share in the symptom-complex. If the tubal exudate drains freely into the recto-uterine culdesac, a true *pelvic abscess* may develop. Pelvic abscesses may rupture spontaneously into the rectum, vagina, loops of intestine, or bladder. The rupture of a pus tube may cause extension of infection into the broad ligament and a broad *ligament abscess* may result. A pus tube rarely ruptures into the abdominal cavity.

31

Salpingitis, in the majority of instances, responds well to nonoperative treatment and, allowed to subside, often does not preclude subsequent pregnancy. Tuberculous salpingitis does not respond to nonoperative measures but demands complete extirpation of all infected tissues.

2. **Ectopic Pregnancy.**—Various anatomical and pathologic conditions hinder the migration of the fertilized ovum to the normal area of implantation on the uterine mucosa: the arborescent system of folds in the tubal mucous membrane, in which the ovum may be sequestered, especially if the folds are swollen and adherent from a catarrhal inflammation (salpingitis follicularis); an abnormally long and excessively tortuous tube; congenital atresia or pathologic atresia after fertilization has taken place; adhesions which may have exerted a distorting influence on the tube; and destruction of the columnar epithelium of the mucosa.

A *tubal pregnancy* is by far the commonest form of ectopic gestation. Pregnancy in both tubes may occur simultaneously or separately. The implantation generally is in the lateral portion of the ampulla, but may be at any point from the fimbriated extremity to the uterine ostium. *Primary abdominal pregnancies* occur very rarely, if ever, and the fertilized ovum is unlikely to be implanted on the ovary (*ovarian pregnancy*), although it may be implanted on the tube and ovary (*tubo-ovarian pregnancy*). Tubo-ovarian pregnancy scarcely ever proceeds to term. The principal cause of the interruption of the pregnancy is hemorrhage which separates the placenta and deprives the embryo of nour-

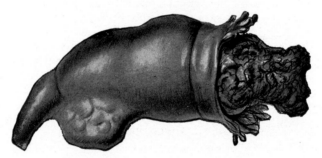

Fig. 486.—Tubal Abortion. (Montgomery.)

ishment. When *pregnancy occurs in the fimbriated extremity of the tube*, the fetus develops partly in the cavity of the infundibulum and partly in the pelvic cavity in that vicinity. The ovum may be arrested near the uterine ostium of the tube and the fetus may develop within the wall of the uterus (*interstitial pregnancy*).

When the fertilized ovum becomes embedded in the wall of the uterine tube (tubal pregnancy), the trophoblastic cells invade the mucosa and musculature of the tube. Because the musculature is thin and there is not an adequate specialized mucosa like the endometrium in the uterus, the continued corrosive action of the trophoblastic cells causes a rupture of the tube. Rupture usually occurs between six and eight weeks after implantation, although it may take place at an earlier or a later period. Extrusion of the fetus into the lumen of the tube is *internal rupture*. A hematosalpinx results. If the fetus is extruded through the abdominal ostium (*tubal abortion*), the fetus dies or may become implanted on the peritoneum (*abdominal pregnancy*). This pregnancy may proceed to full term and a live child be obtained by abdominal section.

In the usual tubal pregnancy, the corrosive action of the trophoblastic cells completely destroys the mucosa and the musculature and *external rupture* occurs, usually accompanied by sharp pain and hemorrhage. Excessive loss of blood may produce shock. The free blood in the peritoneal cavity produces a general peritoneal irritation. Vaginal bleeding usually occurs with the breaking down of the decidua of the uterus. Repeated small hemorrhages may occur until the abnormal gestation is removed by excision of the tube.

3. **Clinical Examination of the Tubes.**—In *bimanual pelvic examination*, a tube of normal size and consistency cannot be palpated.   An acutely inflamed tube becomes enlarged and indurated and usually prolapses into the recto-uterine culdesac, where it is palpated readily and is painful when pressed.   Movement of the cervix from side to side pulls upon the inflamed tubes and causes exquisite pain.   In chronic tubal infection, adhesions about the tubes may be presupposed if the uterus and ovaries lack their normal mobility.   In investigating the causes of sterility, it is important to determine the patency of the tubes.   Several methods are available for this determination.   Gas under known manometric pressure may be passed into the cervical canal, uterine cavity, and uterine tubes (*tubal insufflation*).   Obstruction in the tubes prevents the passage of gas into the abdominal cavity.

The cavities of the uterus and tube may be visualized by the injection of a nonirritating substance (*lipiodol*) opaque to *x*-ray.   The lipiodol outlines the patent structures and normally escapes into the peritoneal cavity.   Operative attempts to restore tubal patency require an exact knowledge of the location of the obstruction.

4. **Salpingectomy and Salpingo-oophorectomy.**—*Salpingectomy* or removal of the uterine tube may be unilateral or bilateral and may or may not be accompanied by removal

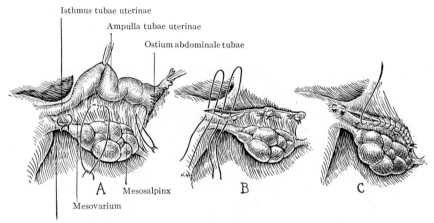

Isthmus tubae uterinae
Ampulla tubae uterinae
Ostium abdominale tubae

A   Mesosalpinx   B   C
Mesovarium

Ligamentum ovarii proprium (utero-ovarian ligament)

Fig. 487.—Salpingectomy.

of the corresponding ovary (salpingo-oophorectomy).   The usual indications for the operation are residual infection and tubal pregnancy.   There may be dense adhesions to the surrounding structures which require blunt or sharp dissection to mobilize the tube. The blood vessels to the tubes, branches of the ovarian vessels, then are clamped in the mesosalpinx and ligated separately to prevent kinking and occlusion of the main vessels. The blood supply to the ovary must be preserved to prevent degeneration of the ovary and the formation of ovarian cysts.   The uterine portion of the tube with a wedge-shaped portion of the cornu of the uterus is excised and the tube is freed from the mesosalpinx. The uterine wedge is closed carefully by suture and the edges of the mesosalpinx are sutured to the peritoneum of the broad ligament below the round ligament to peritonealize the raw surfaces and aid in the suspension of the ovary.

Removal of the tube with the corresponding ovary (*salpingo-oophorectomy*) is simpler than removal of the tube alone.   After exposing the tube and ovary and freeing them from adhesions, ligation of the ovarian vessels in the suspensory ligament of the ovary may be performed.   The uterine portion of the tube is removed as in salpingectomy and the uterine vessels are ligated at or just below the cornu.   The tube and ovary then are removed, with little or no bleeding.

D. OVARIES

1. **Anatomical Summary.**—The ovary or germinal gland of the female is a flattened almond-shaped body projecting from the posterior layer of the broad ligament, which it draws out to form the *mesovarium*. It is brought into connection with the mucosa of the uterine tube by the fimbriae attached to the upper pole of the ovary. The posterior border of the ovary projects backward and medially toward the rectum.

The upper pole of the ovary is connected to the pelvic brim by the *suspensory (infundibulopelvic) ligament*, enclosing the ovarian vessels. This peritoneal fold is derived from the upper and lateral aspects of the broad ligament. The upper pole of the ovary lies within the loop formed by the ampulla of the uterine tube just below the external iliac vessels against the side wall of the pelvis and just behind the pelvic attachment of the broad ligament (ovarian fossa). The lower pole of the ovary is attached to the uterus by a fibromuscular band, the *ovarian (utero-ovarian) ligament*.

2. **Abnormal Positions.**—The ovary, like the testis, originates in the lumbar region. At birth, the ovary is found at the medial border of the psoas muscle; subsequently, it migrates to its permanent site. In multiparae, the ovary lies fairly constantly in the "ovarian fossa." Because of its freedom within the peritoneal duplication of the mesovarium, the ovary is mobile.

The principal conditions causing the ovary to assume an ectopic position are: retroversion and retroflexion of the uterus; failure of the overstretched peritoneum of the broad ligament to return to the normal state after parturition; and ovarian enlargement. Displacement may be temporary, but frequently is permanent because of the development of adhesions. The ovary, in an abnormal position, very often becomes tender and painful.

The ovary may lie behind the ureter and hypogastric vessels in close relationship to the uterosacral fold, or may gravitate into the recto-uterine culdesac (of Douglas). It may occupy an entirely ectopic position in the sac of an inguinal or femoral hernia. It possesses a gubernaculum which sometimes anchors it in the inguinal canal with the round ligament. The descent of the ovary, like that of the testis (p. 292), is accompanied by a tubular process of peritoneum (canal of Nuck), which normally disappears. Persistence of this process affords a sac for a congenital inguinal hernia. Cysts in the inguinal canal and in the labium majus develop from remnants of the primitive peritoneal canal, and their development is analogous to that of vaginal hydrocele and cyst of the spermatic cord (p. 297).

3. **Structure.**—The ovary is divided into a central medullary layer and a peripheral cortical layer. The *medullary zone* is characterized by a profusion of blood vessels within connective tissue, containing strands of smooth muscle and elastic fibers. Small glands, sometimes called medullary cells, are present. To these glands, an endocrine function has been attributed. The *cortical layer*, besides containing connective tissue, contains the essential glandular tissue in the form of graafian follicles in all stages of development. Many graafian follicles may develop incompletely. The persistence of immature follicles may cause an enlargement of the ovary, *cystic ovary*. The condition is asymptomatic and does not require treatment.

The ova are formed and matured in the substance of the cortical ovarian stroma, each in a small cyst (*graafian follicle*). The follicle, by enlargement, reaches the surface of the ovary. The mature follicle bursts as a result of the increasing tension of the fluid filling it. This fluid and the ovum floating within it are discharged into the peritoneal cavity, whence the ovum is directed into the uterine tube by the fimbriae and propagated into the uterine cavity by the cilia and tubal peristalsis. The cavity of the ruptured follicle fills with blood and constitutes a *corpus luteum*. Occasionally, hemorrhage is excessive and produces a corpus luteum hematoma which may be palpable on bimanual examination. If the bleeding continues, the hematoma may rupture and discharge its contents into the peritoneal cavity. The corpus luteum remains active until the onset of the succeeding menstruation, when gradual absorption begins. Absorption continues until only a small white homogeneous body, the *corpus albicans*, remains. This body finally is absorbed completely. When an ovum has been impregnated, the corpus luteum grows for several months.

The cystic forms of ovarian tumors, including by far the greatest number of ovarian new growths, appear, for the most part, to develop from the graafian follicles and there-

A

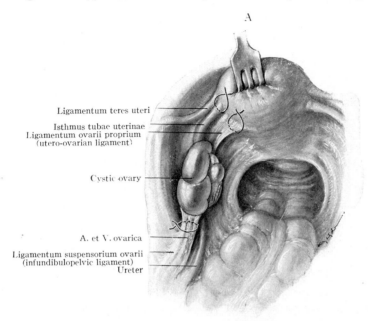

Ligamentum teres uteri

Isthmus tubae uterinae
Ligamentum ovarii proprium
(utero-ovarian ligament)

Cystic ovary

A. et V. ovarica

Ligamentum suspensorium ovarii
(infundibulopelvic ligament)
Ureter

B

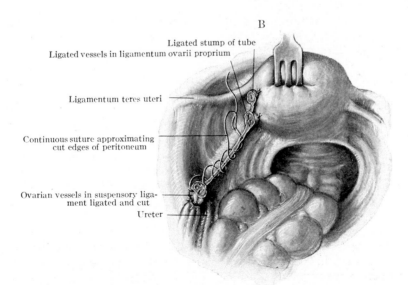

Ligated stump of tube
Ligated vessels in ligamentum ovarii proprium

Ligamentum teres uteri

Continuous suture approximating
cut edges of peritoneum

Ovarian vessels in suspensory ligament ligated and cut
Ureter

FIG. 488.—REMOVAL OF THE UTERINE TUBE AND OVARY.
In A, the uterus is drawn forward and the ligatures are placed; in B, the tube and ovary are removed.

fore in the ovarian cortical zone. Inflammation of the gland involves both the central and cortical zones and causes sterility. The acute pain in ovarian disease is caused by inflammatory involvement of the ovarian nerves

Surgical Considerations

The ovary contains an unusual variety of energetic cellular elements which vary in morphology and functional activity in successive periods of life. The ovary is subject to pathologic processes, and, although involved most frequently during the reproductive period, is by no means exempt from involvement either in infancy or in old age.

1. **Inflammation of the Ovary.**—"Oophoritis" is the result of a direct invasion of the ovary by micro-organisms. An acute involvement is characterized by swelling, congestion, and leukocytic infiltration causing formation of a serous, bloody, or purulent exudate. The most common causative organisms are the gonococcus and the streptococcus. The dense cortical stroma of the ovary is resistant to infection, but the ruptured graafian follicle or a corpus luteum hematoma is a portal of entry for, and a site for development of, infection. Oophoritis occurs only during a severe pelvic infection.

Gonococcal oophoritis is the result of an infection ascending from the involved mucous membrane of the vagina to the uterus, tubes, and finally to the ovary. It is secondary to, and part of, a pelvic peritonitis caused by dissemination of the infection through the fimbriated end of the tube. When infection enters a corpus luteum, a *corpus luteum abscess* is formed. The characteristic results are the formation of dense periovarian adhesions and sclerosed areas in the ovary. Subsequent swelling of the "buried" ovary, as a result of the development of graafian follicles, distends the adhesions and peritoneum and causes "ovarian pain." *Streptococcic infection* usually is puerperal or follows surgery on the genital tract; it is particularly frequent after an infected abortion. The condition is nonoperative, as intervention tends to disseminate infection and cause a generalized peritonitis or a bacteremia.

Tuberculous infection in the ovary is exceedingly rare, as the primary disease usually is in the tube. The condition requires removal of the tube and ovary.

2. **Ovarian Cysts.**—Cyst formation may result from the failure of completion of the normal physiologic processes in the ovary. The multiple development of graafian follicles which fail to mature may produce multiple small cysts (*retention cysts*), from 1 to 2 cm. in diameter. These cysts usually are thin walled and are filled with clear fluid. They occur generally in chronically inflamed and sclerosed ovaries.

Failure of a large corpus luteum hematoma to absorb may result in a *corpus luteum cyst*. These cysts usually are larger than retention cysts and may measure from 8 to 10 cm. in diameter. The thin cyst wall may have a characteristic color from retained carotin, and the cyst contents usually are colored by blood pigments, generally cholesterin. When these cysts are large and filled with blood, they are known as *corpus luteum hematomata*.

Endometrial cysts of the ovary, *endometriomata* (chocolate or Sampson cysts), often are mistaken for corpus luteum hematomata. The endometrial cysts arise from aberrant endometrium which undergoes changes similar to those in the uterus during menstruation. Since there is no egress of blood unless rupture of the cyst occurs, the menstruum progressively distends the cyst.

E. VAGINA

1. **Anatomical Summary.**—The vagina is an anteroposteriorly flattened musculo-membranous tube extending from the cervix to the vestibule in the vulvar cleft. Its anterior and posterior walls are in contact, save above where they are applied over the cervix; its cavity, therefore, is only potential. Most of the vagina lies above the level of the pelvic diaphragm and is surrounded by the visceral pelvic fascia. The lower portion of the vagina is embraced by the levator ani muscles and by the structures of the anterior perineum.

The upper end of the vagina forms the vaginal vault, which is reduced to an annular groove where it surrounds, and is attached to, the cervix. This groove is divided into an anterior and a posterior and two lateral *fornices*. The posterior fornix is a pouchlike depression from 1 to 2 cm. in depth. The anterior fornix is a shallow recess.

The *vaginal mucosa* is thrown into folds or rugae, especially in nulliparae. As the vaginal mucosa is continuous with that of the uterus, vaginitis may be followed by endo-cervicitis and endometritis.

The vagina has a remarkable capacity for dilation, which attains its maximum at parturition and is limited mainly by the resistance of the muscles of the pelvic floor. The vaginal outlet is the narrowest portion of the vagina and may be lacerated by the passage of the fetal head. In prolonged labor, the long-continued compression of the anterior vaginal wall against the pubic arch may be followed by sloughing of the vaginal wall and the adjacent part of the bladder with subsequent establishment of a communication between them (vesicovaginal fistula).

The vagina is maintained in position by its attachment to the cervix, to the extra-peritoneal connective tissue of the pelvis, and to the bladder. The terminal portion of the vagina is supported firmly in the urogenital perineum.

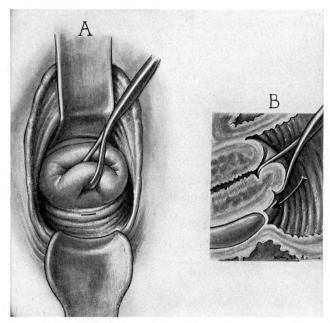

FIG. 489.—POSTERIOR COLPOTOMY FOR RECTO-UTERINE CULDESAC ABSCESS.

In A, the cervix is drawn upward and forward; the horizontal black line marks the incision through the vaginal mucosa; B, a sagittal section which shows the location of the abscess; the arrow indicates the incision for drainage.

2. **Congenital Anomalies.**—When the vagina is absent, the uterus and uterine tubes are rudimentary or absent. A congenital septum, usually of mucous membrane, sometimes occurs in the upper part of the vagina. The cervix may be hidden entirely by the septum and the communication from the vulva to the vaginal vault be but a small orifice on one side. A septum occasionally extends transversely across the entire vagina (*atresia*). If the partition or septum between the müllerian ducts is not absorbed in the fusion, the result is a *septate uterus* and a *double vagina*. The septum of the double vagina usually is falciform in shape, and may extend the whole length of the vagina or be found only in the upper, middle, or lower third. There may be an atresia of one or the other half of the double vagina. The menstrual flow may be retained within a rudimentary vagina lying beside a well-developed vagina. If tension becomes sufficiently great in the vaginal pocket, a small opening may form and allow the fluid to escape into the functioning vagina.

3. **Relations.**—Over its upper two thirds, the anterior vaginal wall is related to the bladder. A midlongitudinal bulge in the forward part of the anterior vaginal wall indi-

cates the course of the urethra. The segment of the vaginal wall lying posterior to the bladder trigone and the urethra is separated from the bladder wall by a layer of loose connective tissue, the *vesicovaginal septum*. This septum affords a cleavage interval between the two organs and helps to retain the bladder in the pelvis. Through this septum, vesicovaginal fistulae present. The lower segment of the anterior vaginal wall is related to the urethra through the dense urethrovaginal septum.

The posterior vaginal wall in the posterior fornix is related to the peritoneum of the recto-uterine culdesac (of Douglas). The segment of the vagina related to the recto-uterine culdesac is made accessible by drawing the cervix anteriorly. This maneuver affords exposure for incision into the pelvic cavity for evacuation of a culdesac abscess (*posterior colpotomy*). Inferiorly, the posterior vaginal wall is related to the anterior surface of the ampulla of the rectum; only a thin layer of connective tissue intervenes.

The most inferior part of the posterior vaginal wall is located in the perineum within the thickness of the urogenital diaphragm (triangular ligament), and is adherent to the fibrous layers which compose it and the muscles which sustain it. A fibromuscular interval (*perineal body*) lies between the perineal portions of the vagina and the rectum. In sagittal section, this body appears as a triangular mass with a cutaneous base, the *vaginorectal triangle* (urethrorectal triangle in the male). The perineal body and the posterior vaginal commissure constitute the least distensible portion of the perineum. If a laceration of the perineum involves the perineal body, the posterior vaginal wall and the rectum may prolapse into the vagina (rectocele). A strain is placed on the anterior vaginal wall which, with the bladder, prolapses gradually (cystocele).

Surgical Considerations

1. **Vesicovaginal Fistulae.**—In difficult and prolonged labor, there is constant pressure of the anterior vaginal wall against the pubic arch. This pressure may cause a sloughing of the vaginal wall and the contiguous portion of the bladder with subsequent estab-

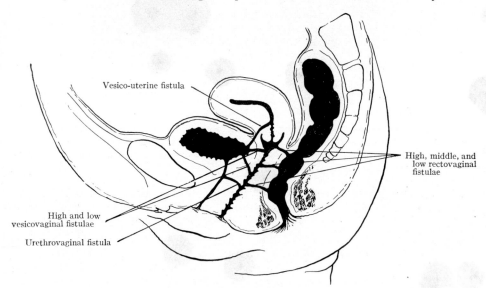

Vesico-uterine fistula

High, middle, and low rectovaginal fistulae

High and low vesicovaginal fistulae

Urethrovaginal fistula

Fig. 490.—Vaginal Fistulae.

lishment of a vesicovaginal fistula. The condition causes much distress because of the continuous flow of urine from the vagina. Fistulous communications are distinguished according to their locations. *High fistulae* occur in the fundus or base of the bladder, are difficult of surgical approach by the vagina, and may require suture through the bladder cavity. *Middle fistulae* involve the trigone and *low fistulae* involve the urethra. The vaginal fistula may involve the ureter (*ureterovaginal fistula*).   *Urethrovaginal fistulae* are distinguished from vesicovaginal fistulae by the fact that they allow urine to escape from the vagina only during micturition.

2. **Rectovaginal Fistulae.**—Rectovaginal fistulae are abnormal channels of communication between the rectum and vagina.   The common cause of fistulae in the upper part of the vagina is an extension of a carcinoma of the cervix to the vagina and into the rectum through the rectovaginal septum.   The fistulae may follow destruction of the septum in severe labor.

During parturition, the posterior commissure of the vagina may be torn and the laceration may involve the skin and superficial tissue as far as the anus.   The posterior wall of the vagina, the perineal body, and the anal sphincters, also, may be involved.

3. **Cystocele.**—Cystocele is a hernia of the bladder through the vesicovaginal septum. Some degree of prolapse of the urethra through the urinary meatus. *urethrocele*, with relaxation of the vesical sphincter usually accompanies it.   Cystocele results from stretching and tearing of the pubocervical connective tissue.   The weakest spot usually is at the vesico-

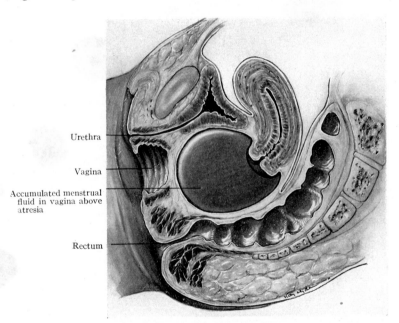

Urethra

Vagina

Accumulated menstrual
fluid in vagina above
atresia

Rectum

Fig. 491.—Hematocolpos from Vaginal Atresia.

cervical junction.   A patient with cystocele complains of a protruding mass.   Urinary incontinence frequently is present.   Sometimes an examination in the standing position is necessary to demonstrate the lesion.   The steps in the surgical repair of the lesion are indicated in Fig. 492.

4. **Perineal Laceration and Rectocele.**—The important perineal muscles related to the vaginal cleft in the urogenital diaphragm are the paired pubococcygeal bands of the anal levators (Fig. 493).   From pubic origin, lateral to the symphysis, these fascia-covered muscles converge on the rectum to insert on the coccyx.   Forward of the rectum, their margins hem the interlevator cleft, through which the vagina, almost exclusively a pelvic structure, emerges.   Injury to and subsequent retraction of these muscles and their clothing and intervening fascia are the result of stretching and tearing.

As a result of this damage to these supporting structures, the rectum may protrude anteriorly through the posterior vaginal wall (*rectocele*).   This is a true hernia, comparable with cystocele in the anterior vaginal wall.   The protruding rectal sac may be near the vulvar orifice or it may be high on the posterior vaginal wall.   Essentially, repair of a

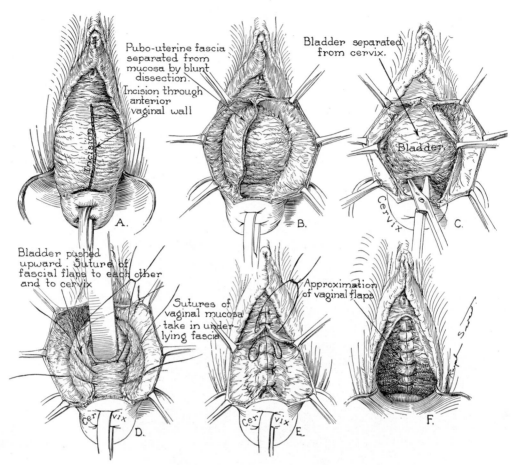

Pubo-uterine fascia separated from mucosa by blunt dissection.

Incision through anterior vaginal wall

Bladder separated from cervix.

Bladder

A.

B.

Cervix

C.

Bladder pushed upward. Suture of fascial flaps to each other and to cervix

Sutures of vaginal mucosa take in underlying fascia

Approximation of vaginal flaps

Cervix

D.

Cervix

E.

F.

FIG. 492.—REPAIR OF CYSTOCELE. (After Curtis.)

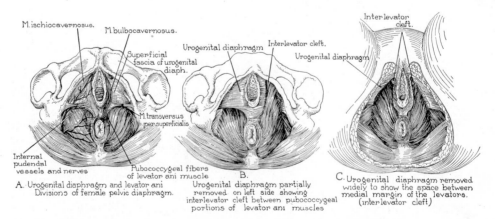

Interlevator cleft.

M.ischiocavernosus.

M.bulbocavernosus.

Superficial fascia of urogenital diaph.

Urogenital diaphragm

Interlevator cleft.

Urogenital diaphragm

M.transversus per.superficialis

Internal pudendal vessels and nerves

Pubococcygeal fibers of levator ani muscle

A. Urogenital diaphragm and levator ani Divisions of female pelvic diaphragm.

B. Urogenital diaphragm partially removed on left side showing interlevator cleft between pubococcygeal portions of levator ani muscles

C. Urogenital diaphragm removed widely to show the space between medial margin of the levators. (interlevator cleft)

FIG. 493.—THE UROGENITAL AND ANAL PORTIONS OF THE PELVIC DIAPHRAGM IN THE FEMALE.

These drawings were made to show the interlevator cleft between the pubococcygeal portions of the levator ani muscles.

The cleft is widened in forcible childbirth, and the fascial coverings of the muscles hemming it are torn. Perineorrhaphy consists in suturing, from within the vaginal orifice, the muscular medial margins of the levator ani muscles which hem the cleft.

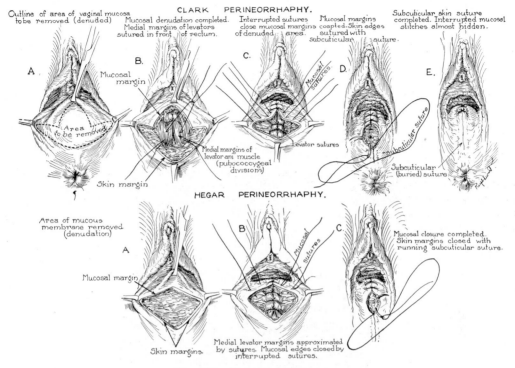

CLARK PERINEORRHAPHY.

Outline of area of vaginal mucosa to be removed (denuded)

Mucosal denudation completed. Medial margins of levators sutured in front of rectum.

Interrupted sutures close mucosal margins of denuded area.

Mucosal margins coapted. Skin edges sutured with subcuticular suture.

Subcuticular skin suture completed. Interrupted mucosal stitches almost hidden.

A B C D E.

Mucosal margin

Area to be removed

Skin margin

Mucosal sutures

Medial margins of levator ani muscle (pubococcygeal divisions)

Levator sutures

Subcuticular suture

Subcuticular (buried) suture

HEGAR PERINEORRHAPHY.

Area of mucous membrane removed (denudation)

A B C

Mucosal margin

Mucosal sutures

Mucosal closure completed. Skin margins closed with running subcuticular suture.

Skin margins.

Medial levator margins approximated by sutures. Mucosal edges closed by interrupted sutures.

FIG. 494.—REPAIR OF RECTOCELE.

cystocele approximates the retracted medial margins of the levators after a flap of posterior vaginal mucosa and connective tissue has been dissected forward to allow operative manipulation (Fig. 494).

MALE PERINEUM AND EXTERNAL GENITALIA

I. MALE PERINEUM

THE perineum is a partition of soft parts extending from one lateral pelvic wall to the other between the pubis and coccyx. It includes the musculomembranous pelvic diaphragm and those soft parts at the pelvic outlet lying inferior to it. At the pelvic outlet, all the boundaries—the pubic symphysis, ischiopubic rami, ischial tuberosities, sacrotuberous ligaments, and coccyx—can be palpated.

The region is subdivided into two triangular portions by a transverse line just anterior to the ischial tuberosities, the midpoint of which lies just anterior to the anal orifice. The area in front of this line is known as the anterior or urogenital triangle, and that behind it, as the posterior or anal triangle. Although the relations of the anal canal to the anal triangle differ but little between the sexes, the urogenital relations differ widely.

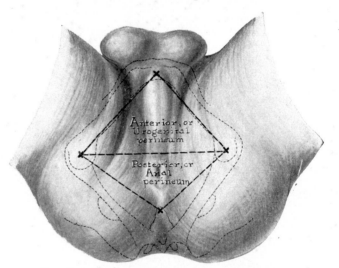

FIG. 495.—TOPOGRAPHY OF THE MALE PERINEUM.

The male perineum, exclusive of the external genitalia, possesses unusual interest for the surgeon because of the relationship it bears to the deeper stages of the urethra, prostate, seminal vesicles, bladder, and rectum. It is divided into the pelvic diaphragm, the anterior or urogenital perineum, and the posterior or anal perineum.

A. PELVIC DIAPHRAGM

The pelvic diaphragm is a musculomembranous partition which forms the lower boundary and floor of the pelvic basin and is the framework for the perineum. Viewed from above, the diaphragm presents the appearance of a hollow cone, at the most dependent part (apex) of which the rectum emerges on the perineum. It is divided into the main pelvic diaphragm, consisting of the levator ani muscles, and the accessory or urogenital diaphragm, composed chiefly of aponeurotic elements.

1. **Main Pelvic Diaphragm.**—The muscles forming the diaphragm, the levator ani and coccygeus, spread like a sling from the walls of the pelvis to the anus. They have a continuous line of attachment to the inner aspect of the pelvic wall from a point near the lower border of the symphysis anteriorly, to the ischial spine posteriorly. From this extensive origin on each side, the muscle fibers blend into a thick sheet and are directed

492

with varying degrees of obliquity toward the median raphe. The more anterior fibers from the pubic bones support the base of the bladder and the prostate as these muscles converge to the central point of the perineum (p. 499). Their mesial margins are hemmed by aponeuroses which adhere to the lateral margins of the prostate and are known as the

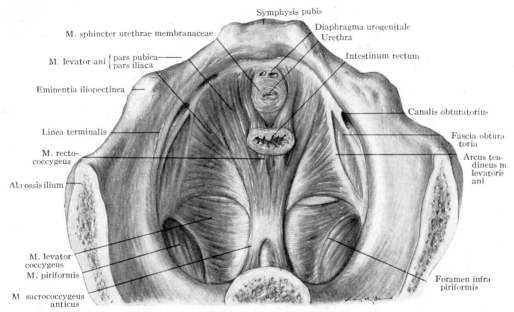

FIG. 496.—MALE PELVIC DIAPHRAGM FROM ABOVE.

lateral puboprostatic ligaments. Because the pubic origin of the levators is considerably lateral to the symphysis, the muscular diaphragm is incomplete anteriorly, leaving a broad anterior hiatus (*interlevator cleft*), against the inferior aspect of which lies the urogenital or accessory pelvic diaphragm.

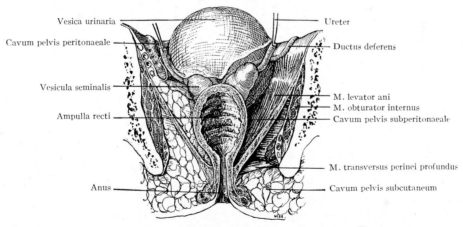

FIG. 497.—FRONTAL SECTION THROUGH THE PELVIC FLOOR AND PERINEUM.

An extension from the *pelvic fascia* invests the upper surface of the diaphragm and furnishes prolongations of an ensheathing character to the structures lying upon the pelvic floor. The lower or perineal aspect of the levator ani muscle is closed by a thin membrane of the inferior levator fascia, while the adjoining aspect of the pelvic wall is clothed by the obturator or parietal layer of the pelvic fascia.

2. **Accessory or Urogenital Diaphragm (Triangular Ligament).**—The urogenital diaphragm is that part of the pelvic floor occupying the pubic angle and separating the soft parts of the perineum from the contents of the pelvis anteriorly. The essentially aponeurotic bundle of fibers, of which it is composed, stretches transversely from one ischiopubic ramus to the other, terminating posteriorly at the level of the ischial tuberosities by a posterior free border. The point in the pelvic floor between the levator margins and the posterior edge of the urogenital diaphragm would be weak were it not for the dense union between these structures anterior to the anus at the tendinous point of the perineum (p. 500). The urogenital diaphragm is composed of superior and inferior layers of fascia separated by various structures (p. 497). The superior layer of the diaphragm is densely adherent to the mesial edges of the levators and, to a great extent, maintains the base of the bladder and the prostate within the pelvic cavity.

3. **Interlevator Cleft.**—The broad hiatus between the mesial margins of the levators anterior to the rectum is known as the interlevator cleft or anterior prostatic space. The floor is the superior fascia of the urogenital diaphragm, and the roof, the base of the bladder. The space contains a quantity of loose areolar tissue, within which run the *middle pubovesical and puboprostatic ligaments*, all derived from the superior division of the pelvic fascia. These ligaments attach anteriorly to the pubes on each side of the symphysis and run backward to insert into the capsule of the prostate and the antero-inferior surface of the bladder.

About the ligaments lie the *anterior prostatic venous plexuses*, definitely superficial to the capsule of the prostate. They are derived from the dorsal vein of the penis, after that vessel has passed anterior to the superior fascia of the urogenital diaphragm, and they terminate in the internal iliac veins. The plexuses are continued backward on each side about the lateral aspects of the prostate and there join the large thin-walled veins lying in the sulcus between the bladder wall and prostate (p. 453). If hemorrhage is to be avoided, only blunt dissection should be used in exposure of the lateral surface of the prostate in radical removal of the gland for carcinoma, or inmanipulatio to free the seminal vesicles.

B. ANTERIOR OR UROGENITAL PERINEULM(TRIAE)NG

The anterior and posterior regions of the perineum should not be considered as isolated in either the male or female. Both regions are related intimately to their common levator substratum, have a common blood supply and innervation by the internal pudendal vessels and nerves, and jointly participate in the formation of the central region of the perineum.

The framework of the anterior perineum is adapted especially to support the anterior pelvic structures and is specialized for, and differentiated by, the passage of the urogenital apparatus, the injuries and diseases of which give the area clinical and operative significance.

1. **Definition and Boundaries.**—The urogenital perineum extends from the pubic symphysis to the central area of the perineum just anterior to the anus, and is limited laterally by the pubic arch. Its contents consist of all the structures located between the anterior portion of the levator diaphragm above and the skin overlying the triangle below.

The space is divided into two compartments by a definite membranous partition, the urogenital diaphragm (triangular ligament), which extends across the pubic arch in somewhat the same way that the mylohyoid muscles extend between the mandibles to separate the floor of the mouth from the sublingual space (p. 138). The divisions formed are the superficial and deep compartments of the urogenital perineum.

2. **Superficial Structures.**—Save for minor branches of the inferior hemorrhoidal (rectal), pudendal, and posterior scrotal vessels and nerves, little of interest attaches to the superficial structures of the anterior perineum except the derivation of the **superficial fascia.** This fascia consists of two strata, the *outer* of which is a fatty layer continuous with the general fatty covering of the body, particularly that investing the scrotum, thighs, penis, and anterior abdominal wall. It contains little fatty tissue except at its peripheral part, but consists of smooth muscle fibers which are continuous anteriorly with the dartos

layer of the scrotum.   The *inner* or *deeper layer*, *Colles' fascia*, is found only over the urogenital region.   It is denser and more membranous in character than the superficial layer and is attached on each side to the periosteum of the pubic arch.   Behind, it is fused with the base of the triangular ligament.   It passes anteriorly over the scrotum and penis and along the spermatic cord to the anterior abdominal wall, where it is continuous with the corresponding deeper layer of the superficial fascia (p. 275).   This continuous layer incloses the penis, envelops the scrotum, and forms a roof for the superficial perineal pouch.   In cases of extensive urinary extravasation or hemorrhage into the space, the actual lines of attachment of the fascia are demonstrated.

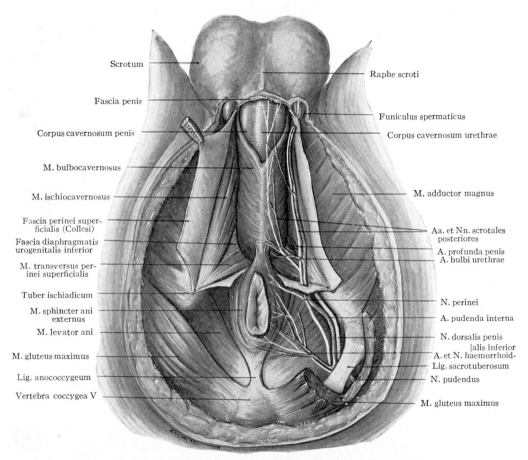

Scrotum

Raphe scroti

Fascia penis

Funiculus spermaticus

Corpus cavernosum penis

Corpus cavernosum urethrae

M. bulbocavernosus

M. ischiocavernosus

M. adductor magnus

Fascia perinei super-
ficialis (Collesi)

Aa. et Nn. scrotales
posteriores

Fascia diaphragmatis
urogenitalis inferior

A. profunda penis
A. bulbi urethrae

M. transversus per-
inei superficialis

Tuber ischiadicum

N. perinei

M. sphincter ani
externus

A. pudenda interna

M. levator ani

N. dorsalis penis
[alis inferior
A. et N. haemorrhoid-

M. gluteus maximus

Lig. sacrotuberosum

Lig. anococcygeum

N. pudendus

Vertebra coccygea V

M. gluteus maximus

FIG. 498.—SUPERFICIAL STRUCTURES OF THE MALE PERINEUM.
The superficial perineal fascia (of Colles) has been incised and retracted to show the contents of the superficial perineal compartment.

3. **Superficial Perineal or Ischiobulbar Compartment of the Urogenital Perineum.**—
The superficial compartment of the urogenital perineum is a space bounded inferiorly by Colles' fascia, and superiorly by the urogenital diaphragm.   It is closed posteriorly and laterally by the fusion of its two walls and their attachment to the pubic arch.   Anteriorly, the space communicates freely with the cellular interval between Scarpa's layer of the superficial fascia of the abdominal wall and the anterior rectus sheath.   The compartment is divided incompletely into two spaces by a median septum extending from the deep aspect of Colles' fascia to the superficial aspect of the bulbocavernosus muscle.   It is evident that the natural outlet of the compartment is anterior, and that it is closed securely both posteriorly and laterally.

4. Contents of the Superficial Perineal Compartment.—Within the superficial perineal pouch are: the roots or fixed portions of the corpora cavernosa of the penis and urethra, their overlying ischiocavernosus and bulbocavernosus muscles, and those branches of the internal pudendal vessels and nerves which pierce the inferior fascia of the urogenital diaphragm to reach the space.

The two roots of the *corpora cavernosa of the penis* arise from the midportion of the ischiopubic rami and run obliquely upward and forward, adhering to the periosteum of the descending rami of the pubes and to the inferior surface of the urogenital diaphragm. Each cavernous body of the penis is covered by the ischiocavernosus muscle. The *corpus cavernosum (spongiosum) urethrae* incloses the urethral canal and is directed forward to form the central body of the penis. Before the cavernous part of the *urethra* engages into its covering, it presents a dilation on its inferior surface, known as the culdesac of the bulb. In passing a urethral sound, the tip of the instrument usually engages in this depression and may be forced into a false passage. This mishap is avoided by following the upper rather than the lower wall of the canal into the membranous and prostatic portions of the

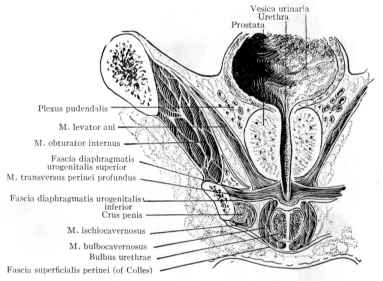

Vesica urinaria
Urethra
Prostata

Plexus pudendalis
M. levator ani
M. obturator internus
Fascia diaphragmatis urogenitalis superior
M. transversus perinei profundus
Fascia diaphragmatis urogenitalis inferior
Crus penis
M. ischiocavernosus
M. bulbocavernosus
Bulbus urethrae
Fascia superficialis perinei (of Colles)

FIG. 499.—FRONTAL SECTION THROUGH THE MALE PELVIS AND PERINEUM.
The formation of the superficial and deep perineal compartments and the homology with the female perineum are shown.

urethra. Gonorrheal urethritis often is chronic in the culdesac of the bulb, and strictures are likely to localize there. In the unsupported cavernous urethra, proximal to a stricture in this location, rupture is likely to occur, resulting in infiltration in the superficial perineal compartment.

The urinary extravasation, limited by Colles' fascia, first distends the posterior part of the superficial perineal pouch, then passes forward, distends the scrotum, and infiltrates the loose cellular tissue of the penis (p. 510). Finally, it passes upward on the anterior abdominal wall, spreading laterally behind Scarpa's fascia (p. 275). Urine is hindered from passing from the abdominal wall down the thighs by the attachment of Scarpa's fascia to the fascia lata.

At the posterior part of the space, the *superficial transverse perineal muscles* pass medially and a little forward from their ischial origin and insert into the central part of the perineum, midway between the bulb and anus. These small muscles lie in the most posterior plane of the superficial compartment and cannot be exposed without incising Colles' fascia; they form an important landmark in perineal surgery. With the elements forming the root of the penis, these muscles help to outline a small triangular area on each side of the median line, the boundaries of which are: the crus laterally; the bulb medially; and the superficial transverse perineal muscle posteriorly. The inferior fascia of the urogenital diaphragm, which extends across the space, forms the deep boundary or floor of these triangular areas.

The perineum on each side of the corpus cavernosum urethrae is traversed by *vessels and nerves*, chiefly small branches of the pudendal trunks. The perineal artery leaves the internal pudendal in the ischiorectal fossa and runs forward toward the pubes.

5. Urogenital Diaphragm.—The urogenital diaphragm is a semirigid musculomembranous structure attached to the ischiopubic rami and stretched tightly across the pubic arch to assist in closing the forward part of the pelvic outlet. It separates the perineum from the pelvis anteriorly. The closed interval, or pouch, separating the layers of the diaphragm, is filled principally with the muscle tissue about the membranous urethra. The two fascial layers blend with one another, with Colles' fascia, and with the central point of the perineum posteriorly, and are attached to the margins of the pubic arch. The *inferior fascia (superficial layer of the triangular ligament)* alone possesses any strength, though it is deficient immediately behind the subpubic angle and ligament. Its ante-

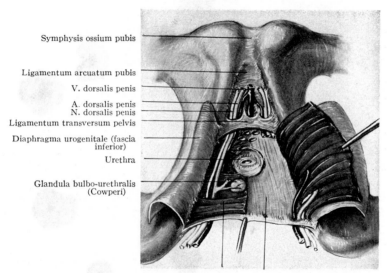

Symphysis ossium pubis

Ligamentum arcuatum pubis

V. dorsalis penis

A. dorsalis penis
N. dorsalis penis

Ligamentum transversum pelvis

Diaphragma urogenitale (fascia inferior)

Urethra

Glandula bulbo-urethralis (Cowperi)

M. Trasversus perinei profundus   Diaphragma urogenitale (fascia superior)

FIG. 500.—CONTENTS OF THE DEEP PERINEAL COMPARTMENT LYING BETWEEN THE FASCIAE OF THE UROGENITAL DIAPHRAGM.

rior free margin is somewhat thickened and is known as the transverse perineal ligament This fascia forms the deep wall of the superficial perineal compartment. The dorsal vessels and nerves of the penis pierce the inferior fascia of the urogenital diaphragm. The *superior layer* of the urogenital diaphragm is an undifferentiated fibrous structure, which really is an extension from the parietal pelvic fascia through the interlevator cleft.

6. Deep Compartment of the Urogenital Perineum.—The space between the two layers of the urogenital diaphragm is known as the deep perineal compartment. It is related on its deep aspect with the pubic recess or anterior prolongation of the ischiorectal fossa (p. 499), the slitlike space on each side between the levator ani and obturator internus muscles. It contains the deep transverse perineal muscle, the membranous urethra and its sphincter, the bulbo-urethral glands (of Cowper), the artery to the bulb, the internal pudendal vessels, and the dorsal nerve to the penis.

The *deep transverse perineal muscle* (of Guthrie) is so interrelated and fused with the superior fascia of the diaphragm as to render it difficult of dissection. Recognition of the muscle is made more difficult because of the tendency of the surrounding tissues to become so infiltrated as to present the appearance of muscle fibers. Each muscle runs from the ramus of the ischium to the midline, where it interlaces in a tendinous raphe with its opposite fellow. It lies on the same plane but behind the striated sphincter of the membranous urethra, and has no attachment to it. The two muscles function as the external sphincter of the urethra (p. 457).

The *membranous urethra*, so-called because it has no strengthening walls, as have the prostatic and cavernous portions, is related on its deep aspect with the pubic recess or anterior prolongation of the ischiorectal fossa. It is the shortest division of the urethra, being about 1 cm. long, and is narrower than any other part save the external orifice. The membranous urethra is fixed firmly to the urogenital diaphragm by fibrous expansions dense enough to rupture it in pubic fracture. The membranous urethra lies about 2.5 cm.

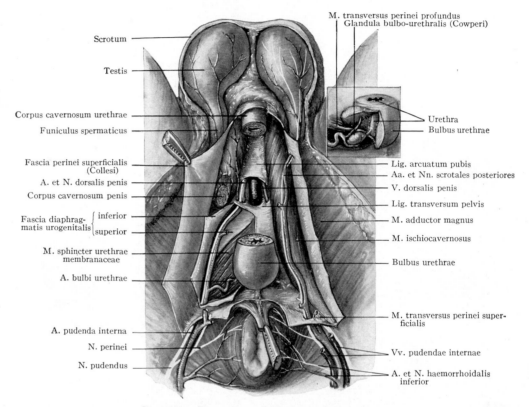

FIG. 501.—DEEP STRUCTURES OF THE PERINEUM.

On the left, the superficial perineal fascia (of Colles) has been incised and retracted to show the contents of the superficial perineal compartment. On the right, the structures of the deep perineal compartment are exposed through an incision in the inferior fascia of the diaphragm. The inset shows the relation of the bulbo-urethral gland and duct to the urethra.

behind the subpubic ligament, against which it may be pressed forcibly and destroyed in a severe fall or blow upon the perineum.

Rupture of the membranous urethra occurs proximal to stricture in the cavernous portion, resulting in extravasation into the deep perineal compartment, whence exit is found only by escaping through one or the other of the fascial leaves of the diaphragm. If urine breaks through the inferior fascia, it passes into the superficial perineal pouch and forward on the abdomen in front of the pubis. If the extension is through the superior fascia, or if there is an extraperitoneal rupture of the bladder, extravasated urine enters the interval about the median puboprostatic ligaments (p. 444), and extends forward into the retropubic space (of Retzius). From there, it ascends in the anterior abdominal wall between the transversalis fascia and parietal peritoneum.

The membranous urethra is surrounded by the *sphincter urethrae (external sphincter)*. This striated muscle (p. 457) is not a complete sphincter about the apex of the prostate, but does encircle the membranous urethra with a cuff of muscle 5 mm. thick. It may or may not be fused with the deep transverse perineal muscles.

The deep perineal pouch contains the *bulbo-urethral glands* (of Cowper) in the midst of the deep transverse perineal muscles. The excretory ducts of these glands are about 2.5 cm. long. Each pea-sized gland receives a branch of the bulbo-urethral artery, and each duct pierces the inferior fascia of the diaphragm to open by a minute orifice on the floor of the cavernous urethra. Not infrequently, these glands are involved in gonorrheal inflammation of the cavernous urethra, and may give rise to abscesses which can be felt through the rectum and evacuated through the perineum.

Between the leaves of the urogenital diaphragm run the *internal pudendal vessels* and the *dorsal nerve* of the *penis*. The internal pudendal artery is the terminal branch of the hypogastric artery which leaves the pelvis by the greater sciatic notch (p. 417), winds

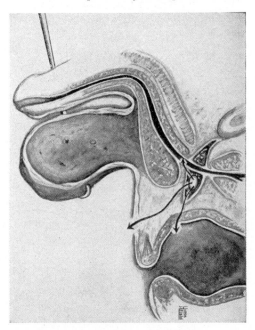

FIG. 502.—POSITION OF COWPER'S GLAND BETWEEN THE LAYERS OF THE UROGENITAL DIAPHRAGM. Arrows indicate the directions in which suppuration of the gland may evacuate into the urethra, the rectum, or the perineum. (Bickham, "Operative Surgery.")

about the ischial spine, and is located on the lateral wall of the ischiorectal fossa (Alcock's canal). After traversing the anal perineum, where it gives off branches to the superficial pouch, it pierces the base of the urogenital diaphragm and runs forward in the lateral part of the deep perineal pouch on the medial surface of the ischiopubic ramus. Within the pouch, it gives off an important artery to the bulb, which runs medially, piercing the inferior fascia of the diaphragm near the midline, and the dorsal artery of the penis. The dorsal vein of the penis runs into the prevesical plexus.

7. Anterior Prolongation of the Ischiorectal Fossa.—The anterior extension of the ischiorectal fossa is the deepest space in the anterior perineum. It runs forward toward the pubes between the superior fascia (deep layer) of the urogenital diaphragm, the anterior portion of the levator ani, and the mesial surface of the obturator internus muscle.

8. Central Point of the Perineum.—The central point of the perineum, a fibromuscular node lying between the anorectal junction and the apex of the prostate, serves as a point of origin for the external and internal anal sphincters and the bulbocavernosus muscle. It also is a point of insertion for the recto-urethral and superficial transverse perineal muscles and for the levator fibers which support the prostate. In the female, the tendinous region lies between the anorectal junction and the posterior vaginal commissure, and is termed the *perineal* body (p. 527).

This area is the key region of the perineum, for it not only unites the urogenital diaphragm and anus with their common substratum, the levators, but also affords the logical perineal approach to the deeper pelvic structures.

SURGICAL CONSIDERATIONS

1. Perineal Approaches for Drainage of Periprostatic and Prostatic Abscesses.—Intraprostatic abscess is one of the results of acute prostatitis (p. 458). Periprostatic abscesses are found in the immediate vicinity of the prostate. Abscesses about the prostate localize most frequently in the area anterior to the rectum, and are likely to rupture into the rectum or the membranous urethra, or upon the perineum. Those lying lateral to the gland tend to invade the ischiorectal fossae, while those superior to the prostate tend to localize between the seminal vesicles.

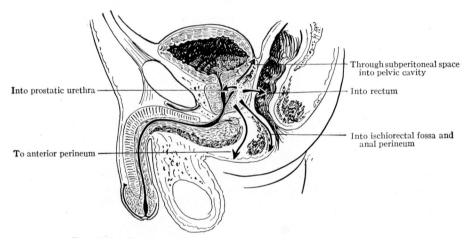

Into prostatic urethra

Through subperitoneal space into pelvic cavity

Into rectum

Into ischiorectal fossa and anal perineum

To anterior perineum

FIG. 503.—PATHS OF EXTENSION FROM PROSTATIC ABSCESS.

The abscess may extend through the subperitoneal space into the pelvic cavity; into the rectum; into the ischiorectal fossa and anal perineum; into the prostatic urethra.

The usual methods of evacuating these abscesses group themselves under two heads: stab incisions through the perineum and incisions after exposure by careful dissection. Abscesses should be opened before tissue is destroyed extensively or rupture into the peritoneum occurs.

The best of the **stab incisions** is that in the *prerectal perineum*, since the finger in the rectum may be utilized to guide the knife as well as to reveal the point of maximum fluctuation of the abscess. The knife is entered behind the bulb, about 2.5 cm. anterior to the anus. The blade is passed deeply into the interval between the bulb and ampulla of the rectum toward the tip of the intrarectal finger and the main mass of the abscess A finger carried through the incision into the abscess enlarges the path for drainage and breaks down any septa in the abscess cavity.

A stab incision in the *lateral perineum* may be guided by a finger in the rectum and a sound in the urethra. The knife is entered about 1 cm. lateral to the median perineal line, about 2 cm. anterior to the anus. The incision is deepened toward the abscess and the wound is stretched or enlarged until the finger can explore the cavity.

The membranous urethra and periprostatic space are reached by careful **dissection** through the *classical incision for perineal prostatectomy* (p. 461). This approach is the most orderly for any prostatic or periprostatic abscess and should be selected in cases uncertain in nature or likely to be complicated. The urethra is opened on a sound, which is withdrawn, and the finger is introduced into the membranous urethra and carried into the prostatic urethra. A narrow-bladed knife or hemostat is passed alongside the finger and made to enter the abscess cavity through the normal prostatic tissue. A periprostatic abscess is evacuated before the prostate is reached. If the abscess lies superior and posterior to the prostate, blunt dissection will evacuate its contents into the wound.

C. POSTERIOR OR ANAL PERINEUM

1. **Definition and Boundaries.**—The posterior or anorectal perineum is the triangular area behind the line joining the ischial tuberosities, and is peculiarly adapted to support the terminal rectum. Its base is the superficial transverse perineal musculature which lies on the posterior margin of the urogenital diaphragm; its apex, the tip of the coccyx; and its lateral margins the gluteus maximus muscles. It is subdivided into two ischiorectal fossae by the bulbo-anococcygeal raphe.

2. **Superficial Structures.**—The perianal skin is thick save about the anus, where it thins out, is pigmented, moist, densely adherent to the subjacent tissue, and continuous, without demarcation, with the anal mucosa. It contains hairs and sweat glands which are the points of origin of *perianal abscesses*. The anal orifice presents folds which penetrate the anal canal, between which longitudinal excoriations (*anal fissures*) occur and produce exquisite pain. The subcutaneous tissue is in free communication with the fatty areolar tissue of the ischiorectal fossa, and within it a perianal abscess may remain localized and later open laterally or into the anal canal.

3. **Ischiorectal Fossa.**—Each ischiorectal fossa or inferior pelvirectal space lies between the mesial aspect of the obturator internus muscle and the levator ani muscle. The *lateral wall* is vertical and is formed by the ischium and obturator internus muscle with its aponeurosis. The internal pudendal vessels and nerves are applied intimately to the wall, and their branches supply the fossae and their contents. The oblique fibers of the levator ani, as they run from the pelvis to the rectum, form the *mesial wall*, the boundary being the bulbo-anococcygeal raphe. In the course of an extensive ischiorectal abscess, this musculofibrous barrier may be broken down and the infection be spread to the opposite fossa, resulting in a large horseshoe-shaped abscess, embracing, in whole or in part, the anal portion of the rectum. In the midline is the external sphincter which surrounds the anal canal. The gluteus maximus muscle and sacrotuberous ligament form the *posterior wall*. The superficial transverse perineal muscles and free margin of the urogenital diaphragm mark out the *anterior boundary* of the region superficially. The fossa is related to the extraperitoneal cellular space of the pelvis (superior pelvirectal space) through the levator ani and its enveloping aponeuroses. An ischiorectal abscess may perforate the levator ani and gain access to this space. More frequently, a large abscess in the ischiorectal fossa pushes the levator upward against the rectum, obliterating the extraperitoneal space so that the abscess ulcerates into the rectum without seriously contaminating the pelvic spaces.

There are two important pouches in each fossa. An *anterior prolongation* or *pubic recess* (p. 499) continues the fossa forward. It is a wedgelike interval between the forward portion of the obturator internus muscle and the superior fascia of the urogenital diaphragm. A *posterolateral prolongation* lies between the levator ani and gluteus maximus muscles.

The obturator internus and inferior levator ani fasciae line the walls of the fossa. These, with the superior fascia of the levator, constitute the two divisions of the pelvic fascia which diverge from their origin at the tendinous arch (p. 429).

4. **Contents of the Fossa.**—The *ischiorectal fat* is very abundant and is loculated by fibrous septa derived from the inferior levator fascia. Similar to the fat in the orbit, it persists in patients who otherwise are very emaciated. It is destroyed rapidly in suppuration and is reproduced slowly. The yielding character of the fat readily permits the dilation of the rectum at defecation.

Before the *internal pudendal artery and nerve* penetrate the urogenital diaphragm, they are applied by a duplication of fascia (Alcock's canal) against the obturator internus aponeurosis   Inferior hemorrhoidal branches leave the parent trunks within the fossa and **are**

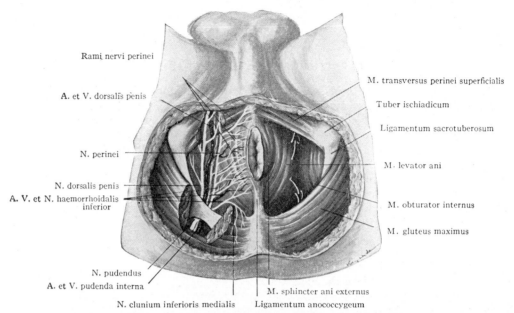

Rami nervi perinei

A. et V. dorsalis penis

N. perinei

N. dorsalis penis

A. V. et N. haemorrhoidalis inferior

M. transversus perinei superficialis

Tuber ischiadicum

Ligamentum sacrotuberosum

M. levator ani

M. obturator internus

M. gluteus maximus

N. pudendus
A. et V. pudenda interna

N. clunium inferioris medialis

M. sphincter ani externus
Ligamentum anococcygeum

FIG. 504.—BOUNDARIES, CONTENTS, AND PROLONGATIONS OF THE ISCHIORECTAL FOSSA.

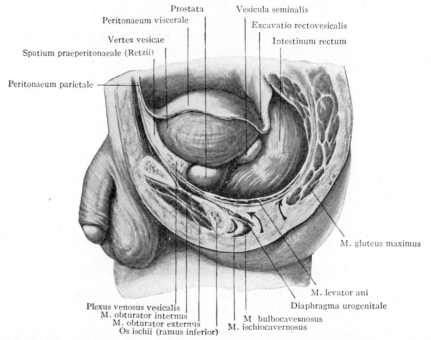

Prostata
Peritonaeum viscerale

Vertex vesicae

Spatium praeperitonaeale (Retzii)

Peritonaeum parietale

Vesicula seminalis

Excavatio rectovesicalis

Intestinum rectum

M. gluteus maximus

M. levator ani
Diaphragma urogenitale

Plexus venosus vesicalis
M. obturator internus
M. obturator externus
Os ischii (ramus inferior)

M. bulbocavernosus
M. ischiocavernosus

FIG. 505.—PARAMEDIAN SAGITTAL SECTION THROUGH THE PELVIS AND PERINEUM TO SHOW THE ANTERIOR AND POSTERIOR PROLONGATIONS OF THE ISCHIORECTAL FOSSA.

distributed to the ischiorectal fat and external anal sphincter.   The perineal artery branches from the internal pudendal in the anterior part of the region to supply portions of the anterior perineum.

5. **Anal Portion of the Rectum.**—The anal canal, about 4 cm. in length, passes downward and backward to connect the rectal ampulla with the exterior. The sides of the canal are related to the fat pads of the ischiorectal fossa and are liable to involvement in any infection in the fossa. Anteriorly, the anal canal is related to the central tendinous point of the perineum, the membranous part of the urethra, and the bulb. Advantage is taken of these relations in passing an instrument through a difficult stricture of the urethra. With a forefinger in the rectal ampulla, the beak of the entering instrument can be controlled and prevented from making a false passage.

The **anal canal** presents four landmarks: (1) the anocutaneous line (anal verge or rima); (2) Hilton's line (palpable more than visible); (3) the pectinate (dentate) line; and (4) the anorectal line.

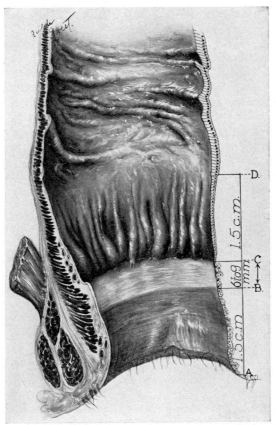

Fig. 506.—Divisions and Landmarks of the Anal Canal Viewed in Frontal Section.
A, The anocutaneous line (anal verge); B–C, pecten band; C, pectinate (dentate) line; D, anorectal line (James W. Morgan, Surg., Gynec. and Obst., Nov., 1934.)

The *anocutaneous line* marks the lower end of the gastro-intestinal tract. It is the external margin of the walls of the anus in its normal state of apposition. The epithelium superior to this line usually is thrown into folds by the action of an involuntary muscle, sometimes termed the "corrugator of the anal skin."

Hilton's white line in the living subject is decidedly blue in color and is palpable rather than visible. It marks the linear interval between the internal and external sphincters. This interval lies halfway between the anal verge and the pectinate line.

The band of tissue between the intersphincteric space and the pectinate line has a smooth surface and a glossy, shining appearance. It may be likened to a circular saw-blade, with the teeth pointing upward. These dentations interdigitate with the rectal columns of Morgagni to form the anal papillae. The appearance of this area with its dentations led Stroud to call this region the *pecten* from its resemblance to a comb (L. pecten). Miles emphasizes the significance of the pecten by describing the heavy deposit of fibrous tissue underlying it as the pathological result of inflammation, "pectenosis." He believes that it is necessary to cut this stenosing ring of fibrous tissue (pectenotomy) to cure anal fissure. The pecten is an important anatomic and clinical landmark. It is the mucocutaneous junction, and is the divide over which prolapsing masses of mucosa fall through the sphincter region. Immediately proximal to this area lies the internal hemorrhoidal ring where internal hemorrhoids develop. Caudal to this line, external hemorrhoids develop. The pecten also is the lymphatic watershed of this region. The mucous membrane and bowel above this line drain into pelvic lymph nodes. The skin distal to this line drains into the subinguinal glands by lymphatics which run around the root of the thigh. The territories of the cerebrospinal and the sympathetic nerves also meet here.

The *anorectal line* lies about 1.5 cm. proximal to the pectinate line, and between the two are the columns and crypts of Morgagni. The anorectal junction, so formed, lies 1½ inches proximal to the anocutaneous line when the canal is empty.

The muscles of the anal canal are developed strongly into **sphincters.** The circular muscle fibers of the rectum are continued downward to form the *internal sphincter* which encloses the upper two thirds of the canal. The fibers constituting the *external sphincter* are attached to the tip of the coccyx and the anococcygeal raphe behind the central point of the perineum. When the anal canal is obliterated, *i. e.*, its muscles in a state of contraction, much of the external sphincter lies distal to the internal, definitely overlapping it. When the canal is distended by digital examination, or by the passage of a formed stool, the sphincters occupy a more truly internal and external position. Even then, the lower margin of the internal sphincter is definitely proximal to the lower margin of the external sphincter. The external sphincter can be palpated easily as a definite roll of muscular tissue. The *mucosa* is attached loosely to the muscle walls, particularly in the upper part, where it is disposed in a number of vertical folds, the rectal columns of Morgagni. At their lower ends, these columns are united by semilunar folds, the anal valves. An anal fissure is produced by the tearing downward of one of the anal valves by a hard fecal mass.

The main **arterial supply** to the anal canal is from the inferior hemorrhoidal arteries, branches from the internal pudendal. The superior, middle, and inferior hemorrhoidal *veins* form an internal hemorrhoidal plexus in the submucous and subcutaneous tissue of the anal canal. This plexus presents a distinct band of dilated veins, forming what is termed the hemorrhoidal ring. Minute clusters of thin-walled veins comprising the ring lie within the columns of Morgagni. In the recesses between the columns is what is known as the hemorrhoidal zone. The superior hemorrhoidal veins pierce the muscle coat to unite in the sigmoid mesocolon in a common trunk tributary to the inferior mesenteric vein. The middle hemorrhoidal veins empty into the hypogastric (internal iliac) vein, and the inferior hemorrhoidal veins join the internal pudendal vein.

The **lymphatics** of the rectum and anal canal have a plexiform arrangement in the mucous and submucous coats. Those located above the mucocutaneous line drain into lymph glands lying on the posterior surface of the rectum, and their efferents ascend along the superior hemorrhoidal artery to end in the sacral and lumbar lymph nodes. The lymph vessels from the lower part of the canal pass to the medial group of the subinguinal nodes, whence efferent trunks pass through the femoral ring to empty into the external iliac lymph glands.

Surgical Considerations

1. **Transperineal Approach to the Membranous (Deep) Urethra, Prostate, and Seminal Vesicles.**—An exaggerated lithotomy position with the perineum parallel to the floor is the ideal position in all operations on the membranous (deep) urethra, prostate, and seminal vesicles, the purpose being to keep all tissues on a tension so that with each cut the exposure is increased. It is vital that the recto-urethralis muscle (p. 433) be kept tense.

A sound introduced into the bladder serves as a guide, and a curved incision with a forward convexity is made about 2.5 cm. anterior to the anus. By blunt dissection, the anterior prolongations of the ischiorectal fossa are opened so that, with a finger in each, the sound in the urethra can be felt between them. With bifid retractors, the transverse perineal muscles and bulb are pulled upward and the rectum downward in order to put the *central tendon* under tension. As the central tendon is cut, the recto-urethral muscle presents and in turn is severed. If tension on the recto-urethral muscle is relaxed, there is danger of entering the rectum.

The membranous urethra, prostate, seminal vesicles, and vasa deferentia can be exposed much more readily if the region about the neck of the bladder be levered into the wound by Young's intravesical retractor.

2. **Ischiorectal Abscess.**—A submucosal or subcutaneous infection about the anal canal may open into the canal or upon the skin surfaces at the margin of the anus, or extend into the ischiorectal fossa. Abscesses in the ischiorectal fossae occur for various

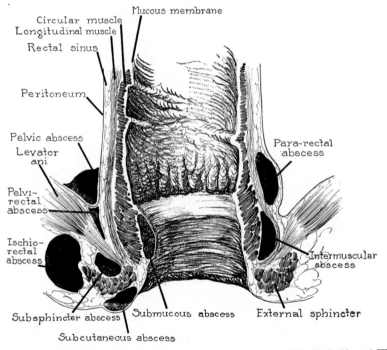

FIG. 507.—ABSCESS FORMATION IN THE ANORECTAL REGION. (M. S. Woolf, Calif. and West. Med.)

anatomical reasons. The fossa is contiguous with the rectum and anal canal which are laden with septic contents and are prone to laceration. The poorly vascularized, fatty, areolar tissue in the fossa is involved readily from the sweat glands and hair follicles in the perineal skin, a region constantly exposed to infection, trauma, and marked temperature change. The levator ani, with its upper and lower fascial coverings, usually is a sufficient barrier to intrapelvic extension of an abscess. Extension of an ischiorectal abscess follows the path of least resistance to the surface of the perineum or spreads mesially into the anal canal below the level of the levator floor. Lateral extension is limited by the obturator internus muscle and fascia and the ischial tuberosity. The abscess may open upon the perineal skin and into the anal canal, forming a complete fistulous tract. An ischiorectal abscess should be opened early to forestall the formation of fistulae and the development of extraperitoneal pelvic cellulitis from extension through the levators. Abscesses above the levators are by no means always of perineal or rectal origin, but may arise from disease of neighboring structures, such as osteitis of the sacrum and coccyx, or infection in or about the prostate and seminal vesicles which reaches the ischiorectal fossae by perforating the levator at the side of the rectum. Ischiorectal infection has been known to erode the levator ani, spread extraperitoneally, and cause perinephric abscesses (p. 406).

3. **Fistula-in-ano.**—At the anus, the skin overlaps the mucous membrane in a serrated margin, the pectinate line, which consists of the papillae of Morgagni. Between these pillars lie the anal crypts, little culdesacs surrounded by lymphoid tissue, which are subject to the same trauma as other parts of the rectal outlet. Trauma producing a break in the tissues about the anal crypts forms a point of entrance for infection. The infectious process burrows in the tissues adjacent to the anus and usually passes either through the substance of the external sphincter, or between the internal and external sphincters into the ischiorectal tissues, where an abscess develops. When the sinus tract of the infectious process has passed through or between the muscles, sphincter spasm probably prevents a return of pus to the anal canal, and the abscess may extend into the soft tissues of the buttocks, the ischiorectal space, or the extraperitoneal space of the pelvis. With increase in size, the abscess, depending upon its location, ruptures either onto the skin or into one

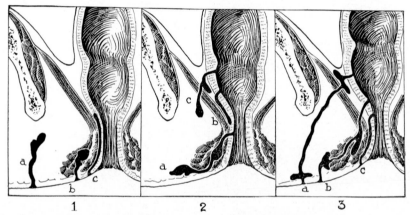

FIG. 508.—SCHEMATIC FRONTAL SECTION TO SHOW VARIETIES OF SINUSES AND FISTULAE-IN-ANO.

1, Blind external sinuses, *a*, extrasphincteric; *b*, intrasphincteric; *c*, submucous; 2, blind internal sinuses, *a*, intrasphincteric toward ischiorectal fossa; *b*, submucous; *c*, pelvirectal communicating with ischiorectal fossa through the levator ani muscle; 3, complete fistulae; *a*, extrasphincteric from above levator through ischiorectal fossa to perineal skin; *b*, transsphincteric; *c*, submucocutaneous.

of the pelvic viscera. With the appearance of a secondary opening, irrespective of its situation, a fistula is formed.

It has been customary to describe as fistulae-in-ano the "blind internal" and "blind external" fistulae which properly are sinuses and are relatively uncommon. The *external sinus* is, in the majority of instances, a fistula whose internal opening has not been demonstrated. The *internal sinus* is the beginning of almost every case of true fistula. It is improbable that more than 2 to 5 per cent of fistulae are caused by tuberculosis.

Successful *treatment* of fistulae is dependent upon finding the internal opening which is the source of trouble. When this is found, an attempt should be made to probe it; the incision should be made from this point laterally through the wall of the fistula, including any part of the anal sphincters external to the tract. When this continuity cannot be established, incision of the tract should be begun externally and the tract be followed upward to the opening into the bowel.

4. **Hemorrhoids.**—Hemorrhoids, or piles, are varicosities or dilatations of the veins of the anal canal. Those arising from the radicles of the middle hemorrhoidal vein, usually the anterior or right and left groups, are situated in the lower rectum and upper anal canal above the external sphincter in the area occupied by the columns of Morgagni. They

are called *internal hemorrhoids* to distinguish them from the dilatations of the plexuses of the inferior hemorrhoidal veins which are covered with skin: these are called *external hemorrhoids*.

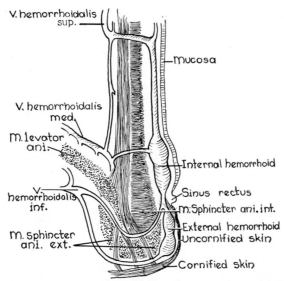

FIG. 509.—HEMORRHOIDAL VEINS SHOWING INTERNAL AND EXTERNAL HEMORRHOIDS. (R. I. Hiller.)

Digital examination for internal hemorrhoids may reveal only thickened folds of mucous membrane, but proctoscopic examination reveals three to five bluish-red longitudinal folds. When internal hemorrhoids become large, they sometimes are carried through the anus in defecation and become extremely painful. They may be so constricted by the external sphincter as to present areas of sloughing and gangrene. Bleeding

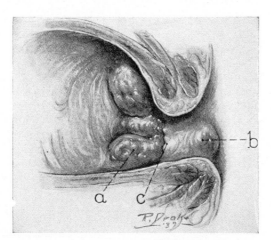

FIG. 510.—GROSS DISTINCTION BETWEEN INTERNAL AND EXTERNAL HEMORRHOIDS.
A, Internal hemorrhoid covered by mucous membrane; b, external hemorrhoid covered by skin; c, pectinate line separating two types of hemorrhoids. (Buie.)

from the eroded surface of such veins is a common occurrence and is likely to produce a severe anemia. Pain may be relieved by returning the everted varicosities through the anal orifice, but permanent relief is obtained only by their removal. The methods available for this purpose are: injection of sclerosing chemicals, excision, and clamping with cauterization.

External hemorrhoids usually are not painful unless they undergo thrombosis. If thrombosed, and particularly if infected, they form hard painful circumscribed tumors which require incision and evacuation.

5. **Rectal Prolapse and Intussusception.**—Rectal prolapse is the protrusion of part of or the entire thickness of the rectal wall through the anal orifice. In an *incomplete* or *partial prolapse*, the mucous membrane of the perineal or anal part of the rectum protrudes from the anus and fails to retract when defecation ceases. The loose connection between the mucous membrane and muscular coat of the bowel facilitates this form of prolapse. The everted mucosa remains protruded because the relaxed submucosa is unable to draw it back through the canal against the obstructing action of the sphincters. This is exemplified by the prolapse occasionally seen with hemorrhoids, which, because of their size and the traction they exert on the mucous membrane, show a marked tendency to descend and protrude through the anus. For a time, reduction is spontaneous, but becomes increasingly difficult. The prolapsed part usually is of limited extent and may involve but a part of the anal circumference.

Partial prolapse is common in early childhood, when the pelvic rectum is straighter, more vertical, and much more movable than in the adult, since it lacks the support from the fully developed pelvic organs. Prolapse occurs in adults, particularly in old age when the muscle tone of the bowel is weakened. It occurs fairly commonly with urethral stric-

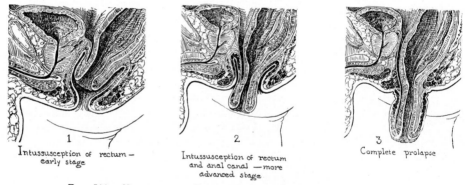

Intussusception of rectum — early stage

Intussusception of rectum and anal canal — more advanced stage

Complete prolapse

FIG. 511.—VARIETIES OF RECTAL INTUSSUSCEPTION AND PROLAPSE.

ture, enlarged prostate, and chronic bronchitis, in all of which there is a sudden and frequently recurrent increase in intra-abdominal pressure.

The comparative rarity of *complete prolapse* is accounted for by the secure manner in which the rectum is held in position. Weakening of the pelvic floor and anal sphincter, or relaxation of the rectal suspensory apparatus, including the pelvic mesocolon and its contained vessels, are predisposing causes.

The prolapsed part consists of two concentric cylinders, the outer of which is continuous above with the anal skin. The inner or enclosed cylinder ascends within it through the anus into the pelvis, where it is continuous with the pelvic colon. When a complete prolapse attains large dimensions, the peritoneum of the rectovesical or rectovaginal pouch descends and forms a distinct culdesac anteriorly between the inner and outer cylinders. Into this pouch, a loop of small intestine or piece of omentum may find its way and become incarcerated, causing a sudden or marked increase in the size of the prolapsed part. A peritoneal pouch is not formed posteriorly since the pelvic mesocolon and contained vessels descend but to a limited extent. The prolapse may assume a decided backward curve because of the resistance these structures offer to a descent of the bowel.

Prolapse may be associated with *intussusception*, wherein the invagination of some higher part of the rectum into the immediately adjoining segment below emerges through the anus. Intussusception originating in the colon, or even in the cecal segment (p. 380), may present through the anus in a similar manner. In true prolapse, the base of the outer cylinder always is continuous with the skin. In intussusception, a slitlike interval exists all around between the intussuscepted part and the anal mucous membrane.

6. Pilonidal Cyst.—A pilonidal cyst is a common congenital anomaly consisting of an epithelium-lined pocket sometimes containing hair and epithelial elements. It is located at the tip of the coccyx, generally where the neurenteric canal opens onto the skin, and usually is not recognized until brought to attention by infection, when it may assume considerable proportions and present redness, tenderness, and swelling. It ordinarily discharges through a small sinus in the midline well behind the anus.

Effective treatment consists in wide excision in order to remove all of the sinus ramifications, from any one of which the condition may recur. Complete extirpation is facilitated by delineating the tract by the injection of a dye.

7. Congenital Anomalies of the Lower Rectum and Anal Canal.—A description and explanation of the commoner congenital malformations of the lower rectum and anal canal are given under the pelvic rectum.

8. Lymphopathia Venereum (Lymphogranuloma Inguinale).—Lymphopathia venereum usually is characterized in the acute stage by mild febrile reaction, and by an inguinal adenitis which follows a minute, evanescent, and often unnoticed, primary lesion. The inguinal nodes break down soon and one or more chronic, draining sinuses result. The anus and rectum often are involved primarily or secondarily, and the commonest lesion is inflammatory rectal stricture. Surgical anatomic interest in rectal involvement in this disease lies in the lymphatic paths of extension between the external and internal genitalia and the rectum.

If the initial lesion occurs at any point on the external genitals of either sex, regional inguinal adenitis (bubo) usually results from a direct spread of infection. Inguinal involvement is more common in the male because external genital lesions are the rule, and the lymphatic extension is direct. Rectal stricture is the usual secondary manifestation in the female because the initial lesion in the female commonly is at some point along the posterior vaginal wall or on the cervix, implanted there from the lesion on the male external genital. Lymphatic drainage from these areas traverses the uterosacral ligaments which skirt the lateral walls of the rectum. The rectal lymphatics then are involved by direct anastomosis. A more direct invasion of the rectal lymphatics leading to rectal stricture is by way of the lymph vessels of the rectovaginal septum.

Explanation of the frequent involvement of the rectum in the male, and of the occasional involvement of the rectum in the female when no genital lesion, external or internal, has been demonstrated, is not so clear. Extension of the disease from the male anterior urethra to the posterior urethra eventually may involve the rectal lymphatics and cause stricture. This we believe, is an unusual method of spread. In most of our cases of rectal stricture in the male, abnormal practices (pederasty) account for the direct implantation of the virus into the rectal mucosa. A primary anal lesion may spread to the rectum by way of the anorectal lymphatics. The end-result of this invasion is perirectal fibrosis, with subsequent stricture of the rectum.

II. External Genitalia

A. PENIS

1. Definition and Division.—The penis is composed of a posterior fixed part or root, and an anterior mobile part or body. The parts constituting the *root* of the *penis* are discussed in the superficial perineal pouch of the urogenital region (p. 496).

The *body* of the *penis*, formed by the union of the cavernous bodies, begins at the apex of the urogenital diaphragm beneath the pubic angle, and is attached firmly to it by connective tissue bands. The corpora cavernosa of the penis lie side by side on the dorsum, and the corpus cavernosum of the urethra lies in the ventral groove. The corpus cavernosum urethrae at its anterior termination expands into a conical enlargement, the *glans penis*, which spreads out as a cap over the blunt anterior extremities of the corpora

cavernosa of the penis. The posterior part of the corpus cavernosum urethrae terminates posteriorly in a large, free, bulbous extremity, the *bulb* of the *urethra*. This considerably overlaps the junction of the membranous and cavernous divisions of the urethra posteriorly. The prominent margin of the glans, the *corona*, projects dorsally and laterally beyond the extremities of the corpora cavernosa penis.

2. Superficial Structures.—The skin of the penis is thin, loose, free from hair, and freely movable over the body of the organ. At its neck, the skin is folded back to form a cuff or hood, the *prepuce* or covering for the glans. Within the cavity of the prepuce, the modified skin contains the sebaceous glands secreting the smegma. Since this secretion is an admirable culture medium for micro-organisms whose normal habitat is the preputial cavity, there often occurs about the corona of the glans a more or less active inflammation of the apposed surfaces of the glans and prepuce (balanoposthitis).

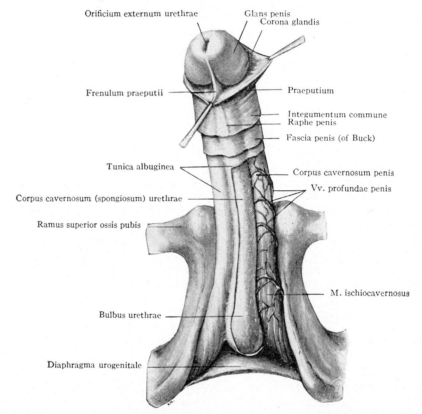

Orificium externum urethrae

Glans penis
Corona glandis

Frenulum praeputii

Praeputium

Integumentum commune
Raphe penis

Fascia penis (of Buck)

Tunica albuginea

Corpus cavernosum penis

Vv. profundae penis

Corpus cavernosum (spongiosum) urethrae

Ramus superior ossis pubis

M. ischiocavernosus

Bulbus urethrae

Diaphragma urogenitale

FIG. 512.—STRUCTURE OF THE PENIS AND ITS RELATIONSHIP TO THE SYMPHYSIS PUBIS.

This infection may establish adhesions between the prepuce and glans and obliterate the preputial cavity. On the under aspect of the glans, a well-marked fold of skin, the *frenum*, passes forward and is attached to the prepuce.

The *subcutaneous tissue* in the penis is very loose in texture, devoid of fat, and traversed by the superficial dorsal vein. It is the laxness of this tissue that gives mobility to the penis and explains the urinary and bloody extravasations producing enormous distention in the organ. The *superficial lymphatics* accompany the superficial dorsal vein and enter the subinguinal nodes. They are involved in infection about the prepuce and glans and form tender hard knots over the dorsum of the organ. Beneath the subcutaneous layer, the penis is invested by a thin, fibrous membrane, the *fascia* of the *penis* (*Buck's fascia*), which extends anteriorly to the free margin of the prepuce and is continued backward in the perineum to the posterior margin of the triangular ligament. It is difficult

at times to differentiate Buck's fascia from the tunica albuginea. Beneath Buck's fascia
are the deep dorsal nerves and vessels.

3. **Tunica Albuginea and Subjacent Erectile Tissue.**—Each erectile body is surrounded
by a distensible, elastic, resistant, fibrous envelope, the **tunica albuginea,** the trabeculae
of which surround blood spaces or areolae. Where the corpora of the penis are applied

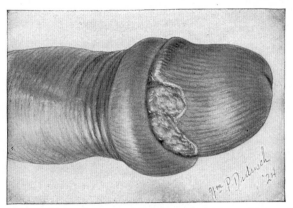

FIG. 513.—CHANCRE IN THE USUAL LOCATION IN THE CORONARY SULCUS. (Young, "Practice of Urology.")

against one another, the albuginea forms a median septum or partition, the *septum* of the
penis. The areolae or blood spaces, which form the hypertrophied vascular layer of the
urethral mucosa, are dilated and more highly developed in the corpora of the penis than
in the corpus of the urethra. The number of areolae explain why injuries to the penis are
accompanied by abundant hemorrhage, and why such hemorrhage is stopped easily by

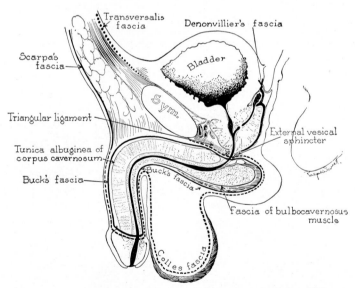

FIG. 514.—PERINEAL FASCIAE AND LINES OF URINARY EXTRAVASATION. (Hinman after Wesson.)

compression. In certain cases of gonorrhea, the blood spaces in the cavernous body of the
urethra are involved, and as a result, elasticity and dilatability may be lost to the extent
that there is a downward curved erection of the penis and acute pain, a condition known
as *chordee*. Wounds involving the erectile tissue, if transverse and extensive, are followed
by scar tissue formation and loss of erectile power over the region distal to the injury

Fracture may occur when the bodies have undergone calcification or are subjected to violence in a state of erection.

4. **Vessels.**—The vessels and nerves to the erectile organs are the deep and main supply to the penis. The *arteries* supplying the erectile tissue are the terminal branches of the

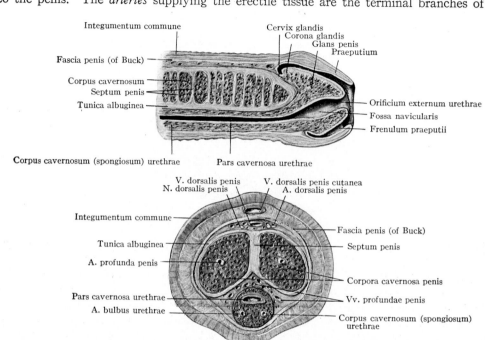

FIG. 515.—SAGITTAL AND CROSS SECTIONS THROUGH THE ANTERIOR PART OF THE URETHRA.

internal pudendal, the paired bulbo-urethral, dorsal, and cavernous arteries. The dorsal arteries to the penis lie on the corpora of the penis, deep to the fascia and lateral to the deep dorsal vein. The cavernous arteries penetrate the corpora of the penis at their posterior extremities and run axially postero-anteriorly.

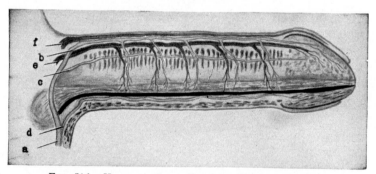

FIG. 516.—VESSELS OF THE PENIS IN SAGITTAL SECTION.

a, Internal pudendal artery; *b*, dorsal artery of the penis; *c*, cavernous branch of the dorsal artery; *d*, artery of corpus spongiosum urethrae; *e*, deep dorsal vein; *f*, superficial dorsal vein. (Bickham, "Operative Surgery.")

The *veins* returning the blood from the erectile tissue lie deep to the fascia and empty mainly into the deep dorsal vein.

The penile *lymphatics* are collected into two main groups, an extensive one from the glans and a network from the skin. Both of these groups empty into large lymphatic trunks which follow the dorsal vein of the penis and, at the root of the organ, pass to the inguinal

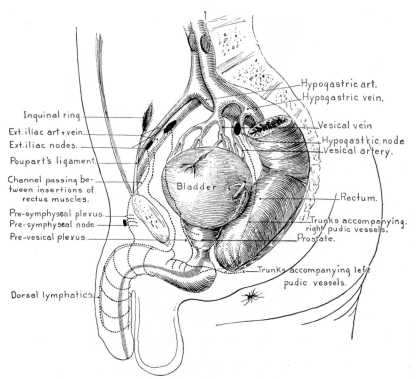

Fig. 517.—Diagram Showing the Course Taken by the Lymphatic Channels Draining the Urethra.

Lymphatics from the penile portion form part of the dorsal lymphatics. They do not enter the sub-inguinal nodes. Some drain to a small channel passing between the insertions of the right and left rectus muscles to enter the external iliac node. There are anastomoses beneath the symphysis with the lymphatics of the bulbar and membranous portions of the urethra. The bulbar lymphatics drain mainly into trunks accompanying the internal pudic vessels to enter the hypogastric nodes. At the apex of the prostate there are anastomoses with the prevesical lymphatic plexus, with the prostatic plexus, and doubtless with the lymphatics of the ejaculatory ducts and vasa deferentia. (Young, "Practice of Urology.")

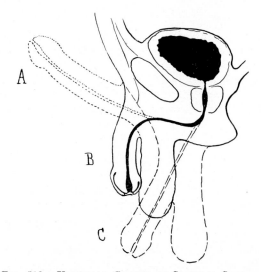

Fig. 518.—Urethral Curves in Sagittal Section.

A, During erection; B, in repose; C, penis drawn down to admit straight instrument.

and iliac lymph glands. The group of lymphatics from the skin empties into the superficial subinguinal nodes, while the group from the glans passes to the deep subinguinal nodes and thence to the external iliac lymph glands through the femoral canal. It is evident that operations for carcinoma of the penis cannot be satisfactory unless undertaken before lymphatic involvement has extended from the deep inguinal nodes through the femoral canal to the iliac nodes.

5. Cavernous, Penile, or Mobile Urethra.—The cavernous division of the urethra, about 18 to 20 cm. long, is by far the longest portion and extends from the inferior or superficial layer of the urogenital diaphragm to the external meatus. After piercing the urogenital diaphragm, the urethra enters the bulb about 1 cm. in front of its rounded posterior extremity. In traversing the cavernous body of the urethra, the urethra lies nearer the dorsal than the ventral aspect. The bulbous portion of the urethra usually is capacious and forms the most dependent part of the perineal curve. The *bulbo-urethral glands* (of Cowper) (p. 499) open into the urethra at its lower or posterior wall. The external orifice is the narrowest part of the canal and may require incision to permit the passage of instruments which then pass readily through the remainder of the canal.

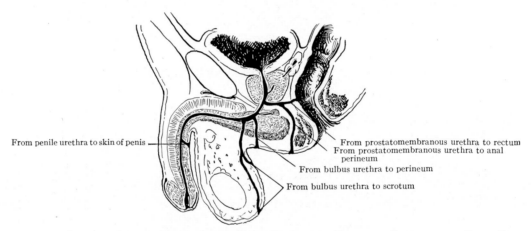

From penile urethra to skin of penis

From prostatomembranous urethra to rectum
From prostatomembranous urethra to anal perineum
From bulbus urethra to perineum
From bulbus urethra to scrotum

FIG. 519.—SAGITTAL SECTION THROUGH THE MALE PELVIS AND EXTERNAL GENITALIA TO SHOW URETHRAL FISTULAE.

Strictures may occur at any point in the cavernous urethra and, when several are present, the one first encountered must be dilated to full size before the next is dealt with. The passage of a sound along a normal urethra into the bladder presents no difficulty if the beak is kept in contact with the roof of the urethra after the navicular fossa has been passed. It then will find its way more readily into the membranous portion. Once this level is reached, little difficulty is encountered in entering the bladder, save in certain cases of enlarged prostate where the corresponding segment of the urethra becomes elongated and acquires a much accentuated anteroposterior curve.

SURGICAL CONSIDERATIONS

1. Phimosis and Circumcision.—When an excessively long narrow prepuce, because of its constriction, cannot be drawn back over the glans, the condition is known as *phimosis*. Adhesions between the deep surface of the prepuce and superficial surface of the glans may prove partly causative. The narrow preputial orifice hinders urinary outflow and causes straining. The redundant prepuce sometimes forms a sort of reservoir into which part of the voided urine settles, to be discharged subsequently through the narrow aperture. Decomposing urine is likely to set up infection of the apposed surfaces of the glans (*balanitis*) and the prepuce (*posthitis*), which may be succeeded by a retrograde urethritis and cystitis.

Circumcision is indicated whenever an obvious phimosis exists. Adhesions of the prepuce to the glans must be freed, and the prepuce be pulled back over the corona of the glans before circumcision is begun. When the prepuce is cut away, the outer skin of the cuff retracts, but the deep layer remains in contact with the glans. The deep layer of the prepuce is trimmed off the glans to a point one half of the distance back to the coronary sulcus, special care being taken to preserve the frenum. The tributaries of the dorsal vein and arteries require ligation, as may the small artery of the frenum. The cut edge of the skin is sutured to the deep layer of the prepuce.

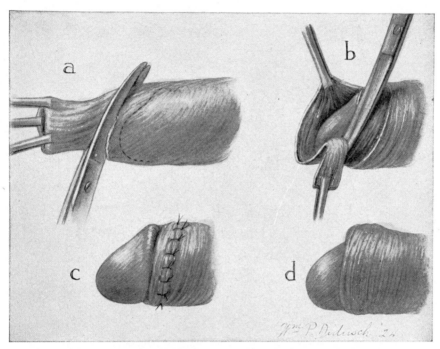

FIG. 520.—CIRCUMCISION.
a, The prepuce is drawn down and the redundant skin is excised. A long clamp usually is applied proximal to line of excision to avoid injury to the glans; *b*, the redundant inner (mucous membrane) layer of prepuce is excised; *c*, the closure is by interrupted sutures; *d*, this shows the partial covering of the glans when the proper amount of prepuce is removed. (Young, "Practice of Urology.")

2. Paraphimosis.—Paraphimosis results when the prepuce, having been drawn back to uncover the glans, cannot be drawn forward again, but forms a constricting band behind the corona. The glans may become edematous and engorged, but the prepuce, because of its laxity of structure and the obstruction to the return of its venous flow, swells to such a degree as to form an edematous collar surrounding the neck of the penis. Behind this constricting band, there often is a deep excoriated sulcus and a second edematous band less marked than the first. The penis seems to take an upward bend at the neck, the appearance being caused mainly by the large amount of swelling about the frenum. When the tense edge of the preputial ring exerts an unusual amount of constriction, circulation is seriously interfered with and ulceration, or even gangrene, of the foreskin and head of the penis may occur. Except for the rich blood supply of the glans, this complication would be much more frequent.

Treatment consists in replacing the prepuce by exercising heavy pressure on the glans with the thumbs, while maintaining traction on the prepuce with the encircling fingers. In advanced stages, the constricting preputial ring must be incised.

3. Amputation of the Penis.—Carcinoma of the penis is the usual condition for which amputation of the organ is required. Removal may be partial or complete, depending upon the amount of involvement.   For *partial amputation*, a skin flap may be fashioned from the ventral aspect of the organ and folded over the end of the stump to provide a satisfactory covering.   Particular attention should be paid to the removal of Buck's fascia from the stump as far back as the suspensory ligament (Young).   The inguinal lymph nodes should be removed on both sides as thoroughly as are the axillary nodes in operation for cancer of the breast.   The dissection should be carried through the saphenous opening, and the glands occupying the femoral canal (p. 703) also should be removed.

For recurrent epithelioma of the penis or an original growth extending more than 2.5 cm. behind the corona, it is imperative to perform a *complete amputation*.   This operation should be combined with bilateral excision of the inguinal glands.   The operation has

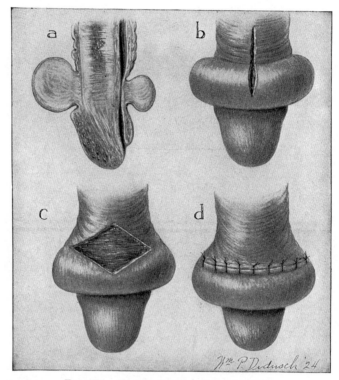

FIG. 521.—OPERATION FOR PARAPHIMOSIS.

a, The longitudinal section shows the point of constriction proximal to the swelling; *b*, longitudinal incision divides the constricting band; *c, d*, show plastic procedure to eradicate the constricting band.   The edema disappears later.   (Young, "Practice of Urology.")

the advantage that not only the primary growth and inguinal glands are removed, but also the whole of the cutaneous lymphatic tract.

Incision for this operation is made down the midline from the penoscrotal junction to the central point of the perineum and deepened until the corpus cavernosum urethrae is reached and defined.   After separation of the corpus from the urethra at the urogenital diaphragm, attention is turned to the crura, which are traced from the main body of the penis to their attachments to the ischiopubic rami.   Each crus is dissected completely from the bone.   The suspensory ligament of the penis is incised and the penis is dissected downward.   After the dorsal vessels are secured where they pierce the diaphragm, the whole organ may be removed.   The operation is completed by removing the inguinal glands on each side.   The divided urethra then is brought down into the perineum, cut off to an appropriate length, and stitched to the lips of the wound just anterior to the anus.

B SCROTUM AND SPERMATIC CORD

1. Scrotum.—The scrotum is of the nature of a bag, within which are lodged the testes and the lower portions of the spermatic cords. Originally, it consists of two folds, one on each side of the urogenital furrow. Later, these fuse and a vestige of the fusion remains as the median raphe, continued into the perineal skin behind the scrotum and along the lower aspect of the penis, anteriorly. Its homologue in the female remains permanently separated as the labia majora.

The *scrotal skin* is of delicate texture, usually darker in color than that in the adjoining regions, and is semitransparent and distensible. Contraction of the subjacent dartos causes it to present a wrinkled or corrugated appearance. The *dartos* tunic is a smooth, thin layer of involuntary muscle lying immediately beneath the skin and intimately adhering to it (skin-dartos layer). It is prolonged backward into the superficial perineal fascia (of Colles) (p. 495). This platysma-like muscle contracts with cold and relaxes with heat; its tonicity decreases with age. At the median raphe, the dartos gives off a sagittally disposed septum dividing the scrotum into right and left pouches, each of which forms a distinct sac containing the corresponding testicle and its coverings. This partition limits a scrotal effusion to one or the other space.

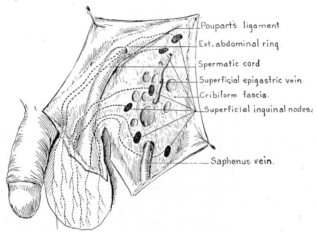

FIG. 522.—DIAGRAM OF THE LYMPHATIC DRAINAGE OF THE SCROTUM.

There are about six main trunks. The anterior trunks run well up on the base of the penis. None pass under the spermatic cord. All drain into the subinguinal nodes. None pass through into the deep nodes or the iliac nodes. Deep dissection of femoral triangle is not necessary in excision of these glands. (Young, "Practice of Urology.")

The dartos layer is connected to the subjacent testicles and their envelopes by *subdartos connective tissue (Cowper's fascia)*. This tissue is sufficiently loose to permit the testis, epididymis, and cord to move about freely beneath the skin and to allow their easy enucleation when the skin-dartos layer is sectioned. Within the potential spaces of this loose tissue, which is freely continuous with the cellular tissue of the perineum, penis, and abdominal wall, hematomas and urinary extravasations readily localize. This tissue is traversed by numerous small vessels which must be ligated carefully to prevent postoperative scrotal hemorrhage. The *scrotal lymphatics* form an exceedingly rich network, the main stems of which drain to the medial group of subinguinal glands.

The *cremaster muscle* (p. 290), with its looplike fibers, forms a partial investment for the testis and cord. As these thin muscle strands reach the gland, they thin out and are fused to the parietal layer of the tunica vaginalis, in company with a fibrous layer derived from the internal spermatic (infundibuliform) fascia (p. 294). By the contractions of this musculofibrous layer, the testis is drawn toward the subcutaneous inguinal ring. Scratching the skin of the medial aspect of the thigh produces a strong cremasteric contraction, the *cremasteric reflex*

2. **Tunica Vaginalis Testis.**—The tunica vaginalis testis, derived from the vaginal process of the peritoneum (p. 292), lines the inner aspect of the scrotum and sheathes most of the testis and epididymis. The remainder of the funicular or upper portion of the process (vaginal ligament) (p. 294) extends from the internal ring to the epididymis and lies among the elements of the spermatic cord.

As is true of all serous cavities, the tunica vaginalis has a visceral and a parietal leaf with a potential cavity between them. The *visceral layer* is closely adherent to the fibrous covering of the testis and epididymis (tunica albuginea), and dips in between the upper part of the testis and epididymis to form a pouch, the digital fossa or sinus of the epididymis. The visceral serosa extends for a short distance upward along the cord, covering it upon each side and in front. The part of the testis not covered by the visceral layer of the tunica vaginalis corresponds to the posterior border of the hilum of the gland, where its vessels enter and leave and where the excretory duct (vas deferens) passes upward into the cord. The *parietal layer* is separated from the scrotum by a thin layer of extravaginal cellular tissue. It is resistant, but may be distended by accumulation of fluid in a vaginal hydrocele.

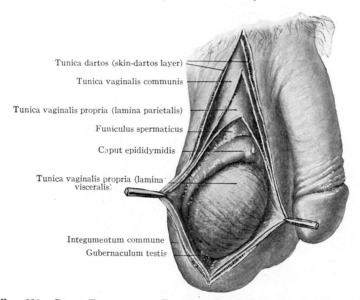

Tunica dartos (skin-dartos layer)
Tunica vaginalis communis
Tunica vaginalis propria (lamina parietalis)
Funiculus spermaticus
Caput epididymidis
Tunica vaginalis propria (lamina visceralis)
Integumentum commune
Gubernaculum testis

Fig. 523.—Right Testicle and Terminal Portion of the Spermatic Cord with Their Coverings.

3. **Epididymis and Testis (Testicle).**—The term "testicle" in this discussion includes the spermatic gland (testis) and its mass of collecting tubules (epididymis). The testicle, loosely suspended by the spermatic cord and its investing tunics, is in contact with the posterior wall of the scrotum and is attached to its base by the *scrotal ligament* (p. 293).

The **epididymis** is a crescent-shaped body connected with, and surmounting, the posterior border of the testis. It is composed mainly of an elaborately coiled tube connected at the upper pole of the testis with the ducts (vasa efferentia) emerging from the superior pole of the gland. By its lower extremity, the epididymis is continued into the *ductus* (*vas*) *deferens*. The epididymis consists of three parts: an upper expanded portion, the *globus major* or *head*, which surmounts the upper pole of the testis; a smaller, lower extremity, the *globus minor* or *tail;* and an intervening portion, the *body*. Most of the epididymis is invested by the tunica vaginalis. Occasionally, it is connected less intimately with the testis than usual, the connection taking the form of a duplication of the tunica vaginalis. In *epididymectomy*, an anterior approach should be used and the epididymis be very carefully disengaged from the testis to avoid injury to the testicular vessels.

Each lobule of the **testis** consists of greatly convoluted *seminiferous tubules*, from the epithelial cells of which the spermatozoa are formed. As the tubules approach the mediastinum of the testis, they unite to form a number of ductlike passages which converge at the upper extremity of the gland into the *efferent ductules*. These ductules form the mass of the globus major and open separately into a single canal, the duct of the epididymis, which forms an exceedingly tortuous passage, continued into the vas deferens at the lower extremity of the gland.

The pearly white *tunica albuginea* surrounding the testis and epididymis is a fibrous layer somewhat resembling in appearance the sclerotic layer of the eyeball. From the deep aspect of this covering, numerous fibrous septa pass radially backward to the connective tissue at the hilum of the testis (*mediastinum testis*).

A knowledge of the normal relationships between the testis and epididymis is important in conducting the examination of these parts. The normal testis is smooth, firm, and elastic. Squeezing it beyond a certain point causes a peculiarly nauseating pain, normal testicle sensation. The different portions of the epididymis may be differentiated readily, particularly the globus major. Inflammatory enlargement of the testis and epididymis is produced by tuberculosis, gonorrhea, and syphilis.

Epididymitis is commonly of tuberculous, gonorrheal, or pyogenic origin. Theoretically, if the globus minor is involved first, a descending infection is responsible, either gonococcal or nonspecific pyogenic. If the globus major is involved first, tuberculosis is responsible Whether the primary focus of genital tuberculosis is in the seminal vesicles or in the testis is debatable, since infection may travel directly or by the blood stream and

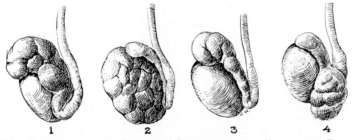

Fig. 524.—Location of the Principal Lesions of the Testis and Epididymis.

1, Acute epididymitis; 2, acute orchitis; 3, chronic tuberculous epididymitis; 4, chronic gonorrheal epididymitis. (Testut and Jacob.)

lymphatics. When the inflammatory process involves bilaterally the duct of the epididymis or the beginning of the vas deferens, sterility is the inevitable consequence. Because of the intimate connection between the epididymis and testis, reciprocal infection is common (epididymo-orchitis). A gradual enlargement of the testis, accompanied by diminished testicle sensation, suggests syphilis; rapid enlargement of the testis, in the absence of an inflammatory lesion or injury, suggests malignancy.

4. Spermatic Cord.—The spermatic cord begins at the posterosuperior margin of the testicle, to which organ it supplies a supporting pedicle within the scrotum, and ends at the abdominal inguinal ring. The structures comprising the cord are the deferent duct and the vessels and nerves of the testicle. These structures are united by loose cellular tissue within a common sheath (p. 294). The *scrotal course* of the spermatic cord ascends almost vertically to the front of the pubic crest, where it can be palpated readily through the scrotal tissues. After running an *inguinal course* to the deep inguinal ring, the constituent elements run in various directions in the pelvic extraperitoneal space. The size of the cord occasionally is increased by a hydrocele (p. 297), an encapsulated mass of fat (lipoma), or a group of varicose veins (varicocele).

The *deferent duct* (*vas*) begins in the tail of the epididymis, of which it is the prolongation and with the pathologic changes of which it is allied. A thickened vas deferens with tuberculous epididymitis indicates upward extension of the disease. The firm consistency of the muscular wall of the vas is recognized readily among the other elements of the cord.

Normally, the vas is bluish-white resembling cartilage, smooth, and supple; when inflamed by tuberculosis, it is elongated and presents a rosary-like appearance. It is related anteriorly to the anterior or spermatic group of veins surrounding the testicular artery and to the remains of the vaginal process of peritoneum. Because of the latter relationship, the sac of a congenital inguinal hernia usually is found anterior to the vas. Posteriorly, the vas is related to the deferent group of veins.

The *arteries* of the cord are the testicular (internal spermatic) artery of the vas and external spermatic artery from the inferior epigastric. The testicular artery branches from the abdominal aorta in the lumbo-iliac region and engages the cord at the abdominal

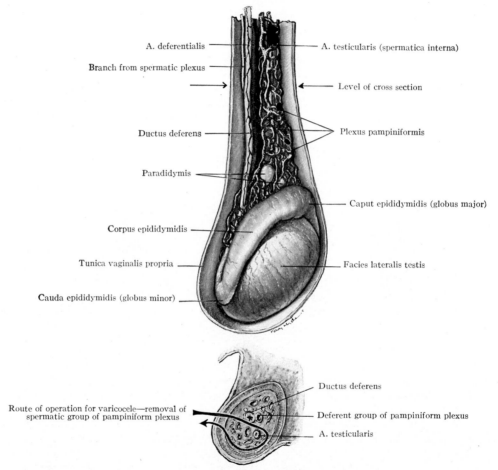

A. deferentialis

A. testicularis (spermatica interna)

Branch from spermatic plexus

Level of cross section

Ductus deferens

Plexus pampiniformis

Paradidymis

Caput epididymidis (globus major)

Corpus epididymidis

Tunica vaginalis propria

Facies lateralis testis

Cauda epididymidis (globus minor)

Ductus deferens

Route of operation for varicocele—removal of spermatic group of pampiniform plexus

Deferent group of pampiniform plexus

A. testicularis

FIG. 525.—LATERAL VIEW AND CROSS SECTION OF THE RIGHT SPERMATIC CORD AND TESTICLE.
Cross section illustrates the removal of the spermatic group of veins of the pampiniform plexus for varicocele.

inguinal ring. Within the cord, it is so surrounded by the anterior or spermatic group of veins as to be masked in the course of operation. The artery of the vas deferens is a branch of the superior vesical artery and accompanies the duct to its origin, being everywhere adherent to it and loosely incorporated within its sheath. Because of the free anastomosis between the testicular artery and the artery of the vas, division of the former is devoid of serious consequences if the integrity of the artery to the vas is preserved.

The *veins* of the cord arise in the testis and epididymis and are remarkable for their number, size, and tendency to become varicose. Those emerging from the testis are joined by others from the globus major and all ascend within the cord in a plexiform manner (pampiniform plexus). They are alluded to surgically as an anterior or spermatic group about the testicular artery and a posterior or deferent group intimately associated with the deferent duct. The anterior group is more prone to become varicose.

The *lymphatics* of the cord and testicle follow the spermatic vessels throughout their course and terminate in the external iliac glands or lumbar nodes about the aorta and vena cava.

In addition to the elements just enumerated, the external spermatic (cremasteric) artery and genital (external spermatic) branch of the genitofemoral nerve accompany the structures of the spermatic cord.

Surgical Considerations

1. **Anomalies in the Position of the Testicle.**—Abnormalities in the position of the testicle usually are of a congenital nature and result from some defect in the descent of the testis into the scrotum.

In *inversion*, the testicle reaches the scrotum, but occupies a variety of twisted or inverted positions within it, designated according to the position of the epididymis. In the superior type of inversion, the epididymis surmounts the testicle and runs horizontally forward. The inversion is anterior if the epididymis is anterosuperior rather than posterosuperior, the testicle having rotated forward 180 degrees through its transverse axis.

Torsion of the entire testicular mass may occur within the scrotum so that the cord is twisted in its extravaginal portion. To allow twisting to occur, the loose areolar connections between the outer surface of the tunica vaginalis and the skin-dartos layer of the scrotum must be broken. A *lateral* torsion is lateral or medial accordingly as the epididymis lies on its lateral or medial aspect. When the tunica vaginalis furnishes an abnormally long mesentery-like duplication to the testis and epididymis, torsion may be intravaginal. Twisting effectively occludes the veins but not the arteries to the gland, so that the tissue distal to the twist becomes a hemorrhagic infarct.

In *irregularities in the descent of the testicle* (*retained or undescended testicle*), the gland may not reach the scrotum, but be retained somewhere in its normal course of descent between the abdominal position and the scrotum. Strictly speaking, the term *cryptorchidism* applies to those cases in which one or both of the testes are hidden from view, but it has come to include all varieties of retention. The testicle may lie in contact with the posterior abdominal wall (abdominal or supravaginal retention), in the iliac fossa (iliac retention), or at some point between the subcutaneous inguinal ring and the upper part of the scrotum. An incompletely descended testicle often is associated with a patent vaginal process (peritoneovaginal canal) and a congenital inguinal hernia (p. 295).

Not only may the testicle fail to reach the scrotum and be retained at some point along the line of normal descent, but it may migrate to an aberrant or *ectopic position* outside the normal course. It may miss the inguinal canal and emerge by way of the femoral opening to an anterior position on the thigh (femoral ectopia). More frequently, the testicle, after traversing the inguinal canal, descends beyond its normal position and comes to lie in the perineum, anterior to the anus (perineal ectopia). The testicle has been found in the true pelvis (intrapelvic ectopia) beneath the bladder.

2. **Varicocele and Its Operative Treatment.**—In varicocele, there is dilation, elongation, and tortuosity of the veins of the spermatic cord (pampiniform plexus). It is much more common on the left than on the right side, and is accentuated just above the testis. In some instances, the normal veins are increased greatly in size with no appreciable increase in number, while in others, the number of veins is increased markedly. When the patient stands, the veins form curious loops and coils within the cord which suggest to the touch a "bag of worms." The bulk of the mass of veins belongs to the anterior group surrounding the testicular artery. When the patient lies down, the veins empty themselves and the varicocele disappears.

Among the many explanations of the cause of varicosity in the spermatic veins are lack of external support, great length and tortuosity of the veins, and imperfect development of the valves. The union of the left spermatic vein with the left renal vein at a right angle,

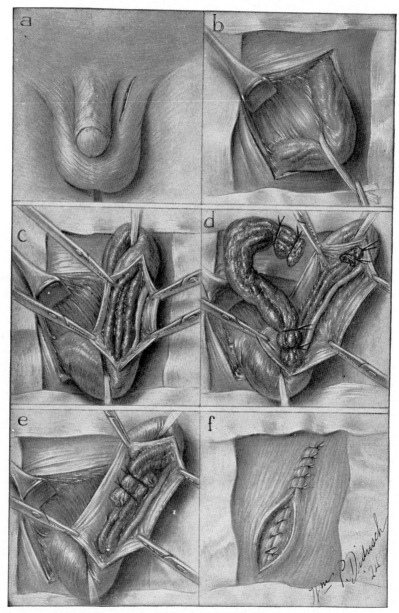

FIG. 526.—OPERATION FOR VARICOCELE.

a, High scrotal incision; *b*, cord freed and drawn out; *c*, covering of the cord opened, exposing veins and vas; *d*, resection and removal of redundant veins; double ligature of stump with catgut; veins, vas, and artery of vas preserved; *e*, ends of veins bound together to elevate and support testis; *f*, closure of skin-dartos layer and sheath of cord. (Young, "Practice of Urology.")

together with the fact that it is overlain by the sigmoid colon, the weight of which, in cases of constipation, may impede the venous return, are judged to impede venous flow. These theories do not explain the occurrence of varicocele in the young and its comparative absence in the old, in whom conditions supposedly are ideal for its development.

The approach for *excision of a varicocele* is through the skin-dartos layer in a low inguinal or high scrotal position. The finger is hooked around the cord to draw it outward into the wound. After division of the sheath of the cord and lateral retraction of the margins, the vessels are exposed and the anterior or spermatic group of veins is carefully sepa-

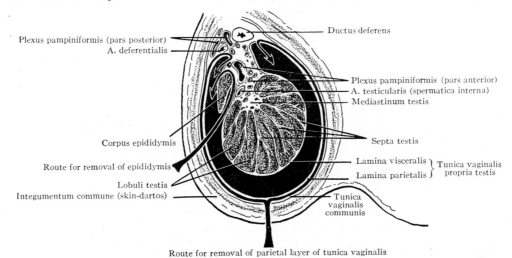

Plexus pampiniformis (pars posterior)
A. deferentialis
Ductus deferens
Plexus pampiniformis (pars anterior)
A. testicularis (spermatica interna)
Mediastinum testis
Corpus epididymis
Septa testis
Route for removal of epididymis
Lamina visceralis ⎤ Tunica vaginalis
Lamina parietalis ⎦ propria testis
Lobuli testis
Integumentum commune (skin-dartos)
Tunica vaginalis communis
Route for removal of parietal layer of tunica vaginalis

FIG. 527.—SECTION THROUGH THE MIDDLE OF THE RIGHT TESTIS, EPIDIDYMIS, AND SCROTUM. One arrow indicates the route to anterior resection of the epididymis; the other that for excision of the parietal layer of the tunica vaginalis for hydrocele.

rated from the posterior or deferent group which is recognized easily by its close relation with the vas. One inch or more of the isolated group of varicose veins is excised between ligatures and the proximal and distal extremities of the divided vessels are approximated and sutured. This supports the testis and keeps it from falling to the bottom of the

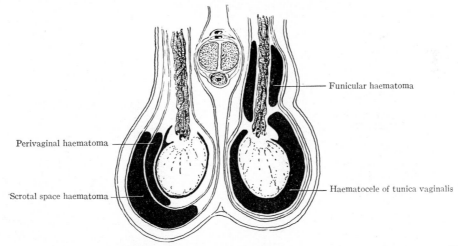

Funicular haematoma
Perivaginal haematoma
Scrotal space haematoma
Haematocele of tunica vaginalis

FIG. 528.—SCHEMATIC FRONTAL SECTION OF SCROTUM AND CONTENTS TO SHOW THE LOCATION OF HEMORRHAGIC EFFUSIONS.

scrotum. As the testicular artery and nerves are associated inextricably with the corresponding veins, they, of necessity, are included in the mass excised.

3. **Hydrocele.**—A hydrocele is a circumscribed collection of fluid usually occupying the cavity of the tunica vaginalis (vaginal hydrocele), but sometimes occurring in the spermatic cord. In the more common **primary form,** *vaginal hydrocele*, the fluid collects

slowly, unaccompanied by pain or evident distress. This hydrocele occasionally attains an enormous size, greatly distending the scrotum. A type frequently seen is that associated with incomplete obliteration of the funicular part of the vaginal process above the tunica vaginalis (*funiculovaginal hydrocele*). This variety may extend superiorly to any

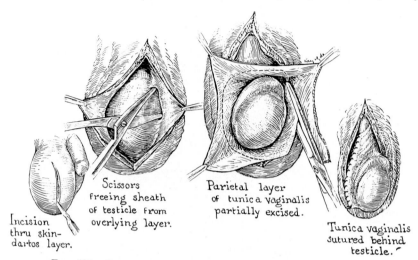

Incision thru skin-dartos layer.

Scissors freeing sheath of testicle from overlying layer.

Parietal layer of tunica vaginalis partially excised.

Tunica vaginalis sutured behind testicle.

FIG. 529.—OPERATION FOR HYDROCELE OF TUNICA VAGINALIS.

level in the spermatic cord and reach even the internal abdominal ring. This condition resembles closely an inguinal hernia. The contents of a hydrocele cannot be returned to the abdominal cavity.

The acute or **secondary form** of *vaginal hydrocele* is associated with **inflammation of** the testis and epididymis.

FEMALE PERINEUM AND EXTERNAL GENITALIA

I. FEMALE PERINEUM

A. ANTERIOR PERINEUM

1. Superficial Compartment of the Urogenital Diaphragm and Its Contents.—The superficial compartment of the urogenital diaphragm in the female is the homologue of the penile compartment in the anterior perineum of the male. It contains the roots of the corpora cavernosa of the clitoris, the bulb of the vestibule, and the vulvovaginal or major vestibular glands (of Bartholin). The inferior wall of the pouch is an exceedingly thin perineal fascia and the roof, the inferior fascia of the urogenital diaphragm. The urethra and vaginal orifice traverse the compartment.

The *clitoris* lies so buried within the subcutaneous tissue and labia that only the glans appears when the labia are separated. The body forms a sharp downward bend from the

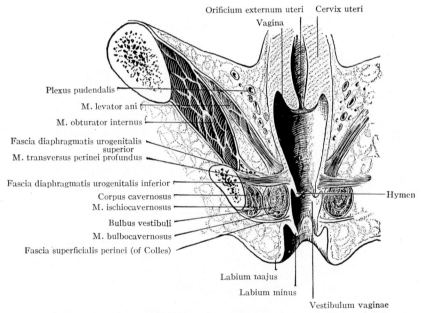

Orificium externum uteri Cervix uteri
Vagina

Plexus pudendalis

M. levator ani

M. obturator internus

Fascia diaphragmatis urogenitalis
superior
M. transversus perinei profundus

Fascia diaphragmatis urogenitalis inferior

Corpus cavernosus
M. ischiocavernosus

Bulbus vestibuli
M. bulbocavernosus

Fascia superficialis perinei (of Colles)

Hymen

Labium majus

Labium minus

Vestibulum vaginae

FIG. 530.—DIAGRAMMATIC FRONTAL SECTION THROUGH THE FEMALE PELVIS AND UROGENITAL PERINEUM TO SHOW HOMOLOGY WITH THE MALE PERINEUM (Fig. 499).

fixed diverging crura and is fixed to the lower part of the symphysis by a diminutive suspensory ligament.

The *bulb of the vestibule* is an imperfectly developed mass of erectile tissue about the vaginal orifice, corresponding to the erectile tissue in the corpus cavernosum urethrae of the male. In the female, the fusion of the two halves of this structure is not nearly so complete as in the male, for the vagina and urethra divide the bulb into two lateral portions which are connected only slightly anteriorly by a narrow intermediate part. The divisions of the bulb rest on the inferior fascia of the urogenital diaphragm, and their presence about the urethra explains the vascularity of tumors about the urinary meatus (caruncles). The intimate connection of the vestibular glands (of Bartholin) with the bulb explains the hemorrhage sometimes following extirpation of these glands. The trauma of labor may rupture the bulb and cause extensive hematomas which undergo thrombosis.

The *major vestibular glands* (of Bartholin) lie one on each side of the vaginal orifice deep to the bulb, but superficial to the urogenital diaphragm. They are located superficially in the posterior extremities of the labia majora. Enlarged glands, palpated between the thumb placed over the labium majus and the forefinger in the vagina, have the resistance of an indurated lymph node. The duct runs through the base of the labium minus to open in the groove separating the labium minus from the hymen at the junction of the posterior and middle thirds of the depression. By incising the labium minus a little lateral to this

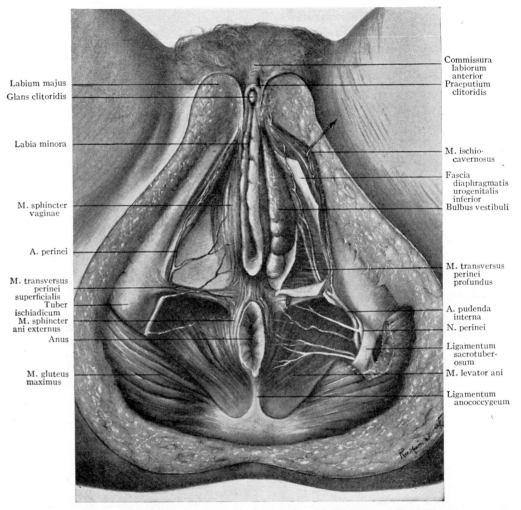

Labium majus
Glans clitoridis

Labia minora

M. sphincter
vaginae

A. perinei

M. transversus
perinei
superficialis
Tuber
ischiadicum
M. sphincter
ani externus
Anus

M. gluteus
maximus

Commissura
labiorum
anterior
Praeputium
clitoridis

M. ischio-
cavernosus

Fascia
diaphragmatis
urogenitalis
inferior
Bulbus vestibuli

M. transversus
perinei
profundus

A. pudenda
interna
N. perinei

Ligamentum
sacrotuber-
osum
M. levator ani

Ligamentum
anococcygeum

FIG. 531.—SUPERFICIAL AND DEEP STRUCTURES OF THE FEMALE PERINEUM.
On the right the elements of the superficial perineal compartment are exposed; on the left the inferior fascia of the urogenital diaphragm is incised to show the structures of the deep perineal compartment.

groove, the vascular bulb can be avoided and the gland located on the inferior fascia of the urogenital diaphragm. These glands are functionally active during sexual excitement, their secretion acting as a lubricant. Infection, almost exclusively gonococcal, reaches their branching tubules through the ducts, patent during intercourse, and may lie dormant, later to result in abscess or cyst formation. An abscess should be incised downward. Cysts or chronically infected glands are best treated by complete excision.

2. **Urethra.**—Owing to its relations to the external genitalia, the urethral orifice is exposed constantly to infection from without. Its position under the resistant pubic arch

renders the urethra liable to damage from prolonged pressure in labor or in pelvic tumors. It is well protected from external injury by its position between the thighs.

An important barrier to bacterial infection of the urinary tract by way of the urethra are the delicate mucous folds, the urethral labia, which meet over the urethral orifice. These are seen best when the hymen is intact, or in multiparae. They are developed in association with the hymen and project beyond the urethral orifice somewhat as the labia minora cover the introitus.

The urethra measures 3 to 4 cm. in length and has an average caliber of 2 to 8 mm., but is easily dilated. The external orifice lies between the labia minora immediately anterior to the vaginal opening and posterior to the clitoris.

On either side of the midline, close to the posterior margin of the urethral orifice, lie the minute openings of the *para-urethral ducts* (of Skene). They are from 1 to 2 cm. long and are the common excretory passages for small groups of tubular *para-urethral glands* located within the wall of the urethra. They are the homologues of the prostatic ducts in

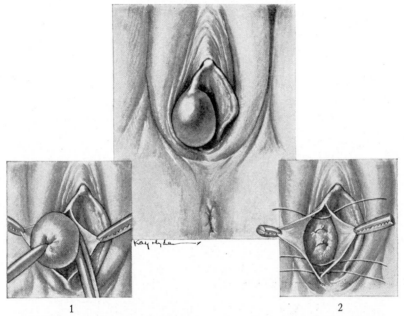

FIG. 532.—BARTHOLIN'S GLAND CYST AND THE STEPS IN ITS REMOVAL.
1, Cyst enucleated; 2, pedicle ligated—sutures placed for closure of incision.

the male, and sometimes open into the posterior urethral wall just inside the external urinary orifice.

The urethra has pelvic and perineal divisions. The *intrapelvic portion*, about 2 to 3 cm. long, begins at the vesical orifice 2 to 3 cm. behind the symphysis, and terminates where the canal penetrates the urogenital diaphragm. At the vesical neck, the internal vesical sphincter (which controls urination) surrounds the urethra. The intrapelvic portion is in relation anteriorly with the vascular tissue between the vagina and pubes.

The *perineal portion* is about 1 cm. long and traverses the urogenital diaphragm about 1 to 2 cm. below the subpubic angle. It is related anteriorly with the transverse ligament of the pubes, which separates the canal from the dorsal vein of the clitoris. The urethra opens into the vaginal vestibule about 2 cm. posterior to the clitoris.

3. **Central Point of the Perineum.**—The central point of the perineum is a fibromuscular tendinous mass formed from the criss-crossing fibers of the anal sphincters, constricting muscles of the vagina, transverse perineal muscles, and the levator ani muscles. In pregnancy, because of the inherent elasticity of this composite, it gradually distends to

sustain, direct, and support the fetus. When the elasticity is insufficient, or the exerting force too strong or too precipitous, the perineal body ruptures. The tear may involve only the superficial muscle layers and leave the vulva and skin intact. More frequently, the fourchette of the vagina is destroyed and the laceration extends toward the anus

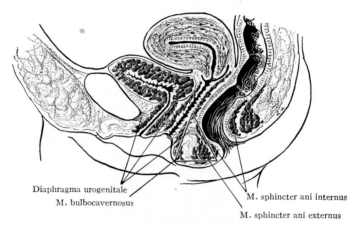

Diaphragma urogenitale
M. bulbocavernosus

M. sphincter ani internus

M. sphincter ani externus

FIG. 533.—MIDSAGITTAL SECTION THROUGH THE FEMALE PELVIS AND PERINEUM TO SHOW THE STRUCTURES INJURED IN PERINEAL TEARS.
The structures within the obstetrical perineal triangle frequently are lacerated.

(incomplete tear). Infrequently, the laceration may extend from the vagina into the anal canal (complete tear). When the tear involves the rectovaginal septum and weakens the pelvic floor, it relaxes the pelvic outlet and predisposes to a rectocele or prolapse.

SURGICAL CONSIDERATIONS

1. **Prolapse of the Urethral Mucosa.**—Occasionally, the urethral mucosa becomes loosened from its submucosal attachment and a part protrudes through the external orifice, forming a small, pale, bluish mass which may become edematous and sometimes gangrenous. This protruding mass is covered on all sides by sensitive, easily bleeding mucous membrane.

2. **Urethritis.**—Inflammation of the urethra is a common and often overlooked condition in women, frequently misdiagnosed as cystitis. In acute gonococcal infections, urethritis tends to disappear spontaneously with the disappearance of the disease elsewhere, unless it persists in and recurs from a chronically infected para-urethral gland (of Skene). A purulent exudate at the urethral meatus usually is indicative of "skenitis." When inflammation in the para-urethral glands is overlooked, treatment of the accompanying leukorrhea may be misdirected toward the cervix. A persistent infection in these glands should be treated by cauterization through the ducts.

3. **Urethral Caruncle.**—A caruncle is a connective tissue tumor (polyp), rich in blood vessels and nerve filaments, attached to the margin of the urethral orifice by a broad base. These tumors are intensely red, exquisitely tender, and difficult to distinguish from prolapsed urethral mucous membrane, save by tissue examination. Effective treatment of this excrescence requires complete extirpation. Anything short of complete removal almost always is followed by recurrence.

B. EXTERNAL GENITALIA

The female external generative organs lie within the pubic arch superficial to the urogenital diaphragm. They include the labia majora with the mons pubis (veneris), the labia minora and enclosed vestibule of the vagina, bulb of the vestibule, and orifices of the urethra and vagina. Of these structures, collectively termed the *vulva*, usually little more than the mons pubis and labia majora is visible.

1. **Labia Majora.**—The labia majora are two prominent fleshy skin folds projecting backward from the rounded eminence of the mons pubis, enclosing between their mesial surfaces the urogenital cleft. Their posterior tapering extremities blend with the perineum anterior to the anus to form the *posterior commissure* of the *vulva*. In the center of each labium is a well-defined mass of fat and strands of connective tissue, into which the fibers

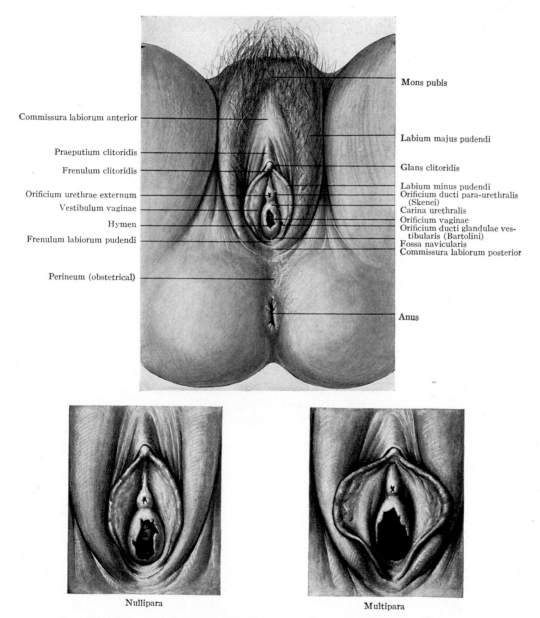

Commissura labiorum anterior

Praeputium clitoridis

Frenulum clitoridis

Orificium urethrae externum

Vestibulum vaginae

Hymen

Frenulum labiorum pudendi

Perineum (obstetrical)

Mons pubis

Labium majus pudendi

Glans clitoridis

Labium minus pudendi
Orificium ducti para-urethralis (Skenei)
Carina urethralis
Orificium vaginae
Orificium ducti glandulae vestibularis (Bartolini)
Fossa navicularis
Commissura labiorum posterior

Anus

Nullipara

Multipara

FIG. 534.—PERINEAL REGION IN THE FEMALE TO SHOW THE EXTERNAL GENITALIA.

of the round ligament of the uterus insert. The congenital process of peritoneum which accompanies the round ligament into the labium may fail to become obliterated and be the seat of a congenital hernia or of a hydrocele.

2. **Labia Minora.**—The labia minora (nymphae) are two thin folds of delicate skin, concealed between the larger labia, and enclosing the vestibule of the vagina. The size of

34

the labia may vary from scarcely noticeable structures to flaps a centimeter or more in length. They are said to be hypertrophied in masturbation. At their anterior extremities, the labia divide into folds which form a prepuce for the free end of the clitoris. The mesial margins of the posterior extremities of the labia are connected by a transverse crescentic fold or *frenulum* (*fourchette*).

3. **Vestibule of the Vagina.**—The vestibule of the vagina is enclosed between the labia minora and extends from the clitoris anteriorly to the frenulum posteriorly. In its floor are the urethral and vaginal orifices, the minute openings of the para-urethral ducts (of Skene), and the ducts of the major vestibular glands (of Bartholin). The *urethral orifice* occupies a conspicuous elevation (urethral papilla) which lies about 2 cm. behind the clitoris. The *vaginal orifice* in the virgin is narrowed by a duplication of mucous membrane, the *hymen*, which, after rupture, is represented by irregular projections into the vaginal orifice, the *hymeneal caruncles*.

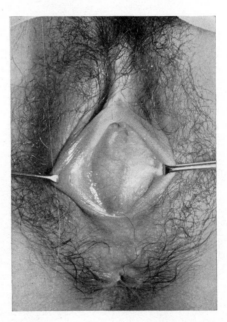

FIG. 535.—IMPERFORATE HYMEN WITH HEMATOCOLPOMETRASALPINX.   (C. L. Callander)

4. **Imperforate Hymen.**—Imperforate hymen may not be recognized until puberty, at which time the patient may experience all symptoms of menstruation save the escape of menstrual flow from the genital canal. The menstrual fluid dilates the vaginal canal. The first symptom may be urinary retention from pressure of the dilated vagina on the urethra. Further accumulation may cause dilatation of the uterine canal and even of the uterine tubes, with escape of menstrual products into the peritoneal cavity.

The accumulation of the menses in the vagina is termed *hematocolpos;* if the menstruum then dilates the uterine cavity, the condition is termed *hematocolpometra.* If the tubes also become dilated, the condition is termed *hematocolpometrasalpinx.* The treatment is free incision of the hymen.

THE VERTEBRAL COLUMN, VERTEBRAL CANAL, AND SPINAL CORD

I. VERTEBRAL COLUMN

THE spinal column is the central pillar of the body through which many varied and complicated motions are combined. It functions as two segments: the *superior*, long, flexible portion supports the head and carries the thorax and abdomen; the *inferior*, short, rigid, pelvic portion carries the lower extremities. Through the pelvic portion, the weight of the body and the effect of shock are transmitted to the lower extremities.

The spinal column is comprised of the vertebrae, enveloped and bound together by a series of well-distributed and strongly resistant ligaments, and balanced one upon the other by strong active musculature. The vertebrae articulate anteriorly through their bodies by the interposition of fibrocartilaginous disks and posterolaterally through articular processes. The column has a very considerable range of movement, but movement beyond its normal range unduly compresses the vertebral disks and may permit fracture of the related bodies, with consequent injury to the spinal cord or its root nerves.

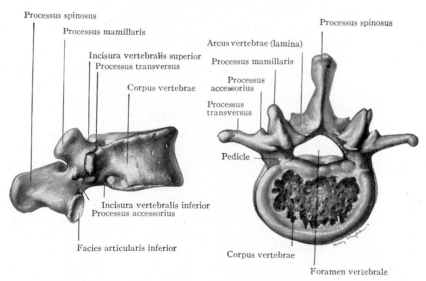

FIG. 536.—LATERAL AND SUPERIOR VIEWS OF A LUMBAR VERTEBRA.

The *visceral, anterior,* or *flexor surface* of the pillar presents in the midline a cylindrical column comprised of the superimposed vertebral bodies. This surface is in relation throughout with the viscera and supports and protects them and their vessel and nerve supply; it is separated from them by a cellular layer which occupies the prevertebral space. Into and along this space extend abscesses from Pott's disease; the course of extension depends upon the anatomy of the various regions. The abscess may bulge into or present at the pharynx (p. 151), descend into the neck, bulge into the supraclavicular fossa, or follow the nerve plexuses into the axilla. It may extend into the mediastinum and follow intercostal nerves into the thickness of the chest wall; it may open into the abdomen or into the rectum, or other abdominal viscus, or extend into the gluteal region and thence into the posterior region of the thigh and the popliteal space.

The *posterior* or *extensor surface* of the pillar descends along the midline of the body posteriorly. It is made up of the superimposed spinous processes, laminae, transverse processes, pedicles, and articular processes of the vertebrae with their retrospinal soft

531

parts. The bony part of this posterior portion, covered only by the skin and a single heavy layer of muscles, is relatively superficial and therefore is accessible to clinical examination and surgical intervention. For the same reason, these bony structures are exposed to direct trauma, buckling, and crushing. The products of tuberculous inflammation in these bony parts present or localize promptly at the skin.

Between these two surfaces is the *spinal (vertebral) canal* which encloses the spinal cord and its coverings. Between each pair of vertebrae, on either side, are apertures, the intervertebral foramina, for the transmission of spinal vessels and nerves. Fractures of the

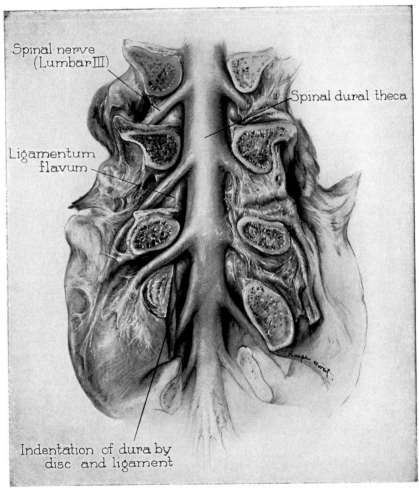

FIG. 537.—POSTERIOR VIEW OF THE LUMBAR AREA OF THE VERTEBRAL CANAL WITH ITS CONTENTS. (Naffziger, Inman, and Saunders, Surg., Gynec. and Obst., Feb. 15, 1938.)

bodies, arches, or their processes may injure the cord or its nerve roots. Hemorrhages consequent upon fracture may cause pressure on the cord, with resulting paralyses.

1. **Vertebral Characteristics.**—The central bony pillar or spine extends from the base of the skull to the inferior extremity of the trunk. It is divided into four topographical regions: the cervical, thoracic, and lumbar, embraced in the superior segment, and the sacrococcygeal in the inferior segment. The component vertebrae are morphologically equivalent and conform to a real type.

Each vertebra consists of two portions, an anterior mass of spongy bone, the *body*, and a posterior portion, the *arch*. The arch comprises two pedicles and two laminae, from which various processes project. The pedicles, one on each side, project backward from the upper portion of the body and are indented deeply, superiorly and inferiorly, into intervertebral notches. The notches of each contiguous pair of bones form the intervertebral foramina which transmit the spinal nerves and blood vessels. The broad plates of the laminae complete the neural arch and enclose the spinal foramen. From the junction of the two laminae, the spinous process projects backward and serves as an attachment for muscles and ligaments. The articular processes, two on each side spring from the union of the pedicles with the laminae. The superior processes, in general, are directed backward, while the inferior processes are directed forward. The two transverse processes, one on each side, project from the point of union of the articular processes with the pedicle.

2. **Development.**—Each vertebra is developed through three *primary centers* of ossification, one for the body and one for each half of the vertebral arch. The two halves of the neural arch unite posteriorly in the first year. This process of union, beginning in the cervical region at the end of the first year, progresses consecutively to the other regions and is completed in the sacrum toward the tenth year. The vertebral body is separated from the ventral part of the arch by a bar of cartilage (neurocentral synchondrosis) which disappears about the third or fourth year. Occasionally, this may persist, particularly in the lumbar region, so that in interpreting x-rays of the vertebral column, this anomaly may be mistaken for a fracture (see Spondylolisthesis, p. 536).

Five *secondary centers* appear at puberty, and the epiphyses they form add upper and lower plates, or disks, to the bodies and tips to the spinous and transverse processes. These epiphyses unite about the twentieth to the twenty-fifth year.

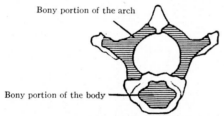

FIG. 538.—VERTEBRAL DEVELOPMENT.

Faulty or arrested development of the primary centers may result in incomplete closure of the vertebral arch behind, with herniation of portions of the cord and membranes into the breach (*spina bifida*). Faulty or arrested development of the epiphyseal plates of the secondary centers results in curvature, the *scoliosis* of *adolescence*. Developmental abnormalities may present in the transverse processes of the sixth and seventh cervical vertebrae and in the first lumbar vertebra in the form of cervical and lumbar ribs.

3. **Landmarks.**—It is necessary in the study of pathologic conditions in the spine to differentiate and locate the vertebrae numerically. The cervical spinous processes are obscured by the thick overlying ligamentum nuchae. From the tip of the seventh vertebra (*vertebra prominens*), to the inferior extremity of the spine, the spinous processes are palpable. A line running through or joining their tips normally is median, so that a plumb line dropped from the prominent spinous process of the seventh cervical vertebra is in the line of the crease of the buttocks. Irregularities in this line of processes, whether lateral or anteroposterior, constitute the spinal deformities of scoliosis, kyphosis, and lordosis, and call for a study of causes.

On each side of the line of spinous processes, which is represented on the strongly muscled subject as a groove, lies the longitudinally placed spinal musculature. In the thoracic region, this musculature is limited laterally by the palpable line of the angles of the ribs. Forward bending shows the spinous processes in detail. Undue prominence of either line of rib angles indicates a structural spinal curvature with rotation of the vertebrae.

When the arms are at the sides, certain *transverse lines* joining recognized landmarks designate definite vertebrae and are aids in vertebral localization. Of these, the line joining the mesial extremities of the spines of the scapulae marks the spinous process of the third thoracic vertebra; that joining the inferior angles of the scapulae is in the line of the transverse process of the seventh thoracic vertebra; that at the level of the umbilicus

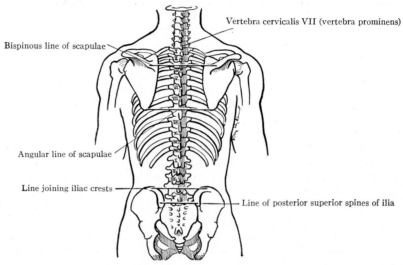

FIG. 539.—LANDMARKS OF THE BACK.

usually locates the transverse process of the third lumbar vertebra. The level of the summits of the iliac crests crosses the spinous process of the fourth lumbar vertebra; and the line joining the posterosuperior iliac spines marks the middle of the second sacral vertebra.

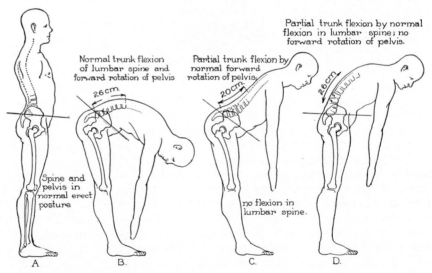

FIG. 540.—FLEXION OF THE TRUNK IN STANDING POSITION.
The straight line between the anterior superior and the posterior superior iliac spines indicates the degree of flexion of the pelvis. In full lumbar spine flexion, the distance between the eleventh thoracic and first sacral vertebrae is increased 6 cm. in the change of position from the erect posture to full lumbar flexion. (After Brahdy.)

4. **Normal Curvatures of the Spine.**—The vertebral column normally presents alternately placed anteroposterior curves. The curves of the cervical and lumbar regions are convex anteriorly and the curves of the thoracic and sacrococcygeal regions are concave anteriorly. The thoracic and sacrococcygeal curves suspend the thoracic and pelvic cavi-

ties and add greatly to their depth. The curves of the cervical and lumbar regions are compensatory. The lumbar curve forms a sloping shelf for the support of the heavy upper abdominal viscera. By directing the downward thrust of these organs forward against the lower abdominal musculature, the lumbar curve shields and protects the pelvic viscera. To its curves, the spine owes much of its elasticity and its resistance to trauma acting in the line of the column. The curves are made possible by the shape of the intervertebral disks. The disks of the cervical and lumbar segments are thicker anteriorly, while those of the thoracic region are thicker posteriorly.

The normal curvatures vary according to age. In the newborn, the vertebral column shows two *primary curves*, both concave forward. Of these, the upper extends from the head to the pelvis and the lower affects the sacral region. As the child begins to sit erect and to elevate its head, *secondary curves* appear, the first of which is a forward convexity in the cervical region. As the child begins to stand and later to walk, a forward convexity appears in the lumbar region. The development of these secondary curves enables the column to transmit the weight of the trunk to the pelvis in such a way that little or no muscle effort is needed to maintain the erect attitude. As old age comes on, the spine tends to assume one great curvature with an anterior concavity. The cause of this is the atrophy of the intervertebral disks. The column then is shaped as it is when the individual vertebrae are articulated without disks. In females, the lumbar curve is greater than it is in males, making a marked anterior prominence at its junction with the sacrum.

5. **Movements.**—The spinal column, although made up of superimposed vertebral bodies, firmly joined articular processes, and reinforcing ligaments, is capable of a wonderful degree of flexibility. It executes a great variety of movements, forward, lateral, and backward bendings, rotation, and even circumduction. A large number of these movements is made possible by the compressibility of the intervertebral fibrocartilages. The greatest degree and widest range of movement is in the segments which have the best developed disks.

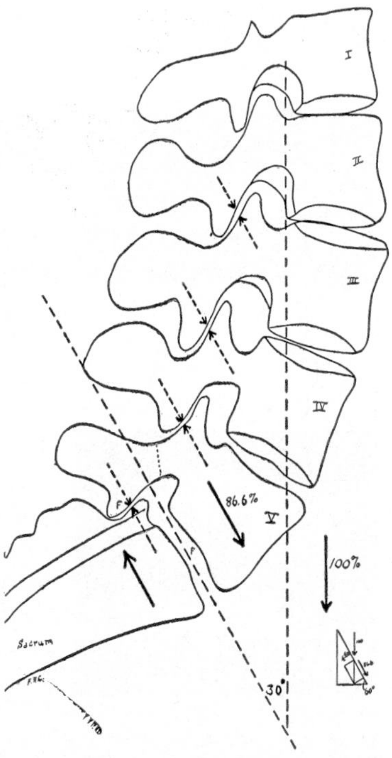

Not all segments of the spine permit the same variety of movement. In general, the greatest mobility occurs where one type of vertebra changes to another (cervicodorsal and dorsolumbar junctions). The vertebrae at these levels are most liable to injury. The

Fig. 541.—Diagram Showing the Forces Acting on the Interarticular Area (Isthmus) of the Laminae of the Fifth Lumbar Vertebra. (F. Chandler, Surg., Gynec. and Obst., Sept., 1931.)

cervical segment is very mobile and permits a wide range of all movements. The thoracic region permits little movement in anterior and posterior flexion, which adds to thoracic stability and preserves respiratory function. In the lumbar segment and through the lumbosacral articulation, anterior, posterior, and lateral flexion are extensive. In the sacro-iliac synchondrosis, there is only the very slight mobility characteristic of such joints (*e. g.*, sternoclavicular, symphysis pubis) which later in life become synarthroses.

These normal movements and curvatures are modified by inflammation, the deformities of paralysis, and fracture. In Pott's disease, there is muscle spasm to maintain the spine rigid and to serve as a protective mechanism to lessen pain. A list of the trunk on the pelvic girdle may be assumed for relief of pain and tenderness in sacro-iliac strain or in sciatica from whatever cause.

6. Lumbosacral Joint and Spondylolisthesis.—The accompanying diagram indicates the tremendous shearing action exerted by the vertebral column on the *lumbosacral joint* and upon the interarticular areas of the lowermost lumbar vertebrae when the body is in the upright position. The potential force of weight-bearing exerted on these areas is increased almost unbelievably when activated by the inertia of motion, leverage, and muscle spasm resulting from sudden strains and falls. Increase in the normally sharp lumbosacral angle further lessens the security of the region.

Spondylolisthesis designates the slipping forward of a vertebral body. It occurs most commonly when the fifth lumbar vertebral body rides forward on the sacrum. The fourth lumbar body may slip forward on the fifth. What usually allows a vertebral body to slip forward is a break in continuity in the interarticular area of one or both laminae. The term "isthmus" is applied to this region of the neural arch because it connotes a narrowing between two larger parts. The isthmus is at the point of maximum shearing force. Moreover, it often is the location for a congenital cleft or incomplete fissure. This marks out the

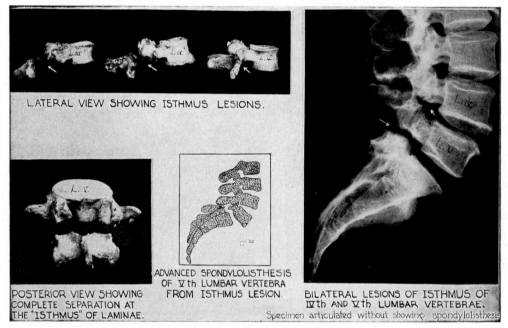

FIG. 542.—LESIONS OF THE "ISTHMUS" OF THE LAMINAE OF LUMBAR VERTEBRAE. (Fremont Chandler. Surg., Gynec. and Obst.)

interarticular area as one of defective ossification. Complete division of the isthmus with separation of fragments must be attributed to trauma. When rupture occurs through the isthmus, fibrous or cartilaginous tissue and not bone is severed. These separate and stretch under strain until the fifth lumbar vertebra, having lost its bony anchorage to the sacrum, slips forward to an amount allowed by the ligaments which unite the vertebral body to the sacrum, and those which unite the two portions of the defective arch. In a severe case, the spinous process and attached laminae of the fifth lumbar vertebrae present dorsally as a single fragment and are seen as a tumor at the lumbosacral junction.

An operation which produces bony fusion between the third and fourth lumbar vertebrae and the sacrum is the logical procedure to stabilize a spondylolisthetic spine.

7. The Intervertebral Disk (Fibrocartilage) and Its Protrusion. (See Fig. 554.)—Between each two vertebrae there is a shock absorber in the form of the intervertebral disk. In the aggregate, these disks form one fourth of the movable part of the spine. Each disk is attached intimately to the compact rim of the super- and subjacent vertebral bodies, and is connected loosely to the limiting cartilaginous plates over their sievelike surfaces. It is composed of an intricately planned mass of fibrocartilage (annulus fibrosus) surrounding the nucleus pulposus. The nucleus is a highly elastic, semifluid, indistensible tissue mass.

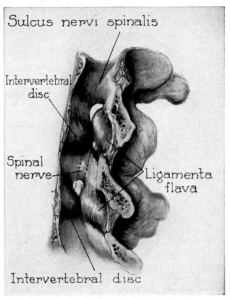

FIG. 543.—RIGHT THIRD AND FOURTH LUMBAR INTERVERTEBRAL FORAMINA VIEWED WITHIN THE VERTEBRAL CANAL.

The apposition of the intervertebral disk and the ligamentum flavum may obliterate the inferior half of the bony foramen. The spinal nerve leaves through the upper half of the bony foramen. (Naffziger Inman, and Saunders, Surg., Gynec. and Obst., Feb. 15, 1938.)

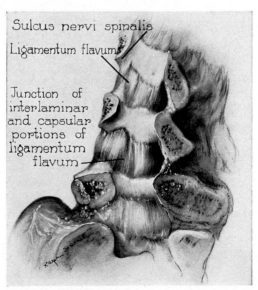

FIG. 544.—SAGITTAL SECTION THROUGH LUMBAR AREA OF VERTEBRAL CANAL TO SHOW LIGAMENTA FLAVA. (Naffziger, Inman, and Saunders, Surg., Gynec. and Obst., Feb. 15, 1938.)

The annulus fibrosus forms the major part of the disk. The nucleus pulposus lies rather more posteriorly than centrally. The annulus fibrosus gives form, size, and strength to the disk, and is its main weight-bearing portion.

When the spinal column is subjected to ordinary strain and stress, the disk bulges in all directions but returns to its normal position after the force producing the stress has ceased to operate. It is maintained in its position principally by the anterior and posterior longitudinal vertebral ligaments, the posterior ligament being the weaker of the two. Following unusual strain to the column, the disk itself, or its center, the nucleus pulposus, may be extruded beyond its normal limits and fail to return to position. Slight posterior protrusions may cause root pain because of pressure of the disk on one or more spinal nerve roots. More marked protrusion may cause symptoms and signs similar to those in transverse lesion of the cord or of the cauda equina. Thus, the lesion may resemble intraspinal neoplasm. The protrusion may occur at any level in the movable part of the column. The most common location is low in the lumbar region, and the most frequent symptom is sciatic pain. Protrusion of the disk through the cartilage plates of the superjacent and subjacent vertebral bodies and thence into their spongy interior occurs commonly.

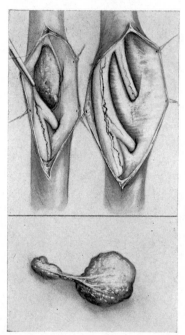

Fig. 545.—Transdural Exposure of Herniated Fibrocartilage.
Cartilage removed. (Naffziger, Inman, and Saunders, Surg., Gynec. and Obst. Feb. 15, 1938.)

Lesions which present objective neurologic findings are not difficult to diagnose. When there is motor weakness and sensory loss, the level of compression of the root or cord is determined by neurological examination. The patient in whom pain is the only symptom presents a different diagnostic problem. The diagnosis then depends on fluoroscopic and roentgenographic examination of the spinal canal after injecting a radiopaque oil (lipiodol) into the subarachnoid space. If protrusion of the disk is present, it will impinge on the column of lipiodol and indent or displace it posteriorly or laterally because the protruded fragment of the disk is extradural. Complete obstruction to passage of the oil has been observed.

The therapy of choice for protruded disk is laminectomy with the removal of the extruded part of the disk, provided that the protruded disk corresponds to the level of the root pain.

8. **Hypertrophy of the Ligamentum Flavum.**—Hypertrophy of the ligamentum flavum is one of the more recently recognized intraspinal lesions which produce neurologic signs and symptoms by pressure on the cord, nerve roots, or cauda equina.

The ligamenta flava, composed normally of yellow elastic tissue, connect the laminae of contiguous vertebrae and blend with the interspinous ligaments. They help form the capsules between the articular facets, and their lateral edge forms the posterior margin of the intervertebral foramina. In some patients, one or more of these ligaments, probably from continued trauma, undergoes hyperplastic change and becomes so thick that it encroaches on the spinal canal and compresses its contents. The ligament or ligaments usually thickened connect the laminae of the fourth and fifth lumbar vertebrae so that the nerve elements compressed are the fibers of the cauda equina.

Low back pain, radiating down one or both thighs, motor weakness, and objective sensory phenomena are the usual findings in an advanced case. There usually is a history of trauma. Fluoroscopic examination of the spinal canal after subarachnoid injection of a

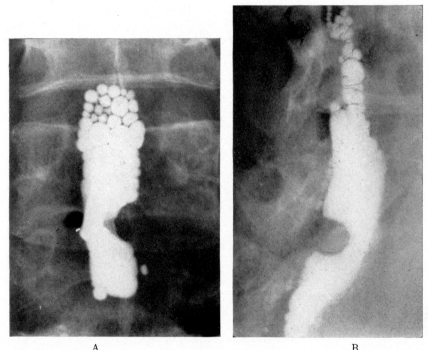

A B

FIG. 546.—DIAGNOSTIC SUBARACHNOID LIPIODOL INJECTION TO OUTLINE DISK PROTRUSION.
A, Postero-anterior view in prone position; B, prone oblique view. (H. A. Brown and J. W. Cox.)

radiopaque oil (lipiodol) locates the lesion. The characteristic filling defect is at the fourth lumbar interspace.

Treatment consists of the removal of the involved ligament or ligaments and the adjacent laminae. Spinal fusion may not be necessary. The tissue removed is a mass of dense fibrous material, different from the normally soft, pliable ligamentum flavum. Frequently, the adjacent laminae are thickened markedly.

SURGICAL CONSIDERATIONS

1. Abnormal Curvatures.—Deviations from the normal curvatures of the vertebral column occur either in the anteroposterior or the lateral direction. Deviations in the anteroposterior plane ordinarily are exaggerations of the normal curves.

The basic factors in these deviations range from faulty attitudes or postures to traumatic and diseased processes. In sickly children and debilitated adolescents, the body may grow too rapidly to be supported by its muscles. Instinctively, these patients adopt attitudes to relieve the overworked muscles and transfer the strain to the ligaments about the intervertebral joints. The ligaments upon which the strain is thrown are overstretched by habitual adoption of a compensatory attitude, and the opposing ligaments become shortened. Thus there is a tendency for the faulty attitude to be maintained. With improper alignment of the column, the muscle balance is upset and one group of muscles attains a mechanical advantage over the corresponding antagonistic group to the end that the latter becomes overstretched.

Kyphosis or increased backward curvature of the spine commonly results from tuberculosis of the spine (Pott's disease) and occurs most often in the thoracic segment. The destruction of the vertebral bodies causes forward compression of the bodies and backward knuckling of the spinous processes. The same deformity presents in compression fracture of the spine.

Lordosis, or exaggerated forward curvature in the lumbar segment, usually is compensatory to abnormal flexion or fixed flexion at the hip joint. It is exemplified in cases of double congenital dislocation of the hip where the support of the pelvis is not through the acetabulum but posterior to it. This increases the inclination of the pelvis and carries the lumbar spine into abnormal anterior convexity. Spondylolisthesis is another cause of marked lumbar lordosis.

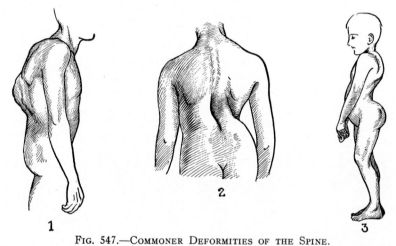

FIG. 547.—COMMONER DEFORMITIES OF THE SPINE.
1, Thoracolumbar lordosis caused by Pott's disease; 2, left thoracolumbar scoliosis; 3, lordosis in double congenital dislocation of the hips.

Scoliosis, or lateral curvature, is the commonest of the spinal deviations and occurs primarily in the thoracic region. In the curve of scoliosis, all or a series of the spinous processes show a constant deviation from the median line. A careful study of the spine in its movements, checked by x-ray findings, is essential.

In *junctional scoliosis*, the convexity of the curve almost always is to the left. The spinous processes usually deviate about 1 cm., and seldom more than 2.5 cm., from the median line. The left shoulder is carried high and forward and the right shoulder downward and backward. Forward bending produces a prominence on the concave side of the curve. The prominence is the evidence of rotation of the vertebrae and is the result of bending the anteroposteriorly curved spine in more than one plane. It is produced by the rib angles. The curvature may be a sign of poor muscle tone or of faulty standing.

In *transitional scoliosis*, the characteristics of functional scoliosis are observed except that a prominence presents at some level on the convex side of the curve. The usual prominence on the concave side of the curve is present at all other levels.

Structural scoliosis is a constant lateral deviation of the spine, characterized by changes in the vertebrae and in the surrounding muscles and ligaments. Forward bending produces a prominence on the convex side of the curve, because of the rotation of the vertebral bodies away from the point of greatest weight and pressure. If the curve is double, there are two prominences, each of which is on the convex side of the curve. There are associated changes in the form and shape of the thorax, abdomen, and pelvis.

Round back (stooped shoulders) is an exaggeration of the convexity of the whole dorsal and even the lumbar segment. In some cases, it is mechanical only, and in others, may present marked bony changes. In old age, a fixed round back is characteristic, because of the atrophy of the disks. In the **hollow back,** the lower part of the dorsal curve may be decreased or reversed and the head be thrust forward. In **flat back,** the physiologic curves of the dorsal and lumbar segments are lost.

2. **Tuberculosis of the Spine.**—Tuberculosis of the spine, or Pott's disease, like tuberculosis in other bones and joints, is a local manifestation of blood-borne tuberculosis, characterized by bone destruction with but slight tendency to bone regeneration. It is accompanied by localized swelling, atrophy of tissues, and painful weight bearing and movement. The spinal muscles maintain, as far as possible, a relieving or protective rigidity, and the pain caused by the return of muscle spasm following relaxation in sleep is responsible for night cries; these may be the initial sign of the disease. In the later stages, there may be abscess formation with kyphos deformity and possible nerve root irritation, or even cord injury with paralysis of the lower extremities. Invasion by way of the upper and lower epiphyseal plates is commonest in childhood. It occurs by extension from paravertebral abscesses, usu-

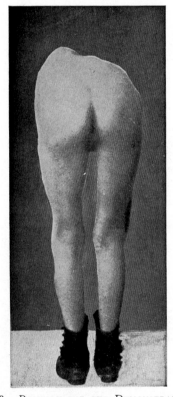

Fig. 549.—Position for the Demonstration of Rotation in Lateral Curvature.

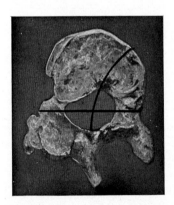

Fig. 548.—Distorted Sagittal Plane of a Scoliotic Vertebra. (Riedinger.)

The left dorsal scoliosis causes a backward prominence of the left side of the thorax. (Lovett.)

ally at the center of the anterior portion of the vertebral body. The process sometimes begins in the synovial cavity of an intervertebral disk. Rarely, it begins in the transverse processes, spinous processes, and in the posterior articulations.

The tuberculous process invades the vertebrae in a variety of ways. As the concavities of the physiologic curves carry the great stress of weight bearing, disease of the bodies in the cervical or lumbar regions tends to less destruction than does disease in the thoracic region. Involvement in the thoracic bodies is formidable and is marked by serious deformity. Destruction of the intervertebral disks, especially in the thoracic curve, leads to collapse of the diseased tissues and results in the deformity of angular posterior projection of the spinous processes, the typical kyphos of Pott's disease. Thinning or destruction of the disk usually is the earliest x-ray finding.

The points of accumulation and paths of extension of pus from abscess formation in Pott's disease depend upon the spinal segment involved. In the *cervical region*, the abscess may bulge into the pharynx, obstructing respiration, and even rupturing into the mouth,

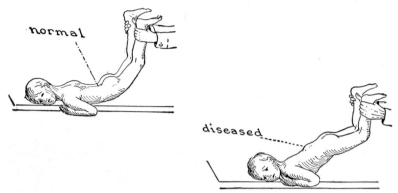

FIG. 550.—METHOD OF DEMONSTRATING THE RIGIDITY OF THE SPINE IN VERTEBRAL TUBERCULOSIS. (Babcock, "Textbook of Surgery.")

suffocating the patient; it may accumulate in the deep tissues of the neck or, rarely, break into the spinal canal. It commonly extends laterally into the floor of the supraclavicular area. Either the body or the odontoid process of the second cervical vertebra (axis) may

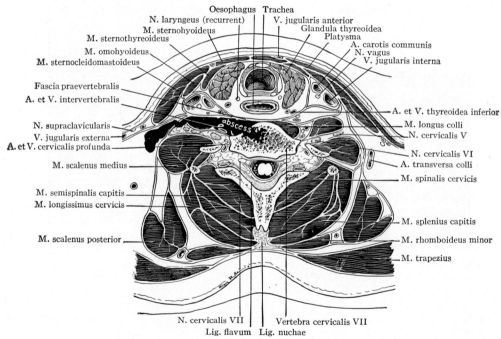

FIG. 551.—CROSS SECTION THROUGH THE NECK AT THE LEVEL OF THE SEVENTH CERVICAL VERTEBRA TO SHOW TUBERCULOUS EROSION OF THE VERTEBRAL BODY AND THE LATERAL EXTENSION OF THE RESULTING TUBERCULOUS ABSCESS INTO THE SUPRACLAVICULAR REGION BEHIND THE PREVERTEBRAL FASCIA.

be involved. From the odontoid process (dens), pus may extend forward and infect the joint between the dens and atlas, or backward and involve the bursa between the dens and the transverse ligament. When the dens is eroded or the transverse ligament is destroyed, the dens slips backward into the medulla, resulting in death, since cord injury occurs above the level of the origin of the phrenic nerve. These joints are supplied by branches from the first two cervical nerves which also supply the muscles rotating the head. Irritation of the joints sets up reflex phenomena in the cutaneous and muscle distribution of the nerves and the head is kept rigid from muscle spasm.

When the third or the fourth cervical vertebra is involved, the same rigidity from muscle spasm is present and there is pain over the distribution of the third and fourth cervical nerves. The symptoms are caused by pressure on the nerves themselves as they emerge from the vertebral canal, in contradistinction to the reflex symptoms noted in involvement of the joints between the articular processes.

When the *lower cervical* and *upper thoracic vertebrae* are affected, the corresponding part of the vertebral column is held rigid in muscle spasm, giving rise to the "military attitude" in walking, as well as to the typical habit of sitting with the elbows upon the table and supporting the chin to relieve the spastic muscles. The distribution of the referred pain may help to localize the exact site of the disease. When there is abscess formation, the pus tends to travel downward behind the anterior longitudinal ligament or prevertebral fascia into the mediastinum.

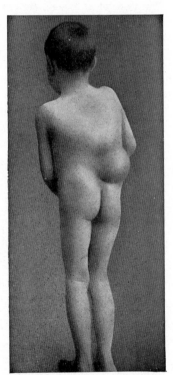

FIG. 552.—LUMBAR ABSCESS FROM DORSAL VERTEBRAL TUBERCULOSIS. (Lovett.)

When the disease occurs in the *midthoracic segment*, muscle spasm occurs in the sacrospinalis muscle and sometimes in the abdominal muscles. Pain commonly is referred to the anterior abdominal wall, where it may lead to errors in diagnosis. Abscesses in connection with the involved vertebrae may gravitate downward behind the medial lumbocostal arch (internal arcuate ligament) and subsequently descend under the fascial covering of the psoas major muscle. Since modern treatment of these lesions usually is recumbency in hyperextension, these abscesses commonly gravitate upward. They form large paravertebral collections which may require evacuation by *costotransversectomy* (rib resection and the removal of the corresponding transverse process), if they are infected secondarily or cause pressure symptoms on the spinal cord

In involvement of the *lower thoracic* and *lumbar regions*, pain may be present in the back, lower anterior abdominal wall, and the thigh or leg. The usual course of an abscess in these regions is along the psoas muscle on one or both sides to present in the groin, loin, or buttock. There is associated spasm of the psoas muscle and resulting flexion of the thigh.

Spinal cord involvement by caries may occur in any portion of the vertebral column, but usually takes place in the dorsal spine. The paraplegia which may result usually is not caused by bony deformity but by backward extension of the disease into the vertebral canal. Although the angular bony deformity may be so great as to cause actual compression, the condition arises so slowly that it may not lead to paralysis.

3. **Injuries of the Spine.**—Injuries of the spine constitute a considerable number of industrial compensation cases. Difficulties are encountered not only in arriving at the correct interpretation of the results of the injury, the type and duration of treatment, the time of partial disability, and the degree of permanent disability, but also the amount of compensation warranted. Injury to an already existing deforming arthritis offers many serious difficulties in diagnosis and treatment. Many fractures are overlooked because of the relatively slight trauma necessary to produce them. Slight injuries to the column may cause serious results because of the delicate nature of the spinal cord and the nerve roots housed

therein. The cord and its membranes may escape laceration and suffer concussion only, or any or all parts may be damaged, even to complete severance of the cord. The membranes may be torn and hemorrhage may accumulate, causing pressure. Injuries to the cervical region are common because of the great freedom of movement permitted there.

Fracture is particularly common near the union of the flexible with the more fixed regions, and most frequently results from violent exaggerated flexion. The trauma is spent on the large cancellous vertebral body, tending to produce compression fracture. Resistance is offered by the components of the neural arch, chiefly by the articular processes. If the posterior parts give way, subluxation may take place with less likelihood of compression fracture. Hyperextension is the proper treatment of compression fracture of the vertebral bodies.

A useful test for the diagnosis of fracture of the spine is the following (R. Soto-Hall): "The patient is placed flat on his back without pillows. The examiner, with one hand, exerts gentle pressure upon the sternum so that no flexion can take place in the lumbar or thoracic regions of the spine. The examiner's other hand then is placed under the occiput and the head and neck are flexed upon the sternum slowly but forcibly. This movement produces a progressive pull upon the posterior spinous ligaments, starting at the ligamentum nuchae, and this pull is transmitted downward along the interspinous ligaments until it reaches the spinous process of the injured vertebra. The pull acts as a lever which gently compresses the injured vertebral body and which localizes pain accurately. The usefulness

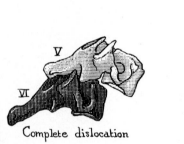 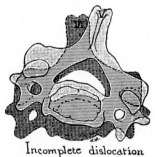

Complete dislocation   Incomplete dislocation

FIG. 553.—COMPLETE AND INCOMPLETE DISLOCATIONS IN THE CERVICAL REGION.

of this sign rests upon the ability to localize fractures without moving the patient and without examining the injured area locally."

Dislocation without fracture of the vertebrae is rare, unless it occurs in the atlo-axoid junction where the cord structures may escape damage because of the space afforded by the large vertebral canal, or between the fourth and fifth and between the fifth and sixth cervical vertebrae.

Dislocation in the cervicodorsal region occurs most commonly where the flexible cervical segment meets the rigidly splinted thoracic segment. Unilateral dislocation of an articular process may come from a sudden twist or bend. The inferior articular process slips forward past the superior articular process of the vertebra next below and readily compresses the emerging spinal nerve, causing pain over its cutaneous distribution. The injury may bruise the cord directly or cause extravasation of blood into and around it with consequent sensory and motor changes, depending upon the extent and location of the lesion. Bilateral dislocations always are serious, and, if they destroy the spinal medulla in any of the four upper segments, death occurs from paralysis of the diaphragm and the accessory muscles of respiration.

4. Surgical Approach to the Cord (Laminectomy).—It may be necessary, for a variety of reasons, to expose the spinal cord in the vertebral canal. Laminectomy is the procedure whereby the canal is opened widely to expose the dural sac, cord, and nerve roots. By this procedure, pressure from bony fragments, tumors, or blood clots may be relieved:

laceration in the cord membranes may be repaired or operations on the nerve roots or the cord be performed to relieve intractable pain.

The incision for laminectomy is made from the tip of the spinous process, superior to the one or two processes to be removed, to the tip of the next inferior process. The muscles are separated subperiosteally from the sides of the spinous processes and laminae, exposing the articular processes on either side. The bleeding at this step of the operation is controlled by packing tightly with gauze and retracting the muscle masses laterally. The interspinous and supraspinous ligaments are cut away. The spinous processes and then the laminae are removed with bone forceps, taking care not to injure the dura through the fat-filled extradural space. Just beneath the laminae and connecting them on their under surfaces is the tough ligamentum flavum which is removed with the laminae. The subsequent procedure depends upon whether the tumor, blood clot, fracture fragment, or foreign body is extradural or intradural. The dura is incised and, as the arachnoid may be injured at the same time, subarachnoid fluid is likely to escape at once. When the operation has been completed, the cut edges of the dura are united carefully and the thick muscle flaps are replaced.

5. Spinal Fusion Operations.—Spinal fusion operations are designed to immobilize certain areas of the spinal column by an artificial ankylosis (arthrodesis). The indications for stabilizing operations on the spine are: vertebral tuberculosis, spinal injuries or deformities with persistent weakness and pain, and scolioses that tend to recur after correction is obtained by traction and casts.

Hibbs' fusion is an osteoplastic operation for immobilizing the spinal column. It accomplishes arthrodesis of the intervertebral joints by destruction of the articular processes. It also builds bony bridges into the solid bone plates which embrace the vertebral arches of a succession of vertebrae, usually two above and two below the diseased vertebrae. The skin and subcutaneous tissue are incised from above downward, exposing the tips of the spinous processes of the vertebrae which are to be fused. Their periosteum and inter-

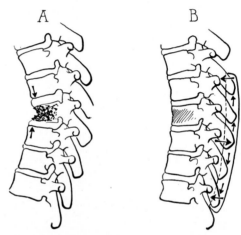

FIG. 554.—INLAY GRAFT METHOD OF CORRECTING KYPHOTIC ANGULATION IN VERTEBRAL TUBERCULOSIS.

In A, the arrows indicate the direction of the lines of the force which influence the crushing of the vertebral body; in B, the arrows indicate the line of force directed to and from the graft inlay in the line of the spinous processes.

spinous ligaments are split, the dissection is carried down subperiosteally through that plane and is continued over the laminae to the articular and transverse processes, exposing the entire posterior aspect of the neural arches. Oozing of blood is controlled by gauze packs. The spinous processes are laid bare to their bases at the neural arch. The ligamenta flava are dissected from their attachments to the laminae and adjacent articular processes. The articulations of the pairs of articular processes are destroyed (arthrodesed). Bone flaps, hinged laterally, are raised from the adjacent laminae and applied as bridges across the spaces between the laminae. The spinous processes are nicked at their bases, allowing the processes to be broken down so that their tips contact the raw places of the bases of the spinous processes below. Bony bridges are formed in this way, one in the midline and one on each side of the midline. In a variation of Hibbs' technic, long osteoperiosteal strips may be removed from the tibia and be placed along the laminae before closure of the soft parts. The components of the bony bridges are maintained in contact with denuded bone by suturing the overlying periosteum The skin, subcutaneous tissue. and muscle flaps are replaced and sutured.

The *Albee fusion* is an implantation of a bone graft along the channel of split spinous

35

processes. The incision is carried through the skin and subcutaneous tissue, exposing the tips of the spinous processes. The supraspinous and interspinous ligaments are split in this line. With a wide chisel, the processes are split into halves to a depth of from 1 to 2 cm. The halves on one side are broken back and crowded laterally so as to present throughout a channel for the graft, which is taken from the crest of the tibia. The leg prepared for the taking of the graft is flexed on the thigh, incision is made over the tibial crest, and the anterior surface of the bone is exposed. The measurement for the graft is noted and marked on the exposed tibia. By means of a twin saw, the graft is removed with the periosteum intact. This is placed in the channel made for it along the split spinous processes and is secured there by through-and-through chromic sutures.

II. VERTEBRAL OR SPINAL CANAL

The collective vertebral foramina make a continuous central canal in the spinal column. The anterior wall is closed uniformly by the posterior surfaces of the bodies of the vertebrae and their intervertebral disks, and the common posterior longitudinal ligament passes over it. The posterior and lateral walls are made up of the superimposed bony arches, the interspaces of which are spanned behind by the ligamenta flava and left open laterally as

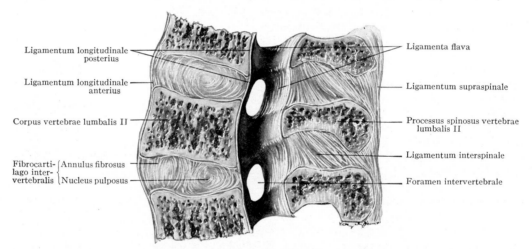

Ligamentum longitudinale posterius
Ligamentum longitudinale anterius
Corpus vertebrae lumbalis II
Fibrocarti- [Annulus fibrosus
lago inter- {
vertebralis [Nucleus pulposus

Ligamenta flava
Ligamentum supraspinale
Processus spinosus vertebrae lumbalis II
Ligamentum interspinale
Foramen intervertebrale

FIG. 555.—SAGITTAL SECTION THROUGH THE SPINAL COLUMN IN THE LUMBAR REGION TO SHOW THE VER-
TEBRAL CANAL AND THE INTERVERTEBRAL FORAMINA.

the intervertebral foramina. The whole is lined smoothly by periosteal and ligamentous surfaces. The well-housed cord and its coverings and the spinal nerve roots may be invaded by pathologic processes through the intervertebral foramina or through the less protected interlaminar spaces, by extruded portions of an intervertebral disk, or by a thickened ligamentum flavum.

The form of the vertebral canal, although presenting some individual variations, is fairly constant. It is approximately circular where it is continuous with the foramen magnum, assumes a triangular form through the cervical region, becomes round through the thoracic region, and again assumes the triangular form in the lumbar region. Within the sacrum, the canal flattens and expands laterally in the form of a crescent. In the flexible cervical and lumbar regions, the canal has distinct enlargements to accommodate the cervical and lumbar enlargements of the cord.

1. Spinal Meninges, Their Spaces and Fluid.—The spinal meninges are the direct downward continuation of the cranial meninges. In the cranial cavity, the *dura mater* consists of two layers, the outer constituting the lining periosteum of the skull, and the inner investing the brain and, by its duplications, forming the cranial venous sinuses (p. 28). At the foramen magnum, the outer dural layer blends with the periosteal and ligamentous lining of the vertebral canal. The inner layer is tough and fibrous and forms the dural sac investing the more delicate meninges and cord and the emerging nerve roots.

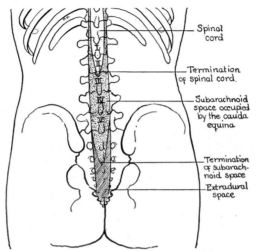

Spinal cord

Termination of spinal cord.

Subarachnoid space occupied by the cauda equina

Termination of subarachnoid space

Extradural space

FIG. 556.—DIAGRAM OF THE VERTEBRAL AND SACRAL CANALS TO SHOW THE LEVELS OF THE INFERIOR EXTREMITY OF THE SPINAL CORD PROPER AND THE LOWERMOST LIMIT OF THE SUBARACHNOID SPACE.

The diagram shows that spinal puncture in the lumbar area cannot injure the cord proper; the needle can contact only the fibers of the cauda equina; the diagram indicates that the transsacral and caudal types of anesthesia are extradural in their location.

It also sends out expansions over the spinal nerves emerging through the intervertebral foramina.

Between the dural sac and the walls of the vertebral canal is the *extradural space*. This is filled loosely with fatty areolar tissue and venous plexuses, and the whole is sup-

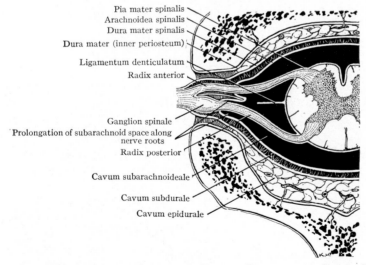

Pia mater spinalis
Arachnoidea spinalis
Dura mater spinalis
Dura mater (inner periosteum)
Ligamentum denticulatum
Radix anterior
Ganglion spinale
Prolongation of subarachnoid space along nerve roots
Radix posterior
Cavum subarachnoideale
Cavum subdurale
Cavum epidurale

FIG. 557.—SCHEMATIC TRANSVERSE SECTION THROUGH THE SPINAL CORD AND SPINAL MENINGES.

ported by connective tissue bands holding the dural envelope to the anterior and posterior walls of the vertebral canal. Spinal puncture may injure an extradural vein and bloody spinal fluid may be withdrawn. Laminectomy without injury to the dural sac and cord is possible because of the extradural space, but is complicated if the extradural veins are injured, since only compression arrests the bleeding. The inflammatory products of vertebral tuberculosis may invade the extradural space and cause cord symptoms from pressure.

The spinal *arachnoid*, a delicate, nonvascular sac lining the dural tube and intimately connected with it, is the continuation of the cranial arachnoid. The dura and arachnoid move freely upon one another; the space between them is a potential cavity. The delicate arachnoid sac invests the cord loosely, and its deep space forms the outer limit of the subarachnoid space.

The *subarachnoid space* is filled with cerebrospinal fluid, since it is in direct continuity with the subarachnoid cisterns surrounding the base of the brain and medulla. In lumbar puncture, this space is entered when the needle penetrates the resistant dura and its subjacent thin arachnoid lining.

The *pia mater* is a delicate vascular membrane closely attached to the fissures and surfaces of the cord and carrying blood vessels to its substance. It gives off numerous lateral

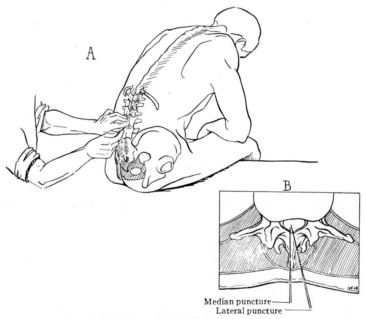

FIG. 558.—TECHNIC OF LUMBAR PUNCTURE.

A, The left forefinger locates the area between the fourth and fifth lumbar spinous processes; B is a cross section at this level to show the median and lateral insertion of the needle into the subarachnoid space.

septal prolongations to the arachnoid and adheres closely to the nerve roots, investing them with delicate sheaths which accompany the nerves across the subarachnoid space to blend with the dural sheath. The denticulate ligament is a frontally disposed sheet of membrane attached to the pia mater midway between the anterior and posterior nerve roots from the epistropheus (axis) to the first lumbar vertebra. Its lateral border is serrated; the serrations are attached to the dura in the intervals between the emerging nerve roots.

SURGICAL CONSIDERATIONS

1. **Subarachnoid Anesthesia.**—Intraspinal or subarachnoid anesthesia is nerve root block produced by the injection of a local anesthetic into the subarachnoid space. The anesthetic is administered by spinal puncture, performed with the patient in the sitting or in the lateral recumbent position. The fourth lumbar interspace is a favorite site for injection, since it is located readily on a line joining the crests of the ilia, and because the space is accessible by reason of the direct posterior projection of the lumbar spinous proc-

esses. At this level, there is no danger of striking more than the fibers of the cauda equina as the body of the spinal cord terminates at a higher level (p. 551).

The interspinous space is located by palpation and the needle is thrust through it in the median line. The resistant interspinous ligament is traversed and the needle is inserted until it perforates the dense and somewhat elastic dura and the underlying arachnoid. Upon removal of the obturator, spinal fluid escapes. The injection of anesthetizing fluid is made slowly and with uniform pressure. Anesthesia produces almost complete loss of conduction of sensory and, to a lesser degree, of motor nerve impulses.

2. Sacral Anesthesia.—Sacral anesthesia is extradural and is designed to reach the nerves within the sacral canal, where the anesthetizing solution saturates the sacral nerves and produces anesthesia in the parts supplied by them. When 30 cc. of the solution are injected, the extradural space is invaded as far as the lower lumbar region (Farr). Anesthesia is afforded the structures of the perineum and the external genitalia.

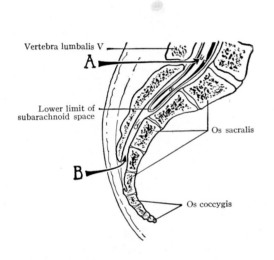

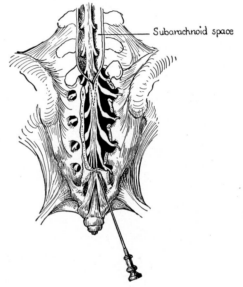

FIG. 559.—MEDIAN SAGITTAL SECTION THROUGH THE FIFTH LUMBAR VERTEBRA AND THE SACRUM TO INDICATE AREAS FOR SUBARACHNOID AND EXTRADURAL INJECTIONS.

A shows the point of injection into the subarachnoid space through the superior aperture of the sacral canal. B indicates the point of injection for caudal extradural anesthesia.

FIG. 560.—SACRAL NERVES EXPOSED IN THE SACRAL CANAL. THE CAUDAL TYPE OF SACRAL EXTRADURAL ANESTHESIA IS INDICATED.

The needle penetrates the posterior sacrococcygeal ligament to enter the inferior aperture of the sacral canal.

In the *caudal type* of sacral anesthesia, the patient is placed in the prone position, the sacral hiatus is located, and the overlying structures are anesthetized. Puncture is made into the sacral hiatus through the resistant sacrococcygeal ligament with a fine long needle, the hub of which is depressed until the shaft passes upward along the axis of the sacral canal for a distance of 3 or 4 cm. Fifty cc. of a 2 per cent solution of procaine is deposited in the canal, where it bathes the emerging sacral and coccygeal nerves. The needle point, if improperly directed, fails to enter the canal, but travels upward posterior to the sacrum.

Transsacral (posterior sacral) anesthesia is accomplished by direct injection of an anesthetizing fluid into the sacral canal and about the sacral nerves by way of each of the posterior sacral foramina. The first sacral foramen lies about 3 cm. lateral to the line of sacral spinous processes, and the foramina of each side are from 2 to 2.5 cm. apart. As practical landmarks, the posterosuperior spines of the ilia should be located. About 1 cm. mesial to, and just below, these spines lie the second sacral foramina. Usually, infiltration of only the lower four pairs of sacral nerves is made. The first pair of sacral foramina are located on a line directly opposite the tip of the transverse process of the fifth lumbar vertebra. Because of the greater thickness and forward inclination of the sacrum above, it is necessary to introduce the upper needles a greater distance than the lower. The efficiency of this method may be augmented by caudal injection of the sacral canal.

For the administration of *presacral anesthesia*, the patient is placed in the exaggerated lithotomy position where the sacral plexus can be reached anterior to the sacrum alternately at the right and left of the sacrococcygeal joint. The points of entrance are about 1.5 to 2 cm. from the median line. On each side, the needle travels upward and laterally along the anterior surface of the sacrum, the nerves being anesthetized by the infiltration block method. As the needle encounters the anterior surface of the sacrum, the anesthetizing

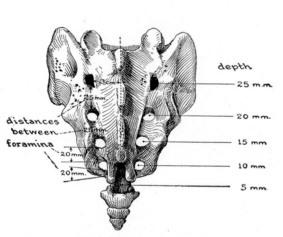

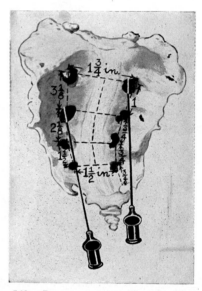

FIG. 561.—POSTERIOR VIEW OF THE SACRUM AND THE POSTERIOR SACRAL FORAMINA.

The diagram indicates the depth of the foramina from the surface and the distances between the foramina. These measurements are aids in the injection of sacral anesthesia by the transsacral route. (Babcock, "Text-book of Surgery.")

FIG. 562.—POSITIONS OF THE NEEDLES USED IN THE INJECTION OF PRESACRAL ANESTHESIA.

The needles are shifted to conform to the shape of the sacrum as they pass from the sacrococcygeal junction to the higher sacral vertebra. The distances between the foramina are indicated. (Bickham, "Operative Surgery.")

fluid is allowed to escape rapidly in advance of the needle until a large amount of the fluid is deposited in the hollow of the sacrum. The fluid forces the rectum forward out of danger.

3. **Paravertebral Anesthesia.**—In paravertebral anesthesia, an effort is made to anesthetize the spinal nerves a short distance from their emergence from the column. The special field for this anesthesia lies in the abdominal and thoracic regions. The needle may be introduced from 2 to 3 cm. lateral to the midline until the vertebral arch is touched. It then is passed 1 cm. deeper between the transverse processes, where it encounters the nerves as they emerge from the intervertebral foramina. Although anesthesia may be obtained in this manner, it is almost impossible to reach all the emerging nerves. For infiltration block, the needle may be introduced obliquely inward somewhat farther from the median line, from 3 to 4 cm. lateral to the point between the transverse processes.

III. Spinal Cord and Nerve Roots

The spinal cord or medulla spinalis, when freed from its coverings and attached nerves, presents the general form of an elongated cylinder, compressed anteroposteriorly. The foramen magnum defines the level at which the cord is continuous with the medulla oblongata. The relations of the cord and vertebral column differ markedly in the fetus, infant, and adult. Up to the third month of intra-uterine life, the cord occupies the entire length of the vertebral canal. After the third intra-uterine month, the column lengthens more rapidly than the cord, so that the cord appears to shrink upward in the vertebral canal. At birth, the lower end of the cord is opposite the body of the third lumbar vertebra. In the adult, the lower level of the cord is opposite the lower level of the first or the upper level of the second lumbar vertebra. From the inferior limit of the spinal cord (conus medullaris), a glistening thread, the terminal filament, is prolonged downward within the vertebral canal; it anchors the medulla to the coccyx.

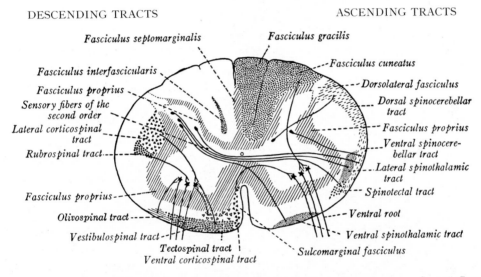

DESCENDING TRACTS   ASCENDING TRACTS

Fasciculus septomarginalis — *Fasciculus gracilis*

Fasciculus interfascicularis — *Fasciculus cuneatus*

Fasciculus proprius — *Dorsolateral fasciculus*

Sensory fibers of the second order — *Dorsal spinocerebellar tract*

Lateral corticospinal tract — *Fasciculus proprius*

Rubrospinal tract — *Ventral spinocerebellar tract*

Fasciculus proprius — *Lateral spinothalamic tract*

Olivospinal tract — *Spinotectal tract*

Vestibulospinal tract — *Ventral root*

Tectospinal tract — *Ventral spinothalamic tract*

Ventral corticospinal tract — *Sulcomarginal fasciculus*

Fig. 563.—Diagram Showing the Location of the Principal Fiber Tracts in the Spinal Cord of Man. Ascending Tracts on the Right Side, Descending Tracts on the Left.

The fibers of the corticospinal tract that supply the cervical segments of the cord lie in its medial portion, those supplying lumbar segments lie laterally with fibers to thoracic segments between (Walker, 1940).

1. **Gray Matter of the Cord.**—Cross section of the cord shows the gray matter on either side of the midline arranged in a comma-shaped mass with well-defined columns which project anteriorly and posteriorly lateral to the connecting gray commissure. The *anterior column*, short, broad, and blunt at its extremity, contains the motor cells which give origin to the fibers of the anterior nerve roots. The *posterior column* is pointed, and near its tip the posterior nerve roots enter the spinal cord. The cord levels with the largest amount of gray matter are the cervical and lumbar enlargements, whence emerge the great nerve trunks forming the large limb plexuses. In the thoracic region, the amount of gray matter is reduced, corresponding with the smaller size of the thoracic nerves.

2. **White Matter of the Cord.**—The white matter of the cord is seen on cross section as the field between the gray column and the cord periphery. The milky-white color is that of the medullary substance about the transversely cut nerve fibers. These fibers, although indistinguishable anatomically, differ functionally, part being motor and part sensory.

The **posterior (dorsal) area** of white matter is divided by the posterior median septum into a right and left column or funiculus. Each of these funiculi is divided by a paramedian septum into a mesial tract, the *fasciculus gracilis* (of Goll), and a lateral tract, the *fasciculus cuneatus* (of Burdach). The sensory fibers of which these tracts are composed enter the gray matter by the posterior nerve roots and are the centrally directed axones of nerve cells which lie in the spinal ganglia. The majority of these fibers pursue an uncrossed upward course along the mesial side of the posterior column of gray matter. Most of the impulses conducted in these fasciculi are transformed into impressions of muscle and joint sensation. Destruction of the nerve cells in the spinal ganglia, which give rise to these long ascending

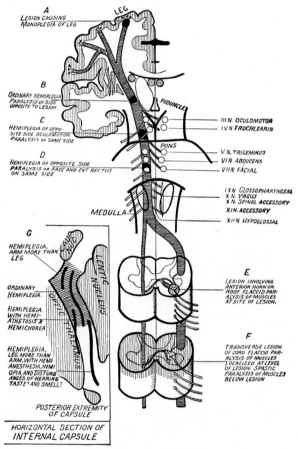

Fig 564.—Effect of Lesions in the Motor Path of the Brain and the Spinal Cord. Lesions
Are Indicated by Circles.
G, Internal capsule lesions and the variations in symptoms caused by the different anteroposterior locations
of the lesions. (Butler.)

fibers, causes degeneration of the fibers and prevents the muscle and joint sensations essential for equilibrium from reaching the brain centers; ataxic movements result. This destruction is the essential and constant lesion of tabes dorsalis.

The remaining mass of white matter is designated roughly as the **anterolateral column,** most of which consists of nerve fibers springing from nerve cells in the gray column. These fibers form an intrinsic system which links different levels of the spinal cord.

The more important systems of fibers are the lateral cerebrospinal (crossed motor or pyramidal) tract, the anterior cerebrospinal (uncrossed motor or direct pyramidal) tract, the dorsal and ventral spinocerebellar tracts, and the spinothalamic and spinotectal tracts.

The *lateral cerebrospinal (crossed motor or pyramidal) tract* is the great motor connection bringing the spinal motor apparatus under control of the brain. It lies anterior and lateral to the posterior column of gray matter and its fibers arise from the pyramidal cells in the motor area of the cerebral hemisphere. Most of the fibers cross the median plane (decussate) in the medulla. Destruction of these fibers as they descend in the brain substance causes paralysis in the muscles supplied by the motor nerves in the opposite side of the cord. In each spinal segment which the fiber bundle traverses, numerous fibers enter the anterior column of gray matter and ramify about the motor cells from which the fibers of the corresponding anterior nerve root are derived.

The *anterior cerebrospinal* (*uncrossed motor or direct pyramidal*) *tract* is a small motor nerve strand lying near the anterior median sulcus of the cord. It arises in the motor area of the cortex and continues down the cord on the same side. While the bundle as a whole does not decussate as it enters the cord from the brain, the fibers at each point along the downward course cross to the opposite side and ramify about the motor cells in the opposite gray matter.

The *dorsal spinocerebellar fasciculus* (of Flechsig) and the *ventral spinocerebellar fasciculus* (of Gower) convey sensations from the muscles and overlying skin which aid muscle coordination between the cord and the cerebellar centers of coordination. *Spinothalamic* and *spinotectal* tracts carry sensations of pain and temperature.

3. Spinal Nerve Roots, Ganglia, and Nerves.—An anterior and a posterior nerve root attach each spinal nerve to the cord. The *anterior* (*ventral*) *nerve roots*, which are purely motor, emerge in series from the anterior column of gray matter. The *posterior* (*dorsal*) *nerve roots*, which are purely sensory, enter the spinal cord in series on its posterolateral aspect On each posterior root is a *ganglion*, the cells of which give origin to central and peripheral fibers. The ganglia of all save the sacral and coccygeal nerves occupy the intervertebral foramina. Those of the sacral and coccygeal nerves lie within the vertebral canal. Within or near the intervertebral foramen, each pair of nerve roots unites to form a *spinal nerve*, which almost at its formation divides into an anterior and a posterior branch or primary division. Both divisions are mixed (sensory and motor) nerves. Just distal to the division, the spinal nerve gives off a minute recurrent branch to the meninges and cord, after uniting with a branch from the sympathetic trunk.

Each nerve root receives an investment from the pia mater and another from the arachnoid just before the root meets the dura. Within the subarachnoid space, the roots are bathed in cerebrospinal fluid. Outside the space, the nerves are encased in a tubular sheathing of dura which includes the ganglion on the posterior root.

4. Path of Sensory Conduction.—The path of sensory conduction is more complicated than that of motor conduction. It is composed of at least three sets of neurons disposed one above the other. The cells of the *lowest set* of *sensory neurons* lie in the ganglia of the posterior nerve roots. The axon of a ganglion cell divides in such a manner that one portion runs to the spinal cord and the other to the periphery of the body. The peripherally disposed sensory fibers make up the peripheral sensory nerves and conduct sensory impulses toward the ganglion cells from various specialized end-organs. The centrally disposed fibers enter the cord by the posterior roots and are the true axones of the nerve cells. They conduct sensory stimuli to the cord. The axones terminate in the cord in a variety of ways; many terminate about the cell bodies of the lower motor neurons to complete the reflex pathway; others divide into ascending and descending branches which travel in the white matter. Some of the ascending branches run upward to the medulla to end about cells in the cuneate and gracilis nuclei of the dorsal column. Other fibers (pain and temperature), after traveling two to three segments up the cord, cross to the opposite side and ascend in anterolateral tracts.

The cells lying in the nuclei of the dorsal column with their centrally directed axones form the *middle sensory neurons*. These axones, after decussating, do not run to the sensory cortex directly, but end in cells in the thalamus.

The cutaneous fields corresponding to the peripheral sensory nerve distribution are well known. The site and outline of the segmental cutaneous fields represented by the dorsal roots are known less accurately, but aid in determining the level of cord and dorsal root lesions.

SURGICAL CONSIDERATIONS

1. Diagnosis of Lesions in the Motor Pathway.—Abnormality of motion usually is the most important localizing sign of lesions in the motor pathway. The character of the impaired function varies according to whether an upper or a lower motor neuron is involved.

Degeneration which follows a destructive lesion in the *lower (spinomuscular) motor neuron* involves the axis-cylinders which run in the peripheral nerves. The muscles in

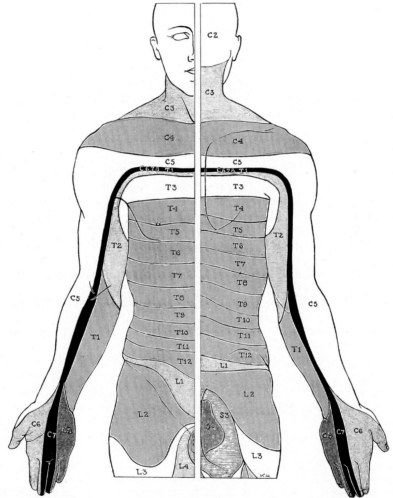

FIG. 565.—SPINAL CORD SEGMENT DISTRIBUTION TO THE SKIN OVER THE TORSO AND THE UPPER EXTREMITY.

which they end are weakened or paralyzed. With an irritative lesion, the muscles supplied by the nerve involved are thrown into abnormal contractions. The muscles of a paralyzed limb become small and flabby, the limb hangs helplessly, and the joints are relaxed because the articular processes no longer are held in close apposition by tonic contracture of the muscles about them. The muscle reflexes and tonus which depend upon the integrity of the reflex arc, of which the lower motor neuron is the efferent limb, are lost.

A lesion in the lower motor neuron causes paralysis of a few muscles only, or at the most, of a group of muscles. Sensory symptoms which may accompany the paralysis assist in making an accurate diagnosis. If paralysis with characteristic signs of a lower motor neuron lesion involves a group of muscles supplied by one nerve, and the anesthetic area of skin belongs to that nerve, the lesion obviously is in the nerve itself. If the paralyzed muscles are not supplied by a single nerve, but are represented together in the cord and the anesthetic area corresponds to that segment or segments, it is clear that the lesion must be in the cord itself or in a nerve root.

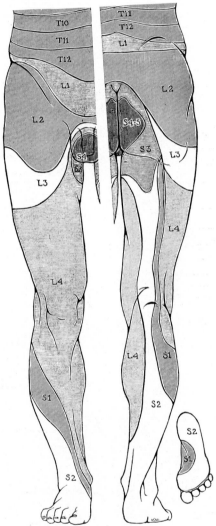

FIG. 566.—SPINAL CORD SEGMENT DISTRIBUTION TO THE SKIN OVER THE LOWER ABDOMEN AND THE LOWER EXTREMITY.

The *upper (corticospinal) motor neurons* are wedged into a small space, and a small lesion may cause paralysis of many muscles. The compact motor fiber bundle, the pyramidal tract, may have enough fibers involved in the internal capsule to produce paralysis of most of the muscles of the opposite side of the body (hemiplegia). The tract descends as a compact bundle, most of the fibers of which decussate in the medulla. The pyramidal tract gives off fibers to the motor nuclei at successive levels. A lesion anywhere in its course results in paralysis of all the muscles the spinal centers of which lie below the level of the lesion. Above the internal capsule, the fibers are separated somewhat so that in the cerebral cortex the centers controlling different sections of the body are comparatively far apart (p. 42).   A sharply localized cortical lesion causes a limited paralysis in a limb or a segment of a limb (cerebral monoplegia).

Destructive lesions in the upper (corticospinal) motor neuron cause paralyses with distinctive characteristics.   The paralysis is accompanied by a spastic condition, exaggerated muscle reflexes, and increased muscle tension.   All the muscles of a limb are in-

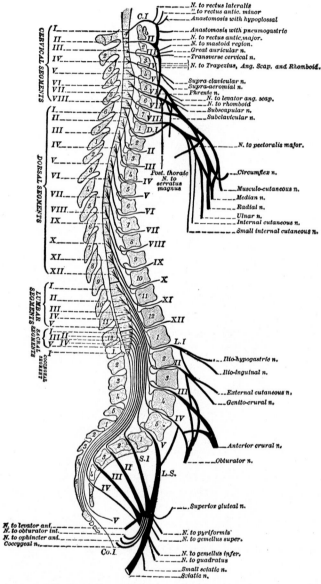

Fig. 567.—Relations of the Segments of the Spinal Cord and Their Nerve Roots to the Bodies and Spinous Processes of the Vertebrae.   (Déjerine and Thomas, modified by Starr.)

volved about equally.   The limb is stiff and can be moved only slowly and with difficulty because of muscle rigidity.   The muscles are hypersensitive to irritation so that tapping a muscle tendon elicits a quick muscle response.   The muscles atrophy somewhat.

In complete transverse section of the cord, the paralyzed muscles are flaccid and their reflexes are absent.

2. **Diagnosis of Lesions in the Sensory Pathway.**—A destruction of the sensory pathway in any part of the body deprives that part of all qualities of sensation.   Sensory loss

occurs most frequently from a lesion of the sensory neurons in the peripheral nerves; the anesthetic area depends upon the nerve involved. Unilateral lesions in the cord or in the higher sensory centers cause disturbances in sensation on the opposite side of the body. As a rule, destructive lesions do not involve all the paths of sensory conduction and the loss of sensibility usually is not complete. Astonishingly slight disturbances may be consequent upon fairly extensive lesions. Pain and temperature sensation may be lost and touch sensation remain normal, or muscle sense may be lost and the stereognostic sense (ability to recognize an object by the sense of touch) remain unimpaired. The distribution rather than the character of sensory loss is of consequence, and even distribution may give but insecure localization of the lesion. A combination of paralysis and sensory changes affords the most secure diagnosis.

3. **Vertebromedullary and Radicular Topography.**—The careful determination of the height at which a vertebral body or a cord segment is injured is a point of primary importance in the diagnosis and surgical treatment of cord and vertebral body disease. There can be no direct operative approach until a proper segmental diagnosis pointing to the site for laminectomy has been made.

The cord reaches inferiorly only to the level of the second lumbar vertebra, so that each of the cord segments is smaller than the corresponding vertebral body, and its nerve roots cannot leave the column at the same height as they leave the cord. The nerve roots run an appreciable distance downward within the vertebral canal before reaching the intervertebral foramina through which they pass. As a consequence of discrepancy between the length of the spinal cord and that of the vertebral column, the farther down the cord, the greater the distance between the attachment of the individual nerve roots to the cord and their emergence through the intervertebral foramina.

In order to determine the vertebral level at which a spinal cord lesion occurs, the exact difference in the levels of vertebral and cord segments must be known. The discrepancy in level between the numerically corresponding cord segments and vertebrae is measured roughly in vertebral bodies. It becomes progressively greater from above downward. In the cervical and upper thoracic regions, the cord segments lie one or two vertebral bodies higher than the numerically corresponding vertebrae; that is, cord segment C_7 lies at the level of vertebral body C_5. In the lower thoracic and upper lumbar regions, the cord segments lie two or three vertebral bodies higher; cord segment T_{12} is at the level of vertebral body T_{10}. In the lower lumbar and upper sacral regions, cord segments lie four or five vertebral bodies higher; cord segment L_5 is at the level of vertebral body T_{12} or L_1.

4. **Cord Injuries.**—Early examination and careful observation of cord injuries are essential to proper treatment. If a partial lesion gradually becomes more extensive, it is evidence of advancing change in the cord which should be investigated by laminectomy and exploration of the vertebral canal. Signs of a complete cord lesion which appear at the moment of injury usually indicate complete destruction of the cord. Complete cord lesions rarely are improved by operation. Occasionally, however, removal of a bony fragment pressing on the cord is followed by improvement.

Spinal puncture and the Queckenstedt test are helpful in determining the method of treatment. The *Queckenstedt test* utilizes manometric readings of spinal fluid pressure. The contents of the cranium are packed so economically within the skull that any increase in intracranial volume raises intracranial pressure, an increase which is transmitted to the cerebrospinal fluid system. Compression of both internal jugular veins above the sternal ends of the clavicles dams back blood in the skull and thus raises intracranial pressure. When a tumor completely obstructs the spinal canal, and, therefore, the flow of the cerebrospinal fluid, that part of the subarachnoid space superior to the tumor is cut off from that part below it. An increase in pressure in the fluid system above the tumor will not be transmitted to that part of the system below the tumor.

To perform this test, a lumbar puncture is made in the low lumbar region and the needle is connected to a manometer. The jugular veins then are compressed. If there is no increase in pressure in the fluid in the manometer, there is a block in the subarachnoid space somewhere between the needle and the skull. Thus, immediately after injury, pressure may show free communication between the cranial and lower spinal fluid spaces. A few hours later, manometric readings may indicate a complete block. These findings indicate increasing pressure on the spinal cord and call for laminectomy as a means of exploring and decompressing the cord.

A *complete transverse lesion of the cord* is followed by total sensory and motor loss in the regions innervated by the cord segments below the lesion. This is characterized by a flaccid paralysis and an abolition of all reflexes below the level of the injury. Voluntary control of the bladder and rectum is lost, but sometimes these organs regain an automatic power of evacuation. This is especially true if the cord lesion is above the third and fourth sacral segments, where the centers for the bladder and rectum are located. If the cord lesion occurs in these segments, complete bladder and rectal retention is more likely to occur.

A complete cord lesion at the level of the fourth cervical segment (second cervical vertebra) usually is fatal because paralysis of the phrenic nerve at its origin in the fourth cervical segment results in paralysis of the diaphragm. Frequently, lesions even one or two segments below the fourth cervical segment involve the phrenic nerve because of edema of the cord above the injury.

Lesions involving the cauda equina show usually patchy nerve involvement below the level of injury, with partial paralysis and sensory impairment. The sphincter power may or may not be lost, depending upon the completeness of the injury.

Partial injuries of the cord manifest spastic paralyses of varying degrees below the level of injury. Sensation is decreased, but not abolished, reflexes are increased, the great toe reflex is positive, and there may be complete loss of sphincter control.

Hemisection of the cord results in complete paralysis of the muscles innervated by the segments below the lesion, on the same side of the body as the lesion. There also are sensory changes, the locations of which are dependent upon the sensory tracts involved. Those fibers which carry pain and temperature sensations cross the median line immediately on entering the cord. Therefore, hemisection interrupts pain and temperature sensations only on the side opposite the lesion. The fibers carrying pressure sensation and tactile discrimination pass upward in the cord without crossing, so that hemisection interrupts pressure sensation and tactile discrimination only on the side of the lesion. Posture and movement sensations, however, are lost only in the paralyzed limb, as they are carried in fibers which ascend on the same side until they reach the medulla where they decussate. A narrow zone of anesthesia is present at the upper limit of the motor paralysis where the sensory fibers are involved as they enter the cord. The position of the anesthetic strip is a certain indication of the site of the lesion.

5. **Rhizotomy and Cordotomy.**—If intractable pain cannot be relieved by ordinary measures, section of the sensory nerve roots, rhizotomy, or section of the pain tracts in the cord, cordotomy, may be resorted to.

Rhizotomy is the operation of preference in the neck because cordotomy may injure fiber tracts to the brachial plexus and phrenic nerve. *Cordotomy*, or section of the anterolateral columns in the spinal cord, is effective in the relief of pain on the side opposite the incision. For relief of pain below the costal margins, cordotomy is more effectual than rhizotomy. Exposure for either operation is gained through a laminectomy at a point well above the foraminal entrance of the involved spinal nerves. In cordotomy, traction is made on the denticulate ligament lateral to the cord in such a manner that the cord is rotated dorsally and laterally. A knife then is inserted straight into the cord just ventral to the denticulate ligament to a depth of 3 mm. An incision made ventrally and laterally from this point should interrupt the pain and temperature tracts and cause anesthesia on the side opposite the incision. Section may be unilateral or bilateral. Great care must be taken to avoid injury to the pyramidal tract fibers to prevent paralysis and loss of sphincter control. It is advisable to perform the operation under local anesthesia so that sensory tests may be made to indicate the amount of anesthesia obtained. The results in either procedure are variable and the anesthesia produced may not effect abolition of pain.

UPPER EXTREMITY

I. SHOULDER

THE shoulder is differentiated topographically into four divisions: the axillary, posterior scapular, and deltoid regions, and the bones and joints.

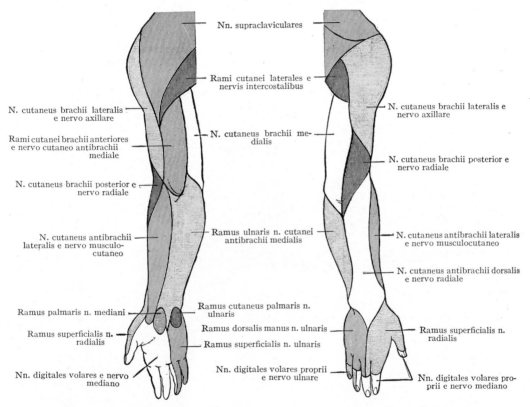

Nn. supraclaviculares

Rami cutanei laterales e nervis intercostalibus

N. cutaneus brachii lateralis e nervo axillare

Rami cutanei brachii anteriores e nervo cutaneo antibrachii mediale

N. cutaneus brachii posterior e nervo radiale

N. cutaneus antibrachii lateralis e nervo musculocutaneo

Ramus palmaris n. mediani

Ramus superficialis n. radialis

Nn. digitales volares e nervo mediano

N. cutaneus brachii medialis

Ramus ulnaris n. cutanei antibrachii medialis

Ramus cutaneus palmaris n. ulnaris

Ramus dorsalis manus n. ulnaris

Ramus superficialis n. ulnaris

Nn. digitales volares proprii e nervo ulnare

N. cutaneus brachii lateralis e nervo axillare

N. cutaneus brachii posterior e nervo radiale

N. cutaneus antibrachii lateralis e nervo musculocutaneo

N. cutaneus antibrachii dorsalis e nervo radiale

Ramus superficialis n. radialis

Nn. digitales volares proprii e nervo mediano

FIG. 568.—AREAS OF CUTANEOUS NERVE DISTRIBUTION IN THE UPPER EXTREMITY.

A. AXILLARY REGION

The axilla is the space situated between the upper lateral aspect of the chest wall and the proximal part of the upper limb. It is shaped like a pyramid with a blunted apex. The apex or inlet of the space transmits the large vessels and nerves which pass between the upper limb and the root of the neck. With the arm at rest along the thorax, the muscle walls of the region are relaxed and the examining hand can palpate the full extent of the fossa and examine the head of the humerus and the thoracic walls as far as the second rib. When the arm is in right angle abduction, the fossa becomes a groove with the anterior and posterior walls in apposition. In exaggerated abduction, the axillary fossa is obliterated and its structures are made tense.

1. **Walls of the Axilla.**—The axilla presents for examination an anterior or clavipectoral wall, a posterior or scapular wall, a mesial or costal wall, and a lateral or humeral wall

The **anterior wall** consists of two main strata. The pectoralis major muscle with its enveloping fascia forms the outer stratum, and the pectoralis minor muscle with the costocoracoid membrane of the clavipectoral fascia forms the deeper stratum. When the super-

559

ficial structures have been removed, the *pectoral fascia* is seen to enclose the pectoralis major muscle. This fascia attaches above to the clavicle and mesially to the sternum. It closes the superficial deltopectoral (infraclavicular) triangle laterally and is continuous below with the fascial covering of the serratus anterior and external oblique muscles. It blends with the axillary fascia in the floor of the axilla and with the fascia of the arm. Because the fascia contains many efferent mammary lymphatics, its removal is necessary in carcinoma of the breast (p. 235).

Division and reflection of the pectoralis major muscle in the anterior wall of the axilla exposes the *coracoclavicular (clavipectoral) fascia* which extends from the clavicle above to the axillary fascia below. The incision for the evacuation of an abscess under the coracoclavicular fascia is the same as that employed for infraclavicular ligation of the first portion of the axillary artery (p. 565).

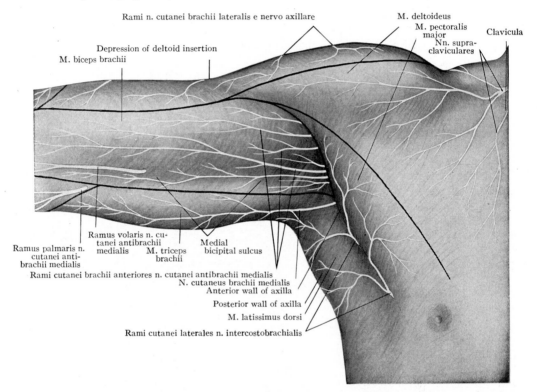

Rami n. cutanei brachii lateralis e nervo axillare

M. deltoideus
M. pectoralis major
Nn. supra-
claviculares
Clavicula

Depression of deltoid insertion
M. biceps brachii

Ramus volaris n. cu-
tanei antibrachii
Ramus palmaris n.   medialis   M. triceps   Medial
cutanei anti-   brachii   bicipital sulcus
brachii medialis

Rami cutanei brachii anteriores n. cutanei antibrachii medialis
N. cutaneus brachii medialis
Anterior wall of axilla
Posterior wall of axilla
M. latissimus dorsi
Rami cutanei laterales n. intercostobrachialis

FIG. 569.—SURFACE ANATOMY AND THE AREAS OF CUTANEOUS NERVE DISTRIBUTION IN THE AXILLARY REGION.

After enveloping the pectoralis minor muscle, the clavipectoral fascia descends to meet the axillary fascia in its stretch from the anterior to the posterior axillary folds. Between the two strata of the anterior wall of the axilla is a cellulo-areolar interval, the interpectoral compartment, in which vessels and nerves to the pectoral muscles ramify, and in which an interpectoral abscess sometimes is formed.

The **medial (costal) wall** of the space corresponds to the five upper ribs and their intervening spaces which are concealed by the upper digitations of the serratus anterior muscle. The serratus anterior arises from the lateral surfaces of the upper eight ribs, a short distance in front of the midaxillary line. Its fibers pass backward, closely applied to the chest wall, and are inserted into the ventral aspect of the vertebral border of the scapula. The serratus anterior pulls the scapula forward, and, when opposed by the rhomboid muscle, steadies the scapula in the movement of forward pushing. By acting with the trapezius muscle to rotate the scapula, it enables the arm to be raised above the head. The long thoracic nerve (of Bell) (C$_5$, $_6$, $_7$) appears from behind the axillary vessels and enters the serratus anterior muscle on its superficial aspect.

The **lateral wall** of the axilla, to which the important axillary vessels and nerves are related, is formed by the coracobrachialis and biceps brachii muscles, the proximal part of the shaft of the humerus, and the mesial aspect of the shoulder joint.

The **posterior (scapular) wall** is composed of the subscapularis muscle on the anterior surface of the scapula, and the latissimus dorsi (p. 312) and teres major muscles. The subscapularis arises from the subscapular fossa and converges toward the head of the humerus, where it is inserted by a thick tendon into the lesser tubercle of the humerus and into the capsule of the shoulder joint. The posterior wall of the axilla approaches the anterior wall closely at the level of the intertubercular sulcus of the humerus; the

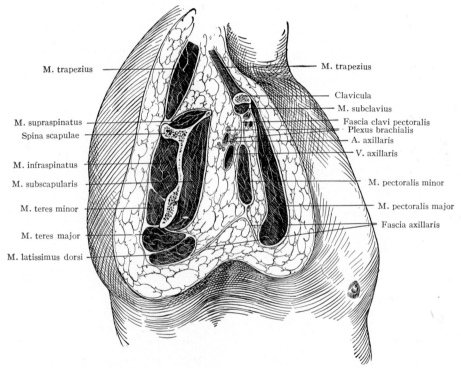

FIG. 570.—SAGITTAL SECTION THROUGH THE AXILLARY FOSSA TO SHOW THE CONTENTS AND THE MUSCULAR AND FASCIAL WALLS.

angular interval separating the two is occupied by the long and short heads of the biceps and the coracobrachialis muscles. The axillary vessels and nerves lie in close relationship with the medial aspect of these muscles.

The structures constituting the **floor** of the axilla are the skin, subcutaneous tissue, and axillary fascia. The axillary fascia is an ill-defined, resistant membrane. Because of its great strength, deep abscesses rarely perforate it.

The **apex** of the axilla is in communication with the supraclavicular fossa along the axillary vessels and nerves and the surrounding areologlandular tissue.

2. Axillary Vessels and Nerves.—The axillary sheath is a downward and lateral prolongation of the prevertebral fascia from the neck. It encloses the axillary vessels and nerves, as well as a few apical lymph glands, and is lost upon the neurovascular elements as they pass outward from the axilla. In axillary dissection for carcinoma of the breast the apical nodes are removed by excising part of the sheath.

The **axillary artery** is the direct continuation of the subclavian artery; it extends from the outer margin of the first rib to the lower border of the teres major muscle, beyond which it is known as the brachial artery (p. 592). Throughout its course, it is accompanied closely by the axillary vein and has very intimate, although changing, relationships with the nerves of the brachial plexus. The artery is divided into three stages corresponding to the parts of the vessel situated proximal, behind, and inferior to the pectoralis minor muscle.

The *first division* of the artery lies behind the clavipectoral fascia and the clavicular head of the pectoralis major muscle.

The *second division* of the artery, that behind the pectoralis minor muscle, is the shortest. About it are arranged the medial, lateral, and posterior cords of the brachial plexus, exactly as their names indicate.

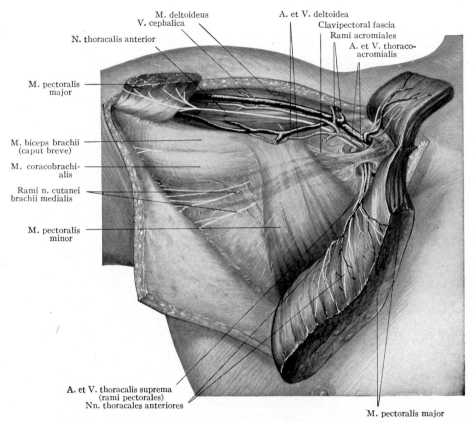

FIG. 571.—FRONT VIEW OF THE AXILLARY REGION WITH THE PECTORALIS MAJOR PORTION OF THE ANTERIOR WALL OF THE AXILLA REMOVED.

The *third division* of the artery at first is overlain by the pectoralis major muscle, but becomes superficial before reaching its termination. The terminal nerves of the brachial plexus are arranged about it, two on each side. Laterally, lie the musculocutaneous nerve and the lateral head of the median nerve; anteriorly, are the medial head of the median nerve and the medial cutaneous (internal) nerve of the forearm; mesially, between the axillary artery and the axillary vein, is the ulnar nerve; and posteriorly, lie the radial (musculospiral) and axillary (circumflex) nerves. The axillary nerve leaves the artery at the lower border of the subscapularis muscle and passes backward through the quadrilateral space (p. 567). The subscapular artery from the third division of the axillary is the largest branch.

The axillary artery is related to the capsule of the shoulder joint and therefore is exposed to pressure from anterior dislocation of the head of the humerus, especially if the dislocation is extreme and the head is mesial to the coracoid process. The artery may be injured in delayed reduction of shoulder dislocations. Where the artery lies over the subscapularis tendon and the fusion of the tendon with the capsule of the shoulder joint, it is exposed to lacerations from fracture of the surgical neck of the humerus and from epiphyseal separation.

The **axillary vein** is formed from the union of the basilic and the two brachial veins. Its principal affluent is the cephalic vein, which enters it a short distance below the clavicle through the crease between the pectoralis major and deltoid muscles (deltopectoral infraclavicular triangle). The subscapular tributaries of the axillary vein possess a wide anas-

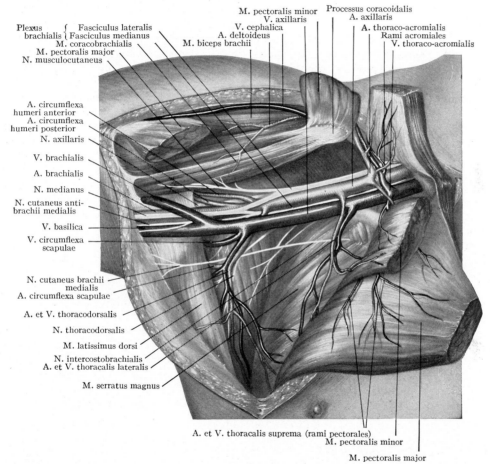

FIG. 572.—VASCULONEURAL CONTENTS OF THE AXILLA AFTER REMOVAL OF THE ANTERIOR OR PECTORAL WALL OF THE AXILLARY FOSSA.

tomosis with the veins of the thoracic wall, and, as these tributaries are associated with the axillary lymph nodes, they must be removed along with the nodes as a routine measure in radical removal of the breast for carcinoma. With the arm in abduction, the vein lies anterior to the artery, hiding it from view. The intimate relations of the artery to the vein explain the frequency of traumatic arteriovenous aneurysm. A wound in the upper part of the axillary vein is particularly dangerous, not only because of profuse hemorrhage, but also because of the risk of air entering the vessel, the walls of which tend to be held apart by the fibrous expansions thrown over the vessel by the coracoclavicular (clavipectoral) fascia. It is advisable in all axillary operations to clear the axillary vein as soon as possible to avoid wounding it in the course of subsequent dissection.

It is important to be able to identify the various **nerves** of the brachial plexus as they surround the third division of the axillary artery (see Fig. 205). The *median nerve* is recognized by its great size and its two heads of origin. Because of its superficial position, it is the nerve most frequently involved in wounds of the axilla. The *musculocutaneous nerve* is smaller than the median and occupies a lateral position where it reaches and pierces the coracobrachialis muscle. The *ulnar nerve* may be difficult to distinguish from the *medial (internal) cutaneous nerve* of the forearm, since both arise from the median cord and are overlain by the axillary vein at their origin. The ulnar is the larger and more posterior. The *radial (musculospiral) nerve* is the direct continuation of the posterior cord and differs from the ulnar nerve by its posterior position and greater size. In the axilla, the radial nerve is exposed to pressure in improper use of a crutch. From the posterior cord arises the *axillary (circumflex) nerve* which runs a posterolateral course upon the neck of the humerus. It may be lacerated or contused by dislocation of the head of the humerus or by fracture fragments. Injury of this nerve (p. 667) causes atrophy of the deltoid muscle, loss of the rotundity of the shoulder, and an area of cutaneous anesthesia over the deltoid.

3. **Axillary Lymph Glands** (see Fig. 224).—The axillary lymph glands are embedded in the areolo-adipose tissue occupying the axillary space. They are arranged in several groups. The *anterior or pectoral (thoracic) group* lies in the mesial part of the axilla, against the serratus anterior muscle and between the posterior surface of the pectoralis major muscle and the coracoclavicular (clavipectoral) fascia. An abscess arising from these glands tends to point at the upper or lower margin of the pectoralis major muscle. This group drains not only the outer part of the breast, but also the superficial layers of the anterior abdominal wall above the umbilicus, and the side of the chest. The *lateral (brachial) group* accompanies the axillary vein on the lateral wall of the axilla, receives the lymphatics from the upper limb, and is the first group of axillary glands to be involved in lymphangitis of the hand and forearm.

The *posterior (subscapular) glands* are arranged about the posterior axillary fold upon the subscapularis muscle and are associated with the subscapular vessels and the thoraco-dorsal nerve. They drain the superficial layers of the back of the chest and some of the anterior pectoral glands. The *apical nodes* lie high up in the axilla behind the coraco-clavicular fascia. They drain the pectoral, subscapular, and lateral groups of glands and are connected with the infraclavicular nodes in the superficial deltopectoral (infraclavicular) triangle. In carcinoma, the apical glands may become adherent to the axillary vein, thereby necessitating excision of a part of that vessel. The glands sometimes obstruct the cephalic vein as it pierces the coracoclavicular fascia. Efferents from this group of glands open into the lymph channels at the root of the neck.

SURGICAL CONSIDERATIONS

1. **Axillary Abscesses.**—Axillary abscesses occur in the pectoral region or in the axillary space. A *pectoral or interpectoral abscess* from involvement of the anterior pectoral glands cannot extend upward into the neck as it is confined between two layers of fascia, both of which are attached to the clavicle. As a rule, the abscess is not large and becomes superficial either in the infraclavicular fossa or at the level of the anterior axillary fold.

An *abscess within the axillary space* usually is of lymphatic origin, the causative infection draining from a neighboring source, particularly from the fingers. It may occur from infection within the shoulder joint or in one of the upper ribs. A common source is infection spreading down an axillary hair follicle. If the suppurative process is not checked, the whole axilla may be converted into an abscess cavity. In the presence of abscess the normally concave floor of the axilla bulges convexly downward. Because of the free communication between the apex of the axilla and the supraclavicular fossa, the abscess readily extends upward behind the clavicle into the root of the neck. Its backward progress is checked by the attachment of the serratus anterior muscle to the scapula. Extension of the abscess into the arm along the great vessels occasionally is observed.

The proper *treatment* of axillary abscesses is early evacuation of their contents and the establishment of free drainage. The incision should be directed between and parallel to the anterior and posterior axillary folds to avoid injury to the lateral thoracic and subscapular vessels. An abscess from infection of the apical group of lymph glands lies behind the coracoclavicular fascia, and the incision for drainage is the same as that employed for infraclavicular ligation of the first portion of the axillary artery.

2. **Axillary Aneurysm and Injury to the Axillary Artery.**—The comparative frequency of *axillary aneurysm* may result from the free range of mobility of the artery and its close proximity to the heart. The presence of an aneurysm usually is revealed by a fluctuant swelling in the axilla. If the upper divisions of the artery are implicated, the tumor tends to project forward below the clavicle through the infraclavicular fossa. When the aneurysm springs from the third stage of the vessel, the anterior axillary fold is raised, the hollow of the armpit disappears, and a soft pulsating mass presents. Because of the laxity of the tissue about the artery, the aneurysm meets with little resistance and its growth usually is rapid. Pressure of the aneurysm on the nerves of the brachial plexus causes pain and, subsequently, a loss of cutaneous sensibility in certain areas of the upper limb. Loss of power in the upper extremity may result from interference with the motor nerves, and edema of the arm and hand from compression of the axillary vein.

Injury of the axillary artery sometimes occurs in the reduction of old dislocations at the shoulder joint while breaking down adhesions between the axillary vessels and the tissue about the dislocated head of the humerus.

3. **Ligation of the Axillary Artery.**—Ligation of the axillary artery is performed either in the first division of the vessel (above the pectoralis minor muscle) or in the third division (below the pectoralis minor muscle) where it lies on the tendon of the latissimus dorsi.

Infraclavicular ligation of the first division of the axillary artery is difficult because of the depth of the vessel, the many small vessels encountered in reaching it, and the narrow confines of the space in which the manipulations are conducted. After the shoulder is drawn backward and upward, a curved incision is made from a point mesial to the coracoid process to a point just below the sternoclavicular joint. The clavicular portion of the pectoralis major muscle is exposed and is divided the full length of the wound. The pectoralis minor muscle then is identified and retracted downward. The coracoclavicular (clavipectoral) fascia, now exposed, is divided close to the coracoid process, care being taken not to wound the thoraco-acromial artery and the lateral anterior thoracic nerve emerging at this level. As the axillary vein comes into view behind the membrane, it is retracted mesially and the artery is exposed. To accomplish the ligation, it may be necessary to bring the arm down to the side, as the vein tends to overlie and conceal the artery when the arm is abducted at right angles to the trunk. The collateral circulation for ligation of this division of the artery is similar to that forced into play when the subclavian artery is ligated in its third division.

The third division of the axillary artery is superficial and is the site of election for ligation. The incision for *ligation of the artery in the third division* is made through the outer part of the armpit parallel to the course of the vessel. After the superficial tissues have been divided, the coracobrachialis muscle is exposed and drawn outward with the musculocutaneous nerve. The axillary artery lies in the depth of the wound, surrounded by the large brachial nerves. Probably the best site to apply the ligature is between the origin of the subscapular artery and the two circumflex arteries, but the vessel may be tied immediately proximal to the origin of the subscapular artery. In the latter instance, the collateral circulation is carried on by the anastomosis between the intercostal, lateral thoracic, transverse cervical, transverse scapular (suprascapular), and thoraco-acromial arteries proximal to the ligature, and by the subscapular and humeral circumflex arteries on the distal side of the ligature. When the axillary artery is tied between the subscapular and circumflex branches, anastomosis between the humeral circumflex arteries and the branches of the

thoraco-acromial and transverse scapular arteries reestablishes the circulation. When the
subscapular and humeral circumflex vessels arise by a common trunk and a ligature is
applied distal to the vessel, the collateral anastomosis follows the same course as in ligation
of the brachial artery proximal to the origin of the (superior) profunda artery (p. 592).

B. POSTERIOR OR SCAPULAR REGION

The scapula with its embracing musculature occupies the posterior part of the shoulder
and affords valuable protection to that part of the chest wall to which it is applied. It
serves to connect the humerus with the trunk and to increase greatly the range of movements of the upper extremity, so that, even with a firmly ankylosed shoulder joint, con-

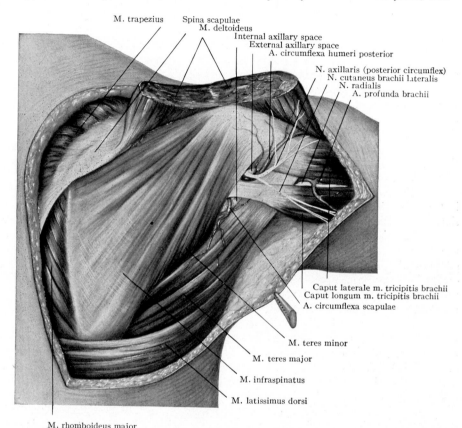

FIG. 573.—SUPERFICIAL STRUCTURES OF THE SCAPULAR REGION.

siderable mobility is retained. The infrequency of fracture of the body of the scapula
results mainly from the protective action of the many muscles which clothe it.

1. **Landmarks.**—The posterior aspect of the scapula is divided by the scapular spine
into an upper or supraspinous and a lower or infraspinous area. The *scapular spine* extends
upward and laterally from the vertebral margin of the bone opposite the third thoracic
spinous process to become continuous with the *acromion*. The spine, acromion, *vertebral
border*, and *inferior angle* of the scapula are palpated easily, especially when the shoulder
is retracted with the elbow drawn out from the side. In wasting diseases, these bony
landmarks become very prominent.

An important action of the serratus anterior muscle is the maintenance of the scapula
in close contact with the chest wall. As a sequel of paralysis of the serratus anterior
muscle from injury to the long thoracic nerve (of Bell) in operations in the axilla or from

a blow or undue pressure upon the shoulder, the vertebral border and inferior angle of the scapula lose contact with the chest wall and project from it like a wing (*winged scapula*). This deformity is rendered more striking by pressing forward against a wall with the arms extended at shoulder level.

2. **Superficial Structures.**—The skin over the scapula is thick and is bound down closely to a dense subcutaneous tissue. Over the intrinsic scapular musculature pass the trapezius, deltoid, and latissimus dorsi muscles. These are intrinsic in adjoining regions and, with their enveloping aponeuroses, form a powerful musculofibrous layer.

3. **Posterior Scapular Muscles.**—The *supraspinatus muscle* (N. suprascapular, $C_4, _5, _6$) arises from the supraspinous fossa and the deep surface of the dense overlying aponeurosis. It runs outward under the acromion into the deltoid region where it inserts on the uppermost of the three facets on the greater tuberosity of the humerus and blends with the capsule of the shoulder joint. When the arm is in abduction, the supraspinatus rotates it slightly outward; its primary function is to initiate lateral elevation of the arm.

The infraspinatus, teres major, and teres minor muscles lie in and about the infraspinous fossa under the dense infraspinous aponeurosis which blends laterally with the overlapping deltoid sheath. The *infraspinatus muscle* (N. suprascapular, $C_4, _5, _6$) arises from the infraspinous fossa and runs upward and laterally to insert into the middle facet on the greater tuberosity of the humerus. It is a lateral rotator of the arm. The *teres minor muscle* (N. axillary, $C_5, _6, _7$) arises just below the infraspinatus muscle from the axillary margin of the scapula and inserts on the inferior facet of the greater tuberosity. It acts as a lateral rotator and adductor of the arm; its power of external rotation is increased proportionately as the arm is abducted. The *teres major muscle* (N. subscapularis, $C_5, _6$) arises from the inferior angle of the scapula and inserts into the mesial border of the intertubercular sulcus (bicipital groove). It adducts the arm and rotates it medially. The anterior scapular muscles are described with the costal and scapular walls of the axilla (p. 559).

The sheathing of the posterior scapular muscles within dense fascial and osteofibrotic compartments explains the clinical findings in the region. *Hemorrhage* from scapular fracture appears on the surface as trifling ecchymosis, and *tumors* from the fascial coverings may be mistaken for bony growths. The dense, overlying fascia is weakened above the transverse scapular (suprascapular) ligament where the transverse scapular (suprascapular) vessels enter the region. *Infection in the supraspinous fossa* generally passes through the scapular notch and points under the anterior border of the deltoid muscle near the coracoid process, or gravitates into the infraspinous fossa. The fascia is thin also at a point midway down the axillary margin of the scapula where the circumflex scapular (dorsal scapular) vessels pass to the dorsum of the scapula. An *abscess in the infraspinous fossa* is prevented from extending backward by the dense overlying fascia; hence, pus follows the circumflex scapular vessels, gravitates downward, and points at the lower part of the posterior fold of the axilla. Infection in either fossa may escape outward toward the muscle insertions.

4. **Vertebroscapular Muscles.**—The *levator scapulae muscle* ($C_3, _4$) is inserted into the medial (superior) angle of the scapula. The *major and minor rhomboid muscles* (C_5) arise from the upper thoracic spines and insert into the vertebral margin of the scapula. The dorsal scapular nerve (to the rhomboids) passes down along the vertebral border of the scapula under these muscles. The vertebroscapular muscles are the antagonists of the trapezius and serratus anterior muscles; they rotate the scapula so that the lower angle passes backward and mesially. In paralysis of the rhomboid muscles, the scapula on the injured side lies below its normal level and its inferior angle is farther than normal from the median plane.

5. **Intermuscular Vasculoneural Pathways.**—The downward passage of the long head of the triceps muscle (p. 591) between the teres minor and major muscles forms two obliquely transverse intermuscular spaces. The quadrilateral *external axillary space* is bounded by the humerus, the long head of the triceps, and the minor and major teres muscles.

Through the space pass the posterior humeral circumflex branch of the axillary artery and the axillary (circumflex) nerve. The triangular *medial axillary space* is bounded at the side by the long head of the triceps muscle, above by the teres minor, and below by the teres major. Through it emerges the circumflex scapular branch of the axillary artery. Below the teres major muscle is a *triangular triceps interspace* between the two heads of the triceps, through which run the superior profunda artery and the radial nerve These interspaces are the posterior exits of axillary infection.

6. **Vessels and Nerves.**—The arteries to the scapular region are derived from two widely separated sources, the proximal subclavian, and the terminal axillary arteries. They form an important collateral pathway which restores circulation to the upper extremity after ligation of either the subclavian or axillary trunks. The *transverse scapular*

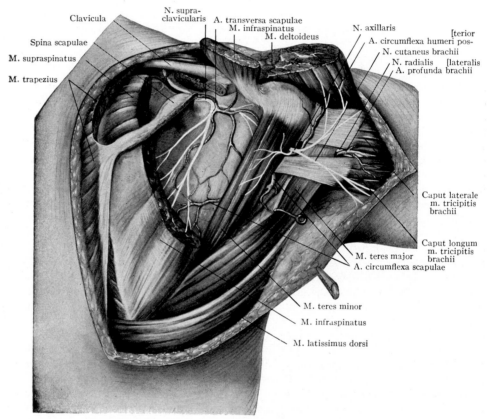

FIG. 574.—DEEP STRUCTURES OF THE SCAPULAR REGION.
Parts of the trapezius, supraspinatus, infraspinatus, and deltoid muscles have been removed.

(suprascapular) artery is a branch of the thyrocervical trunk of the subclavian artery (p. 210). It reaches the region through the scapular incisura and ramifies over the posterior surface of the scapula. The *circumflex scapular (dorsal scapular) artery* from the axillary emerges through the medial axillary space and is distributed over the inferior part of the posterior surface of the scapula.

The nerves are the suprascapular, axillary, and radial. The *suprascapular nerve* runs with the transverse scapular artery and innervates the muscles of the scapular fossae. The *axillary (circumflex) nerve* leaves the axilla through the external axillary space with the posterior humeral circumflex artery and passes laterally upon the surgical neck of the humerus to supply the deltoid muscle. It gives branches to the teres minor muscle and the shoulder joint, and forms the lateral cutaneous nerves of the arm. The *radial nerve* passes downward with the profunda artery of the arm, supplies the long head of the triceps muscle, and gives off the posterior cutaneous nerve of the arm.

7. **Fractures of the Scapula.**—Fracture of the scapula is rare because of the protective action of its intrinsic muscles and those connecting it with the trunk, and because of its mobility and the elasticity of the underlying chest wall. The most common variety is *transverse fracture of the body* of the scapula through the infraspinous fossa. Overlapping and angular projection of the fragments are prevented by the muscles which invest the bone and act as splints. An old method of examination suited to demonstration of fracture of this kind consists in gripping the acromion and outer end of the clavicle with one hand, drawing the shoulder backward, and grasping the prominent lower angle of the scapula with the other hand, and endeavoring to obtain preternatural mobility and possible crepitation. This procedure is unnecessary if a good x-ray examination can be obtained.

When fracture occurs in the *scapular neck*, which extends from the scapular notch to the upper part of the axillary border, almost parallel to the glenoid articular surface, the spine and acromion may be grasped with one hand and the proximal end of the humerus with the other. Crepitus sometimes can be elicited by moving the head of the humerus forward and backward. The degree of displacement of the detached fragment necessarily is limited because of the strong ligamentous connection interposed between the coracoid process and the clavicle. The *acromion process*, notwithstanding its exposed position, rarely is the site of fracture, but when fracture does occur there is little tendency toward displacement because of the dense fibrous investment of that part of the scapula. It must be borne in mind that the acromial epiphysis may fail to unite with the spine of the scapula and be connected with it only by a layer of cartilage. The two may be connected by a distinct joint. When the presence of a movable acromion, especially with a history of trauma, suggests a fracture, the finding of bilateral ununited epiphyses is of great value in differential diagnosis. Normally, the acromial epiphysis begins to ossify about the fifteenth year and joins the spine at about the twenty-fifth year.

Because of its sheltered position under the clavicle, the *coracoid process* seldom is injured. It may be broken off by an inward dislocation of the head of the humerus (p. 580). There is little displacement of the fragments unless the coracoclavicular ligament sustaining the process is broken. The ligament is steadied mesially by the pectoralis minor muscle. The distal fragment tends to be drawn downward by the weight of the arm and by the attachment of the coracobrachialis muscle and the short head of the biceps muscle to its tip. A sling for the forearm and a circular bandage about the chest usually are sufficient *treatment* for scapular fractures with little displacement.

8. **Rupture of the Supraspinatus Tendon.**—To understand the pathologic change and the symptoms produced by rupture of the supraspinatus tendon, it is necessary to recall that the capsule of the shoulder joint in its superior and posterior portions blends with, and becomes indistinguishable from, the flat expanded tendons of the supraspinatus, infraspinatus, and teres minor muscles as they pass to their insertions on the greater tuberosity of the humerus. The supraspinatus tendon lies above and forms the roof of the shoulder joint. It also forms a part of the floor of the subacromial bursa, which is interposed between the tendon and the acromion process and extends outward nearly 2.5 cm. between the greater tuberosity and the deltoid muscle. The function of the bursa is to facilitate movement of the greater tuberosity under the acromion in abduction of the shoulder.

Rupture of the supraspinatus tendon commonly takes place close to the greater tuberosity. The muscle then retracts, enlarging the separation and creating an opening of greater or less extent through which there is direct communication between the overlying bursa and the shoulder joint. In addition to large complete ruptures, there probably are many small tears which involve only a few fibers of the tendon. Codman considers injuries of this type to be the most common cause of traumatic subdeltoid bursitis. Wilson is of the opinion that gradual deterioration of the tendon takes place from excessive use and is attenuated by age, and that there probably is defective tendon circulation. It is likely that these changes precede and pave the way for rupture of the tendon; this view explains rupture occurring under normal use.

Meyer has described many examples of attrition affecting bursae, ligaments, and tendons. He has described fraying and rupture of the tendon of the long head of the biceps, and occasionally in cadaver dissection has found the upper half of the shoulder joint destroyed. In these cases, the supraspinatus tendon probably has been ruptured. Rupture of this tendon commonly is a lesion of late adult life and occurs in persons who have done heavy work. The rupture probably is produced in one of two ways, either by muscle strain when the arm is abducted or by a direct blow upon the shoulder.

There may be only a small amount of pain associated with the tear. The history of a painful snap in the shoulder followed by noticeable weakness should suggest the possibility of supraspinatus tendon rupture. Continued disability following a fall on the shoulder, or the sudden onset of disability of the shoulder, should be regarded as suspicious of tendon rupture. Examination reveals atrophy of the shoulder muscles, most marked

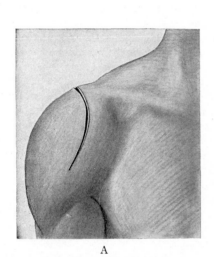

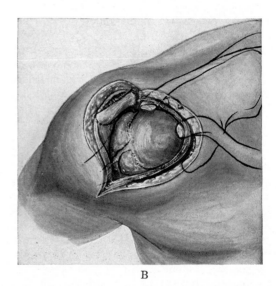

A   B

FIG. 575.—ANTEROSUPERIOR APPROACH TO THE SHOULDER JOINT BY THE CODMAN "SABER-CUT" INCISION.
A is the incision through the soft parts of the shoulder; B is the exposure of the shoulder joint. The acromioclavicular joint has been incised and the base of the acromion has been divided. Lateral retraction of the flap containing the acromion process and the deltoid muscle exposes the superior aspect of the shoulder joint.

in the supraspinatus and infraspinatus regions. Palpation usually reveals a point of sharply localized tenderness over the tip of the greater tuberosity of the humerus, or just medial to it under the acromion. This may disappear when the tuberosity passes under the acromion. As the arm is moved actively through its range of motion, coarse crepitation in the region of the bursa is noted; this crepitation may be under the acromion. As the arm is moved passively forward and backward or in rotation, an unusual bony prominence can be felt to move under the examining fingers in the region of the subacromial bursa. This prominence is the greater tuberosity which stands out prominently because of the gap in the supraspinatus tendon. A common finding is a lack of or weakness in active abduction, which is initiated by the supraspinatus muscle and completed by the deltoid muscle. Contraction of the supraspinatus pulls the greater tuberosity under the acromion and abducts the arm through the first 15 degrees, from which level the deltoid muscle can complete the movement. The supraspinatus muscle also has the power of pulling the head of the humerus inward and fixing and stabilizing it in the glenoid fossa in active motion.

Operative *treatment* should be undertaken whenever function is reduced materially. It is possible to approximate the ruptured tendon by abducting the shoulder and pulling the tendon outward under considerable tension. The tuberosity usually is bare of tissue and a firm point of attachment for the tendon can be secured only by drilling holes in the bone or grooving it to form broad contact with the flat sheet of tendon. It is necessary to provide a smooth floor for the new bursa so that movement of the tuberosity under the acromion will not cause pain.

Codman's "saber-cut" incision affords the exposure necessary. It passes posteriorly from the acromioclavicular joint over the top of the shoulder. The joint is opened and the base of the acromion is cut through with an osteotome or Gigli saw. The outer flap, which includes the tip of the arch of the shoulder girdle, and the attached deltoid muscle are retracted laterally. This affords a wide exposure of the capsule and tendons overlying the humeral head, and the extent of the rupture of the supraspinatus tendon can be determined. The healed fibrous edge of the opening is excised sufficiently to expose sound tendon tissue. With the arm in abduction, the edge of the tendon may be drawn outward to approximate the greater tuberosity without undue tension. With an osteotome, a channel is cut in the anatomical neck of the humerus just proximal to the greater tuberosity to provide a bed for the edge of the tendon. Holes are drilled through the lateral edge of this groove. Sutures of fascia lata lace the tendon to the groove, leaving a smooth floor for the subacromial bursa and providing means for the tendon to become fixed to the bone throughout the length of the channel. The superficial structures are closed in layers, after the parts have been fitted back normally. The shoulder should be fixed in 90 degrees abduction, since recovery of function in the atrophied muscles is favored in a position of muscle relaxation.

9. Congenital Elevation of the Scapula (Sprengel's Deformity).—The congenital deformity of elevation of one scapula usually is associated with some degree of scoliosis. There may be associated anomalies of the face and skull, wryneck, or absence of bones and muscles. A bridge of bone sometimes connects the scapula with the vertebral column, or a piece of bone, which does not articulate with the spine, may project upward from the superior border of the scapula.

Because the scapula is elevated, the shoulder is carried high; the neck on the affected side is short and thick and the trapezius muscle is prominent; the function of the arm is not impaired seriously. The superior border of the scapula is prominent and suggests the presence of an exostosis. The deformity may be bilateral.

C. DELTOID REGION

The deltoid or lateral region of the shoulder is important functionally because of its powerful abductor mechanism. The region is outlined by the deltoid muscle and consequently is triangular in shape. It is bounded above at its base by the outer third of the anterior margin of the clavicle, the apex and lateral border of the acromion, and the lower border of the spine of the scapula. It is limited below by a shallow depression, a little above the middle of the shaft of the humerus, which marks the insertion of the deltoid muscle. Surgical interest in the region lies in the access it affords to the shoulder joint and the frequency of the involvement of the subacromial (subdeltoid) bursa.

1. Surface Anatomy.—The lateral margin of the acromial end of the clavicle is directed backward and overrides slightly the articular surface of the acromion. The *acromion process*, which forms the shoulder cap, is defined easily by palpation, and, where there has been much wasting of the tissue, stands out very distinctly. Laxity of the acromioclavicular joint allows separation of the articular surfaces. The *coracoid process* of the scapula lies under cover of the anterior border of the deltoid muscle, but can be felt on direct downward and backward pressure 2.5 cm. below the clavicle, anterior to the outer curve. The *apex of the acromion* lies a little anterior to the acromioclavicular joint. The continuation of its lateral margin can be traced backward for about 5 cm. where it joins the inferior border of the scapular spine which it meets at the sharp *acromial angle*.   The small *acromial tubercle* at the angle is a useful landmark in taking measurements of the arm.   The comparison of the distance between the acromial angle and the lateral condyle of the humerus on the two sides discloses any difference in the length of the humerus.

The normal rounded contour of the shoulder is maintained by the proximal end of the humerus. over which the deltoid muscle is applied closely.   In joint effusion (serous or purulent synovitis), the deltoid area is abnormally full and prominent, but fluctuation may be difficult to detect because of the overlying muscle.   When the head of the humerus is dislocated mesially beneath the coracoid process or inferiorly beneath the glenoid fossa, the deltoid muscle no longer is prominent, but descends vertically from its upper to its lower attachment; the acromion is unduly prominent, and the shoulder is flattened.

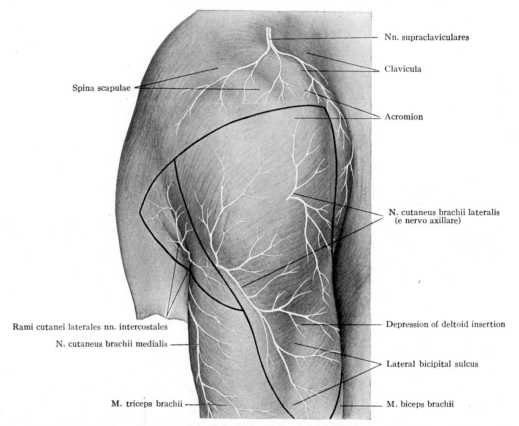

Spina scapulae

Nn. supraclaviculares

Clavicula

Acromion

N. cutaneus brachii lateralis (e nervo axillare)

Rami cutanei laterales nn. intercostales

N. cutaneus brachii medialis

Depression of deltoid insertion

Lateral bicipital sulcus

M. triceps brachii

M. biceps brachii

FIG. 576.—SURFACE ANATOMY AND AREAS OF CUTANEOUS INNERVATION OF THE DELTOID REGION.

Under normal conditions, the head of the humerus is related closely to the under surface of the acromion and is felt rotating beneath it when the arm is moved   In deltoid paralysis and in deep anesthesia, the interval between the acromion and humerus is increased, and the tip of the finger can be thrust into the intervening gap.

2. **Deltoid Muscle.**—The deltoid muscle arises from an extensive V-shaped attachment from the anterior margin of the lateral part of the clavicle, the lateral border of the acromion, and the lateral border of the scapular spine.   It overlies and conceals the shoulder joint and gives the shoulder a smooth, convex contour.   It converges to a pointed insertion on the *deltoid tuberosity* halfway down the lateral aspect of the humerus.

The deltoid muscle continues and maintains abduction of the humerus after its initiation by the supraspinatus.   In complete abduction, the arm is raised to an angle of about 180 degrees, the first 15 degrees of which is effected by the supraspinatus, the next

75 by the deltoid, and the remainder by rotation of the scapula by the trapezius and the serratus anterior muscles. The clavicular fibers of the deltoid are flexors and mesial rotators of the arm; the posterior fibers have an opposite action.

3. **Vessels and Nerves.**—The *posterior circumflex artery* and the *axillary* (*circumflex*) *nerve* reach the deltoid region through the external axillary space. They pursue a horizontal course forward beneath the deltoid, their path being indicated by a transverse line passing a little above the middle of the muscle. Incisions for approach to the shoulder joint should be made near the anterior border of the deltoid muscle to minimize damage to the axillary nerve. Results of injury to the axillary nerve are characteristic (p. 667).

4 **Subacromial (Subdeltoid) Bursa.**—The subacromial bursa lies between the deep surface of the deltoid muscle, the acromial arch, and the lateral surface of the shoulder joint. It has subacromial and subdeltoid divisions which may be separated by a thin

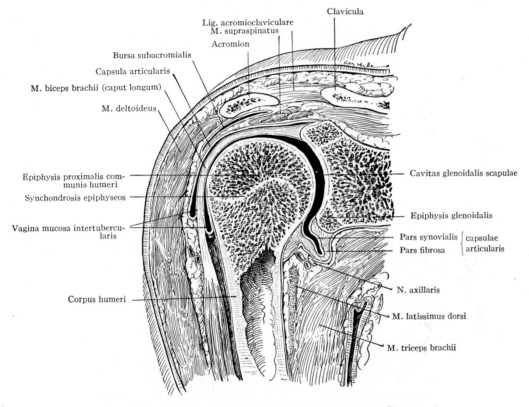

Lig. acromioclaviculare
M. supraspinatus
Acromion
Clavicula
Bursa subacromialis
Capsula articularis
M. biceps brachii (caput longum)
M. deltoideus
Epiphysis proximalis communis humeri
Synchondrosis epiphyseos
Vagina mucosa intertubercularis
Corpus humeri
Cavitas glenoidalis scapulae
Epiphysis glenoidalis
Pars synovialis ⎰ capsulae
Pars fibrosa ⎱ articularis
N. axillaris
M. latissimus dorsi
M. triceps brachii

FIG. 577.—FRONTAL SECTION THROUGH THE SHOULDER REGION.

partition, but they so frequently communicate that the bursa should be considered as a single space. The subacromial division lies between the deep surface of the acromion above and the insertion of the tendon of the supraspinatus muscle below. The supraspinatus tendon, which is fused into the superior part of the capsule of the shoulder joint, forms much of the floor of this division of the bursa. The bursa almost disappears under the acromion when the arm is abducted to a right angle.

The supraspinatus and other tendon attachments to the greater tuberosity of the humerus may be torn in sudden motions or lesions about the shoulder. These lacerations tear the subacromial bursal floor and produce serious disability.

Inflammation of the subacromial bursa, *subacromial bursitis*, causes painful abduction and outward rotation of the arm. The painful stage of abduction is that which marks the passing of the greater tuberosity under the acromion, when the bursa is impinged against.

Since an injury to the bursal floor brings the bursa into communication with the shoulder joint, the excess joint fluid remains in the joint when the arm is adducted and the effusion cannot be detected. When the arm is abducted, the fluid is forced into the bursa and forms an appreciable swelling beneath the deltoid muscle (Codman).

Any tear of the supraspinatus tendon renders abduction weak, except for that part of the motion performed by the deltoid muscle. If the laceration is extensive, abduction cannot be initiated with the arm hanging at the side. Complete abduction, obtained passively, cannot be maintained against feeble downward pressure on the arm. This weakness is explained by the fact that the deltoid muscle cannot initiate abduction, or maintain it unless the supraspinatus tendon holds the humeral head firmly in the glenoid fossa.

Bursitis uncomplicated by tear of the infraspinatus tendon is treated by immobilization with the arm in abduction until the acute symptoms in the bursa subside. Active motion is begun gradually as early as possible.

5. **Anterior Approach to the Shoulder Joint.**—The anterior approach to the shoulder joint is described in the region of the bones and joints of the shoulder (p. 578). The anterior approach to the shoulder joint through Codman's saber-cut incision is described under rupture of the supraspinatus tendon (p. 571).

D. BONES AND JOINTS

The bones and joints of the shoulder include the glenohumeral or true shoulder joint and the coraco-acromioclavicular arch, under which the shoulder joint functions.

1. **Acromioclavicular Joint and the Clavicle.**—The articular surfaces of the **acromioclavicular joint** are oval and flat and their axes are directed backward. They do not lie in the sagittal plane, but are directed obliquely so that the clavicular facet rests upon that of the acromion. The joint surfaces sometimes are separated by an interarticular cartilage. The joint margins are embraced by a weak *capsule*, thickened above and below by the *superior* and *inferior acromioclavicular ligaments*. A sliding anteroposterior movement exists in this joint so that, when the shoulder is thrust forward, the angle between the clavicle and acromion becomes smaller.

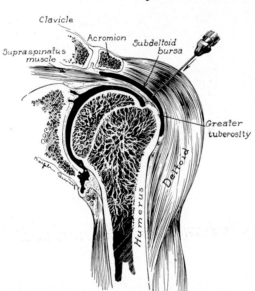

The joint is strengthened by the *coracoclavicular ligament* which binds the upper surface of the coracoid process to the under surface of the clavicle near its acromial end. Much of the weight of the upper extremity is conveyed to the clavicle by this ligament. The joint is strengthened further by the *coraco-acromial ligament* which contributes to the formation of a strong arch above the shoulder joint and to prevention of upward dislocation of the head of the humerus.

Fig. 578.—Frontal Section Through Left Deltoid Area at Level of Supraspinatus Tendon (Haldeman and Soto-Hall, Jour. Amer. Med Assoc., June 29, 1935.)

A factor contributing to the security of this joint against trauma from above is the degree of obliquity with which the clavicular facet rests upon and is supported by the acromion. This arrangement very effectively prevents downward displacement of the acromial end of the clavicle. The slope of the articular surfaces explains also the common injury of *upward dislocation* of the *clavicle*. A force directed downward and mesially on the acromion thrusts it beneath the clavicle, tearing the reinforcing ligaments of the joint.

An exaggerated upward displacement of the clavicle indicates rupture of the coracoclavicular ligament. The reduction of the dislocation is simple, but maintenance of proper position is extremely difficult. Any means by which the acromion can be drawn upward into its natural relations with the clavicle should be utilized. In an extreme form of this injury, some form of operative treatment designed to draw the clavicle down to the coracoid process and maintain it in this position is indicated, as the coracoclavicular ligament usually is torn.

The **clavicle** functions as a prop and keeps the acromion and shoulder joint at a distance from the trunk. The trapezius muscle supports the acromial end of the clavicle and helps to counteract the downward pull of the weight of the arm.

2. **Articular Extremities of the Shoulder Joint.**—The glenoid cavity of the scapula articulates with the head of the humerus in a ball and socket joint. The joint surface of the *articular extremity of the scapula* consists of the shallow glenoid fossa covered with

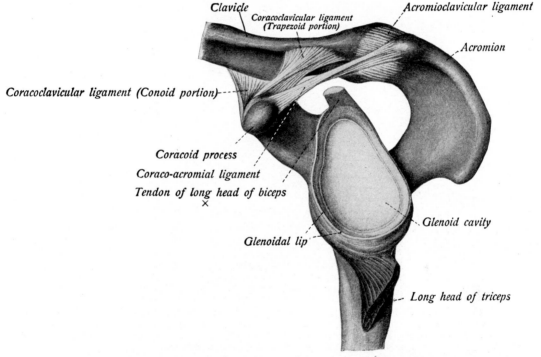

FIG. 579.—SOCKET OF THE LEFT SHOULDER JOINT AFTER REMOVAL OF THE ARTICULAR CAPSULE AND THE TENDON OF THE BICEPS MUSCLE. (Sobotta and McMurrich.)

cartilage and surrounded and deepened by the glenoid labrum (glenoid ligament). Between the glenoid fossa and the body of the scapula is a constricted portion, the neck, marked by superior and inferior glenoid tubercles for the attachment of the long head of the biceps muscle and the triceps muscle

The joint surface of the *upper extremity of the humerus* is almost hemispherical and is directed upward, mesially, and slightly backward. Its cartilaginous surface is large in comparison with that of the scapula; consequently, only a small part remains in contact with the glenoid fossa at any one time. The head of the humerus is separated from the rest of the bone by a shallow groove or constriction, the anatomical neck, which encircles the articular margin. The anatomical neck is distinguished from the surgical neck which is the cylindrical and somewhat constricted part of the shaft intervening between the tubercles and the insertions of the axillary muscles, the pectoralis major, the latissimus dorsi, and the teres major.

Lateral and anterior to the head of the humerus are the greater and lesser tubercle, (tuberosities). The greater tubercle continues downward as the lateral surface of the shafts and the lesser tubercle looks directly forward. Into the greater tubercle insert the supraspinatus, infraspinatus, and teres minor muscles; to the lesser tubercle attaches the subscapularis muscle.

At birth, the upper extremity of the humerus is entirely cartilaginous. The *center of ossification* for the articular head appears during the first year; that for the greater tubercle in the second year, and that for the lesser tubercle at the end of the third year. These three centers unite during the seventh year to form the proximal epiphysis of the humerus. The epiphysis is concave on its under aspect and overlies the cone-shaped proximal end of the diaphysis like a cap. It fuses with the diaphysis between the eighteenth and twenty-fifth years. The epiphyseal line is partly intracapsular and passes distal to the tubercles, but coincides medially with the margin of the articular head of the bone.

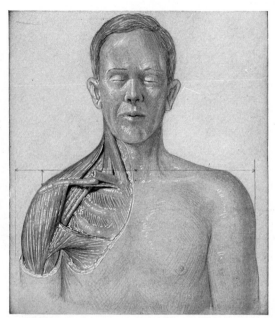

FIG. 580.—USUAL DISPLACEMENT IN FRACTURE OF THE CLAVICLE.

In the usual displacement, the proximal fragment is tilted up by the sternocleidomastoid muscle and the distal fragment is depressed and carried inward by the weight of the arm and contraction of the pectoral teres major, and latissimus dorsi muscles. (Babcock, "Textbook of Surgery.")

Between the tubercles, the intertubercular sulcus (bicipital groove) is prolonged down the shaft; it lodges the tendon of the long head of the biceps and has attached to its crests the tendons of the pectoralis major, latissimus dorsi, and teres major muscles.

3. **Reinforcing Tendons and the Capsule of the Shoulder Joint.**—The capsule of the shou der joint is not exposed fully until the tendons of the infraspinatus and teres minor muscles are separated or dissected away. These tendons fuse with and strongly reinforce the capsule. The subscapularis muscle differs from these muscles by being separated from the capsule by a large subscapular bursa. At the level of this bursa the capsule presents a deficiency of variable extent, through which a small pouch of synovia protrudes. The long tendon of the biceps muscle is an important accessory support of the joint. It is invested by a fold of joint synovia which is carried in the form of a tubular prolongation into the intertubercular sulcus and ends blindly opposite the insertion of the pectoralis major muscle.

The *capsule*, when divested of overlying tendons, appears very large and remarkably loose, and is adapted to a wide range of joint movement, especially abduction. The scapular attachment of the capsule is applied to the bony rim of the glenoid fossa and to the labrum. The presence of the mesial part of the epiphyseal line within the joint capsule explains the frequent extension of osteomyelitis of the shaft into the joint cavity. Because of the mode of capsular attachment, a separated epiphysis may carry with it a small portion of the shaft.

4. **Joint Synovia.**—The synovial membrane lines the capsule throughout and is attached to the articular margins. The long head of the biceps muscle arises from the uppermost point of the glenoid margin and traverses the joint. Although a portion of the tendon of the long head of the biceps is intracapsular, it remains extrasynovial. The synovial sheath and tendon are retained in the intertubercular sulcus by the transverse ligament which is attached to both tubercles and bridges the sulcus. When this ligament is torn, the tendon of the long head of the biceps is displaced to the mesial side of the lessert ubercle.

In a thin person, an *effusion* within the joint may be distinguished along the long head of the biceps where the fluid gravitates along the synovial prolongation surrounding the tendon, and points opposite the tendon of the pectoralis major muscle or lower down on the inner aspect of the extremity. Joint suppuration may establish a fistula through the synovial prolongation. The joint may be aspirated just lateral to the tip of the coracoid process by directing the needle posteriorly, superiorly, and laterally. The great vessels and nerves and the subacromial bursa thus are avoided.

5. **Stability of the Shoulder Joint.**—The stability of the shoulder joint depends upon several factors. The *short capsular muscles*, which are connected intimately with the capsule, are important in maintaining the joint surfaces in contact. When they are severed, the head of the humerus falls away from the glenoid fossa. The stability provided by the *coraco-acromioclavicular arch* compensates, in a large measure, for the discrepancy in the sizes of the articular surfaces. On its under aspect, the arch presents a smooth concave surface with which the tendons of the short capsular muscles are in contact, and against which, through the intermedium of the subacromial bursa, they play in the various shoulder movements. The most important function of the arch is to protect the head of the humerus and prevent its upward displacement. The arch also prevents forward or backward displacement, since the coracoid and acromion processes descend lower than the summit of the head of the humerus. The *long head of the biceps*, which crosses the head of the humerus a little mesial to its center, acts as a steadying brace. It prevents any sudden impact between the head of the humerus and the overlying arch. If air enters the capsule, the cavity is converted from a potential to an actual one, and the laxity of the capsule allows the joint surfaces to fall widely apart.

6. **Movements.**—Movements at the shoulder joint are very free, flexion, extension, abduction, adduction, circumduction, and rotation being possible. They show a remarkable adaptability of structure to function. In *flexion*, the arm can be moved forward through a semicircle from its position of rest beside the trunk. *Extension* has a limited range which is restrained by the anterior part of the capsule and by the contact of the head of the humerus with the coracoid process. Flexion and extension depend in large measure upon the mobility of the scapula. When the arm is flexed, the upper angle of the scapula moves backward and its inferior angle forward. Reverse movements occur in extension. These movements are favored by lax acromioclavicular ligaments and are restrained by the coracoclavicular ligaments. *Adduction* of the arm is prevented by contact with the side; adduction forward and medially is present, but is limited by the chest wall. *Abduction* is free and, like flexion, enjoys a semicircular range; the limit of abduction is reached with the arm vertically over the head and parallel to the long axis of the trunk. Contact of the humerus with the acromion limits the movement, as does the tension on the lower part of the capsule against which the joint surface of the humerus is brought into forcible contact In all injuries about the shoulder, abduction and external rotation are the motions to be guarded. The large articular surface of the humeral head and the small glenoid socket favor *circumduction*. *Rotation* of the humeral head normally approximates 180 degrees.

37

Surgical Considerations

1. **Surgical Approaches to the Shoulder Joint.**—The *anterior approach* to the shoulder joint is through a vertical incision through the anterior fibers of the deltoid muscle midway between the coracoid and the acromion processes. This incision does little damage to the deltoid muscle or to its nerve supply. By rotating the arm mesially and laterally, it is possible in joint resection to elevate the scapular muscles from the tubercles, either subcortically or subperiosteally. The external rotator muscles, the supraspinatus, infraspinatus, and teres minor, are detached subperiosteally from the greater tubercle. The long

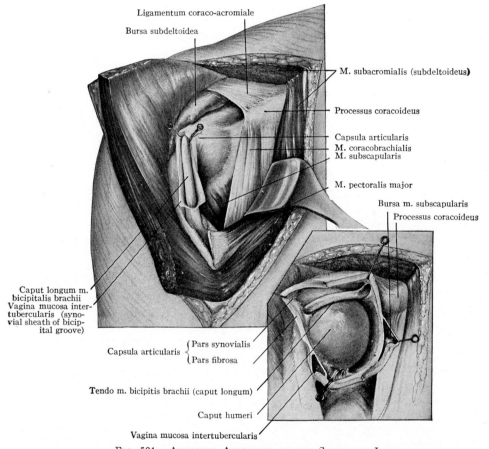

Ligamentum coraco-acromiale
Bursa subdeltoidea
M. subacromialis (subdeltoideus)
Processus coracoideus
Capsula articularis
M. coracobrachialis
M. subscapularis
M. pectoralis major
Bursa m. subscapularis
Processus coracoideus
Caput longum m. bicipitalis brachii
Vagina mucosa inter-tubercularis (synovial sheath of bicipital groove)
Capsula articularis { Pars synovialis / Pars fibrosa
Tendo m. bicipitis brachii (caput longum)
Caput humeri
Vagina mucosa intertubercularis

Fig. 581.—Anterior Approach to the Shoulder Joint.
Much of the insertion of the deltoid muscle along the clavicle has been divided to expose the joint more adequately.

head of the biceps muscle is retracted from its groove and drawn medially, and the subscapularis tendon is detached subperiosteally from the lesser tubercle.

The upper extremity of the humerus may be excised through the opening afforded in this way. The exact line of bone section depends upon the exigencies of the case. The favorite site of section is at the anatomical neck; section may have to traverse the tubercles or, occasionally, the surgical neck. Section through the surgical neck entails the loss of the fulcrum action of the humerus against the glenoid cavity, with loss of power in ele. vating the limb. With the biceps, coracobrachialis, pectoralis major, latissimus dorsi, and teres major muscles preserved, the arm can perform most of its movements. Subperiosteal resection gives the best functional results. Removal of the glenoid fossa for tuberculosis is not easy by the anterior route.

Greater access than can be obtained by vertical incision of the deltoid muscle is procured by detaching the deltoid from its origin along the lateral third of the clavicle and from the acromion and drawing it downward. Hemorrhage during this operation comes from division of the acromial branches of the acromiothoracic artery and that branch of the anterior circumflex artery running in the intertubercular sulcus.

The disability occasioned by the detachment of the muscles in major resection is so great that the operation rarely is performed. Because internal rotation is performed mainly by the subscapularis muscle and external rotation by the infraspinatus and teres minor muscles, loss of their attachments produces a flail joint. The muscles of the axillary fold in no wise compensate for the loss of the rotators attached to the tuberosities.

Arthroplasty of the shoulder joint rarely is indicated because of the more favorable results attending arthrodesis, in which a wide range of motion is attainable in the arm through the action of the scapulothoracic muscles, provided the humerus be ankylosed in abduction.

The *posterior approach* (of Kocher) is more difficult than the anterior, but gives freer access to, and more extensive exposure of, the joint. The approach is made by freeing the deltoid and trapezius muscles from the spine of the scapula, sawing or chiseling through the spine obliquely, and drawing the acromion process and deltoid muscle forward and laterally over the head of the humerus. Reflecting the acromiodeltoid flap laterally makes

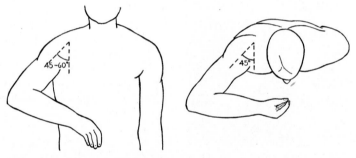

Fig. 582.—Optimum Position of the Arm in Ankylosis of the Shoulder Joint.
A, Position viewed from above; B, position viewed from in front. (Modified from McGregor.)

the head of the humerus, covered by the external rotator tendons, accessible in its upper, lateral, and posterior aspects. The joint is opened from above where subsequent weakness matters least.

The approach to the bones and joint of the shoulder by the *saber-cut incision* has been described in the deltoid region (p. 571).

2. **Arthrodesis of the Shoulder.**—The principal indication for an artificial bony union between the humerus and the glenoid (arthrodesis of the shoulder) is a flail arm which is not benefited by transplantation of the shoulder muscles to the humerus. The shoulder girdle has muscles capable of carrying the arm through its necessary ranges of movement if the joint between the humerus and scapula is obliterated. Arthrodesis is the procedure of preference in correction of the paralyses of the upper arm caused by anterior poliomyelitis (infantile paralysis) if the principal muscles which rotate the scapula are not paralyzed. The deltoid muscle usually is paralyzed and there is no substitute for its action since the supraspinatus muscle is too weak to carry out abduction. Ordinarily, the trapezius muscle is not paralyzed because of the high level of its innervation, and the serratus anterior muscle generally is spared. These two muscles are the main rotators of the scapula and effect abduction if there is fixation of the glenohumeral joint. The main area of stability in this arthrodesis is that between the greater tuberosity of the humerus and the acromion process. This fusion materially strengthens the bony fixation in the glenohumeral joint.

The optimum position for the arm in an ankylosed shoulder is abduction of about 45 degrees. The arm should be 45 degrees forward of the frontal plane. The younger the patient, the greater should be the abduction angle.

3. Effusion in the Shoulder Joint.—Effusions in the shoulder joint may result from injury or disease. They may be confused with accumulations of fluid in the subacromial bursa (p. 573). As the tension of the accumulating fluid increases, the arm is held in abduction to enable the capsule to accommodate it, and it is in this position that fluctuation can be elicited. Fluid frequently follows the long head of the biceps muscle and forms a palpable swelling on the anterior surface of the arm. The effusion tends to escape through the weak areas of the capsule. It may communicate with the subacromial bursa and cause it to become distended.

A purulent effusion may work its way under the deltoid muscle and point on the skin at the anterior and posterior borders of the muscle or at the fold of the axilla. To avoid this complication, it is advisable to institute through-and-through drainage by way of the anterior approach. An instrument is passed through the joint so that it projects posteriorly below the tendon of the teres minor muscle; horizontal incision then is made over the instrument to avoid injury to the axillary (circumflex) nerve.

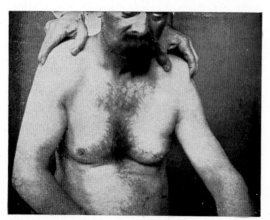

FIG. 583.—SUBCORACOID DISLOCATION OF THE LEFT HUMERUS.

Note the change in the axis of the left humerus and the method of palpating under the acromion, demonstrating the hollow on the left caused by absence of the humeral head from the glenoid fossa. (Scudder, "Treatment of Fractures.")

4. Dislocation at the Shoulder Joint.—Glenohumeral dislocation is the commonest dislocation in spite of the stability of the shoulder joint. Several factors contribute to the incidence of dislocations at this joint: it frequently is exposed to injury by falls on the outstretched hand, the elbow, or the point of the shoulder, thrusting the head of the humerus against the capsule; the glenoid fossa is shallow and small in comparison with the hemispherical surface of the humeral head, making the joint union insecure; and the violence causing dislocation is unexpected so that the reinforcing effect of the well-braced capsular muscles cannot be brought into play. Were it not for the great freedom of movement of the scapula on the chest wall and a considerable degree of motion at the acromioclavicular joint, dislocation at the shoulder joint would occur more frequently.

In childhood, the capsule and reinforcements are stronger than the union between the epiphysis and diaphysis, and epiphyseal separation is more usual than dislocation. As age advances and joint stability is sacrificed for mobility, joint strength depends upon muscle support and the common injury is dislocation.

The acromion usually forms the fulcrum for dislocation when the arm is in abduction. The shaft of the humerus forms the long arm of the lever and the upper extremity of the humerus forms the short arm. In the production of the dislocation, the long lever arm is thrust upward until it impinges against the acromion and causes the humeral head to tilt downward against the inferior part of the capsule, the only area not supported by tendons. The capsule gives way and the humeral head passes through the tear and lies, for a time at least, below the glenoid fossa. It presses against the external (quadrilateral) space and comes into relationship with the axillary nerve (p. 564), which may be bruised or even ruptured. The head of the humerus may come to occupy an inferior, posterior, or anterior position with reference to the glenoid fossa.

After rending the capsule below the subscapularis tendon and anterior to the triceps tendon, the head of the humerus may come to rest in the **inferior (subglenoid) position** below and mesial to the glenoid fossa. The inferior margin of the glenoid fossa rests in the groove of the anatomical neck.

In **posterior dislocation,** the head of the humerus passes through the posterior part of the capsule and comes to rest on the posterior margin of the glenoid fossa, against the neck of the scapula under the acromion (subacromial), or in the infraspinous (subspinous) fossa anterior to the infraspinous muscle. The nature of the rotation of the humerus depends upon whether the subscapularis muscle is or is not ruptured.

Although most dislocations at first are subglenoid, the flexor and adductor muscles of the shoulder usually draw the head of the humerus into **anterior and medial dislocation.** The head of the humerus is thrust through the anterior part of the capsule beneath the subscapularis muscle. The capsule is weak anteriorly and usually presents a small aperture through which the joint synovia communicates with the bursa beneath the subscapularis muscle (p. 561). In anterior displacement, the head of the bone may occupy several positions. As the humeral head leaves the glenoid fossa, it descends a little to pass beneath the coracoid process. If displacement is arrested at this point, the dislocation is *subcoracoid,* and the humeral head lies beneath the subscapularis tendon and anterior to the neck of the scapula. The humerus is rotated laterally because of the stretching of the infraspinatus and teres minor tendons. The posterior part of the capsule is stretched taut against the posterior rim of the glenoid fossa, and the posterior part of the anatomical neck rests against the forward border of the glenoid.

The head of the humerus may be carried still further mesially and for the most part lie to the mesial side of the coracoid process. The anatomical neck rests upon the anterior surface of the neck of the scapula or against the forward part of the glenoid rim as in the last instance, but with more medial rotation of the humerus. There usually is a concomitant marked deflection of the biceps ten-

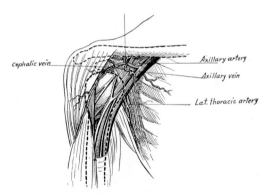

FIG. 584.—RELATION OF THE BLOOD VESSELS AND NERVES TO THE HEAD OF THE HUMERUS. (Moorhead, "Traumatic Surgery.")

don downward and medially from its normal course. The lateral rotators of the arm are overstretched, and, if they do not give way the whole or a part of the greater tubercle may be torn away (fracture dislocation). The subscapularis muscle in these dislocations is stretched or lacerated by the head of the humerus. Displacement further medially occasionally is observed when the head of the humerus is carried more completely into the axilla and upward toward the clavicle into the interval between the serratus anterior and pectoral muscles. The *subclavicular* variety of dislocation ordinarily is associated with extensive tearing of the capsule and the capsular muscles.

In all forward displacements, the normal, rounded contour of the shoulder is lost. The humeral head is drawn mesially so that the deltoid muscle no longer is molded over the greater tubercle but drops straight downward from the acromion. The outer margin of the acromion, now the outermost bony point of the shoulder, becomes prominent and a ruler can be made to touch both the acromion process and the lateral condyle of the humerus. In extreme forward and mesial displacement, the head of the humerus produces a rounded elevation in the superficial infraclavicular area.

The displaced humeral head may press upon the axillary vessels, causing an edematous or gangrenous condition of the limb. In old unreduced dislocations, the axillary vessels may adhere to the fibrous tissue about the humerus and be injured in subsequent attempts at reduction. The axillary nerve is exposed to pressure injury because of its proximity to the neck of the humerus.

In an examination for dislocation, it is well to remember that the range of movement upon the affected side is decreased, and that there is inability to place the palm of the injured extremity upon the opposite shoulder with the elbow applied to the side of the chest.

5. **Reduction of Dislocation of the Shoulder Joint.**—The **direct method** of reduction of an uncomplicated shoulder dislocation is effected by direct traction of the arm against the pull of the strong muscles maintaining the head of the humerus out of position. In this method, an assistant steadies the patient's chest and exerts countertraction, while the operator exerts traction on the arm and manipulates the humerus with his foot in the patient's axilla. The initial steps consist of gentle abduction and slow, steady, firm traction on the arm to draw the head of the humerus free from the scapula, relax the deltoid and supraspinatus muscles, and stretch the subscapularis tendon and the lower part of the capsule. If the tear is through the anterior part of the capsule, reduction may occur without further manipulation; if it is through the inferior aspect of the capsule, the articular head is brought into contact with it by medial rotation. By continued traction on the arm, the subscapularis tendon is stretched tightly over the head of the humerus, pressing it through the rent in the capsule.

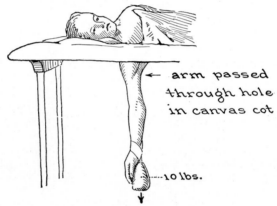

FIG. 585.—STIMSON'S POSTURAL METHOD OF REDUCTION OF AN ANTERIOR DISLOCATION AT THE RIGHT SHOULDER JOINT.

The **indirect method** of reduction (of Kocher) is executed in four maneuvers. In the *first maneuver*, the arm is held as closely as possible against the side and drawn downward, fixing the distal end of the humerus so that the subsequent manipulations exert their maximum action on the head of the bone. For the *second maneuver*, the patient's wrist is grasped so that the flexed forearm may be used as a lever to produce lateral rotation of the humerus, which is effected by carrying the forearm away from the chest until it lies almost in the frontal plane. The motion is performed slowly to overcome gradually the restraining muscle spasm of the adductors of the arm. This maneuver elevates the anatomical neck from the glenoid margin and brings the posterior aspect of the greater tubercle against the articular surface of the glenoid fossa, from which it is separated by a part of the capsule. If the tear involves the anterior part of the capsule, the subscapularis tendon, made tense by the extreme outward rotation, may press the head back into place.

If reduction has not occurred, a *third maneuver* is used. The elbow is carried mesially across the chest; lateral rotation of the arm is maintained by the position of the forearm. This movement of flexion and adduction of the arm stretches the capsule by tilting the greater tubercle backward and usually causes the head to drop into place. If reduction then has not taken place, a *fourth maneuver* is performed. The forearm is pressed rapidly over to the opposite shoulder to cause mesial rotation of the humerus. By elevating the elbow slightly during this movement, the humeral head descends as it rotates mesially and passes through the rent in the inferior part of the capsule.

Shoulder **dislocation complicated by avulsion of the greater tubercle** sometimes occurs The difficulty of treating this combined lesion lies, not in the reduction of the dislocation, but in the maintenance of the arm in abduction to obtain satisfactory healing of the fracture. Abduction is definitely unfavorable to the repair of the torn capsule and, as a compromise, the arm is kept in adduction for sufficient time to assure repair of the capsule; abduction then is begun gradually to restore motion at the shoulder joint. **Dislocation with fracture of the surgical neck** of the humerus almost always must be reduced by open operation, as the small proximal fragment assumes a position that renders manipulative reduction impossible. If the bony fragment torn away includes the supraspinatus insertion, the fragment may be drawn upward under the acromion process and subsequently limit abduction. In longstanding dislocations with fibrous adhesions, the lateral rotation in Kocher's method of reduction exerts a powerful twist on the humerus and may cause a spiral fracture of the surgical neck. In the direct method of reduction with the foot in the axilla, the reducing force is exerted along the long axis of the shaft, and, therefore, incurs little danger of fracture.

6. **Fracture of the Clavicle.**—The clavicle is fractured more frequently than any other bone in the body. The bone is fixed at its sternal extremity by strong ligaments and may be compressed by indirect violence exerted along its long axis until it gives way at its weakest point. Fracture sometimes is caused by direct trauma. The usual location of fracture is at the junction of the middle and outer thirds of the bone; it is therefore mesial to the coracoclavicular ligaments (Fig. 581). As a rule, the fragments are displaced markedly by the combined effect of muscle pull and the weight of the extremity. The displacement is confined chiefly to the outer fragment, which is drawn downward and medially. The trapezius muscle, acting on the shoulder girdle, one arch of which is broken, is unable to support the weight of the upper extremity. The mesial displacement of the outer fragment is increased by the mesial pull of the axillary muscles.

Fracture may occur lateral to the ligament, and the medial fragment be elevated slightly above the lateral, but the up and down displacement is not conspicuous. The anteroposterior displacement may be marked and the lateral fragment be tilted sharply medially at the site of fracture, even forming a right angle with the medial fragment. When fracture occurs between the two components of the coracoclavicular ligament, there is little displacement. Complications rarely attend these fractures unless they are comminuted and a fragment is driven into the subclavian vessels or into the brachial plexus.

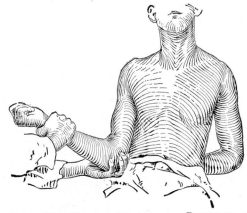

FIG. 586.—Kocher Method of Reducing a Subcoracoid Dislocation of the Humerus.

The first maneuver is fixation of the elbow against the chest and the second is external rotation of the arm. (Babcock, "Textbook of Surgery.")

The *treatment* of clavicular fractures is troublesome because there is no way of splinting the broken bone directly; closed reduction can be made only by pushing the shoulder backward until the two fragments come into apposition and anatomical alignment. Reduction of the fracture in the recumbent position best brings about accurate replacement because the muscles are relaxed and the weight of the arm does not act to produce displacement. A good ambulatory treatment may be carried out by applying a clavicular cross so that the shoulders are pulled upward, backward, and outward.

7. **Fractures of the Proximal End of the Humerus.**—In injuries about any articular extremity, the plane of the epiphysis and the attachment of the joint capsule must be considered. In the humerus, the epiphyseal line passes distal to the tubercles, but on the

medial side it coincides with the margin of the humeral head. The capsule is attached to the anatomical neck, except at the mesial margin where it embraces a small part of the shaft.

In **fractures of the anatomical neck of the humerus,** which occur chiefly in the aged, the proximal fragment may embrace a portion of the tubercles or varying amounts of

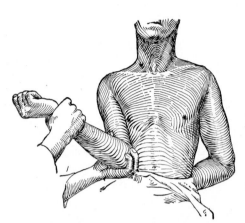

FIG. 587.—KOCHER METHOD OF REDUCING A SUB-CORACOID DISLOCATION OF THE HUMERUS.

With the arm in lateral rotation, the elbow is carried forward on the chest. (Babcock, "Textbook of Surgery.")

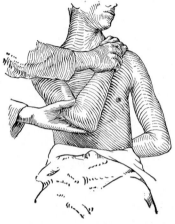

FIG. 588.—KOCHER METHOD OF REDUCING A SUB-CORACOID DISLOCATION OF THE HUMERUS.

The arm is elevated across the chest and the forearm is rotated medially. (Babcock, "Textbook of Surgery.")

the surgical neck. The shaft usually is driven into the head of the bone with considerable impaction, because the most common cause of the fracture is a fall upon the shoulder. If impaction does not occur and the joint capsule is detached completely from the upper fragment, necrosis of the fragment results since there is no direct blood supply to the

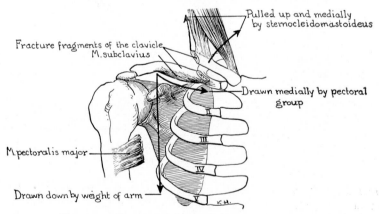

FIG. 589.—MECHANISM OF FRAGMENT DISPLACEMENT IN FRACTURE OF THE CLAVICLE JUST LATERAL TO THE ATTACHMENT OF THE STERNOCLEIDOMASTOID MUSCLE.

head of the humerus. Usually a portion of the periosteum and part of the capsule on the inner side of the fragment remain so that a blood supply is maintained and union occurs.

Treatment is directed toward regaining the use of the shoulder rather than toward care of the fracture. It is important to prevent the breaking-up of an impaction with possible consequent elimination of the blood supply of the proximal fragment.

In **fracture of the tubercles** uncomplicated by dislocation of the head of the humerus, the arm is drawn in the direction of the pull of the intact muscles. With the *greater tubercle torn away*, the supraspinatus, infraspinatus, and teres minor muscles draw the fragment upward and backward out of control, and the arm is rotated mesially by the pull of the intact subscapularis muscle. To secure approximation of the separated fragments, the arm must be brought into abduction and external rotation. In uncomplicated *avulsion of the lesser tubercle*, the tendency to abduction and external rotation, caused by the action of the muscles inserting on the greater tubercle, is corrected readily by bringing the arm to the side, rotating it mesially, and securing it comfortably to the side of the chest.

The surgical neck of the humerus is that considerable expanse of bone extending from the lower limit of the tuberosities to the insertion of the axillary muscles into the intertubercular sulcus. **Fracture of the surgical neck** often results from indirect violence, such as a fall upon the elbow with the arm abducted. When the muscles and ligaments are sufficiently strong to maintain the humeral head in the socket, undue stress falls upon the surgical neck. The acting force is that which ordinarily would cause a shoulder dislocation

The proximal fragment of the fracture is abducted slightly by the supraspinatus muscle but is rotated laterally only to the degree that the lateral rotators attached to the greater tubercle overcome the pull of the subscapularis muscle attached to the lesser tubercle. The distal fragment is adducted and rotated mesially by the muscles inserted into the intertubercular sulcus (bicipital groove), and is drawn proximally (to the extent of arm shortening) by the biceps, triceps, coracobrachialis, and deltoid muscles. To reduce the fracture, the distal fragment must be drawn downward, abducted, manipulated into apposition with the proximal fragment, and brought into that degree of lateral rotation which will bring the tip of the external condyle into the normal straight-line relationship with the greater tubercle and the acromial angle. Without restoration of normal bony relationships, union occurs with considerable deformity and limitation of motion.

8. Separation of the Upper Epiphysis of the Humerus.—Separation of the upper epiphysis of the humerus usually occurs at some period before the twenty-fifth year (p. 575). Since the epiphysis includes the tubercles to which the scapular cone of rotator muscles is attached, complete separation causes abduction and forward tilting of the distal end of the head. The shaft rides past the head mesially. To reduce the deformity, the arm is abducted and pressure is made on the proximal end of the shaft to turn it into its conical socket in the epiphysis. This injury may be followed by permanent shortening of the limb through premature ossification of the epiphyseal cartilage.

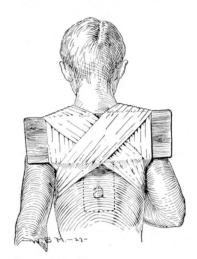

FIG. 590.—FRACTURE OF THE CLAVICLE TREATED BY THE CLAVICULAR CROSS.

A vertical extension, indicated by *a*, sometimes is used. The cross should be well padded. (Babcock, "Textbook of Surgery.")

9. Disarticulation of the Humerus at the Shoulder Joint; Amputation Through the Surgical Neck of the Humerus.—The same incision is used in shoulder joint disarticulation as for amputation through the surgical neck of the humerus. An anterior racket incision is made with the arm in moderate abduction and lateral rotation. The incision marking out the handle of the racket begins immediately below and to the lateral side of the tip of the coracoid process and passes downward between the anterior fibers of the deltoid muscle and the tendon of the pectoralis major muscle. Just below the anterior axillary fold, the incision curves horizontally outward across the anterior aspect of the limb through the superficial tissues and lower part of the deltoid muscle to meet the posterior axillary fold. Starting again at the queue of the racket with the arm in extreme abduction, a second

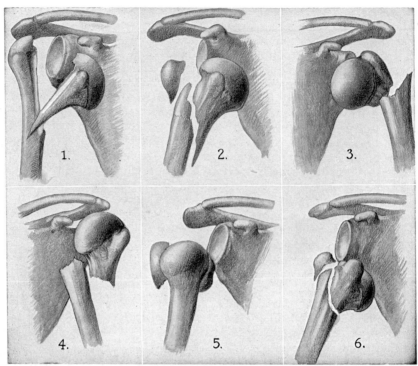

FIG. 591.—VARIOUS FRACTURES OF THE UPPER END OF THE HUMERUS, ASSOCIATED WITH DISLOCATION OF THE HEAD OF THE HUMERUS.

1, Split fracture of the shaft of the humerus with subcoracoid dislocation of the head; 2, oblique fracture of the upper end of the humerus with subcoracoid dislocation and separation of the greater tuberosity; 3, fracture of the surgical neck of the humerus, with dislocation of the head; 4, fracture of the surgical neck of the humerus, with upward displacement of the head and medial displacement of the shaft; 5, subglenoid dislocation of the humerus, with separation of the greater tuberosity to the lateral side and of the lesser tuberosity to the medial side; 6, subglenoid dislocation of the humerus with fracture of the anatomical neck and separation of the greater tuberosity.   (Robert Jones.)

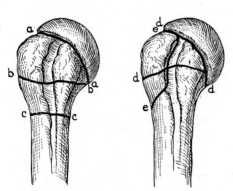

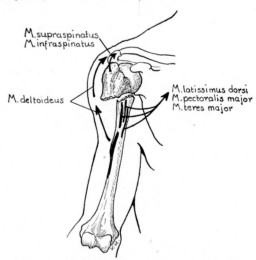

FIG. 592.—COMMONEST FRACTURES ABOUT THE UPPER END OF THE HUMERUS.

a–a, Fracture of the anatomical neck; *b–b,* transverse fracture through the tubercles; *c–c,* fracture of the surgical neck; *d–d–d,* Y fracture; *e–e,* fracture of the greater tubercle.

FIG. 593.—FRACTURE OF THE HUMERUS THROUGH THE SURGICAL NECK.

The proximal fragment is abducted slightly by the supraspinatus muscle. The distal fragment is adducted and rotated mesially by the axillary fold muscles which insert into the intertubercular sulcus.

incision is made continuing the lower extremity of the vertical limb of the first incision. The second incision is carried horizontally across the inner aspect of the limb and along the axilla to meet the horizontal portion of the first incision. The incision forming the queue of the racket is deepened to the bone, and the outer or deltoid flap, containing the axillary (circumflex) vessels and nerves, is raised from contact with the humerus. The axillary vessels, median basilic vein, and acromiothoracic artery are ligated and divided where they emerge beneath the pectoralis minor muscle. The terminal nerves of the brachial plexus are drawn downward, ligated, divided, and allowed to retract into the apex of the axilla or behind the clavicle.

In *disarticulation of the humerus*, the coracobrachialis muscle and the short head of the biceps muscle are divided near their origin at the coracoid process. By abducting and rotating the arm, using internal and external rotation alternately, the capsular muscles, the long head of the biceps, the subscapularis, and the joint capsule can be divided and the head of the humerus be disarticulated. While the arm is held away from the side, the attachments of the latissimus dorsi and teres major muscles and the long and short heads

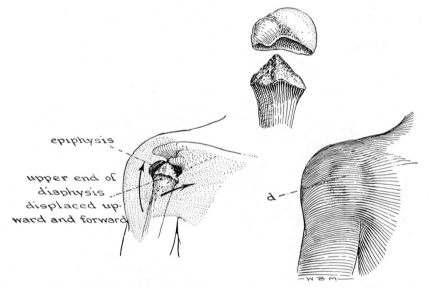

epiphysis

upper end of diaphysis displaced upward and forward

d

FIG. 594.—SEPARATION OF THE UPPER EPIPHYSIS OF THE HUMERUS.
The inset shows the normal cup and cone formed by the epiphysis and the shaft of the humerus. This conformation may render reduction difficult, but retention after reduction easy; *d*, the prominence from the displaced diaphysis. (Babcock, "Textbook of Surgery.")

of the triceps muscle on the posterior aspect of the limb are divided. The tendons of the pectoralis major and the latissimus dorsi muscles with the intrinsic scapular muscles are sutured into the margins of the glenoid fossa. The deltoid muscle flap is refashioned to fill the space from which the humeral head is removed.

In *amputation of the humerus through the surgical neck*, the pectoralis major muscle is cut from its humeral attachment and the axillary and thoraco-acromial vessels and median basilic veins are ligated. The nerves are divided as for disarticulation. With the arm well abducted, the teres major and latissimus dorsi muscles are cut at their insertions into the intertubercular sulcus. The biceps, triceps, and coracobrachialis muscles are cut to retract to the saw line at the surgical neck. The deltoid muscle flap is sutured over the bone end and the latissimus dorsi and pectoralis major muscles are sutured into the stump posteriorly.

Amputation through the surgical neck, although having no stump length and no value from a prosthetic standpoint, is preferable to disarticulation because there is less danger incident to dead space, and less atrophy in the shoulder girdle.

II. Arm or Brachial Region

1. **Surface Anatomy.**—The arm in strong adult males is flattened from side to side, because of the grouping of the arm muscles anterior and posterior to the humerus. The varying degree of fullness anteriorly corresponds to the fleshy belly of the *biceps brachii muscle.* When the biceps is thrown into action by forcible flexion of the arm at the elbow, the fullness is accentuated. The upward slope of the fullness is lost under the anterior surface of the deltoid muscle. Below the center of the arm, the biceps narrows sharply into a rounded tendon which dips backward into the antecubital fossa anterior to the elbow. The lateral margin of the biceps tendon is the more distinct, as the medial margin is somewhat obscured by the lacertus fibrosus which binds it to the deep fascia of the forearm.

The fullness over the posterior aspect of the arm is most marked at its center and is the fleshy mass of the *triceps brachii muscle.* Below this fullness, the surface of the arm

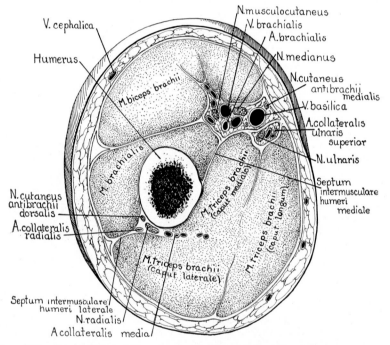

Fig. 595.—Cross Section Through the Middle Third of the Right Arm.
The flexor compartment is separated from the extensor compartment by the intermuscular septa.

presents a flattened appearance which corresponds to the triceps tendon. With the elbow in forcible extension against resistance, the lateral head of the triceps muscle causes a definite prominence, parallel to and below the posterior border of the deltoid muscle. The long head of the triceps can be made out as it emerges from beneath the posterior border of the deltoid muscle. The muscle mass on the posteromesial aspect of the arm is the medial head of the triceps.

The *medial bicipital sulcus* begins in front of the posterior axillary fold and descends along the inner aspect of the arm as far as the lower third where it inclines obliquely forward, terminating at the center of the bend of the elbow. It separates the coracobrachialis and biceps muscles in front from the triceps muscle behind and, toward its termination, defines the line of separation between the biceps and the pronator teres. Superiorly, the groove is obscured by the coracobrachialis muscle, which can be brought into relief when the abducted arm is adducted against resistance. The sulcus indicates the course of the basilic vein toward the axillary vein and is the superficial guide to the brachial vessels and the median nerve (p. 595).

The *lateral bicipital sulcus*, shorter and less distinct than the medial, begins at the depression in the middle of the arm, which marks the insertion of the deltoid muscle, and ends anterior to the bend of the elbow. The groove, in its lower part, separates the brachio-radialis (supinator longus) muscle and the radial extensor muscles from the biceps muscle. The cephalic vein ascends in this sulcus to its upper extremity and then follows the anterior border of the deltoid muscle.

The course of the *brachial artery* and the *median nerve* lies along a line, drawn on the inner aspect of the abducted arm, from a point anterior to the posterior axillary fold to the center of the bend of the elbow (antecubital fossa). The *ulnar nerve* follows the course of the artery in the upper third of the arm, but beyond this point it inclines backward and

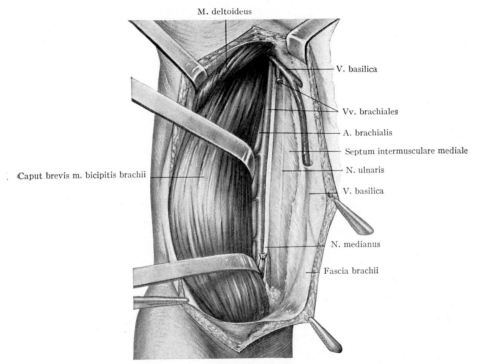

M. deltoideus

V. basilica

Vv. brachiales

A. brachialis

Septum intermusculare mediale

N. ulnaris

V. basilica

N. medianus

Fascia brachii

Caput brevis m. bicipitis brachii

FIG. 596.—STRUCTURES IN THE ANTERIOR COMPARTMENT OF THE RIGHT ARM.
The biceps muscle is retracted laterally, exposing the brachial vessels and the median nerve. The ulnar nerve is shown as a transparency through the medial intermuscular septum.

downward behind the medial condyle of the humerus. The *radial nerve* follows the brachial artery a short distance distal to the posterior axillary fold. Its further course is indicated by an oblique line descending outward across the posterior aspect of the arm, where it meets the lateral bicipital sulcus about 2.5 cm. below the deltoid insertion (Fig. 597). From this point, the trunk of the radial nerve follows the lateral bicipital sulcus to the front of the lateral epicondyle of the humerus, where it divides into superficial and deep branches (p. 602).

The depression on the lateral aspect of the arm marking the *deltoid insertion* is a valuable landmark indicating the level at which the main nutrient artery enters the humerus and the radial nerve crosses the posterior surface of the bone. It also marks the level of the insertion of the coracobrachialis muscle into the medial aspect of the humerus.

The neurovascular relationships at the medial bicipital groove, at the back of the medial condyle of the humerus, along the distal part of the lateral bicipital groove, and at the posterior aspect of the arm just below the level of the deltoid insertion are contra-indications to bold incision in these areas.

2. **Enveloping (Deep) Fascia of the Arm and the Intermuscular Septa.**—The deep fascia furnishes a complete investment for the arm and is continuous with the deep fascia of the forearm. From the deep surface of this ensheathing layer are derived the lateral and medial intermuscular septa, strong, fibrous partitions extending from the ensheathing layer to the shaft and epicondylar ridges of the humerus and dividing the arm into anterior and posterior osseo-aponeurotic compartments. These compartments, in a measure, limit the extravasation of hemorrhage and the spread of infection. The *medial intermuscular*

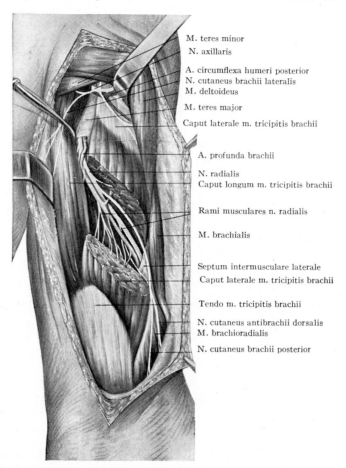

M. teres minor
N. axillaris

A. circumflexa humeri posterior
N. cutaneus brachii lateralis
M. deltoideus

M. teres major
Caput laterale m. tricipitis brachii

A. profunda brachii

N. radialis
Caput longum m. tricipitis brachii

Rami musculares n. radialis

M. brachialis

Septum intermusculare laterale
Caput laterale m. tricipitis brachii

Tendo m. tricipitis brachii

N. cutaneus antibrachii dorsalis
M. brachioradialis
N. cutaneus brachii posterior

FIG. 597.—DEEP DISSECTION OF THE POSTERIOR COMPARTMENT OF THE ARM.
Removal of the section from the lateral head of the triceps muscle shows the path of the radial nerve and the accompanying vessels.

septum extends from the medial epicondyle to the insertion of the coracobrachialis muscle, and the *lateral intermuscular septum* extends from the lateral epicondyle to the deltoid insertion.

The *anterior (flexor) compartment* contains the coracobrachialis, biceps, and brachialis (anticus) muscles, the brachial artery and veins, the basilic vein, and the median, musculo-cutaneous and median antibrachial cutaneous nerves. The *posterior (extensor) compartment* contains the triceps brachii muscle. Several structures are common to both compartments: the radial nerve, profunda (superior profunda) artery, ulnar nerve, superior ulnar collateral (inferior profunda) artery, and the inferior ulnar collateral (anastomotica magna) artery.

3. **Muscles of the Brachial Compartments.**—The biceps brachii, coracobrachialis and brachialis (anticus) muscles occupy the anterior brachial or flexor compartment. The *biceps muscle* (N. musculocutaneus $C_5, _6$) occupies most of the compartment. It arises by a short head from the tip of the coracoid process and from a long head attached to the upper margin of the glenoid fossa, and inserts into the posterior part of the tuberosity of the radius. Its tendon is separated from the anterior part of the tuberosity by a bursa. Its primary function is flexion and supination of the forearm, but it acts also as a suspensory mechanism for the humerus and aids in flexion and adduction of the arm at the shoulder. "It puts the corkscrew in and pulls the cork out." Its mesial border is the guide to the brachial artery. Either of the heads of the belly of the muscle, or the muscle body itself, may be ruptured by violent muscle effort. Weakness in flexion and forced supination of the forearm result

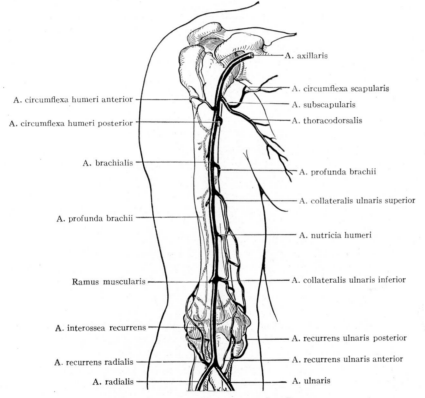

FIG. 598.—BRACHIAL ARTERY AND ITS BRANCHES.

From an origin in the coracoid process, the *coracobrachialis muscle* (N. musculocutaneus C_7) runs parallel to the short head of the biceps and inserts into the middle portion of the mesial margin of the humerus. It aids in flexion and adduction of the arm. The *brachialis (anticus) muscle* arises from the distal half of the anterior surface of the humerus and the adjacent intermuscular septum, and passes anterior to the elbow joint to insert into the coronoid process of the ulna. It is supplied by the musculocutaneous ($C_5, _6$) and radial nerves and is a powerful flexor of the elbow. In fracture of the shaft of the humerus, a portion of the brachialis muscle may be interposed between the fragments and cause nonunion.

The posterior or extensor compartment compactly encloses the *triceps brachii muscle* (N. radial $C_6, _7, _8$). The medial head of this muscle arises from all the posterior surface of the shaft of the humerus distal to the radial groove and from the medial intermuscular septum. The lateral head arises from all the surface of the humerus proximal to the groove and from the lateral intermuscular septum. The long head arises by a tendon from the inferior surface of the glenoid fossa. From these varied origins, the fibers are inserted into the proximal surface of the olecranon.

4. **Brachial Artery, Its Branches and Collateral Anastomoses.**—The **brachial artery,** the continuation of the axillary artery, extends from the lower border of the teres major muscle to the antecubital fossa just distal to the skin crease at the bend of the elbow. Opposite the neck of the radius, it bifurcates into the radial and ulnar arteries.

The *proximal third* of the brachial artery lies upon the medial aspect of the limb anterior to the long and medial heads of the triceps muscle, and may be compressed laterally against the humerus. In operative exposure, the artery is found beneath the deep fascia, bordered laterally by the coracobrachialis muscle and partly separated from it by the median nerve. The medial (internal) cutaneous nerve of the forearm and the ulnar nerve separate it from the basilic vein.

The *middle third* of the artery inclines gradually forward and outward, and, in operative exposure, is found overlapped by the medial border of the biceps muscle; it is overlain by the median nerve which crosses it obliquely. The medial cutaneous nerve and the basilic vein are separated from the artery by the deep fascia. An incision carried too far toward the medial aspect of the arm may expose the ulnar nerve with the ulnar collateral (inferior profunda) artery where they diverge from the brachial artery to reach the medial intermuscular septum.

The *distal third* of the artery is overlapped by the medial border of the biceps muscle, but near its termination lies medial to the biceps tendon, overlain by the lacertus fibrosus (bicipital fascia). Medial to it lies the median nerve.

The brachial artery has several **branches.** The *(superior) profunda artery* arises from the posterior and inner aspect of the main trunk near its origin and passes backward. It is associated with the radial (musculospiral) nerve which it accompanies in the radial groove to the front of the external condyle of the humerus, anastomosing there with the radial recurrent artery (p. 624). The principal *nutrient artery* of the humerus sometimes arises from the profunda in the radial sulcus, but usually has its origin in a muscle branch near the middle of the arm. It may be injured in fractures and delay union. The *superior ulnar collateral (inferior profunda) artery* arises near the middle of the arm and accompanies the ulnar nerve to the groove on the posterior surface of the medial epicondyle, where it anastomoses with the dorsal (anterior) ulnar recurrent artery (p. 623). The *inferior ulnar collateral (anastomotic) artery* arises from the brachial artery near the elbow and forms a rich anastomotic network on the mesial aspect of the elbow.

The branches of the brachial artery form **collateral anastomoses** about the elbow which connect the parent trunk with the arteries of the forearm. Communications are established between the profunda artery and the superior and inferior collateral arteries superiorly and the radial and ulnar recurrent arteries and dorsal interosseous recurrent artery inferiorly.

When the brachial artery is ligated above the origin of the profunda artery, the blood flow in the limb is reestablished through an anastomosis between the circumflex and axillary arteries proximally, and the ascending branches of the profunda artery distally. When the brachial artery is ligated below the level of the profunda artery and above the superior ulnar collateral artery, anastomotic connections are established between the profunda artery proximally and the radial recurrent, dorsal ulnar recurrent, and inferior ulnar collateral arteries, distally.

5. **Radial, Musculocutaneous, Median, and Ulnar Nerves.**—Below the teres major muscle, the *radial nerve* lies between the long head of the triceps muscle and the shaft of the humerus. After supplying the triceps muscle, the nerve enters the radial groove with the profunda branch of the brachial artery and supplies the medial and lateral heads of the triceps muscle, between which it lies. In the radial groove, the nerve passes distally and laterally across the back of the arm, where it traverses the lateral intermuscular septum and enters the anterior brachial compartment. The point at which the nerve pierces the

septum may be located at the union of the proximal and middle thirds of a line joining the lateral epicondyle and the insertion of the deltoid muscle.

In the anterior compartment, the radial nerve lies at the lateral margin of the brachialis muscle and is overlain proximally by the brachioradialis (supinator longus) muscle, and distally by the extensor carpi radialis longus muscle. Anterior to the lateral epicondyle, the radial nerve divides into superficial (radial) and deep (posterior interosseous) nerves.

The radial nerve may be involved in fractures of the shaft of the humerus, either between the fragments themselves or in the callus deposited by the fracture, and may necessitate operative interference. The nerve may be located in the anterior compartment of the arm in the interval between the brachioradialis and the brachialis muscles (Fig. 609). Because of the absence of a definite demarcation between these muscles, the interval separating them is not easy to determine. If the cleft between the brachialis and biceps muscles is opened inadvertently, the musculocutaneous nerve is exposed and may be mistaken for the radial nerve. The radial nerve can be identified where it pierces the lateral intermuscular septum and may be traced upward by cutting through the musculotendinous roof of the radial groove.

The *musculocutaneous nerve*, upon deviating from the axillary artery (p. 564), supplies and then pierces the coracobrachialis muscle. It then runs distally between the biceps and brachialis muscles, supplying both, and emerges at the elbow along the lateral margin of the biceps tendon.

The *median nerve* runs along the medial bicipital furrow in close relationship with the brachial artery. At first it lies lateral to the artery, then, at the middle of the arm, it crosses over, or occasionally under, the artery and descends along the mesial side to the elbow.

In the proximal half of the arm, the *ulnar nerve* lies medial to the brachial artery and anterior to the triceps muscle. In the distal half of the arm, it deviates from the brachial artery and passes behind the medial intermuscular septum. It passes into the elbow region between the medial epicondyle of the humerus and the olecranon.

6. **Shaft of the Humerus.**—The shaft of the humerus consists of a central medullary canal and a thick, dense cortex. Near the middle of the inner border of the shaft is an opening for the principal *nutrient canal*, which is directed obliquely downward for a long course through the cortex before opening into the medullary cavity. Occasionally, the nutrient foramen lies in the radial groove. The rough eminence at the center of the medial aspect of the shaft is marked by the *radial sulcus* which descends obliquely downward and outward, curving around the bone until it reaches the lateral margin of the humerus about 2.5 cm. below the deltoid eminence. In its middle, the shaft of the bone is prismatic; distally, it is flattened anteroposteriorly and curves slightly forward. The medial and lateral margins of the distal part of the shaft, especially the lateral margin, are strong and form stout supporting columns, *supracondylar ridges*, continued directly into the epicondyles. The lateral intermuscular septum is attached to the lateral ridge, and the medial intermuscular septum to the medial ridge.

The *relations* between the humerus and the muscles differ above and below the level of the deltoid insertion. In the upper or deltoid segment, much of the shaft is devoid of muscle attachment, and, because of this, the deltoid, biceps, and coracobrachialis muscles and the long head of the triceps muscle retract freely when divided. In the lower or subdeltoid segment, the muscles invest and are attached to the humerus so that excessive retraction of the divided muscles is prevented. Since the biceps muscle has no point of direct attachment to the humerus save where the capsular and synovial expansions bind the tendon of the long head to the intertubercular sulcus, there is a wide interval of separation when the tendon is severed.

SURGICAL CONSIDERATIONS

1 **Medial Approaches to the Structures of the Arm.**—The *mediai vasculoneural approach* follows the medial bicipital sulcus and affords surgical access to the brachial vessels

38

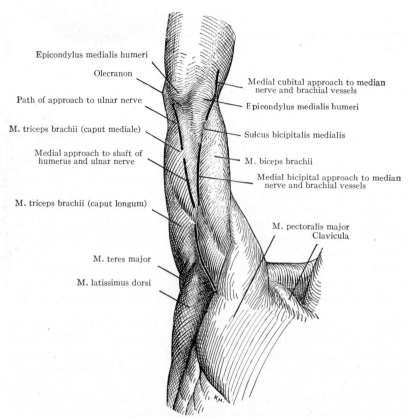

Epicondylus medialis humeri

Olecranon

Path of approach to ulnar nerve

M. triceps brachii (caput mediale)

Medial approach to shaft of
humerus and ulnar nerve

M. triceps brachii (caput longum)

M. teres major

M. latissimus dorsi

Medial cubital approach to median
nerve and brachial vessels

Epicondylus medialis humeri

Sulcus bicipitalis medialis

M. biceps brachii

Medial bicipital approach to median
nerve and brachial vessels

M. pectoralis major
Clavicula

FIG. 599.—MEDIAL BRACHIAL AND MEDIAL HUMERAL ROUTES TO THE STRUCTURES OF THE ARM.

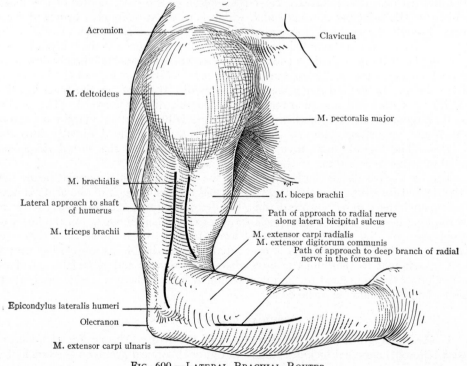

Acromion

Clavicula

M. deltoideus

M. pectoralis major

M. brachialis

M. biceps brachii

Lateral approach to shaft
of humerus

Path of approach to radial nerve
along lateral bicipital sulcus

M. triceps brachii

M. extensor carpi radialis
M. extensor digitorum communis
Path of approach to deep branch of radial
nerve in the forearm

Epicondylus lateralis humeri

Olecranon

M. extensor carpi ulnaris

FIG. 600.—LATERAL BRACHIAL ROUTES.

and median nerve. It extends along a line connecting the apex of the axilla with the medial septum. In exposure of the ulnar nerve in the upper third of the arm, an incision over the medial bicipital groove exposes the nerve mesial to the brachial vessels. In the middle third of the arm, the nerve lies at the level of, or just behind, the origin of the medial

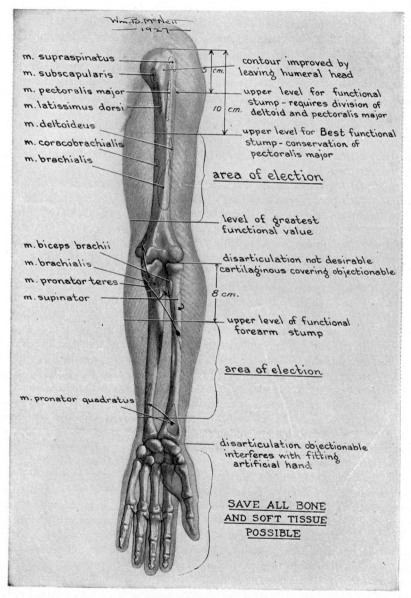

Fig. 601.—Amputation Levels in the Arm, Forearm, and Hand with Relation to Function. (Babcock, "Textbook of Surgery.")

intermuscular septum. In the lower third of the arm, the ulnar nerve lies directly behind the medial intermuscular septum.

In the upper and middle thirds of the arm, *access to the shaft of the humerus* is gained by retracting the medial head of the triceps muscle backward, after separating it from the medial intermuscular septum. The lower third of the shaft is exposed through the interval between the triceps muscle and the deep surface of the medial intermuscular septum.

2. Lateral Approaches to the Structures of the Arm.—The lateral brachial routes consist of a lateral bicipital path for exposure of the radial nerve in the middle of the shaft and a lateral humeral path for exposure of the shaft of the humerus.

The incision for the *lateral approach to the radial nerve* begins at the deltoid insertion and descends two fingerbreadths immediately anterior to the lateral intermuscular septum. It runs obliquely forward and downward toward the crease of the elbow. After incision of the deep fascia over the interval between the brachioradialis and brachialis muscles and separation of the muscles, the radial nerve is exposed on a level with the superior fibers of the brachioradialis muscle and is traced upward. When it is necessary to follow the nerve into the radial sulcus, the lateral intermuscular septum is exposed further and the dissection is carried backward through the entire thickness of the triceps muscle. This approach, combined with the retrodeltoid approach, gives adequate exposure to the radial nerve in its humeral course.

The *lateral approach to the shaft of the humerus* follows the lateral intermuscular septum from the posterior border of the deltoid muscle to the external epicondyle of the humerus. The brachialis (anticus) muscle and the radial nerve are retracted forward and the triceps and brachioradialis muscles backward.

3. Retrodeltoid Approach to the Proximal Part of the Humerus.—The incision in the retrodeltoid approach to the proximal part of the humerus is made parallel to the posterior border of the deltoid muscle about a thumbbreadth mesial to it, and extends to the margin of the humerus at the attachment of the lateral intermuscular septum. Lateral retraction of the deltoid muscle exposes the longitudinal fibers of the long head of the triceps muscle and the external axillary (quadrilateral) space (p. 567). Through this space, the axillary nerve and the posterior circumflex vessels pass backward in close relationship with the surgical neck of the humerus. In the interval between the origin of the lateral head of the triceps muscle and the deltoid insertion, the humerus is devoid of muscle attachments and permits direct surgical access.

4. Posterior Brachial Approach to the Radial Nerve (Fig. 597).—The posterior brachial approach gives direct access to the radial nerve as it leaves the axilla. The incision begins at the middle of the posterior border of the deltoid muscle and continues downward toward the olecranon. After incision of the deep fascia, the space between the long and lateral heads of the triceps muscle is sought by blunt dissection. Through this space, the radial nerve and the profunda artery emerge from the axilla and run in the radial groove. By division of the lateral head of the triceps muscle, the nerve may be followed throughout the groove and along the lateral intermuscular septum to the lateral region of the arm.

5. Amputation Through the Arm.—In *amputation through the lower third* of the arm, equal anterior and posterior rounded flaps are fashioned. If the saw line is made through the condyles, the biceps, brachialis, and triceps muscles are cut from their insertions and are allowed to retract to the saw line. The forearm muscles arising from the supracondylar ridges are cut to retract to the saw line. The biceps tendon is sutured to the brachialis (anticus) muscle, which is brought over the end of the bone and sutured to the triceps muscle. If the supracondylar saw line is selected, the muscle and fascial flaps are cut higher up, the biceps and brachialis muscles are sectioned to retract to the saw line, and the triceps muscle is divided at its insertion into the olecranon process. The triceps muscle is brought forward over the humerus and sutured into the brachialis and biceps muscles.

In *amputation above the lower third* of the arm, all bone should be saved to give as much leverage as possible for an artificial limb. Equal anterior and posterior flaps of skin and fascia are employed and a thin muscle flap is cut from the posterior or the anterior brachial muscles (preferably the triceps muscle) and is carried across the end of the bone. The biceps muscle retracts considerably more than the brachialis and triceps muscles because it has no humeral attachment. When the saw line is above the deltoid insertion, the power of abduction is lost, unless the deltoid muscle is fixed to the end of the stump.

6. Fractures of the Shaft of the Humerus.—Fractures in the shaft of the humerus occur in those parts of the bone which are protected least by muscles. Reference is made

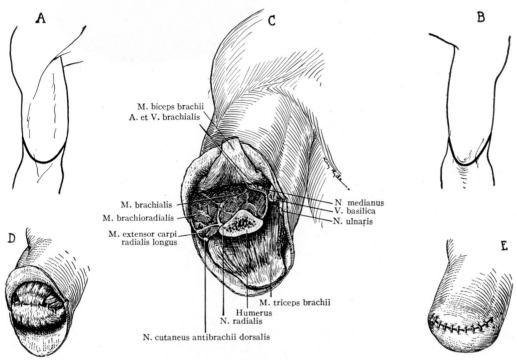

M. biceps brachii
A. et V. brachialis

M. brachialis
M. brachioradialis
M. extensor carpi radialis longus

N. medianus
V. basilica
N. ulnaris

M. triceps brachii
Humerus
N. radialis

N. cutaneus antibrachii dorsalis

FIG. 602.—AMPUTATION THROUGH THE LOWER THIRD OF THE ARM

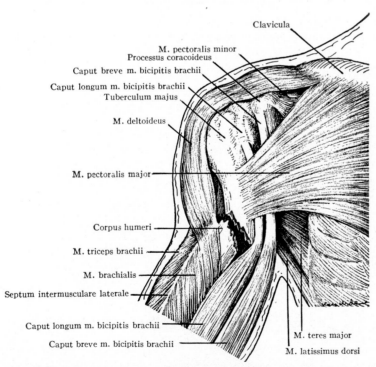

Clavicula

M. pectoralis minor
Processus coracoideus
Caput breve m. bicipitis brachii
Caput longum m. bicipitis brachii
Tuberculum majus

M. deltoideus

M. pectoralis major

Corpus humeri
M. triceps brachii
M. brachialis
Septum intermusculare laterale

Caput longum m. bicipitis brachii
Caput breve m. bicipitis brachii

M. teres major
M. latissimus dorsi

FIG. 603.—FRACTURE OF THE SHAFT OF THE HUMERUS BETWEEN THE DELTOID INSERTION AND THE INSERTIONS OF THE AXILLARY FOLD MUSCLES.

The proximal fragment is drawn medially by the pectoralis major, the latissimus dorsi, and teres major muscles. The distal fragment is drawn upward by the deltoid, coracobrachialis, biceps, and triceps muscles, and outward by the deltoid muscle.

to the common sites of fracture because of the displacement of the fragments caused by muscle pull, although the important factor in determining the displacement of fragments is not so much the muscle action as the force which causes the fracture. Displacement is favored by obliquity of the fracture line.

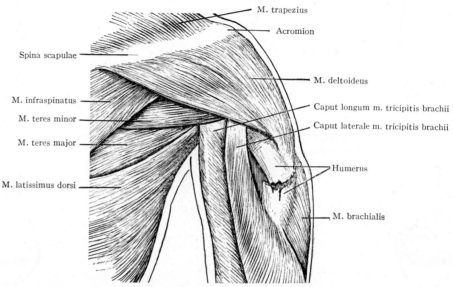

FIG. 604.—FRACTURE OF THE HUMERUS JUST DISTAL TO THE DELTOID INSERTION.
The deltoid muscle tilts the distal end of the proximal fragment outward.

When the line of fracture is *between the insertions of the axillary muscles and the deltoid insertion*, the distal end of the proximal fragment is drawn mesially by the axillary muscles.

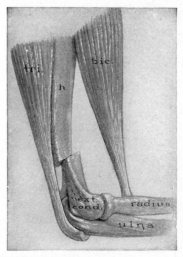

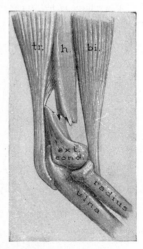

FIG. 605.—FLEXION FRACTURE OF THE LOWER THIRD OF THE SHAFT OF THE HUMERUS. (Babcock, "Textbook of Surgery.")

FIG. 606.—EXTENSION FRACTURE OF THE LOWER THIRD OF THE HUMERUS. (Babcock, "Textbook of Surgery.")

The distal fragment is pulled upward by the deltoid, coracobrachialis, biceps, and triceps muscles and outward by the deltoid muscle. In fracture *distal to the deltoid insertion* (near the center of the shaft), the tendency for the muscles to cause displacement is not so marked, but the deltoid muscle tends to tilt the distal end of the proximal fragment outward. The distal fragment may be drawn proximally and mesially by the pull of the biceps and triceps muscles acting through their insertions at the elbow. The upward pull is overcome partly by gravity if the elbow is not supported.

Fracture of the humerus *near the articular end* (*supracondylar fracture*) usually is transverse or somewhat oblique to the long axis of the shaft. In the resulting displacement, the distal fragment is drawn up behind the proximal fragment by the triceps muscle. The distal end of the proximal fragment may project forward above the level of the crease of the elbow, penetrate the brachialis muscle, and even injure the brachial artery.

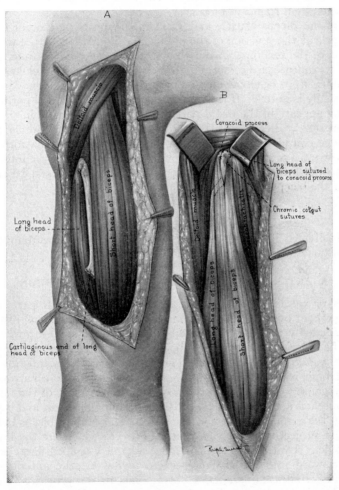

FIG. 607.—RUPTURE AND REPAIR OF THE TENDON OF THE LONG HEAD OF THE BICEPS MUSCLE.

A is condition at operation which shows the tendon of the long head of the biceps completely torn from the cartilaginous lip of the glenoid fossa and turned over on itself in a jack-knife fashion; B shows the tendon sutured to the coracoid process and to the short head of the biceps. (E. L. Gilcreest; courtesy of Jour. Amer. Med. Assoc.)

Fracture by muscle action is more common in the shaft of the humerus than in the shaft of any other bone. As a rule, it results from a forcible effort in throwing, and occurs most frequently just below the deltoid insertion. The contraction of the deltoid muscle arrests the bone suddenly and the impetus acquired by the lower end of the humerus produces the fracture.

Failure of the broken fragments to unite, *pseudo-arthrosis*, is observed frequently. The presence of muscle tissue between the fragments, lack of muscle attachment, inadequate blood supply, and the difficulty of immobilization are important etiologic factors. Injury to the nutrient artery where it enters the bone near the middle of the shaft may injure the blood supply to the humerus and favor nonunion.

The most frequent *complication* is paralysis of the extensor muscles of the forearm and "wrist drop" following damage to the radial nerve. The close proximity of the nerve to the bone in the radial groove renders it prone to injury in displacement of the fragments, or later by compression from the callus formed at the site of fracture. Injury to the brachial artery is rare, but the vessel may be stretched by the displaced fragment so as to occlude its lumen; thrombosis may occur from excessive bruising of its coats; or it may be perforated by a fragment of bone.

7. Rupture of the Biceps Muscle and Tendon.—Rupture may occur in the substance of the biceps muscle at the junction of the muscle and its tendon, in the tendons, or at the origin or insertion of the tendons. A muscle which has degenerated from any debilitating process is prone to rupture; a normal muscle may give way under violent strain. Sharp pain in the shoulder, arm, or elbow may or may not be felt. Progressive weakness in the use of the arm usually is noted. If the rupture occurs in the proximal portion of the biceps muscle, a swelling appears in the distal part of the arm; if it occurs in the distal portion, the swelling is proximal. Because of the rich blood supply to the muscle, partial or complete tears produce considerable bleeding and subsequent hematoma formation. Extensive rupture necessitates repair. If the tendon of the long head of the muscle is torn from its attachment to the lip of the scapular glenoid, the tendon should be sutured both to the short head of the biceps muscle and to the coracoid process.

III. Elbow

The elbow is divided into three regions: anterior or vasculoneuromuscular, posterior or olecranon, and bones and joints.

A ANTERIOR OR VASCULONEUROMUSCULAR REGION

The anterior or vasculoneuromuscular region includes the soft parts anterior to the plane of the elbow joint over an area three fingerbreadths proximal and distal to the joint.

1. Surface Anatomy and Muscle Landmarks.—When the forearm is supinated and extended fully, the anterior aspect of the elbow presents three muscular projections. The *median muscular projection* is made by the lower extremity of the tapering biceps muscle on the subjacent brachialis muscle. The biceps is condensed into a narrow tendon which dips into the antecubital fossa and inserts into the posterior part of the radial tuberosity. The brachialis muscle is attached directly to the underlying humerus and inserts by a short thick tendon into the coronoid process of the ulna. The median biceps bulge is set apart from the muscular projections which flank it by grooves which are the lower extremities of the bicipital sulci. By the coalescence of the sulci, a V-shaped figure is formed which is continued downward into the shallow median furrow on the anterior surface of the forearm. The *medial muscular projection* corresponds to the pronator teres, flexor carpi radialis, and palmaris longus muscles. The *lateral muscular projection* consists of the brachioradialis (supinator longus) and the radial extensor muscles.

These masses of muscle bound the *antecubital fossa*, a triangular depression distal to the intercondylar line. The finger may be inserted easily into the depression between the biceps tendon and the brachioradialis muscle. Medial to the tendon, the sharp upper margin of the *lacertus fibrosus* can be felt as a membranous septum extending over the hollow of the cubital fossa and blending with the deep fascia of the medial aspect of the forearm (Fig. 608). This septum prevents examination between the biceps tendon and the pronator radii teres muscle. The pulsations of the brachial artery are felt by inserting the finger beneath the proximal margin of the septum.

The *joint line* anteriorly is not easily recognized because of its obliquity and the amount of overlying muscle. It is represented fairly accurately by a line crossing the elbow from a point about 1 cm. below the external epicondyle to a point about 2.5 cm. below the internal epicondyle.

2. **Cubital (Antecubital) Fossa and Contents.**—The cubital fossa is a triangular depression anterior to the elbow. Its base is an imaginary line connecting the humeral condyles, and its sides are the converging borders of the pronator teres and brachioradialis muscles. After reflecting the superficial veins and deep fascia, the *brachial artery* and venae comites are exposed at the mesial side of the biceps tendon. The *median nerve* lies a short distance mesial to the brachial artery. These structures are surrounded by a quantity of areolo-adipose tissue, continuous above with the connective tissue planes of the arm. The floor of the space is the brachialis (anticus) muscle. Within the muscular interval at the lateral aspect of the biceps tendon, the *radial nerve* divides into its terminal branches

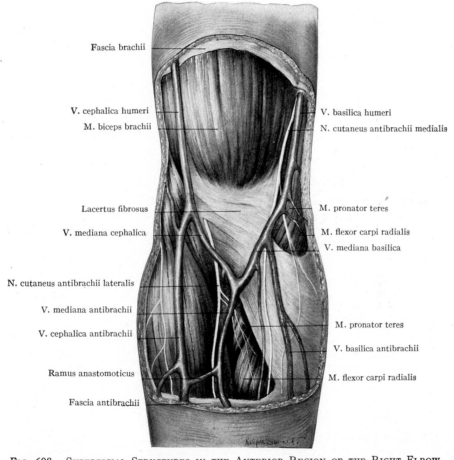

Fascia brachii

V. cephalica humeri
M. biceps brachii

V. basilica humeri
N. cutaneus antibrachii medialis

Lacertus fibrosus
V. mediana cephalica

M. pronator teres
M. flexor carpi radialis
V. mediana basilica

N. cutaneus antibrachii lateralis
V. mediana antibrachii
V. cephalica antibrachii

M. pronator teres
V. basilica antibrachii

Ramus anastomoticus
Fascia antibrachii

M. flexor carpi radialis

FIG. 608.—SUPERFICIAL STRUCTURES IN THE ANTERIOR REGION OF THE RIGHT ELBOW.
The brachial and antebrachial fascia have been removed, but the superficial veins are *in situ.*

3. **Vessels and Nerves.**—The *brachial artery* enters the region in the medial bicipital groove where it lies on the brachialis muscle. It traverses the cubital fossa under the lacertus fibrosus and divides into the radial and ulnar arteries at the level of the coronoid process of the ulna and the neck of the radius. The *radial artery* continues in the direction of the brachial trunk and runs along the border of the pronator teres muscle to the brachioradialis muscle, the mesial border of which it follows through the forearm into the wrist. At the elbow, the radial artery gives off the radial recurrent artery. The *ulnar artery* is the larger terminal branch, but the less direct continuation, of the brachial artery. It runs in the forearm deep to the muscles arising from the mesial epicondyle. About the

elbow, it gives off the posterior ulnar recurrent, the anterior ulnar recurrent, and the common interosseous arteries.   The anatomical steps in ligation of the brachial artery have been described (p. 592).

The *median nerve* enters the region in the medial bicipital groove, mesial to the brachial artery.   It passes into the forearm between the two heads of the pronator teres muscle and is separated from the ulnar artery by the deep head of that muscle.   At the elbow it gives off a branch to the pronator teres, flexor carpi radialis, palmaris longus, and flexor digitorum sublimis muscles.   The results of injury to the median nerve are characteristic (p. 669).   Under cover of the brachioradialis muscle at the level of the external humeral condyle, the *radial nerve* divides into superficial (radial) and deep (posterior interosseous)

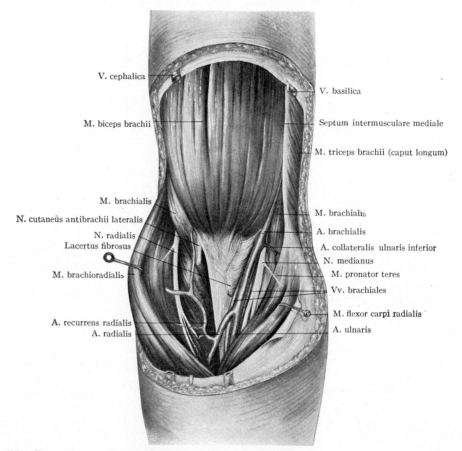

V. cephalica

V. basilica

M. biceps brachii

Septum intermusculare mediale

M. triceps brachii (caput longum)

M. brachialis

M. brachialis

N. cutaneus antibrachii lateralis

A. brachialis

N. radialis

A. collateralis ulnaris inferior

Lacertus fibrosus

N. medianus

M. pronator teres

M. brachioradialis

Vv. brachiales

M. flexor carpi radialis

A. recurrens radialis

A. ulnaris

A. radialis

Fig. 609.—Deep Vasculoneural Structures in the Anterior Region of the Right Elbow. The brachial and antebrachial fasciae and the lacertus fibrosus have been removed.   The muscular latera walls of the cubital fossa are retracted.

branches.   The superficial branch is entirely sensory and descends in the forearm deep to the brachioradialis muscle.   The deep branch crosses the joint line and is directed downward and backward into the supinator (brevis) muscle in close relation with the head of the radius, where it is subject to trauma in fracture or in operative exposure of the lateral aspect of the elbow joint.   Mesial rotation (pronation) of the forearm by the pronator teres muscle carries the nerve away from the radiohumeral joint and lessens the danger from operative injury.

4. **Medial and Lateral Bicipital Approaches to the Structures about the Elbow.**— In the *medial bicipital approach*, the median basilic and basilic veins are retracted and ligated and the free upper margin of the lacertus fibrosus is incised.   Retraction of the

edges of this fascia carries the biceps muscle laterally and the pronator teres muscle mesially. This path affords surgical access to the brachial artery and its bifurcation, and to the median nerve lying mesial to it. The nerve can be traced between the two heads of the pronator teres muscle by resection and mesial retraction of the head of the pronator teres which is attached to the coronoid process of the ulna. A deep abscess may be evacuated through this incision.

In the *lateral bicipital approach*, the interval between the brachioradialis muscle and biceps tendon is exposed. Lateral retraction of the brachioradialis muscle exposes the recurrent radial artery and the radial nerve with its bifurcation into superficial and deep branches. The lateral condyle of the humerus, the joint line, and the head and neck of the radius also may be exposed.

B. POSTERIOR OR OLECRANON REGION

The posterior or olecranon region embraces the posterior soft parts of the elbow and affords easy access to the elbow joint and to the ulnar nerve. The joint coverings are thin and the articular extremities of the bones are superficial.

1. **Surface Landmarks.**—A knowledge of the normal relations of the bony prominences of the region is indispensable to correct diagnosis of the dislocations and fractures

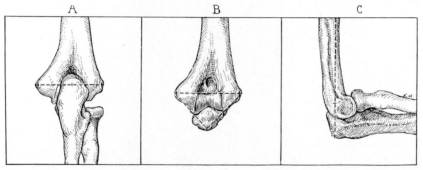

FIG. 610.—RELATIONS OF THE BONY PROMINENCES OF THE ELBOW IN FLEXION AND EXTENSION.
The three points mark a straight line in extension and a triangle in right angle flexion. Side view and right angle flexion show these points to lie in a plane parallel with the posterior surface of the humerus.

occurring in it. Both epicondyles of the humerus are subcutaneous and readily palpable, but the *medial epicondyle* is the more prominent. A narrow, but rather deep, medial para-olecranon groove separates the epicondyle from the olecranon. The ulnar nerve usually can be felt as a cord on the posterior aspect of this groove. The *lateral epicondyle* is palpated most easily with the arm in semiflexion; with the arm in full extension, the

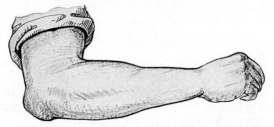

FIG. 611.—SWELLING RESULTING FROM OLECRANON BURSITIS ("MINER'S ELBOW").

condyle is hidden in a small depression bounded by the anconeus muscle mesially and the radial extensor muscles laterally. The lateral epicondyle lies farther from the olecranon than does the medial epicondyle. The surface of the intervening lateral para-olecranon groove is comparatively flat. The joint capsule and synovia are nearest the surface in the para-olecranon grooves. In joint effusions or with excessive synovial thickening, the olecranon no longer is prominent, but lies in the depth of a shallow depression in the swollen tissues.

When the forearm is extended, the *intercondylar line* is horizontal and passes through the proximal border of the *olecranon*. When the forearm is flexed, the olecranon gradually becomes prominent and sinks below the horizontal level of the intercondylar line. In right angle flexion of the forearm, it lies on the same plane as the posterior surface of the shaft of the humerus and represents the apex of an inverted equilateral triangle, the base

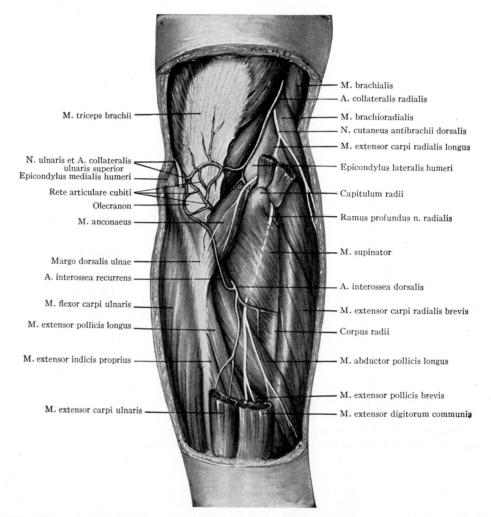

M. triceps brachii

N. ulnaris et A. collateralis ulnaris superior
Epicondylus medialis humeri

Rete articulare cubiti

Olecranon

M. anconaeus

Margo dorsalis ulnae

A. interossea recurrens

M. flexor carpi ulnaris

M. extensor pollicis longus

M. extensor indicis proprius

M. extensor carpi ulnaris

M. brachialis
A. collateralis radialis
M. brachioradialis
N. cutaneus antibrachii dorsalis
M. extensor carpi radialis longus
Epicondylus lateralis humeri
Capitulum radii
Ramus profundus n. radialis
M. supinator
A. interossea dorsalis
M. extensor carpi radialis brevis
Corpus radii
M. abductor pollicis longus
M. extensor pollicis brevis
M. extensor digitorum communis

FIG. 612.—VASCULONEURAL AND MUSCULAR STRUCTURES IN THE POSTERIOR REGION OF THE RIGHT ELBOW.

angles of which are located at the epicondyles of the humerus. In full flexion of the forearm, the olecranon tip is carried farther downward and lies anterior to the articular end of the humerus; the triceps tendon can be traced down to it.

Immediately distal to the lateral epicondyle and the depression marking the humero-radial joint, is the projecting *head of the radius*, the rotary movements of which are detected readily by pronating and supinating the forearm alternately. When the forearm is flexed, the head of the radius lies 2.5 cm. anterior to the lateral epicondyle, the interval separating them being occupied by the capitulum of the humerus. When the forearm is in complete extension, a finger may be inserted into the distinct depression immediately proximal to the head of the radius; this depression corresponds to the lateral and posterior parts of the radiohumeral joint. A joint effusion obliterates the depression.

2. **Superficial Structures.**—The skin over the back of the elbow is thicker than that over the front, and, because of an excessively loose subcutaneous tissue, moves with great freedom over the subjacent parts. The *olecranon bursa* lies between the dorsal surface of the olecranon process, the tendinous expansion of the triceps muscle, and the skin. It is exposed to injury and infection from falls upon the elbow and abrasions of the skin. The bursa may be very painful from constant bruising of the elbow, as from using a tool in a confined space ("miner's elbow") (Fig. 611). Suppuration within the bursa sometimes ulcerates through the bursal wall and sets up a diffuse cellulitis throughout the connective tissue on the back of the forearm. The treatment of olecranon bursitis presents no unusual problems, as the bursa can be excised readily.

3. **Posterior Muscles about the Elbow.**—Proximal to the joint line is the expansive tendon of the *triceps brachii muscle* which inserts into the summit, margins, and posterior surface of the olecranon. Of the extensor group of muscles arising from the lateral epicondyle and the epicondylar ridge, the anconeus is the only muscle which belongs properly

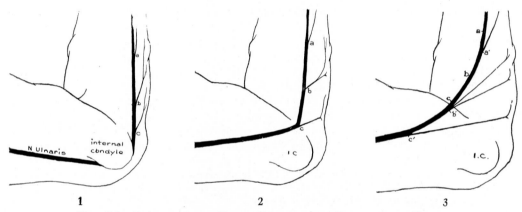

1 **2** **3**

FIG. 613.—REROUTING THE ULNAR NERVE TO THE FRONT OF THE ELBOW.

Illustrating the greater length of slack to be obtained by splitting the sheath of the nerve and stripping back the muscular branches; this enables the nerve to assume a more anterior position at the elbow; 1, ulnar nerve at the elbow with muscle branches, *a, b, c;* 2, ulnar nerve dislocated in front of the medial condyle; the transplantation is restricted by the binding effect of branches *b* and *c; 3,* the sheath of the ulnar nerve has been split, permitting the branches *b* and *c* to leave the nerve at a higher level and the nerve to be dislocated in front of the elbow, thus gaining several additional centimeters of slack. (Babcock, "Textbook of Surgery.")

in the region. The *anconeus muscle* throughout its extent lies in the posterior region of the elbow and is palpable in the lateral olecranon groove. From its origin on the lateral epicondyle, it spreads out to insert over the lateral surface of the olecranon and the posterior border of the ulna; it covers the posterior aspects of the radiohumeral joint. The *flexor carpi ulnaris muscle* (p. 619) arises from the medial epicondyle and the medial surface of the olecranon.

4. **Vessels and Nerves.**—The *arteries* at the back of the elbow are part of a periarticular network, made up of the collateral branches of the brachial, radial, and ulnar trunks, which serves as a collateral anastomosis in obstruction or ligation of the brachial trunk.

The *ulnar nerve* reaches the elbow behind the medial intermuscular septum and can be palpated as a round cord in the medial olecranon groove. It lies in contact with the periosteum under the deep fascia of the arm and under an expansion of the triceps tendon which fuses mesially with the deep fascia of the forearm. The nerve leaves the paraolecranon region between the heads of origin of the flexor carpi ulnaris muscle, and may be injured in any trauma to the medial epicondyle or to the attachments of the flexor carpi ulnaris muscle. The nerve may be drawn from its bed and brought forward around the medial epicondyle to a more protected position on the anterior surface of the elbow. This maneuver affords greater length to the nerve, a point of practical importance in ulnar nerve grafts.

SURGICAL CONSIDERATIONS

1. **Posterolateral Approach (of Kocher) to the Elbow Joint.**—The incision advised by Kocher for resection of the elbow joint begins over the lower part of the lateral supracondylar ridge, about 4 to 5 cm. above the joint level. It extends downward behind the lateral intermuscular septum and radial collateral ligament between the triceps, brachioradialis, and radial extensor muscles. The incision crosses the humeroradial joint and then curves downward along the distal border of the anconeus muscle to the ulna; thus it is J-shaped, the upper portion being straight and the lower curved. It has the merit of dividing no muscle tissue or nerve of importance.

The soft tissues are reflected from the posterior aspect of the joint by subperiosteal exposure. The flap elevated consists of the fascia, the triceps and anconeus muscles, and the periosteum of the humerus and ulna. The subperiosteal elevation is continued until the ulnar and radial collateral ligaments are freed and the extensor muscles are detached from the lateral epicondyle. The bones of the forearm are luxated laterally and the elbow joint is exposed. The ulnar collateral ligament is exposed from within the joint and can be detached from the olecranon and coronoid processes of the ulna and from the internal condyle of the humerus. A synovectomy or an excision of the articular extremities may be performed as the occasion demands.

The ulnar nerve is not exposed if subperiosteal excision is employed. In freeing the radius at its neck for removal of the radial head, the deep (posterior interosseous) branch of the radial nerve must be avoided where it passes through the supinator (brevis) muscle.

Shortening of the limb as a result of removal of the elbow epiphyses is not as serious as might be expected, since growth is most active and prolonged at the shoulder and wrist.

2. **Posteromedian Approach.**—A straight posteromedian incision, 10 cm. long, is made half above and half below the tip of the olecranon. The upper half of the incision splits the triceps tendon vertically and penetrates the joint cavity; the lower half of the incision descends upon the posterior border of the shaft of the ulna. The tissues are peeled off the bones as cleanly as possible and the ulnar nerve is drawn from its bony groove behind the internal epicondyle. If the approach is for joint resection, the structures removed from the outer aspect of the elbow are the anconeus muscle, the outer half of the triceps muscle, and the common origin of the extensor muscles from the lateral epicondyle. The lower articular extremity of the humerus, when denuded, is protruded forcibly and divided transversely. The level of the section depends upon the circumstances of the case. The articular extremities of the radius and ulna are protruded, and the line of bone section is carried through the base of the olecranon process, through the coronoid process of the ulna, and through the head of the radius. In the process of stripping the tissues from the radius, the supinator (brevis) muscle may require dissection from the neck of the bone; the proximity of the deep (posterior interosseous) branch of the radial nerve must be borne in mind.

3. **Bilateral Approach to the Elbow Joint.**—Bilateral epicondylar incisions are convenient for drainage of the elbow joint. Incision in the lateral aspect of the radiohumeral joint involves no important structures, but the mesial incision requires careful regard for the ulnar nerve and, therefore, should be close to the olecranon. Simple para-olecranon incisions suffice for joint drainage.

4. **Medial Approach to the Elbow Joint.**—Molesworth and Campbell advise removing the medial epicondyle of the humerus to expose the elbow joint. The elbow is flexed to a right angle and an incision is made over the medial epicondyle from a point 5 cm. below to a point 5 cm. above the elbow joint line. The ulnar nerve is isolated in the medial para-olecranon groove, is dissected free, and is retracted posteriorly. The medial epi-

condyle is cleared of all surrounding soft parts except the common tendinous origin of the flexor muscles of the forearm.   The medial epicondyle with its muscle attachments is chiseled off the humerus and is turned inferiorly and posteriorly.   Blunt dissection frees the massive flexor group of muscles without injury to their small nerves.   The medial aspect of the coronoid process is dissected free, the medial wall of the joint capsule is incised, and the periosteum with the anterior and posterior parts of the capsule is stripped from the humerus sufficiently to afford exposure of the interior of the joint.   The forearm then can be levered laterally with the lateral part of the capsule as a hinge.   The elements of the elbow joint thus become accessible to inspection and operation.

C. BONES AND JOINTS

The distal extremity of the humerus, the proximal extremity of the ulna, and the head of the radius form the elbow joint and the proximal radio-ulnar joint.   The elbow is a perfect hinge joint and depends for its stability upon the shape of the articular sur-

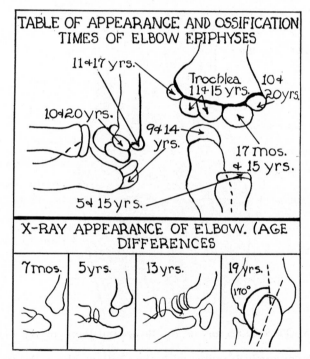

Fig. 614.—Table of Appearance and Ossification Times of Elbow Epiphyses. (Modified from Camp and Cilley, Amer. Jour. of Roent.)

faces.   These surfaces are disposed in such a fashion as to render their mutual displacement very difficult.   The joint between the humerus and ulna is shaped so as to allow flexion and extension only; that between the humerus and the head of the radius is a ball and socket joint, allowing pronation and supination through rotary movement of the radius.

1. **Articular Extremities.**—The **distal extremity of the humerus** is flattened anteroposteriorly into the widest part of the bone.   At its junction with the shaft, this portion bends forward until its plane is angulated 45 degrees on the shaft.   It consists of the *trochlea* and *capitulum* (*capitellum*) for articulation with the semilunar notch (greater sigmoid cavity) of the ulna and the proximal surface of the head of the radius respectively. The articular portion is bounded laterally by the epicondyles.   The *medial epicondyle* is the longer and more prominent; its superior margin is about 2.5 cm. from the inner border of the trochlea.   This greater length produces the lateral deflection of the forearm known

as the "carrying angle." The *lateral epicondyle* forms a conical projection immediately adjoining the capitulum. Each epicondyle may be traced proximally into an *epicondylar ridge*.

At the junction of the articular extremity with the shaft, the humerus is hollowed out posteriorly into one fossa and anteriorly into two fossae. The anterior or *coronoid* and the *radial fossae* are occupied by fatty tissue covered by joint synovia. In full flexion, the coronoid process of the ulna and the head of the radius come into close relationship with these fossae. The posterior or *olecranon fossa* is deep and receives the summit of the olecranon when the forearm is in full extension.

The *ossification* of the distal extremity of the humerus begins in the second or third year, when a center for the capitulum and outer half of the trochlea appears. At about the fifth year, there develops a center for the medial epicondyle. At this time, the medial and distal parts of the diaphysis grow downward and separate the medial epicondyle from the remainder of the epiphysis. The center for the remainder of the trochlea appears about the seventh year, and coalesces with the other two centers to form the true lower

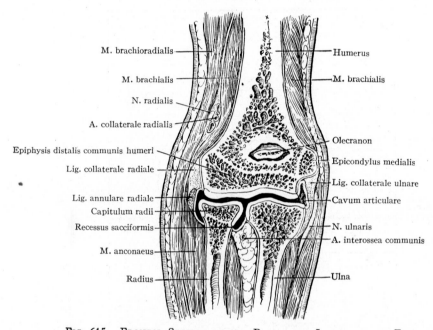

M. brachioradialis — **Humerus**

M. brachialis — **M. brachialis**

N. radialis — **Olecranon**

A. collaterale radialis —

Epiphysis distalis communis humeri — **Epicondylus medialis**

Lig. collaterale radiale — **Lig. collaterale ulnare**

Lig. annulare radiale — **Cavum articulare**

Capitulum radii —

Recessus sacciformis — **N. ulnaris**

M. anconaeus — **A. interossea communis**

Radius — **Ulna**

F<small>IG</small>. 615.—F<small>RONTAL</small> S<small>ECTION OF THE</small> B<small>ONES AND</small> J<small>OINTS OF THE</small> E<small>LBOW</small>.

epiphysis of the humerus which unites with the shaft at about the twelfth year. The medial epicondyle has a separate epiphysis which appears in the fifth year, but remains separate from the other centers; it joins the shaft in the eighteenth or nineteenth year. Separation at the epiphyseal line does not involve the medial epicondyle, which, even as late as the twentieth to twenty-fifth year, may be separated alone and be carried distally by its attached musculature. A fracture involving the epiphysis of the medial epicondyle is extra-articular.

The growth at the inferior humeral epiphyseal line is relatively less important than that at the superior or fertile epiphysis which is responsible for four fifths of the growth of the arm. Resection of the elbow performed in early youth limits the possibility for growth of the humerus to the upper epiphyseal line.

The **proximal extremity of the ulna** is the heaviest part of that bone. The projecting *olecranon* and *coronoid processes* forming it are hook shaped, the concavity of the hook being the semilunar notch which revolves upon the trochlea of the humerus. The coronoid process presents a small concave facet, or *radial notch* (lesser sigmoid cavity) which, with the annular (orbicular) ligament, helps to form the socket within which the head of the radius rotates in the movements of pronation and supination. At the anterior surface of the base of the coronoid process is the *tuberosity of the ulna* for the attachment of the brachialis (anticus) muscle.

The *development* of the olecranon and coronoid processes of the ulna takes place almost entirely from a primary ossification center in the shaft where growth continues during childhood. A secondary nucleus for the proximal part of the olecranon, to which the triceps muscle attaches, appears about the tenth year and unites with the shaft about the seventeenth year. Because the bony prominences which produce a strong bony joint in the adult are developed only partially in childhood, elbow dislocations at that time are common.

The upper surface of the **head of the radius** is concave and rests against the capitulum of the humerus. The circular periphery of the head is covered with a band of cartilage for

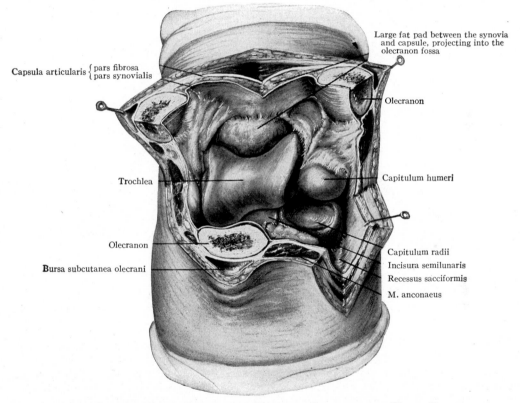

FIG. 616.—DEEP STRUCTURES OF THE POSTERIOR REGION OF THE RIGHT ELBOW.

movement in the radial notch of the ulna, but it is not attached to the annular (articular) or the capsular ligaments; it has no stabilizing tendinous or ligamentous attachments. Fracture of the head not only may derange and flatten this rotating wheel surface, causing pain in pronation, but also may cause a mechanical block to flexion or extension.

The *development* of the upper extremity of the radius takes place largely from a secondary center which appears between the fifth and sixth year and forms the disk-shaped proximal epiphysis. It is united to the shaft between the eighteenth and twentieth years. The proximal epiphysis and part of the neck of the metaphysis are intra-articular. The epiphyseal line is almost transverse.

2. **Carrying Angle.**—The transverse axis of the lower articular extremity slants medially and downward, forming an acute angle with the intercondyloid axis, the direc-

tion of which is at right angles to the shaft of the bone. This obliquity is responsible for the lateral deflection of the forearm and the obtuse carrying angle of the forearm in complete extension and supination. The transverse axis of the olecranon forms an outside angle of less than 90 degrees with the shaft of the ulna, a factor which contributes to the lateral angulation of the forearm. Midpronation masks the carrying angle by allowing the radius to come into direct line with the humerus, and is the position of the forearm in which the hand is used most frequently. When the midsupinated forearm is flexed acutely, the corresponding surfaces of the arm and forearm are applied accurately to one another.

When the supinated forearm is flexed fully with the arm at one side, the fingers lie over the medial half of the clavicle and not over the apex of the shoulder. This does not imply medial rotation of the humerus, but illustrates that its anterior surface is directed medially as well as forward. To align the arm and forearm correctly after fracture about the elbow and to reproduce the carrying angle accurately, the fingers should lie in front of

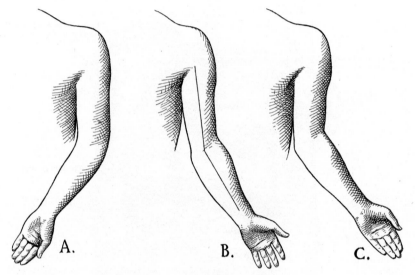

FIG. 617.—VARIATIONS IN THE CARRYING ANGLE AT THE ELBOW.
A, Cubitus varus deformity; B, normal carrying angle; C, cubitus valgus deformity. (Eisendrath in "Keen's Surgery.")

the inner half of the clavicle when the arm is flexed fully and supinated almost completely. An increase in the carrying angle is known as *cubitus valgus*, and a decrease as *cubitus varus*.

3. **Ligaments and Synovia of the Elbow and Proximal Radio-ulnar Joints.**—The ligaments about the humerus and the bones of the forearm form a complete capsular invest- ment for the elbow joint and the proximal radio-ulnar joint. The anterior and posterior parts of the *capsule* are relaxed into culdesacs in the respective positions of flexion and extension. In joint effusion, the synovia bulges markedly into these pouches.

The *anterior* and *posterior ligaments* of the elbow are the anterior and posterior thick- enings of the capsule. They are not strong, but are reinforced by the brachialis and triceps tendons. The *annular ligament* surrounds the head of the radius and is attached to the anterior and posterior margins of the radial notch of the ulna.

The *radial collateral (external lateral) ligament* extends fanwise from the lateral epi- condyle into diverging bundles which pass over the head and neck of the radius. The *ulnar collateral (internal lateral) ligament* extends fanwise from the medial epicondyle. Its fibers pass to the coronoid process and the margin of the semilunar notch.

The *synovia*, applied throughout to the deep surface of the capsule, pouches down- ward at the distal margin of the annular ligament for a varying distance around the neck of the radius.   The pads of fat which fill the coronoid, radial, and olecranon fossae are intracapsular but extrasynovial.   The fat pad occupying the radial fossa may become fibrocartilaginous, project into the joint, and cause locking and effusion.

Presence of fluid in the joint is manifest first in the para-olecranon groove on each side of the tendon of the triceps because of the weakness of the posterior part of the capsule in these areas.   The deep fascia over the front of the elbow, reinforced by the lacertus fibrosus, is especially strong and, if sinuses develop in connection with joint suppuration, they usually will be found on one or the other side of the triceps tendon.   The joint may be *aspirated* from the lateral side by inserting a needle immediately proximal to the head of the radius.

4. **Bursae about the Elbow Joint.**—The *radiohumeral bursa* lies over the radiohumeral joint between the extensor digitorum communis and the supinator brevis muscles.   *Radio-ulnar bursitis* may occur from the irritation of repeated or violent extension of the wrist with the hand pronated, "tennis elbow."   The lesion causes tenderness over the region

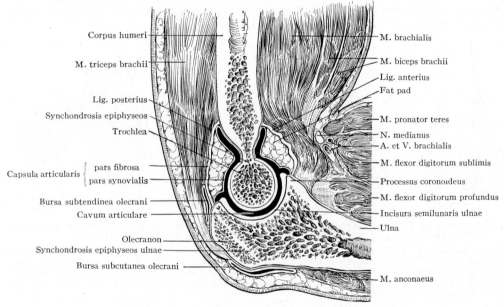

FIG. 618.—SAGITTAL SECTION THROUGH THE ELBOW REGION.

of the radio-ulnar joint and marked disability.   The bursitis may recur even after a long period of rest from irritation.   The bursa may require excision or curettement.

The *interosseous bursa* is related laterally to the tendon of the biceps and medially to the ulna.   It lies behind the supinator (brevis) muscle.   The *bicipitoradial bursa* lies between the tuberosity of the radius and the insertion of the biceps muscle.   Thus, the biceps tendon runs between these two bursae, either or both of which may be irritated in engagements requiring violent movements at the elbow.   When these bursae are diseased, they are painful upon contracture of the biceps muscle, especially if associated with supination of the forearm.

SURGICAL CONSIDERATIONS

Injuries and infections about the elbow may involve only the soft parts which include the cubital vessels, the muscle fibers, and the capsule with its reinforcing ligaments.   Hemorrhage with consequent periarticular fibrosis may occur about the joint, producing adhesions and causing impairment of the joint action.   When the trauma causes intra-articular fracture and actual joint derangement, joint motion may be blocked and the faulty alignments bring about a synovial effusion.   Continued mild trauma may induce chronic synovial irritation with a predisposition to the formation of loose bodies or attached tags of synovial fringes within the joint.

Pyogenic infection disintegrates the joint, inflames the synovia, erodes the cartilage, and roughens the articular extremities. Intra-articular adhesions and a resistant, thickened capsule result. The degree of joint destruction determines whether function can be restored or whether ankylosis with loss of all free motion will occur.

1. **Examination of an Injured Elbow.**—Often the diagnosis of lesions involving the elbow joint or the articular ends of the bones forming it is extremely difficult. In the light of the faulty functional results and unsightly deformities sometimes obtained, an injured elbow is a source of genuine perplexity and anxiety. A systematic examination should be made of the four bony prominences about the joint: the two epicondyles, the olecranon, and the head of the radius. Both the active and passive motions of the joint should be tested. Unless the joint is examined very soon after injury, the attendant difficulties are increased greatly by the swelling which rapidly supervenes and masks all landmarks. Without careful use of the x-ray, many forms of fracture and dislocation are reduced improperly, so that by the time the swelling has subsided, the resulting deformity may lead to ankylosis of the joint or a diminished range of movement.

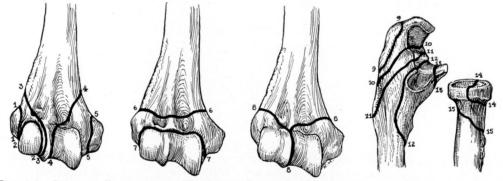

FIG. 619.—LINES OF FRACTURE AND EPIPHYSEAL SEPARATION ABOUT THE DISTAL EXTREMITY OF THE HUMERUS, AND THE PROXIMAL EXTREMITIES OF THE RADIUS AND ULNA.

1–1, Fractura epicondyli externi; 2–2, fractura capituli; 3–3, fractura condyli externi; 4–4, fractura condyli interni; 5–5, fractura epicondyli interni; 6–6, fractura supracondylica; 7–7, epiphyseal separation; 8–8–8, Y fracture; 9–9, fractura olecrani (summit); 10–10, fractura olecrani (middle); 11–11, fractura olecrani (base); 12–12, fractura coronoideae (base); 13–13, fractura coronoideae (tip); 14–14, fractura capitis radii; 15–15, fractura colli radii.

2. **Separation of the Distal Epiphysis of the Humerus.**—Separation of the distal epiphysis of the humerus is one of the commonest of the more severe elbow injuries occurring in childhood and adolescence. After union of the epiphysis, supracondylar fracture may occur with a corresponding amount of trauma. Epiphyseal separation often is accompanied by fracture across the distal part of the diaphysis. Separation of the epiphysis may occur before the sixteenth or seventeenth year, at which time the detached fragment usually includes the trochlea, capitulum, and external epicondyle. The medial epicondyle, which develops from a separate center of ossification, is independent of the epiphysis proper and is extra-articular. Up to the age of five years, the entire humeral cartilaginous extremity with its four developing centers may be torn from the shaft, and the lesion may simulate supracondylar fracture in deformity, swelling, discoloration, and mobility of the fragments. The epiphysis sometimes carries away a small part of the humeral diaphysis. Up to the age of sixteen or seventeen years, epiphyseal separation may be associated with posterior dislocation.

The displacement observed most commonly in epiphyseal separation is that in which the epiphysis is carried backward with the forearm bones. The deformity then somewhat resembles posterior dislocation of both bones of the forearm. Because the periosteum is attached firmly to theepiphyseal cartilage, it is carried with the epiphysis and is stripped up from the posterior part of the diaphysis for a varying distance. Unless the reduction is accurate, the stripped periosteum lays down new bone behind the humerus, which subsequently interferes with complete extension of the forearm. The difficulty in effecting reduction and in maintaining the parts in accurate apposition is very great. To maintain reduction, the forearm is immobilized in full flexion.

Since the cartilaginous extremity is translucent to the x-ray, the condition is difficult to diagnose in children under three years of age, in whom the secondary centers of ossification are not yet developed.

3. Fractures Involving the Distal Extremity of the Humerus.—The distal extremity of the humerus is exposed to injury from falls on the outstretched hand because of the transmission of the force through the bones of the forearm. In children, these injuries occur in a great variety and number, and it is difficult in any case to ascertain the exact nature and direction of the fracturing force. It is not possible by examination and palpation alone to distinguish the exact nature of the fracture. The increased width of the humerus at this level, its flattened shape, its lessened strength resulting from the presence of the olecranon, coronoid and radial fossae, and the superficial position of the epicondyles account for the frequency of fractures.

The *medial epicondyle*, because of its prominent position at the medial aspect of the elbow, may be detached and subsequently displaced downward and forward by the flexor and pronator muscles of the forearm. The ulnar nerve, which is in close proximity to the bone, often is injured in this accident.

A more extensive fracture of the *medial part of the distal extremity of the humerus* starts from the medial supracondylar ridge and descends obliquely downward and outward through the olecranon and coronoid fossae and through the trochlea into the cavity of the elbow joint. The detached fragment, with the ulna, may rise above the normal level and produce inward deflection of the forearm. This deflection obliterates the carrying angle, carries the forearm into a cubitus varus position (p. 610), and interferes materially with the function of the limb. In the reduction of this fracture, care must be taken to avoid excessive mesial deflection of the forearm.

Fracture of the lateral epicondyle alone rarely is detected because of the small size and slight projection of the fragment. A much more common lesion is a *fracture extending from the lateral epicondylar ridge into the elbow joint* through the capitulum or between the capitulum and trochlea. The lesion may be produced by a fall on the palm of the hand in which the force is transmitted through the head of the radius. The usual cause of this fracture is direct violence to the elbow, and a common complication is cubitus valgus (p. 610).

The displacement in *transverse supracondylar fracture* is in the anteroposterior direction. The long fragment overrides the distal fragment which, with the elbow, is carried backward by the pull of the triceps muscle. The deformity resembles that of posterior dislocation. Careful examination shows that the relation of the condyles to the olecranon is unchanged. This lesion has been described as an extension fracture, in contradistinction to the far less common flexion fracture caused by a blow on the back of the flexed elbow. In the latter, the distal elbow fragment and the forearm are driven forward anterior to the proximal fragment. Supracondylar fractures frequently radiate downward through one of the fossae into the joint, resulting in so-called T-*shaped or* Y-*shaped (transverse diacondylar) fractures.* The displacement is the same as that in transverse fracture. Callus usually encroaches on the anterior and posterior fossae and limits the range of motion in the joint.

Successful treatment of these fractures consists in accurate reposition of the fragments and in operative reduction for serious displacement. Acute flexion is maintained after the reduction of almost all these fractures, since in this position the lower end of the humerus is splinted by the tightening of the triceps tendon, the forearm muscles are relaxed, and the elbow is in a position from which function is regained most readily, as gravity and exercises subsequently bring back extension. If limitation of motion then occurs, whatever motion remains is of functional value. Although acute flexion is the surest way of holding the fragments in position, it is subject to serious risk, for, should there be hemorrhage and edema within the deep fascia, the flexion has so tightened the fascia and muscles that venous return may be cut off and a Volkmann contracture may occur (p. **617**).

Deformities from unsatisfactory reduction of fractures of the distal end of the humerus are exceedingly common. Many of these fractures enter the joint and distort the articular surfaces. Because of the complex nature of the joint, there is limitation of motion when only moderate displacement remains. Joint motion frequently is limited by adhesions within the muscles about the joint and by ossifying myositis.

4. **Fracture of the Olecranon Process.**—The olecranon process, like the patella, surmounts the extensor surface of a joint and receives the pull of a powerful extensor muscle. In many respects, olecranon fracture resembles patellar fracture. The site of fracture of the olecranon varies; it may lie near the extremity of the process or cross it so that the proximal fragment includes the proximal half of the semilunar notch, thereby involving the joint cavity. As a rule, the fracture is caused by the direct violence of a fall upon the point of the elbow. Muscle action probably plays an important rôle in producing the break, as the triceps muscle is likely to be in contraction at the time of the fall, thus throwing a great strain upon the bone. Muscle action alone may cause fracture. In this type of fracture the proximal fragment usually is a small piece of bone holding the triceps insertion.

In all fractures involving the olecranon, the triceps muscle tends to draw the detached fragment upward. This action is opposed by the lateral tendinous expansions investing the sides of the bone, by the ulnar collateral ligament which often remains untorn, and by the ulnar periosteum, the anconeus muscle, and the common ulnar periosteum. The degree of separation depends upon the extent to which these structures are torn. When wide separation occurs, difficulty is experienced in keeping the fragments in apposition. It usually is necessary to expose the site of fracture, empty the joint of clots, and suture the fragments into position. After surgical reduction, the arm need not be placed in full extension, as is required when the fragments are reduced by manipulation.

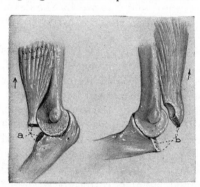

FIG. 620.—FRACTURE ABOUT THE ELBOW FROM MUSCLE ACTION.

Contraction of the brachialis muscle has torn away the coronoid process of the ulna, *a;* contraction of the triceps has fractured the olecranon process, *b.* (Babcock, "Textbook of Surgery.")

5. **Fracture of the Neck of the Radius.**—The head of the radius is in the direct line of force applied through the hand and radius to the humerus. The radial head and neck also receive the brunt of rotary and torsion strains on the forearm. Fracture through the neck is fairly common. Displacement of the head may be forward, backward, or lateralward; forward displacement is the most common. When the anterior ligament of the elbow joint and the annular (orbicular) ligament give way, the head moves forward anterior to the humerus and interferes seriously with the range of elbow movements. Flexion is limited at or near **90** degrees by the contact of the misplaced head with the forward surface of the inferior extremity of the humerus. Rotation is resisted strongly, pronation less so, and the hand is rendered useless for many purposes. Rotary movements can occur only at the shoulder.

The head of the radius lies as an unattached fragment in the elbow joint, produces an unusual fullness on the anterolateral aspect, and is subject to faulty union or nonunion. It should be removed, preferably through a dorsal incision between the extensor carpi ulnaris and anconeus muscles. Removal of the head of the radius does not imply any disability or loss of function, provided the annular ligament is preserved or repaired.

6. **Subluxation of the Radius (Pulled Elbow).**—In young children, sudden traction on, or torsion of, the hand or wrist may result in an anterior displacement of part of the

head of the radius. The bone first is pulled downward through the annular ligament. The child cannot use the elbow and carries the forearm in partial pronation, since supination is painful. Forcible supination screws the partially dislocated radial head back into position.

7. **Dislocation at the Elbow Joint.**—In spite of its structural stability, exposure of the elbow to severe trauma causes dislocation to occur at the elbow joint with a frequency second only to that of the shoulder joint. The resistance offered by the bony elements of the joint sometimes is responsible for accompanying fractures. The forearm bones may be dislocated posteriorly, anteriorly, laterally, or medially, and the dislocation in any direction may be partial or complete. The dislocated ulna carries the radius with it.

Posterior dislocation of both bones of the forearm is the most common dislocation at the elbow. It results from a fall upon the outstretched hand with the forearm abducted and extended. As the line of force passes upward behind the transverse axis of the elbow joint, the forearm is hyperextended and the anterior ligament and anterior part of the collateral ligaments are overstretched and give way. The articular surface of the humerus is pried from the semilunar notch and pushed forward over the coronoid process. The fibers of the brachialis muscle, which are attached to the coronoid process, are overstretched or torn. The dislocation is incomplete if the free edge of the coronoid process rests against the lower part of the trochlea, and complete if the coronoid process passes backward and upward and rests in the olecranon fossa.

In complete dislocation, the head of the radius lies behind the lateral epicondyle, and the distal end of the humerus sinks into the cubital fossa. The arm and forearm are held in semiflexion and meet at an angle of about 120 degrees. The forearm appears shortened, the depth of the elbow is increased, and the olecranon projects posteriorly. The relations between the humeral epicondyles and the olecranon are altered. The olecranon lies above and behind its normal level, and its posterior projection is increased by attempts at flexion of the forearm. All movements, however slight, are painful.

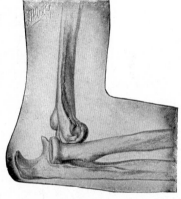

FIG. 621.—POSTERIOR DISLOCATION OF BOTH BONES OF THE FOREARM. THE ELBOW IS FLEXED TO A RIGHT ANGLE. (Scudder, "Treatment of Fractures.")

Anterior dislocation of both bones of the forearm is the rarest of the elbow dislocations and arises from trauma applied to the olecranon from behind when the elbow is flexed. In this position, the olecranon lies anterior to the trochlea. If the acting force continues, the olecranon may be torn away from its ligamentous connections with the humerus and be driven forward, carrying the radius with it. The dislocation is incomplete if the summit of the olecranon comes to rest anterior to the trochlea, and complete if it comes to rest anterior to the distal end of the humeral shaft.

Lateral and medial dislocations occur from falls on the pronated outstretched hand. The direction of dislocation depends upon whether the line of force is directed lateral or medial to the midpoint of the transverse axis of the elbow. Lateral dislocation usually is complete. In its least accentuated form of dislocation, the head of the radius rests beneath the lateral epicondyle of the humerus, and the sharp free margin of the coronoid process lies in the groove between the trochlea and capitulum. In a more advanced stage of dislocation, the radial head is lateral to the humerus, and the semilunar notch of the ulna lies beneath the capitulum and lateral epicondyle. In complete dislocation, both forearm bones lie to the lateral side of the humerus. The forearm usually is rotated medially in such a way that the radius is directed forward and the ulna backward. Lateral dislocation occasionally is associated with posterior dislocation of the radius and ulna.

Medial dislocation almost always is incomplete. Its rare occurrence is explained by the marked downward projection of the medial lip of the trochlea. When the ulna clears this projection, the semilunar notch rests beneath the trochlea.

8. **Resection of the Elbow for Tuberculosis.**—Resection of the elbow by the postero-lateral approach (of Kocher) and by the posterior longitudinal approach is described in the olecranon region.

Tuberculosis in the elbow joint spreads from a focus in the fertile growing diaphysis of the lower end of the humerus. The infection may spread through the epiphyseal cartilage, or it may spread toward the medullary cavity and result in tuberculous osteomyelitis. If the infection spreads in all directions, the periosteum lining the humeral fossae is eroded. The lesion at this stage is intracapsular, but extrasynovial, and is in direct relation with the fat areas (p. 608) in the humeral fossae. There is rapid extension through the joint synovia with joint involvement (tuberculous arthritis).

If one elbow is to become ankylosed, it is best that it be fixed at a right angle. If both elbows are fixed, the right should be ankylosed at something greater than a right angle, and the left at something less than a right angle. The right hand then can be brought to the mouth. The left can be used for cutting food, and also can reach the trouser pocket. In all cases, the forearm is put in a position midway between pronation and supination.

9. **Arthroplasty of the Elbow.**—Arthroplasty of the elbow (formation of an artificial joint) is indicated for ankylosis in an unsuitable position, such as complete extension.

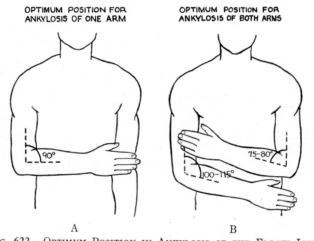

FIG. 622.—OPTIMUM POSITION IN ANKYLOSIS OF THE ELBOW JOINT.
A, Position of choice when one elbow is ankylosed; B, position of choice when both elbows require fixation.

If one elbow is ankylosed in flexion and the other in extension, an arthroplasty should be performed on the elbow in extension. If both elbows are ankylosed at a right angle or less, mobilization of one elbow is indicated.

The J-shaped incision (of Kocher) and the posterior longitudinal incision (p. 606) afford satisfactory access to the joint. After the ulnar nerve is dissected free, a transverse incision is made through the soft parts and periosteum at the base of the olecranon. When the olecranon is sawed through, the whole joint may be broken open. The fascias, capsule, and ligaments are dissected from the bones and the anteroposterior surface of the joint comes into view. If the joint is fused, the bony union is broken. After the articular ends are brought out through the incision, they are remodeled to articulate as smoothly as possible. Sufficient bone should be removed to allow free motion. An area of fascia lata is cut from the thigh, fashioned about the newly modeled humeral condyles, and sutured to the capsule. The detached portion of the olecranon process then is sutured to the ulna and the wound is closed. Absorption of the tissue interposed between the bone ends results in the formation of a bursa-like structure which permits joint mobility.

10. **Complications of Injuries about the Elbow.**—The complications of elbow injuries may involve any of the surrounding soft parts. *Injury to the ulnar nerve* may occur in any

of the dislocations at the elbow, and particularly in fracture of the medial epicondyle which extends into the trochlea, especially when the distal fragment is forced backward across the course of the nerve.

Myositis ossificans, or the abnormal growth of bone in muscle, occurs near the brachialis and triceps insertions and is common after fracture or dislocation. The bone deposited interferes materially with flexion and extension.

In *Volkmann's (ischemic) contracture*, there is a boardlike hardening of the forearm from fibrosis of the muscles which are shortened and adherent to each other. Use of the fingers is lost and there are sensory and motor changes. The contracture has been ascribed to compression of the arteries and anemic necrosis from immobilization in flexion or from applying splints and bandages too tightly. The condition actually is caused by edema and hemorrhage beneath the deep fascia which obstruct venous return and produce venous congestion. This blocks the drainage of the waste products of metabolism in the muscle and leads to an actual replacement of the muscle tissue by fibrous tissue.

Circulatory disturbances below the elbow or severe pain following an injury at the elbow warrant incision of the deep fascia to relieve tension in the antecubital fossa. In the treatment of this condition about the elbow or in the forearm, the criterion for releasing bandages or altering the angle of flexion should not alone be inability to feel the radial pulse and circulatory changes in the hand. Volkmann's contracture can occur without these signs being present. Pain here, as elsewhere, is an important symptom and demands careful investigation.

IV. FOREARM

A. ANTERIOR AND POSTERIOR REGIONS OF THE FOREARM

1. **Definition and Boundaries.**—Topographically, the forearm extends from an imaginary horizontal line three fingerbreadths below the level of the elbow to the bend of the wrist. The forearm is considered in the supine position with the palm of the hand looking forward. The *anterior* or *volar region* contains all structures anterior to the plane of the radius and ulna, and includes the antero-internal and antero-external muscle groups arising from the medial and lateral epicondyles and the epicondylar ridges. The *posterior* or *dorsal region* contains the soft parts posterior to the shafts of the radius and ulna and their interosseous membrane. The extensor muscle group, which composes the bulk of this region, is limited mesially by the posterior border of the ulna and laterally by the septum of the deep fascia of the forearm which separates the extensors of the carpus from those of the hand.

2. **Surface Anatomy.**—In full supination, the forearm appears as a cone flattened anteroposteriorly. The increase in the transverse diameter near the elbow is caused by masses of muscle arising from the epicondyles of the humerus. The lessened bulk of the distal half of the forearm marks the transition of the fleshy portions of the muscles into their respective tendons. Distally, the shafts of the radius and ulna are superficial and their contour is defined readily. The distal end of the radius, in passing from full supination to full pronation, carries with it the carpus and hand and revolves about the head of the ulna in such a way that the surfaces of the forearm become reversed.

The surfaces of the forearm present elevations separated by linear depressions which correspond to the subjacent muscles and the interstices and fascial septa between them. In children and in females, in whom the muscles are not prominent and in whom there is abundant subcutaneous fat, the forearm presents a uniform aspect with an almost cylindrical contour.

The anterior surface of the forearm is traversed by a shallow furrow which begins above at the level of the biceps tendon, and inclines slightly laterally as it descends to the medial side of the radial styloid. This groove marks the line of separation between the antero-external group of muscles composed of the brachioradialis and the radial extensors, and the antero-internal group of muscles composed of the pronator (radii) teres and the flexor muscles. When flexion of the elbow is resisted, this groove is defined more clearly and the brachioradialis muscle stands out prominently at the lateral aspect of the forearm. The groove marks the direction of the course of the radial artery. The vessel may be palpated readily in the lower part of the radial sulcus because of its superficial position and its proximity to the bone. The radial artery lies between the prominent tendons of the brachioradialis and flexor carpi radialis muscles.

Proximally, the individual flexor and pronator tendons cannot be distinguished easily under the deep fascia. Distally, their tendons are important surgical landmarks. By volar flexion of the hand against resistance, certain of the volar tendons at the wrist become unusually distinct. The tendon of the flexor carpi ulnaris lies nearest the medial border of the forearm where it may be gripped between the fingers and thumb opposite the distal extremity of the ulna and be traced to its insertion into the pisiform bone. The ulnar vessels and nerves lie immediately to its lateral side. The tendon of the flexor carpi

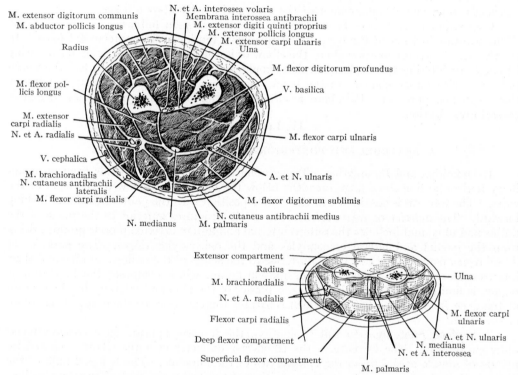

FIG. 623.—HORIZONTAL SECTION THROUGH THE MIDDLE OF THE LEFT FOREARM.
The inset shows the fascial spaces and vessels and nerves.

radialis lies just mesial to the navicular tubercle and the radial vessels lie just lateral to it. The palmaris longus tendon stands out to the ulnar side of the flexor carpi radialis tendon and is the guide to the median nerve which lies just beneath it or to its radial side.

The posterior aspect of the forearm is narrower than the anterior aspect, but the contour is more rounded because of the longitudinal bulge representing the extensor and flexor musculature of the posterior region. The muscle mass of the flexor group is distinguished readily from the protrusion made by the brachioradialis and radial extensor muscles. The common boundary line of the two groups of muscles is the dorsal border of the ulna, which is subcutaneous throughout its entire length and can be followed distinctly from the olecranon to the styloid process. The lateral boundary of the extensor group is less distinct, as it is formed by the lateral margin of the radius. In a muscular limb, the lateral boundary is indicated by the linear sulcus which lies along a line drawn from the lateral epicondyle to the dorsal radial tubercle and separates the radial extensor muscles from the extensor communis digitorum muscle.   The abductor and the extensor muscles of the thumb cross the lateral surface of the radius obliquely below its center and form a soft rounded projection.

The tendons and much of the muscle mass of the mesial or flexor muscle group pass forward around the ulna to the anterior or volar region of the forearm.

3. **Deep Fascia of the Forearm.**—The deep antibrachial fascia invests the forearm completely and is continuous with the deep fascia of the arm and hand.   It is especially strong along the dorsal surface, and is attached to the olecranon process and the humeral epicondyles.   It is strengthened around the elbow by expansions from the triceps brachii muscle.   The deep fascia is reinforced anteriorly by the lacertus fibrosus (bicipital fascia) (p. 608), an expansion from the biceps tendon.   At the wrist, the deep fascia is continuous with the *transverse* and *dorsal carpal (annular) ligaments* (p. 631).   From its deep surface, the fascia furnishes attachment to several muscles and sends *intermuscular septa* to the radius and ulna.

4. **Muscles of the Forearm.**—The forearm muscles are separated into three groups: antero-internal, antero-external, and posterior.

The **antero-internal** or **flexor-pronator group** of muscles lies in a mesial, deep, fascial space and includes the pronators and flexors arising from the medial epicondyle and the epicondylar ridge.   The more superficial of these, extending medially from the midline of the forearm, are the pronator teres, flexor carpi radialis, palmaris longus, flexor digitorum sublimis, and flexor carpi ulnaris muscles.   With the exception of the flexor carpi ulnaris muscle, they are supplied just beyond the elbow joint by branches of the median nerve (C_6).   The *pronator teres muscle* (N. median C_6) has, in addition, a deep head of origin from the coronoid process of the ulna.   The muscle is inserted into the middle of the lateral surface of the radius and is a powerful pronator as well as a flexor of the forearm. The *flexor carpi radialis muscle* is inserted into the bases of the second and third metacarpals and causes flexion and radial deviation of the hand at the wrist.   If it acts in conjunction with the radial extensors, it effects radial deviation only.   The *palmaris longus muscle* (N. median C_6) terminates in a long, slender tendon which passes anterior to the transverse carpal (anterior annular) ligament to an insertion into the palmar fascia.   The *flexor digitorum sublimis muscle* (N. median $C_{7,\,8}$, T_1) lies deep to the preceding tendons. Its individual tendons arise in the distal third of the forearm and pass behind the transverse (anterior annular) carpal ligament.   It acts primarily as a flexor of the proximal interphalangeal joints, and secondarily as a flexor of the metacarpophalangeal, wrist, and elbow joints.   The *flexor carpi ulnaris muscle* (N. ulnar C_8, T_1) descends along the ulnar border of the forearm to a principal insertion on the pisiform bone.   If the flexor carpi ulnaris acts with the flexor group, it aids in flexing the wrist and elbow joint; if it acts with the extensor carpi ulnaris, it produces ulnar deviation of the hand.

The deep set of antero-internal muscles includes the flexor digitorum profundus, flexor pollicis longus, and pronator quadratus.   These muscles are supplied by the volar interosseous branch of the median nerve ($C_{7,\,8}$, T_1), except for that part of the flexor digitorum profundus (N. ulnar C_8, T_1) controlling the ring and small fingers.   The *flexor digitorum profundus muscle* arises from the volar and median surfaces of the ulna and from the interosseous membrane, and terminates in tendons which pass beneath the transverse carpal ligament, along with the tendons of the flexor digitorum sublimis muscle, to enter the digital sheaths of the four fingers (p. 662).   These tendons are inserted into the bases of the terminal phalanges; their primary action is to flex the terminal phalanges and, continuing this action, to flex the remaining phalanges and, finally, the hand.   The *flexor pollicis longus muscle* (N. median C_8, T_1) arises mainly from the volar surface of the radius and the interosseous membrane.   Its tendon passes along the volar surface of the thumb to an insertion at the base of its terminal phalanx.   The *pronator quadratus muscle* (N. median C_8, T_1) is flat and quadrangular; it extends across the lower portions of the radius and ulna in the distal fourth of the forearm.

The **antero-external** or **radial group** of muscles springs from the lateral humeral epicondyle and includes the brachioradialis (supinator longus) and the extensor carpi radialis longus and brevis muscles. Under these muscles, the upper part of the radial shaft is invested by the *supinator brevis muscle*.

The *brachioradialis (supinator longus) muscle* (N. radial C_5, $_6$) arises between the triceps and brachialis muscles from the lateral margin of the humerus, the lateral intermuscular septum, and the lateral epicondyle. It is attached by a long, thin tendon to the styloid

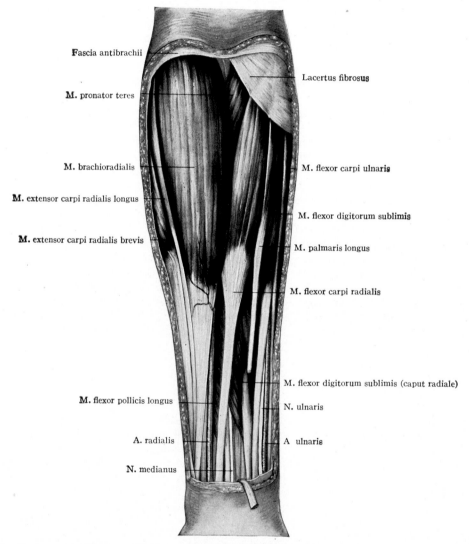

Fascia antibrachii

Lacertus fibrosus

M. pronator teres

M. brachioradialis

M. flexor carpi ulnaris

M. extensor carpi radialis longus

M. flexor digitorum sublimis

M. extensor carpi radialis brevis

M. palmaris longus

M. flexor carpi radialis

M. flexor digitorum sublimis (caput radiale)

M. flexor pollicis longus

N. ulnaris

A. radialis

A ulnaris

N. medianus

FIG. 624.—SUPERFICIAL MUSCLES, VESSELS, AND NERVES ON THE ANTERIOR REGION OF THE RIGHT FOREARM.

process of the radius and flexes and somewhat supinates the forearm. The *extensor carpi radialis longus* and *brevis muscles* have a common origin from the lateral epicondyle and lateral intermuscular septum. Their tendons are inserted into the bases of the second and third metacarpals and extend the hand. The long extensor muscle is supplied by the deep division of the radial nerve (C_6, $_7$); the short extensor muscle by the dorsal interosseous branch of the radial nerve (C_6, $_7$). The *supinator (brevis) muscle* (deep branch of the radial nerve, C_6, $_7$, $_8$) is concealed almost wholly by the foregoing superficial muscles.

It arises mainly from the lateral epicondyle of the humerus and the supinator crest and fossa of the ulna, and its diverging fibers are inserted into the posterior, lateral, and anterior surfaces of the radius.

The **posterior** or **dorsal group** of muscles is arranged in a superficial and a deep layer. The superficial members of the group include the extensor digitorum communis extensor digiti quinti proprius, and extensor carpi ulnaris.   The anconeus muscle (p. 605) belongs in the proximal part of this region.   With the exception of a small branch of the radial nerve to the anconeus muscle, the deep ramus of the radial (posterior interosseus) nerve

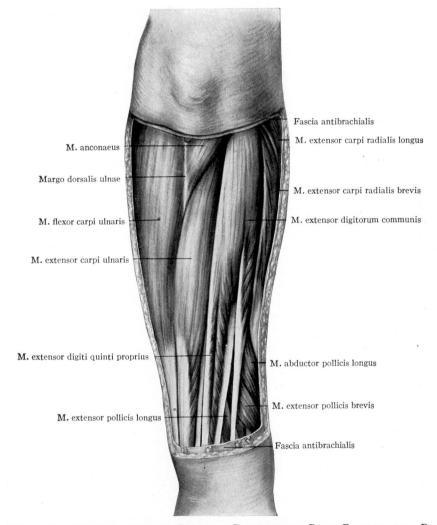

M. anconaeus

Margo dorsalis ulnae

M. flexor carpi ulnaris

M. extensor carpi ulnaris

M. extensor digiti quinti proprius

M. extensor pollicis longus

Fascia antibrachialis

M. extensor carpi radialis longus

M. extensor carpi radialis brevis

M. extensor digitorum communis

M. abductor pollicis longus

M. extensor pollicis brevis

Fascia antibrachialis

FIG. 625.—SUPERFICIAL MUSCULATURE IN THE POSTERIOR REGION OF THE RIGHT FOREARM AFTER REMOVAL OF THE ANTIBRACHIAL FASCIA.

($C_6, _7, _8$) supplies all the muscles in the posterior group.   The *extensor digitorum communis muscle* arises mainly from the lateral epicondyle of the humerus and the deep fascia of the dorsal part of the forearm.   Its four tendons are inserted into the bases of the middle and terminal phalanges of the four fingers.   The *extensor digiti quinti proprius muscle* arises in common with the preceding muscle and accompanies its tendon to the little finger.   The *extensor carpi ulnaris muscle* arises with the adjacent superficial extensors from the lateral epicondyle and the dorsal antibrachial fascia.   Its tendon is inserted into the base of the fifth metacarpal.

The deep group of extensors springs from the dorsal surfaces of the radius and ulna and is supplied by the deep branch of the radial nerve (C_6, $_7$, $_8$). The group includes the abductor pollicis longus, extensor pollicis brevis, extensor pollicis longus, and extensor indicis proprius muscles. The *abductor pollicis longus* (extensor ossis metacarpi pollicis) muscle is inserted into the base of the metacarpal of the thumb. The *extensor pollicis longus* and *brevis muscles* are inserted into the bases of the second and first phalanges respectively. The *extensor indicis proprius muscle* is inserted with the tendon of the common extensor which passes to the index finger.

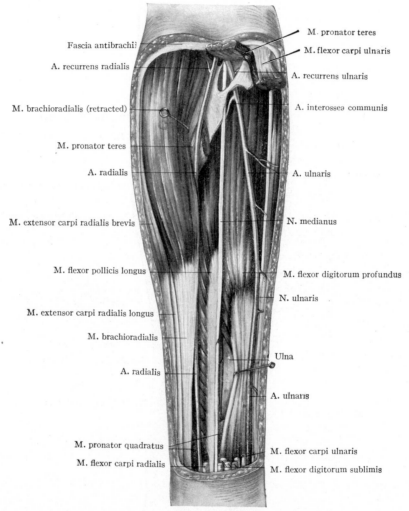

Fascia antibrachii

A. recurrens radialis

M. brachioradialis (retracted)

M. pronator teres

A. radialis

M. extensor carpi radialis brevis

M. flexor pollicis longus

M. extensor carpi radialis longus

M. brachioradialis

A. radialis

M. pronator quadratus

M. flexor carpi radialis

M. pronator teres

M. flexor carpi ulnaris

A. recurrens ulnaris

A. interossea communis

A. ulnaris

N. medianus

M. flexor digitorum profundus

N. ulnaris

Ulna

A. ulnaris

M. flexor carpi ulnaris

M. flexor digitorum sublimis

FIG. 626.—DEEP MUSCLES, VESSELS, AND NERVES OF THE ANTERIOR REGION OF THE RIGHT FOREARM.

5. Arteries of the Forearm and Their Ligation.—The **ulnar artery** is the larger of the two terminal trunks of the brachial artery. From its origin (p. 592) at the neck of the radius, it descends through the anterior surface of the forearm and crosses the transverse carpal ligament on the radial side of the pisiform bone. In the *lower two thirds* of the forearm, the course of the artery is straight and is indicated by a line drawn from the front of the medial epicondyle to the radial surface of the pisiform bone with the forearm in full supination. The artery lies upon the flexor digitorum profundus muscle between the flexor carpi ulnaris muscle mesially and the flexor digitorum sublimis muscle laterally. It gradually becomes superficial toward the wrist. In the *upper third* of the forearm, the vessel is placed deeply between the superficial and deep layers of the antero-internal musculature. This part of its course is indicated by a slightly curved line beginning 2.5 cm. below the bend of the elbow at the center of the limb and extending mesially to meet the vertical course at the junction of the upper and middle thirds of the forearm.

The *volar* and *dorsal ulnar recurrent branches* are given off near the origin of the ulnar artery. The *common interosseous artery* arises farther distally.

Ligation of the ulnar artery usually is performed near the wrist or at the junction of the upper and middle thirds of the forearm where its curved and vertical portions meet. With the arm fully supine, the artery may be ligated in the upper forearm through an incision beginning a palmbreadth below the medial epicondyle. After exposure of the deep fascia, the wound margins are retracted and the white line nearest the ulnar border of the limb is located. This line indicates the interspace between the flexor carpi ulnaris and flexor digitorum sublimis muscles, between and beneath which the artery lies. The ulnar nerve is more medially placed.

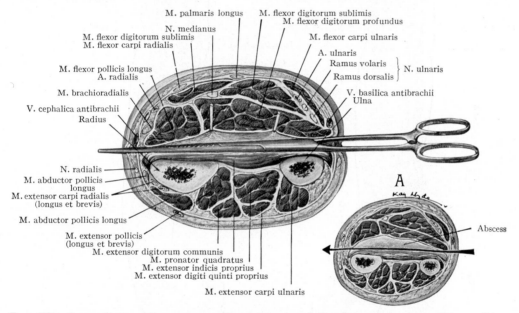

FIG. 627.—CROSS SECTION THROUGH THE LEFT FOREARM 7 CM. PROXIMAL TO THE RADIAL STYLOID PROCESS. A SHOWS THE PATH FOR INCISION OF AN ABSCESS IN THE ANTERIOR REGION OF THE LOWER FOREARM, EXTENDING FROM INFECTION IN THE CARPAL SYNOVIA.

A hemostat is inserted transversely in juxtaposition to the radius and ulna through the anterior interosseous space; incision can be made here without injuring important vessels and nerves and the abscess can be evacuated; note the amount of tissue between the radial artery and the hemostat. (After Kanavel.)

In ligation of the artery at the wrist, incision is made through the deep fascia 2.5 cm. proximal to the flexion fold, in the interval between the flexor carpi ulnaris and the flexor digitorum sublimis muscles. Near the wrist, the ulnar artery lies in the same relation to the ulnar nerve as it does in the upper forearm.

The **radial artery** runs a fairly straight course through the forearm. As it descends, it inclines laterally gradually, and, after reaching a point mesial to the radial styloid, enters its carpal course (p. 633) by passing beneath the extensor tendons of the thumb. Its course is indicated by a line drawn from the termination of the brachial artery (p. 592) to the navicular tubercle. In its *upper two thirds*, it lies under cover of the brachioradialis muscle and crosses the supinator muscle. The superficial (sensory) branch of the radial nerve approaches it on the lateral side. In the lower half of the forearm, it lies between the brachioradialis and flexor carpi radialis muscles. Save where it is overlapped by the fleshy fibers of the brachioradialis muscle, the artery occupies a superficial position. The *distal third* of the artery is subcutaneous and lies on the radius and on the flexor pollicis longus muscle.

The radial artery gives off two large branches in the forearm, the *radial recurrent artery* near its origin, and the *superficial volar artery* in the distal part of the forearm. The *superficial volar artery* runs through the short muscles of the thumb to meet the ulnar artery and complete the superficial palmar arch.

Because the artery is superficial, *ligation of the radial artery* is performed readily at any part of its course in the forearm. In ligation in the upper third of the forearm, the artery is found deep to the interval between the brachioradialis and pronator teres muscles.

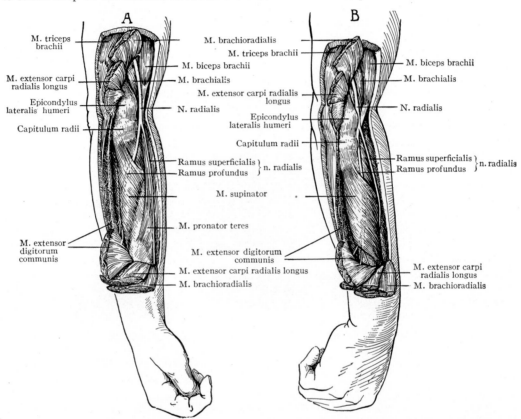

FIG. 628.—RELATIONS BETWEEN THE DEEP BRANCH OF THE RADIAL NERVE AND THE RADIOHUMERAL JOINT AND PROXIMAL PART OF THE SHAFT OF THE RADIUS.

In A, the forearm is in full supination; in B, the forearm is pronated. With the forearm in pronation, the radial nerve is not so likely to be injured in operations upon the proximal third of the radius.

For ligation of the artery at the wrist, an incision is made over the artery midway between the outer border of the radius and the tendon of the flexor carpi radialis. The vessel lies upon the pronator quadratus muscle.

6. **Nerves of the Forearm.**—The nerves of the forearm are the median, the ulnar, and the superficial and deep branches of the radial.

The **median nerve** enters the forearm between the superficial and deep heads of the pronator teres muscle (p. **619**) and is separated from the ulnar artery by the deep head of that muscle. It runs an approximately median course along the axis of the forearm. In the forearm, it lies between the superficial and deep flexors of the fingers and is attached firmly to the deep surface of the flexor digitorum sublimis.

The median nerve supplies all the superficial group of antero-internal muscles of the forearm, save the flexor carpi ulnaris which is supplied by the ulnar nerve. By its *volar interosseous branch*, it supplies all the deep group of antero-internal muscles except that part of the flexor digitorum profundus which controls the small and ring fingers; it is supplied by the ulnar nerve.

The **ulnar nerve** enters the forearm between the two heads of the flexor carpi ulnaris. It descends almost vertically upon the flexor digitorum profundus muscle and is overlapped by the flexor carpi ulnaris muscle. Its *course* is indicated by a line drawn from the medial epicondyle to the lateral margin of the pisiform bone. In the upper part of the forearm, the nerve is almost subcutaneous and can be rolled against the ulna. It is exposed by a vertical incision through the deep fascia over the medial para-olecranon groove, where it lies in contact with the mesial side of the elbow joint. In violent flexion of the elbow, the deep fascia over the nerve sometimes is torn, allowing the nerve to slip forward around the medial epicondyle. This nerve dislocation may require operative replacement (p. 605). In the forearm, it supplies the flexor carpi ulnaris muscle and the medial part of the flexor digitorum profundus muscle.

The **superficial (sensory) branch of the radial nerve** descends beneath the brachioradialis muscle from an origin anterior to the lateral epicondyle. It approaches the radial artery and lies close to its lateral wall in the middle third of the forearm. About a palmbreadth from the radial styloid, the nerve leaves the artery, pierces the deep fascia, and runs to the dorsum of the wrist and hand.

The **deep (dorsal interosseous) branch of the radial nerve** reaches the back of the forearm by winding around the neck of the radius through the substance of the supinator muscle (p. 620). On reaching the lateral side of the shaft of the radius, the nerve occupies the interspace between the superficial and deep muscles of the back of th e forearm, and innervates them.

B. SHAFTS OF THE RADIUS AND ULNA; INTEROSSEOUS MEMBRANE

1. **Shafts of the Radius and Ulna.**—The radius and ulna differ in certain important features. The *ulna* is strongest and most massive in its proximal extremity. It is connected securely with the humerus, stabilizes the elbow joint, and is essential to flexion and extension. The shaft gradually tapers downward to its distal extremity which plays only a minor rôle in the wrist joint.

The *radius*, in contrast, is weakest at its proximal extremity where its articulation with the humerus is one chiefly of contact, and its presence is not essential to elbow movement. The shaft becomes stronger and wider toward its distal extremity where it forms almost the entire forearm articulation at the wrist. At the middle of the forearm, the radius and ulna are about equally strong and their dimensions correspond closely.

With the forearm in supination, the radius and ulna enclose the elliptical interosseous space, which is bridged by the *interosseous membrane (ligament)*. With increasing pronation, the interosseous space gradually becomes narrower and the interosseous ligament is relaxed until the two bones come into contact. In the thumb-up, semiprone position, the interosseous space is widened. This position favors muscle relaxation, coaptation of fragments in the fracture of one or both of the bones of the forearm, and the restoration of pronation and supination after immobilization for fracture. The range of pronation is increased considerably by internal rotation of the humerus at the shoulder joint. Partial or complete loss of pronation and supination is a common result of fractures and dislocations involving the bones of the forearm and the wrist and elbow joint, and is a serious disability.

2. **Combined Fracture of the Shafts of the Radius and Ulna.**—Fracture of both bones of the forearm, usually in the middle or the lower third, occurs from direct or indirect violence. Falls upon the hand are the usual cause. Only a small part of the shock is transmitted directly to the ulna; the greater part is transmitted to the distal extremity of the radius and up the shaft of the humerus. The radius transmits only a small amount of the shock to the ulna by the interosseous membrane, the fibers of which are directed downward and mesially. The fracture lines usually are transverse, but may have varying degrees of obliquity

40

Displacement from overlapping of the fragments occurs when the fracture lines are oblique, and lateral displacement is likely to occur when fractures are transverse. There may be an angular displacement of both bones forward, backward, or to either side, or the fragments may be approximated. Green-stick, incomplete, or subperiosteal fractures of both bones are common, especially in children. In incomplete fracture in children, the bones undergo a variable amount

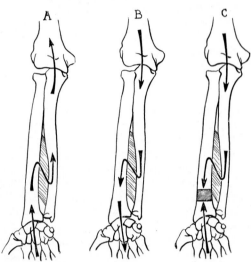

FIG. 630.—RÔLE OF THE INTEROSSEOUS MEMBRANE IN THE PATHOGENESIS OF FRACTURE OF THE RADIUS.

A shows how the force of a blow is transmitted to the arm through the radius, the interosseous membrane, and through the shaft of the ulna; B shows how force, acting through the arm, is transmitted to the hand. The force follows the ulna, the interosseous membrane, and then the radius; C shows the forces from below and above acting simultaneously, such as occurs in a fall upon the hand. The two forces meet in the shaded area in the distal extremity of the radius. (After Testut and Jacob.)

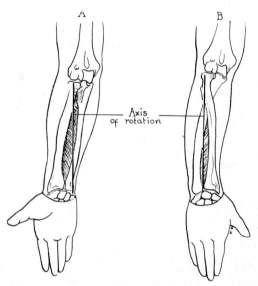

FIG. 629.—RADIUS AND ULNA AND INTEROSSEOUS MEMBRANE IN THE POSITIONS OF SUPINATION AND PRONATION.

A, Supination; B, pronation.

of bending, which produces an angular deformity of the forearm. The deformity should be overcome by straightening the limb forcibly while it is in the supine position. The forearm is grasped with both hands and pressure is exerted by the thumbs against the

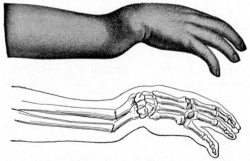

FIG. 631.—FRACTURE OF BOTH FOREARM BONES NEAR THE WRIST.

Note that the deformity is a considerable distance proximal to the wrist joint. (Helferich.)

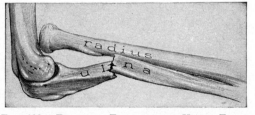

FIG. 632.—FRACTURE THROUGH THE UPPER THIRD OF THE SHAFT OF THE ULNA, COMPLICATED BY ANTERIOR DISLOCATION OF THE HEAD OF THE RADIUS.

The proximal fragment is flexed by the brachialis muscle. The distal fragment is drawn toward the radius by the pronator quadratus muscle. (Babcock, "Textbook of Surgery.")

projecting angulation. Lateral pressure should be avoided as it tends to drive the forearm bones together and to lessen the interosseous space. While rotation is being effected, digital pressure is exerted in the interosseous area to separate the bones as widely as possible

Certain tendencies to displacement should be borne in mind; the two bones are approximated by the action of the pronating muscles; the pull of the extensor and flexor muscles of the wrist, which arise from the humerus, tends to cause overriding of the fragments and shortening of the forearm and, even with accurate reposition of the fragments, to cause bowing at the point of fracture. Fractures in the distal part of the shaft usually are attended by overriding, the proximal fragments, as a rule, being anterior. The fragments of a fracture in the distal part of the shaft tend to be drawn together by the pronator quadratus muscle.

3. **Fracture of the Shaft of the Ulna.**—Fracture of the shaft of the ulna alone usually is transverse and is caused by direct violence, such as is sustained in warding off a blow directed at the head. The direction of the force producing the fracture determines the displacement, which usually is not great. The fracture may occur from indirect violence from a fall upon the ulnar border of the hand; in this case, it usually occurs in the distal

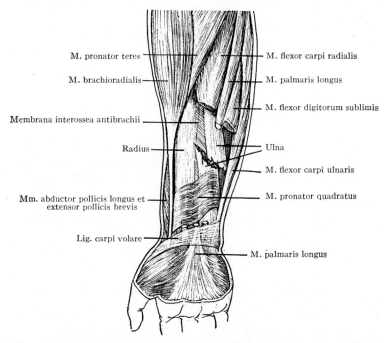

FIG. 633.—FRACTURE BELOW THE MIDDLE OF THE SHAFT OF THE ULNA.
The distal fragment is drawn toward the radius by the pronator quadratus muscle.

third of the shaft where the tendons replace the attached muscle masses. The fracture often is compound because the dorsal margin of the bone is subcutaneous throughout its extent. Marked displacement of the fragments is not common because of the splinting action of the intact shaft of the radius, but there is a tendency to a narrowing of the interosseous space, either from the displacement from the blow or from the pull of the pronator quadratus muscle upon the lower fragment.

Fracture of the upper part of the ulnar shaft may be associated with dislocation of the head of the radius, for the force which fractures the ulna may be so violent as to act upon the radius and tear the annular (orbicular) ligament. Possible radial dislocation should be suspected in all fractures of the upper part of the ulnar shaft.

4. **Fractures of the Shaft of the Radius.**—An isolated fracture of the radius usually presents little overlapping or shortening because of the splinting action of the interosseous membrane and the ulnar shaft. Fracture occurs from direct or indirect violence, and not uncommonly from thrusts and torsion strains at the wrist. The displacement is deter-

mined by the direction of the force producing the fracture. Marked deformity accompanying fractures of either the radius or ulna indicates a ligamentous tear at the proximal or distal radio-ulnar joint. Few fractures occur at the upper extremity of the radial shaft where it is well protected against direct violence. The majority of them occur in the weak midportion of the bone and in the lower third, where the transition from dense bone to cancellous bone takes place.

In fracture between the radial tuberosity and the insertion of the pronator teres, the small proximal fragment is flexed and supinated by the biceps and supinator muscles, and the action of the pronator muscles draws the lower fragment into pronation. The proximal fragment, because of its small size, is difficult to control in reduction of the fracture; hence it becomes necessary to bring the distal fragment into proper alignment with it by flexing the elbow and supinating the hand. If union takes place with rotary displacement, that

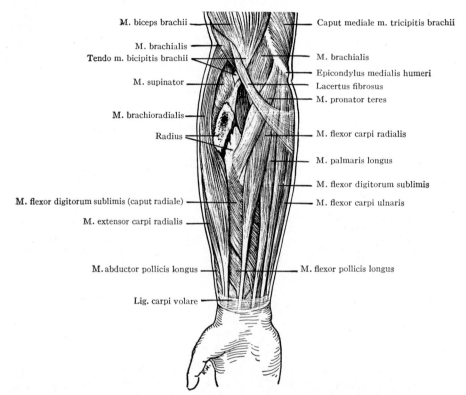

M. biceps brachii — Caput mediale m. tricipitis brachii
M. brachialis — M. brachialis
Tendo m. bicipitis brachii — Epicondylus medialis humeri
M. supinator — Lacertus fibrosus
— M. pronator teres
M. brachioradialis — M. flexor carpi radialis
Radius — M. palmaris longus
— M. flexor digitorum sublimis
M. flexor digitorum sublimis (caput radiale) — M. flexor carpi ulnaris
M. extensor carpi radialis —
M. abductor pollicis longus — M. flexor pollicis longus
Lig. carpi volare —

FIG. 634.—FRACTURE OF THE SHAFT OF THE RADIUS BETWEEN THE RADIAL TUBEROSITY AND THE INSERTION OF THE PRONATOR TERES MUSCLE.

The proximal fragment is rotated outward by the biceps and supinator muscles.

is, with the lower fragment in pronation and the upper fragment in supination, the power of supination of the hand is lost permanently.

In fracture immediately distal to the insertion of the pronator teres muscle, the proximal fragment is adducted and flexed slightly in midpronation. The supinating action of the biceps and supinator muscles is counteracted by the pronator teres muscle which acts at a greater mechanical advantage. The distal fragment is pronated and drawn toward the ulna by the pronator quadratus muscle. The proximal fragment in this fracture is sufficiently long to be controlled so as to prevent rotary displacement. For reduction, the forearm is placed in the thumb-up midprone position, that is, with the palm of the hand facing the chest. This attitude insures correct apposition of the fragments and is the most comfortable position.

5. **Surgical Approaches to the Bones of the Forearm.**—The *ulna* may be exposed readily throughout all its extent, without injury to any important structure, by incision along its posterior margin which lies between the extensor and flexor carpi ulnaris muscles.

Anterior exposure of the entire shaft of the radius may be obtained by a volar vertical incision along the anterior margin of the brachioradialis muscle. After division of the deep fascia, the brachioradialis muscle and the superficial branch of the radial nerve are drawn laterally and the flexor carpi radialis muscle and the radial vessels, medially. The radial origin of the flexor digitorum sublimis muscle and the insertion of the pronator teres muscle are divided at the radius. The supinator muscle is reflected upward and laterally from its area of attachment on the radius and, subsequently, the flexor pollicis longus and the pronator quadratus muscles are detached from the bone and are retracted mesially.

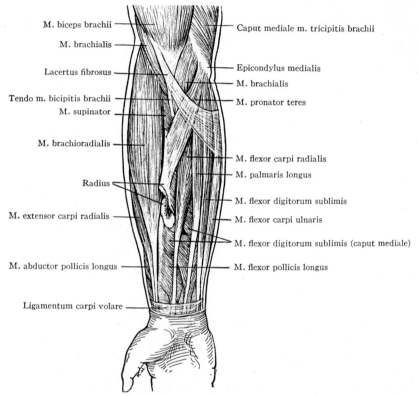

FIG. 635.—FRACTURE OF THE RADIUS IMMEDIATELY DISTAL TO THE INSERTION OF THE PRONATOR TERES MUSCLE.

The proximal fragment is placed directly forward in a position midway between supination and pronation.

Exposure of the upper extremity and *proximal third of the radius* is obtained by cleaving the interspace between the extensor digitorum communis muscle and the radial extensor muscle of the wrist. The supinator muscle is exposed and is divided distal to and parallel with the deep (dorsal interosseous) branch of the radial nerve. The cartilaginous head of the radius, with the epiphysis, if it has been formed, may be removed with the upper part of the shaft by subperiosteal resection, as the head is attached only to the synovia and lacks ligamentous joint connections.

The proximal third of the radius may be approached by an incision along the lateral epicondylar ridge and across the line of the humeroradial joint and the head of the radius. The incision follows the groove between the anconeus and the extensor digitorum communis muscles. In separating the supinator muscle from the neck and upper part of the shaft, care must be taken not to injure the deep branch of the radial nerve which traverses the muscle obliquely in its course to the dorsum of the forearm (Fig. 628).

The *middle third of the radial shaft* may be exposed posteriorly where it occupies a superficial position between the extensor digitorum communis muscle mesially and the brachioradialis and radial extensor muscles laterally. This is above the level at which the outer border of the radial shaft is crossed by the extensor muscles of the thumb and the superficial branch of the radial nerve.

The posterior incision for approach to the *distal third of the radius* exposes the abductor pollicis longus and the extensor pollicis brevis muscles where they cross the tendons of the radial extensors of the wrist. The extensor digitorum communis muscle on the ulnar side of the incision is retracted mesially. Retraction of the lateral muscles and tendons exposes the distal part of the radial shaft where it is devoid of muscle attachments.

6. Amputation Through the Forearm.—It is advisable, in all cases of amputation, to save as much of the forearm as possible to facilitate the subsequent wearing of an artificial limb. Supination and pronation should be preserved whenever possible. If the bone is divided below the level of the insertion of the pronator teres muscle, rotary movement is possible.

Amputation at the junction of the middle with the lower third gives the best stump from a prosthetic and surgical standpoint. The circulation in the skin at this level is good, the skin is tough, the subcutaneous layer is thick, and there is much muscle substance. Pronation and supination are preserved if the bone ends and the interosseous tissues and periosteum are dealt with to prevent excessive callus formation.

V. WRIST

The wrist is the mobile, flexible link between the forearm and hand. It may be said to include the soft parts and bones and joints over an area embracing not only the carpus, but the bony extremities of the radius and ulna and the bases of the metacarpals articulating with it. It includes the radiocarpal, midcarpal, and carpometacarpal joints. In the wrist, the forearm tendons and their synovial sheaths proceed to their insertions in the carpus. They are maintained in close contact with the wrist bones by specialized thickenings of the deep fascia, an arrangement insuring strength and graceful contour, and permitting the remarkable freedom of movement essential to the marvelously intricate functions of the hand.

A. SOFT PARTS OF THE WRIST

1. Surface Anatomy.—The relative positions of the important *tendons, vessels,* and *nerves* on the flexor surface of the wrist are very important because of the frequency of lacerating wounds at this level. By flexing the wrist forcibly, or against resistance, the tendons stand out prominently. Starting where the radial pulse is felt and palpating mesially, the important tendons can be identified. The first tendon encountered is that of the flexor carpi radialis (p. 619) as it passes to its insertion on the bases of the second and third metacarpal bones. The tendon of the palmaris longus, which lies in the midline of the wrist and inserts into the palmar fascia, is felt mesial to it. Next in succession are the tendons of the flexor digitorum sublimis. The median nerve lies between the palmaris longus and flexor carpi radialis tendons. The flexor carpi ulnaris tendon occupies the ulnar side and terminates on the pisiform bone. The ulnar nerve and vessels lie between this tendon and those of the flexor digitorum sublimis, and occupy a superficial position. The flexor digitorum profundus and flexor pollicis longus lie on a deeper plane and are concealed on superficial inspection. Abscesses which originate in the digital (p. 662) and palmar (p. 650) synovia point between these structures; they may be propagated to the carpal synovia about the flexor tendons at the wrist.

A deep laceration anteriorly in the wrist divides one or more of the flexor tendons and possibly the median and ulnar nerves and the radial and ulnar vessels. Unless the divided tendons and nerves are identified and sutured accurately, the movements of the hand are impaired seriously.

A number of *bony prominences* of the anterior wrist are important landmarks. Laterally, the expanded distal extremity of the radius is palpable. Its lateral border projects distally into a strong styloid process, at the base of which is a prominent ridge for the attachment of the brachioradialis tendon. The radial styloid process is more prominent, descends lower, and lies on a more anterior plane than the ulnar styloid process. The ulnar styloid is felt most readily at the mediodorsal side of the wrist with the forearm in lax pronation. It marks the radiocarpal joint level fairly accurately. A line joining both styloid processes crosses the wrist obliquely and is considerably below the highest point of the curve described by the joint line. The head of the ulna sometimes stands out in strong relief, rendering the otherwise graceful contour of the wrist somewhat unsightly. When there is lateral bowing of the lower end of the radius, deflecting the hand toward the radial side, the head of the ulna forms a prominence on the dorsal surface of the wrist (Madelung's deformity). The hand is carried ventrally on the articular surface of the radius.

The tubercle of the navicular (scaphoid) bone may be palpated at the radial side of the distal skin crease, and the pisiform bone occupies a corresponding position on the ulnar side. The latter bone is identified readily by allowing the hand to hang in the flexed position to relax the pull of the flexor carpi ulnaris muscle. The hook of the hamate (unciform) bone lies a little distal to the pisiform on a line with the ulnar margin of the metacarpal of the ring finger. The ridge on the multangulum majus (trapezium) lies immediately distal to the navicular tubercle.

On the dorsolateral aspect of the wrist, a shallow triangular depression, the *anatomical snuff-box*, is visible when the thumb is extended. The tendons of the abductor pollicis longus and the extensor pollicis brevis muscles bound the fossa on the radial side of the wrist, and the tendon of the extensor pollicis longus forms the boundary on the ulnar side. The floor of the depression contains the apex of the styloid process of the radius, the navicular (scaphoid), multangulum majus (trapezium), and base of the metacarpal of the thumb. The floor is crossed by the radial artery coursing from the front of the wrist posteriorly to the proximal extremity of the first interosseous space. Direct pressure in the floor of the fossa elicits tenderness when there is a fractured navicular (p. 642).

2. **Transverse Carpal (Anterior Annular) Ligament; Carpal Canal and Its Contents.**— The *transverse carpal (anterior annular) ligament* is a specialized portion of the deep fascia of the forearm. It is a tough, fibrous, anterior band stretched across the arch formed by the carpal bones, making a canal or tunnel for the conveyance of the flexor tendons and the median nerve from the anterior compartment of the forearm into the central compartment of the palm. On the radial side, the ligament is attached to the tubercle of the navicular (scaphoid) and the ridge on the multangulum majus (trapezium), which together form the radial eminence. It is attached on the ulnar side to the ulnar eminence which consists of the pisiform and the hook of the hamate. The ligament is continuous along its proximal margin with the deep fascia of the forearm, and it merges distally into the palmar fascia.

The palmaris longus tendon expands anterior to the transverse carpal ligament and inserts into the central part of the palmar aponeurosis. The ulnar nerve and artery cross the ligament into the palm immediately to the radial side of the pisiform bone. Laterally, the ligament is crossed by a superficial volar branch of the radial artery which extends into the palmto help form the superficial palmar arch.

The flexor tendons passing through the *carpal canal* under the transverse carpal ligament are provided with two synovial sheaths, one for the flexor pollicis longus muscle, and another for the closely grouped tendons of the flexor digitorum sublimis and profundus muscles. Their sheaths (carpal synovia) extend proximally beyond the transverse carpal ligament and distally into the palm and fingers (palmar and digital synovia). The median nerve is very superficial at the wrist and is injured by minor lacerations. It enters the carpal canal lateral to the flexor digitorum sublimis muscle.

3. **Dorsal Carpal (Posterior Annular) Ligament.**—The dorsal carpal (posterior annular) ligament is a thick derivative of the deep fascia of the forearm which crosses the

back of the wrist obliquely upward and medially. It occupies a more proximal level than the transverse carpal ligament. Laterally, it is attached to the lateral margin of the lower extremity of the radius and its styloid process, and mesially to the styloid process

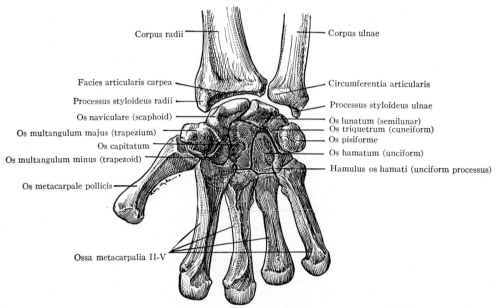

Corpus radii —   — Corpus ulnae

Facies articularis carpea —   — Circumferentia articularis

Processus styloideus radii —   — Processus styloideus ulnae

Os naviculare (scaphoid) —   — Os lunatum (semilunar)

Os multangulum majus (trapezium) —   — Os triquetrum (cuneiform)

Os capitatum —   — Os pisiforme

Os multangulum minus (trapezoid) —   — Os hamatum (unciform)

Os metacarpale pollicis —   — Hamulus os hamati (unciform processus)

Ossa metacarpalia II-V —

FIG. 636.—ANTERIOR VIEW OF THE DISTAL EXTREMITIES OF THE RIGHT RADIUS AND ULNA AND THE CARPUS AND METACARPUS.

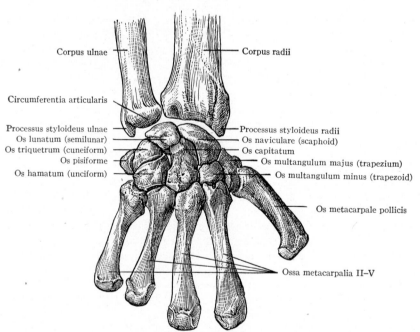

Corpus ulnae —   — Corpus radii

Circumferentia articularis —

Processus styloideus ulnae —   — Processus styloideus radii

Os lunatum (semilunar) —   — Os naviculare (scaphoid)

Os triquetrum (cuneiform) —   — Os capitatum

Os pisiforme —   — Os multangulum majus (trapezium)

Os hamatum (unciform) —   — Os multangulum minus (trapezoid)

Os metacarpale pollicis

Ossa metacarpalia II–V

FIG. 637.—POSTERIOR VIEW OF THE DISTAL EXTREMITIES OF THE RIGHT RADIUS AND ULNA AND THE CARPUS AND METACARPUS.

of the ulna and the ulnar border of the carpus. Septal processes or partitions pass from the deep aspect of the dorsal carpal ligament to ridges on the subjacent radius and ulna, forming separate osteofascial tunnels for the extensor tendons and their synovial sheaths

As these tendons pass beneath this ligament, they cross the very thin posterior ligament of the radiocarpal joint (p. 637). In places, this underlying ligament is so thin that, when the extensor tendons are deflected from their grooves, small protrusions of the radiocarpal synovia are brought into evidence as the hand is flexed and extended. An abscess on the dorsum of the wrist may penetrate the ligament and involve the radiocarpal and carpal joints.

4. **Vessels and Nerves.**—The *radial artery* at the wrist lies superficially under the deep fascia of the forearm on the flexor pollicis longus and pronator quadratus muscles and the lower expanded extremity of the radius. It enters the wrist in a groove between the brachioradialis tendon laterally and the flexor carpi radialis tendon mesially. At the level of the radial styloid, it gives off a superficial volar branch which passes distally over the ball of the thumb and the transverse carpal ligament to aid in the formation of the superficial palmar arch (p. 649). Distal to the radial styloid process, the main trunk of the artery winds over the radial collateral (external lateral) ligament under cover of the abductor pollicis longus and extensor pollicis brevis muscles, and reaches the triangular

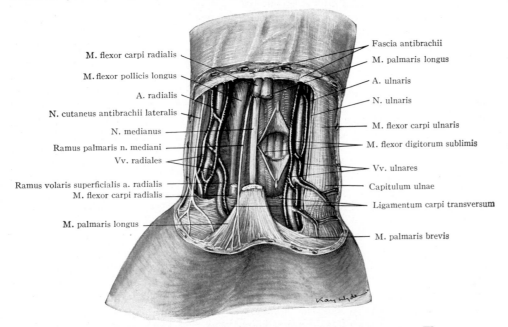

M. flexor carpi radialis
M. flexor pollicis longus
A. radialis
N. cutaneus antibrachii lateralis
N. medianus
Ramus palmaris n. mediani
Vv. radiales
Ramus volaris superficialis a. radialis
M. flexor carpi radialis
M. palmaris longus

Fascia antibrachii
M. palmaris longus
A. ulnaris
N. ulnaris
M. flexor carpi ulnaris
M. flexor digitorum sublimis
Vv. ulnares
Capitulum ulnae
Ligamentum carpi transversum
M. palmaris brevis

FIG. 638.—DEEPER STRUCTURES OF THE ANTERIOR REGION OF THE WRIST.

depression (anatomical snuff-box) at the lateral and dorsal aspect of the wrist. After reaching the proximal extremity of the first interosseous space, the artery passes between the two heads of the first interosseous muscle to reach the palm where it takes part in the formation of the deep palmar arch (p. 649).

The *ulnar artery* enters the region at the radial side of the pisiform bone where it is held on the transverse carpal ligament by a fascial expansion. The pisiform bone is a guide to ligation of the artery at this point. The artery divides into a superficial and a deep branch. The superficial branch continues the course of the parent artery and helps to form the superficial palmar arch. The deep branch passes through the transverse carpal ligament to contribute to the deep palmar arch.

About a handbreadth proximal to the radial styloid, the *superficial* or *sensory branch of the radial nerve* leaves the path of the radial artery to gain access to the dorsum of the wrist by passing under cover of the brachioradialis muscle. It is a purely sensory nerve and terminates on the back of the hand. Injuries to the nerve produce characteristic findings (p 668).

The *median nerve* is superficial in the wrist and is exposed in minor lacerations. It enters the region between the tendons of the palmaris longus and flexor carpi radialis muscles and lies to the radial side of the tendons of the flexor digitorum sublimis muscle, which it accompanies into and through the carpal canal under the transverse carpal ligament.

The *ulnar nerve* enters the wrist in company with and mesial to the ulnar artery and its satellite veins. With these vessels, it is contained within a thin fascial investment which is bound down to the transverse carpal ligament on the radial side of the pisiform bone.

B. BONES AND JOINTS

The wrist includes the distal extremities of the radius and ulna, the two rows of carpal bones, and the bases of the metacarpals. These bones are arranged into a series of joints: the radiocarpal, midcarpal, and carpometacarpal, which act as an extremely flexible unit to enable the hand to perform its specialized functions.

On their volar surfaces (Fig. 636), the bones and joints are arranged in a spreading groove, narrow proximally and widening out into the palm. The carpal groove is converted into an osteofibrous canal by the transverse carpal ligament which extends across the anterior surface of the carpus from the radial to the ulnar eminence.

1. **Distal Extremity of the Radius.**—The expanded distal extremity of the radius is large and well-developed to support and control the hand in its variety of movements. The spongy tissue is encased within a thin layer of compact bone. The pronator quadratus muscle is attached to its slightly flattened anterior surface, and over it the forearm structures pass into the carpal canal without obstruction. The *posterior surface* is ridged and grooved to accommodate and direct the extensor tendons to the dorsum of the hand. The styloid process is the distal prolongation of the *lateral surface*, and into its base the tendon of the brachioradialis is inserted. The *mesial surface* presents a concave articular facet for the reception of the articular surface of the head of the ulna, and a narrow ridge, to which the base of the triangular fibrocartilage, the articular disk, is attached. The disk is attached by its apex to the base of the styloid process of the ulna (Fig. 641).

The *elliptical distal articular surface* that receives the proximal row of carpal bones is concave from side to side and anteroposteriorly. On the ulnar side, the concave surface is roughly quadrilateral for the play of the convex surface of the lunate (semilunar) bone. Toward the radial styloid, the surface is triangular with still greater concavity to accommodate the movements of the navicular (scaphoid) bone. The anterior and posterior margins of this surface project downward and deepen the articular surface, giving attachment to the corresponding ligaments of the wrist joint. The dorsal margin of the articular surface extends farther distally than the volar margin. As a consequence, the plane of the radial articular surface faces distally and slightly toward the volar aspect. This plane must be maintained in the reduction of fractures about the lower end of the radius.

The radial styloid extends distally farther than does the ulnar styloid. The bistyloid line roughly parallels the radial articular surface. Therefore, the radial articular surface faces distally and slightly toward the ulnar side.

The *center of ossification* for the distal end of the radius appears about the third year and is developed fully by the fifteenth year. The *epiphyseal line* is about 1 cm. proximal to the joint margin and is extra-articular. Bony union is complete between the twentieth and twenty-fifth years; this is the fertile radial epiphysis where bone growth is greatest and most prolonged. Radial osteomyelitis which begins in the metaphysis does not involve the radiocarpal joint, but may invade the distal radio-ulnar joint.

2. **Distal Extremity of the Ulna and the Articular Disk.**—The *distal extremity of the ulna* is expanded only slightly from the neck into a small rounded head. The distal surface of the head is flat for articulation with the articular disk. The narrow circumference of the head, save where the ulnar styloid projects, is an articular arc applied to the radial notch, affording a wide range of rotation in the distal radio-ulnar joint. The base of the styloid process is roughened for the attachment of the apex of the *articular disk*. This

attachment and that of the ulnar collateral ligament explain the frequent wrenching away of the ulnar styloid in wrist trauma. The distal articular surface of the disk participates in the more elaborate radiocarpal joint.

The *center of ossification* for the distal extremity of the ulna appears between the sixth and ninth years and the epiphysis is fused with the shaft by the twentieth year. The *epiphyseal line* lies at a higher level than that of the radius, but is intrasynovial with respect to the distal radio-ulnar joint.

3. **Carpal Bones.**—Each of the carpal bones is composed of close-meshed cancellous bone within a shell of compact bone. Their joint surfaces are covered with cartilage, but the remaining surfaces are roughened for the attachment of their periosteocapsular covering. The dorsal surface of the carpal mosaic is slightly convex, but the palmar surface is markedly concave with its margins elevated into radial and ulnar eminences for the attachment of the transverse carpal ligament and the formation of the carpal canal (p. 637).

The **bones of the proximal row** in order from the radial to the ulnar side are: the navicular (scaphoid), lunate (semilunar), and triquetrum (cuneiform). The pisiform lies on the volar surface of the triquetrum, with which it articulates.

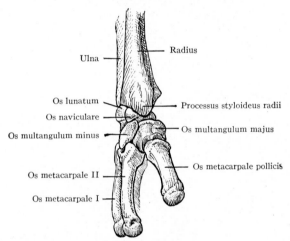

FIG. 639.—LATERAL VIEW OF THE BONES OF THE LEFT WRIST WHICH RESEMBLES THE APPEARANCE IN AN *x*-RAY.

The *navicular*, because of its curved shape and obliquely curved axis, is not adapted to withstand the indirect blow it receives in falls upon the palm with the hand in radial deviation. If the fall occurs with the hand in ulnar deviation, only the proximal part of the bone is exposed to trauma. The navicular is the most commonly fractured carpal bone. The *lunate*, the middle bone of the row, presents distally a moon-shaped articular surface which, with a part of the distal navicular articulation, lodges the head of the capitate bone (os magnum). It is the carpal bone most subject to dislocation. After traction on the hand, it sometimes may be reduced manually. The *triquetrum* (cuneiform) presents part of its proximal surface for articulation with the articular disk and part for articulation with a specialized surface on the ulnar collateral ligament. This mechanism permits the triquetrum, with the *pisiform* on its volar aspect, to glide toward the ulna in ulnar flexion. The remainder of its proximal surface is nonarticular. The distal concavities of the triquetrum, navicular, and lunate bones make a deep depression, into which the capitate and hamate bones are lodged.

The proximal row of bones presents an elongated, markedly convex joint surface for articulation with the radius and with the articular disk. The pisiform bone does not enter into the radiocarpal joint. The distal articular surface of this unit is uneven. The navicular bone presents like a prow to articulate with the two multangular bones.

The **bones of the distal row** in order from the radial to the ulnar side are: the mult-angulum majus (trapezius), multangulum minus (trapezoid), capitate (os magnum), and hamate (unciform). The *capitate* is the central, most prominent, and strongest bone of

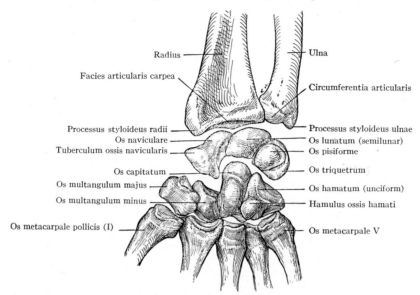

Radius — Ulna

Facies articularis carpea

Circumferentia articularis

Processus styloideus radii

Os naviculare

Tuberculum ossis navicularis

Os capitatum

Os multangulum majus

Os multangulum minus

Os metacarpale pollicis (I)

Processus styloideus ulnae

Os lunatum (semilunar)

Os pisiforme

Os triquetrum

Os hamatum (unciform)

Hamulus ossis hamati

Os metacarpale V

FIG. 640.—ROWS OF CARPAL BONES AND THE BONES WITH WHICH THEY ARTICULATE

this row. The force of a fall upon the hand is distributed to the radius through the head of the capitate, which articulates in the saddle formed by the navicular and lunate. The capitate articulates distally with the base of the third metacarpal

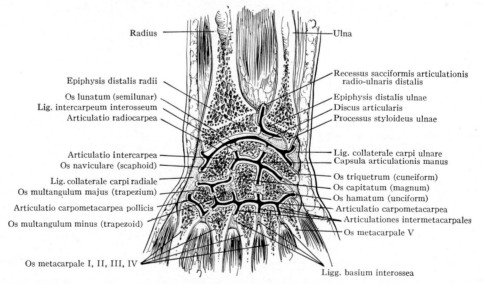

Radius — Ulna

Epiphysis distalis radii

Os lunatum (semilunar)

Lig. intercarpeum interosseum

Articulatio radiocarpea

Articulatio intercarpea

Os naviculare (scaphoid)

Lig. collaterale carpi radiale

Os multangulum majus (trapezium)

Articulatio carpometacarpea pollicis

Os multangulum minus (trapezoid)

Os metacarpale I, II, III, IV

Recessus sacciformis articulationis radio-ulnaris distalis

Epiphysis distalis ulnae

Discus articularis

Processus styloideus ulnae

Lig. collaterale carpi ulnare

Capsula articulationis manus

Os triquetrum (cuneiform)

Os capitatum (magnum)

Os hamatum (unciform)

Articulatio carpometacarpea

Articulationes intermetacarpales

Os metacarpale V

Ligg. basium interossea

FIG. 641.—FRONTAL SECTION THROUGH THE FOREARM AND HAND TO SHOW THE BONES, JOINTS, AND LIGAMENTS.

Within the first year, *ossification centers* appear for the capitate and the hamate. In the third year, a center appears for the triquetrum; in the fifth, for the lunate; in the sixth, for the greater multangular and the navicular; in the seventh, for the lesser multangular; and, about the tenth, for the pisiform. The rule that each carpal bone ossifies from one center has many exceptions. A bone may ossify from two or even three centers, a confusing condition in an x-ray study of carpal injuries. The navicular presents this variation most frequently.

4. Bases of the Metacarpals.—The bases or carpal extremities of the metacarpal bones as a unit present a fairly even joint surface for the distal row of carpal bones. They are broad and cuboidal, and articulate with each other in the carpal mosaic type of compact arrangement.

5. Distal Radio-ulnar Joint.—A triangular fibrocartilage, the articular disk, excludes the ulna from the radiocarpal joint. The disk is attached by its apex to the base of the styloid process of the ulna and by its base to the ulnar margin of the distal end of the radius. The joint capsule, which fuses distally with the articular disk, is lax and weak and permits pronation and supination. In these motions, the ulna is stationary and is the axis about which the radius rotates. The synovia bulges upward between the radius and ulna beyond the level of the distal epiphyseal lines. Volar and dorsal radio-ulnar ligaments maintain a close-fitting but very movable joint. If the disk is perforated, the synovia is continuous with that of the radiocarpal joint.

6. Radiocarpal Joint or Wrist Joint Proper.—The lower extremity of the radius in conjunction with the articular disk and the proximal row of carpal bones forms the radiocarpal joint. Their articular surfaces are united by a capsule reinforced by dorsal, volar, and lateral ligaments.

The volar and dorsal radiocarpal ligaments possess little strength, but, of the two, the volar is the stronger. They are reinforced by the flexor and extensor tendons. The radial collateral (external lateral) ligament extends from the radial styloid to the navicular bone and is crossed by the carpal portion of the radial artery. The ulnar collateral (internal lateral) ligament is attached above to the ulnar styloid and below to the triquetrum (cuneiform) and pisiform bones. The strength of the joint depends largely upon these collateral ligaments.

Aspiration of the joint may be performed immediately distal to the tip of the styloid process of the ulna between the flexor and extensor carpi ulnaris tendons.

7. Carpal Joints.—The junction of the two rows of carpal bones forms the *midcarpal joint*. This joint is surrounded by a complete capsule, strengthened by dorsal, volar, and lateral ligaments, and is reinforced by fibers derived from the tendons. The midcarpal joint has an extensive synovial cavity which corresponds not only to the interval between the two rows of the carpus, but also extends upward and downward between the bones of each row. It frequently communicates with the synovia of the *carpometacarpal joints*. The carpometacarpal joint of the thumb and the joint between the triquetrum and pisiform bones maintain separate synovial cavities which do not communicate with the midcarpal synovial cavity.

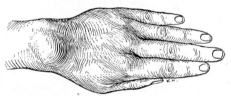

FIG. 642.—GANGLION OF THE CARPUS.

Prolongations of joint synovia sometimes present on the dorsum of the wrist as synovial cysts or *ganglia*. These circumscribed cystic swellings are of a firm elastic consistency, hemispherical or spherical in outline. Sometimes they are cystic protrusions of the synovial sheaths of the extensor tendons at the wrist, but they may arise independently of the joint or tendon synovia as cystic degenerations of connective tissue. Their contents are of a gelatinous character; treatment consists of careful excision.

8. Movements.—The main movements at the wrist joint are executed through the transverse and anteroposterior axes. Forward (volar) flexion and backward (dorsal) flexion are effected through the transverse axis and adduction (radial deviation) and abduction (ulnar deviation) through the anteroposterior axis. A combination of these movements and pronation and supination allows circumduction of the hand. Exaggeration of these movements causes rupture of the ligaments.

The slight projection of the two styloid processes facilitates radial and ulnar deviation, whereas, in contrast, the projecting malleoli of the tibia and fibula almost prohibit lateral movements of inversion and eversion. Of the lateral movements at the wrist, ulnar deviation has the more extensive range. Radial deviation is checked by the ulnar collateral ligament and by contact of the greater multangular with the radial styloid process, which projects downward to a considerably lower level than the ulnar styloid. Dorsal and volar flexion, particularly volar flexion, are enhanced by the gliding movements between the proximal and distal rows of carpal bones at the midcarpal joint. Exaggerated movements in volar and dorsal flexion rupture the volar or dorsal carpal ligaments and may result in carpal dislocation with or without associated fracture of the navicular and dislocation of the lunate. The numerous intercarpal joints give elasticity to the hand and thereby increase its ability to withstand the effects of severe shocks, such as falling upon the outstretched palm. Any lateral displacement in the midcarpal joint is resisted strongly by the concavo-convex configuration of the joint.

SURGICAL CONSIDERATIONS

The close relations between the bones and joints of the wrist and the overlying ligaments, tendons, synovial sheaths, vessels, and nerves explain the varying degrees of disabling and deforming arthritis, periarthritis, and tenosynovitis which may occur after trauma.

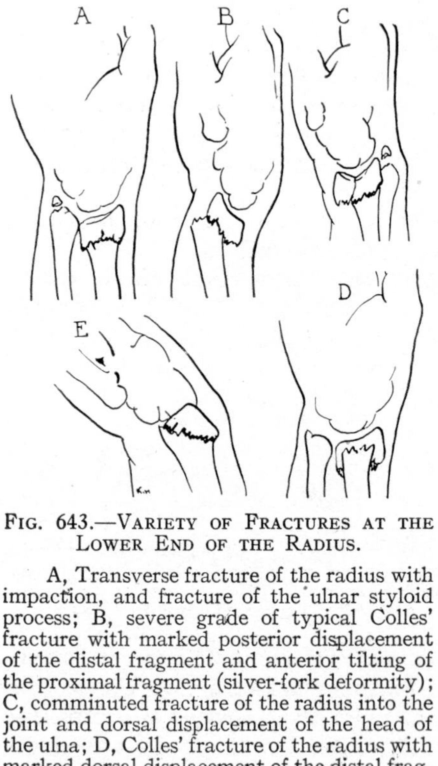

FIG. 643.—VARIETY OF FRACTURES AT THE LOWER END OF THE RADIUS.

A, Transverse fracture of the radius with impaction, and fracture of the ulnar styloid process; B, severe grade of typical Colles' fracture with marked posterior displacement of the distal fragment and anterior tilting of the proximal fragment (silver-fork deformity); C, comminuted fracture of the radius into the joint and dorsal displacement of the head of the ulna; D, Colles' fracture of the radius with marked dorsal displacement of the distal fragment; shortening of the forearm is indicated by the bistyloid line transverse to the long axis of the forearm; E, fracture of the posterior margin of the articular surface of the radius (Barton's fracture).

1. **Colles' Fracture.**—The radius, through the rigidly bound carpus, bears the brunt of shocks transmitted through the hand. If the reinforcing ligaments and tendons resist this trauma, the usual occurrence is a transverse fracture of the lower extremity of the radius, Colles' fracture. The *fracture line* usually is located within 3 cm. of the radiocarpal joint, and when the fracture occurs proximal to this level, it partakes of the characteristics of fracture of the shaft (p. 628). The most frequent cause of Colles' fracture is a fall upon the outstretched hand. It is probable that when the impact is received upon the palm, the long axis of the forearm is inclined to the ground at an angle of less than 60 degrees. The line of force passes through the distal end of the radius instead of passing upward along the bone, as it would were the forearm at an angle of more than 60 degrees. A great strain is thrown upon the front of the wrist which overstretches the anterior ligaments. The line of force drives the carpus against the radius with the result that the lower extremity of the radius is broken. It is evident that the resisting power of the ligaments is greater than that of the lower end of the radius where the expansion of bone is not accompanied by corresponding increase in strength.

The *usual displacement* in Colles' fracture is one in which the distal fragment is carried backward, or backward and upward, since the line of force tends to thrust it proximally; there may or may not be an associated impaction. The distal fragment carries with it the rigidly attached carpus and hand.

There may be displacement of the distal fragment without impaction. In addition to dorsal displacement of the distal fragment and hand, there may be rotation about the transverse axis so that the radial articular surface and styloid process look dorsally as well as distally (p. 634). In this rotation, the distal fragment hinges upon the articular disk, the radial styloid rises to the same level or even higher than the styloid of the ulna, and the hand is thrown into radial deviation. If the traumatizing force is excessive and continues to act, the strain it throws upon the articular disk may bring about fracture of the ulnar styloid. If the disk, ulnar collateral ligament, and ligaments of the inferior radio-ulnar joint are torn, the lower extremity of the ulna may protrude through the skin.

In a typical fracture with the displacements just noted, the diagnosis can be made at a glance by the characteristic deformity of the wrist, which has been compared aptly to the outline of a silver fork. Sometimes the degree of displacement is slight and there are no symptoms or objective findings at the wrist other than pain and swelling; the injury easily may be mistaken for a sprain.

There may be impaction of the distal fragment into the proximal fragment. The impaction may be such as to cause the whole circumference of the compact bone of the proximal fragment to penetrate the lower fragment, or the compact bone of the proximal fragment to overlap the corresponding layer of the distal fragment. The most common variety of impaction is that in which the distal fragment, with or without being displaced backward, hinges upon the proximal fragment so that there is impaction of the dorsal portions of both fragments. The carpal articular surface of the distal fragment then looks dorsally as well as distally.

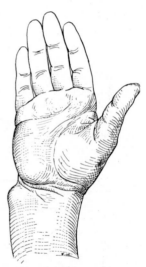

FIG. 645.—RADIAL DEVIATION OF THE HAND IN FRACTURE OF THE RADIUS.

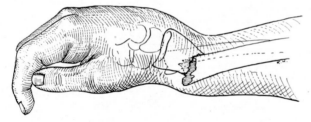

FIG. 644.—SILVER-FORK DEFORMITY OF THE FOREARM AND HAND IN FRACTURE OF THE RADIUS.

The diagram illustrates the dorsal displacement of the distal fragment and the volar displacement of the proximal fragment.

Colles' fractures require immediate reduction under relaxing anesthesia to obtain perfect alignment. When reduction has been accomplished, the surface markings, even in the presence of swelling, can be palpated and seen. There must be a restoration of the normal relations between the styloid processes, a uniform dorsal plane along the forearm through the wrist to the hand, and a normal axial relation of the hand and wrist to the forearm. By correct reduction, deformities, stiff joints, and limited movement with associated loss of power are avoided. The hand and wrist are immobilized in a position of volar flexion and ulnar deviation for a few days. Volar flexion overcomes the backward tilt of the distal radial fragment. The hand soon can be brought into the functional position of slight dorsiflexion at the wrist and ulnar deviation. A strain to the shoulder joint with the possibility of subsequent stiffening should not be overlooked. In many older patients, it is not discovered until removal of the forearm cast that the trauma to the shoulder and the enforced immobilization of the arm often have caused as much disability as that arising from the wrist injury.

It has been demonstrated (Abbott and Saunders) that median nerve injury in fracture of the radius sometimes results from pressure of the nerve between the sharp proximal margin of the transverse carpal ligament and the prominent anterior border of the lower end of the radius. Nerve pressure is especially likely to occur when palmar hyperflexion is chosen as the position of fixation after fracture reduction.

2. **Reversed Colles' Fracture (Smith's Fracture).**—The reversed Colles' frac ure (Smith's fracture) usually is caused by a fall on the back of the hand with the wrist fl ꝗ ed. The line of force passes through the anterior surface of the distal end of the radius a nd the distal fragment is displaced forward and proximally.

After reduction of the deformity, the alignment of the fragment is maintained by immobilization in a cocked-up, pistol-grip position with slight ulnar deviation of the hand.

3. **Epiphyseal Separation.**—Epiphyseal separation at the *lower extremity of the radius* is an extremely frequent injury any time before the twentieth year. It is especially com-mon in children. The resulting de-formity resembles Colles' fracture, but radial deviation of the hand is not so marked and reduction is more difficult. There usually is no joint involvement because the synovial membrane does not reach the level of the epiphyseal line. When the separated epiphysis is reduced, the two styloid processes maintain their normal relationships and there is little if any deviation of the distal articular surface of the radius. Many injuries described as Colles' fracture probably are epiphyseal separations.

Separation of the *distal epiphysis of the ulna* is rare because the radius

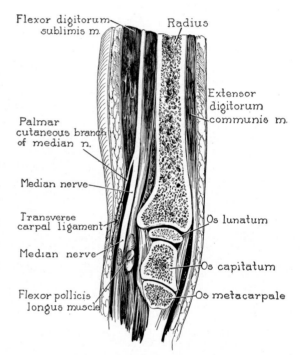

FIG. 647.—SAGITTAL SECTION THROUGH THE RIGHT WRIST TO ILLUSTRATE THE VULNERABLE POSITION OF THE MEDIAN NERVE BETWEEN THE PROMINENT ANTE-RIOR MARGIN OF THE DISTAL EXTREMITY OF THE RADIUS AND THE TRANSVERSE CARPAL LIGAMENT. (Abbott and Saunders, Surg., Gynec., and Obst., Oct., 1933.)

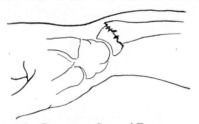

FIG. 646.—REVERSED COLLES' FRACTURE OR SMITH'S FRACTURE.
The fracture occurs with the wrist in flexion; the distal fragment is displaced vol-arward and the proximal fragment projects dorsally.

bears the brunt of falls upon the hand. Since most of the growth of the ulna is from the inferior epiphyseal line, it is important that this injury be recognized and corrected.

4. **Dislocations at the Radiocarpal and Inferior Radio-ulnar Joints.**—*Dislocation at the radiocarpal joint* is rare because the violent shocks transmitted from the hand to the wrist are diffused throughout the carpal joints and because the anterior ligaments at the wrist joint are strong. Many supposed dislocations are fractures of the radius. True disloca-tion, however, does occur from great violence, and the inferior ends of the radius and ulna may protrude on the dorsal or volar surface of the wrist.

In dorsal dislocation of the carpus, the deformity resembles that of Colles' fracture, except that the palmar swelling in radiocarpal dislocation extends farther down the hand because the displacement occurs at the radiocarpal joint rather than at some point above it. In dislocation, the dorsal bulb has an abrupt upper edge which is not present in fracture, and both styloid processes remain attached to their shafts.

Anterior dislocation of the carpus may occur from trauma, but usually is the result of disease about the wrist. Both the radius and ulna become prominent on the dorsal surface of the wrist with associated depression over the volar surface of the forearm just above the hand.

Dislocation of the ulna at the inferior radio-ulnar joint may be anterior or posterior, but more commonly is posterior. Neither form is seen commonly except with fracture of the radius. The articular disk and the ulnar collateral ligament usually remain attached to the ulna, which projects markedly on the dorsum of the wrist (Madelung's deformity). Early reduction of the dislocation usually can be accomplished by direct pressure on the epiphysis and rotation of the hand under traction as in reduction of dislocation of the radiocarpal joint.

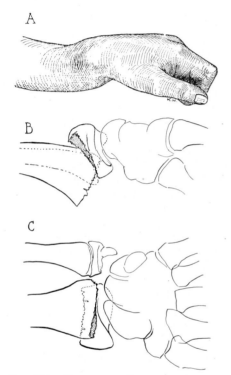

A

B

C

Fig. 648.—Epiphyseal Separation of the Radius with Dorsal Displacement of the Epiphysis.

A shows the silver-fork deformity simulating Colles' fracture; B is a sketch of the *x*-ray finding in lateral view; C is the sketch of an anteroposterior *x*-ray view.

5. **Carpal Injuries.**—The force of a fall upon the palm is directed mainly through the third metacarpal to the capitate bone and thence to the navicular and lunate; it causes a variety of injuries to the carpus. Whether a fracture of the navicular or a dislocation of the lunate is sus-

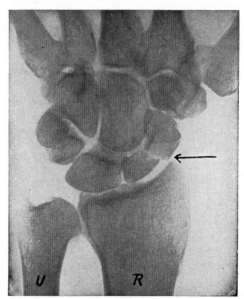

Fig. 649.—Transverse Fracture of the Navicular Bone.

The arrow points to the fracture line. (Scudder, "Treatment of Fractures.")

tained, depends largely upon whether the extended hand is held in radial or ulnar flexion. With the hand in radial flexion, the navicular is brought into a position directly under the radius and is fractured by the direct impact of the capitate. In ulnar flexion, all but the proximal part of the navicular glides out of the way and the lunate is exposed to trauma between the radius and the capitate. The other bones occasionally are fractured and the capitate sometimes is dislocated dorsally.

x-Ray has made possible the recognition of these injuries, which are potential of great disability. When a wrist, after a definite history of trauma, fails to function properly, *x*-ray examination often reveals evidences of old carpal fracture or dislocation. If injury to a carpal bone or a fragment thereof cuts off the blood supply entering through the periosteocapsular cuff, the bone dies. The bone may become revascularized or undergo cystic degeneration (Kienböck's disease)

41

In *fracture of the navicular*, the tubercle to which the radial collateral ligament is attached may be torn away. If the bone lies in the articular concavity of the radius at the time of impact, a compression fracture may result. If the hand is in forced dorsiflexion and radial deviation, the distal part of the navicular is driven against the radius by the greater multangular. At the same time, the capitate thrusts the proximal end of the navicular against the radius, and the combined result of the two pressures is a transverse fracture beginning at the convexity of the navicular.

Lunate (semilunar) dislocation occurs because the bone is the least securely anchored of all those of the carpal mosaic. The ligaments binding the lunate to the radius are its strongest attachment; therefore, dislocation usually takes place through its weaker carpal attachments. The dislocation occurs with the hand in forced extension, and usually is forward. The notch on the distal surface of the lunate lodges the capitate. When the lunate is in an anterior luxation, a lateral x-ray shows it to be volar to the capitate, with its saddle concavity or crescent shadow plainly visible. The direction of the concavity determines the degree of lunate rotation. Not only is bone circulation disturbed by the periosteal injury resulting from the displacement forward into the carpal canal, but the median nerve is compressed. A dislocation of the lunate rarely can be reduced and maintained in reduction by the closed method. It is far better to remove or replace it through a volar median incision.

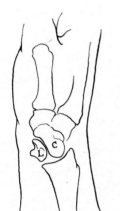

FIG. 650.—ANTERIOR DISLOCATION OF THE LUNATE (SEMILUNAR) BONE.

The capitate (os magnum) lies almost against the articular surface of the radius.

6. **Tuberculosis of the Carpal Bones.**—Tuberculosis of the carpus often is extensive and interferes with or abolishes the movements of the wrist and hand. It often begins in the carpus and spreads rapidly throughout the carpal joints. Occasionally, although rarely, it extends to the radiocarpal joint through a deficiency in one of the interosseous ligaments connecting the proximal row of carpal

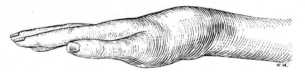

FIG. 651.—TUBERCULOSIS OF THE CARPAL AND WRIST JOINTS.

bones. In an advanced stage of the disease, the carpal bones are carious, the articular spaces are occupied by granulation tissue, and the ligaments of the joint soften and relax. Because of their proximity to the diseased parts, the sheaths of the flexor and extensor tendons frequently are involved. The result is an invading tenosynovitis in which masses of granulation tissue distend the sheaths and surround the tendons completely. The wrist and metacarpus are swollen until the normal landmarks disappear. The tapering and stiffened fingers and wasted forearm give the diseased area a characteristic spindle-shaped outline. When suppuration becomes established, sinuses may appear upon the dorsum of the wrist.

Excision of the wrist removes the tuberculous areas. The carpus, the lower articular extremities of the radius and ulna, and the proximal extremities of the metacarpal bones are removed. Removal of all the affected tissues is difficult because of the number of bones and joints involved and the danger of injuring the important vessels, nerves, and tendons surrounding them. Interference with the tendon sheaths may cause stiffness, loss of power, and pain in the hand.

Excellent drainage for suppuration in the radiocarpal joint is established by *ulnar incision* into the joint along the extensor carpi ulnaris tendon. Maintenance of the hand in the semiprone position allows dependent drainage.

7. **Arthrodesis of the Wrist.**—An arthrodesis, or operative production of a bony ankylosis, is indicated for a flail wrist, for ankylosis of the wrist in faulty position, for paralytic wrist drop, and for some arthritic conditions. Thirty degrees' extension with ulnar deviation is the functional position for the hand, since the flexors and extensors of the wrist are in muscle equilibrium in this position.

Through a dorsal incision, the tendons and the capsule with its reinforcing dorsal ligament are exposed. The capsule is incised longitudinally and stripped from the insertion on the forearm bones until these bones and the proximal row of carpal bones are exposed. A wedge is removed from the radius and from the adjoining portions of the navicular and lunate bones. The wedge is of sufficient size to permit the hand being fixed in 25 to 30 degrees of extension. Radical carpal arthrodesis does not eliminate motion in the carpus since the movement between the proximal and distal rows of carpal bones is not disturbed. Pronation and supination are sacrificed.

8. **Disarticulation Through the Radiocarpal Joint.**—Disarticulation through the radiocarpal joint rarely is performed because it gives an unsatisfactory stump from both the surgical and prosthetic standpoints. The stump end is irregular and both styloid processes are prominent and sensitive. The skin covering is thin and its circulation is poor. The stump is more difficult to fit than one low in the forearm, and a prosthesis tends to make the extremity longer than normal. Pronation and supination are retained in radiocarpal disarticulation, but few prostheses make use of this function. If disarticulation at the radiocarpal level is selected, both styloid processes should be removed and the radius and ulna should be rounded. The base of the radial styloid should be preserved to save the attach-

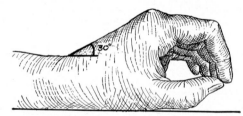

FIG. 652.—OPTIMUM POSITION FOR ANKYLOSIS OF THE WRIST.

ment of the brachioradialis tendon which aids materially in supination and flexion of the forearm. A long palmar flap brings portions of the short muscles of the thenar and hypothenar eminences over the stump, and the line of closure is on the dorsal aspect of the stump. As these tissues are very vascular, they bear pressure well. Circular amputation has the disadvantage of causing a terminal scar and of forming only a scant covering for the bones.

9. **Disarticulation at the Carpometacarpal Joint.**—The carpus makes a fair functional stump when covered with healthy skin and subcutaneous tissue from a long convex palmar flap. When the flexor and extensor tendons are sutured into the stump, a good range of motion is obtained.

The skin incision for the palmar flap begins 1 cm. below the radial styloid and extends down the palmar surface of the hand along the line of the second metacarpal nearly to the middle of the palm, gradually swinging across the palm to its middle. Another skin incision begins 1 cm. below the ulnar styloid and extends down the palmar surface of the hand along the fifth metacarpal to meet the radial incision in the middle of the palm. A straight dorsal incision, or an incision with a slight proximal convexity, is made across the carpus to form the short dorsal flap. The incision is deepened to the bone. The long palmar flap composed of skin and palmar fascia is dissected back to the carpometacarpal joint. The flexor tendons are cut long and are freed from the carpometacarpal joint on the palmar aspect. The dorsal extensor tendons which have been cut are secured to the carpus to prevent retraction. The metacarpals are disarticulated from their carpal attachments. The median, ulnar, and radial nerves are secured, ligated, and injected with absolute alcohol before they are allowed to retract. A sufficient number of the flexor and extensor tendons are sutured into the periosteocapsular tissue of the stump to assure flexion and extension. A palmar cock-up splint prevents palmar flexion at the radiocarpal joint.

If the amputation includes the bases of the metacarpals, suture of the flexor and extensor tendons into the stump is not necessary as the carpal flexors and extensors inserting into the metacarpal bases control the stump and give good power.

VI. THE HAND

The hand is an organ of prehension and exquisite sensibility. The sensory function is dependent upon the fact that the terminals of the digital nerves are connected with specialized end-organs (tactile corpuscles) in the papillary layer of the skin. These end-organs are developed particularly well over the palm and volar aspect of the terminal phalanges. Tactile sensibility probably is keenest at the extremities of the fingers. In the blind, who judge objects by touch, tactile sensibility attains a remarkable acuity and, in a considerable measure, compensates for the loss of sight.

The prehensile function is dependent upon the fact that the hand modifies its shape and strength of action to suit the conformation and consistency of the object grasped, like a marvelously adapted pair of forceps. The thumb, with its strong, mobile metacarpal, forms one blade of the forceps, and the remaining fingers, individually or collectively, form the other. The property of apposition cannot be overestimated, for the functional capacity of the hand depends largely upon the integrity of the thumb. Viewed mechanically, a hand deprived of the thumb is little more than a hook, and loses its usefulness to a degree out of all proportion to that which results from the loss of any of the other digits. In injury or disease of this digit, effort should be made to preserve it entirely, or as much of it as is possible.

The hand, directed by the will and guided in a large measure by the eyes, can perform a great variety of delicate and complicated movements through the highly coordinated action of its extrinsic and intrinsic muscles and its complicated system of joints. This is witnessed in the marvelous dexterity acquired by musicians, magicians, and skilled mechanics

The hand is divided into a palmar region, a dorsal region, and the phalanges.

A. PALMAR REGION

The palm is roughly quadrilateral in outline and comprises all the soft parts in front of the metacarpal bones and the volar interosseous muscles. The triangular central part is depressed into the "hollow of the hand" and is bounded on each side by a well-defined projection of muscle. That on the radial side, the thenar eminence, formed by the short muscles of the thumb, and that on the ulnar side, the hypothenar eminence, formed by the short muscles of the little finger, approximate each other as they approach the wrist. Their line of junction is indicated by a shallow median groove which leads across the wrist toward the tendon of the palmaris longus.

1. **Surface Anatomy.**—The *superficial palmar arch* lies at the level of the deep transverse crease made by metacarpophalangeal flexion. The common volar digital arteries emerge from this arch and divide into their proper digital arteries about 1 cm. proximal to the webs of the fingers. The *deep palmar arch* lies about 2 cm. nearer the wrist than the superficial arch, and its center corresponds fairly closely with the apex of the hollow of the hand.

With the fingers in complete extension, a series of shallow longitudinal *grooves* extend from the roots of the fingers toward the palm, with the intervals between the furrows occupied by raised areas in the skin. The furrows correspond to the digital slips of palmar fascia which overlie the flexor tendons, and the intervening prominences or masses of fatty tissue are smoothed out when the tendons are stretched. Within the projections of tissue, the digital vessels, nerves, and lumbrical muscles are directed toward the webs of the fingers.

The metacarpophalangeal joints are located fairly accurately on a line 2 cm. proximal to the webs of the fingers.

2. **Superficial Structures.**—The skin over the thenar eminence is thinner than that over the heads of the metacarpal bones and that of the hypothenar eminence. Over the central areas of the palm, the skin is rendered extremely tight and resistant by fibrous septa which bind it to the palmar aponeurosis (deep palmar fascia). These septa are a distinctive feature of the subcutaneous tissue in this region. The close connection between the skin and the resistant palmar fascia enables the center of the palm to withstand great

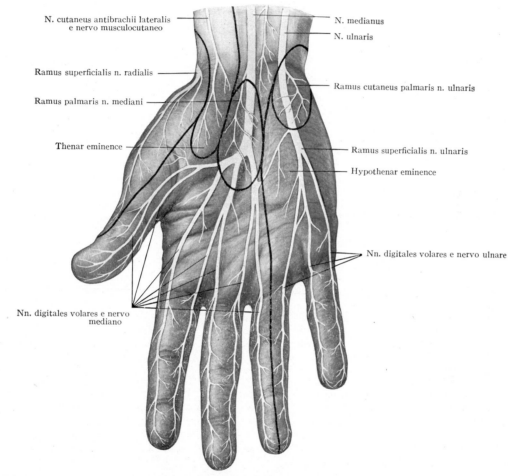

N. cutaneus antibrachii lateralis
e nervo musculocutaneo

N. medianus

N. ulnaris

Ramus superficialis n. radialis

Ramus cutaneus palmaris n. ulnaris

Ramus palmaris n. mediani

Thenar eminence

Ramus superficialis n. ulnaris

Hypothenar eminence

Nn. digitales volares e nervo ulnare

Nn. digitales volares e nervo
mediano

FIG. 653.—SURFACE ANATOMY AND AREAS OF CUTANEOUS NERVE SUPPLY OF THE PALMAR REGION.

pressure. For the same reason, pus cannot accumulate in any quantity superficial to the palmar fascia but makes its way upward through the skin and collects under the epidermis.

3. **Palmar Aponeurosis.**—The palmar aponeurosis (deep fascia) consists of a strong central portion and two weaker lateral portions which overlie the thenar and hypothenar eminences. The central portion or palmar aponeurosis proper is an exceedingly dense white ligamentous structure which prevents the outward spread of pus or blood. The longitudinal fibers are most numerous and are derived from the tendon of the palmaris longus muscle. From the radial and ulnar margins, fibrous septa pass backward to wall off the muscles of the thenar and hypothenar eminences. Proximally, the aponeurosis blends with the transverse carpal ligament (p. 631); distally, it widens out and divides into four slips at the level of the head of the inner four metacarpal bones. These slips

blend with the corresponding fibrous digital sheaths and lateral ligaments of the meta-carpophalangeal joints and insert into the sides of the bases of the proximal phalanges, which they assist in flexing. The digital arteries and nerves lie between these slips en route to the webs of the fingers.

All the superficial lymph vessels of the fingers and palm, save a few running up the front of the forearm, pass to the dorsum of the hand where they become associated with

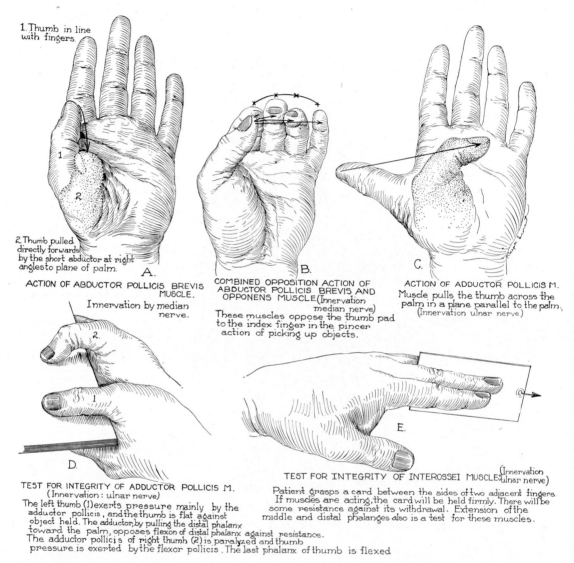

1. Thumb in line with fingers.

2. Thumb pulled directly forwards by the short abductor at right angle to plane of palm. A.

ACTION OF ABDUCTOR POLLICIS BREVIS MUSCLE.
Innervation by median nerve.

B.

COMBINED OPPOSITION ACTION OF ABDUCTOR POLLICIS BREVIS AND OPPONENS MUSCLE.(Innervation median nerve)
These muscles oppose the thumb pad to the index finger in the pincer action of picking up objects.

C.

ACTION OF ADDUCTOR POLLICIS M.
Muscle pulls the thumb across the palm in a plane parallel to the palm.
(Innervation ulnar nerve)

D.

TEST FOR INTEGRITY OF ADDUCTOR POLLICIS M.
(Innervation: ulnar nerve)
The left thumb (!) exerts pressure mainly by the adductor pollicis, and the thumb is flat against object held. The adductor, by pulling the distal phalanx toward the palm, opposes flexon of distal phalanx against resistance. The adductor pollicis of right thumb (2) is paralyzed and thumb pressure is exerted by the flexor pollicis. The last phalanx of thumb is flexed.

E.

TEST FOR INTEGRITY OF INTEROSSEI MUSCLE. (Innervation ulnar nerve)
Patient grasps a card between the sides of two adjacent fingers. If muscles are acting, the card will be held firmly. There will be some resistance against its withdrawal. Extension of the middle and distal phalanges also is a test for these muscles.

FIG. 654.—TESTS FOR THE ACTION OF THE MUSCLES OF THE THENAR EMINENCE AND OF THE INTEROSSEI.
(Modified from MacGregor.)

the superficial veins. These vessels are joined by the deep lymph vessels of the palm, an arrangement which explains the frequency of edema and metastatic infection on the dorsum of the hand from infection of the fingers and palm.

4. Palmar Muscles.—The palm contains not only the tendons of the superficial deep flexor muscles of the fingers which descend into it from the anterior surface of the forearm, but three intrinsic groups of short muscles. The external group embraces the thumb muscles and forms the thenar eminence; the internal group is composed of the muscles of the little finger and forms the hypothenar eminence; and the middle group consists of the lumbrical muscles.

The *thenar eminence* has four muscles, the abductor pollicis brevis, flexor pollicis brevis, opponens pollicis, and adductor pollicis. The first three muscles lie at the radial side of the tendon of the flexor pollicis longus, and all are supplied by the median nerve (C_8, T_1). They lie in a separate compartment which is shut off from the central space of the palm by a fascial sheet that passes dorsally from the radial margin of the central division of the palmar aponeurosis. When pus forms among these muscles, it is

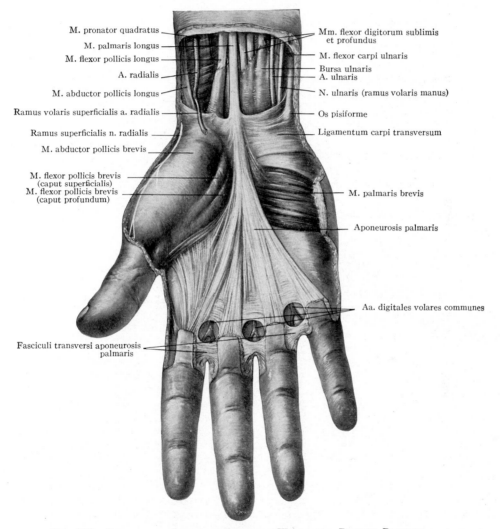

M. pronator quadratus

M. palmaris longus

M. flexor pollicis longus

A. radialis

M. abductor pollicis longus

Ramus volaris superficialis a. radialis

Ramus superficialis n. radialis

M. abductor pollicis brevis

M. flexor pollicis brevis (caput superficialis)
M. flexor pollicis brevis (caput profundum)

Fasciculi transversi aponeurosis palmaris

Mm. flexor digitorum sublimis et profundus

M. flexor carpi ulnaris

Bursa ulnaris
A. ulnaris

N. ulnaris (ramus volaris manus)

Os pisiforme

Ligamentum carpi transversum

M. palmaris brevis

Aponeurosis palmaris

Aa. digitales volares communes

FIG. 655.—SUPERFICIAL STRUCTURES OF THE WRIST AND PALMAR REGIONS.

localized definitely and manifests no tendency to spread backward or medially. Incision for drainage should be made over the distal part of the first metacarpal on the radial side of the eminence in order to avoid the nerve supply which enters the eminence mesially. The adductor pollicis (N. ulnar C_8, T_1) is a fan-shaped muscle which lies in the depth of the palm and possesses an oblique and a transverse head. Its base is attached to the third metacarpal and its apex to the base of the first phalanx of the thumb. It has considerable surgical importance as the floor of the thenar fascial space (p. 652). By its oblique and transverse heads it draws the thumb across the palm in a plane parallel to the palm

The abductor pollicis brevis pulls the thumb directly forward from the palm in a plane at right angles to the palm. The opponens pollicis enables the pad of the terminal phalanx of the thumb to be placed against that of any other finger. The abductor pollicis brevis and the opponens together are responsible for the action of rotating the thumb opposite the other fingers in the pincer action of picking up objects.

The *hypothenar eminence* is made up of the abductor, opponens, and flexor digiti quinti brevis muscles, all of which are supplied by the deep branch of the ulnar nerve (C_8. T_1). When an abscess forms in that area which is shut off from the central space of

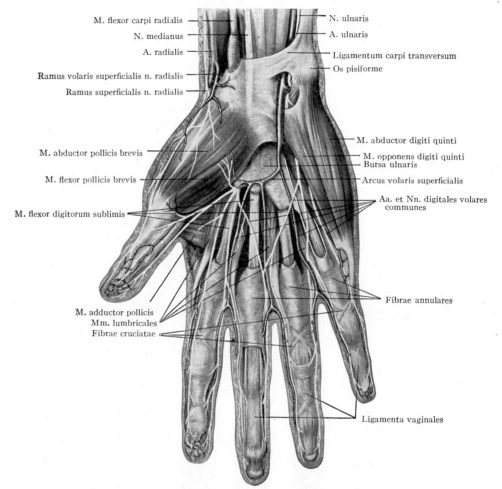

M. flexor carpi radialis
N. medianus
A. radialis
Ramus volaris superficialis n. radialis
Ramus superficialis n. radialis
M. abductor pollicis brevis
M. flexor pollicis brevis
M. flexor digitorum sublimis
M. adductor pollicis
Mm. lumbricales
Fibrae cruciatae

N. ulnaris
A. ulnaris
Ligamentum carpi transversum
Os pisiforme
M. abductor digiti quinti
M. opponens digiti quinti
Bursa ulnaris
Arcus volaris superficialis
Aa. et Nn. digitales volares communes
Fibrae annulares
Ligamenta vaginales

FIG. 656.—STRUCTURES OF THE PALM AFTER REMOVAL OF THE PALMAR APONEUROSIS.
In this drawing, the superficial volar arch is located at an unusually high level and the arches are not complete.

the palm by the fibrous partition passing dorsally from the ulnar side of the palmar aponeurosis, the infection points readily on the surface of the eminence. Incision for draining the abscess is made at the ulnar side of the fifth metacarpal, dorsal to the pisiform. This approach does not endanger the digital branches of the superficial volar arch and the ulnar nerve which run distally in front of the flexor digiti quinti brevis muscle to the ulnar side of the small finger.

The four long, thin *lumbrical* (L. earthworm) *muscles* arise from the tendons of the flexor digitorum profundus in the palm, and are inserted into the radial side of the fibrous expansions of the long extensor tendons and the adjoining parts of the proximal phalanges of the medial four digits They flex the fingers at the metacarpophalangeal joints, but extend them at the interphalangeal joints through the extensor expansions. The lumbrical muscles of the small and ring fingers are supplied by the deep branch of the ulnar nerve, and those of the index and middle fingers by the median nerve.

5. **Arteries of the Palm.**—The radial and ulnar arteries form two anastomotic arches in the palm from which the terminal digital arteries are distributed. The *superficial volar (palmar) arch* is the palmar continuation of the ulnar artery which enters the palm on the radial side of the ulnar nerve, and lies just to the radial side of the pisiform and the hook of the hamate (unciform). It runs obliquely, distally, and laterally to reach the midpoint of the palm in relation to the proximal transverse crease, and describes a variable curve toward the web of the thumb where it lies deep to the palmar fascia. It crosses immediately in front of the flexor tendons and their sheaths and the digital branches of the median nerve. The arch varies in its mode of termination, but always is joined by a superficial branch of the radial artery (superficial volar princeps pollicis or radialis indicis).

The arch gives off four palmar digital branches, one to the ulnar side of the little finger and the other three in the second, third, and fourth intermetacarpal spaces, to the webs of the fingers. In their course, they overlie the second, third, and fourth lumbrical muscles and often receive communicating branches from the deep arch. About 1 cm. proximal to the web, each artery divides into collateral digital branches which run along the palmar sides of the adjacent fingers.

The deep branch of the ulnar artery, given off in the wrist, enters the palm to supply the hypothenar eminence and, with the main trunk of the radial artery, forms the *deep volar (palmar) arch*. On leaving the wrist, the radial artery winds about the radial side of the radial collateral ligament and enters the palm between the bases of the metacarpals of the thumb and the index finger at the proximal end of the first interosseous space. From its position between the transverse and oblique heads of the adductor pollicis muscle. it passes forward across the palm to the fifth metacarpal where it receives the deep branch from the ulnar artery to form the deep volar (palmar) arch. The arch lies deep to the flexor tendons and their palmar synovial sheaths on the volar interosseous muscles and the bases of the metacarpal bones. If hemorrhage from the arch cannot be controlled by pressure. recourse may be had to ligation of the radial and ulnar arteries. The circulation is reestablished by the volar and dorsal interosseous arteries. From the deep arch, branches are given off proximally to the arterial network about the wrist (volar carpal arch) and metacarpal branches are given off distally to join the digital arteries.

6. **Nerves of the Palm.**—The *median nerve* enters the palm deep to the transverse carpal (anterior annular) ligament, where it lies upon the flexor tendons. At the lower border of the ligament, it breaks up into lateral and medial terminal divisions. The lateral division at once supplies the thenar muscles and gives off digital branches to both sides of the thumb and the radial side of the index finger. It also supplies the first lumbrical and second, or lateral lumbrical muscles. The medial terminal division supplies the cleft between the index and middle fingers and between the middle and ring fingers.

The *ulnar nerve* pierces the deep fascia at the wrist and crosses the transverse carpal ligament immediately at the radial border of the pisiform bone. It divides into superficial and deep branches opposite the hook of the hamate (unciform). The superficial branches of the nerve supply digital branches to the little finger and to the ulnar side of the ring finger. The deep branch of the nerve is accompanied by the deep branch of the ulnar artery. It supplies the short muscles of the little finger and the two inner lumbricals. All the interosseous muscles, the adductor pollicis, and part of the flexor pollicis brevis undergo atrophy after section of the ulnar nerve (p. 668). This nerve supplies most of the small muscles of the hand and, therefore, is mainly responsible for most of the fine movements of the hand. On that account, it has been called "the musician's nerve." The lumbricals once were known as the "fiddler's muscles."

7. **Central Compartment of the Palm.**—The central compartment of the palm is bounded superficially by the palmar aponeurosis and deeply by the aponeurosis which

invests the interosseous muscles.   Laterally, the compartment is shut off from the thenar and hypothenar eminences by the union of the two aponeuroses.   The compartment narrows proximally where it becomes continuous with the carpal canal under the transverse carpal ligament.   It widens out below and continues along the flexor tendon sheaths into the subcutaneous stratum of the fingers.

The central portion of the palm contains the lumbrical sheaths, the superficial volar arch and its branches, and the median nerve and its branches.   Between the deep flexor tendons and the fascia over the interossei are potential fascial spaces where palmar infections sometimes localize (p. 652).   Under the fascia covering the interosseous muscles lie the deep palmar arch and the deep division of the ulnar nerve.

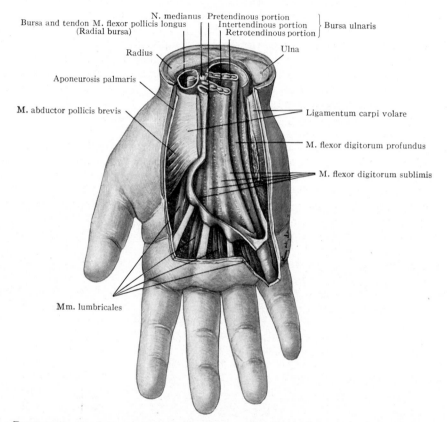

Fig. 657.—Diagram of the Arrangement of the Radial and Ulnar Bursae in the Wrist and Palm.

8. **Flexor Tendons and Their Palmar Synovial Sheaths.**—The **flexor tendons** passing beneath the transverse carpal ligament are provided with two synovial sheaths, one for the flexor pollicis longus muscle and the other for the closely grouped tendons of the flexor digitorum sublimis and profundus muscles.   These synovial investments are arranged in a somewhat complicated manner.

The synovial sheath for the tendon of the flexor pollicis longus extends distally to the insertion of the tendon and proximally to a point two fingerbreadths proximal to the upper margin of the transverse carpal ligament.   This sheath sometimes is known as the **radial bursa** because of its upward extension into the distal part of the radial side of the forearm.   It is made up of a visceral layer which closely invests the tendon, and a parietal layer which lines the wall of the cavity in which the tendon plays.   The arrangement is one which would obtain if the tendon were invaginated into the side of a cylindrical synovial tube with a mesotendon throughout the entire length of the sheath.   The mesotendon degenerates in places but persists as the vinculum breve and vinculum longum. The first vinculum is a triangular fold attaching the terminal part of the tendon to the floor of the synovial cavity, and the second connects the tendon and floor at several more proximal levels. Between the levels of mesotendon attachment, the synovia-covered tendon lies free.

In the wrist and palm, the synovia for the flexor digitorum sublimis and profundus tendons forms a common sheath, the **ulnar bursa,** which extends proximally as far as does the bursa for the flexor pollicis longus muscle. Distally, the limit is oblique, and reaches a lower level on the ulnar than on the radial side. The part of the sheath nearest the ulna runs distally over the tendons of the little finger to their insertion.

From a transverse section through the proximal part of the palm, it is evident that the tendons of the superficial and deep flexor muscles have invaginated the common sheath from the side nearest the thumb, so as to subdivide it into three pouches, all of which

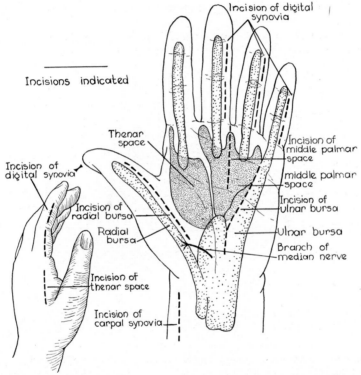

FIG. 658.—LOCATION OF DIGITAL, PALMAR, AND CARPAL SYNOVIA, AND OF FASCIAL SPACES OF THE HAND. Surgical paths of approach to these structures are indicated. (Modified from Kanavel and Mason.)

intercommunicate freely at the ulnar side of the sheath. That division of the ulnar bursa between the four sublimis tendons and the volar aponeurosis (palmar fascia) is the *pre-tendinous pouch;* the one between the sublimis and profundus tendons is the *intertendinous pouch.* The deepest carpal division, that between the profundus tendons, the floor of the carpal canal, and the floor of the central compartment of the palm, is the *retrotendinous pouch.* The prolongations of the ulnar bursa which correspond to the tendons of the index, middle, and ring fingers do not extend beyond the middle of the palm. The prolongation of the tendons of the little finger, as a rule, reaches the base of the terminal phalanx.

Several variations in the sheaths are noteworthy. The flexor pollicis longus sheath sometimes is in two separate parts, palmar and digital. The sheath for the flexor pollicis longus very frequently communicates freely with the common palmar sheath. The index tendon of the profundus sometimes possesses a palmar sheath. The digital sheath of the small finger frequently fails to communicate with the common sheath.

A *compound palmar* **ganglion** is a tuberculous synovitis of the common palmar sheath. It causes an hour-glass swelling extending from the distal part of the forearm into the palm, with the constriction at the transverse carpal ligament. The entire sheath may have to be excised, a procedure usually resulting in damage to the flexor tendons and the median and ulnar nerves.

The *median nerve* lies between the sheath of the flexor pollicis longus (radial bursa) and the common palmar sheath (ulnar bursa). Between the common palmar sheath and the palmar aponeurosis is a fatty areolar layer in which the superficial volar arch lies. Between the common sheath and the volar interosseous aponeurosis are the deep fascial spaces of the palm.

9. Deep Fascial Spaces of the Palm and Their Modes of Infection.—Deep to the flexor tendons and the lumbrical muscles is a large fascial space which is divided into midpalmar and thenar spaces by a fibrous septum attached along the shaft of the middle metacarpal bone. This partition usually is strong enough to prevent the spread of pus from one space to the other.

The *middle palmar space* lies between the middle metacarpal bone and the radial side of the hypothenar eminence, from which it is separated completely by a fibrous partition.

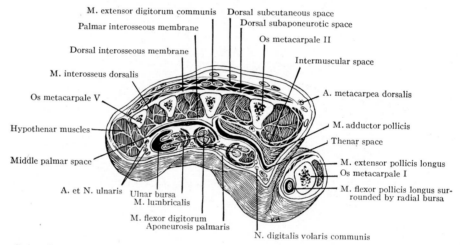

Fig. 659.—Cross Section Through the Right Hand to Show the Fascial Spaces in the Anterior and Posterior Regions of the Hand; Also the Radial and Ulnar Synovial Bursae. (After Kanavel.)

Its dorsal boundary is the volar interosseous aponeurosis which covers the volar interossei in the third and fourth intermetacarpal spaces. It is bounded anteriorly by the tendons of the little, ring, and middle fingers and their lumbrical muscles. This space may be infected directly by puncture wounds or by compound fractures of the third, fourth, and fifth metacarpals, or secondarily by superficial infections in the corresponding fingers. It may be involved by the spread of infection from the closed proximal ends of the digital synovial sheaths of the middle and ring fingers. Pus in this space, unless evacuated early, spreads distally along the lumbrical tendons and points at the webs of the fingers. Rarely, it may extend proximally behind the flexor muscles into the forearm.

The *thenar space* is located deep to the tendons of the index finger and the first lumbrical muscle between the middle palmar space and the tendon of the flexor pollicis longus. It is bounded behind by the adductor of the thumb. Direct infections may result from puncture wounds, or, rarely, from compound fracture of the shaft of the second metacarpal. Pus within the space may spread backward between the two heads of the adductors of the thumb, or, as more usually is the case, over the distal free border of the transverse head to point on the dorsal surface of the web of the thumb. Rarely, the pus may spread proximally into the forearm or distally into the web between the index and middle fingers.

Surgical Considerations

1. **Routes to the Palmar Synovia of the Ulnar and Radial Bursae.**—An *incision into the common palmar sheath* or *ulnar bursa* extends from the base of the small finger at the distal crease of the palm to the apex of the palm toward the carpal canal. A director may be inserted into the sheath at this point and be carried along it. To facilitate drainage of the pretendinous, intertendinous, and retrotendinous pouches, the tissue between the sheath and skin is incised as far to the ulnar side of the sheath as possible. If infection has reached the transverse carpal ligament, pressure over the forearm prolongation of the sheath forces pus downward into the sheath below the ligament. If forearm involvement is diagnosed, incision low in the forearm is indicated (p. 623). It may be necessary to divide the transverse carpal ligament to avoid the danger of necrosis of the tendons. This should be done as far to the ulnar side as possible.

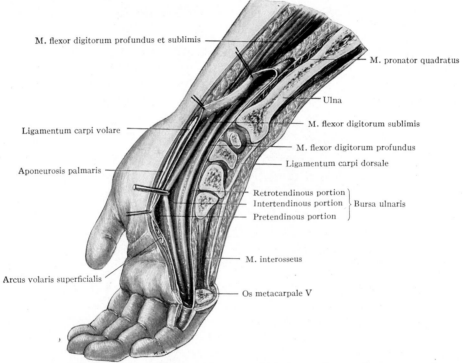

M. flexor digitorum profundus et sublimis

M. pronator quadratus

Ulna

M. flexor digitorum sublimis

Ligamentum carpi volare

M. flexor digitorum profundus

Ligamentum carpi dorsale

Aponeurosis palmaris

Retrotendinous portion ⎫
Intertendinous portion ⎬ Bursa ulnaris
Pretendinous portion ⎭

M. interosseus

Arcus volaris superficialis

Os metacarpale V

Fig. 660.—Longitudinal Section Through the Hand, Wrist, and Lower Forearm to Show the Extent and Divisions of the Ulnar Synovial Bursa.

Attention is called to the carpal and forearm divisions of the common palmar sheath (ulnar bursa); this drawing explains the rationale of draining all the pouches of the ulnar bursa through an incision on the ulnar aspect of the palm. (After Kanavel.)

An *incision into the sheath of the long flexor tendon of the thumb* or *radial bursa* is made on the flexor surface of the proximal phalanx, and is extended upward along the bursa through the margin of the thenar eminence. It should be kept in mind that the tendon lies nearer the hollow of the palm than would be expected, and that, therefore, the mass of thenar muscles lies to the radial side of the incision. The dissection is carried only to within a thumbbreadth of the lower margin of the transverse carpal ligament, for the branch of the median nerve to the thenar muscles (p. 647) passes across the sheath between this point and the lower edge of the transverse carpal ligament. Damage to the flexor tendon of the thumb is the preferable alternative to destruction of this nerve and paralysis of the short thumb muscles which it supplies. Drainage of the proximal or forearm extremity of the radial bursa is obtained best by the method described for evacuation of an abscess in the corresponding location in the ulnar bursa (p. 647).

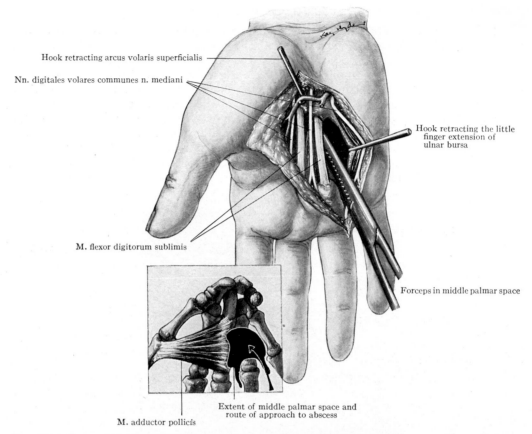

Hook retracting arcus volaris superficialis

Nn. digitales volares communes n. mediani

Hook retracting the little
finger extension of
ulnar bursa

M. flexor digitorum sublimis

Forceps in middle palmar space

Extent of middle palmar space and
route of approach to abscess

M. adductor pollicis

FIG. 661.—DISSECTION OF THE STRUCTURES ABOUT THE MIDDLE PALMAR SPACE AND AN INSET TO SHOW
THE PATH OF SURGICAL DRAINAGE OF THE SPACE.   (After Kanavel.)

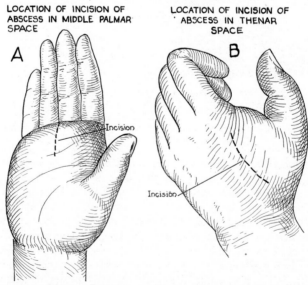

LOCATION OF INCISION OF
ABSCESS IN MIDDLE PALMAR
SPACE

LOCATION OF INCISION OF
ABSCESS IN THENAR
SPACE

A

B

Incision

Incision

FIG. 662.—INFECTIONS IN THE MIDDLE PALMAR AND THENAR SPACES AND SURGICAL PATHS OF APPROACH.
A, Infection in the middle palmar space; concavity of palm lost; incision to space indicated between
middle and ring fingers. B, Infection of the thenar space; thenar area ballooned out and thumb slightly
flexed and pushed away from the hand.   (Redrawn from Kanavel and Mason.)

2. **Routes to the Fascial Spaces of the Hand.**—An *abscess of the middle palmar space* should not be opened upon the ulnar side for fear of infecting the common palmar sheath (ulnar bursa). The least injury and the most efficient drainage are secured through a web incision along the lumbrical tendon between the small finger and the ring finger. It is possible also to incise along the lumbrical tendon between the ring finger and the middle finger. The incision between the ring and middle fingers best avoids injury to the ulnar bursa. The incision is carried a thumbbreadth and a half into the palm. An artery clamp is thrust beneath the group of flexor tendons and affords a path for satisfactory drainage.

In *infection of the thenar space*, the pus usually lies anterior to the transverse head of the adductor muscle of the thumb, but may lie dorsal to it as well. The most available

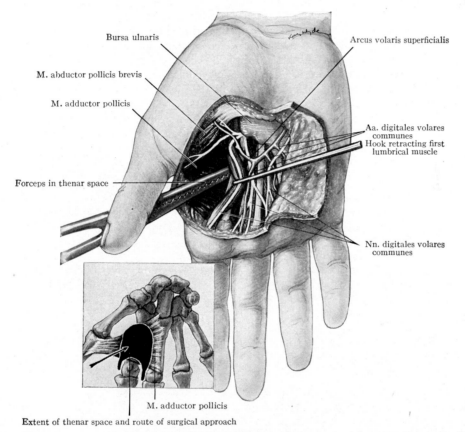

Bursa ulnaris

Arcus volaris superficialis

M. abductor pollicis brevis

M. adductor pollicis

Aa. digitales volares communes

Hook retracting first lumbrical muscle

Forceps in thenar space

Nn. digitales volares communes

M. adductor pollicis

Extent of thenar space and route of surgical approach

FIG. 663.—DISSECTION OF THE STRUCTURES ABOUT THE THENAR SPACE AND AN INSET TO SHOW THE PATH OF SURGICAL DRAINAGE OF THE SPACE.

The inset is a diagram of an abscess in the thenar space lying on the adductor pollicis muscle. (After Kanavel.)

site for incision is the radial side of the index metacarpal opposite its distal half and on a level with its flexor surface. A hemostat is thrust into the space across the flexor surface of the index metacarpal. From this location, a collection of pus, either in front of or behind the transverse adductor, is entered readily. The hemostat should not be carried beyond the middle metacarpal lest the infection be spread to the middle palmar space.

3. **Collar-button Abscess.**—A collar-button abscess is located at the distal edge of the palm under the dermal or epidermal tissues. Its occurrence in workmen may be attributed to the fact that the distal palmar epidermis becomes hypertrophied into a dense sheet, under which infection spreads. Pus in the subdermal tissue passes through

the dermis to the epidermis where a second division of the abscess forms, producing a collar-button-shaped accumulation of pus. Infection may occur in the epidermis, erode through the dermis, and produce the same condition. When pus accumulates in this manner over the distal end of the palmar aponeurosis, where the sheath may be very thin in places, it spreads very easily into the web of the finger. When the palmar aponeurosis is deficient, the abscess enters the cellular tissue of the web and points on the dorsum of the hand between the bases of the fingers, forming a complicated abscess in three layers.

4. **Localized Abscess in the Thenar and Hypothenar Regions.**—Within the thenar and hypothenar eminences, several minor and indefinite spaces lie beneath the fascia overlying the muscles. Because these spaces are superficial, they are infected by puncture wounds more frequently than are the deeper fascial spaces. A minor infection within the superficial tissues of the thenar or of the hypothenar area may be associated with great edema of the dorsum of the hand. This edema may be mistaken for evidence of pus in the palmar spaces. The fascia overlying the eminences localizes infection at the site of implantation. Infection is drained by simple incision.

5. **Dupuytren's Contracture.**—Dupuytren's contracture depends upon an insidious, interstitial fibrotic retraction of one or more of the digital slips or processes of the palmar aponeurosis and of the fibrous bands connecting these with the overlying skin. The progressive retraction of these fibers puckers the skin of the palm and the sides of the fingers into an obstinate flexion It occurs most frequently in the little and ring fingers

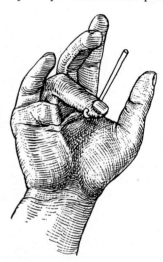

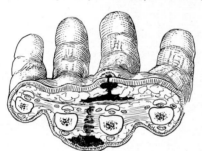

FIG. 664.—COLLAR-BUTTON ABSCESS OF THE PALM.

The pus has penetrated through the interosseous muscles to the back of the hand, forming a complicated abscess with three divisions. (After Homans.)

FIG. 665.—DUPUYTREN'S CONTRACTURE

but particularly in the latter and causes the hand to assume the position of "the Papal Benediction." Flexion occurs at the metacarpophalangeal joint. After the fibrosis has involved the weak areas in the fibrous sheaths opposite these joints, the phalanges are flexed slightly. In this deformity, further flexion is attainable, but normal extension of the finger on the metacarpus is impossible. With forcible efforts to straighten the finger, the shortened band stands out as a rigid cord beneath the skin, to which it appears to adhere very closely. In an advanced contracture, the dense fibrous cord passes downward from the center of the palm to the level of the base of the proximal phalanx of the contracted finger, and has been found in dissected specimens to have attachments to the periosteum of the lateral aspects of the phalanx.

The treatment is operative. The thinnest and most adherent skin is removed and the fascia is excised, including that part of the fascia which passes to the adjoining fingers. For a satisfactory closure, a free full-thickness graft sometimes may be required.

B. DORSAL REGION AND BONES AND JOINTS

1. **Surface Anatomy.**—The extensor tendons and their lateral expansions are visible and palpable on the dorsum of the hand. The metacarpal bones are subcutaneous and

can be felt over their entire length. The muscle prominence on the dorsum of the hand which is seen when the thumb and forefinger are approximated is formed by the contraction of the first dorsal interosseous muscle. The radial artery passes between the two heads of this muscle and enters the palm. When the thumb is extended, the "anatomical snuff-box" becomes evident. When the fingers are flexed, the prominence of the knuckles represents the distal ends (heads) of the metacarpal bones. The interosseous spaces, although normally leveled out by the dorsal interosseous muscles, are very conspicuous when these muscles are atrophied.

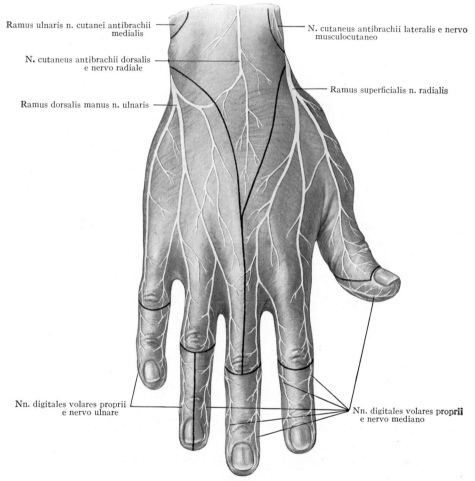

Ramus ulnaris n. cutanei antibrachii medialis

N. cutaneus antibrachii dorsalis e nervo radiale

Ramus dorsalis manus n. ulnaris

N. cutaneus antibrachii lateralis e nervo musculocutaneo

Ramus superficialis n. radialis

Nn. digitales volares proprii e nervo ulnare

Nn. digitales volares proprii e nervo mediano

FIG. 666.—SURFACE ANATOMY AND AREAS OF CUTANEOUS NERVE DISTRIBUTION OF THE POSTERIOR REGION OF THE WRIST AND HAND.

2. **Superficial Structures.**—The dorsal, in contrast to the palmar surface of the hand, is covered with skin of fine texture studded with short hairs and provided with sebaceous glands. The presence of hairs, sebaceous glands, and columns of fat under the dermis predisposes to furuncle and carbuncle formation. The *dorsal subcutaneous space* is an extensive area of loose tissue without definite boundaries, which allows pus to spread over the entire dorsum of the hand.

3. **Dorsal Subaponeurotic Space.**—On the dorsum of the hand, the extensor tendons of the fingers are united by oblique bands, forming an aponeurotic sheet which is a continuation of the fascial sheath over the carpus. This is attached on each side to the borders of the second and fifth metacarpals. The dorsal aponeurotic space lies between this sheath

42

the dorsal surfaces of the middle four metacarpals, and the interosseous muscles. It contains loose connective tissue. An infection in the space generally is secondary to wounds on the dorsum of the hand. When pus collects, it is limited by fibrous partitions distally at the metacarpophalangeal joints and proximally by similar partitions at the bases of the metacarpals.

4. **Dorsal Tendons and Muscles.**—The radial and ulnar extensor muscles of the carpus insert, in this region, into the second, third, and fifth metacarpal bones, and the extensor muscles of the thumb and fingers traverse this region to insert into the phalanges. The

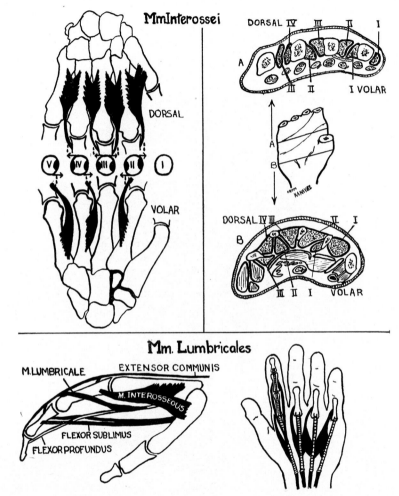

Fig. 667.—Arrangement of Intrinsic Musculature of the Hand. (McNealy and Lichtenstein Surg., Gynec. and Obst., Dec., 1932.)

characteristic sound of "creaking of new leather" in tenosynovitis of the dorsum of the wrist and hand results from inflammation of the visceral and parietal layers of the tendon sheaths. The radial extensor tendons are affected most frequently.

The *interosseous muscles* are intrinsic in this region. The three volar interossei arise from the metacarpal bones and adduct the little, ring, and index fingers toward the middle finger (see Fig. 667). The four dorsal interossei abduct the ring and index fingers from the middle finger. In addition to these actions, they assist the lumbrical muscles in flexing the fingers at the metacarpophalangeal joints, and, by reason of their insertion into the bases of the proximal phalanges and into the dorsal extensor expansions, aid in extending the fingers at the interphalangeal joints. The interossei are innervated by the deep branch of the ulnar nerve (C_8, T_1).

5. **Metacarpal Bones.**—The metacarpal bones, one for each digit, articulate through their bases with the distal row of the carpal bones at the carpometacarpal joints (p. 637). Their heads and the proximal phalanges constitute the metacarpophalangeal joints. The shafts are small as compared with the extremities and, therefore, frequently are fractured.

All the flexor and extensor muscles of the wrist overlie the carpus and have their ultimate attachment to the metacarpal bones. The tendon of the flexor carpi radialis (p. 618) is inserted on the palmar surface of the index metacarpal, that of the flexor carpi

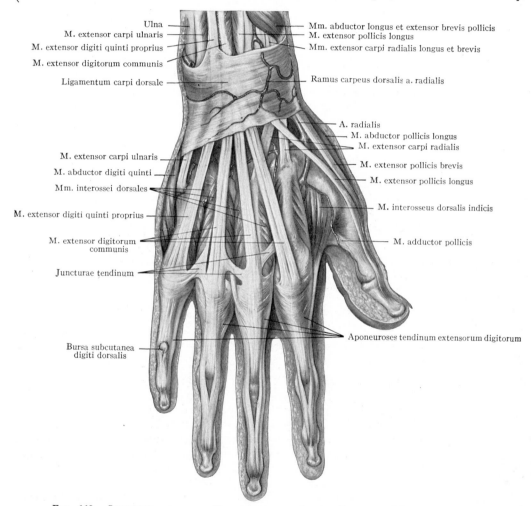

Ulna
M. extensor carpi ulnaris
M. extensor digiti quinti proprius
M. extensor digitorum communis
Ligamentum carpi dorsale
Mm. abductor longus et extensor brevis pollicis
M. extensor pollicis longus
Mm. extensor carpi radialis longus et brevis
Ramus carpeus dorsalis a. radialis
A. radialis
M. abductor pollicis longus
M. extensor carpi radialis
M. extensor carpi ulnaris
M. abductor digiti quinti
Mm. interossei dorsales
M. extensor digiti quinti proprius
M. extensor digitorum communis
Juncturae tendinum
M. extensor pollicis brevis
M. extensor pollicis longus
M. interosseus dorsalis indicis
M. adductor pollicis
Aponeuroses tendinum extensorum digitorum
Bursa subcutanea digiti dorsalis

FIG. 668.—STRUCTURES ON THE DORSUM OF THE LOWER FOREARM, WRIST, AND HAND.

ulnaris is inserted into the base of the fifth metacarpal, and the extensor carpi radialis longus into the dorsal surface of the base of the index metacarpal. The extensor carpi radialis brevis attaches to the middle metacarpal.

The metacarpal of the thumb ossifies from a primary center in the distal extremity (head), but each of the other metacarpals ossifies from a primary center for the base and shaft and has a separate epiphysis for the head, which ossifies at about three years of age and unites with the diaphysis at twenty years of age.

6. **Fractures of the Metacarpals.**—The metacarpals are fractured, as a rule, from a blow upon the knuckles when the first is clenched. *Fracture of the base of the first meta-*

carpal (Bennet's fracture) is a disabling injury which results from a blow upon the interphalangeal knuckle of the thumb, or from a blow received on the end of the extended thumb. The large distal fragment is drawn proximally and backward into a decided prominence by the combined action of the flexor and extensor muscles of the thumb. The small proximal fragment which usually lies a little to the ulnar side of the shaft is displaced only slightly. Crepitus and abnormal mobility are hard to obtain, and the proximal fragment is difficult to immobilize in proper position because of its small size. The fracture often is mistaken for a sprain at the metacarpophalangeal joint.

Reduction and skeletal (wire) maintenance of position is effected best by the use of traction incorporated into a plaster wristlet.

In *fracture of the metacarpal shaft*, the bone usually is bent into a dorsal angulation, accounted for by the greater strength of the flexor muscles of the hand. The break is oblique and the bone may be shortened noticeably so that the knuckle recedes from the knuckle line. Failure to correct the fracture leaves a marked deformity and may interfere with the action of the interosseous and lumbrical muscles in extending the terminal phalanx. Displaced fractures require continuous extension by elastic traction. For fractures without displacement or with palmar angulation, the hand may be bandaged about a rounded

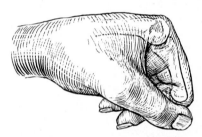

FIG. 669.—SHOWING HOW THE PROMINENCES OF THE KNUCKLES, WITH THE FINGERS FLEXED, ARE FORMED BY THE HEADS OF THE METACARPAL BONES.

Attention is directed to the ease with which a blow on the clenched knuckles opens the metacarpophalangeal joint. Without immediate recognition and adequate drainage, this lesion often causes loss of the finger.

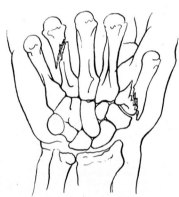

FIG. 670.—FRACTURE OF THE THIRD METACARPAL BONE WITH MODERATE SHORTENING AND FRACTURE OF THE BASE OF THE THUMB METACARPAL.

object grasped in the palm. Compound fractures may lead to infection of the palmar fascial spaces (p. 652).

Developmentally, the hand begins as a flapper-like broadening of the end of the limb. The fingers become separated by four vertical grooves. These grooves deepen until the flapper becomes separated into five parts, which form the thumb and fingers. The thumb is the first to separate; therefore, it is never found webbed. Failure of separation (*webbed fingers* or *syndactylism*) may occur between two or more adjacent processes. As the fingers separate at their distal ends first, the failure may be partial or complete. If partial, two adjacent digits may be united at their bases; if complete, the adjacent digits are united their entire length.

C. FINGERS

The thumb and the four fingers are of the same anatomical construction, except that the thumb has two phalanges and the fingers have three. The short thick metacarpal of the thumb makes for its strength and mobility. The shafts and distal extremities of the phalanges ossify from primary centers. The proximal ends are formed from separate epiphyses which ossify at three years of age and unite with the diaphyses at twenty years of age.

1. Surface Anatomy.—The transverse flexor creases mark off slightly elevated volar prominences, but do not designate the exact position of the joint lines. The distal trans verse crease is somewhat proximal to the distal interphalangeal joint; the middle crease is opposite the interphalangeal joint line; and the proximal crease is a considerable distance distal to the metacarpophalangeal joint. The interphalangeal skin creases are bound down closely to the underlying flexor tendon sheaths. A slight laceration in a skin crease easily may involve the digital synovia and result in synovitis.

2. **Superficial Structures.**—The skin of the flexor surface is thick, relatively immobile, and entirely devoid of hair follicles and sebaceous glands. That over the dorsum is thin and mobile, has little subcutaneous fat, and permits free movement over the underlying deep fascia. The *subcutaneous tissue* over the flexor surface is a meshwork of fibrous septa

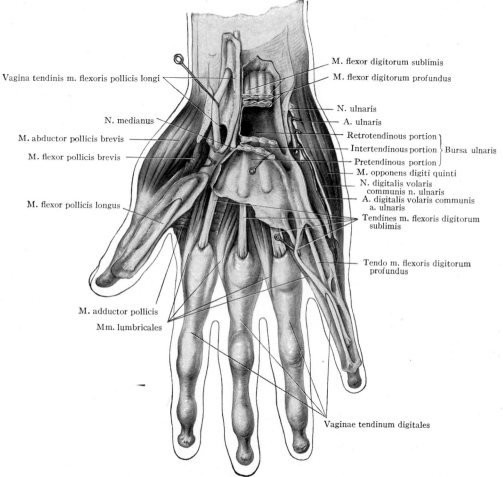

Fig. 671.—Digital and Palmar Synovia of the Anterior Region of the Hand and Fingers.

enclosing small columns of fat. These septa bring the thick skin into intimate relationship with the fibrous layers of the tendon sheaths, and, in the terminal phalanges, with the periosteum. Within the subcutaneous tissue run the digital vessels and nerves.

3. **Sheaths of the Flexor Tendons.**—Deep to the skin and subcutaneous tissue is a resistant fibrous layer whose reflections and attachments to the phalanges form an osteofibrous sheath for the two flexor tendons to each finger. The sheath is strong and resistant over the shafts of the phalanges, but is thin at the level of the interphalangeal joints to allow of free flexion. Through these thin areas, the digital synovia herniates into the subcutaneous tissue, where it is exposed to infection. The *fibrous sheaths* of the thumb and little finger are similar in structure to those of the index, middle, and ring fingers, and are

continuous in the palm with the palmar sheath for the thumb flexor (radial bursa) and with the common palmar sheath (ulnar bursa). *Synovial sheaths* which invest the flexor tendons within the osteofibrous canals extend distally to the insertions of the profundus tendons and into the palm a thumbbreadth proximal to the metacarpophalangeal joints. Each sheath is divided into visceral and parietal layers, as is the synovia of the flexor pollicis longus tendon. The digital synovia of the thumb is a continuation of the radial bursa, and that for the little finger is continuous with the palmar synovia of the ulnar bursa. The digital synovia of the other fingers is closed proximally.

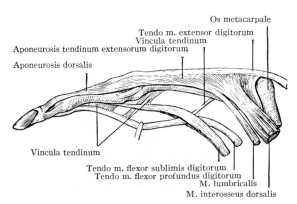

FIG. 672.—DISTAL EXTREMITIES OF THE FLEXOR AND EXTENSOR TENDONS OF THE RIGHT MIDDLE FINGER SEEN FROM THE RADIAL SIDE.

The relations of the lumbrical and dorsal interosseous muscles to the aponeurosis of the extensor tendon are emphasized.

Occasionally, a condition within the tendon sheath exists in which the tendon cannot be flexed after it is extended, or cannot be extended after it is flexed. The patient usually straightens or closes the fingers with the other hand, the action occurring with a sudden recoil (*trigger finger*). This is due to a localized disparity between the tendon and the sheath. There is either a local enlargement of the tendon, or a constriction of its sheath. Any of the fingers may be affected.

4. Insertion of the Flexor Tendons.—In the proximal portion of each digital sheath, the sublimis and profundus flexor tendons are superimposed. Opposite the base of the

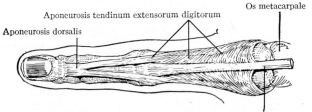

FIG. 673.—DORSAL VIEW OF THE EXTENSOR TENDON OF THE FINGER.

proximal phalanx, the sublimis tendon divides into two slips through which the tendon of the profundus passes to its insertion into the volar aspect of the base of the distal phalanx. The slips of the sublimis tendon continue distally to an insertion into the volar surface of the base and sides of the middle phalanx.

5. Insertion of the Extensor Tendons.—The common extensor tendons form strong fibrous expansions on the dorsal surfaces of the knuckles and the proximal phalanges; these expansions fuse with the capsules and lateral ligaments of the metacarpophalangeal joints. On the dorsum of each proximal phalanx, the tendon expansion splits into three parts.

The central part is inserted into the base of the second phalanx, and the two lateral slips, after receiving the insertions of the lumbrical muscles (p. 648) and a part of the insertions of the interosseous muscles (p. 658), insert into the bases of the distal phalanges. The remaining portions of the tendons of the interossei, which move the fingers toward and from one another, are inserted into the bases of the proximal phalanges. This specialized tendon expansion is unique in its action on the digits. The insertion on the base of the proximal phalanx subserves the function of extension of the fingers at the metacarpophalangeal joints, and the extensor action of the two terminal phalanges is reinforced by the pull of the interosseous and lumbrical muscles.

The thumb has two separate extensor muscles, the extensor pollicis longus and brevis. On the index and little fingers, the tendon expansions are strengthened by the tendons of the extensor indicis and extensor digiti quinti proprius.

6. **Volar Digital Vessels and Nerves.**—The *common volar digital arteries*, which arise from the convexity of the superficial volar arch, give off the proper digital branches which supply the contiguous sides of the thumb and fingers, and the distal parts of their dorsal surfaces. The proximal part of the dorsum of the fingers is supplied by *dorsal digital arteries* which are the terminations of the dorsal metacarpal arteries from the dorsal carpal arch.

The proper digital arteries are superficial to the corresponding *volar proper digital nerves* which supply the adjoining sides of the fingers and the distal parts of the dorsal surfaces. The *dorsal proper digital nerves* supply the proximal parts of the dorsum of the fingers.

The *superficial lymphatics* are numerous over the flexor surface of the fingers and form a mass of anastomotic channels which follow the superficial veins. The *deep lymphatics* accompany the digital vessels. The main branches of the lymphatic network collect into the trunks about the roots of the fingers; these trunks run dorsally toward the wrist and forearm.

SURGICAL CONSIDERATIONS

1. **Dislocations and Fractures of the Phalanges.**—Dislocations of the phalanges at the metacarpophalangeal joints occur with moderate frequency because of their ball and socket arrangement. Each joint has volar and collateral ligaments, but the dorsal ligament is replaced by the expansion of the extensor tendon. The volar accessory (glenoid) ligament is a fibrocartilaginous plate which is attached firmly to the proximal phalanx but connected weakly with the metacarpal.

The usual *dislocation of the thumb* at the metacarpophalangeal joint occurs in forcible dorsiflexion of the thumb as produced by a fall upon the hyperextended hand. A great strain is thrown upon the front of the joint so that the glenoid ligament gives way at the metacarpal attachment and allows the phalanx to pass backward, carrying the ligament with it. The phalanx comes to rest on the dorsal aspect of the metacarpal head. The head of the metacarpal projects anteriorly, and great difficulty sometimes is encountered in effecting reduction. If traction is put upon the thumb in the direction of the axis of the metacarpal, the tendency for the volar accessory ligament and the head of the phalanx is to become wedged more and more firmly against the metacarpal. To overcome this difficulty, the dislocated thumb is dorsiflexed still further until it forms a right angle with the dorsal surface of the metacarpal. While held in this position, the base of the phalanx is carried steadily toward the head of the metacarpal. As soon as it is thought to have cleared it, and while traction is maintained, the phalanx is flexed abruptly and carried medially toward the palm. This maneuver first disengages the volar accessory ligament and sesamoid bones and subsequently restores the articular surfaces to their normal position.

Dislocations and fractures of the middle and distal phalanges frequently occur when the tip of the finger is struck while the phalanx or phalanges are hyperextended. These dislocations are reduced fairly easily, but dislocation often recurs with deformity if there is an accompanying fracture. It is not uncommon to find the extensor tendon ruptured at its insertion into the base of the terminal phalanx. This causes the terminal phalanx to remain in partial flexion (dropped finger). A fragment of bone usually is torn from the

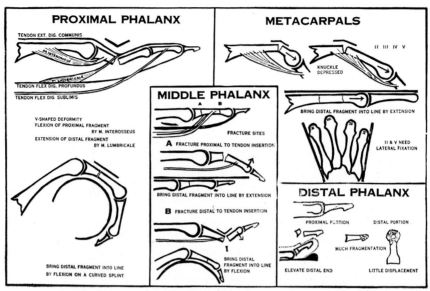

FIG. 674.—MECHANISM OF DEFORMITIES IN SIMPLE FRACTURES OF THE METACARPALS AND PHALANGES Means to overcome these deformities are suggested. (McNealy and Lichtenstein, Surg., Gynec. and Obst., Dec., 1932.)

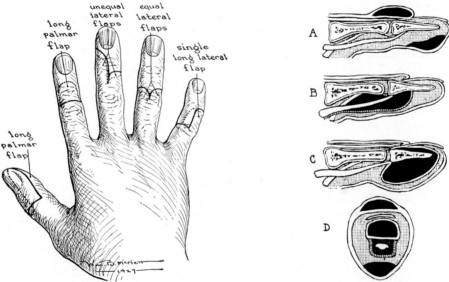

FIG. 675.—INCISIONS FOR AMPUTATIONS THROUGH THE FINGERS AND THUMB.
A palmar flap is preferred. (Babcock, "Textbook of Surgery.")

FIG. 676.—VARIETIES OF INFECTION ABOUT THE TERMINAL PHALANX.
A shows an infection under the epidermis and under the dermis; B is an infection within the tendon sheath; C is an infection of the terminal phalanx under the periosteum; D shows the four varieties of infection in cross section. (After Forgue.)

edge of the articular surface. Immobilization in hyperextension often is all that is required to secure union of the tendon. The tendon does not retract because of the attachment of its lateral expansion.

Fractures of the phalanges frequently are compound and the finger may require amputation. Fracture of the proximal phalanx requires a splint extending well into the palm, or traction from a banjo splint. For fractures of the distal and middle phalanges, splints are not necessary. The pull of the interosseous and lumbrical muscles through their attachments into the extensor tendon may tend to draw the distal fragment dorsally.

2. **Infections of the Fingers.**—The infection termed a *felon* (whitlow) begins in the skin of the palmar surface of the distal phalanx and rapidly involves the tissues beneath. The connective tissue framework is such as to produce an anterior closed space comprising the distal part of the phalanx. When pus develops in this closed sac, it has no means of free exit or spread as in other connective tissue spaces so that its pressure shuts off the blood supply and causes bone necrosis. The base of the phalanx, the epiphysis in the young, gets its blood supply through vessels which do not traverse this dense tissue. Therefore, it does not necrose like the rest of the bone. Treatment consists in immediate incision into the infected area. The incision should be made at the side and not in the midline of the tactile part of the finger pad. Usually the diaphysis, rarely the epiphysis, is involved.

A *paronychia* begins as an acute infection in the subepithelial tissue at the side of the nail. This forms a small abscess, which, if opened, promptly makes a complete recovery. If the infection is neglected, the pus spreads along the side of the nail and back to the base, forming a "run-around." Pus may be expressed from beneath the overlying epithelium (eponychium) and a little later is found under the posterior overhanging edge of the nail. It extends around the nail groove, under the nail, and lifts the soft and delicate root off the nail bed, even when the distal part of the nail still is attached firmly to the matrix (subungual abscess).

The proper *treatment* is to allow the escape of the unexpressed pus. A longitudinal incision is made along the edge of the nail, going back toward the base as far as the sulcus. The detached edge of the nail with as much of the root as has been separated from the matrix is cut off with scissors. After removal of this portion of the nail, the elevated flap of overhanging cuticle is lifted up and a

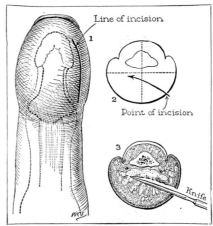

Fig. 677.—Incision for Drainage of Infection in Anterior Closed Space of Terminal Phalanx (Felon) (Koch, Jour. Amer. Med. Assoc., April 6, 1929.)

pack is inserted beneath it to insure drainage. If more than half of the base of the nail becomes involved, a second incision is made upon the other side of the nail. The flap made is elevated as before, exposing the entire nail groove. The loosened portion of the nail, often comprising the entire nail root, is removed, leaving the distal part of the nail attached to the matrix. The nail requires about three months to regenerate.

3. **Spread of Infection from the Digital Synovia.**—The three cardinal signs of infection from the digital synovia are: excessive tenderness over the course of the sheath and limited to it; a flexion attitude of the involved finger; and severe pain, most marked at the proximal end, on extending the finger. In addition to swelling in the infected finger, there is swelling of the adjacent digits and of the back of the hand.

An infection in the sheath of the tendon of the little finger may be limited to the finger. In a case where there is continuity between the sheath of the little finger and the common palmar sheath (ulnar bursa), infection may extend rapidly into the palm and wrist. The most conspicuous and valuable sign is the extension of tenderness into the areas involved. The infection from the ulnar bursa may extend into the radial bursa or may rupture through the proximal end of the sheath and extend along the intermuscular spaces of the forearm. At this time, pus may collect subcutaneously above the wrist as a result of lymphangitis.

One of the commonest sites of extension is along the lumbrical muscles into the palmar fascial spaces. Extension into the midpalmar spaces may occur from rupture of the ulnar bursa. The extension of infection from the synovia of the index, middle, and ring fingers commonly is along the lumbricals into the palmar fascial spaces. Infection from the middle and ring fingers drains into the middle palmar space.

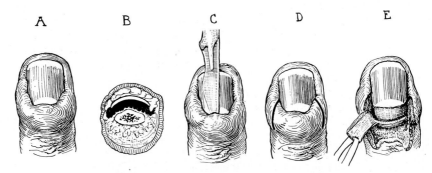

FIG. 678.—PARONYCHIA AND ITS TREATMENT.

A, Appearance of paronychia; B, cross section of a paronychia, showing the elevation of the root of the nail by the pus sac; C, evacuation of an early paronychia by separating the overlying skin from the nail by a thin knife; D, the incisions for operation of a fully developed paronychia; E, removal of the root of the nail after turning back the skin flap. (After Homans and Babcock.)

The seriousness of the spread of a tenosynovitis of the flexor pollicis longus should be recognized fully. The infection spreads easily into the palmar synovia (radial bursa) and may rupture through the closed proximal end into the intermuscular spaces of the forearm, or into the ulnar bursa.

The first incision for drainage of digital tenosynovitis is made at the side of the sheath at the site of known infection. The incision then is carried along the shaft of the proxima or middle phalanx, leaving the part over the joint uncut to prevent prolapse of the tendon

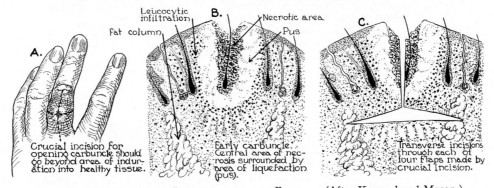

FIG. 679.—TREATMENT OF CARBUNCLE OF THE FINGER. (After Kanavel and Mason.)

unless there is doubt of free drainage. If there is complete involvement of the synovia, a similar incision is made over the proximal or middle phalanx. No incision, as a rule, is necessary over the distal phalanx. If the palmar synovia is known to be involved by tenosynovitis in the small finger or in the thumb, the ulnar and radial bursae require drainage.

VII. EFFECTS OF INJURY OF THE LARGE NERVES OF THE UPPER LIMB

Injuries to, and disease affecting, the nerves of the upper limb are manifested by paralysis of muscles or groups of muscles and by loss of sensation. The loss of sensation with involvement of the large nerves often is less than would be expected, in view of their anatomical distribution, since the terminal branches of neighboring nerves overlap widely and may be able to maintain the sensibility of the part. When one of the large nerves alone is involved, the interpretation of the loss of power and sensation usually is easy; when more than one of the nerves is affected, some confusion may arise.

1. **Nerve Injuries and Their Effects.**—The nerves most likely to be injured individually are the axillary, radial, musculocutaneous, ulnar, and median.

The **axillary nerve,** because of its location close to the head of the humerus, often is damaged in dislocation at the shoulder (p. 580), in severe contusions in the deltoid region, by fragments in fracture of the surgical neck of the humerus (p. 585), or by the upward pressure of a crutch. The resulting loss of innervation to the teres minor muscle does not interfere materially with external rotation of the arm. Loss of innervation to the deltoid muscle causes atrophy of the muscle with loss of sensation over its distal part. Abduction of the arm then is performed by the supraspinatus muscle. Deltoid atrophy attributable to nerve involvement must be differentiated from the wasting of disuse in shoulder joint disease.

The **radial nerve** most frequently is injured individually because of its course and relationships in the arm. It is in intimate contact with the humeral shaft over an area which is exposed to much trauma. It is likely to be injured in fractures of the distal two

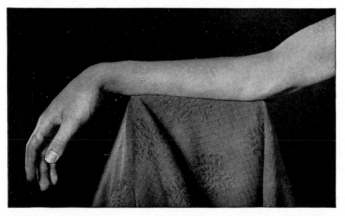

FIG. 680.—WRIST DROP FROM PARALYSIS OF THE RADIAL NERVE. (Dr. Joseph Scattergood.)

thirds of the shaft of the humerus by being caught and crushed by the fragments at the time of accident, or by being compressed by the ensheathing callus (p. 593). It often has been injured in open operations on the shaft of the humerus. Prolonged pressure on the nerve also may harm it: for example, "Saturday night paralysis" is sustained when an intoxicated man falls asleep with his arm hanging over the back of a bench. The pressure of a crutch may injure the nerve in the upper part of the arm where it lies against the shaft of the humerus. Injury usually occurs beyond the origin of the nerve supply of the triceps and anconeus muscles, so that all the remaining muscles supplied directly by the radial nerve and by its deep posterior interosseous branch are paralyzed and the characteristic deformity of *wrist drop* develops. With this lesion, the wrist or fingers cannot be extended voluntarily but, with the tips of the fingers supported in the effort of extension, the interosseous and lumbrical muscles, which insert into the extensor expansions, extend the fingers at the interphalangeal joints. In the wrist drop occurring in lead poisoning, the extensor carpi radialis muscle is affected, but the brachioradialis is not. The elbow is brought against the side in an attempt to rotate the humerus outward to compensate for the loss of the supinator muscles.

The *dorsal interosseous branch* may be injured in dislocation or fracture of the head of the radius (p. 614) or in operations which incise the supinator brevis muscle. In injury to the dorsal interosseous nerve, the motor symptoms are as described for wrist drop, except that the brachioradialis and extensor carpi radialis muscles are spared. The wrist can be extended, but the movement is weak. The *superficial branch* of the radial nerve may be injured in lacerations about the dorsal and radial aspects of the wrist, but, unless other nerves are injured, sensory changes often are not apparent on account of the communications (overlap) with other nerves.

Separate injury to the trunk of the **musculocutaneous nerve** is rare, but one of its divisions or branches may be cut in wounds of the forearm. Injury to the main trunk of this nerve paralyzes the biceps and coracobrachialis muscles and weakens the brachialis (anticus) muscle. Flexion of the forearm when the hand is supine still can be performed by the brachialis muscle and the superficial flexors of the forearm. With the hand in the prone or midprone position, flexion is aided by the extensor carpi radialis longus and brachioradialis muscles. The motor paralysis is accompanied by disturbance in sensation over the radial half of the forearm. Division of the cutaneous branch of the musculocutaneous nerve causes the same sensory signs as those of injury to the parent trunk. Because of nerve overlap, section of the volar or dorsal branch causes no changes in sensation.

The **ulnar nerve** rarely is injured in the upper arm, but may be damaged in fracture or dislocation at the elbow, or operations about it, because of the superficial position of the nerve and its close proximity to the medial epicondyle of the humerus (p. 606). It is

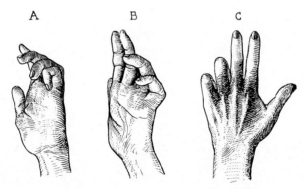

Fig. 681.—Appearance of the Hand in Paralysis of the Ulnar Nerve.
A, Ulnar paralysis of five months' duration. B, Prolonged ulnar paralysis; the index and middle fingers are hyperextended. C, Atrophy of the interosseous muscles. Thumb is abducted because adductor action (ulnar) is lost.

liable to injury from deeply incised wounds at the wrist where the nerve is superficial. In *severance of the nerve at the wrist*, all of the intrinsic muscles of the hand are paralyzed save those supplied by the median nerve. Immediately after section of the nerve, the injury may be overlooked when no tendons are cut because on superficial examination most of the movements of the fingers apparently are performed. It is essential to determine whether or not the patient can separate the fingers, and his inability to do so indicates paralysis of the dorsal interosseous and abductor digiti quinti muscles. The power of adduction of the thumb is lost, the little finger is more or less paralyzed in all its movements, and there is wasting of the muscles of the hypothenar eminence. The action of the interosseous muscles is lost completely, as is evidenced by inability to flex the fingers at the metacarpophalangeal joints or extend them at the interphalangeal joints. This loss of power is less evident in the index and middle fingers than in the ring and small fingers since the lumbrical muscles to the index and ring fingers are innervated by the median nerve. The paralyzed muscles atrophy, and the fingers are extended at the metacarpophalangeal joints since the balance between the flexors and extensors is upset because of the paralysis of the interosseous muscles. In the small and ring fingers, the flexor and extensor equilibrium is upset further by the loss of the lumbrical muscles. As their action on the dorsal extensor expansions is lost, hyperextension of the fingers at the metacarpophalangeal joints and flexion at the interphalangeal joints occur because the common extensor of the fingers can extend the fingers at the metacarpophalangeal joints only The result is a clawlike hand, "main en griffe."

If *injury to the ulnar nerve occurs at the elbow*, there is, in addition, paralysis of the flexor carpi ulnaris muscle, attended by deviation of the hand to the radial side and limited extension and ulnar flexion. That part of the flexor digitorum profundus muscle which controls the ring and little fingers also is paralyzed. As a result, the terminal phalanges of these fingers are not flexed as acutely as they are in severance of the nerve at the wrist.

The **median nerve** rarely is injured alone in the upper arm but occasionally is damaged by a penetrating wound. The nerve is endangered most in incised wounds of the forearm or wrist, especially in the latter location where it lies between the tendons of the palmaris longus and the flexor carpi radialis at the upper margin of the transverse carpal ligament (p. 633). In injury to the nerve, the tendons of the forearm often escape injury.

When the nerve is *severed at the wrist*, the abductor and flexor pollicis brevis, opponens pollicis, and the first and second lumbricals are the only muscles affected. Most of the power of abduction of the thumb is lost, although abduction can be performed partially by the abductor pollicis longus muscle, supplied by the radial nerve. There also is difficulty in apposing the thumb to the tips of the other fingers, although the movement of apposition may be imitated by the flexor pollicis longus, supplied by the median nerve in the forearm. In addition to paralysis, there usually is marked wasting of the muscles of the thenar eminence. In attempts to close the hand tightly, the index and middle fingers lag behind the other two since the balance between the extensors and flexors is disturbed by the lumbrical paralysis. Hyperextension of the index and middle fingers at the metacarpophalangeal joint is not always present, but adduction of the thumb is characteristic when the hand is at rest, because action of the adductor pollicis (ulnar nerve) is unopposed. In a lesion of the nerve at the wrist, there is no loss of the power of flexing the wrist and the fingers. As in the case of injury to the radial nerve, the extent of loss of sensation is subject to great variability.

When the nerve is *severed proximal to the elbow*, the extent of the paralysis is increased greatly, as the injury occurs proximal to the origin of the branches supplying the muscles of the anterior forearm. The power of true pronation of the forearm is lost, but the brachioradialis muscle is capable of producing a midprone position. The loss of power is compensated for to some extent by rotating the humerus inward while carrying the elbow away from the side and allowing the weight of the forearm to complete the action. Attempts at flexing the wrist result in the hand being deviated toward the ulnar side. Flexion is accomplished by the flexor carpi ulnaris muscle and the ulnar half of the flexor digitorum profundus muscle. The thumb is adducted, but its terminal phalanx is extended because of the loss of the flexor pollicis longus muscle. The index and middle fingers are useless because no flexion is possible at the interphalangeal joints and the interosseous muscles at best are feeble flexors at the metacarpophalangeal joints when they must initiate the movement. The ring and little fingers are weakened only by the loss of the flexor sublimis tendons.

LOWER EXTREMITY

I. HIP

The lower extremity is bound to the pelvis by many powerful muscles which are grouped about the hip joint in the pelvifemoral region. This region is subdivided into the gluteal region and the hip joint.

A. GLUTEAL REGION

1. Definition and Boundaries.—The gluteal region is the roughly quadrilateral area of soft parts corresponding to the prominence of the buttocks. It is bounded above by

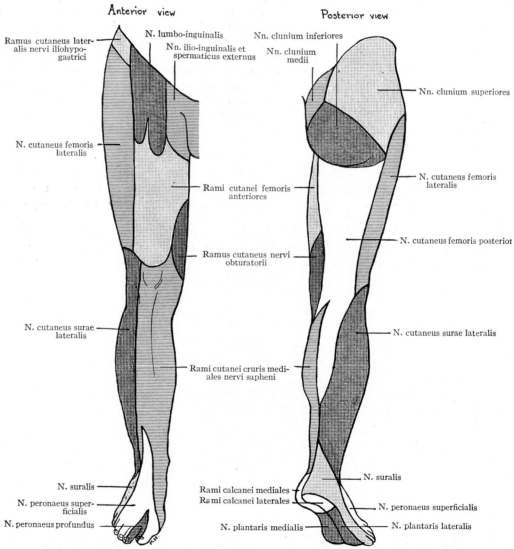

Anterior view

Posterior view

Ramus cutaneus lateralis nervi iliohypogastrici

N. lumbo-inguinalis

Nn. ilio-inguinalis et spermaticus externus

Nn. clunium inferiores

Nn. clunium medii

Nn. clunium superiores

N. cutaneus femoris lateralis

N. cutaneus femoris lateralis

Rami cutanei femoris anteriores

N. cutaneus femoris posterior

Ramus cutaneus nervi obturatorii

N. cutaneus surae lateralis

N. cutaneus surae lateralis

Rami cutanei cruris mediales nervi sapheni

N. suralis

N. suralis

N. peronaeus superficialis

N. peronaeus profundus

Rami calcanei mediales

Rami calcanei laterales

N. plantaris medialis

N. peronaeus superficialis

N. plantaris lateralis

FIG. 682.—AREAS OF CUTANEOUS NERVE DISTRIBUTION IN THE LOWER EXTREMITY.

the iliac crest, which separates the region from the posterolateral abdominal wall (p. 310); below, by the deep horizontal furrow of the transverse gluteal fold; medially, by the lateral margin of the sacrum and coccyx; and laterally, by the tensor fasciae latae muscle.

2. **Landmarks.**—Abnormal fullness of the buttocks occurs with pathologic conditions such as subgluteal abscess, tumor, or dislocation of the head of the femur. The thick superficial fascia ordinarily obscures the muscle landmarks of the buttocks, but the outline of the *gluteus maximus muscle* sometimes can be seen. The lower margin of the muscle runs downward and laterally, crosses the middle of the gluteal fold obliquely, and is lost in the general contour of the lateral aspect of the thigh. In active mesial rotation of the thigh, a muscle prominence appears just below and lateral to the anterior superior iliac

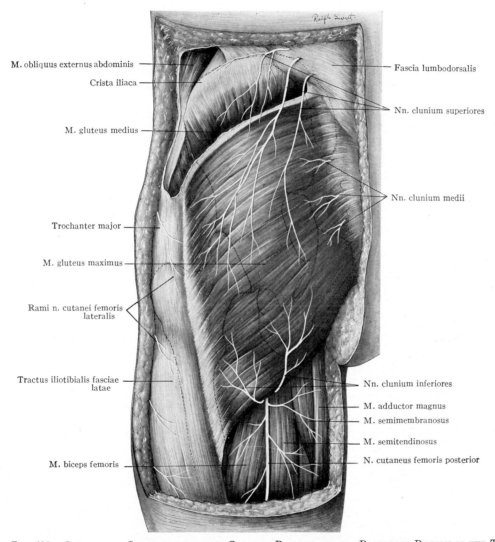

M. obliquus externus abdominis

Crista iliaca

M. gluteus medius

Trochanter major

M. gluteus maximus

Rami n. cutanei femoris lateralis

Tractus iliotibialis fasciae latae

M. biceps femoris

Fascia lumbodorsalis

Nn. clunium superiores

Nn. clunium medii

Nn. clunium inferiores

M. adductor magnus

M. semimembranosus

M. semitendinosus

N. cutaneus femoris posterior

FIG. 683.—SUPERFICIAL STRUCTURES OF THE GLUTEAL REGION AND THE POSTERIOR REGION OF THE THIGH

spine. This prominence is formed by the *tensor fasciae latae muscle*, superficially, and the *gluteus medius* and *minimus muscles* at a deeper level.

The bony landmarks include the crest of the ilium, the ischial tuberosity, and the greater trochanter of the femur. The prominence of the *iliac crest* varies according to the state of nutrition. It terminates in front at the *anterior superior spine* which is an important landmark in taking measurements of the lower extremity. The crest ends behind at the *posterior superior spine*, the position of which can be determined best by palpating backward along the crest. The posterior superior spine lies at the level of the second sacral spine, a little less than a handbreadth from the median line, deep to a shallow dimple in the overlying skin. It corresponds closely in position with the center of the posterior part of the sacro-iliac joint (p. 421). The *ischial tuberosity* lies vertically below the posterior superior iliac spine; it is covered by the inferior part of the gluteus maximus muscle in the erect attitude, but is not covered by this muscle in the sitting posture.

The summit of the *greater trochanter of the femur* lies a palmbreadth below the iliac crest and very nearly midway between the anterior superior spine and the tuberosity of the ischium. Its position is indicated normally by a flattened depression on the lateral aspect of the upper thigh; in thin or wasted persons, it is a prominent projection when the thigh is adducted. The fascia lata is stretched tightly across the interval between the summit of the trochanter and the iliac crest, but is relaxed by passive abduction of the thigh so that the upper edge of the trochanter becomes well defined. In this position, the greater trochanter can be grasped between the fingers and thumb and its anterior and posterior surfaces can be outlined. The fingers can be thrust into the *trochanteric (digital)*

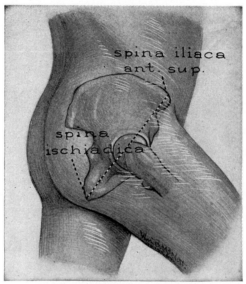

Fig. 684.—Surface Projection of the Skeletal Framework of the Hip to Show the Relations Between the Anterior Superior Iliac Spine, the Tuberosity of the Ischium, and the Summit of the Greater Trochanter.
Nélaton's line extends between the anterior superior iliac spine and the tuberosity of the ischium. (Babcock, "Textbook of Surgery.")

fossa. The depression behind the trochanter overlies the hip joint and the posterior aspect of the neck of the femur. In the depth of the depression between the greater trochanter and the ischial tuberosity, the sciatic nerve can be palpated.

Nélaton's line lies between the anterior superior iliac spine and the ischial tuberosity, and passes through the summit of the greater trochanter when the thigh is flexed partially. When the summit of the trochanter lies above or below this line, there is a deformity of the neck of the femur. The commonest pathologic conditions diagnosed by this criterion are dislocation of the head of the femur backward and upward on the dorsum of the ilium, and intracapsular and extracapsular fractures of the neck of the femur. The use of Nélaton's line in examination of the hip joint often is impractical because of the difficulty in locating the ischial tuberosity accurately.

Bryant's line extends between the highest point on the greater trochanter and a circumferential line or horizontal plane passing through both anterior superior spines. The distance normally is about 5 cm. Shortening of the line, indicating deformity on the side of the shortening, occurs if the tip of the trochanter is elevated, as in fractures of the neck of the femur. *Bryant's (right-angled) triangle* is constructed with the patient lying on his back. One side of the triangle is a perpendicular erected from the table to the anterior superior spine. The second side or base of the triangle (Bryant's line) is a horizontal line drawn from the tip of the greater trochanter to the perpendicular line, and the third side or hypotenuse is that part of Nélaton's line which connects the anterior superior spine and the summit of the trochanter (anterior iliotrochanteric line). In fractures of the neck of the femur, the base of the triangle on the affected side is shortened.

The *anterior iliotrochanteric line* connects the anterior superior spine with the tip of the greater trochanter. It forms an iliotrochanteric angle of about 30 degrees with a circumferential line about the pelvis passing through both anterior superior spines. In dislocation or fracture of the neck of the femur, this angle is reduced in proportion to the shortening. A rough estimation of this angle by palpation usually permits judgment of the degree of shortening from fracture or dislocation without erecting Bryant's triangle.

The *posterior iliotrochanteric line* (of Farabeuf) (Fig. 687) connects the posterior superior iliac spine with the tip of the greater trochanter. It corresponds fairly accurately with the interspace (suprapiriformic foramen) (p. 429) between the gluteus medius and

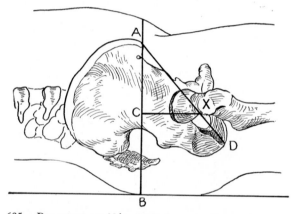

FIG. 685.—RELATION OF NÉLATON'S LINE TO BRYANT'S TRIANGLE.
A perpendicular (ACB) is dropped from the anterior superior spine to the table. Nélaton's line (AXD) extends from the anterior superior spine to the ischial tuberosity. The distance (XC) from the summit of the trochanter to the perpendicular (ACB) is Bryant's line or the base of Bryant's triangle (ACX). In fracture of the neck of the femur, the base (CX) of Bryant's triangle is shorter than normal. (Modified from Scudder.)

piriformis muscles. The junction of the medial and middle thirds of this line is a reliable surface guide to the point at which the superior gluteal artery emerges from the pelvis.

A discussion of the actual and apparent measurements of the lower limbs and the determination of the degree of abduction and adduction at the hip are given under surgical considerations of the hip joint.

3. **Deep Fascia.**—The deep fascia of the buttocks is attached strongly to the iliac crest and, in its anterosuperior position, where it overlies the gluteus medius muscle, it is a strong aponeurotic sheet. At the upper border of the gluteus maximus muscle, the deep fascia splits into two layers which enclose the muscle. The fascia increases in strength at the lateral aspect of the buttock and receives the insertion of most of the fibers of the gluteus maximus and tensor fasciae latae muscles to form the strong iliotibial band.

4. **Gluteal Musculature.**—The superficial muscle layer includes the gluteus maximus and tensor fasciae latae muscles. The *gluteus maximus muscle* (N. inferior gluteal L_5, $S_{1, 2}$) has a rhomboid outline and is the most massive muscle in the body. It passes downward and laterally from the posterior part of the iliac crest and the dorsum of the sacrum to an insertion into the deep fascia (iliotibial band) and the upper and outer part of the shaft of the femur from the great trochanter to the linea aspera. The gluteus maximus

43

covers most of the dorsum of the ilium, the deep layer of the pelvifemoral muscles, the sacrotuberous and sacrospinous (greater and lesser sacrosciatic) ligaments, the suprapiriformic and infrapiriformic spaces, and the vessels and nerves transmitted by these spaces. The large *ischiogluteal bursa* separates the gluteus maximus from the ischial tuberosity and another bursa separates it from the greater trochanter. The gluteus maximus is a powerful extensor and external rotator of the thigh.

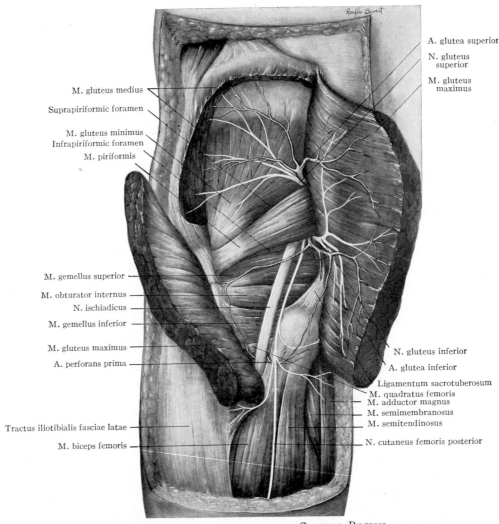

FIG. 686.—DEEP STRUCTURES OF THE GLUTEAL REGION.

A large segment of the gluteus medius muscle is removed to expose the gluteus minimus. Attention is called to the piriformis muscle as the key landmark of the deep structures. All of the important gluteal vessels and nerves emerge through the suprapiriformic and infrapiriformic spaces.

It is very difficult to determine fluctuation through the great bulk of this muscle. The fasciculi composing it are coarse and fibrous and may be separated without damage. Incisions into the buttock are made downward and laterally, parallel to the fasciculi. The areolo-adipose layer under the gluteus maximus sometimes harbors infection spreading from intrapelvic and ischiorectal abscesses.

The *tensor fasciae (femoris) latae muscle* (N. superior gluteal $L_4, _5, S_1$) arises from the forepart of the lateral lip of the iliac crest and the subjacent bony surface and is invested by fascia lata. It lies over the anterior borders of the gluteus medius and minimus muscles and its fibers pass downward and backward to an insertion into the fascia lata a little below the level of the greater trochanter. This part of the fascia lata is known as the *iliotibial band* and is attached below to the lateral condyle of the head of the tibia.

The deep muscle layer is composed of the gluteus medius, gluteus minimus, piriformis, obturator internus, quadratus femoris, and the gemelli muscles. The *gluteus medius* and *minimus muscles* (Fig. 686) are powerful abductors of the thigh. Their forward fibers lie under cover of the tensor fasciae latae and assist in medial rotation.

The *piriformis muscle* ($S_{1, 2}$) emerges from the pelvis through the greater sciatic foramen (p. 417). In passing laterally to the tip of the greater trochanter, the muscle tapers to a narrow tendon which lies on the posterosuperior aspect of the capsule of the hip joint.

Inferior to these muscles and on a somewhat deeper plane are the *obturator internus*, the two gemelli, the *quadratus femoris* muscles, and the sacrotuberous ligament. They rotate the thigh laterally.

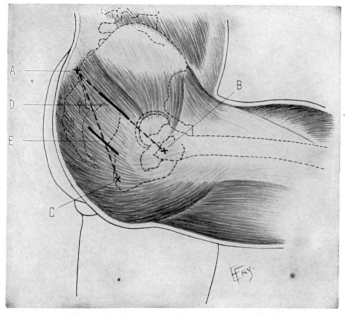

FIG. 687.—LANDMARKS FOR INCISIONS IN THE GLUTEAL REGION.

A, Posterior superior iliac spine; B, greater trochanter; C, tuberosity of the ischium; AB, posterior iliotrochanteric line; D, incision for the exposure of the structures which emerge from the pelvis through the suprapiriformic foramen; E, incision for the exposure of the structures which emerge from the pelvis through the infrapiriformic foramen. (Bickham in "Keen's Surgery.")

5. **Vessels and Nerves.**—Most of the vessels and nerves of the gluteal region traverse the greater sciatic foramen on their way to and from the pelvic cavity. The piriformis muscle passes through this aperture and divides the vessels and nerves into two groups, one above and the other below the tendon. In the **suprapiriformic space** are the superior gluteal vessels and nerves. The *superior gluteal artery*, a branch of the hypogastric artery, enters the gluteal region between the adjoining borders of the gluteus medius and piriformis muscles (Fig. 686). The *superior gluteal nerve* ($L_{4, 5}$, S_1) accompanies the superior gluteal artery. These structures can be reached through an incision along the posterior iliotrochanteric line.

Through the **infrapiriformic space,** a group of important vessels and nerves emerges from the pelvis. These are the inferior gluteal artery with its companion veins and the sciatic and posterior cutaneous (small sciatic) nerves.

The *inferior gluteal (sciatic) artery* appears at the lower border of the piriformis muscle and runs with the sciatic nerve to the interval between the greater trochanter and the tuberosity of the ischium.

The *crucial anastomosis* is an important connection between the external iliac and hypogastric arterial trunks for the reestablishment of the circulation of the lower limb when the external iliac artery is ligated, or when the femoral artery is divided proximal to the origin of the profunda branch (p. 704). The anastomosis consists of branches of the superior and inferior gluteal arteries from the hypogastric artery, branches of the medial and lateral circumflex arteries, and the first perforating artery, all of which are derived from the profunda femoris artery.

The *sciatic nerve* ($L_4, _5, S_1, _2, _3$), the largest nerve in the body, is broad and flat. In its downward course to the back of the thigh (p. 721), it lies nearly midway between the tuberosity of the ischium and the greater trochanter. The nerve may be approached through a vertical incision along the thigh from the center of the line joining the ischial tuberosity to the greater trochanter. Division of the superficial tissues and the deep fascia exposes

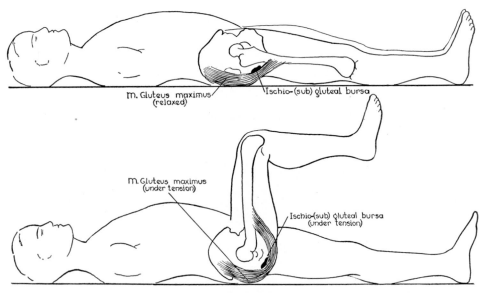

FIG. 688.—EFFECT OF FLEXION OF THE THIGH ON THE ISCHIOGLUTEAL BURSA.
Thigh flexion or trunk flexion exerts painful pressure on an inflamed subgluteal bursa. (Modified from Brahdy.)

the lower margin of the gluteus maximus muscle and the biceps femoris muscle. The nerve lies in the angle between the two muscles and can be hooked up from under cover of the biceps muscle.

The *posterior cutaneous (small sciatic) nerve* ($S_1, _2, _3$) of the thigh runs downward under cover of the gluteus maximus muscle on the surface of the sciatic nerve. At the lower part of the gluteus maximus, it crosses the biceps muscle superficially and runs down the thigh in the midline of the limb just beneath the deep fascia.

The inferior gluteal vessels may be exposed by an incision parallel to the fibers of the gluteus maximus muscle, cutting the line connecting the posterior superior spine and the ischium at the junction of its middle and lower thirds.

SURGICAL CONSIDERATIONS

1. Bursae under the Gluteus Maximus Muscle.—Large bursae separate the gluteus maximus muscle from the tuberosity of the ischium and from the greater trochanter. The *bursa over the tuberosity of the ischium (ischiogluteal bursa)* may become irritated and inflamed in habitual sitting on a hard surface, as tailors, draymen, and horsemen do; hence, the term "tailor's or weaver's bottom." Bursal enlargement is caused by excessive thickening of the bursal wall by layers of fibrous tissue. The bursal cavity usually is not increased in size, but if the swelling becomes large enough to cause inconvenience, the entire bursa may be excised. This bursitis requires differentiation from a gumma or cold abscess, both of which may occur here.

The *trochanteric bursa* frequently is inflamed chronically from tuberculosis. In *ischiogluteal bursitis*, flexion of the thigh puts pressure on the tender bursa and elicits pain referred to the buttock. Flexion of the trunk produces the same pain as thigh flexion, and for the same reason. The inflammation may terminate in suppuration, evacuation of which may produce a chronic sinus. Pus from suppuration in a trochanteric or an ischial bursa may point about the inferior margin of the gluteus maximus muscle and descend under the deep fascia of the thigh. A bursa sometimes is present between the tendon of the gluteus maximus and the vastus lateralis muscles.

2. **Wounds in the Gluteal Region.**—Stab or gunshot wounds in the buttocks may involve intrapelvic structures. The path of the wound usually is directed from behind the greater trochanter through the greater sciatic foramen into the pelvis, and the parts most liable to injury are the gluteal and pudendal vessels, the ureter, and the bladder. If the arteries are divided, there follows an extravasation of blood under the gluteus maximus muscle with the development of a traumatic aneurysm. An injury to the bladder or ureter may result in a urinary fistula on the buttock. An injury to the rectum is likely to produce a fecal fistula. The sciatic nerve may be severed.

3. **Subgluteal Abscesses.**—Abscesses sometimes lie under the gluteus maximus muscle. They reach this location from the pelvis by way of the greater sciatic foramen or the eroded capsule about a suppurating hip joint. Occasionally, they occur from hypodermic injections or from penetrating wounds. The abscess may cause a prominence of the gluteus maximus muscle, making the buttock fuller than normal and the overlying skin smooth and glossy. These deep abscesses, unless evacuated early, gravitate downward, point distal to the inferior border of the gluteus maximus muscle, and obliterate the transverse gluteal fold. Pus may follow the sciatic nerve down the thigh to the back of the knee.

4. **Gluteal Herniae.**—Rarely, a hernia leaves the pelvis through the sciatic foramen and protrudes into the gluteal region. The usual site of appearance of a gluteal hernia is superior to the piriformis muscle and the sac lies under the gluteus maximus muscle. Branches of the superior gluteal artery may spread over the exterior of the sac. If the hernia continues to enlarge, it emerges at the inferior margin of the gluteus maximus muscle. The neck of the sac usually lies in the ovarian fossa (p. 484) of the pelvis in the angle between the hypogastric and obturator arteries. Herniotomy requires an incision in the posterior iliotrochanteric line (p. 673), in the direction of the fibers of the gluteus maximus muscle, sometimes combined with an intrapelvic exposure of the sac.

B. HIP JOINT

In the hip joint, the rounded head of the femur articulates with the cup-shaped acetabulum on the outer aspect of the hip bone. The hip joint is remarkable for its stability in weight-bearing, for its ability to withstand shock, and for its variety and range of motion. It helps maintain the body in erect posture without excessive sustained muscle action. Since the essential characteristic of the hip joint is stability, the chief aim in the treatment of its pathologic conditions is the retention of this stability. If mobility also can be obtained, the result is better, but mobility without stability is useless. The hip joint differs from the shoulder joint in that the bones are heavier and have more prominent processes, and that the muscles surrounding it are larger and more powerful. It often is the seat of fracture, dislocation, and deformity, and frequently is affected by disease.

1. **Acetabulum.**—The acetabulum is a deep hemispheric socket, 3.5 cm. in diameter, located on a high ridge of compact bone connecting the anterior superior iliac spine with the ischial tuberosity. It divides the external surface of the hip bone into an anterior

portion, sloping anteriorly and medially, and a posterior portion, sloping backward.   These slopes influence the direction taken by the head of the femur when it is dislocated.

The ilium, ischium, and pubis share in the formation of the acetabulum and at birth are set apart from each other by a triradiate or Y-shaped bar of cartilage (p. 417).   This cartilage begins to ossify at the twelfth year and the bony segments fuse by the sixteenth or seventeenth year.   Over by far the greater part of its extent, the acetabulum is delimited by a sharp bony rim of compact bone.   The continuity of this rim is interrupted below by a broad deep notch, the *acetabular (cotyloid) incisura*.   The notch extends upward to an irregular rough area in the floor of the acetabulum which lodges and forms an attachment for the *ligamentum teres*, or intra-articular ligament of the hip joint.

The *transverse ligament* bridges over the acetabular notch and completes the circumference of the acetabulum.   The articular cartilage forms a broad strip around the acet-

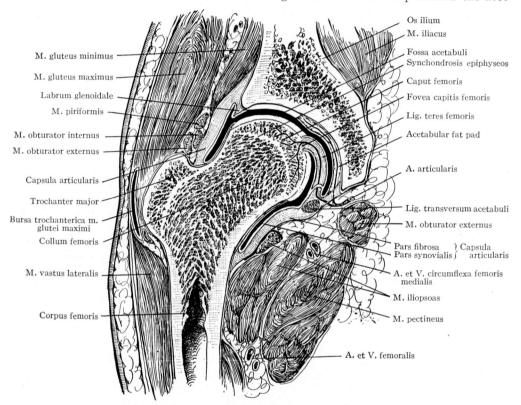

FIG. 689.—FRONTAL SECTION THROUGH THE HIP JOINT.

abulum, but the floor of the cavity and the acetabular (cotyloid) notch are nonarticular. Both the transverse ligament and the margin of the acetabulum are overlain by, and give attachment to, a circular band of fibrocartilage, the *glenoid labrum (cotyloid ligament)*. This structure deepens the socket for the head of the femur and reduces the diameter of the acetabular inlet.   It is pulled around the head of the femur like an air-tight collar so that, even after the joint has been opened, it is not easy to pull the head of the femur out of its socket.

The *floor of the acetabulum* is related internally to the flat surface of the bone which affords attachment to the obturator internus muscle (p. 428) and forms the lateral bony wall of the pelvic cavity.   The bone of the rough nonarticular part of the acetabulum is very thin and may be eroded by destructive hip joint disease or be fractured by the head of the femur.   The latter injury usually is designated as a central dislocation of the head of the femur (p. 692).

The upper part of the acetabulum is very strong and forms part of the powerful buttress which extends upward in front of the greater sciatic notch to the sacro-iliac joint and, in the erect posture, transmits the weight of the trunk to the head of the femur. Another strong buttress extends downward from the inferior and posterior part of the acetabulum to the ischial tuberosity. It transmits part of the weight of the body in the sitting position.

2. Proximal Extremity of the Femur.

—The *head of the femur* forms more than half a sphere. Its globoid surface is covered by cartilage as far as its junction with the neck. A small pitlike depression (fovea capitis), located a little behind the summit of the head, lodges the femoral attachment of the ligamentum teres, through which the head receives a small arterial supply.

In order to increase the power and mobility of the lower limb and to distribute the body weight over a wider base, the *neck of the femur*, which is an upward extension of the shaft, is inclined to the shaft at an angle which varies from 160 degrees in the child, to 125 degrees in

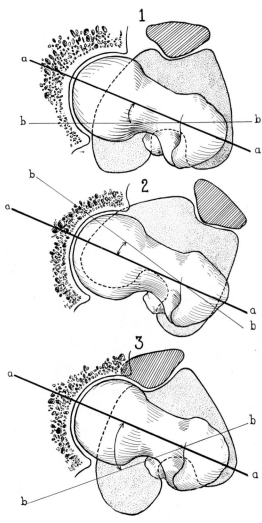

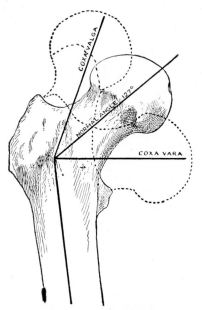

Fig. 690.—Normal and Abnormal Angles of Inclination of the Axes of the Neck and the Shaft of the Femur. (Vertical Neck-shaft Angles.) (Davis after Nifong.)

Fig. 691.—Variations in the Angle of Torsion (Declination) Between the Axis of the Neck of the Femur and the Transverse Bicondylar Axis.

In 1, the axis of the femoral neck normally projects obliquely anterior to the bicondylar axis. In 2, the axis of the femoral neck projects posterior to the bicondylar axis. In 3, the axis of the femoral neck projects far anterior to the bicondylar axis.

the adult (*angle of inclination, vertical neck-shaft angle*). The head and neck of the femur lie on a plane a little oblique to that of the line joining the two condyles. The extent to which the axis of the neck is thrust obliquely ahead of the bicondylar plane determines the *angle of declination* (*torsion, forward neck-shaft angle*).

A knowledge of the angles of inclination and declination is a valuable aid in the diagnosis and treatment of fractures of the upper end of the femur. Stereoscopic *x*-ray examination determines accurately the relation of the fragments and any change in these angles. Abnormal alterations in the angle of inclination may interfere seriously with the mobility of the hip joint. In congenital dislocation of the hip or in early extensive infantile paralysis, the angle of inclination may be increased, because the neck of the femur does not maintain its share of the body weight. Increase in the angle of inclination is known as *coxa valga*. As a result of constitutional diseases, such as rickets and osteomalacia, or following injuries to the neck of the femur during infancy, the body weight may reduce the inclination of the neck to the shaft to 90 degrees or less. This condition is termed *coxa vara*.

The *greater trochanter* is a quadrilateral mass of bone capping the upper and lateral extremity of the shaft of the femur. Its medial surface fuses with the cancellous tissue of the neck and shaft of the femur. The upper posterior portion of the trochanter is free and overhangs the posterosuperior aspect of the neck of the femur, forming with it the deep pit known as the trochanteric fossa. The lateral surfaces and borders of the greater trochanter afford attachment to muscles from the gluteal, obturator, and pelvic regions

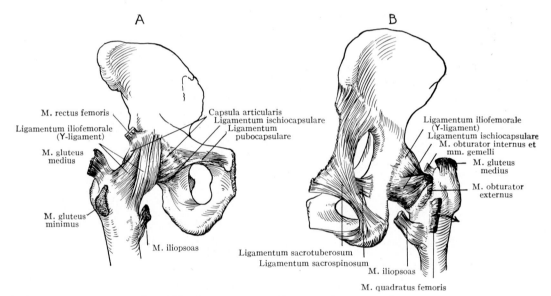

Fig. 692.—Ligaments and Tendons About the Hip.
A, Anterior view. B, Posterior view.

which help control rotation and abduction in the lower extremity. The tip or most prominent point of the greater trochanter is toward its posterior surface opposite the center of the hip joint. The *lesser trochanter* is on the medial and posterior surface of the shaft, at a more inferior level than the greater trochanter. The anterior and posterior intertrochanteric line and crest run in front of and behind the neck of the femur. They are roughened to accommodate the attachments of the various rotators of the hip and for the attachment of the capsular ligament.

At birth, the entire proximal end of the femur is cartilaginous. Development of the head of the femur is from an epiphysis in which a bony nucleus appears in the first year. This epiphysis joins the neck between the eighteenth and twentieth years. The neck is ossified by a proximal extension from the diaphysis. The greater trochanter begins to ossify in the second year and joins the neck and shaft in the eighteenth or nineteenth year. The lesser trochanter has a separate epiphysis which appears about the twelfth year and joins the shaft in the eighteenth year.

3. **Capsule and Its External Reinforcing Ligaments.**—The *capsule* of the hip joint possesses great strength; it is attached proximally to the bony circumference of the acet-

abulum, to the glenoid labrum (cotyloid ligament), and to the transverse ligament. All of the anterior surface and the medial half of the posterior surface of the neck of the femur are intracapsular.

Almost all the blood vessels entering the head of the femur reach it by way of the capsular attachments. A subcapital fracture of the neck of the femur, proximal to the inferior capsular attachment, destroys all the blood supply to the central fragment except that entering through the ligamentum teres. This fragment is dependent on new blood vessels growing in from the femoral neck to supplement this supply. Sclerosis of the proximal fragment often ensues. When some portion of the capsule is attached to the proximal fragment, as occurs in fracture through the base and distal half of the neck, there are better prospects for union.

The capsule is reinforced by certain accessory bands, the iliofemoral, pubocapsular, and ischiocapsular ligaments. The *iliofemoral ligament* (Y-*ligament of Bigelow*), the strongest in the body, thickens the anterior part of the capsule. It passes downward from its origin at the anterior inferior spine and spreads fanlike to an insertion into the anterior intertrochanteric line. The Y-ligament is under tension in all movements at the hip save flexion, and its rôle is of prime importance in the mechanics of dislocation of the hip.

The posterior capsule is reinforced by the *pubocapsular* and *ischiocapsular* ligaments which are much weaker than the iliofemoral ligament. The *ischiocapsular* (*ischiotemoral*) *ligament* lies over the posterior aspect of the capsule and helps to prevent too great a degree of medial rotation.

The *ligamentum teres* is intracapsular but extrasynovial. It is a triangularly flattened band attached proximally to a broad base in the acetabular notch and transverse ligament. By its distal narrow extremity, it is attached to a small depression on the summit of the head of the femur (fovea). It is surrounded completely by a tube of synovial membrane.

The *synovial membrane* of the hip joint covers the deep surface of the capsule. At the distal attachment of the capsule, the synovia is reflected to the femoral neck.

4. Reinforcing Muscles of the Hip Joint.—The strength of the hip joint depends considerably upon the powerful muscles surrounding it. The iliopsoas muscle overlies the capsule anteriorly and inserts into the lesser trochanter. The external rotator muscles are the piriformis, gemelli, obturator, and quadratus femoris muscles, and they pass across the posterior surface of the joint and are inserted into the greater trochanter and into the proximal part of the shaft. The chief internal rotators are the anterior portion of the gluteus medius and the tensor fasciae latae muscles. The gluteus medius and minimus muscles, which are attached to the greater trochanter, are abductors. The length of the neck of the femur and the prominent projection of the greater trochanter afford powerful leverage to the muscles attached to this bony prominence.

5. Movements.—There are all varieties of movement at the hip joint. *Flexion*, especially, has a very free range. When the knee is flexed, the movement is checked only by contact of the thigh with the anterior abdominal wall; when the knee is extended, however, flexion of the hip is much less free, and straight leg-raising (p. 422) cannot be carried beyond a right angle, because of the tension of the hamstring muscles. *Extension* is checked by the iliofemoral ligament when the lower limb reaches a few degrees behind a straight line with the trunk. This stout ligament, stretched over the head and the anterior aspect of the neck of the femur, powerfully braces the front of the joint.

The movement of *abduction* is free until it is checked by the pubocapsular ligament and by the contact of the upper part of the neck of the femur with the acetabular margin. *External rotation* is checked by the iliofemoral ligament when the thigh is extended. *Adduction* of the thigh is very limited because of the limbs coming into contact. The range of adduction is appreciable when the thigh is flexed slightly, but is restricted in this position by the iliofemoral ligament and the upper part of the capsule. *Internal rotation* is limited by the iliofemoral ligament when the thigh is extended, and by the ischiocapsular ligament when the thigh is flexed.

SURGICAL CONSIDERATIONS

1. Examination of the Hip Joint.—The gait may aid in making the diagnosis of hip joint disturbance, so that, if possible, the patient should walk stripped. A limp or a limitation of active movement is observed carefully. The patient then is placed on his back on a hard surface and the bony prominences are outlined and marked. The position of the femoral head is determined. The measurements of both limbs are taken, and the nature and extent of the active and passive motions are studied. Hyperextension is studied with the patient in the prone position, with his pelvis fixed by placing the hand on his sacrum. The distance the thigh may be lifted from the table is measured. The x-ray is a very important adjunct in the diagnosis of injury or disease in the hip.

2. Actual or Bony Measurement of the Lower Limbs.—Comparative measurement of the actual length of the two limbs is essential in the diagnosis and important in the treatment of injury or disease in the hip region. The ability to measure accurately requires knowledge, care, and practice. It is not unusual for the limbs to show trifling differences in length, and a difference not exceeding 1 cm. is disregarded because it does not alter the gait. Bony landmarks are preferable to soft parts in accurate measurements. The bony points must be identified carefully and the measuring tape must be applied accurately. It is essential that the pelvis is not tilted and that the limbs are in corresponding positions. To rule out lateral tilting of the pelvis, it is necessary that a line joining the anterior superior spines be at right angles to the long axis of the body (linea alba).

Measurements are made from the anterior superior spine to the distal margin of the medial condyle of the femur and from that point to the tip of the medial malleolus, or the measurement may be made directly from the anterior superior spine to the medial malleolus across the middle of the patella. The tip of the medial malleolus usually is easy to identify, but the anterior superior spine is not found so readily. The iliac crest is followed forward until its anterior superior spine can be felt distinctly. It is more satisfactory to press the tape firmly upward and backward against the inferior surface of the spine than to rest it upon the skin over the most superficial surface of the spine. The anterior superior spine often is so rounded that it is an uncertain point from which to measure. The deformity in femoral shortening may be ascribed to the shaft or to the surgical neck by comparing the measurements from the tip of the greater trochanter to the distal margin of the lateral femoral condyles, in addition to measuring the distance between the anterior superior spine and the medial malleolus. If the measurements from the trochanter to the condyle are equal, the deformity is in the femoral neck, and if they are unequal, the deformity is in the shaft.

To obtain comparable measurements when one hip is ankylosed, the affected femur is moved with the pelvis until the line joining the anterior superior spines is at right angles to the long axis of the body, and the pelvis is level. The normal limb is placed in a corresponding position.

3. Apparent Measurements of the Lower Limbs.—The abnormal positions assumed by the lower extremities in hip joint disease result from muscle action. Usually, neither abduction nor adduction of the limb is recognized as such by the patient. The usual complaint is that one limb seems longer or shorter than the other. The explanation of apparent lengthening and shortening lies in the degree of tilting of the pelvis and in the degree of adduction or abduction at the hip. The degree of tilting of the pelvis is determined by drawing a line from the anterior superior iliac spine of one side to the anterior superior iliac spine of the other side. The line normally is at right angles to the long axis of the body.

The accompanying diagrams explain the findings. The normal relation of the pelvis to the limbs is shown in the first figure of each diagram. In this position, both lower extremities are nearly at right angles to the pelvis, which is the normal position for standing or walking. If the right leg is fixed by muscle spasm or is ankylosed in an adducted position, the relationships are changed. In order to make the legs parallel for standing or walking, the pelvis is tilted upward on the adducted side. It is apparent that the ele-

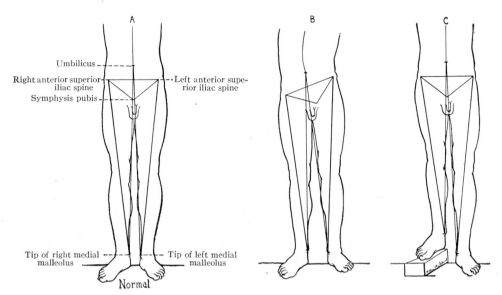

FIG. 693.—DIAGRAMS TO ILLUSTRATE ACTUAL OR BONY SHORTENING OF THE LOWER EXTREMITY.

A shows equal lower extremities, in which measurements from the anterior superior iliac spines to the medial malleoli are identical. In B, the right lower extremity is actually much the shorter. In order to place both feet upon the ground, the pelvis must be tilted down on the short side. The trunk is shifted to the left to maintain balance. In C, a lift is placed under the short leg. This restores the pelvis to the normal horizontal position and brings the trunk upright.

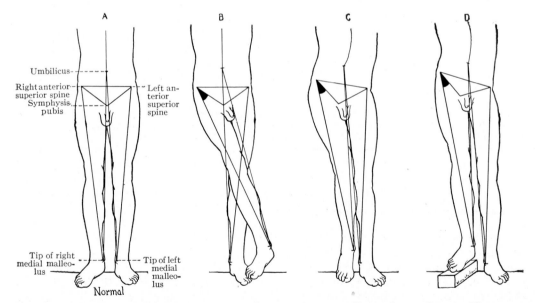

FIG. 694.—DIAGRAMS TO ILLUSTRATE APPARENT SHORTENING IN THE RIGHT LOWER LIMB IN WHICH THE HIP IS FIXED IN ADDUCTION, EITHER BY MUSCLE CONTRACTION OR BY ANKYLOSIS. THERE IS NO BONY SHORTENING OF EITHER LOWER EXTREMITY.

A is a normal individual, in whom there is no actual or apparent shortening. In B, the right thigh is fixed in adduction. The actual or bony measurements of the two lower limbs are equal, but the apparent measurements, taken from the umbilicus to the medial malleoli, show that the adducted limb is apparently shortened. Unless the pelvis is tilted upward on the side of the adducted thigh, the right leg cannot be brought parallel with the left in a walking position. In C, the adducted right extremity is brought parallel with the left extremity by an upward tilting of the pelvis on the adducted side. This maneuver throws the trunk to the left to restore balance. The left thigh is forced into an abduction position. It is obvious that the adducted extremity is apparently shortened and the heel is elevated and the toes are depressed. The actual measurements are the same. In D, a support is placed under the adducted extremity to allow locomotion.

vation of the pelvis on the right carries the right limb upward. To all appearances, the adducted right leg is shorter than the abducted left leg when the patient stands or lies straight. That these differences are apparent only is shown by comparing measurements from the umbilicus to the internal malleoli with those from the anterior superior iliac spines to the internal malleoli.

If the *left leg is fixed in abduction* by muscle spasm or ankylosis, the pelvis must be tilted upward on the sound side to make the legs parallel for standing or walking. The left leg then appears longer than the right. The amount of apparent lengthening depends upon the amount of abduction. The illusion as to the actual inequality in the length of the limbs is dispelled by comparing the measurements taken from the umbilicus to the medial malleoli with those taken from the anterior superior iliac spines to the medial malleoli.

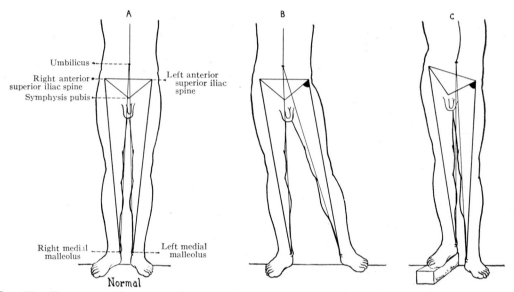

FIG. 695.—DIAGRAMS TO ILLUSTRATE APPARENT LENGTHENING IN THE LEFT LOWER LIMB IN WHICH THE HIP IS FIXED IN ABDUCTION, EITHER BY MUSCLE CONTRACTION OR BY ANKYLOSIS. THERE IS NO ACTUAL OR BONY SHORTENING IN EITHER LOWER EXTREMITY.

A is a normal individual, in whom there is no actual or apparent lengthening. In B, the left thigh is fixed in abduction. The actual or bony measurements of the two lower limbs, taken from the anterior superior iliac spines, are equal, but the apparent measurements, taken from the umbilicus to the medial malleoli, show that the abducted limb is apparently lengthened. It is obvious that the abducted left leg cannot be brought to parallel the right leg in walking, unless the pelvis is tilted upward on the sound side. In C, a block is placed under the sound lower extremity and the pelvis is depressed markedly on the affected side. The apparent lengthening of the abducted leg is very marked.

If the *lower limb is fixed in adduction*, there is, functionally, a shortening of the adducted leg which is caused by upward tilting of the pelvis on the affected side. Locomotion is facilitated by performing an osteotomy on the affected femur and placing it in abduction, or by elevating the adducted limb with a block. Fixation of the lower limb in abduction causes a downward tilting of the pelvis and functionally a lengthening of the affected extremity. Locomotion is made possible by elevating the sound limb with a block. The tilting of the pelvis produces a scoliosis in the lumbar spine.

4. Tuberculosis of the Hip.—Tuberculosis of the hip originates most frequently as an osteomyelitic lesion in the neck of the femur close to the epiphyseal cartilage of the head of the bone, but rarely it may begin in the synovia. Primarily, the disease is intracapsular and almost always is extrasynovial, so that infection of the hip joint occurs with great frequency. In the progress of the disease, the infection reaches the surface of the bone, destroys the periosteum, and invades the synovia. A joint effusion usually accompanies these changes. If effusion develops early, adhesions may form between the synovia lining the capsule and that on the femoral neck, and delay further extension of the disease into the joint. Adhesions cause limitation of motion, which may be the first sign of disease. If adhesions do not form, the lesion erodes the articular cartilage and becomes intrasynovial. The initial lesion very rarely erodes the epiphyseal cartilage without first involving the joint.

The focus may be at the diaphyseal side of the epiphysis of the greater trochanter and may spread down the shaft as an osteomyelitis. The caries may ascend along the neck and ultimately involve the joint or, rarely, may break through the periosteum outside the joint, forming an abscess and, subsequently, a sinus. The tuberculous process may develop in any of the three components of the acetabulum (p. 417). Involvement of the joint is opposed by the articular cartilage only.

The diagnostic symptoms in the course of hip joint tuberculosis present points of anatomical interest. An early diagnostic sign, and one upon which a great deal of reliance may be placed, is the presence of *stiffness in the joint* or of *limitation of motion* when the limb is manipulated. Limitation can be noticed very early in the disease, unless the focus is remote from the joint. The restriction of motion is not the result of adhesions or beginning ankylosis early in the disease, but is caused by a tonic contraction of the muscles which control the joint. Slight degrees of stiffness may be revealed by comparing the resistance in one limb with that in the other, or, particularly, by flexing the thigh at right angles to the body and placing it in extreme abduction and external rotation. A change in the arc of any motion of the joint should arouse suspicion of disease in the joint. In the later stages of tuberculosis, complete stiffness in the joint may occur. Stiffness from muscle spasm disappears, in a measure, under complete anesthesia. Intermittent *limping* is an important sign, but its absence does not exclude hip joint disease.

After the onset of inflammatory changes within the joint, the limb adopts a characteristic attitude. It is flexed moderately, abducted, and rotated outwardly at the hip. This position permits the maximum relaxation and the greatest fluid content of the capsule, and, therefore, is the position of greatest ease. Any attempt to extend the limb is resisted strongly by the contraction of the muscles about the joint, as the effect of extension is to tense the iliofemoral ligament tightly over the front of the joint and to press the head of the femur against the acetabulum. The pressure causes acute pain.

In the standing position, the weight of the body is borne mainly on the healthy limb to avoid pain from weight-bearing on the affected limb. The eversion of the foot is the index of external rotation. The affected leg characteristically is placed in advance of the sound one and there is bending at the groin. Tilting of the pelvis may or may not be apparent, but can be demonstrated by careful examination. There is a change in the gluteal folds and in the buttocks. The gluteal fold on the diseased side is shorter and lower in position as a result of the downward tilt of the pelvis on that side; the buttock is flattened.

The attitude assumed by the patient in lying on a flat surface is characteristic. In order to bring the flexed thigh into contact with the surface, the spine is arched forward in the dorsolumbar region (lordosis) (p. 540). The pelvis on the affected side is tilted downward to bring the affected limb into contact with the sound one. The transverse axis of the pelvis, as indicated by a line through both anterior superior iliac spines, is very oblique. This causes the limb on the affected side to appear longer than the other, although careful measurement reveals no actual difference. The amount of fixed flexion of the limb may be determined by the Thomas test (Fig. 696); the hip and knee of the sound limb are flexed passively until the thigh comes to rest against the abdomen. This maneuver throws the affected thigh into flexion deformity. The angle formed by the axis of the affected thigh with the table denotes the extent of permanent flexion.

If destruction within the joint continues, the attitude of the limb undergoes a change. Flexion at the hip continues, but the limb exchanges a position of abduction and external rotation for one of adduction and internal rotation. The changes in position probably are dependent upon the softening or relaxation of the ligaments, and the destruction of the head of the femur and the acetabulum associated with a weakness of the external rotator muscles, and excessive action of the adductor muscle group. If the patient lies on a flat surface, it is necessary to raise the pelvis on the diseased side in order to bring the adducted limb alongside its fellow. The transverse axis of the adducted limb, as indicated by a line joining the anterior superior spines, is markedly oblique, but the obliquity is inclined in the opposite direction from that noted in the first stage. With the obliquity of the later stage of the disease, the affected limb appears to be shortened, but measurement reveals no actual shortening.

After the disease has caused a dislocation of the partially disintegrated head of the femur and advanced dissolution of the acetabulum, there begins a stage of real shortening of the limb. The head of the femur is dislocated upward and backward on the dorsum of the ilium, while the limb remains flexed, adducted, and rotated medially. This position is assumed by the limb in spontaneous cure. Real shortening is not, of necessity, an indication of dislocation, but may be the result of absorption of the head of the femur and widening of the acetabulum. Eventually, the displaced femur may become ankylosed firmly to the ilium and the acetabular cavity may be filled with granulation tissue.

Pain is a very important, though rarely an early, symptom. It may be in the hip, but very often is referred to the medial or anterior aspect of the knee. This reflex phe-

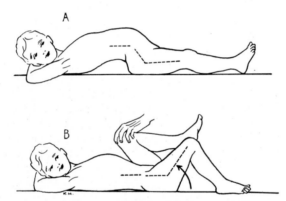

Fig. 696.—Thomas Test for the Degree of Flexion Deformity in Fixation of the Hip in Tuberculosis.

The degree of flexion deformity can be determined only after the compensatory lumbar lordosis has been obliterated; forced flexion of the sound thigh on the abdomen obliterates the lordosis.

nomenon is intelligible when it is recalled that both joints are innervated from the femoral (p. 703) and obturator (p. 711) nerves. In time, the muscle spasm becomes increased to a degree which fixes the disorganized articular surfaces, and relaxes only during sleep. Night cries, typically coming before midnight when sleep is most profound, are caused by the momentary pain resulting from movements of one eroded bone against the other, permitted by the relaxation of sleep. The muscle spasm tends to create permanent deformity, because the position assumed by the limb is not a functional one, but is dictated by the most powerful group of muscles.

5. **Abscesses in Tuberculosis of the Hip and Their Paths of Extension.**—Tuberculosis of the hip almost always becomes intrasynovial; therefore, suppuration in the joint is the rule rather than the exception. The effusion may cause a slight fullness in the femoral triangle (of Scarpa) just inferior to the inguinal ligament and beneath the femoral vessels. The pus eventually perforates the capsule at its weakest points, which are posterolateral and anterior, but it may spread into the pelvis.

If the exit is posterolateral or posterior, the pus at first collects between the gluteal muscles and the lateral surface of the ilium. It apparently finds no obstacle to forward progress, for it usually travels anteriorly deep to the gluteus maximus and tensor fasciae latae muscles to point in the interval between the tensor fasciae latae and the sartorius muscles. The abscess may travel backward, however, and point in the gluteal region at the transverse gluteal fold.

The path taken by pus which has *perforated the anterior part of the capsule* is not constant. If the joint communicates with the iliopsoas bursa, the pus may ascend within the bursa to the iliac fossa or may enter the sheath of the iliopsoas muscle. Pus may descend along the iliopsoas tendon, follow the course of the medial circumflex artery, reach the dorsum of the thigh over the upper border of the adductor magnus muscle, and point at the gluteal fold; or it may pass laterally along the lateral circumflex artery and become superficial near the gluteal fold or near the greater trochanter.

Occasionally, the abscess makes its way through the acetabulum into the pelvis, especially when the tuberculosis originates in the acetabulum. The direction of *intrapelvic spread* depends upon whether the infection pierces the pelvic wall above or below the line of origin of the levator ani muscle (p. 429). In the first instance, the pus erodes the parietal pelvic fascia and is free to extend in the extraperitoneal space of the pelvis. It may travel down along the rectum or fill up the pelvis until it overflows through the obturator foramen or escapes forward into the thigh behind the inguinal ligament. When the hip joint abscess pierces the pelvic wall below the origin of the levator ani, the pus invades the ischiorectal fossa and points near the anus. A collection of pus on the pelvic aspect of the acetabulum may be recognized by digital rectal examination. If the abscess results in sinus formation, the clinical picture becomes one of mixed infection. The x-ray then may show areas of new bone formation and sequestration. These findings are absent in uncomplicated tuberculosis.

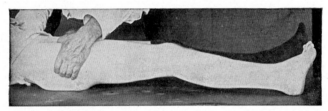

FIG. 697.—METHOD OF PALPATING THE GREAT TROCHANTER. (Scudder, "Treatment of Fractures.")

Pyogenic osteomyelitis, that devastating disease peculiar to shafts at their metaphyseal extremities, must be differentiated from tuberculosis. Pyogenic osteomyelitis frequently invades the neck of the femur, which is the superior and medial continuation of the shaft. The lesion is intra-articular by virtue of the capsular attachment, and is propagated swiftly to the synovia and to the other joint structures. Pyogenic osteomyelitis destroys the joint in a graver and more septic manner than does tuberculosis. It is accompanied by prostration, pyrexia, and marked leukocytosis. The x-ray shows no bony changes in the acute stages but shows areas of new bone formation late in the disease. Very early radical drainage is imperative.

6. **Injuries of the Upper Extremity of the Femur in General.**—In the *infant*, the cartilaginous upper extremity of the femur, which includes the head and neck, may be fractured. The fracture may occur when the infant, held upright, throws itself backward so that the body weight stretches the strong iliofemoral ligament across the anterior surface of the head and neck of the femur. When the limbs are held firmly, the neck of the femur gives way, since the restraining ligament is too strong to yield; if the limbs are not held firmly, the backward thrust of the body weight on the iliofemoral ligament flexes the thigh and relieves the strain.

In a *child*, injury about the upper extremity of the femur may result in a greenstick fracture, as the cartilaginous neck is undergoing ossification. This lesion probably is one of the most frequent causes of coxa vara. In *later childhood*, separation of the epiphysis of the femoral head sometimes occurs. The diagnosis of this condition is very important lest the epiphysis be allowed to unite in a faulty position and result in subsequent limitation of motion.

In vigorous *middle life*, dislocation of the head of the femur is the commonest severe lesion. In *later life*, trivial trauma may cause fracture of the neck of the femur.

7. **Epiphyseal Separation of the Proximal Extremity of the Femur.**—Separation of the capital epiphysis of the femur usually does not occur in childhood when the epiphysis is cartilaginous, but does occur in adolescence when the epiphysis is bony and is uniting with the neck. As a rule, separation occurs from minor trauma and from a stumble in which the leg is hyperextended. Separation frequently occurs in the overweight children of the Fröhlich type (dystrophia adiposogenitalis), in whom ossification is delayed. The iliofemoral (**Y**) ligament holds the neck of the femur forward and the epiphysis is levered from its position. If the displacement is partial, there is a persistent limp, slight shortening, limitation of abduction and internal rotation, and excessive external rotation. *x*-Ray examination shows a coxa vara outline. Complete displacement of the epiphysis resembles fracture of the neck of the femur; there is shortening and eversion of the limb.

An attempt should be made to replace the epiphysis by hyperabduction, extension, and internal rotation. If these maneuvers fail, open reduction is required.

8. **Fracture of the Neck of the Femur.**—Fracture of the neck of the femur usually occurs in persons over sixty, particularly in women. It leads to many fatalities and much chronic invalidism, and may result in extensive deformity, even when considerable function has been restored. When fracture occurs at a high level (subcapital), the blood supply

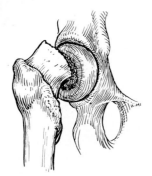

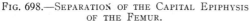

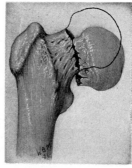

FIG. 698.—SEPARATION OF THE CAPITAL EPIPHYSIS OF THE FEMUR.

FIG. 699.—SUBCAPITAL FRACTURE OF THE NECK OF THE FEMUR. (Babcock, "Textbook of Surgery.")

to the head of the femur from the neck is damaged. The supply by way of the ligamentum teres (p. 679) frequently is inadequate. When fracture occurs at a lower level, part of the posterior capsule usually is left attached to the proximal fragment, affording it, at best, a feeble blood supply. Since the fracture commonly occurs at an age when the cortex of the bone is thinned and its internal structure is weakened, the power of bone repair is diminished.

The cause of fracture may be a stumble, a fall, or, in vigorous adults, a fall upon the greater trochanter. It also may be occasioned by exaggerated movements at the hip joint. The line of fracture may be just below the head, through the middle of the neck, or just above the trochanters. The closer the break is to the head of the femur, the less ligamentous attachment is left upon the proximal fragment and the poorer is the prospect of repair. The more extensive the ligamentous attachment to the proximal fragment, that is, the farther toward the trochanter the neck is divided, the more adequate is the blood supply and the better is the chance of union. The presence or absence of impaction is a significant factor. An efficient impaction at the base of the neck is an aid to union.

In any variety of fracture of the neck of the femur, shortening of the limb is the rule. This is attributed to the tension of the powerful muscles with which the femur is surrounded—the glutei, adductors, hamstrings, iliopsoas, and rectus femoris. The summit of the greater trochanter rises above its normal level, exceeds Nélaton's line, and shortens the base of Bryant's triangle. In fractures near the femoral head, the shortening of the limb is greater than in fractures nearer the trochanter.

When the greater trochanter ascends, following fracture of the femoral neck, that portion of the fascia lata which stretches between this prominence and the iliac crest

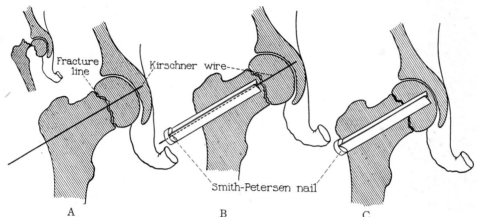

FIG. 700.—USE OF FLANGED-NAIL METHOD (SMITH-PETERSEN) IN INTERNAL FIXATION OF FRACTURE OF THE NECK OF THE FEMUR.

A, Drill guide wire into trochanter, neck, and head of femur; B, flanged nail threaded over wire and driven into anatomic neck; C, nail in position and wire removed. (Henderson, Surg., Gynec. and Obst., Feb. 15, 1935.)

becomes relaxed unduly, so that the tenseness or resistance of the tissues to pressure immediately above the trochanter is less on the injured side than on the sound side. The limb lies in helpless eversion. This depends to some extent on its tendency to roll outward under the influence of gravity and to the action of the external rotator muscles, which are stronger than the medial rotators.

In the *abduction treatment*, complete abduction, hyperextension, and internal rotation are instituted after the shortening has been overcome by traction. The maintenance of the abduction position in fixation

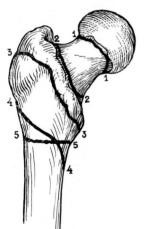

FIG. 701.—LINES OF FRACTURE IN THE UPPER EXTREMITY OF THE FEMUR.

1, Supcapital fracture of the neck of the femur; 2, fracture through the base of the neck; 3, pertrochanteric fracture; 4, oblique subtrochanteric fracture; 5, transverse subtrochanteric fracture.

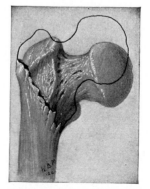

FIG. 702.—PERTROCHANTERIC FRACTURE OF THE FEMUR. (Babcock, "Textbook of Surgery.")

prevents shortening and coxa vara formation, and apposes the fragments in a manner most favorable to bony or fibrous union. In robust individuals, absolute reduction should be obtained, even if an open operation is required, with the insertion of a peg of bone which extends from the trochanter through the neck into the head of the bone.

44

Plastic operations upon the proximal end of the femur are followed by fixation in **ab-duction.**

     9. Intertrochanteric and Pertrochanteric Fractures.—*Intertrochanteric tractures* are similar in cause and displacement to fractures at the base of the femoral neck. The fracture line follows the anterior oblique intertrochanteric line, and usually is impacted with slight displacement of the fragments. The spongy, vascular character of the bone at this level is conducive to bony union, but some degree of coxa vara is likely to ensue. If the fracture is not impacted, the extremity should be immobilized in moderate abduction, extension, and internal rotation.

     A *pertrochanteric fracture* usually passes through the base of the neck or upper part of the shaft, distal to the greater trochanter and proximal to the lesser trochanter. The treatment is similar to that for intertrochanteric fracture.

     10. Traumatic Dislocation of the Hip.—Traumatic dislocation of the hip is comparatively rare because of the great stability the hip derives from its powerful capsule and

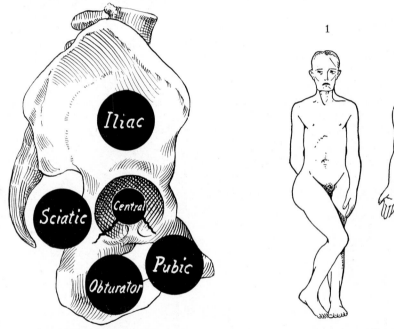

FIG. 703.—LOCATION OF THE HEAD OF THE FEMUR IN THE COMMONER VARIETIES OF DISLOCATION OF THE HIP. (Eisendrath in "Keen's Surgery.")

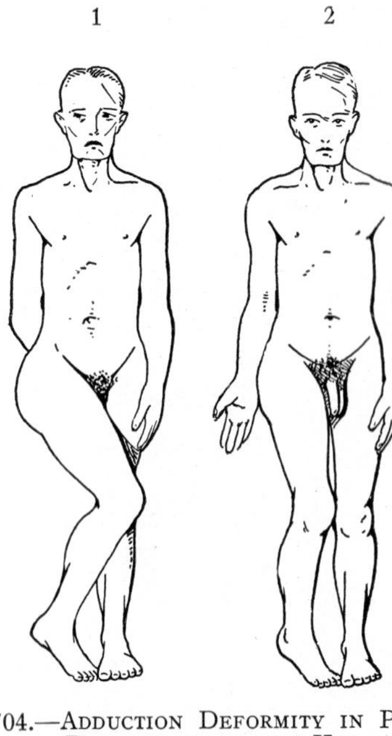

FIG. 704.—ADDUCTION DEFORMITY IN POSTERIOR DISLOCATION OF THE HIP.
1, Dorsal (iliac) dislocation. 2, Ischial (sciatic) dislocation. (Babcock, "Textbook of Surgery.")

from the strong muscles surrounding it. The joint is particularly secure above, in front, and behind, because the socket of the acetabulum is deep and the rim is strong at these points. At its lower part, the acetabular cavity is comparatively shallow and part of its rim is deficient.

     Posterior dislocation is produced by indirect violence applied through the feet, legs, or back when the thigh is flexed, adducted, and rotated medially. The injury often is produced by a heavy weight falling upon the sacrum when the patient is in a stooping position with the lower limbs flexed and rotated medially. In this position, the femoral shaft is the long arm of the lever, the iliofemoral (Y) ligament is the fulcrum and the neck is the short arm of the lever. The head is forced against the posterior part of the capsule, tears it, and passes upward and backward on the dorsum of the ilium, superior to the tendon of the obturator internus muscle; it may occupy an iliac or a sciatic position. The short rotator muscles of the femur, particularly the obturator internus muscle, are liable to injury. The strongest part of the capsule, the iliofemoral (Y) ligament, usually is not ruptured but the posterior capsule is torn widely. The tendon of the obturator internus muscle may be interposed between the neck of the femur and the socket. There may be damage to the sciatic nerve.

In the iliac variety of posterior dislocation, the femoral head lies on the dorsum of the ilium and can be felt in the buttock. The thigh is flexed, adducted, and rotated inward, a position which is determined mainly by the tension of the iliofemoral ligament and the direction of the inclined plane against which the head and neck of the femur rest. The foot is inverted and the heel sometimes rests on the dorsum of the opposite foot. Flexion of the thigh is marked when the femoral head remains low, but is slight when it is high on the ilium (the usual position). With this upward displacement of the femur, shortening always is present; the amount may be estimated readily by noting how far the summit of the greater trochanter projects proximal to Nélaton's line. There is a marked alteration in the contour of the hip; the normal depression behind the trochanter is obliterated; the gluteal fold is raised; there is an unusual fullness of the buttock, and it may be possible to feel the head of the femur or the trochanter beneath the gluteus maximus muscle. Abduction and external rotation of the thigh are impossible. The deformity of *sciatic dislocation* (into the sciatic notch) is similar to, but less noticeable than, dislocation on the dorsum of the ilium, and the mode of production is very similar. Flexion and inversion of the

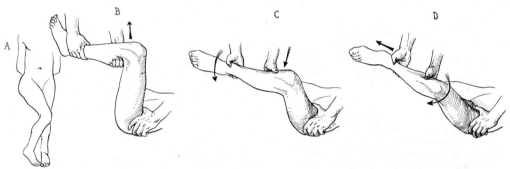

FIG. 705.—BIGELOW'S METHOD OF REDUCTION OF A POSTERIOR DISLOCATION AT THE HIP.
A is the deformity in posterior dislocation. In B, upward traction is exerted upon the flexed limb; the pelvis is steadied by an assistant. In C, the flexed limb is abducted while the pelvis is steadied. In D, the flexed and abducted limb is rotated laterally; the last step consists in extending the limb.

thigh sometimes are more marked in sciatic dislocation, in which the head of the femur rests upon the back of the ischium, close to its spine, partially overlies the two sciatic foramina, and lies below the tendon of the obturator internus muscle.

In the *Bigelow method for the reduction of posterior dislocation of the hip*, the head of the femur is made to retrace its course through the tear in the capsule. The main obstacle to the reduction of posterior dislocation is the tension of the iliofemoral (Y) ligament which keeps the limb flexed and adducted. This tension acts powerfully when an extending force is applied to the limb. To obviate this, the first step in reduction consists in flexing the thigh on the pelvis and adducting the limb, as these movements tend to disengage the head of the femur and enable it to be brought along the inclined plane posterior to the acetabulum toward the opening in the capsule. The thigh then is abducted and rotated laterally to bring the head of the femur opposite its socket. This movement renders the relaxed iliofemoral ligament tense so that it may be used as the fulcrum of the lever, which has the femoral shaft for its long arm and the neck for its short arm. The movement of lateral rotation levers the head forward over the posterior margin of the acetabulum. By completing the circumduction and extending the limb, the head is made to travel medially and upward into the socket.

In *Stimson's gravity or postural method of reduction of posterior dislocation of the hip*, the patient is placed face downward upon a table with his legs projecting beyond the edge of the table. The normal limb is held horizontally by an assistant while the injured thigh extends directly downward. The ankle of the injured limb is grasped and the knee is flexed to a right angle. The weight of the limb, in addition to that of a sand-bag placed upon the flexed half just below the knee, furnishes the necessary traction in the desired direction. The position is maintained until the muscles relax. The bone usually is felt to slip into place with no more manipulation than a slight rocking of the limb.

Anterior dislocation results from violent abduction of the thigh. The head of the femur leaves the inferomedial part of the socket and passes forward and mesially to rest upon the obturator foramen (obturator or thyroid dislocation), or reaches an even more anterior position beneath the pubis (pubic dislocation).

In *dislocation into the obturator foramen*, the femur comes to rest on the obturator externus muscle. The iliofemoral ligament is not torn, and, in conjunction with the iliopsoas muscle, it helps to maintain the limb slightly flexed, abducted, and rotated outward. The great trochanter is depressed and is less prominent than on the sound side, and its upper extremity impinges on the lower border of the acetabulum.

Dislocation upon the pubis is an advanced form of obturator dislocation. From its primary position inferior and slightly anterior to the acetabulum, the head of the femur advances forward and upward in front of the horizontal ramus of the pubis, opposite the iliopectineal eminence. It is impelled in this direction and to this position by a powerful everting action applied to the limb. The head of the femur may cause the iliopsoas muscle to project inferior to the inguinal ligament, carrying forward with it the femoral vessels and the femoral nerve. The iliopsoas and pectineus muscles may be lacerated, and the obturator and femoral nerves may be stretched or torn. The thigh is flexed, abducted, and rotated externally. Flexion results from the contraction of the iliopsoas muscle.

In the *reduction of anterior dislocation*, the thigh is flexed to a right angle and abducted to disengage the head of the femur. The thigh then is lifted, rotated medially, and extended so that the head of the femur may be made to retrace its path to the postero-inferior part of the acetabulum.

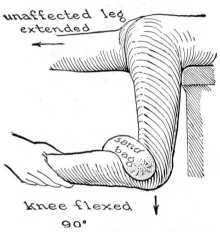

FIG. 706.—STIMSON'S METHOD OF REDUCING A POSTERIOR DISLOCATION OF THE HIP. (Babcock, "Textbook of Surgery.")

Intrapelvic or central dislocation of the head of the femur is a penetrating fracture of the acetabulum. Routine radiographic examination has demonstrated that it is not an unusual injury. The lesion occurs when a fall upon the hip drives the femoral head so violently into its socket as to fracture the acetabulum. It is an accident of vigorous middle age and is unlikely to occur in the elderly, in whom the femoral neck usually fractures before the head can damage the acetabulum. A radiating fracture of the acetabulum occurs with depression of the socket and a bulging inward of its central part. The socket may remain intact and be driven in as a whole. The head of the femur seldom is driven deeply into the pelvis.

The condition must be differentiated from ordinary dislocation and from fractures through and about the femoral neck. An impacted fracture through the neck of the femur or a trochanteric fracture at the base of the neck may resemble closely fracture of the acetabulum with central dislocation. In the latter condition, rectal examination should reveal the characteristic inward displacement of the acetabulum. The fracture dislocation is reduced by downward traction upon the leg, combined with an outward pull upon the upper thigh.

11. Surgical Approaches to the Neck of the Femur.—The horizontal limb of the incision for the *Smith-Petersen approach* to the hip joint begins a little below the midpoint of the iliac crest and extends forward in the direction of the crest to the anterior superior spine of the ilium. From this point, the incision is carried vertically downward between the tendons of the tensor fasciae latae and the sartorius muscles. The horizontal, or iliac crest portion of the incision is deepened through the origins of the gluteus maximus and gluteus medius muscles. The large flap of tissue thus formed is reflected subperiosteally downward and backward, without injuring vessels or nerves, until the anterior and superior surfaces of the joint are exposed.

In the *posterolateral approach (of Kocher)* the patient lies upon his sound side with the affected thigh flexed. The incision is carried from the inferior border of the greater trochanter upward along its anterior border to the anterosuperior angle. From this point, the incision angles upward and backward toward the posterosuperior iliac spine in the direction of the fibers of the gluteus maximus muscle. In the inferior (vertical) portion of the incision, the aponeurotic insertion of the gluteus maximus muscle is divided over the lateral aspect of the greater trochanter to the insertion of the gluteus medius muscle, the fibers of which cover most of the superior border of the trochanter. After locating the interval between the posterior edge of the gluteus medius muscles anteriorly and

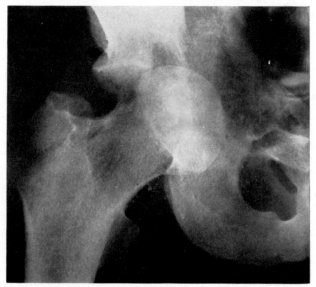

FIG. 707.—*x*-RAY OF INTRAPELVIC OR CENTRAL DISLOCATION OF THE HEAD OF THE FEMUR. (Callander.)

the piriformis muscle posteriorly, the insertions of the gluteus medius and minimus muscles are detached from the trochanter as far as the anterior portion of the intertrochanteric ridge and are carried forward. At this point, the femoral insertion of the iliofemoral ligament may be detached. After the femoral insertion of the piriformis muscle is detached subperiosteally, the external rotator muscles with their periosteal attachments may be retracted downward and backward. The posterior, lateral, and anterior surfaces of the head of the femur and the superior portion of the greater trochanter then are exposed.

The incision for the *posterolateral approach (of Langenbeck)* is a smaller and more laterally placed incision than that of Kocher. It is directed obliquely from the middle of the greater trochanter toward the posterior superior spine of the ilium in line with the long axis of the semiflexed femur. The incision is carried down to the gluteus maximus muscle. The tendon of the gluteus maximus muscle is incised on the trochanter and the muscle is split in the line of the wound. Retraction of the margins of the gluteus maximus exposes the gluteus medius and piriformis muscles. Separation of these muscles exposes the posterior surface of the capsule of the hip joint. The sciatic nerve may be damaged if the incision is carried too far medially.

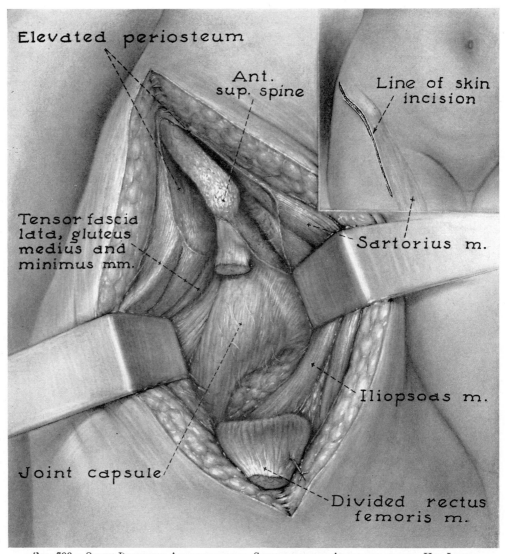

Elevated periosteum

Ant. sup. spine

Line of skin incision

Tensor fascia lata, gluteus medius and minimus mm.

Sartorius m.

Iliopsoas m.

Joint capsule

Divided rectus femoris m.

Fig. 708.—Smith-Petersen Anterolateral Subperiosteal Approach to the Hip Joint.

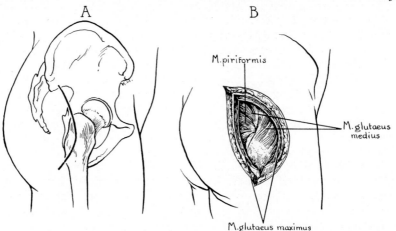

A   B

M.piriformis

M.glutaeus medius

M.glutaeus maximus

Fig. 709.—Kocher's Posterolateral Approach to the Hip Joint.
A, Skin incision and landmarks.   B, Incision through the gluteus maximus muscle.

The *lateral semilunar* (U-*shaped*) *approach* (*of Ollier*) is through a curved incision, the lowest point of which is at the base of the greater trochanter. The incision is carried anteriorly and superiorly between the gluteus medius and tensor fasciae latae muscles,

A   B

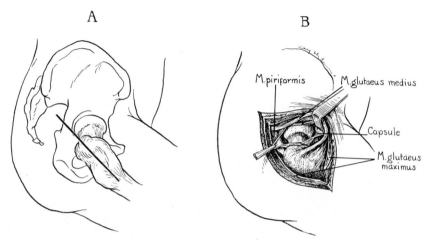

FIG. 710.—LANGENBECK'S POSTEROLATERAL APPROACH TO THE HIP JOINT.
A, Skin incision and landmarks.   B, Exposure of the hip joint.

and posteriorly and superiorly through the fibers of the gluteus maximus muscle. Division and upward retraction of the tendon-bearing greater trochanter exposes the hip joint thoroughly. Upon completion of the surgery within the joint, the trochanter is returned

A   B

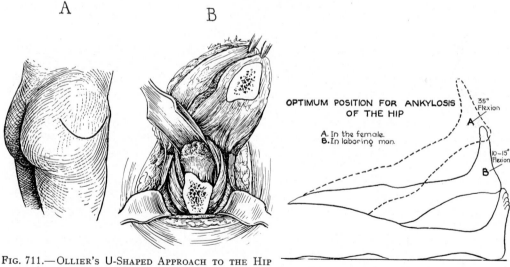

FIG. 711.—OLLIER'S U-SHAPED APPROACH TO THE HIP
JOINT.

A, Skin incision. B, The base of the great trochanter is sectioned and drawn upward and the head and neck of the femur are exposed.

FIG. 712.—OPTIMUM POSITIONS IN ANKYLOSIS OF
THE HIP JOINT.

The thigh is placed in slight abduction and external rotation.

to its normal position and is fixed there. Although this approach is used extensively because of the wide exposure it affords, the incision should be condemned for any purpose except arthrodesis of the hip joint as it divides the terminal branches of the superior gluteal nerve and paralyzes the tensor fasciae latae muscle.

II. THIGH

A. THIGH IN GENERAL

1. Boundaries and Divisions.—The thigh is bounded above and in front by the fold of the groin which corresponds in direction to the inguinal ligament. Its upper limit posteriorly is the transverse gluteal fold. The lower boundary of the thigh is a plane three fingerbreadths above the base of the patella, a level which corresponds to the upper limit of the subquadriceps bursa (p. 751).

The thigh is divided topographically into four regions: the inguinofemoral (root of the thigh); adductor (obturator); anterior (flexor); and posterior (extensor).

2 Landmarks.—The general outline of the limb is conical, and the oblique direction of the long axis is downward and inward. The obliquity is greater in females than in males because of the greater proportional width of the pelvis. In females, the general surface of the thigh is rounded uniformly by the great amount of subcutaneous fatty tissue. In vigorous adult males, well-developed muscles stand out in bold relief.

The sartorius muscle inclines downward and inward across the iliopsoas muscle from the anterior superior spine to its tibial insertion. It is rendered distinct by flexing the limb actively in outward rotation. The femoral trigone (of Scarpa) is the depression inferior to the inguinal ligament. In a well-muscled person, a definite groove extends from the apical extremity of the femoral trigone along the medial aspect of the thigh toward the medial condyle of the femur, especially when the thigh is flexed and abducted. This groove indicates the demarcation between the vastus medialis muscle laterally and the adductor musculature medially. The sartorius muscle descends within this groove; the groove overlies the femoral vessels in the adductor canal. Immediately superior to the patella is the flat tendon of the rectus femoris muscle; medial to the patella is the rounded mass of the vastus medialis muscle. A groove runs upward and medially from the lateral margin of the patella to the middle of the thigh and separates the rectus femoris muscle from the vastus lateralis. On the lateral side of the thigh is a longitudinal depression formed by the iliotibial band of the fascia lata. In this area, the deep fascia sends a partition inward to the linea aspera, the external (lateral) intermuscular septum, which separates the flexor group from the extensor group of thigh muscles. In the upper two thirds of the posterior part of the thigh, the hamstring muscles are grouped closely into a prominent mass. As they diverge toward the knee, the biceps and the semitendinosus tendons become prominent.

3. Deep Fascia (Fascia Lata) and Fascial Spaces.—The sheathing or **deep fascia** of the leg is a well-defined aponeurotic membrane which completely invests the muscles of the thigh. In the lower part of the thigh, it extends over the patella, the quadriceps tendon, and the capsule of the knee joint. It covers the popliteal space and binds together the muscles forming its margins.

The fascia lata varies in strength and thickness. It is unusually strong over the outer aspect of the thigh where it is reinforced by the insertions of the tensor fasciae latae and gluteus maximus muscles. This part of the fascia lata is known as the *iliotibial tract* and stretches from the lateral margin of the iliac crest to the external condyle of the tibia Over the lower part of the front of the thigh and over its medial surface, the fascia is comparatively thin.

It is contended by Ober that a *contracture of the iliotibial band* or of the lateral fascia lata in general causes limitation of motion, muscle spasm, tenderness over the lumbosacral or sacro-iliac regions, limitation of straight leg raising, and functional scoliosis. The abnormal pull on the pelvic bones causes bad posture. The contracted portion lies usually between the crest of the ilium and the anterior aspect of the trochanter. Incision of the fascia lata in this area, when contracture is definite, improves the disturbances mentioned above.

From its deep aspect, sheathing septa extend between the muscles. The *lateral intermuscular septum* is a strong partition which connects the deep fascia with the lateral lip of the linea aspera on the posterior surface of the shaft of the femur. This septum separates the lateral vastus muscle from the femoral (short) head of the biceps muscle and demarcates the extensor and flexor regions of the thigh. The septum begins at the level of the lowermost insertion of the gluteus maximus muscle inferior to the greater trochanter and terminates at the lateral aspect of the knee joint. The *medial intermuscular septum* is not as well defined as the lateral; it extends from the level of the lesser trochanter to the adductor tubercle and separates the adductor and extensor muscle compartments of the thigh.

These septa enclose the thigh muscles in three osteofibrous compartments, each of which has its own nerve. The anterior or extensor group of muscles is supplied by the femoral nerve, the posterior or flexor group by the sciatic nerve, and the medial or adductor group by the obturator nerve.

The arrangement of the fascia lata at the root of the thigh and about the fossa ovalis is described in the section on the inguinofemoral region (p. 701).

It is apparent (Milgram and Prentiss) that there is a large anterolateral *fascial space* which runs the entire length of the thigh. This space communicates superiorly with a large posterior fascial area under the gluteus maximus muscle. In direct continuation with the subgluteal space is the fascial space which extends downward about the diverging hamstring muscles and tendons.

4. **Pathogenesis of Infections Within the Deep Fascial Spaces of the Thigh.**—Infections adjacent to the deep fascial spaces of the thigh may rupture into them. When these potential spaces are infected, pus or extravasations of blood may travel long distances and point in areas remote from the initial lesion.

Hematogenous infection may localize in the fascial spaces of the thigh. Hematomata from fracture of the neck of the femur may become infected, and the resulting abscess cavity may extend upward under the gluteus maximus muscle and downward into the anterior or posterior fascial spaces. Hematogenous infections in the posterior fascial space often have been observed without involvement of the popliteal space. Infected emboli may cause widespread infection of the fascial spaces.

Infections may be introduced directly into the fascial spaces by hypodermic injections and hypodermoclysis. Extraspatial purulent foci may extend into the deep spaces. Tuberculous abscess from the spine or sacro-iliac joint, or retroperitoneal suppurating glands may involve these spaces. These purulent collections follow an anterior route beneath the inguinal ligament or a posterior path through the suprapiriformic and infrapiriformic foramina (p. 429). Lesions of the ilium which perforate the gluteus medius muscle may rupture into the posterior space and point far down the thigh. Lesions of the hip joint, the greater trochanter, or the shaft of the femur may involve either the anterior or the posterior space. Among the intraspatial lesions which burrow down the fascial spaces are infected bursae and lymph glands.

The complications of fascial space infection are: extension from one space to another; persistent draining sinuses from inadequate drainage of the original focus or of the fascial compartment; and involvement of the vasculoneural element in the floors of the spaces. Femoral and sciatic nerve involvement is common, and femoral phlebitis and arterial thrombosis have been observed.

Efficient treatment consists in accurate preoperative localization followed by drainage of the primary focus, and adequate drainage of the fascial space or spaces involved. The anterior fascial compartment may be incised widely through an incision begun behind the greater trochanter, because only the subcutaneous tissue and the deep fascia are encountered. The incision can be extended downward and forward almost the entire length of the thigh.

When the lesion is in the posterior space about the greater trochanter, the upper two thirds of the fibers of the gluteus maximus tendon should be divided near their insertion on the trochanter. Simple splitting of the gluteus maximus muscle is likely to be unsatisfactory as drainage becomes blocked in a short time. The principles and details of the treatment by packing and immobilization are adapted to these infections.

B. INGUINOFEMORAL OR SUBINGUINAL REGION

1. **Definition and Boundaries.**—The inguinofemoral region includes the soft parts at the root of the thigh. It is bounded above by the inguinal ligament, medially by the pectineus muscle, and laterally by the tensor fasciae latae muscle. Its lower boundary is an artificial horizontal line passing through the apex of the femoral triangle (of Scarpa).

2. **Landmarks.**—In a well-muscled male, the muscles in this region are prominent, especially when the hip and knee joints are flexed and the limb is rotated laterally. In this attitude, the surface of the thigh is flattened or depressed for some distance below the inguinal ligament. From the distal part of the flattened area, two muscle prominences diverge upward. The medial prominence corresponds to the pectineus and adductor longus muscles. The medial margin of the adductor longus becomes very distinct when the thigh is adducted against resistance. Its rounded tendon can be felt and traced to the pubic tubercle, even in obese individuals. The sartorius muscle forms the lateral prominence. The area included between these muscles and the inguinal ligament is known as the femoral trigone (of Scarpa).

Within the femoral triangle, the femoral artery and often the superficial subinguinal lymph glands are palpable. The inguinal ligament forms a ridge passing from the anterior superior spine to the pubic tubercle. The location of the tubercle is utilized in differentiating between a femoral and an inguinal hernia. The neck of a femoral hernia lies inferior to the tubercle, while that of an inguinal hernia lies superior to it.

Lateral to the sartorius muscle, and just distal to the anterior superior spine, is a triangular depression, the outer boundary of which is the tensor fasciae latae muscle and the anterior superior spine. This depression overlies the proximal part of the rectus femoris muscle; this in turn overlies the capsule of the hip joint. In forced extension of the thigh combined with outward rotation, a fullness representing the head of the femur projecting against the front of the capsule appears in this depression. Through this depression, the incision for the anterior approach to the hip joint usually is made (p. 708). The surface projection of the femoral artery is a line from the midpoint of the inguinal ligament to the adductor tubercle when the knee is flexed, abducted, and rotated laterally.

3. **Superficial Structures.**—The subcutaneous tissue usually contains a considerable amount of fat within its meshes. Near the inguinal ligament, the subcutaneous tissue is arranged in two layers which are continuous with those over the lower abdominal wall. The three *superficial branches of the femoral artery* arise in this region. The superficial epigastric and the superficial external pudendal arteries have been described. The superficial circumflex iliac artery pierces the deep fascia lateral to the fossa ovalis and passes laterally. These small arteries are accompanied by corresponding veins which join the great saphenous vein close to its termination.

The *great saphenous vein* runs in the superficial fascia on the anteromedial part of the upper thigh and, after receiving numerous tributaries, pierces the cribriform fascia and enters the femoral vein. There sometimes is a venous swelling where the great saphenous vein enters the femoral vein; this may be mistaken for a femoral hernia, since the venous dilation transmits an impulse on straining or coughing, and disappears in the recumbent position. In order to differentiate this condition from a femoral hernia, the patient lies down, and the swelling is reduced and held back by placing the finger on the proximal part of the fossa ovalis. When the patient stands, the swelling, if venous in nature, gradually reappears as the great saphenous vein fills. With the limb in abduction and lateral rotation, the vein may be ligated through a transverse incision through the skin and subcutaneous tissue at the distal margin of the fossa ovalis.

The *superficial subinguinal lymph glands* lie in two groups on the deep fascia inferior to the inguinal ligament. The proximal group is a chain of glands lying just inferior to the inguinal ligament, and roughly parallel to it. To these glands drain efferents from the glands of the perineum, external genitalia, buttocks, and abdominal wall below the umbilicus. The distal group lies about the great saphenous vein and the lateral border of the fossa ovalis, and drains all the superficial lymph vessels of the lower limb save those from the buttocks and lateral side of the foot and leg; the latter drain to the popliteal glands. The efferents of both groups drain into the *deep subinguinal glands*.

4. Structures between the Inguinal Ligament and the Iliopectineal Line.—The space between the inguinal ligament and the iliopectineal line is divided into two compartments

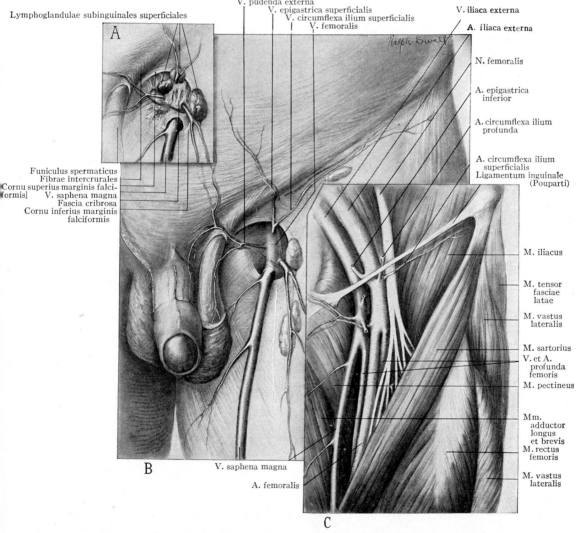

FIG. 713.—LEVELS IN THE DISSECTION OF THE INGUINOFEMORAL REGION.

A indicates the relations of the fossa ovalis to the deep fascia of the thigh, the inguinal ligament, and the superficial vessels. B shows the fossa ovalis cleared of the lymphatic contents and the cribriform fascia. C exposes the contents of the femoral trigone (of Scarpa) after all superficial structures and the deep fascia have been removed.

by a band of iliac fascia which extends from the inguinal ligament to the iliopectineal eminence at the outer side of the femoral artery. The lateral space (*lacuna musculorum*) is somewhat oval in outline; it is occupied by the iliopsoas muscle and the femoral (anterior crural) nerve. The medial smaller compartment (*lacuna vasorum*) is occupied by the femoral vessels and the femoral canal. The extreme lateral portion of the lacuna vasorum is occupied by the femoral artery and the lumbo-inguinal (crural) branch **of the** genitocrural nerve. The femoral vein lies more mesially; most mesial is the **small**

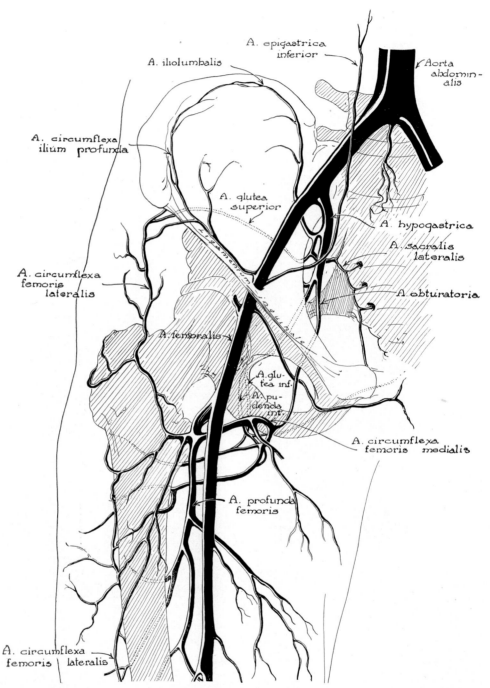

FIG. 714.—COLLATERAL CIRCULATION ABOUT THE ROOT OF THE THIGH. (Mont Reid, Amer. Jour. of Surgery.)

oval femoral ring, which serves as a communication between the abdominal cavity and the thigh.

5. **Deep Fascia.**—The deep fascia in this region is a well-defined structure. Laterally, it encloses the tensor fasciae latae muscle; medially, it is attached to the inguinal ligament and the margin of the subpubic arch as far as the ischial tuberosity.

A gap of some size, the *fossa ovalis* (*saphenous opening*), lies in the deep fascia, distal to the medial extremity of the inguinal ligament. The middle of the opening lies 4 cm. distal and lateral to the pubic tubercle. The fossa is closed partially by the cribriform fascia, a loose and ill-defined portion of the fascia lata, which is pierced by numerous apertures. The fossa as an actual aperture does not exist until the *cribriform fascia* has been removed. The lateral border of the fossa is defined sharply into the falciform ligament which overlies the venous compartment of the femoral sheath. The superior cornu of the ligament arches medially and proximally to the pubic tubercle where it merges into the *lacunar ligament* (of Gimbernat). The well-marked inferior cornu is just distal to the junction of the saphenous and femoral veins. The medial margin of the fossa, formed

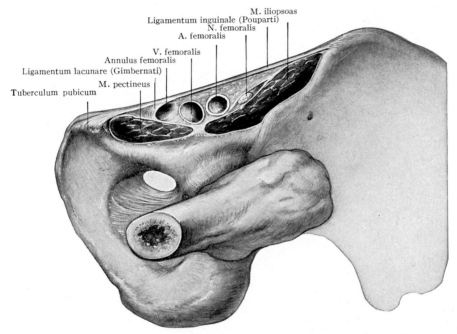

Labels: M. iliopsoas · Ligamentum inguinale (Pouparti) · N. femoralis · A. femoralis · V. femoralis · Annulus femoralis · Ligamentum lacunare (Gimbernati) · M. pectineus · Tuberculum pubicum

FIG. 715.—CONTENTS OF THE FEMORAL ARCH VIEWED FROM THE THIGH.

by the deep fascia overlying the pectineus muscle, is defined poorly. When it is traced laterally, it disappears behind, and fuses with, the posterior layer of the femoral sheath.

6. **Femoral Sheath.**—Within the lacuna vasorum, and for about 4 cm. distal to it, the femoral vessels are provided with a membranous investment, known as the femoral sheath. This sheath is a sleevelike prolongation of the fascial envelopment of the abdomen which passes downward into the thigh behind the inguinal ligament. Lateral to the lacuna vasorum, mainly over the iliopsoas muscle, the transversalis and iliac fasciae are attached firmly to the inguinal ligament. Opposite the vessels, the fascial layers are carried into the thigh to form the femoral sheath. The anterior wall of the sheath is very thin and is continuous with the transversalis fascia lining the deep surface of the anterior abdominal wall; the posterior wall is constituted partly by the iliac fascia which is prolonged downward over the iliopsoas muscle, and partly by the pubic portion of the fascia lata covering the pectineus muscle. The sheath extends downward as far as the origin of the profunda artery, where it fuses with the outer coats of the femoral vessels. Two septa from the femoral sheath divide the lacuna vasorum into arterial, venous, and lymphatic compartments.

The medial compartment is the femoral canal, the entrance of which, the femoral (crural) ring, is an aperture bounded anteriorly by the inguinal ligament, posteriorly by the pectineus muscle and the subjacent pubic ramus, laterally by the femoral vein, and medially by the sharp lateral border of the lacunar ligament (of Gimbernat). The femoral ring is occluded by a fascial septum (septum femorale), and is a weak area in the fascial envelope of the abdomen. It is important surgically because it allows the passage of a femoral hernia into the thigh.

7. **Deep Musculature.**—The floor of the inguino-abdominal region is composed of the tensor fasciae latae, sartorius, iliopsoas, pectineus, and adductor longus muscles. The tensor fasciae latae and sartorius muscles arise from a common origin at the anterior superior iliac spine. The iliopsoas and pectineus muscles are the substratum for the vasculoneural elements of the area, and the adductor longus muscle, which forms the medial boundary of the region, is an element in the adductor region of the thigh (p. 709).

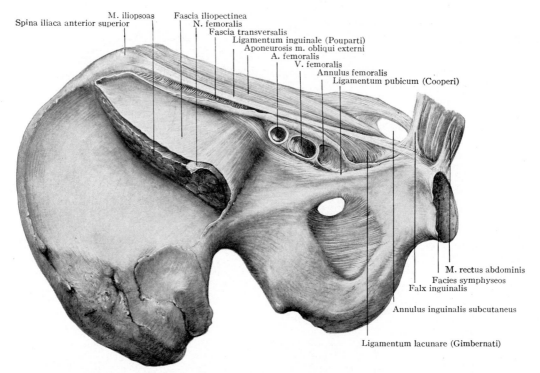

FIG. 716.—CONTENTS OF THE LEFT FEMORAL ARCH VIEWED FROM WITHIN THE PELVIS.

8. **Femoral Trigone (of Scarpa).**—The femoral trigone is a triangular space lying immediately distal to the inguinal ligament. This ligament forms the base of the trigone. The oblique lateral boundary is the medial margin of the sartorius muscle, and the medial boundary is the medial border of the adductor longus muscle. The roof consists of the fascia lata which completely covers the space anteriorly. The floor is made up of two inclined planes, which form a well-marked median groove at their junction. The lateral inclined plane consists of the iliopsoas muscle invested by a thin layer of fascia. The adductor longus and pectineus muscles, both of which are invested with fascia lata, form the medial plane. The most important contents of the prismatic space, included between the fascial roof and floor of the femoral trigone, are the femoral vessels and nerve and their large branches. These structures, the termination of the great saphenous vein, and the deep subinguinal lymph vessels and glands are embedded in a quantity of loose fatty tissue. The efferents from the popliteal gland send in this deep group which sends its

efferent trunks to the external iliac lymph glands. This space communicates with the abdomen through the lacuna vasorum.

9. **Femoral Canal.**—The femoral canal is a narrow space bounded anteriorly by the cribriform fascia, posteriorly by the fascia lata over the pectineus muscle, and laterally by the femoral vein. The proximal aperture or inlet of the canal is the femoral ring, which is directed downward. The lower aperture, or outlet, is the fossa ovalis which faces anteriorly. The canal is angular, with a decided forward curve. It is this curve, probably, which directs a femoral hernia forward and upward. The canal is occupied by the deep subinguinal lymph vessels, areolo-adipose tissue, and one or two lymph glands. It corresponds to the lymphatic compartment of the femoral sheath.

10. **Surgical Relations of the Femoral (Crural) Ring.**—The *spermatic cord* lies superior and medial to the femoral ring. Between the cord and the femoral ring is the *pubic tubercle*, an important surgical landmark. If the hernial protrusion lies in front and to the inner side of this tubercle, it presumably emerges through the subcutaneous inguinal ring (inguinal hernia); if the herniating mass is inferior to, and to the outer side of, the tubercle, it almost certainly has made its way through the femoral canal (femoral hernia).

The obturator artery normally arises from the hypogastric artery (p. 431), but sometimes it is derived from the inferior (deep) epigastric artery. In the latter instance, the obturator artery descends behind the pubis to the obturator foramen, but not always in the same direction, for it may pass either medially or laterally to the femoral ring. When a femoral hernia coexists with an abnormal obturator artery which passes medial to the femoral ring, the artery lies in close relationship with the medial side of the neck of the sac and may be injured when the lacunar ligament is incised to relieve the constriction at the neck of the sac.

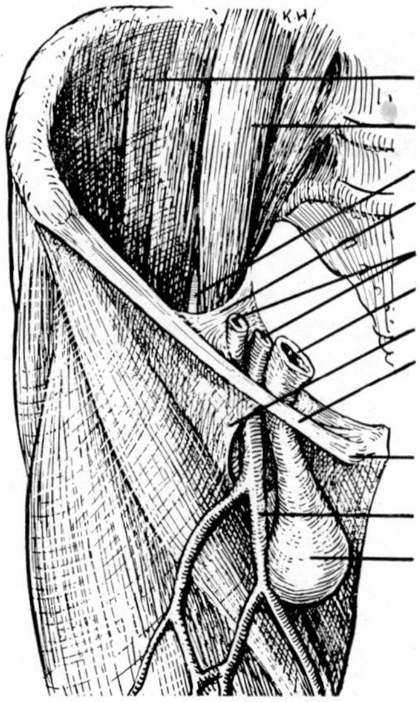

M. iliacus
M. psoas
N. femoralis
Lig. iliopectineum
A. et V. femoralis
Mouth of hernial sac
Margo falciformis fossae ovalis
Lig. inguinale
Tuberculum pubicum
V. saphena magna
Hernial sac

Fig. 717.—Contents of the Femoral Arch with a Hernial Sac Extending Through the Femoral Canal.

11. **Femoral Nerve.**—The femoral nerve ($L_2, _3, _4$) enters the thigh behind the inguinal ligament, 1 cm. lateral to the femoral artery. In the thigh, it lies deep to the fascia lata in the groove between the psoas major and iliacus muscles. The saphenous nerve runs medially and distally toward the femoral artery at the apex of the femoral trigone and accompanies the artery down the adductor canal (of Hunter). Muscle branches supply the sartorius, pectineus, and quadriceps muscles. The nerves to the vastus divisions of the quadriceps muscles give off articular branches to the knee joint, and the nerve to the rectus femoris muscle partially innervates the hip joint. Both the hip and knee joints also receive a nerve supply from the obturator nerve (p. 711). It is very common for the pain of hip joint disease to be referred entirely to the knee.

12. **Femoral Artery.**—The femoral artery, a direct continuation of the external iliac artery, enters the thigh behind the inguinal ligament midway between the anterior superior spine and the pubic tubercle. It extends from this point to the upper and medial part of the popliteal space, which it enters through the tendinous ring in the adductor magnus muscle, a palmbreadth above the adductor tubercle. Between these two points, the artery follows an almost straight course, gradually inclining from the anterior toward the posteromedial aspect of the limb.

The femoral artery is comparatively superficial at its origin but is deeply placed at its termination.   The proximal half of the artery lies immediately behind the deep fascia, covering the femoral trigone.   At a point about 4 cm. below the inguinal ligament, the femoral artery gives off the large profunda branch.   It is convenient to speak of the short portion of the femoral trunk above this branch as the common femoral artery.   The remaining part is termed the superficial femoral artery.

13. **Branches of the Femoral Artery.**—Early in its course, the femoral artery gives off **superficial** branches: the *superficial external pudendal*, the *superficial epigastric*, and the *superficial circumflex iliac arteries.*

The **deep** branches include the deep external pudendal, the profunda, the superior geniculate arteries, and the muscle branches.   The *deep external pudendal artery* is derived from the medial aspect of the femoral artery and courses medially over the pectineus and adductor longus muscles.   After piercing the fascia lata, it is distributed to the scrotal tissues or to the labia majora.

The *profunda femoris artery* usually branches from the common femoral artery about 4 cm. below the inguinal ligament, and in its descent is first lateral, and then posterior, to the superficial femoral vessels.   It soon passes beneath the adductor longus muscle, to which the superficial femoral artery remains superficial; the profunda artery runs in close proximity to the linea aspera of the femur.   It descends toward the popliteal space, pierces the adductor magnus muscle close to the aperture for the femoral artery, and terminates as the fourth perforating artery.

The profunda artery has several important branches.   The lateral circumflex artery sometimes arises from the common femoral artery, but usually is derived from the profunda close to its origin, passing transversely laterally deep to the rectus femoris and sartorius muscles, where it is encountered in the anterior approach to the hip joint (p. 708).   It divides into three terminal branches.   The ascending branch runs upward and laterally beneath the rectus femoris and tensor fasciae latae muscles to the anterior part of the gluteal region.   The transverse branch pierces the vastus lateralis muscle and winds around the posterior surface of the shaft of the femur.   The descending branch descends within the vastus lateralis muscle to join the anastomosis around the knee joint.

The medial circumflex artery, which sometimes arises from the common femoral artery, generally originates from the profunda artery.   It runs posteriorly and medially between the pectineus and psoas major muscles; for the remainder of its course it is contained within the upper part of the adductor region of the thigh (p. 709).   The four perforating arteries arise from the profunda more distally and run to the posterior compartment of the thigh, where they form a regular chain of anastomoses extending from the gluteal region to the popliteal space.   The first perforating artery contributes to the crucial anastomosis about the hip (p. 676), the second usually furnishes the chief nutrient artery to the femur, and the third and fourth, the terminations of the parent stem anastomose freely with branches from the popliteal artery.

The *supreme geniculate (anastomotica magna) artery* arises from the superficial femoral artery in the lower part of the adductor canal (of Hunter).   It divides into a superficial or saphenous branch and an articular branch.   The latter descends on the femur and contributes to the anastomosis about the knee joint.

SURGICAL CONSIDERATIONS

1. **Femoral Hernia.**—In femoral hernia, the abdominal contents push the parietal peritoneum, the extraperitoneal fat, and femoral septum through the femoral ring into the femoral canal.   The protruding mass stretches the thin anterior wall of the femoral sheath and gains another covering.   The sac, with its coverings, emerges through the fascia lata at the fossa ovalis and, following the course of least resistance, bends upward toward the inguinal ligament.   It produces a palpable swelling at the medial part of the root of the thigh, below and to the lateral side of the pubic spine.   There usually is a large amount of extraperitoneal fat about the sac so that even if the sac is small, the protruding mass appears as an elongated, rounded, elastic swelling of considerable size.

The *content* of a femoral hernia usually is a tonguelike piece of omentum which seldom is more than partially reducible. This omental mass, by being converted into a plug of fibrofatty tissue, often loses its normal appearance. In addition, the sac may contain part or all of a coil of intestine. When part of the convex portion of a loop of intestine is nipped within the small space of a hernial ring, a *Richter's hernia* results. A small area of bowel constricted in this manner may become gangrenous and lead to perforation as readily as a larger portion of strangulated bowel. When the bladder is part of the content of a femoral hernia, the herniating portion of the bladder wall usually is preceded through the ring by a mass of the prevesical fat. The viscus sometimes is wounded in high ligation of the neck of a hernial sac. A bladder diverticulum, normal in appearance, incarcerated or strangulated, may lie within the hernial sac.

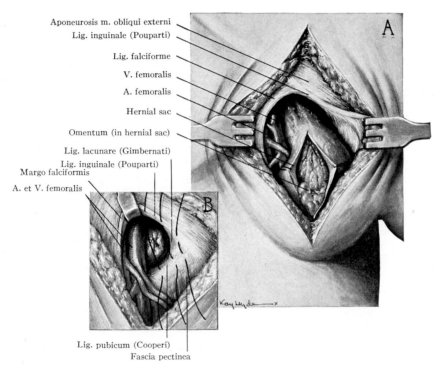

Aponeurosis m. obliqui externi
Lig. inguinale (Pouparti)
Lig. falciforme
V. femoralis
A. femoralis
Hernial sac
Omentum (in hernial sac)
Lig. lacunare (Gimbernati)
Lig. inguinale (Pouparti)
Margo falciformis
A. et V. femoralis
Lig. pubicum (Cooperi)
Fascia pectinea

FIG. 718.—SUBINGUINAL APPROACH FOR THE REPAIR OF A FEMORAL HERNIA IN THE FEMALE.

Vertical incision is made directly over the hernial protrusion. The sac is located in the midst of the superficial fat and the areolar tissue of the cribriform fascia, and it is isolated by blunt dissection. Internally, the sharp edge of the lacunar (Gimbernat's) ligament may require division. Externally, the margin of the falciform may be sectioned to give exposure. After the contents of the sac have been reduced and the sac ligated and excised, the pectineal fascia is sutured to the inguinal and falciform ligaments.

In long-standing femoral herniae, the strata of tissue about the sac are modified very markedly. The layers may be attenuated by stretching, or may acquire such thickness from the accumulation of fat that it is impossible to recognize them individually.

Femoral hernia, in contrast to inguinal hernia, always is acquired, and occurs more frequently in females than in males, probably because of the greater proportional width of the pelvis, the consequent greater size of the femoral ring, and the tendency of pregnancy to produce an overstretched and atonic abdominal wall. If the iliopsoas muscle is not well developed, there is more room beneath the inguinal ligament than is necessary for the passage of the muscle and the femoral vessels, so that the potential space (femoral ring) medial to the vein is enlarged and is more capable of receiving a hernial sac.

The greater incidence of *incarceration* and *strangulation* in femoral hernia than in inguinal hernia is not surprising, considering the narrowness and unyielding character of the femoral ring. In most instances, the lacunar ligament (of Gimbernat) is responsible for the constriction, but the margin of an unduly rigid falciform ligament may be a factor. In attempting to reduce a femoral hernia, the thigh should be flexed and adducted slightly to relax the pectineus muscle, the fascia lata, and the inguinal ligament. The herniating mass should be manipulated gently.

The *differential diagnosis* of femoral hernia from other lesions in the groin is decidedly more important than the distinction between the femoral and inguinal varieties of hernia. The most important and commonest of the lesions to be differentiated are: enlarged inguinal glands, hydrocele of the cord, or of the canal of Nuck, varix of the great saphinous veins at the saphenous opening, and psoas abscess which has gravitated downward

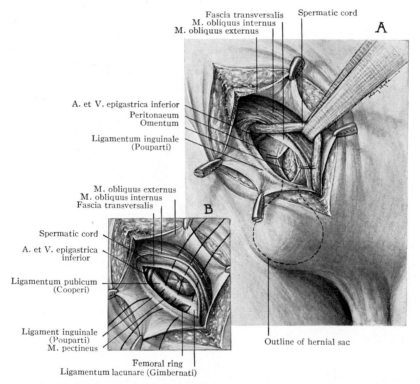

FIG. 719.—INGUINAL APPROACH FOR THE REPAIR OF A FEMORAL HERNIA IN THE MALE.

In A, the inguinal falx and the transversalis fascia are retracted upward. After exposing the peritoneum proximal to the femoral ring, the peritoneum is incised. The hernial contents are seen in the femoral canal. After withdrawal of the contents, the neck of the sac is ligated. If the sac and contents are adherent, an incision must be made over the hernial bulge in the thigh. In B, the hernial contents and the sac have been drawn into the inguinal wound. The contents have been reduced and the sac has been ligated; the inguinal and femoral canals are closed by interrupted sutures, which pass through the inguinal falx, the inguinal ligament, and the pubic ligament (of Cooper) on the iliopectineal line.

beneath the inguinal ligament. The swelling of a psoas abscess is at the lateral side of the femoral sheath because the pus usually enters the thigh through the lacuna musculorum. Examination generally reveals a fluctuant tumor in the iliac fossa; x-ray evidence of an enlarged psoas shadow or of vertebral caries confirms the diagnosis.

2. **Operative Treatment of Femoral Hernia.**—The *subinguinal approach* to a femoral hernia is through an incision parallel with, and just distal to, the medial part of the inguinal ligament or through a vertical incision over the hernial protrusion. After division of the skin, superficial fascia, and superficial vessels, blunt dissection reveals a mass of fat beneath the subcutaneous fatty areolar layer. The coverings of the hernia often cannot be differentiated. Further blunt dissection isolates the neck of the tumor at the femoral ring.

The fatty tissue which is derived from the extraperitoneal tissue, and that distal to it, is incised step by step in the search for the hernial sac. Sometimes the herniating mass is a lipoma arising from the extraperitoneal fat. When the sac is found and its contents are reduced, the sac is ligated and excised.

Many methods are employed to close the femoral ring through the subinguinal incision, but, because of the rigidity of the parts above the ligaments and the constant movements of the parts below them, none of these methods has proved altogether satisfactory. The usual course is to close the ring by sutures which draw the inguinal ligament to the pectineal fascia, or by a strong purse-string suture which puckers the fascia forming the femoral canal. The purse-string suture is passed through the inguinal ligament, the fascia lata, the falciform border of the fossa ovalis, and the fascia over the pectineus muscle. It is difficult, if not impossible, to include in the suture Cooper's ligament, the fibrous thickening on the pectineal line just proximal to the origin of the pectineus muscle. Care must be exercised not to injure the femoral vein.

Because of the tension on the stitches and the impossibility of securing a ligation of the sac flush with the abdominal peritoneum, the inferior approach is not nearly as satisfactory as the *inguinal approach*, which opens the inguinal canal as for the repair of inguinal hernia. After incising the transversalis fascia which forms the floor of the inguinal canal, the neck of the sac can be isolated in the extraperitoneal tissue proximal to the femoral ring. By pressure from below and traction from above, the sac sometimes can be drawn into the inguinal canal where it can be incised and its neck ligated at its emergence from the abdominal cavity. The inguinal incision often must be continued into the thigh over the tumor mass in order to free the sac from the elements of the femoral canal; the sac then can be drawn upward into the inguinal canal. Both the inguinal canal and the femoral ring are closed by sutures which draw the inguinal falx (conjoined tendon) and the inguinal ligament down to Cooper's ligament on the iliopectineal line. In this operation, the inferior (deep) epigastric artery and the external iliac vein must be retracted carefully.

The sac of a *strangulated femoral hernia* is difficult to recognize because of edema and congestion of the elements of the protruding mass. Each layer of the herniating mass must be incised separately through the subinguinal incision until the escape of discolored fluid from within the sac indicates the proximity of the bowel. Before the condition of the bowel at the constricted neck of the sac can be ascertained and reduction effected, the femoral ring must be enlarged. This is accomplished by introducing the knife, guided by the finger, along the medial aspect of the neck of the sac and dividing the free edge of the lacunar ligament (of Gimbernat) until the opening is enlarged sufficiently to permit withdrawal of the bowel for examination. If division of the lacunar ligament does not afford sufficient exposure, the only other alternative is section of the inguinal ligament, which interferes with successful repair of the abdominal wall. Incision of the lacunar ligament by the inguinal approach is a simple procedure and entails no risk of injuring an anomalous obturator artery.

3. **Ligation of the Femoral Artery.**—The superficial position of the femoral artery in the femoral trigone (of Scarpa) renders it liable to injury by lacerations or gunshot wounds at this level. The proximity of the femoral vein to the artery accounts for the readiness with which these vessels are wounded simultaneously. The result of this injury commonly is the establishment of an *arteriovenous fistula (aneurysm)*, of the aneurysmal varix or the varicose type. In the aneurysmal varix, the injured vessels communicate directly and, in the varicose aneurysm, the communication is effected indirectly through the intermedium of a sac formed by the surrounding tissues.

Within the inguinofemoral region, the femoral artery may require ligation immediately below the inguinal ligament (common femoral artery) or at the apex of the femoral trigone (superficial femoral artery).

Ligation of the common femoral artery is not difficult, because of the superficial position of the artery and the ease with which it can be separated from the femoral vein, inasmuch as each vessel occupies a separate compartment within the femoral sheath. The three small superficial branches of the common femoral artery and the occasional origin of the circumflex vessels from this trunk make ligation of the external iliac artery (p. 676) the ligation of choice as a preliminary measure to disarticulation at the hip joint.

After ligation of the common femoral artery, collateral circulation is established through anastomosis between the superior and inferior gluteal branches from the hypogastric artery proximal to the ligature, and the two circumflex branches and the first perforating branch of the profunda distal to the ligature. Another collateral path is the anastomosis of the deep circumflex iliac artery (from the external iliac) with the superficial circumflex iliac artery and the ascending ramus of the lateral circumflex artery (from the femoral).

Ligation of the femoral artery at the apex of the femoral trigone is made through an incision over the course of the vessel. The sartorius muscle is identified and retracted laterally and the artery is exposed just before it enters the adductor canal. The femoral artery is crossed at this level by the medial cutaneous nerve, to which the saphenous nerve

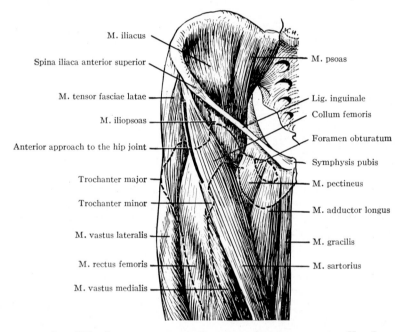

M. iliacus
Spina iliaca anterior superior
M. tensor fasciae latae
M. iliopsoas
Anterior approach to the hip joint
Trochanter major
Trochanter minor
M. vastus lateralis
M. rectus femoris
M. vastus medialis

M. psoas
Lig. inguinale
Collum femoris
Foramen obturatum
Symphysis pubis
M. pectineus
M. adductor longus
M. gracilis
M. sartorius

FIG. 720.—INCISION FOR THE ANTERIOR APPROACH TO THE HIP JOINT.

is either anterior or lateral. Although the femoral vein lies to the medial side of the artery in the proximal part of the thigh, it occupies a position posterior to the artery at the apex of the femoral trigone. For this reason, the sheath of the artery is opened at its anterolateral aspect. Collateral circulation is established by anastomoses around the knee joint, where branches from the profunda femoris artery communicate with the geniculate anastomosis on the proximal side of the ligature and with branches of the popliteal artery on the distal side.

Ligation of the femoral artery in the adductor canal (of Hunter) is described in the section on the anterior region of the thigh (p. 714).

4. **Anterior (Inguinofemoral) Approach to the Hip Joint.**—The anterior approach to the hip joint is through an incision which extends downward from the anterior superior iliac spine in the line of the axis of the femur. The incision develops the interval between the sartorius muscle on the medial side and the anterior margin of the tensor fasciae latae muscle laterally. The wound is deepened in the inverted V-shaped depression between these muscles until the rectus femoris muscle is exposed. After retracting the rectus

femoris medially, the ascending branch of the lateral circumflex artery, which runs beneath it, is divided and the anterior aspect of the joint capsule is identified.

The route sometimes is used for excision of tuberculous tissue in the hip joint (p. 684), and has the advantage that no muscles, nerves, or vessels of importance are sacrificed. The objection to the operation is a wound which is not well situated for drainage, but, when used in conjunction with the posterolateral approach (of Langenbeck) (p. 693), this incision affords ideal through-and-through drainage for acute suppurative arthritis of the hip joint.

5. Abscess in the Root of the Thigh.—*Superficial abscesses* usually originate in suppurating superficial subinguinal lymph glands, the focus for which may be on some part of the limb or buttock, the anus, or the external genitalia.

Deep abscesses often are secondary, invading the thigh from an adjoining region. They manifest a decided tendency to gravitate beneath the deep fascia, since this dense structure is a powerful obstacle to the collection's becoming superficial. The pus, if not evacuated, usually descends along the lateral side of the femoral sheath; from this area, it may be guided by the deep femoral vessels to the back of the thigh. The abscess may point at the medial aspect of the thigh. The path of pus from tuberculosis of the hip joint is alluded to in connection with that joint (p. 684).

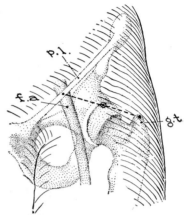

FIG. 721.—LOCATION OF THE POINT FOR ASPIRATION OF THE HIP JOINT.

This point lies midway between the tip of the great trochanter and the point where the femoral artery crosses the inguinal ligament. (Babcock, "Textbook of Surgery.")

C. ADDUCTOR OR OBTURATOR REGION

1. Definition and Boundaries.—The adductor region is a wedge of muscles interposed between the extensor group of thigh muscles in front and the flexor muscles behind. The adductor muscles arise from the margins of the obturator foramen and from the obturator membrane. Within this region is the obturator canal, which is a potential pathway for an obturator hernia. The adductor region is limited medially by the pubic arch, the perineum, and the gracilis muscle; laterally, by the hip joint and shaft of the femur; and above, by the horizontal ramus of the pubis. Its lower boundary is the inferior insertion of the adductor magnus muscle into the adductor tubercle of the femur.

2. Adductor Musculature.—From a restricted area on the pubis, the collective adductor muscles (N. obturator $L_{2, 3, 4}$) and the pectineus and gracilis muscles spread fanwise to the linea aspera along almost the entire length of the femur.

The *pectineus muscle* (N. femoral $L_{2, 3}$) arises from the superior ramus of the pubis, passes distally and laterally, and inserts into the posterior aspect of the proximal part of the femoral shaft just behind and below the lesser trochanter. It also is a constituent muscle of the inguinofemoral region and is an adductor and flexor of the thigh.

The *gracilis muscle*, thin and straplike, extends from the margin of the pubic arch along the medial side of the thigh. Before inserting into the proximal part of the tibia, it runs behind the medial epicondyle of the femur, and acts more powerfully as a flexor of the knee than as an adductor of the thigh. When the hamstring muscles are paralyzed, flexion of the leg may be carried out by the gracilis and sartorius muscles.

The *adductor longus muscle* forms part of the floor of the inguinofemoral region (p. 702) and of the adductor canal (p. 713); therefore, it is a support for a considerable extent of the femoral vessels. The adductor longus is the most anterior of the three adductor muscles and is on the same plane as the pectineus. It inserts into the linea aspera. The *adductor brevis muscle* lies deep to the adductor longus, arises from the inferior ramus of the pubis and inserts into the back of the femur. Its superior margin lies against the obturator externus muscle. The *adductor magnus muscle*, the largest and most posterior of the three adductors, forms a broad triangular floor for the support of the other muscles of the adductor group. It arises from the pubic arch and the ischial tuberosity. Its upper fibers run horizontally to the back of the femur and the lower fibers run downward almost

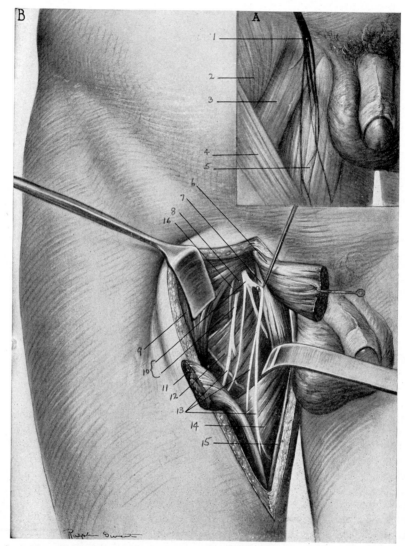

Fig. 722.—Superficial and Deep Structures of the Obturator or Adductor Region of the Thigh.
In A, the obturator nerve is shown in surface projection. In B, the adductor longus muscle is divided and the pectineus and adductor magnus muscles are retracted to show the obturator artery and nerve on the obturator externus and the adductor brevis muscles. 1, N. obturatorius (surface projection); 2, M. pectineus; 3, M. adductor longus; 4, M. sartorius; 5, M. adductor magnus; 6, M. adductor longus; 7, M. adductor magnus; 8, M. obturator externus; 9, M. pectineus; 10, N. obturatorius, ramus anterior, ramus posterior; 11, M. adductor longus; 12, M. adductor brevis; 13, rami musculares; 14, M. adductor magnus; 15. M. gracilis; 16, A. obturatoria.

vertically to insert into the linea aspera and the adductor tubercle. The anterior surface of the upper part of the adductor magnus is covered by the adductor brevis. More inferiorly, the adductor magnus is overlain by the adductor longus; inferior to the adductor longus, it forms the floor of the adductor canal. The adductor magnus, in its inferior part, presents a tendinous hiatus for the transmission of the femoral vessels to the popliteal fossa. Along the insertion of the muscle into the linea aspera are osteo-aponeurotic passages for the perforating branches of the profunda artery. Injuries to the adductor muscles, such as are sustained readily by cavalrymen, may cause hemorrhages which undergo calcification (myositis ossificans).

The *obturator externus muscle* (posterior branch of N. obturator $L_{3, 4}$) arises from the mesial margin of the obturator foramen and from the lateral surface of the obturator membrane; its tendon passes, almost horizontally, laterally to an insertion into the trochanteric fossa of the femur. It is a powerful lateral rotator of the thigh.

3. **Obturator Canal.**—A gap exists at the superior lateral part of the obturator foramen. This opening enters a short oblique tunnel, the obturator canal, which is directed forward and medially from the pelvis and relates the pelvis with the adductor region along the course of the obturator vessels and nerves emerging through it. Its length is from 1 to 2 cm. and its breadth is about 1 cm. The canal is bounded superiorly by the obturator groove of the pubic bone and inferiorly by the obturator membrane and the two obturator

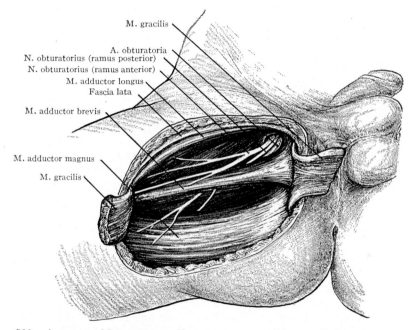

M. gracilis

A. obturatoria
N. obturatorius (ramus posterior)
N. obturatorius (ramus anterior)
M. adductor longus
Fascia lata
M. adductor brevis

M. adductor magnus
M. gracilis

FIG. 723.—ADDUCTOR MUSCULATURE VIEWED FROM THE MESIAL ASPECT OF THE THIGH.

muscles. The internal or *pelvic orifice* of the canal is overlain by the parietal pelvic fascia and the pelvic extraperitoneal space. The external or *superficial orifice* is related to the deep aspect of the pectineus muscle and is slightly medial to the femoral vein.

4. **Obturator Artery and Nerve.**—The *obturator artery* usually arises from the hypogastric artery. It occupies the lateral part of the obturator canal and lies beneath the obturator nerve.

The *obturator nerve* ($L_{2, 3, 4}$), a branch of the lumbar plexus, runs through the psoas muscle over the sacro-iliac joint and along the lateral wall of the pelvis, where it enters the obturator canal. Within the canal, it divides into two branches. The anterior branch passes over the upper border of the obturator externus muscle and descends behind the pectineus and adductor longus brevis muscles. The posterior branch, after piercing the upper margin of the obturator externus muscle, which it supplies, descends between the adductor brevis and adductor magnus muscles. It supplies the adductor magnus and gives off a small branch to the knee joint. Both the artery and the nerve run in a bed of areolo-adipose tissue which connects the extraperitoneal tissue of the pelvis with the corresponding tissue in the upper and inner thigh. This continuity affords a reciprocal path of infection between the regions. Along this path, the pelvic peritoneum may be prolonged and may furnish the sac for an obturator hernia.

5. **Obturator Hernia.**—A hernia of pelvic contents may traverse the obturator canal with the obturator vessels and nerve and present at the upper and medial part of the thigh; its occurrence is extremely rare. Obturator hernia is more common in females than in males. When the conditions are favorable for the formation of a hernia, forcible straining causes a loop of bowel, a diverticulum from the bladder, a portion of omentum, or even an ovary or a tube to become engaged within the narrow internal orifice of the obturator canal.

An obturator hernia usually is small. Since the outer orifice of the canal is located deep to the pectineus and adductor longus muscles, little protrusion is noted externally, and the presence of the hernia may be unsuspected. This condition should be considered as a possible cause of acute intestinal obstruction. Certain diagnostic signs are present in some cases. The protrusion causes pressure on the obturator nerve and tenderness in the adductor muscles, with pain referred to the cutaneous distribution of the obturator nerve on the mesial side of the thigh. The hernia, which usually is strangulated, lies behind the pectineus muscle on the obturator externus muscle and produces a slight fullness in the upper and medial part of the thigh. The thigh is flexed to relieve tension on the pectineus muscle; efforts at extension or adduction cause severe pain, since both movements tend to squeeze the hernia against the external obturator muscle. Mesial rotation of the thigh aggravates the pain by stretching the obturator externus muscle. Rectal or vaginal examination confirms the diagnosis.

The vertical incision for *obturator herniotomy* overlies the interval between the pectineus and adductor longus muscles. The pectineus muscle is drawn laterally and may require partial division close to its pubic attachment. The body of the adductor brevis muscle is retracted distally and medially, and some of the fibers may require division. The relationship of the vessels to the sac is variable, and a free dissection is necessary for adequate exposure of the parts adjacent to the neck of the sac.

D. ANTERIOR OR EXTENSOR REGION OF THE THIGH; SHAFT OF THE FEMUR

1. **Musculature.**—The *tensor fasciae latae muscle* is described in the section on the gluteal region (p. 674). The *sartorius muscle* (N. femoral $L_{3, 4}$) is the lateral boundary of the femoral trigone and forms the roof of the adductor canal. It arises from the anterior superior iliac spine and crosses the thigh obliquely downward and inward. On the medial aspect of the thigh, it descends almost vertically to an insertion into the proximal part of the medial surface of the tibia. It is a flexor and medial rotator of the leg and an abductor, flexor, and lateral rotator of the thigh.

The *quadriceps femoris muscle* (N. femoral $L_{3, 4}$), the powerful extensor of the leg, has four divisions which form a thick muscle mass, embracing the anterior, lateral, and medial surfaces of the shaft of the femur. The manner of insertion of the components of the quadriceps into the base and lateral border of the patella is described in the discussion of the region of the knee (p. 731). The *rectus femoris muscle* arises from a straight head, which originates in the anterior inferior spine of the ilium, and a reflected head from the dorsum of the ilium just above the acetabulum. In the upper part of the thigh, it forms the floor of a depression between the tensor faciae latae and sartorius muscles, and is related closely to the anterior aspect of the capsule of the hip joint. The rectus femoris becomes superficial after it is crossed by the sartorius muscle, and forms a well-marked rounded elevation in the front of the thigh when the knee is extended. The *vastus intermedius muscle* arises from the anterior and lateral aspects of the shaft of the femur. It is overlapped partially by the lateral and medial vasti and is covered by the rectus femoris. The *vastus lateralis* has a linear origin from the linea aspera and the proximal part of the shaft of the femur and constitutes the muscle mass on the lateral aspect of the thigh. The *vastus medialis* arises from the proximal part of the femur and from the linea aspera, and occupies the anterior and medial part of the thigh. On each side of the patella, the knee joint capsule is strengthened by tendinous expansions from the medial and lateral vasti.

    2. Adductor Canal (of Hunter) and Its Contents.—The *adductor canal* is an intermuscular space on the medial aspect of the middle third of the thigh which contains the femoral vessels and the saphenous nerve. The lateral wall is formed by the vastus medialis muscle and the posterior wall by the adductor longus muscle proximally and the adductor magnus muscle distally. The roof of the canal is a layer of deep fascia running from the adductor longus and magnus muscles to the vastus medialis muscle. The sartorius muscle covers

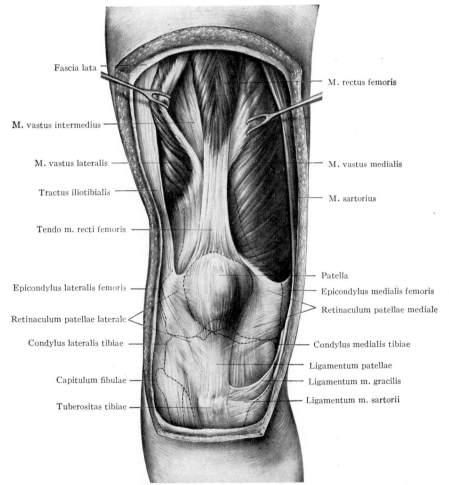

Fascia lata

M. rectus femoris

M. vastus intermedius

M. vastus lateralis

M. vastus medialis

Tractus iliotibialis

M. sartorius

Tendo m. recti femoris

Patella

Epicondylus lateralis femoris

Epicondylus medialis femoris

Retinaculum patellae laterale

Retinaculum patellae mediale

Condylus lateralis tibiae

Condylus medialis tibiae

Ligamentum patellae

Capitulum fibulae

Ligamentum m. gracilis

Ligamentum m. sartorii

Tuberositas tibiae

Fig. 724.—Superficial Musculo-aponeurotic Structures of the Anterior Region of the Thigh and Knee.

the space. The canal runs from the apex of the femoral triangle (of Scarpa) to the tendinous hiatus in the adductor magnus muscle, through which the femoral vessels enter the popliteal fossa.

    The *femoral artery* is bound closely by connective tissue to the femoral vein, which at first lies posterior to and then slightly to the lateral side of the artery. The superior geniculate (anastomotica magna) artery branches from the femoral near its termination.

    The *saphenous nerve* crosses anterior to the femoral artery and diverges from it at the tendinous hiatus. The nerve passes downward under the sartorius muscle to a distribution over the medial aspect of the leg and ankle.

The incision for *ligation of the femoral artery in the adductor canal* is along a line extending from the midpoint of the inguinal ligament to the adductor tubercle. The incision is deepened through the superficial fascia, and the great saphenous vein is retracted. The thin fascia over the sartorius is divided and the muscle is retracted medially. The strong fascial roof of the canal is opened and the femoral artery is exposed with the saphenous nerve on its anterior surface.

After ligation of the femoral artery, collateral circulation is established through the anastomosis between the descending branch of the lateral circumflex artery and the superior

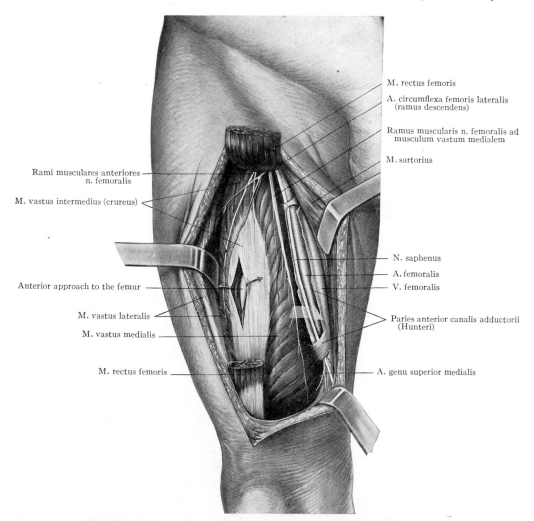

M. rectus femoris

A. circumflexa femoris lateralis (ramus descendens)

Ramus muscularis n. femoralis ad musculum vastum medialem

M. sartorius

Rami musculares anteriores n. femoralis

M. vastus intermedius (crureus)

N. saphenus

A. femoralis

V. femoralis

Anterior approach to the femur

M. vastus lateralis

Paries anterior canalis adductorii (Hunteri)

M. vastus medialis

M. rectus femoris

A. genu superior medialis

FIG. 725.—DEEP STRUCTURES OF THE ANTERIOR REGION OF THE THIGH.
This drawing indicates the structures encountered in the anterior approach to the shaft of the femur.

geniculate (anastomotica magna), and through the connections between the fourth perforating artery and branches of the popliteal artery.

3. **Shaft of the Femur.**—The shaft of the femur is longer and stronger than that of any other bone. It is inclined downward and medially toward the knee; the obliquity is greater in females than in males on account of the proportionately greater width of the female pelvis. The direction of the shaft presents a gentle forward convexity. Its shape is not quite cylindrical because of the pronounced ridge or *linea aspera* which projects from its posterior surface. In the distal third of the femur, the linea aspera bifurcates into

elevations which are continued down to the condyles as the epicondylar ridges.   The **bone** increases in size toward the condyles and assumes an oval outline on cross section.

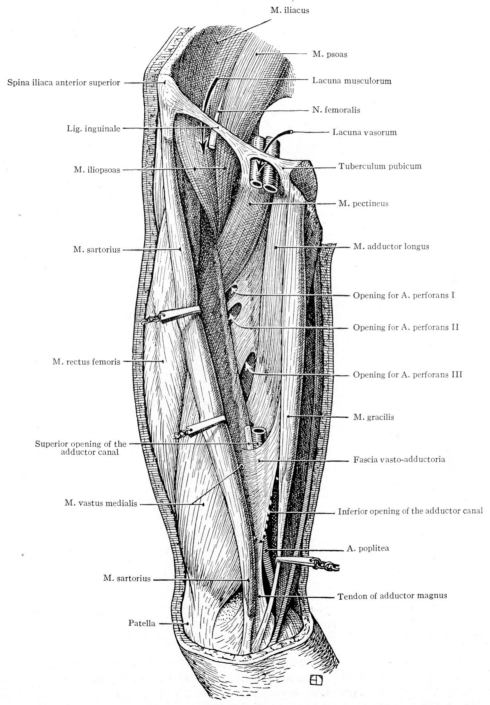

FIG. 726.—DEEP STRUCTURES OF THE ANTERO-INTERNAL REGION OF THE THIGH.   (Corning.)

The shaft is obscured by the muscles covering it so that actual palpation **cannot be** performed and ready surgical approach is rendered difficult.   The depth of the bone from the anterior surface of the thigh is greatest in its proximal part, but diminishes progressively downward. A cross section through the thigh at the junction of the lower and middle thirds shows the femur altogether within the anterior half of the section. The absence of large vessels on the lateral or anterolateral aspect of the thigh permits the deep incision necessary for the repair of fractures or the treatment of osteomyelitis. Incision is made parallel or anterior to the lateral intermuscular septum.

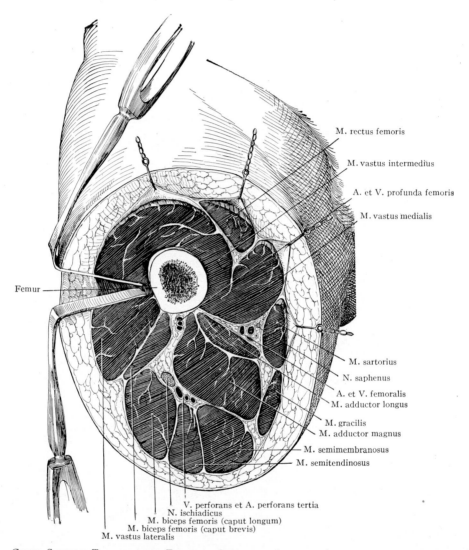

FIG. 727.—CROSS SECTION THROUGH THE THIGH TO SHOW THE LATERAL APPROACH TO THE FEMUR.
The incision does not follow the lateral intermuscular septum, but traverses the vastus lateralis muscle
A better approach follows the intermuscular septum between the vastus lateralis and biceps muscles.

The cortex is a thick layer of compact bone about the central medullary cavity. The thickest part corresponds to the linea aspera. The thickness of the cortex decreases progressively in the lower third of the bone until it is reduced to a thin layer at the condyles. The central canal extends from the base of the lesser trochanter to a point about a palmbreadth above the articular surface of the condyles. The main nutrient artery enters the nutrient foramen on the linea aspera above the middle of the shaft and, after traversing the bone obliquely upward for about 5 cm., enters the medullary canal. A second nutrient foramen may be present farther distally. Of the femoral epiphyses, the lower is the last to unite.

4. **Anterior and Lateral Approach to the Femur.**—The *anterior route* to the femur is through the deep fascia along the mesial border of the rectus femoris muscle. Lateral retraction of the rectus femoris exposes the subjacent vastus intermedius (crureus) muscle which blends with the vastus medialis. The incision can be deepened with scarcely any bleeding to expose the shaft of the femur over an area free from muscle attachments.

The entire diaphysis of the femur is accessible by a *lateral approach* through the fascia lata and vastus lateralis muscle or along the line of the lateral intermuscular septum. Few important structures are encountered along this route. The incision splits the ilio-tibial tract and exposes the vastus lateralis muscle. After deepening the wound through the vastus lateralis, the vastus intermedius is exposed and is retracted forward from the lateral surface of the femur. In the distal part of the shaft, the vastus lateralis is retracted forward from the lateral intermuscular septum. The septum is drawn backward with the short head of the biceps. Hemorrhage in this area comes from injury to the anastomosis between the descending branch of the lateral circumflex and the lateral superior genicular artery from the popliteal. This part of the incision is the approach to the femur used in cuneiform osteotomy for genu varum (p. 754).

5. **Fractures of the Shaft of the Femur.**—Fractures of the femoral shaft present problems somewhat like those involved in fracture of the humerus. There is no splinting

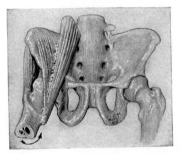

Fig. 728.—Mechanism of the Displacement of the Proximal Fragment in Fracture of the Upper Third of the Shaft of the Femur.
The proximal fragment is flexed by the iliopsoas muscle and is rotated laterally by the lateral rotator muscles of the hip. (Babcock, "Textbook of Surgery.")

bone, and the powerful muscles, some of which span the femur, cause characteristic angulation and overriding.

Although subject to a variety of strains, the femur usually is broken by direct violence. The fracturing force may act indirectly, as it does in a fall upon the knee or in powerful twists, such as may occur when the body is turned to one side with the foot held firm. Fractures from direct violence, as a rule, are transverse, or nearly so; spiral or long oblique fractures are fairly common. Fragment displacement is greater in fractures from indirect violence than in those from direct violence where the break tends to be transverse. The degree of displacement depends upon the direction of the injuring force, the line of fracture, the muscle pull, and the influence of the weight of the limb. The most powerful muscles effecting the displacement are the adductors and hamstrings. The entire femur may be regarded as a rigid arc, subtended by a mass of muscles upon the medial and posterior aspects of the thigh. Consequently, when the shaft breaks, these two groups of muscles tend to approximate the extremities of the bony arc, with the result that the distal fragment is drawn up beneath the proximal fragment. An angular deformity results. The summit of the angle most frequently is directed forward, or forward and laterally. With this deformity, there is a considerable degree of shortening. The correction of shortening is one of the main problems encountered in the treatment of femoral fracture. In spite of the bulk of thigh muscles, femoral fractures frequently are compound.

In *fracture of the proximal third of the femur,* anterior and lateral displacement of the proximal fragment usually is marked, as this fragment is drawn forward by the iliopsoas and pectineus muscles and is abducted and rotated laterally by the muscles attached to the greater trochanter. The forward tilting of the proximal fragment is increased by the forward push of the distal fragment, which is drawn upward behind the proximal fragment by the hamstring and adductor muscles. The distal fragment is rotated laterally by the adductors and the weight of the everted foot.

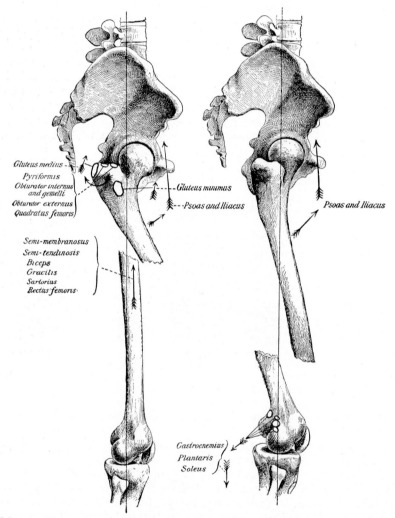

Fig. 729.—Mechanism of the Displacement of the Fragments in Fracture of the Upper and Lower Thirds of the Shaft of the Femur. (Deaver after Nifong.)

The short, deeply placed proximal fragment is difficult to manipulate into position. To correct displacement and bring the distal and proximal fragments into apposition, traction in wide abduction usually is necessary. Skeletal traction from the femoral condyles readily brings the fragments to proper length. The anterior muscles are relaxed by flexion of the thigh on the pelvis and the posterior muscles are relaxed by flexion of the knee on the thigh.

Fracture of the middle third of the shaft is treated more easily than fracture of the proximal third because of the greater length and the more superficial position of the proximal fragment. The displacement is caused by the same forces that act upon fracture through the proximal third and is similar, save that there is less tendency toward over-riding and more toward angulation. As a rule, however, the distal fragment slides upward, behind, and medial to the proximal fragment. In fracture produced by indirect violence, the fragment ends sometimes are pointed and sharp, and become embedded in the muscles and deep fascia, rendering reduction difficult.

Fracture through the middle third usually can be treated successfully by skin traction in a Thomas or Hodgen splint, considerably elevated above the plane of the bed. The distal fragment, which, as a rule, is displaced posteriorly and mesially, is supported in the splint; lateral traction on the distal fragment may be required. In infants and children, skin traction is employed on the leg and thigh, which are flexed at right angles to the trunk; the body weight acts as countertraction.

In *fracture of the distal third of the shaft*, the distal fragment is tilted backward by the gastrocnemius muscle and the nearer the fracture is to the condyles, the more marked is the tilting. This fragment is drawn upward behind the proximal fragment by the quadriceps femoris and hamstring muscles. The popliteal artery and the common peroneal (external popliteal) nerve may be lacerated or may be stretched over the sharp proximal edge of the distal fragment. The artery lies deeper and is more liable to injury. The thigh appears shortened and thickened, and the swelling from hemorrhage soon obscures the bony deformity. Slight rotary movements show that the trochanter fails to move with the distal fragment of the shaft.

Reduction is effected by skeletal traction through the femoral condyles; the knee must be flexed to relax the gastrocnemius muscle and allow the distal fragment to tilt forward to its normal position. Since traction causes a downward tilting of the pelvis on the affected side, and hence a relative abduction of the distal fragment, a genu valgum may be produced. If the fracture is too close to the condyles for the use of skeletal traction on the condyles, reduction is attempted by manipulation; the fragments are immobilized with the knee at a right angle or less, and with the thigh partially flexed on the pelvis. Skeletal traction may be effected with pin or wire passed through the proximal portion of the tibial crest. The knee joint, which is peculiarly prone to stiffening after prolonged fixation, is safeguarded partially when skeletal traction is applied to the femoral condyles, since, in this method of treatment, motion at the knee is not hindered

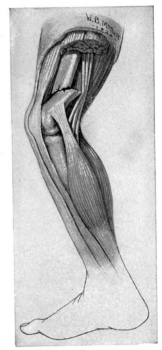

FIG. 730.—FRACTURE OF THE DISTAL THIRD OF THE SHAFT OF THE FEMUR.

The posterior displacement of the distal fragment by the gastrocnemius muscle endangers the popliteal vessels and nerves. (Babcock, "Textbook of Surgery.")

E. POSTERIOR OR FLEXOR REGION OF THE THIGH

1. **Definition and Boundaries.**—The posterior or flexor region of the thigh represents the soft parts behind the plane of the intermuscular septa. It is limited laterally by the lateral intermuscular septum, mesially by the plane of the posterior surface of the adductor muscles, the medial intermuscular septum, above by the inferior border of the gluteus maximus, and below by the upper limits of the popliteal space.

2. **Musculature.**—The posterior compartment of the thigh contains the three hamstring muscles and the sciatic nerve with its two terminal branches, the tibial (internal popliteal) and the common peroneal (external popliteal).

The hamstring muscles arise from the posterior surface of the ischial tuberosity and span the long distance between the pelvis and knee with no attachment to the body of the femur except for the short head of the biceps.   As a result, these muscles retract more after amputation than do the anterior thigh muscles which have femoral attachments.

The *biceps femoris muscle*, which runs distally and laterally, has a second or short head of origin from the linea aspera.   The common tendon is felt easily through the skin.   It descends to an insertion on the head of the fibula, extends the thigh, and is a powerful flexor and a weak lateral rotator of the knee joint.   The *semimembranosus muscle* runs distally along the medial side of the posterior compartment of the thigh to insert into the medial condyle of the tibia.   The *semitendinosus* is muscular above, but tapers distally

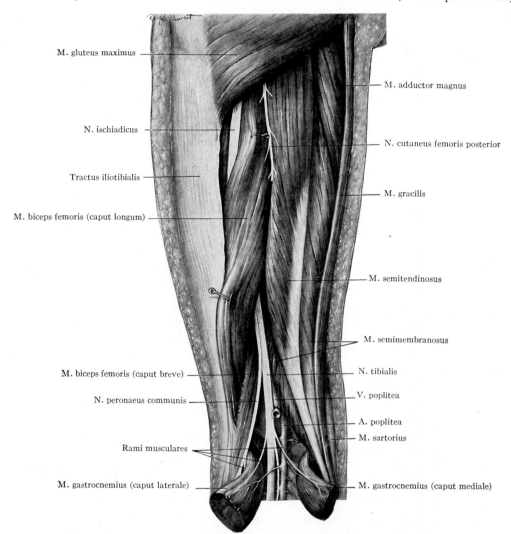

M. gluteus maximus

M. adductor magnus

N. ischiadicus

N. cutaneus femoris posterior

Tractus iliotibialis

M. gracilis

M. biceps femoris (caput longum)

M. semitendinosus

M. semimembranosus

M. biceps femoris (caput breve)

N. tibialis

N. peronaeus communis

V. poplitea

A. poplitea

M. sartorius

Rami musculares

M. gastrocnemius (caput laterale)

M. gastrocnemius (caput mediale)

FIG. 731.—STRUCTURES OF THE POSTERIOR REGION OF THE THIGH AND THE POPLITEAL SPACE.

into a long tendon which lies in a groove on the posterior surface of the semimembranosus. It inserts into the medial surface of the tibia.   Both of these muscles extend the thigh and flex the leg, and, with their medial tibial insertion, produce a slight amount of medial rotation at the knee joint.

The posterior group of thigh muscles is supplied by the sciatic nerve (L_4, $_5$, S_1, $_2$, $_3$), but the nerve to the short head of the biceps may arise from the common peroneal (external popliteal) nerve (L_4, $_5$, S_1)

3. **Vessels and Nerves.**—The perforating branches of the *profunda femoris artery*

(p. 704) enter the posterior portions of the thigh through openings in the adductor magnus muscle, close to its insertion into the linea aspera. They wind posteriorly about the bone to supply the hamstring muscles and much of the vastus lateralis. Hemorrhage from operations on the shaft of the femur is difficult to control because of the depth of the source of the bleeding. The first perforating artery, in addition to forming longitudinal loop-anastomoses, enters into the crucial anastomosis (p. 676). The third and fourth perforating arteries anastomose with the proximal muscular rami of the popliteal artery.

The superficial *lymphatics* drain into the superficial subinguinal lymph nodes, and the deep lymphatics follow the inferior gluteal vessels to the hypogastric lymph nodes in the pelvis. Two nerves run down the axis of the posterior compartment of the thigh. The *posterior cutaneous nerve (small sciatic)* runs deep to the enveloping fascia and its branches supply the overlying skin. The *sciatic nerve (great sciatic)* is the continuation of the flattened band of the sacral plexus and descends between the greater trochanter of the femur and the tuberosity of the ischium. It is overlain proximally by the long head of the biceps muscle, and below is overlapped by the semimembranosus muscle. Early in its course, it supplies the hamstring and the adductor magnus muscles. It terminates in the middle third of the thigh by dividing into the common peroneal and tibial nerves

The *surgical approach to the sciatic nerve* is along the axial line of the femur from a point midway between the greater trochanter and the ischial tuberosity and the apex of the popliteal fossa. In the proximal part of the incision, the inferior margin of the gluteus maximus muscle is exposed and retracted superiorly. The nerve is located in a mass of fatty tissue after retracting the relaxed hamstring muscles medially. In the midportion of the thigh, the groove between the diverging hamstring muscles is identified and the nerve is exposed by retracting the long head of the biceps laterally.

4. **Amputation Through the Thigh.**—Unless there are definite contraindications, the site of election for amputation through the thigh is through the lower third where a stump, admirably adapted to the adjustment of a prosthesis, is obtained. The shortest satisfactory amputation in the upper third of the thigh requires a 7.5 cm. stump, for it is almost impossible to f. t a stump of less length with a prosthetic device.

In thigh amputations, certain anatomical points are of interest. Because of the great mobility of the skin and subcutaneous tissue over the fascia lata, superficial flaps are raised easily at any level of the limb. The muscles, from the viewpoint of amputation, form the principal bulk of the limb and constitute two groups. The first group consists of those which are invested by loose areolar tissue and which have no fixed attachment to the femur. It includes the sartorius, gracilis, and hamstring muscles, with the exception of the short head of the biceps. These muscles lie in the medial and posterior parts of the thigh and retract freely when divided. The second group includes those muscles which are attached to the femur—the quadriceps femoris group and the three adductors. When these are divided they retract to a much less extent than do the muscles of the first group. In transverse sections through the middle third of the thigh, the femoral and profunda vessels are located in the muscles at the inner side of the divided femur. The descending branches of the lateral circumflex vessels, which run downward in the substance of the vastus lateralis muscle, some muscle branches of the femoral vessels, and the perforating branches of the profunda vessels may require ligation. The sciatic nerve is recognized readily in the midst of the hamstring muscles. It is advisable to retract the nerve from the loose connective tissue which surrounds it and to remove enough of it to insure its remaining deeply buried between the muscles when it is released. If it comes sufficiently near the end of the stump to be subjected to pressure, it subsequently develops a painful bulbous extremity, known as an amputation neuroma.

A very successful *amputation through the lower third* of the thigh is that described by the author* as follows. The patient is placed in the dorsal decubitus position, the knee

---

* 1. Callander, C. L.: A New Amputation in the Lower Third of the Thigh, J.A.M.A., **105**: 1746–1753, Nov. 30, 1935. 2. Callander, C. L.: Tendoplastic Amputation Through the Femur at the Knee. (Further Studies), J.A.M.A., **110** (No. 2): 113–117, Jan. 8, 1938.

of the affected extremity is flexed slightly, and the leg is elevated a little above the horizontal on one or two sandbags.   No tourniquet is applied.   The surgeon stands on the

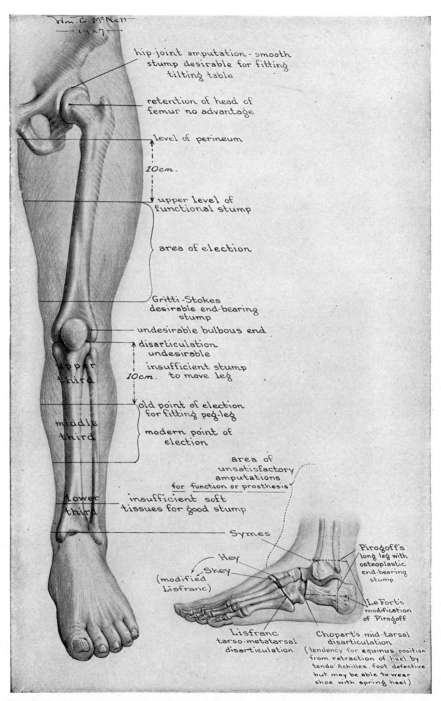

FIG. 732.—AMPUTATIONS IN THE LOWER EXTREMITY.   (Babcock, "Textbook of Surgery.")

side opposite the affected extremity and faces the medial aspect of the thigh and knee to be operated upon.   He maintains this position throughout the operation, because the essential steps are directed through a medial approach to the popliteal space. The operative work on the lateral aspect of the lower part of the thigh and knee is accomplished readily by rotating the knee medially.

The incisions in the skin outlining the slightly unequal anterior and posterior flaps coincide with the incisions that sever all the deeper soft parts. The incision on the medial aspect of the thigh begins at a point three fingerbreadths proximal to the most prominent part of the medial femoral condyle and runs horizontally distally in the palpable groove between the vastus medialis and the sartorius muscles. With the knee in partial flexion, this groove can be defined readily. After the incision has been deepened to the enveloping or deep fascia of the thigh, the adductor tubercle of the medial femoral condyle and the tendon of the adductor magnus muscle, which inserts on it, can be palpated. The incision in the skin continues distally over the medial condyle, sweeps forward and crosses the anterior surface of the tibia at the anterior tibial tuberosity, the point of insertion of the quadriceps extensor tendon.

The thigh then is rotated medially (*i. e.*, toward the surgeon). The incision on the lateral aspect of the leg begins at a point three fingerbreadths proximal to the lateral femoral condyle in the palpable groove between the tendon of the tensor fasciae latae (iliotibial tract) and the biceps femoris muscles. This incision must overlie and split the tensor fasciae latae tendon in order to avoid the muscle fibers of the biceps. Continuing distally over the lateral epicondyle, the incision extends forward to meet the medial incision at the anterior tibial tuberosity, thus outlining the anterior flap of the amputation.

Corresponding incisions from each femoral epicondyle are carried obliquely posteriorly and inferiorly until they meet on the calf of the leg at a point considerably inferior to the level of the anterior tibial tuberosity, at about the midpoint of the belly of the gastrocnemius muscle. This incision for the posterior flap is deepened to the fascia on the gastrocnemius muscle. Thus are outlined two long amputation flaps, the posterior a little longer than the anterior. Each flap partakes not only of the soft parts of the lower thigh, but of a considerable portion of the soft parts of the leg.

Attention then is centered again on the medial aspect of the thigh and knee. The horizontal portion of the medial incision, common to the two flaps (*i. e.*, that portion lying between the vastus medialis and the sartorius muscles) is deepened through the deep fascia of the thigh. Division of this powerful fascial layer, which is the only strong structure in the medial wall of the popliteal fossa at this level, affords ingress to the popliteal space. The left forefinger, now inserted into the superficial popliteal space, by blunt dissection frees the medial hamstring tendons as far as their tibial insertions. At this juncture, these tendons are divided in the order named: sartorius, gracilis, semimembranosus, and semitendinosus. During this dissection, no fleshy portion of any of the medial hamstring muscles nor any part of the vastus medialis muscle need be exposed, much less severed. The severed hamstring tendons retract at once into the aponeurotic and areolar tissue of the posterior flap and are not dealt with again. Further exposure is gained by severing the tendon of the adductor magnus muscle at its attachment to the adductor tubercle. Free access to the vasculoneural contents of the popliteal space thus is afforded. Moderate flexion of the knee relaxes the popliteal vessels and nerves and favors their manipulation. With a finger now inserted more deeply into the popliteal space and kept close to the posterior surface of the femur, the popliteal artery and vein are withdrawn easily to a level flush with, or even outside of, the incision in the skin. Here they are clamped, ligated, and divided as far proximally in the popliteal space as possible. The tibial (internal popliteal) and common peroneal nerves are then drawn readily into the wound as one trunk and are anesthetized, ligated, and divided. Each of the components of the nerve bundle then is injected with absolute alcohol to prevent formation of neuroma, and the stump is allowed to retract into the proximal recess of the popliteal space. Ligation of these three essential structures low down in the popliteal space prevents unnecessary separation of the posterior flap from the femur and minimizes formation of dead space.

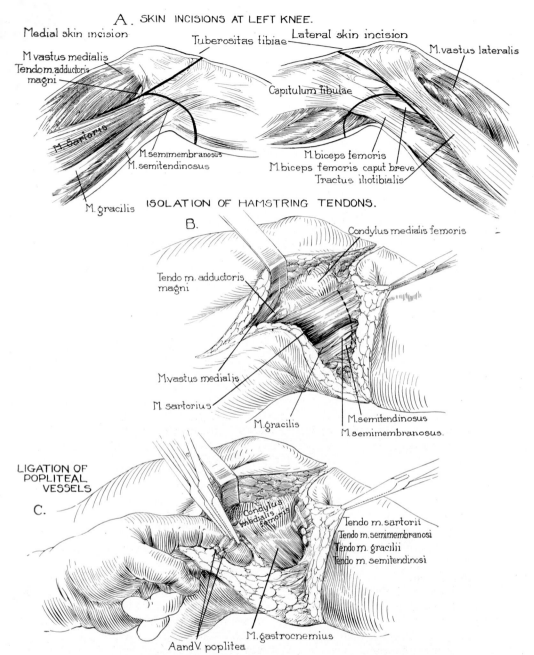

A. SKIN INCISIONS AT LEFT KNEE.

Medial skin incision — Tuberositas tibiae — Lateral skin incision

M.vastus medialis
Tendo m.adductoris magni
M.sartorius
M.semimembranosus
M.semitendinosus
M.gracilis

M.vastus lateralis
Capitulum fibulae
M.biceps femoris
M.biceps femoris caput breve
Tractus iliotibialis

ISOLATION OF HAMSTRING TENDONS.

B.

Condylus medialis femoris

Tendo m. adductoris magni

M.vastus medialis

M. sartorius

M.gracilis

M.semitendinosus
M.semimembranosus.

LIGATION OF POPLITEAL VESSELS

C.

Condylus medialis femoris

Tendo m.sartorii
Tendo m.semimembranosi
Tendo m. gracilii
Tendo m. semitendinosi

M.gastrocnemius

A and V. poplitea

FIG. 733.—AUTHOR'S TENDOPLASTIC AMPUTATION THROUGH THE FEMUR AT THE KNEE.
A. Skin incisions indicate that the skin and subcutaneous tissues of the leg enter into flap formation. It is evident that the hamstring muscles are cut through their tendinous insertions.
B. Fleshy portion of medial hamstring muscles exposed to show anatomic location. Only the tendinous portions are exposed during operation
C. The medial hamstring muscles have retracted after section, exposing the popliteal space widely for ligation of the popliteal vessels.

The partly flexed knee then is rotated toward the operator, and the lateral longitudinal incision is deepened through the more posterior fibers of the tensor fasciae latae tendon. This incision is carried inferiorly as far as the insertion of the biceps muscle on the head of the fibula, where the biceps tendon then is severed. At this stage of the operation, the popliteal space may be opened widely from side to side, since the essential

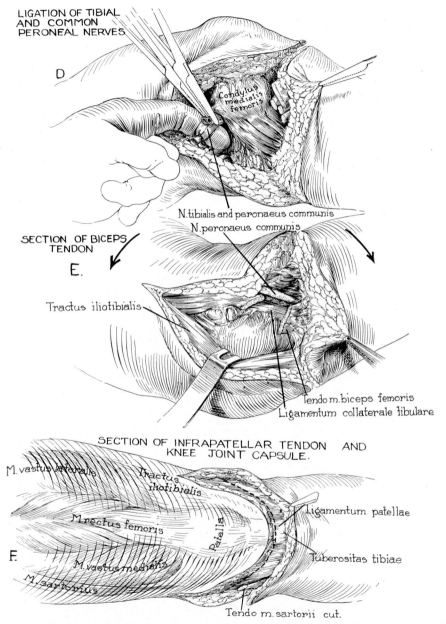

FIG. 733 (*Continued*).—AUTHOR'S TENDOPLASTIC AMPUTATION THROUGH THE FEMUR AT THE KNEE.

D. The tibial and common peroneal nerves are hooked into the wound with the index finger prior to section.

E. The lateral side of the knee is rotated medially toward the surgeon, who always stands throughout the operation on the side opposite to the extremity operated upon. The biceps tendon is sectioned.

F. The quadriceps extensor apparatus is sectioned at its tibial insertion. Incision likewise is carried through the quadriceps aponeurotic expansions.

structures have been divided. Deepening of the incision outlining the posterior flap down to the gastrocnemius aponeurosis and clearing from it the areolo-adipose débris, free the posterior flap.   It is advantageous to leave as much as possible of the fibro-areolar tissue of the popliteal space in contact with the femur as far distally as the level of the ad-

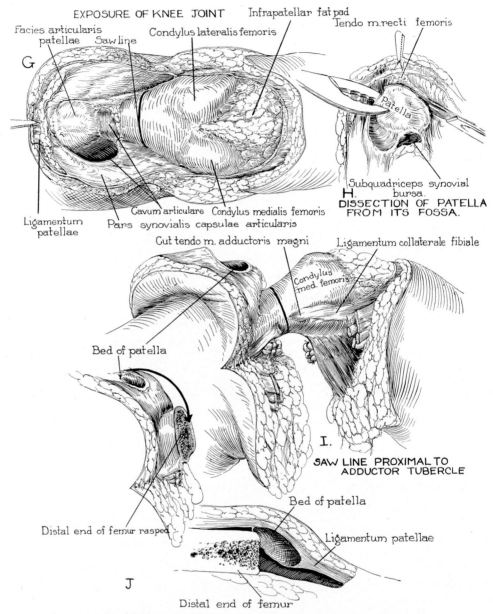

EXPOSURE OF KNEE JOINT

H. DISSECTION OF PATELLA FROM ITS FOSSA.

I. SAW LINE PROXIMAL TO ADDUCTOR TUBERCLE

J ILLUSTRATING HOW FEMUR FITS INTO PATELLAR FOSSA.

FIG. 733 (*Continued*).—AUTHOR'S TENDOPLASTIC AMPUTATION THROUGH THE FEMUR AT THE KNEE.

G. Knee joint exposed and saw-line on the femur indicated.   Saw-line an inch more proximal on the shaft than line indicated gives a shorter stump, and one better adapted to a prosthesis.

H. Patella is removed from its fossa by sharp and blunt dissection.   Removal is easier from the apex to the base.

I, J. Patellar fossa falls naturally over sectioned end of the femur.

ductor tubercle in order that there may be but little dead space between the posterior flap and the femur.

The knee then is extended and the incision marking the distal portion of the **anterior** flap is deepened through the capsule of the knee joint down to the femoral condyles and to the tibia, thereby severing the quadriceps tendon at its insertion into the tibial tuberosity. The anterior flap, containing the patella, is dissected upward off the infrapatellar fat pad and drawn upward on the thigh until the superior synovial recesses of the subquadriceps space are seen. The patella is dissected from the apex to the base from its sesamoid position in the quadriceps tendon, care being taken to preserve the longitudinally disposed tendon of the rectus femoris muscle, which runs over it. Preservation of this tendon adds materially to the end-bearing capacity of the stump after the cut end of the femur is fitted into the socket from which the patella has been removed. The synovia on the anterior flap and on the femur proximal to the condyles is not excised. The femur now is sawed through its cancellous portion just proximal to the adductor tubercle. At this level, the shaft of the femur corresponds in size to the patellar socket in the quadriceps tendon. The cut end of the femur is rounded with a bone-cutting forceps and a rasp until no sharp surfaces and no fringes of periosteum remain.

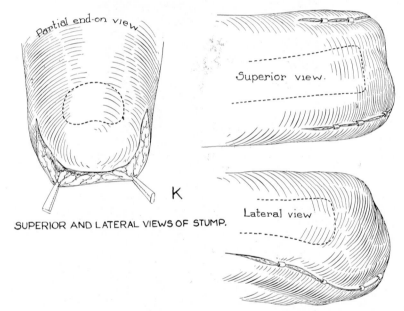

FIG. 733 (*Continued*).—AUTHOR'S TENDOPLASTIC AMPUTATION THROUGH THE FEMUR AT THE KNEE. K. Indicates the redundant amputation flaps and the loose closure of the suture line.

The two large flaps are inspected for small bleeding points. These can be ascertained best by sluicing the surfaces of both flaps with large quantities of warm salt solution. The flushing has the additional advantage of washing away any soft tissue or bone débris. Many small bleeding points may require ligation after this procedure. Inspection of the body of the posterior flap shows no muscle fibers. It does show areolo-adipose tissue and the cut ends of the hamstring tendons, which already are retracted into their aponeurotic beds and scarcely are visible. The flaps now are allowed to fall loosely together.

The coaptation suturing during the operation is limited to the placing of six or eight clips or sutures at such intervals as to keep the flaps in fair apposition. When the edges of the skin are approximated, the aponeurotic edges lie in contact also; mere apposition is sufficient to produce firm union. None of the tendons or aponeuroses of the anterior flap are sutured to the corresponding structures of the posterior flap. In this way, no structure is under any tension, and the trauma and consequent pressure necroses which result from suture of these deeper structures cannot occur. The flaps appear exceedingly long and even extend one or more inches beyond the end of the femur immediately after they are fashioned. To the surgeon accustomed to the routine type of amputation in the lower third of the femur, the flaps appear excessively redundant and clumsy and arouse suspicion that a bulbous stump end and large dead spaces will result. When he notes how wobbly the femur lies between the flaps, he questions whether the end will gain contact with the patellar socket and fuse there. As early as the second or third post-operative day and sometimes even within a few hours after the operation, the reason for

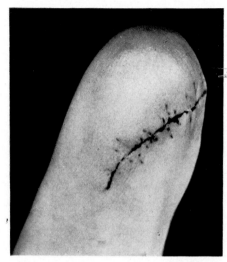

FIG. 734.—HEALED AMPUTATION STUMP.
Note the degree of retraction of the posterior flap. This retraction helps lodge the end of the femur in the patellar fossa. (Callander.)

leaving these flaps under no tension becomes apparent, as the hamstring muscles, severed only at their distal attachment, contract to the degree that the cutaneous suture line lies posteriorly at about the level of the stump end, and the femur is felt in the patellar fossa (Fig. 734).

III. KNEE

The region of the knee is bounded superiorly by a line drawn around the thigh at a level three fingerbreadths superior to the base of the patella. Its inferior limit is at the level of the distal part of the tibial tuberosity. The knee presents three regions: an anterior or quadriceps extensor region, a posterior or popliteal region, and the bones and joint of the knee, including the superior tibiofibular joint.

A. ANTERIOR OR QUADRICEPS EXTENSOR REGION

The anterior or quadriceps extensor region (Fig. 724), composed entirely of soft parts offers protection as well as direct access to the knee joint. It constitutes the terminal part of the extension apparatus of the quadriceps muscle which is homologous to the triceps-olecranon extension apparatus at the elbow.

1. **Landmarks.**—The surface markings over a region as important as the knee require detailed study, since familiarity with them facilitates proper interpretation of the varied and extensive pathologic conditions which alter them. The knee joint is covered thinly on each side and in front; the bones forming it can be examined easily, any deviation from the normal contour is detected readily, and certain forms of articular disease can be diagnosed at a comparatively early stage. The landmarks at the knee vary greatly according to whether the leg is extended or flexed, so that it is necessary to study each attitude separately. The patella, because of the inelasticity of the ligamentum patellae, lies at a constant distance from its insertion into the tibial tuberosity, whether the knee is flexed or extended.

When the leg is extended, it does not lie in the axis of the thigh, but forms an obtuse angle, open laterally. The angle varies considerably, but ordinarily measures about 170 degrees. The angulation is more striking in females, because of the more marked medial obliquity of the femur, and is greatly accentuated in the deformity of genu valgum or knock knee. The *patella* projects prominently in front and its outline is defined readily. When the quadriceps muscle is at rest, the patella enjoys a free range of motion and may be moved from side to side, proximally and distally. The tendon of the rectus femoris muscle may be traced to the upper border of the patella, and the *ligamentum patellae* can be felt from its attachment at the apex of the patella to its attachment at the tuberosity of the tibia. The tendon is about 5 cm. long and its midpoint corresponds to the level of the knee joint. When the joint is distended with fluid, the articular surfaces of the patella and femur are separated. A gentle tap on a "floating patella" causes it to knock against the femur.

Between the lateral margins of the patella and the corresponding femoral condyles are longitudinal depressions, the *lateral and medial parapatellar grooves*. If the subcutaneous fat is abundant, these depressions are obliterated. When the rectus femoris muscle is relaxed, as in passive extension, the lateral grooves are connected by a shallow groove above the base of the patella, giving the bone the appearance of being bounded by a horseshoe-shaped peripatellar groove. Beneath the grooves lie the upper and lateral

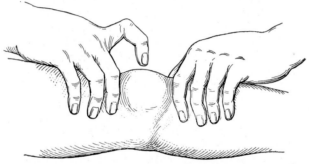

FIG. 735.—ELICITING THE "TAP" OR "CLICK" OF THE FLOATING PATELLA IN SYNOVITIS OF THE KNEE. The hands are used to gather the fluid under the floated patella so that the index finger may percuss and elicit the "tap" or "click." (Moorhead.)

prolongations of the synovial membrane af the knee joint. When the peripatellar groove becomes distended with blood or an inflammatory effusion, the superficial depressions are replaced by a crescentic swelling which almost encircles the patella. Aspiration of the knee joint may be done through any part of this crescent.

The lateral and medial parapatellar grooves are succeeded below by a fullness on each side of the patellar ligament which is accentuated by contraction of the quadriceps muscle. This fullness is caused by the intra-articular, extrasynovial *fat pad* which is wedged into the interval between the patellar ligament, the head of the tibia, and the femoral condyles. When the leg is extended, the fat pad conveys a sense of fluctuation to the examining fingers, especially in the transverse direction, and may be mistaken for an effusion. Another source of swelling in this region is the *infrapatellar bursa* which lies between the patellar ligament and the upper part of the tibia. A fluctuant bursa may project to each side of the ligament.

The *joint line* between the femur and tibia is palpated most readily on each side of the patellar ligament. Laterally, the joint line is indistinct because of the resistance and tenseness of the collateral (lateral) ligaments. By displacing the patella inward or outward, the outer and inner lips and part of the anterior articular surface of the femur can be palpated. Both of these margins become thickened or lipped in certain varieties of arthritis. By flat palpation over the joint line, the degree of thickening of the joint capsule can be determined.

The outer surface of the *lateral condyle of the femur* is crossed by the lower part of the *iliotibial band* of the fascia lata and by the *tendon of the biceps* as it descends to its insertion into the *head of the fibula*. The *common peroneal (external popliteal) nerve*, which follows the medial aspect of the biceps tendon into the popliteal space, becomes superficial at this level and can be rolled under the finger where the nerve passes behind the head of the fibula. The prominent anterior part of the *lateral tibial condyle* can be felt in front of the head of the fibula at a somewhat higher level. The iliotibial band inserts into it.

The prominent *medial condyle of the femur* can be felt on the medial side of the knee. Above and deeply placed, the *adductor tubercle* marks the lower point of insertion of the adductor magnus tendon into the femur. This is an accurate guide to the distal epiphyseal line which runs horizontally just above the trochlear surface of the femur. Behind the medial epicondyle, the *sartorius muscle* and *gracilis tendon* curve about the medial aspect of the condyle, after which they incline almost directly forward and insert into the upper and medial aspect of the tibial shaft. At the knee, these tendons are related closely to those of the semimembranosus and semitendinosus muscles.

In active extension of the leg, the tendon of the *rectus femoris muscle* forms a tense band which is inserted into the proximal border of the patella. The *vastus medialis muscle* forms a prominent elevation on the medial side of the rectus tendon, and the vastus lateralis muscle, a similar bulge on the lateral side at a more proximal level. Disuse atrophy of the vastus muscles calls attention to more or less painful joint conditions with limited joint function. A very evident depression lies distal to the bulge formed by the lateral vastus muscle between the rectus femoris muscle medially and the iliotibial tract laterally. With the leg in relaxed extension, as in reclining, the whole quadriceps apparatus relaxes, the suprapatellar depression is deeper, the bulges of the vasti are less prominent, and the patella can be moved freely.

When the leg is flexed, the patella at first becomes more prominent, but as the movement is continued, it sinks deeply into the hollow of the intercondyloid notch and becomes firmly fixed, the apex corresponding to the joint line. Through the thin layer of tissue above the patella, the upper part of the trochlear surface of the femur may be felt. In flexion, the interval between the tibia and femur anteriorly is increased; the condyles of the femur become more distinct and their curved lower margins are defined more readily. In the kneeling position, the patella protects the joint, and, with the tuberosity of the tibia, supports the superincumbent weight.

2. **Superficial Structures and Deep Fascia.**—The *skin* over the anterior region of the knee is moderately thin and possesses a high degree of mobility. It is very resistant, as is the lamellated layer of *superficial fascia.*

The superficial structure of surgical interest is the **prepatellar bursa** which lies between the skin and the front of the lower part of the patella and patellar ligament. A division of it may be found between the deep fascia and the tendinous covering of the patella or even beneath the tendinous coverings of the patella itself. As a rule, the interior of the bursal space is intersected by fibrous bands. This large bursa allows the skin to glide over the patella and withstand pressure. It especially adapts the patella for use in the Gritti-Stokes amputation through the knee (p. 762).

This bursa, because of its superficial and exposed position, becomes inflamed easily. Effusion may occur within it and terminate in suppuration—*acute, suppurative prepatellar bursitis*. This acute septic bursitis requires prompt drainage by incision on each side of the median line. Failure to institute drainage may result in the escape of the purulent contents of the bursa into the loose subcutaneous tissue about the knee. This diffusion gives rise to a swelling which has the appearance of a knee-joint effusion, but the abscess always is superficial rather than deep to the patella.

If the inflammation follows a chronic course, the bursa usually becomes distended with clear serous fluid which forms a soft fluctuant swelling anterior to the knee. This condition, commonly known as "housemaid's knee," occurs from the irritation caused by frequent and prolonged kneeling on a hard surface. Chronic bursitis requires complete excision of the bursa. A curved incision with upward convexity is made through the superficial tissues at the upper part of the swelling. The superficial tissues are raised from contact with the cystic swelling, which then is dissected completely from the patella and its ligaments. The scar from an incision with the convexity downward sometimes is a source of pain or tenderness from pressure in kneeling.

In those whose occupation requires constant kneeling, a small, subcutaneous **pretibial bursa** sometimes is present in front of the tibial tuberosity and the distal part of the patellar ligament. A bursa related to the deep surfaces of the tendons at the medial aspect of the knee occasionally is enlarged, and forms an ovoid swelling at the medial aspect of the tibia and the tibial collateral (internal lateral) ligament of the knee joint.

The deep aspect of the **enveloping fascia** of the knee is intimately adherent to the subjacent tendinous structures. Laterally, the fascia is adherent to tendinous fibers of insertion of the iliotibial tract. It is attached mesially to the condyle of the tibia, and, inferior to this, is fused to the expanding terminal tendon of the sartorius muscle.

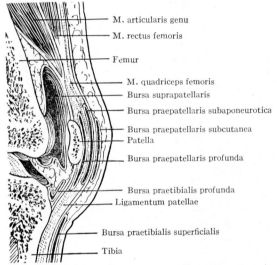

M. articularis genu
M. rectus femoris

Femur

M. quadriceps femoris
Bursa suprapatellaris
Bursa praepatellaris subaponeurotica

Bursa praepatellaris subcutanea
Patella

Bursa praepatellaris profunda

Bursa praetibialis profunda
Ligamentum patellae

Bursa praetibialis superficialis

Tibia

FIG. 736.—SCHEMATIC SAGITTAL SECTION THROUGH THE KNEE REGION TO SHOW THE POTENTIAL DIVISION OF THE PREPATELLAR BURSA AND THE BURSA OVER THE TIBIAL TUBEROSITY.

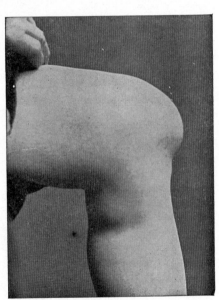

FIG. 737.—PREPATELLAR BURSITIS (HOUSEMAID'S KNEE). (Binnie.)

3. Quadriceps Extension Apparatus.—The musculotendinous suprapatellar segment, the patellar segment, and the patellar tendon are the divisions of the quadriceps femoris extension apparatus which properly belong to the knee region.

The *suprapatellar segment* has the combined strength of its four component muscles, which is exerted through their tendons of insertion into the base and borders of the patella. The direction of the pull on the patella is not in a straight line along the thigh, but along the most direct course to the insertion into the tibial tuberosity. Hence, contraction of the quadriceps muscle tends to dislocate the patella laterally out of the trochlear groove (p. 755).

The rectus femoris muscle is inserted in the median line into the anterior border of the base of the patella by a thin layer, and the most of its fibers continue over the bony surface to form the infrapatellar ligament. The fibrotendinous layer is attached to the rough longitudinal striae of the patella. On each side of the rectus femoris tendon are the prominent muscle bulges and short common tendons of the medial and lateral vasti. These muscles are inserted mainly into the base of the patella posterior to the flattened attachment of the rectus femoris muscle and to the lateral and mesial margins of the bone in its upper third. In the median line, deep to the tendon of the rectus femoris, is the vastus intermedius (crureus) muscle which is inserted more posteriorly into the base of the patella. The suprapatellar arrangement clasping the upper third of the patella is in three superimposed layers: a superficial layer, formed by the tendon of the rectus femoris; a middle layer, consisting of the tendons of the vasti; and a deep layer, made of the tendon of the vastus intermedius. The insertions of this suprapatellar complex at different levels explain the rupture of one or more of the components of the quadriceps extension apparatus.

The *patella* or bony part of the quadriceps apparatus is a true sesamoid bone. Part of the suprapatellar structures pass over and by it to form the *infrapatellar ligament* which fixes the patella in definite relation to the tibia.

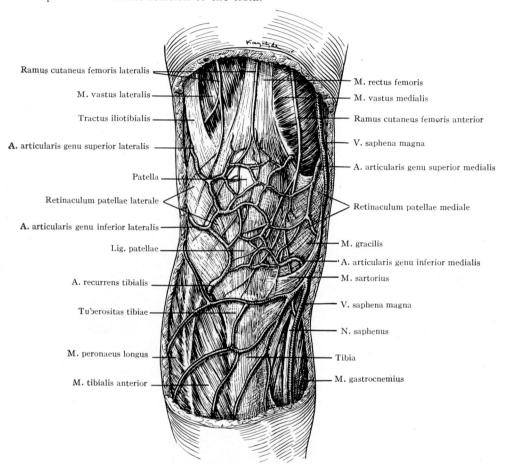

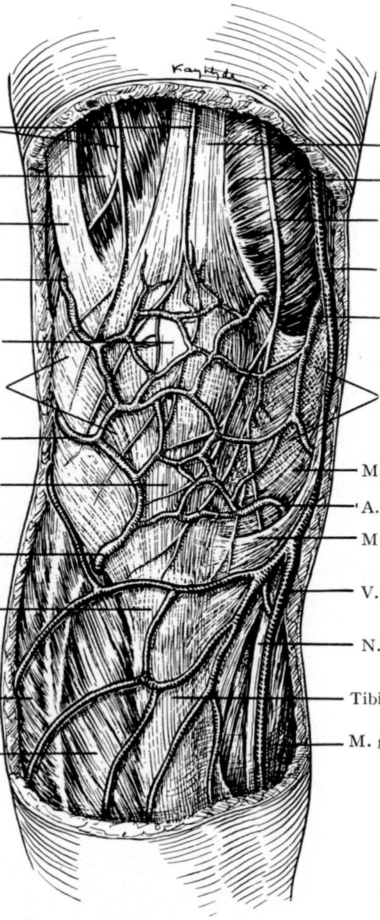
Ramus cutaneus femoris lateralis
M. vastus lateralis
Tractus iliotibialis
A. articularis genu superior lateralis
Patella
Retinaculum patellae laterale
A. articularis genu inferior lateralis
Lig. patellae
A. recurrens tibialis
Tuberositas tibiae
M. peronaeus longus
M. tibialis anterior
M. rectus femoris
M. vastus medialis
Ramus cutaneus femoris anterior
V. saphena magna
A. articularis genu superior medialis
Retinaculum patellae mediale
M. gracilis
A. articularis genu inferior medialis
M. sartorius
V. saphena magna
N. saphenus
Tibia
M. gastrocnemius

FIG. 738.—VASCULONEURAL AND APONEUROTIC ELEMENTS IN THE ANTEROLATERAL REGION OF THE KNEE

Fibrotendinous (*quadriceps*) *expansions* (Fig. 724) from the inferior margins of the vastus muscles criss-cross over the anterior surface of the patella, superficial to the patellar fibers of the rectus femoris muscle. These expansions diverge on each side and anchor the quadriceps muscle and the patella to the enveloping fascia, making for stability of the patella, and reinforcing the capsule of the knee joint.

The *lateral and mesial retinacula* (*accessory patellar ligaments*) are strong, resistant, fibrous supports connecting the margins of the patella near its apex with the margins of the tibial plateaus and the anterolateral surfaces of the tibial condyles as far back as the collateral ligaments. Their purpose is to fix the apex of the patella to prevent dislocation, which can occur only after these supports are stretched and lacerated. The stronger and more expansive mesial retinaculum overcomes the tendency to lateral displacement.

4. Vessels.—The *arteries* of this region are branches from the popliteal, the supreme geniculate (anastomotica magna), femoral (descending branch of the lateral femoral circumflex), and the recurrent branch of the anterior tibial. Their terminals in the subcutaneous tissue form a rich network over the bones, ligaments, and tendons, known as the articular rete of the knee. This network is arranged in three well-defined arterial arches on the anterior aspect of the joint. The uppermost of these arches lies in the midst of the superficial fibers of the quadriceps muscle near the upper border of the patella. The two lower arches are directed transversely through the fatty tissue behind the patellar ligament. After ligation of the popliteal artery, the circulation in the leg is maintained through these collateral anastomoses. The *lymphatics* follow the course of the great saphenous vein and drain into the inguinal nodes.

Surgical Considerations

1. Dislocation of the Patella.—Dislocation of the patella is exceedingly uncommon; it is opposed by the normally prominent outer lip of the trochlea of the femur and by the strong medial tendinous expansion of the vastus medialis muscle and the medial patellar retinaculum. Displacement almost always is lateral; it may be caused by direct violence or by exaggerated muscle action with the leg in extension. In that position, and even in moderate flexion, the patella stands out prominently and the tendinous expansions of the vasti are relaxed. If the lateral femoral condyle is underdeveloped, or if considerable "knock knee" exists, there is a predisposition to dislocation which, having occurred once, tends to recur. Occasionally, with direct violence, the patella undergoes a rotary displacement and is twisted around through a right angle, with the result that one of its lateral margins lies in contact with the groove of the trochlea, while the other is directed forward. Reduction can be effected only after complete relaxation of the quadriceps muscle.

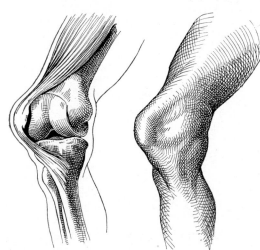

FIG. 739.—Lateral Dislocation of the Patella. (Hoffa.)

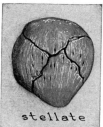

Fig. 740.—Stellate Fracture of the Patella from Direct Violence.

Since the tendinous expansions are not torn, there is no separation of the fragments. (Babcock, "Textbook of Surgery.")

A satisfactory *operative treatment* for recurrent dislocation consists in transplanting the outer half of the patellar ligament under the mesial half, and suturing it to the periosteum and sartorius expansion over the medial condyle of the tibia (Goldthwaite). This procedure shifts the pull of the quadriceps muscle medially, and the shortening of the tendon holds the lateral margin of the patella against the lateral femoral condyle.

2. Fracture of the Patella.—The connections and relations of the patella reveal its disadvantageous position as regards exposure to trauma. It is interposed as a shield between the knee joint and the exterior, and is suspended between the quadriceps muscle and the patellar tendon, where it undergoes great longitudinal strain.

Two types of injury to the patella are recognized according to the nature of the violence which causes them. The patella is exposed to *direct violence* from falls or severe blows upon the knee. In a fall, the principal part of the impact is borne by the tuberosity of the tibia. Fractures of the patella so produced usually are comminuted in a stellate fashion, but the tendinous expansions of the vasti generally remain untorn, so that there is, as a rule, little separation of the fragments.

Fractures from *indirect violence* usually are caused by pure muscle contraction, and commonly by attempted extension with the leg in flexion, as in forcible muscle effort to prevent falling backward. When the quadriceps muscle undergoes a sudden contraction with simultaneously increased flexion at the knee, a great strain is thrown upon the patella. The base of the patella is held against the femoral condyles which act as a fulcrum, and the unsupported distal portion is drawn backward by forced flexion of the leg. Not only is the patella fractured transversely, but the tendinous expansions of the vasti are torn widely. The usual fracture of the patella opens into the joint, which soon fills with blood. The distal or apical extremity of the bone is not of necessity intra-articular, as it is separated from the joint by some fatty tissue and a layer of synovial membrane. Patellar fracture ordinarily results in a separation of the fragments, the edges of which are covered

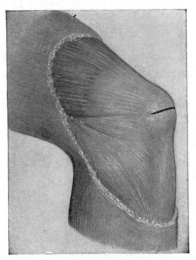

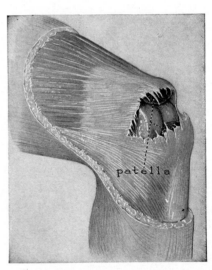

FIG. 741.—TRANSVERSE FRACTURE OF THE PA-
TELLA BY DIRECT VIOLENCE.
There is little separation of the fragments because the lateral tendinous expansions have not been torn. (Babcock, "Textbook of Surgery.")

FIG. 742.—TRANSVERSE FRACTURE OF THE PA-
TELLA BY INDIRECT VIOLENCE.
There is marked separation of the fragments because the lateral tendinous expansions have been torn extensively. (Babcock, "Textbook of Surgery.")

by frayed fibers of the quadriceps tendon. The intervening gap may be slight, but may amount to 5 cm. or more. Its extent depends upon the traction exerted by the quadriceps muscle upon the proximal fragment, and is influenced largely by the degree of tearing of the tendinous expansions of the vasti muscles.

A patellar fracture in which the lateral capsular reinforcements are torn is immediately disabling, for, although the weight can be balanced upon the passively extended foot, no active movement can be made in extension.

Fractures resulting from indirect violence, in which there is definite separation of the fragments, demand early *operative treatment*. A horseshoe-shaped flap, with its convexity upward, is raised from the front of the joint and the site of the fracture is exposed fully. The joint cavity is emptied of blood clots, any soft tissue interposed between the bony fragments is removed, and the fractured surfaces are brought into close and accurate apposition by stitches taken through the covering of the bone or through drill holes in the bone. The lateral tears in the tendinous expansions must be sutured carefully, or most of the advantage of the operation is lost. A snug suture of the lateral expansions usually holds the patellar fragments in apposition without sutures through the bone. Unless the tendinous fringes which have dropped between the fracture fragments are removed before the fragments are approximated, the bony surfaces cannot be brought into immediate contact, and the union is of a fibrous character, especially as the patella is a sesamoid bone without periosteum and bone repair can take place only from the fractured surfaces.

In *conservative treatment*, the leg is elevated in extension to relax the quadriceps, and the thigh is flexed at the hip to relax the rectus femoris still further. Fibrous if not actual bony union, with slight degrees of separation of the fragments, may be expected if there is no obvious tearing of the expansions of the quadriceps.

3. **Suprapatellar and Infrapatellar Rupture of the Quadriceps Muscle.**—The pull exerted by the longitudinal strain of quadriceps muscle contraction may cause, instead of fracture of the patella, a rupture of the suprapatellar portion of the muscle or of the patellar ligament, or a tearing away of the tibial insertion of the tendon.

Any or all of the suprapatellar divisions of the quadriceps, which insert at different levels into the base and margins of the bone, may rupture close to their attachments. The adjacent capsule may be torn and the joint be exposed. If normal function is to be restored, the gap must be repaired by accurate suturing of the lacerated structures. Rupture of the patellar tendon by muscle action is rare.

Avulsion of the tibial tuberosity occurs in youth before the epiphysis of the tibial tubercle is ossified, and usually is caused by excessive muscle strain from the quadriceps. Minor degrees of the accident cause loosening and partial separation of the tubercle. The condition becomes chronic if untreated; extension of the leg no longer can be performed fully, and soreness, lameness, and swelling develop. To rest the quadriceps muscle and permit the tubercle to become fixed firmly, the knee must be immobilized. In the less severe cases, where only slight separation of the epiphysis occurs, adhesive strapping limits extension and steadies the tuberosity until healing takes place.

Osgood-Schlatter's disease is an epiphysitis (osteochondritis) of the tibial tuberosity. The condition is analogous to deforming osteochondritis of the hip (Legg-Perthes' disease) and to epiphysitis of the tarsal scaphoid (Köhler's disease). Roentgenograms show the bony epiphysis to be altered in shape, fragmented, and without the normal trabeculation Views of both tuberosities may be required to differentiate this condition from avulsion of the normal tibial tuberosity. Epiphysitis of the tibial tuberosity frequently is bilateral.

B. POSTERIOR OR POPLITEAL REGION

The posterior aspect of the knee coincides with the region known as the popliteal space. This space, with an osteofibrous floor, rigid musculotendinous walls, and a strong posterior aponeurosis, affords a protected passage for the neurovascular trunks passing from the thigh to the leg. As a flexor area, it occupies the same sheltered position as the analogous flexor region of the elbow.

1. **Boundaries and Divisions of the Popliteal Fossa.**—The muscles, which bound the popliteal fossa laterally, circumscribe a lozenge-shaped space consisting of an upper, or femoral, and a lower, or tibial, triangle. The lateral boundaries of the **femoral triangle** are recognized easily through their superficial coverings. The *lateral wall* consists of the combined long and short heads of the biceps muscle. A septum of the overlying deep fascia is applied to the mesial surface of the biceps, binding it down to the lateral lip of the linea aspera of the femur. The strong rounded tendon of the biceps passes slightly posterior to the lateral condyle of the femur and divides to surround the fibular attachment of the fibular collateral (external lateral) ligament. The *mesial wall* of the upper triangle is composed of a complex of four muscles: the semitendinosus, semimembranosus, sartorius, and gracilis. These are held together in a common bundle by a septum of deep fascia which binds this bundle down to the mesial lip of the linea aspera. Through an interval in this septum, which is directly continuous with the adductor ring (p. 713) in the adductor magnus tendon, the neurovascular trunks of the thigh enter the popliteal space. The semimem-

branosus forms the bulk of this mesial mass of muscles, and its tendon passes behind the medial condyle of the femur and inserts into the medial condyle of the tibia. The posterior surface of the semimembranosus is grooved by the tendon of the semitendinosus, which is the prominent palpable tendon in this wall. The tendons of the gracilis and sartorius pass forward more anteriorly to insert into the medial surface of the tibia.

The **lower** or **tibial triangle,** which is much smaller, has its lateral boundaries formed by the two heads of the gastrocnemius muscle, which, in turn, is embraced by the muscles forming the lateral boundaries of the femoral triangle. The space within the triangle is very narrow, so that the two heads of the gastrocnemius not only form the two lateral boundaries, but, to a large extent, cover the posterior aspect of the joint. The origin of the soleus muscle is at the apex of this triangle. Through the tendinous arch of the soleus,

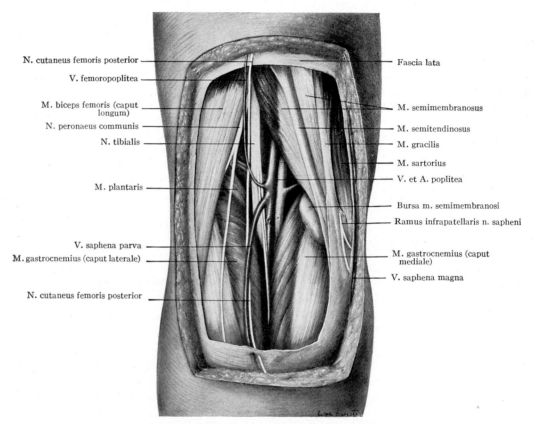

FIG. 743.—LEFT POPLITEAL SPACE AND ITS CONTENTS.
The roof of the investing fascia has been removed.

the popliteal vessels enter the calf of the leg. This pathway allows the reciprocal spread of infection between these adjoining regions.

The *roof* of the two triangles forming the popliteal space is a thin strong sheet of deep fascia which is pierced near its center by the small saphenous vein. The *floor* of the space is the popliteal surface of the femur, inclosed between the diverging lines of bifurcation of the linea aspera. The lower part of the floor is the posterior surface of the posterior ligament of the knee joint with the related posterior part of the joint capsule. This is overlain by the *popliteus muscle* which arises within the capsule of the knee joint from the lateral femoral condyle. The muscle passes distally and medially across the back of the knee joint and inserts into the proximal part of the posterior surface of the tibia. Near its origin, the popliteus is surrounded by a bursa lying between the lateral meniscus (semilunar cartilage) and the fibular collateral ligament. The popliteus muscle is a flexor of the leg, but acts as a medial rotator of the tibia when the knee is flexed. It is supplied by the tibial (internal popliteal) nerve (L_4, $_5$, S_1).

The resistant fascia roofing the fossa unites with the tendons and muscles forming the walls of the space and covers a well-delimited cavity, incapable of great distention. If the cavity contains a purulent collection, a cyst, a hernia of the capsule, or a popliteal aneurysm, pressure is exerted on the nerves, causing intense pain.

2. **Landmarks.**—When the *knee is extended*, the muscles forming the lateral boundaries of the space and the deep fascia by which it is covered are rendered very tense, and the cutaneous surface appears full and slightly rounded from side to side. Because of the unyielding character of the tissues, it is not possible to make out any details of the space and its contents. A proximal relief or bulge, representing the neurovascular structures, occu-

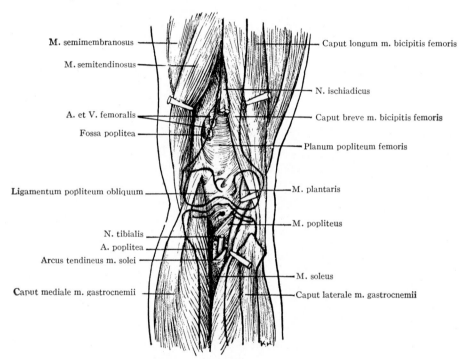

FIG. 744.—FLOOR OF THE RIGHT POPLITEAL SPACE.
The lateral walls of the fossa are retracted and the vasculoneural contents of the space are removed. (After Corning.)

pies the long axis of the space. Extension places the contents of the space on a tension, and is the position which most favors operative procedures.

When the *knee is flexed*, the muscle boundaries and deep fascia of the part are relaxed and the popliteal space can be palpated as a vertical median furrow extending from the lower part of the thigh downward beyond the knee joint line. The semitendinosus tendon on the mesial aspect and the biceps tendon on the lateral aspect are unmistakable landmarks. On deep palpation, the fingers slip into the upper part of the space and identify the triangular interval on the back of the femur and the popliteal vessels and tibial (internal popliteal) nerve. The popliteal artery, which runs close to the bone, can be palpated and compressed easily, and is damaged readily in fracture of this part of the femur (p. 719). The common peroneal (external popliteal) nerve is distinctly palpable first under cover of, and then posterior to, the biceps tendon before the nerve winds about the head of the fibula to enter the peroneal or lateral compartment of the leg (p. 766).

3. **Popliteal Bursae.**—The extensive play of the muscles and tendons about the knee

demands their protection by multiple bursae; the rôle of these bursae in knee injuries justifies their enumeration.   As a group, they are subject to irritation from undue strain and overexercise and must be considered a cause of disability in this region.

Of the *posteromedial bursae*, the semimembranosus bursa, which lies on the medial head of the gastrocnemius muscle, is most extensive; it reaches the joint line and often communicates with the joint cavity.   The bursa for the medial head of the gastrocnemius muscle facilitates play of the capsule over the medial femoral condyle.   It often is in communication with the semimembranosus bursa and with the joint.   Bursae separate the tendons of the sartorius, gracilis, and semitendinosus from each other at their insertions and from the tibial collateral (internal lateral) ligament.

The *posterolateral bursae* are related to the important structures playing across the joint line and to the outer bony prominences, the biceps tendon, the fibular collateral (external lateral) ligament, and the popliteus and gastrocnemius muscles.   The bursa of the biceps lies on the head of the fibula deep to the tendon, and, when swollen, simulates enlargement of the fibular head.   Another biceps bursa is interposed between the tendon

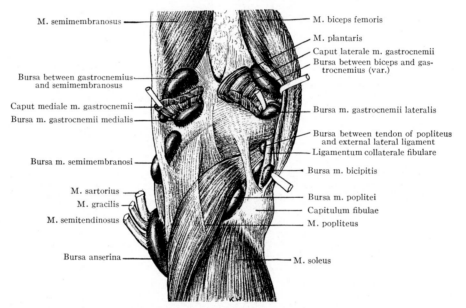

FIG. 745.—IMPORTANT BURSAE ABOUT THE RIGHT POPLITEAL SPACE.

of that muscle and the fibular collateral ligament.   The bursa for the popliteus muscle regularly communicates with the joint (p. 751).   The origin of the popliteus from the lateral femoral condyle is intracapsular, and winds obliquely downward and behind the joint line and lateral meniscus.   The popliteal bursa, which sometimes is a tubal extension of the knee-joint synovia, extends downward and outward beneath the popliteal muscle. A diverticulum of synovia lies between the tendon and the lateral meniscus, so that the meniscus has little attachment to the tendon and capsule.   This arrangement allows the meniscus free movement on the tibia, which probably accounts for its relative freedom from injury.   The inferior diverticulum of the bursa often communicates with the superior tibiofibular joint.   A bursa is situated between the lateral head of the gastrocnemius and the capsule covering the lateral femoral condyle; it sometimes communicates with the knee joint.

Infrequently, small *posterior synovial diverticula* herniate through the fibers of the oblique posterior ligament of the knee joint.

4. **Popliteal Artery and Veins.**—The **popliteal artery** enters the superior and medial part of the popliteal space through the tendinous arch in the adductor magnus muscle.

it is a continuation of the femoral artery. As the popliteal artery passes through the popliteal space, it inclines laterally along the outer border of the semitendinosus muscle until it reaches the middle of the limb; it then descends vertically to the distal border of the popliteal muscle and terminates by dividing into the anterior and posterior tibial arteries. It lies at first along the lateral border of the semimembranosus muscle, but gradually inclines laterally and gains the midline of the limb at the level of the intercondyloid notch of the femur and occupies a median position for the remainder of the course. The popliteal artery throughout its course is placed deeply and lies in direct contact with the posterior ligament of the knee joint.

Three pairs of branches are given off by the popliteal artery at three different levels and are distributed mainly about the bony part of the knee. The *superior genicular arteries*,

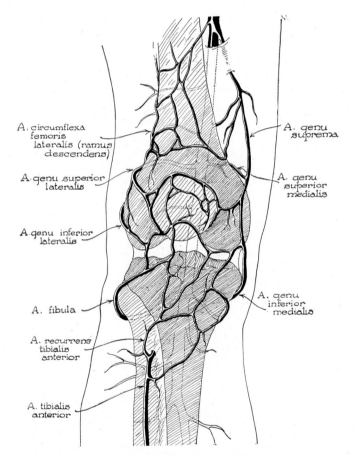

A. circumflexa
femoris
lateralis (ramus
descendens)

A. genu superior
lateralis

A. genu inferior
lateralis

A. fibula

A. recurrens
tibialis
anterior

A. tibialis
anterior

A. genu
suprema

A. genu
superior
medialis

A. genu
inferior
medialis

FIG. 746.—COLLATERAL CIRCULATION ABOUT THE KNEE   (After M. Reid, Amer. Jour. of Surg.)

lateral and medial, originate at the level of the femoral condyles and wind about the femur proximal to the condyles. They are in close contact with the bone and anastomose with each other anteriorly. They anastomose also with the inferior genicular arteries, the descending branch of the lateral circumflex artery, and the articular branch of the superior geniculate (anastomotica magna) artery. The last anastomosis establishes circulation in the leg after ligation of the popliteal artery in its proximal portion.

The *middle genicular arteries* enter the knee joint through the posterior ligament. They are chiefly muscular and articular, and are distributed to the gastrocnemii and the structures within the capsule. The *interior genicular arteries*, lateral and medial, wind around the front of the knee, pass under cover of the tibial and fibular collateral (internal and external lateral) ligaments, and anastomose with each other deep to the patellar ligament. By communicating with the superior genicular arteries, they contribute to the important anastomoses about the knee. No branches are given off in the upper course of the popliteal artery; in this portion, the artery is accessible for ligation. Should obstruction occur in the branches, the circulation is carried on through the intact collateral path, but if the obstruction is low down and close to the openings of all the important genicular arteries, collateral circulation is interfered with and the possibility of gangrene impends.

The anterior and posterior tibial veins unite to form the **popliteal vein** in the lower part of the space. The popliteal vein lies superficial to the artery, mesial to it distally, and lateral to it proximally. The **small saphenous vein,** which runs over the calf of the leg on the enveloping fascia, pierces the deep fascia in the lower part of the popliteal space and divides into two branches, one entering the popliteal vein and the other the great saphenous vein. The popliteal vein and artery are bound wall to wall in a resistant connective tissue sheath, a relationship which explains their simultaneous injury and the formation of an arteriovenous fistula.

5. **Tibial (Internal Popliteal) Nerve.**—The tibial and common peroneal nerves are the terminal branches of the sciatic nerve at the upper angle of the popliteal space. The tibial (internal popliteal) nerve (L_4, $_5$, S_1, $_2$, $_3$) continues the direction of the popliteal nerve and runs a straight course to the lower angle of the space superficial to the popliteal vessels, just beneath the deep fascia. As the vessels pursue an oblique lateral course, the nerve lies at first to their lateral side. Opposite the intercondyloid notch of the femur, the nerve lies immediately over both vessels, and at the lower angle of the space, to their medial side. At the distal border of the popliteus muscle, the tibial nerve passes deep to the soleus muscle and enters the posterior compartment of the leg.

While traversing the popliteal fossa, the tibial nerve distributes muscular, cutaneous, and articular branches. The *muscular branches* supply both heads of the gastrocnemius muscle and the plantaris, popliteus, and soleus muscles. The *cutaneous branch* or medial cutaneous nerve of the calf (ramus communicans tibialis) descends along the back of the leg and pierces the deep fascia in its middle third. It is joined by a corresponding branch of the common peroneal (external popliteal) nerve and the peroneal anastomotic (ramus communicans fibularis) nerve. The last two branches form the sural (external saphenous) nerve (S_1, $_2$). Three small *articular branches* supply the knee joint. The intimate relations between the popliteal vessels and the tibial nerve and its branches explain the nerve involvement in popliteal aneurysm.

6. **Common Peroneal (External Popliteal) Nerve.**—The common peroneal (external popliteal) nerve (L_4, $_5$, S_1, $_2$) passes distally and laterally in close relation to the medial aspect of the biceps tendon, which forms the outer boundary of the femoral subdivision of the space. It accompanies the biceps tendon to its insertion, and leaves the popliteal fossa between that tendon and the lateral head of the gastrocnemius muscle. The relation of this nerve to the biceps at its insertion must be borne in mind in biceps tenotomy for knee joint contracture (p. 742). From this region, the nerve descends behind the head of the fibula just beneath the deep fascia and winds around the lateral aspect of the fibular neck, piercing the origin of the peroneus longus muscle. The nerve ends by dividing into the superficial (musculocutaneous) and deep peroneal (anterior tibial) nerves.

The common peroneal nerve gives off no muscle branches, but supplies small articular twigs to the knee joint.

7. **Popliteal Lymph Glands.**—The popliteal lymph glands form a superficial and a deep group. The superficial lymph glands surround the small saphenous vein where it pierces the deep fascia. Their afferent branches drain the lateral aspect of the leg and the foot and their efferents drain to the deep group of popliteal glands. The deep lymph glands lie in the fatty tissue about the popliteal vessels. Their afferents proceed from the deep tissues of the calf and sole of the foot and receive the efferents from the superficial glands. Many of the efferents from the calf and sole of the foot drain directly into the deep subinguinal nodes.

SURGICAL CONSIDERATIONS

1. **Popliteal Abscesses.**—Following infection of the leg or toes, popliteal abscesses may arise in the popliteal lymph glands, and, because of their depth, are difficult to detect at an early stage. The infection is unusually painful because of the unyielding character of the walls of the fossa. For the same reason, and because of the fatty areolar tissue in which they are embedded, these abscesses are slow to heal when drained.

The next most frequent source of popliteal abscess is acute suppurative osteomyelitis of the lower end of the femur. Popliteal abscess may occur as a sequel to suppuration within the knee joint The space may be invaded by way of the communicating popliteal bursae. Because of the dense and unyielding character of the deep fascia roofing the space, pus may remain unnoticed until the tissues of the space have become infiltrated extensively and the space has been converted into a large abscess cavity, within which the popliteal vessels and nerve lie free. Rarely the pus may burrow upward into the thigh through the

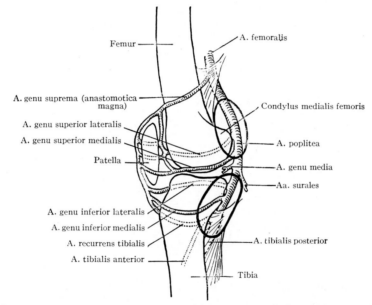

FIG. 747.—EFFECT OF ANEURYSM UPON THE ANASTOMOSING CHANNELS WITHIN AND ABOUT THE POPLITEAL SPACE.

The upper circle indicates the location of an aneurysm in the upper portion of the popliteal artery. Since it obliterates only a few branches, an efficient collateral circulation can be established. The lower circle indicates an aneurysm in the lower part of the popliteal artery where branches are numerous. The resulting tumor is a serious obstacle to collateral circulation and may cause gangrene of the leg. (Modified after Testut and Jacob.)

ring in adductor magnus muscle. Eventually, the coverings of the space are eroded by ulceration, allowing the abscess to point. Not infrequently, thigh amputation must be performed because of intractable suppuration in the space from femoral osteomyelitis.

Incision for popliteal abscess is made best from the lateral aspect of the space anterior to the biceps tendon. When the deep fascia is divided, a hemostat is passed between the biceps tendon and the femur, and the pus is evacuated without injury to the large vessels and nerves.

2. **Popliteal Aneurysm.**—The incidence of popliteal aneurysm approaches that of aneurysm of the thoracic aorta. The longitudinal strain thrown upon a normal artery during extension of the leg produces no untoward effect, but may rupture the coats of a diseased vessel and result in the development of an aneurysm. Popliteal aneurysm enlarges with marked rapidity because of its location in the midst of very loose tissue and because of the absence of the muscle support common to the other vascular trunks of the

extremity. The obliquely curved course of the popliteal artery distributes pressure irregularly in the artery, and the bifurcation tends to increase the tension in the main trunk.

If aneurysm develops proximal to the joint line, only a few of the collateral branches entering into the anastomosis about the knee are involved. If aneurysm develops distal to the joint line, it involves the mouths of the more numerous collateral branches which present there, introducing the danger of gangrene. The presence of aneurysm may be accompanied by stiffness and pain in the knee, not unlike that of chronic arthritis. The leg is maintained in the semiflexed position and can be straightened only with difficulty. When aneurysm develops toward the superficial aspect of the space, its progress usually is rapid, as it meets with very little resistance. Pressure on the nerves produces great pain and muscle weakness. When aneurysm develops toward the deep aspect of the space, it may erode the bones and the joint.

Rupture of a popliteal aneurysm almost certainly leads to gangrene of the leg, as the venous return and, eventually, the arterial flow of the leg are interrupted by the pressure within the space. A pulsatile swelling within the space is not necessarily an aneurysm, inasmuch as cystic or other tumors in the vicinity may transmit the pulsations of the popliteal artery.

3. Popliteal Cysts.—The cystic tumors commonly found in the popliteal space arise from the popliteal bursae and projections of synovial membrane from the knee joint. The bursa between the medial head of the gastrocnemius muscle and the posterior ligament of the knee joint is irritated frequently, may attain a considerable size, and may form a fluctuant swelling at the back of the knee. The cyst outline usually may be determined readily with the leg in flexion. When cysts communicate with the knee joint synovia, it sometimes is possible to diminish their volume by continued pressure, the reduction of the mass being dependent upon the character of the fluid contained and the size of the aperture into the knee joint. Popliteal pulsation may be transmitted to these swellings, but the pulsation is not expansile. A large cyst is a source of inconvenience in movements of the knee, and may require operative removal. Excision is most satisfactory through an approach over the most prominent part of the swelling.

4. Flexion Contractures at the Knee.—Contracture of the posterior soft parts of the knee, with resulting flexion deformity, is common where flexion is maintained over a considerable period of time. The fact that the main origin of the hamstring muscles is on the pelvis, that the insertion is on the tibia, and that there is only a negligible attachment to the femur over the intervening space, favors the production of this deformity.

The stretching of the extensor muscles militates against easy correction of the contracture. If the contracture is neglected, retraction of other structures about the joint occurs. The posterior joint capsule and popliteal artery are shortened to the degree that mechanical manipulation may do irreparable harm. A neglected flexion contracture, if associated with a chronic joint lesion, immobilizes the joint by fibrous and even bony ankylosis. Mobilization may be accomplished only by prolonged traction, tenotomy, and posterior capsuloplasty.

The principal difficulty in *tenotomy of the hamstring tendons* is encountered in the division of the biceps tendon, as the common peroneal (external popliteal) nerve, which descends in close relation with the inner border of that tendon, may be injured. If the biceps muscle is made tense by applying an extending force to the leg, its tendon can be recognized readily. Free incision over the tendon with a full view of the operative field is preferable to subcutaneous tenotomy. Tenotomy should be performed from 3 to 4 cm. proximal to the tendon insertion on the head of the fibula. The division of the semitendinosus and semimembranosus tendons presents little difficulty, as no noteworthy anatomical structures are endangered.

5. Posterior Capsuloplasty.—Posterior capsuloplasty is performed to correct flexion deformity at the knee. The essential feature in the operation is lengthening of the posterior capsule of the knee by stripping away its superior attachment from the posterior surface of the femur. Lengthening of the biceps tendon is combined with capsuloplasty because the biceps muscle is responsible for much of the subluxation and lateral rotation of the tibia on the femur. The iliotibial band is divided because it definitely limits extension at the knee.

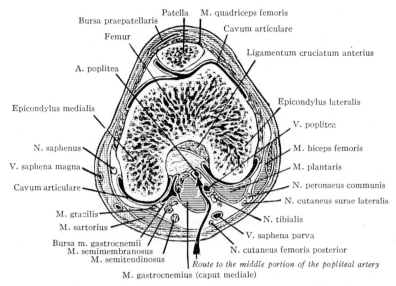

Patella M. quadriceps femoris
Bursa praepatellaris
Femur
Cavum articulare
Ligamentum cruciatum anterius
A. poplitea
Epicondylus medialis
Epicondylus lateralis
V. poplitea
N. saphenus
M. biceps femoris
V. saphena magna
M. plantaris
Cavum articulare
N. peronaeus communis
N. cutaneus surae lateralis
M. gracilis
M. sartorius
N. tibialis
Bursa m. gastrocnemii
M. semimembranosus
V. saphena parva
M. semitendinosus
N. cutaneus femoris posterior
Route to the middle portion of the popliteal artery
M. gastrocnemius (caput mediale)

FIG. 748.—TRANSVERSE SECTION THROUGH THE RIGHT KNEE, PASSING THROUGH THE FEMORAL CONDYLES TO SHOW THE SURGICAL APPROACH TO THE POPLITEAL ARTERY IN THE MIDDLE OF ITS COURSE.

An incision 12 cm. long made over the lateral aspect of the knee, extending from just above the femoral condyle to the head of the fibula, exposes the iliotibial band and the biceps tendon. The iliotibial band is divided transversely at a level 5 cm. proximal to the

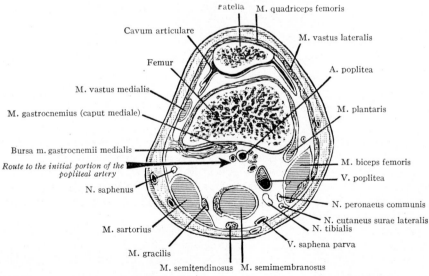

Patella M. quadriceps femoris
Cavum articulare
M. vastus lateralis
Femur
A. poplitea
M. vastus medialis
M. gastrocnemius (caput mediale)
M. plantaris
Bursa m. gastrocnemii medialis
M. biceps femoris
Route to the initial portion of the popliteal artery
V. poplitea
N. saphenus
M. sartorius
N. peronaeus communis
N. cutaneus surae lateralis
N. tibialis
M. gracilis
V. saphena parva
M. semitendinosus M. semimembranosus

FIG. 749.—TRANSVERSE SECTION THROUGH THE RIGHT KNEE IN THE UPPER PART OF THE POPLITEAL SPACE TO SHOW THE SURGICAL APPROACH TO THE INITIAL PART OF THE POPLITEAL ARTERY.

joint interval. After retracting the common peroneal (external popliteal) nerve, the biceps tendon is isolated and freed as far as its insertion into the head of the fibula. The biceps tendon is lengthened by division with a Z-shaped incision. The lateral portion of the knee joint capsule is exposed. The capsule is incised at the posterior border of the articular margin of the lateral condyle of the femur and the posterior compartment of the knee joint is opened. A periosteal elevator is introduced into the joint and the posterior capsule is stripped upward subperiosteally from the back of the femur. Subperiosteal dissection is carried to the midline of the femur and upward 8 cm. from the joint line.

A second incision is made over the medial aspect of the knee from the adductor tubercle to slightly below the joint line. Incision of the capsule at the posterior margin of the joint opens the posterior compartment. The subperiosteal stripping of the posterior capsule now is performed from the medial side. The medial dissection, carried upward and laterally, meets the dissection from the lateral side. It usually is necessary to free subperiosteally the tight capsular structures which remain attached to the femur around the intercondyloid notch. The capsule then is closed. The extremities of the divided biceps tendon are sutured and the leg can be extended and immobilized (Wilson).

6. **Lateral and Median Popliteal Approaches.**—The *lateral popliteal approach* offers access to the common peroneal nerve and to bursal cysts about the lateral confines of the space. It follows the posterior margin of the biceps tendon over the lateral femoral condyle to the head of the fibula. The common peroneal nerve lies immediately beneath the deep fascia under cover of the biceps tendon and lateral to the lateral head of the gastrocnemius muscle.

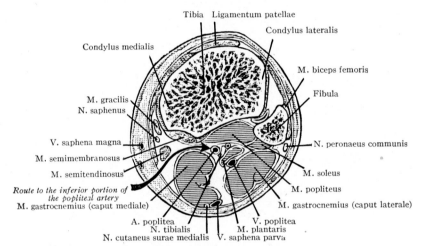

Fig. 750.—Transverse Section Through the Right Knee at the Level of the Tibial Condyles and the Head of the Fibula to Show the Surgical Access to the Terminal Part of the Popliteal Artery.

The *median popliteal approach* leads to the tibial nerve and the popliteal vessels. The incision is carried through the deep fascia, avoiding the posterior femoral cutaneous nerve which lies in the midline just deep to the fascia. In the lower part of the incision, the small saphenous nerve lies deep to the fascia between the heads of the gastrocnemius muscle. The tibial nerve lies mesial to these structures in the fatty areolar tissue and is more superficial than the popliteal vessels.

7. **Ligation of the Popliteal Artery.**—Ligation of the popliteal artery may be performed for aneurysm or wounds of this vessel. The artery is reached most readily at the upper and medial part of the popliteal space. A medial popliteal incision is made parallel to and just behind the tendon of the adductor magnus. In dividing the superficial tissues and deep fascia, the great saphenous vein and the saphenous nerve are exposed. These structures and the sartorius muscle are retracted backward. The tendon of the adductor magnus is defined and drawn forward. Care is taken to avoid injury to the deep branch of the superior geniculate (anastomotica magna) artery. Upon displacing the semimembranosus muscle backward and deepening the interval between that muscle and the adductor magnus tendon, the popliteal artery, surrounded by loose fatty tissue, and the

popliteal vein to its lateral side, are found lying in close contact with the femur. The vasculoneural sheath is incised carefully on its medial aspect and the popliteal and tibial veins, which lie posterolaterally, are avoided.

In the inferior part of this approach, a cleavable interspace separates the gracilis tendon from the mesial head of the gastrocnemius muscle. By deepening this cleft, the gastrocnemius can be retracted from the popliteus muscle and the origin of the soleus muscle which covers the bone. The popliteal artery may be ligated after it pierces the soleus ring and before it bifurcates into its two terminal branches. The combined incision affords adequate drainage for abscess in the space.

C. BONES AND JOINTS

The skeletal structures of the knee include: the lower extremity of the femur, the upper extremity of the tibia, the patella, and the head of the fibula. These structures form the knee joint proper and the superior tibiofibular joint. The knee joint includes the articulation of the patella with the trochlear of the femur.

1. **Lower Extremity of the Femur.**—The lower extremity of the femur is expanded laterally into the two *condyles*, which are prominent articulating eminences, elongated anteroposteriorly and relatively narrow laterally. The condyles are adapted to anteroposterior rocking in the shallow concavities of the tibial head. The somewhat obliquely placed medial condyle is narrower and shorter anteroposteriorly than is the outer. The articular surface of the lateral condyle is directed in a sagittal plane. When the shaft of the femur is vertical, the medial condyle extends farther downward than the lateral condyle, but when the shaft is inclined medially with its normal degree of obliquity, the plane of the lower surface of each condyle is almost horizontal. Both condyles are roughened medially and laterally for the attachment of ligaments, and are surmounted by *condylar ridges* which are readily palpable when the leg is flexed, but are difficult to palpate when it is extended.

The cartilage-covered surfaces of the condyles are continuous in front and form the *trochlea*, a shallow depression for articulation with the patella when the leg is extended. The lateral surface of the trochlea is more prominent and ascends to a higher level than the medial surface. The portion of the femur immediately above the trochlea is perforated by large vascular foramina and is covered by a layer of synovial membrane and a quantity of subsynovial fat which supports the proximal two thirds of the patella when the leg is extended.

Nearer to the posterior than to the anterior part of each condyle is the irregular prominence of the *epicondyle* for the attachment of the collateral ligaments. Proximal to the medial epicondyle is the small, bony projection of the medial condyloid ridge, the *adductor tubercle*, or point of insertion for the tendon of the adductor magnus muscle. Below the lateral epicondyle is a depression marking the origin of the popliteus muscle and lodging its tendon.

The condyles are separated posteriorly by a deep fossa, the *intercondyloid notch*, within which the crucial ligaments are lodged and to the walls of which their upper extremities are attached. In the femur, as in long bones generally, the thick cortex of the shaft thins out into a shell of compact bone which embraces the cancellous structure of the condyles. The compact cortical bone is thickest over the margins of the intercondyloid fossa to strengthen the areas of attachment of the crucial ligaments. The condyles are so separated and weakened by the trochlear groove and the intercondyloid notch that lines of fracture often extend up the base of the fossa.

The lower extremity of the femur *develops* from a single center of ossification which appears in the cartilage during the ninth month of fetal life. The finding of this center in a stillborn infant has been accepted as proof that the fetus has come to term. In accordance with the general rule that the epiphyses ossifying early unite late, union of the distal femoral epiphysis with the diaphysis takes place in the twenty-first year. The distal *epiphyseal line* is roughly transverse and corresponds anteriorly to the proximal border of the trochlea and posteriorly to the intercondyloid line. On the medial side, the epiphyseal line is on a level with the adductor tubercle. While the line lies at some distance from the capsule laterally, it may lie within the capsule in front and behind. Juxta-epiphyseal infections of the diaphysis (acute osteomyelitis) invade the joint in front and behind more readily than laterally, but the epiphyseal line is a strong barrier against distal spread of the infection.

In resection of the knee joint during the period of growth, very little of the condyles can be removed without causing arrest of growth. Growth continues longest in this, the more active epiphysis, which, therefore, is a favorite site for infection or malignancy. Excessive growth at one or the other extremity of the epiphyseal line leads to the deformities of genu varum and genu valgum.

2. Proximal Extremity of the Tibia.—The upper or condylar end of the tibia is its most expanded part and presents an *articular surface*, commensurate with those of the femoral condyles. The articular surface of the two closely united tibial condyles forms a nearly horizontal plateau. This articulation presents two oval, slightly concave facets which are deepened by the menisci (semilunar cartilages) into fossae or sockets for the femoral condyles. The margins of the articular surfaces are depressed into a slight groove for the attachment of the menisci.

Between the two articular surfaces is a rough area surmounted by the *intercondylar eminence*, from which the double-spurred prominence of the tibial spine projects upward. Anterior and posterior to this eminence are flattened areas for the attachment of the corresponding crucial ligaments and the extremities of the menisci. A thumbbreadth distal to the anterior articular margin is the *tuberosity of the tibia;* the broad, flat, intervening area is occupied by the infrapatellar bursa, bridged over by the ligamentum patellae. The head of the tibia slopes downward and forward to the tuberosity which is the upper limit of the anterior tibial crest. A flat facet on the posterolateral surface of the lateral condyle articulates with the head of the fibula.

The upper extremity of the tibia *develops* from one center of ossification which appears a short time before birth and unites with the shaft at about the twentieth year. From it are developed the two condyles and the tuberosity. The tuberosity may be formed from a separate center of ossification which fuses with the shaft at a later date. This sometimes is avulsed partly or wholly (p. 735). The upper extremity of the tibia is the active epiphysis and the favorite site for osteosarcoma. In a young child, the *epiphyseal line* is very close to the joint, so that in joint excision not more than a few millimeters should be removed.

3. Patella.—The patella is a sesamoid bone developed within the tendon of the quadriceps muscle. It is irregularly triangular in shape and is flattened anteroposteriorly. Its posterior surface is covered almost entirely by cartilage and is divided by a vertical ridge into two surfaces, which slope a little away from each other to the femoral condyles. The lateral of these surfaces is the larger. Frequently both surfaces are subdivided by two transverse ridges, so that three smaller faceted areas are observed on each side of the vertical median ridge. The rough inferior part of the posterior surface of the patella is extra-articular and is related closely to the fat pad of the knee. The anterior surface of the patella is rough and is united intimately with the patellar tendon (ligamentum patellae). When the patella is fractured, the edges of the fragments may be covered with a veil formed by the torn outer fibers of the patellar tendon. Because the patella is practically without periosteum, the repair of fracture takes place chiefly in the bony substance.

In full flexion of the leg, the patella glides into a position between the projecting femoral condyles and is seated partly in the intercondyloid fossa. When the leg is extended, only the inferior part of the patella is in contact with the trochlea.

The patella is cartilaginous at birth and *ossifies* from a single center which appears about the third year. Ossification usually is complete by the fifteenth year.

4. Head of the Fibula.—The head of the fibula is thickened and pyramidal. Into the styloid process are inserted the fibular collateral ligament and the tendon of the biceps. *Ossification* begins about the third year from a single center and forms an epiphysis which unites with the shaft from the nineteenth to the twenty-second year. Separation of the proximal epiphysis is a very unusual injury, but when it does occur, may involve the common peroneal (external popliteal) nerve. Tuberculosis originating in the fibular diaphysis near the epiphyseal cartilage usually does not spread to the proximal tibiofibular joint, since the epiphyseal cartilage is entirely extracapsular. If, however, the disease originates in the proximal and lateral part of the tibial diaphysis, the proximal tibiofibular joint may be involved, for its capsule is attached partly to the tibial diaphysis.

5. **Knee Joint.**—The knee joint, the largest and most complex of all the joints, combines strength and stability with a wide range and variety of motion, qualities seldom associated. It comprises the articulation between the patella and the trochlea, and the femorotibial joint. The femorotibial joint may be subdivided into medial and lateral

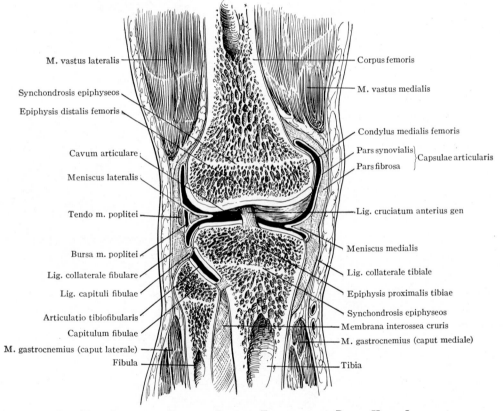

FIG. 751.—SCHEMATIC FRONTAL SECTION THROUGH THE RIGHT KNEE JOINT.

femoro-menisco-tibial divisions, which are set apart by the incomplete partition formed by the ligamentum mucosum and the fat pad. Each condylar or femoro-menisco-tibial joint may be considered as composed of femoromeniscal and meniscotibial divisions, for the synovial cavity on each side extends peripherally to the capsule, both above and below each meniscus.

The strength and varied function of the joint are the result of the complex formation and the powerful ligamentary structures uniting the bones and reinforcing the capsule. The tibiofibular joint stabilizes the knee by reinforcing the lateral tibial condyle and furnishing a firm point of attachment for the fibular collateral ligament.

From a brief examination of the joint, one might be led to believe that its security was not great, considering how imperfectly the articular surfaces are adapted to one another, and taking into account the powerful leverage brought to bear upon the joint by the femur and the tibia, two of the longest and most powerful bones in the body. These apparent sources of weakness are more than overcome by the powerful ligaments which maintain the bone ends in contact and by the strong muscles with which they are surrounded. The proof of the strength of the joint is attested by the extreme rarity of traumatic dislocation of the head of the tibia, no matter how extreme the causative violence may be.

6. **Ligaments of the Knee Joint.**—The ligaments about the knee are divided into an extra-articular and an intra-articular group. The **extra-articular ligaments** include the capsule, the quadriceps muscle and its tendinous expansions, the two collateral ligaments, and the oblique popliteal ligament.

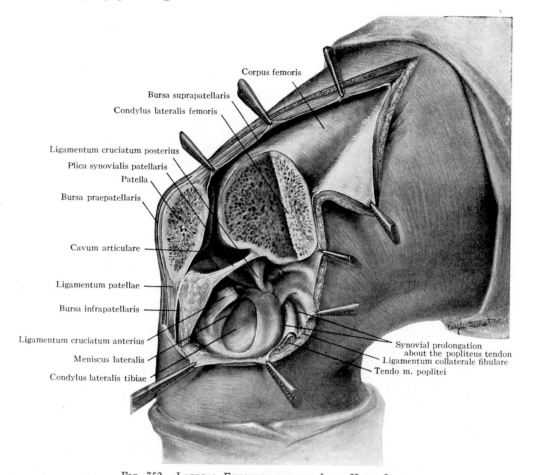

Corpus femoris

Bursa suprapatellaris

Condylus lateralis femoris

Ligamentum cruciatum posterius

Plica synovialis patellaris

Patella

Bursa praepatellaris

Cavum articulare

Ligamentum patellae

Bursa infrapatellaris

Ligamentum cruciatum anterius

Meniscus lateralis

Condylus lateralis tibiae

Synovial prolongation about the popliteus tendon

Ligamentum collaterale fibulare

Tendo m. poplitei

Fig. 752.—Lateral Exposure of the Left Knee Joint.
The lateral condyle of the femur has been removed and the leg has been forced medially to enlarge the cavity of the knee joint.

The *capsule* of the knee joint, which invests the bony ends of the joint as with a cuff, is a somewhat ill-defined structure anteriorly, where it stretches between the condyles of the femur and the head of the tibia on each side of the patella and the patellar ligament. The proximal line of attachment of the capsule includes the epiphyseal line on the lateral and medial condyles of the femur, but remains at least 1 cm. distant from the margin of the articular surface. It is reinforced strongly by the patellar and infrapatellar portion of the quadriceps tendon. The capsule is overlain by, and is incorporated with, the tendinous expansions of the lateral and medial vasti (p. 732) which, in turn, are invested by the fascia which extends over the joint and fuses with the deep fascia of the leg. Proximal to the patella and over the area occupied by it, the capsule is entirely deficient. Posteriorly, it is more clearly defined than elsewhere, and extends from the proximal margin of the articular surfaces and the intercondylar line to the posterior border of the head of the tibia; the femoral attachment coincides approximately with the epiphyseal line. This part of the capsule is supported powerfully by the hamstring and gastrocnemius muscles. It is strengthened further by the *oblique popliteal ligament* which extends obliquely across the back of the joint from the semimembranosus insertion to the medial border of the lateral femoral condyle. Many small spaces interrupt the continuity of the posterior capsule. A small aperture often is present in the part overlying the medial femoral condyle, through which the bursa beneath the medial head of the gastrocnemius communicates with the joint. On the lateral and medial aspect, the capsule is short and strong.

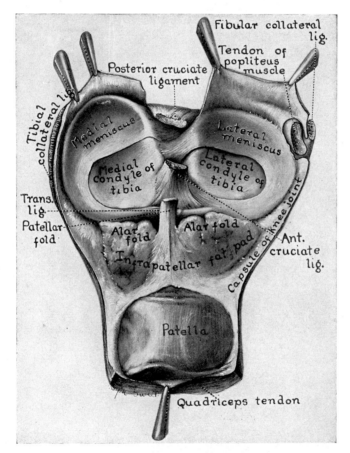

FIG. 753.—STRUCTURES ON THE SUPERIOR ARTICULAR SURFACE OF THE LEFT TIBIA.

The *quadriceps muscle*, its *tendinous expansions*, and the *infrapatellar tendon* have been described (p. 731).

The *tibial collateral (internal lateral) ligament* is a broad, flattened, straplike band which strengthens the capsule on its medial aspect. It is attached proximally to the medial condyle of the femur near the adductor tubercle and crosses the medial aspect of the joint, where it is attached firmly to the peripheral border of the corresponding meniscus. The ligament is attached distally to the medial border of the shaft of the tibia behind the attachment of the semitendinosus tendon. The *fibular collateral (external lateral) ligament* is a distinctly palpable rounded band attached to the lateral epicondyle of the femur, about 1 cm. proximal to the articular margin and the groove of origin of the popliteus tendon, over which it plays. As the ligament crosses the lateral aspect of the knee joint, it is separated from the joint by the popliteus tendon and its associated bursa. The ligament is attached distally to the head of the fibula. At its insertion, the two slips of attachment of the biceps tendon, with an interposed bursa, embrace it. The ligament is overlain by an expansion of the fascia lata prolonged backward from the iliotibial band.

Either of the collateral ligaments may be strained or torn by the same violent movement that causes injury to the menisci. When the collateral ligaments are torn, there is point tenderness over them; when the menisci are damaged, the tenderness is most marked over the joint line in the triangular depressions at the sides of the patellar ligament.

The more important of the **intra-articular ligaments** are the cruciate ligaments and the menisci.

The *cruciate ligaments* are strong cordlike structures which extend from the intercondylar fossa of the femur to attachments in front of and behind the intercondylar eminence on the plateau of the tibia. The two cruciate ligaments, which may be termed the

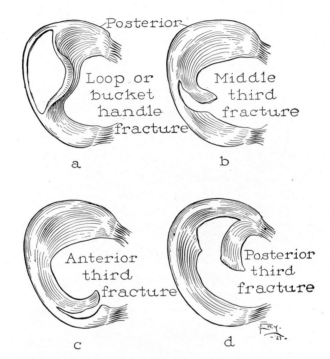

FIG. 754.—COMMON TYPES OF FRACTURE OF THE MEDIAL SEMILUNAR CARTILAGE. (Henderson, M. S. Surg. Clin. North America, Dec., 1927.)

collateral ligaments of the bicondylar joints, cross each other in the center of the knee joint, and are a powerful stabilizing mechanism. They are intracapsular, but extrasynovial. The anterior cruciate ligament is attached to the tibia anterior to the intercondylar eminence and passes upward and backward to an extensive insertion over the posterior part of the medial aspect of the lateral femoral condyle. Since its points of attachment are farther from one another when the knee joint is freely extended, the ligament is tense in this position of the limb and bears the brunt of the strain of forced extension. The collateral ligaments and the thickened posterior part of the capsule, combined with the anterior cruciate ligament, are sufficient to prevent hyperextension of the joint, unless undue force is acting. In addition to preventing hyperextension of the knee, the anterior cruciate ligament prevents the tibia from moving forward on the femur in passive extension of the joint. If, after injury, anterior movement of the tibia on the femur is obtained, a rupture of the anterior cruciate ligament is suspected. The posterior cruciate ligament is attached to the posterior part of the base of the intercondylar eminence of the tibia, and extends upward and forward to the lateral surface of the medial condyle of the femur. It is relaxed in extension of the leg, but is tightened in flexion. It prevents backward movement of the tibia on the femur. In a severe strain of the knee, one or both cruciate ligaments may be ruptured without causing actual dislocation of the joint.

The *menisci* (*semilunar cartilages*) are two sickle-shaped fibrocartilaginous wedges which form a circumferential investment for the head of the tibia and are interposed, wedgelike, between the tibial plateau and the head of the femur. Each cartilage is attached by its thick peripheral border to the deep aspect of the joint capsule. In addition, the peripheral borders of the cartilages are attached to the margins of the tibial condyles by short fibrous bands, known as coronary ligaments. The free medial margins of the cartilages are directed toward the joint cavity; their superior surfaces are concave and their inferior surfaces are comparatively flat; both surfaces are invested by the synovial membrane of the joint. The menisci cover about two thirds of the articular surface of the tibia and accommodate themselves to the changing position of the joint by changes in their shape and position. They slide on the articular surfaces, and adjust themselves to the required weight-bearing demands of the femoral condyles. They glide backward in flexion and forward in extension, and, in the movements of rotation and torsion, one is carried forward and the other backward. The lateral meniscus is the smaller of the two; it is very nearly circular in outline, and its two extremities are in close relationship, the anterior to the front of the intercondylar eminence (tibial spine), and the posterior to the interval between the tubercles of the eminence and to the posterior cruciate ligament. The lateral meniscus is related by its lateral and posterior aspect to the tendon of the popliteus muscle; a bursa intervenes, so that the synovial membrane of the knee joint projects laterally, both above and below it. It has no direct relation to the fibular collateral ligament. This arrangement perhaps more than any other factor is responsible for this cartilage possessing great freedom of movement and, consequently, little likelihood of derangement.

The medial meniscus forms almost a half circle, and its extremities are widely separated from one another. The anterior extremity is attached to a depression in front of the intercondylar eminence and the posterior to a depression behind the eminence. The peripheral margin of the medial meniscus is firmly adherent to the broad and powerful tibial collateral ligament and on this account is not freely movable. This fact explains the relative frequency of derangement of the medial meniscus in knee-joint strain or injuries involving the tibial collateral ligament. The menisci are attached to each other anteriorly by the slender transverse ligament, which may be looked upon as the continuation of the peripheral fibers of each meniscus. This may be torn when a meniscus is deranged.

7. **Synovial Membrane of the Knee Joint and the Infrapatellar Fat Pad.**—The synovial membrane lining the knee joint is the most extensive of its kind in the body, and its arrangement is complicated by the presence of the intra-articular ligaments and menisci. It lines the deep aspect of the capsule of the joint, covers the infrapatellar fat pad and the femoral and tibial surfaces of the menisci, and helps to attach their peripheral margins to the tibia. A large synovial pouch balloons upward between the quadriceps muscle and the shaft of the femur, where it forms the subquadriceps (suprapatellar) bursa. This bursa may be infected by stabs or punctures and thereby initiate joint infection, or it may be involved by fracture of the lower end of the femur and result in hemarthrosis. The synovia forms culs-de-sac about the lateral surfaces of the condyles, covering them for a third of their anteroposterior depth. The popliteus tendon is in contact with the synovial membrane in the intra-articular part of its course. It is through the medium of the bursa between this tendon and the posterior aspect of the head of the fibula that the knee-joint synovial membrane often is brought into connection with the synovial membrane of the proximal tibiofibular joint. A communication sometimes exists between the knee-joint synovial membrane and the bursa beneath the inner head of the gastrocnemius. In the posterior part of the joint, the cruciate ligaments push the membrane forward from the capsule into a synovial duplication. The membrane thus covers both cruciate ligaments in front and on each side, rendering them extrasynovial.

The large, pyramidal **infrapatellar fat pad** lies distal to the apex of the patella and behind the superior portion of the patellar tendon.   It is extra-articular and extrasynovial, and is thickest in its *body* which lies in the median plane.   From the body extend lateral free margins or processes, known as *alar folds* (*ligamenta alaria*).   Because of its semifluidity, the fat pad conforms to the shape of the trochlea and intercondylar spaces.   The *patellar synovial fold* (*ligamentum mucosum*) extends upward from the centrally placed apex of the pad to the intercondyloid notch of the femur.   A portion of the main fat pad on its lateral or superior prolongation frequently is the seat of hypertrophy (*lipoma arborescens*), in which grapelike proliferations may become detached and form loose bodies in the joint

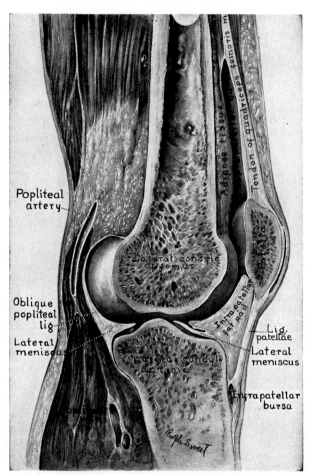

FIG. 755.—SAGITTAL SECTION THROUGH THE KNEE.

cavity.   Similar hypertrophy may affect the fat pad lying between the femur and the suprapatellar bursa.

A vertical parapatellar incision close to the patella encounters the pad in its thick portion.   An incision placed more laterally admits easier access to the joint, since only the thin alar fold is encountered.   The pad and its alar and patellar synovial folds obstruct exploration from one side of the joint to the other.

8. **Movement at the Knee Joint.**—The principal movements at the *emorotibial joint* are flexion and extension.   The mechanism by which these movements are effected differs from that in a true hinge joint, since the changes of attitude are accompanied by a slight gliding movement of the head of the tibia backward and forward on the condyles of the femur and by a certain degree of torsion or rotation (screw movement) of the tibia about its

longitudinal axis. Because of the gliding movement between the femur and the tibia, the socket formed by the articular surface of the tibia and the menisci does not revolve upon a fixed transverse axis passing through the femoral condyles, but upon axes that vary with the different attitudes of the knee.

In semiflexion, there is allowed the greatest amount of rotary movement, and this is the position of greatest instability. In complete extension of the leg, as in standing, the joint is locked strongly against lateral and rotary motion; the femur rotates a little mesially as a terminal stabilizing movement. Further extension is opposed by the tension of the anterior cruciate, collateral, and posterior ligaments and the hamstring muscles.

In passing from the extended to the flexed position, the slight lateral rotation of the tibia accompanying extension disappears before semiflexion is reached. In full flexion, the collateral and posterior ligaments are relaxed and a slight amount of rotary movement of the tibia upon the femur is possible. Excessive medial rotation is checked by the cruciate ligaments, and lateral rotation is checked by the lateral ligaments.

Adduction, abduction, and lateral sliding of the tibia occur at the knee only under abnormal circumstances and are the result of torn collateral and cruciate ligaments. Since movements are at their minimum in extension of the leg, clinical examination should be made with the knee joint in that position.

In considering the *movements at the patellofemoral joint*, it will be found that complete coaptation between the two articular surfaces does not occur, but that, as the knee passes ... first contact with the troch- ... part.

of the trochlea. When flexion is carried still further, the superior patellar facets lie against the most inferior part of the trochlea, and in complete flexion, most of the articular surface of the patella is apposed to the intercondylar notch.

SURGICAL CONSIDERATIONS

1. Genu Valgum or Knock Knee.—Under normal conditions, a line dropped from the center of the head of the femur passes between the femoral condyles at the knee joint. In this way, the superincumbent weight is transferred to the foot through the center of the knee, the tibial shaft, and the center of the ankle joint. In rickets, because of irregular growth and ossification at or near the epiphyseal line, there may take place an abnormal degree of downward growth in the medial part of the distal extremity of the femoral diaphysis; this results in the thrusting of the medial part of the epiphysis downward, backward, and laterally instead of straight downward. Thus, there arises the condition known as genu valgum or inward bowing of the knee. There is, in addition, bending of the femur and tibia close to the joint, so that a line dropped from the femoral head passes lateral to the

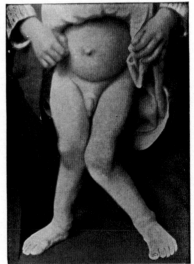

FIG. 756.—GENU VALGUM (KNOCK KNEE). (Lovett in "Keen's Surgery.")

center of the knee joint. The outward deflection of the leg may be such that the angle between the long axes of the femur and tibia, normally about 170 degrees, may approach a right angle. In addition, the foot usually is everted into the splay-foot deformity of talipes valgus.

In some instances, flat foot may be the cause and not the result of genu valgum. Many young adolescents with pronated feet adopt a position of rest in which the feet are everted and separated widely, while the knees are flexed and the thighs adducted. In this position, the medial condyle of the femur is tilted off the tibia and the tibial collateral ligament is stretched. The body weight is borne by the lateral femoral condyle which brings

48

about a diminished pressure on the medial part of the epiphyseal cartilage. As a result of this postural defect, the medial distal part of the femoral diaphysis undergoes an abnormal growth, and the apparent genu valgum of rest becomes a true genu valgum.

When knock knee occurs from infantile paralysis, there often exists a certain amount of flexion and lateral rotation of the leg and some contracture of the hip joint. An important factor in producing this deformity is the powerful pull on the tibia exerted by the iliotibial band which, through its pelvic and thigh attachments, summarizes the power of the gluteus maximus and medius and the tensor fasciae latae muscles. In advanced genu valgum, the femur requires osteotomy; the tibia is osteotomized to correct torsion and the iliotibial band is divided to correct hip and knee flexion. These operative procedures are supplemented by suitable apparatus to maintain the corrections.

The disability caused by genu valgum may be relieved by medial cuneiform oteotomy of the femur, and, in exaggerated cases, by transplanting the tibial tuberositys and the insertion of the patellar tendon into the medial aspect of the tibia.

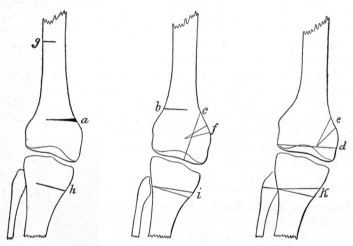

FIG. 757.—LINES OF OSTEOTOMY ABOUT THE KNEE.

　　a, Transverse wedge-shaped osteotomy of the medial femoral condyle; *b*, linear osteotomy superior to the lateral condyle; *c*, linear osteotomy of the medial femoral condyle; *d*, linear osteotomy of both femoral condyles; *e*, *f*, oblique wedge-shaped osteotomies of the medial femoral condyle; *g*, linear osteotomy of the femoral shaft; *h*, linear osteotomy of the medial tibial condyle; *i*, wedge-shaped osteotomy of the medial tibial condyle; *k*, wedge-shaped osteotomy of the medial condyle of the tibia and linear osteotomy of the head of the fibula. (Warbasse.)

In *supracondylar wedge osteotomy*, an incision down to the femur is made over the medial aspect of the thigh, a fingerbreadth inferior to the most proximal part of the femoral trochlea and the same distance in front of the tendon of the adductor magnus. No vessel is encountered, save possibly the supreme geniculate (anastomotica magna) artery, which usually lies more posteriorly. The femur is divided transversely with an osteotome above the epiphyseal line for a distance of two thirds or more of the thickness of the bone, and a wedge of bone is removed; the remaining part is fractured by bending the limb forcibly. An osteotomy of the femur may be performed from the lateral surface of the limb, the incision for which readily avoids the epiphyseal line and the superior geniculate and superior articular arteries. Linear or simple osteotomy on the lateral aspect of the femur is indicated in genu valgum, and lateral wedge osteotomy may be performed for genu varum.

Osteotomy of the tibia below the condyles may be required to complete the remedy of the knock-knee deformity. The bone is exposed on its medial surface just below the tuberosity and is divided with an osteotome. As in osteotomy of the femur, two thirds or more of the bone is cut and the remainder is fractured forcibly. To obviate the danger to the common peroneal nerve by forcible stretching, the cuneiform type of osteotomy should be performed.

2. **Genu Varum (Bowlegs).**—Overgrowth of the lateral part of the distal extremity of the diaphysis of the femur, or of the superior part of the tibial diaphysis, is one of the features of rickets. This results in outward bowing of the legs or genu varum. The weight of the body contributes to the deformity by causing bending in the bones of the thigh and leg. The point of greatest bending may be near the ankle or near the knee joint, but will be lateral to the center of the ankle joint. Consequently, the body weight is distributed mainly over the lateral part of the foot which is well adapted to bear the increased strain and little disability is encountered.

If the child is kept off his feet, the bones usually regain their normal shape after the rachitic softening disappears and the bones become more brittle. Designed fracture (osteoclasis) or cuneiform osteotomy may be necessary to overcome the deformity. Dietetic treatment and corrective-pressure methods assist the natural tendency toward self-correction, and usually are sufficient to restore the condition to normal.

3. **Dislocation at the Knee Joint.**—The knee rarely is dislocated and then only by extreme trauma or following severe infection. In traumatic dislocation, the tibia may be luxated forward, backward, or to either side, or it may be rotated upon the femur. The

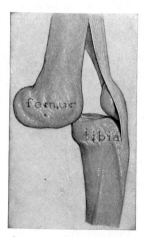

FIG. 758.—ANTERIOR DISLOCATION OF THE TIBIA AT THE KNEE JOINT. (Babcock, "Textbook of Surgery.")

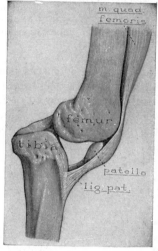

FIG. 759.—POSTERIOR DISLOCATION OF THE TIBIA AT THE KNEE JOINT. (Babcock, "Textbook of Surgery.")

usual mechanism of dislocation is extreme hyperextension and torsion. The laceration of the soft tissues may be so extensive as to rupture the popliteal vessels and require amputation. If the luxation is caused by the weakening of the knee joint by disease, the powerful hamstring muscles tend to pull the tibia backward, producing a deformity very difficult to correct.

4. **Injuries of the Menisci.**—The menisci rarely become detached in their entirety, but a portion of one of them may be torn (Fig. 754) partly or completely loose and be caught between the tibial and femoral articular surfaces, causing characteristic symptoms. Forcible extension of the leg, accompanied by a forcible rotation of the flexed or semiflexed knee, such as occurs in certain occupations and in violent sports, is a common cause of an accident of this sort. Catching the foot in a hole while running is a frequent cause. The accident may occur when the tibia is rotated on the flexed femur, or when the femur is rotated on the flexed tibia. The medial meniscus is much more likely to be injured than is the lateral meniscus. The comparative immunity of the lateral meniscus probably is the result of its greater range and freedom of movement.

When the femur is rotated laterally on the fixed tibia suddenly and violently, the lateral meniscus readily follows the lateral femoral condyle and, in so doing, throws a strain on the anterior extremity of the medial meniscus through the transverse ligament. The anterior part of the medial meniscus may be split or its forward extremity may be torn from its tibial attachment and be dragged toward the center of the joint. Violent flexion of the knee, combined with medial rotation of the femur on the tibia, may tear away the anterior or anterolateral attachments of the medial meniscus. The most common lesions are a

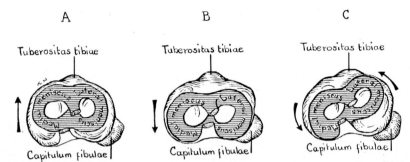

Fig 760.—Gliding Movements of the Menisci on the Tibial Plateau in Flexion, Extension, and Medial Torsion of the Leg.

A, The menisci glide forward in extension. B, The menisci glide backward in flexion. C, Movements of the menisci in medial rotation; the lateral meniscus moves forward and the medial meniscus backward. (After Forgue.)

transverse tear of the meniscus near the collateral ligament, detachment of the anterior insertion, and partial concentric splitting. Occasionally, the capsule of the knee joint becomes sufficiently relaxed to permit a slight amount of abduction and adduction; this predisposes to meniscal injury, since the slight separation between the femur and tibia renders the menisci more likely to be caught between the articular surfaces.

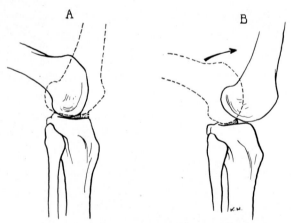

Fig. 761.—Diagram to Show the Anterior and Posterior Gliding of the Menisci on the Tibial Plateau and One Mechanism of Meniscus Injury.

A, The meniscus in accommodating the femoral condyles glides backward in flexion. The femur in dotted lines shows how the meniscus is pressed forward in extension. B, The diagram illustrates how the meniscus may be caught between the femur and the tibia in a rapid movement from flexion to extension. (After Forgue.)

If a part of the cartilage actually is displaced, the joint cannot be extended completely and often fills with fluid. There is likely to be acute localized tenderness at some palpable point along the joint line, especially over the tibial margin medial to the patellar tendon. Use of the limb is extremely painful until the cartilage is released. Derangement of the knee joint from an injured cartilage is subject to recurrence from trivial causes. Removal of the cartilage entails no ill effects.

5. **Tuberculosis of the Knee Joint.**—Tubercle bacilli and the organisms of pyogenic osteomyelitis usually lodge in the ends of the diaphyses about the knee joint. Direct tuberculous infection of the synovial membrane from the blood stream undoubtedly occurs, and occasionally the process begins in the epiphysis itself (epiphysitis). The knee joint is second only to the hip joint in the frequency of tuberculous involvement.

Tuberculosis of the distal end of the femur begins in the distal part of the diaphysis, nearer the posterior than the anterior surface. The focus may spread proximally along the diaphysis or pass directly outward toward the surface. In the latter instance, it usually spreads backward and breaks through the cortical bone of the popliteal surface of the femur, causing a popliteal abscess. Tuberculosis from this focus may involve the joint, but usually does not since the lesion is extracapsular and the infection finds less difficulty in passing to the popliteal fossa than in eroding the epiphysis and entering the joint.

When *tuberculous involvement begins in the proximal end of the tibial diaphysis*, it is entirely extracapsular and may spread distally along the shaft. The focus may spread circumferentially and finally involve the joint, either at the reflexion of the synovia, or by eroding the epiphysis and the articular cartilages. Occasionally, the disease may extend directly through the articular cartilage and involve the proximal tibiofibular joint. If this joint communicates with the knee joint by the popliteus bursa, the knee joint is infected secondarily.

When the infection is communicated to the synovial membrane, a reaction is set up and fluid is secreted. As the involvement of the membrane increases, it becomes the seat of an extensive growth of granulation tissue. The newly formed tissue fills the available space within the joint, giving it the appearance of a traumatic synovial effusion, a condition with which it may be confused. The articular cartilages of the femur, patella, and tibia are destroyed gradually, and the subjacent cancellous tissue of these bones then becomes the seat of a fungating caries. A noteworthy feature of a tuberculous lesion, in contrast to a lesion caused by pyogenic infection, is that the cartilaginous surface is preserved for a considerable period as a thin shell. This tendency, detected in *x*-ray films, is of some differential diagnostic import. The intra-articular and extra-articular ligaments become progressively infiltrated, softened, and weakened to the degree that the joint acquires an abnormal lateral and antero-posterior mobility. The granulation tissue undergoes

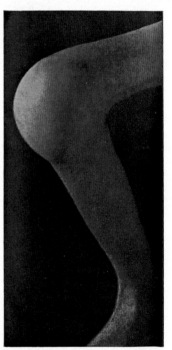

FIG. 762.—TUBERCULOSIS OF THE KNEE JOINT WITH FLEXION DEFORMITY AND SINUS FORMATION. (Lovett in "Keen's Surgery.")

coagulation necrosis, and chronic abscesses may make their way to the surface. Their ultimate evacuation, spontaneous or surgical, frequently is succeeded by persisting sinuses.

While these changes are occurring within the joint, the thigh and leg muscles undergo marked wasting until the knee assumes a spindle-shaped outline. Unless suitable precautions are taken, the knee joint becomes more and more flexed; the tibia may be subluxated backward and rotated laterally by the action of the hamstring and biceps muscles. The action of the hamstring muscles in pulling the tibia backward is facilitated by the degeneration of the ligaments in and about the knee.

6. **Surgical Approaches to the Knee Joint.**—Aspiration of the joint may be required to relieve pressure, obtain fluid for bacteriological study, evacuate a recently extravasated bloody effusion, or irrigate the joint cavity. The site for puncture should be somewhat proximal and lateral to the patella through the tendinous part of the vastus lateralis muscle rather than through the corresponding area on the medial aspect where the fleshy vastus

medialis is encountered.   The needle or trocar is carried distally toward the middle of the joint.

Arthrotomy or incision into the knee joint is performed through a variety of incisions. The *longitudinal parapatellar incision* may be made on either side of the patella from a point two fingerbreadths proximal to its base or just below its apex.   The incision is carried through the capsule and the capsular reinforcement supplied by the quadriceps expansion. The synovial membrane then is incised and the joint is exposed.   Bilateral parapatellar incisions may be employed, but this may not furnish adequate drainage of the posterior part of the joint, owing to the complicated arrangement of the synovial membrane; hence, a small posterolateral *counter-incision* may be made on each side.   These counter-incisions can be made most easily by carrying a hemostat backward through each anterior incision, across the corresponding surface of the femoral condyle, and into the posterior synovial pouch.   By making pressure from within outward on the posterolateral and posteromedia soft parts, th ese structures are steadied for counter-incision.   In the posterolateral regionl the hemostat is made to point just anterior to the biceps tendon to avoid the common,

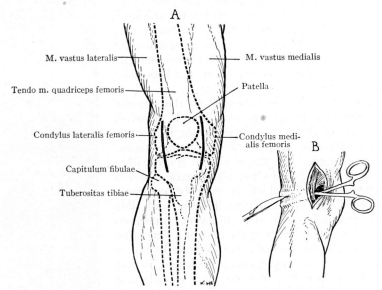

FIG. 763.—LONGITUDINAL PARAPATELLAR INCISIONS FOR ARTHROTOMY OF THE KNEE JOINT.
The inset illustrates the mechanism of counter-drainage.

peroneal nerve.   In the posteromedial region, the hemostat is carried into the hamstring tendons where a counter-opening is made.

Thorough exploration of the joint may be accomplished with little damage through the *lateral J-shaped incision* (of Kocher) or through a similar medial incision.   The lateral incision is directed a little obliquely downward and medially upon the lateral aspect of the knee joint and is curved medially at its inferior extremity to cross the tibial crest somewhat below the tibial tuberosity.   The incision begins over the vastus lateralis muscle, a palm-breadth above the base of the patella and a fingerbreadth from its lateral margin.   It descends vertically over the femoral and tibial condyles and curves forward to a point about 3 cm. below the tibial tuberosity.   The structures divided include the subcutaneous tissue, fascia lata, the lower fleshy fibers of the vastus lateralis and its aponeurosis, and the capsule overlain by the quadriceps expansions.   The incision is carried through the synovial membrane and alar portion of the fat pad, but the capsular attachment to the meniscus is not disturbed.   At this point, an offending meniscus may be removed by dissecting it from its capsular and tibial attachments.   Freer access is gained by elevating the insertion of the infrapatellar tendon from the tibia.   In the adult, the tuberosity of the tibia is chiselled off. In a child, the ligament is freed by removing a layer of cartilage from the tibial tuberosity. In neither instance should the periosteum at the distal margin of the tuberosity be divided, since it retains the tuberosity in place after the operation. The patella with the quadriceps, the patellar tendon, and the tibial tuberosity then may be rotated through more than a right angle and displaced medially, fully exposing the joint. Through this incision, either synovectomy or excision of the joint may be performed. The *medial* J-*shaped incision* suffices for thorough exploration of the joint and, of the major knee-joint incisions, does the least amount of damage. The patella can be dislocated laterally without removing the tibial insertion of the patellar ligament.

In the *median longitudinal approach*, the suprapatellar part of the quadriceps muscle, the patella, and the infrapatellar ligament are sectioned vertically and the joint is exposed for thorough exploration. Small pieces of the articular borders loosened by trauma sometimes are found in the synovial pouches. Small bits of synovial fringes and folds which have undergone cartilaginous changes also may become detached.

7. **Excision of the Knee Joint.**—Excision of the knee joint is performed most frequently for tuberculosis, and the best surgical access is afforded by a large U-shaped incision. The vertical trunks of the incision descend immediately anterior to the collateral ligaments, and the transverse limb is midway between the patella and the tibial tuberosity. The incision divides the superficial tissues, the capsule and its reinforcements, and the infrapatellar tendon, opening the knee joint. The joint may be exposed widely by flexing the knee.

The aim of the operation is the removal of the articular extremities of the femur, tibia, and patella, and the excision of the diseased synovial membrane as thoroughly as possible. The ultimate result of the operation is a rigid joint.

Frequently, the most extensive area of disease is located beneath the quadriceps muscle in the subquadriceps bursa. This bursa reaches a palmbreadth above the patella and is continuous with the synovial membrane overlying the superficial aspect of the femoral condyles. This large synovial pouch is dissected carefully from the overlying muscle and the underlying fat pad on the anterior surface of the femur.

The removal of the cruciate ligaments facilitates the dissection of the synovial membrane from the lateral and medial parts of the posterior division of the capsule. In these situations, synovial pouches extend upward behind the condyles and, if they are not removed, the disease may recur. In dissecting diseased synovial membrane from the posterior part of the joint, the proximity of the popliteal artery makes caution necessary. The point at which the synovial membrane comes most intimately into relation with the vessel is opposite the posterior part of the tibial plateau. The middle genicular artery may be ligated where it enters the joint after piercing the posterior popliteal ligament.

After resection of the cruciate ligaments, a stable and movable joint cannot be obtained and, since stability is of paramount importance, bony ankylosis in slight flexion is essential. This result is achieved by removing the articular cartilage and a layer of bone from the tibial and femoral condyles and from the patella. The anterior articular surface of the femoral condyles should be removed to render ankylosis more secure. When the disease lies mainly in the synovial membrane, and the bone is not involved seriously, only that thickness of bone should be removed which will assure osseous union. In adults, the line of bone section of the femur should be below the upper margin of its trochlear surface, which is at a point just distal to the attachment of the collateral ligaments. In order to gain proper thigh-to-leg alignment, the line of section of the femoral condyles should be parallel to the joint line and not at right angles to the long axis of the bone. The tibial section should be parallel to the articular surface of the bone, and the segment removed will vary from 0.5 to 1 cm. in thickness. After fixing the femoral condyle against the tibial condyles and fixing the patella against both bones, the anterior flap of skin and fascia is replaced and sutured.

The amount of actual permanent shortening usually is small but serves to keep the foot from dragging on the ground when the patient walks again.

In young people and in those whose skeletal growth is not yet complete, it is obviously undesirable to perform an extensive resection of these bones as this leads to a shortened and poorly developed limb. It is of the greatest importance, therefore, that the line of bone section should be upon the articular sides of the epiphyseal cartilages. In children, the safest course is to shave off only the articular cartilages and to remove the diseased parts of the bones with a gouge, leaving as much of the epiphysis as possible.

8. Injuries to the Lower Extremity of the Femur and Upper Extremity of the Tibia.— *Separation of the lower epiphysis of the femur* usually occurs in young boys, from violent overextension and rotation of the leg. A common mechanism is for the leg to be twisted

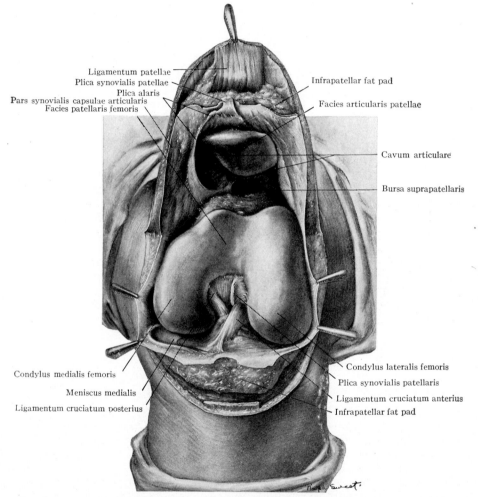

FIG. 764.—WIDE EXPOSURE OF THE LEFT KNEE JOINT THROUGH A U-SHAPED INCISION.

between the spokes of a revolving wheel (wagon-wheel fracture). The movement throws a severe strain on the posterior part of the capsule, which is strong and does not give way The strain, therefore, is transmitted to the distal femoral epiphysis; fracture separation takes place through that part of the metaphysis which abuts on the epiphyseal cartilage. The displacement may be slight, but when considerable, thrusts the femoral shaft backward into the popliteal space behind the epiphysis; the gastrocnemius muscle remains attached to the epiphysis. The injury often is complicated by injury to the popliteal vessels so extensive as to require amputation. Reduction is obtained under full anesthesia by flexing the knee and drawing the lower fragment downward by downward traction on the foot and forward traction on the upper tibia. By lifting the femur forward, the fragments come together much as in a dislocation. Future growth depends on the accurate reposition of the epiphysis.

Supracondylar fracture of the femur (p. 719) sometimes is converted into a T-*shaped intercondylar fracture* by a vertical splitting of the distal fragment. The knee is broadened by the spreading of the distal fragments by the gastrocnemius muscle. The thigh muscles, acting on the leg, drag it and the attached distal fragment of the femur proximally until the distal fragment overlies the proximal fragment in front. There is usually a considerable effusion into the joint.

Manipulations to restore the proper alignment are carried out with the knee flexed to relax the gastrocnemius muscle. If these fail, traction treatment with a Steinmann pin passed through the crest of the tibia is required to align the fragments. In a T-shaped fracture, the distal fragments may be approximated by pressure against the femoral condyles with the knee in flexion.

Fracture of the tibial condyles almost invariably invades the knee joint and deforms the tibial articular surface. The injury ordinarily results from the shearing force of one or the other femoral condyle. One whole side of the tibial plateau may be driven downward,

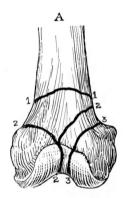
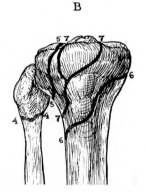

FIG. 765.—COMMONER FRACTURE LINES IN THE DISTAL EXTREMITY OF THE FEMUR AND THE PROXIMAL EXTREMITIES OF THE TIBIA AND FIBULA.

A, Fracture lines in the distal extremity of the femur. B, Fracture lines in the upper extremities of the tibia and fibula. 1-1, Supracondylar fracture of femur; 2-2-2, intercondylar Y-fracture; 3-3, fracture of medial condyle of femur; 4-4, fracture of neck of fibula; 5-5, fracture of lateral condyle of tibia; 6-6, infracondylar fracture of tibia; 7-7-7, intercondylar Y-fracture of tibia.

leaving the joint asymmetrical. A strong lateral strain upon the knee, as produced by a blow from an automobile bumper, may drive the lateral tibial condyle downward and impact it (bumper fracture). Occasionally, an intercondylar fracture occurs in which the tibial shaft is driven upward between the lateral fragments or the femoral shaft is driven downward between the split condyles. The articular surface is broadened and one or the other articular surface may be so depressed as to cause genu varum or genu valgum. Treatment is designed to restore the normal place and shape of the articular surface. A depressed condylar fragment may require open reduction.

In *infracondylar fracture of the tibial shaft*, proper alignment is of great importance to prevent the deformity of genu recurvatum.

Fracture of the intercondylar eminence of the tibia occasionally occurs from forcible extension of the femur upon the fixed and medially rotated tibia. In a similar way, forcible extension of the femur with the tibia fixed causes the lateral femoral condyle to fracture the lateral tubercle of the eminence. Absolute rest in the extended position usually produces a good result; open operation may be necessary. The best exposure is obtained through the median longitudinal incision (p. 759), which splits the patella vertically.

Separation of the tibial tuberosity has been described (p. 735).

9. **Gritti-Stokes Supracondylar Amputation.**—In the Gritti-Stokes amputation, the articular surface of the patella is removed. The patella, with its covering of soft parts and attached quadriceps tendon, then is fitted to the sawed end of the femur. The supracondylar saw line is a thumbbreadth proximal to the adductor tubercle of the femur. The U-shaped incision for the long anterior flap begins in the midlateral long axis of the femur, just above the lateral condyle, and curves downward across the anterior surface of the leg midway between the patella and the tuberosity of the tibia. A corresponding incision on the medial aspect of the knee joins this incision. The incision for the posterior short flap begins and ends at the upper extremities of the preceding incision and passes with a downward convexity across the posterior surface of the thigh. The anterior incision is deepened, cutting across the middle of the patellar tendon and opening the knee joint. The soft parts in the flap are dissected back to the saw line. All structures in the posterior flap are cut to retract to the saw line. The femoral vessels are caught and ligated. The sciatic nerve is isolated, ligated, and injected with absolute alcohol, sectioned, and allowed to retract. The femur then is sawed through. The patella is grasped in lion-jawed forceps and held so that the articular surface can be removed with a thin saw. The sectioned patella is placed over the end of the sawed femur, and the patellar tendon is sutured to the periosteum of the posterior surface of the femur. The flaps are refashioned and approximated. The suture line falls behind the stump end. The amputation provides an excellent end-bearing stump.

IV. LEG

The skeletal structure of the leg is made up of the tibia and fibula. The tibia is constructed strongly and bears most of the weight of the body through its articulation with the femur above and the talus below. The fibula is slender and lies behind and to the lateral side of the tibia. The bones of the leg furnish insertions to the thigh muscles and attachments to the leg muscles which control the foot. The muscles spanning the knee and ankle are largely responsible for the contractures at these joints and increase the difficulty of maintaining fracture fragments in position. Fractures of the leg bones, therefore, require immobilization of the thigh and foot.

In topographic study, the upper limit of the leg is defined as the horizontal plane at the level of the inferior part of the tuberosity of the tibia, and the lower limit as a plane through the bases of the malleoli.

1. **Bony Landmarks.**—The well-developed leg is conical in outline, smooth and uniformly rounded in children and females, but is irregular in males because of muscle development. The muscles may be brought prominently into relief if made to contract, as they do in the effort to stand on tip-toe.

The *tuberosity of the tibia* is a prominent bony landmark. The *medial surface of the tibia*, below the level of the insertion of the sartorius and semitendinosus muscles, is covered by the skin and superficial fascia only, and can be palpated throughout its entire length. The finger passed over it readily detects any irregularity on its surface. The sharp anterior border or *crest of the tibia*, "the shin," is a distinct landmark which begins at the tibial tuberosity and descends in a slightly curved fashion to the talocrural (ankle) joint. In the lower third of the bone, the crest loses its sharpness and merges into the evenly rounded tibial shaft. The medial margin of the tibial shaft, although less distinct than the anterior margin, can be palpated throughout its entire length.

The *shaft of the fibula* in its upper three fourths is concealed by the anterior and lateral groups of leg muscles and cannot be palpated directly, but the indefinite resistance of the shaft can be felt on deep palpation. Pressing the fibula against the tibia elicits pain over a fibular fracture area. The lateral surface of the distal quarter of the fibula is subcutaneous and is palpable between the lateral and anterior groups of leg muscles. It continues into the *lateral malleolus*. The *head of the fibula* is a prominent landmark.

2. **Regional Subdivisions and Muscle Landmarks.**—The general surface of the leg is subdivided by natural landmarks into a bony region and three separately functioning

muscle regions, the boundaries of which can be made out readily in muscular limbs free from excess fat. Their boundaries are the crest of the tibia and two vertically directed grooves on the anterolateral aspect of the leg, known as the anterior and posterior sulci. These grooves define anterior and posterior intermuscular (peroneal) septa which pass from the investing deep fascia of the leg to the anterior and lateral margins of the shaft of the fibula. These septa separate the peroneal or abductor muscle group from the flexors of the ankle and extensors of the toe in front, and the calf muscles behind.

The four subdivisions of the leg are arranged as follows: the anteromesial area which overlies the exposed shaft of the tibia; the anterolateral region, situated between the tibial crest and the anterior intermuscular septum; the lateral region which corresponds to the area included between the two intermuscular septa; and the posterior and most extensive region which embraces the area between the posterior intermuscular septum and the mesial border of the shaft of the tibia.

The **anteromesial area** over the exposed shaft of the tibia is traversed over much of its extent by the *great saphenous vein* in its upward course to the mesial side of the knee and thigh. Pathologic changes dependent upon varicosities of this vessel and its tributaries localize here. The skin over this surface may appear to be in a state of chronic

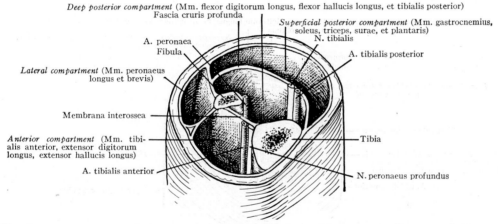

Deep posterior compartment (Mm. flexor digitorum longus, flexor hallucis longus, et tibialis posterior)
Fascia cruris profunda
Superficial posterior compartment (Mm. gastrocnemius, soleus, triceps, surae, et plantaris)
N. tibialis
A. peronaea
Fibula
A. tibialis posterior
Lateral compartment (Mm. peronaeus longus et brevis)
Membrana interossea
Anterior compartment (Mm. tibialis anterior, extensor digitorum longus, extensor hallucis longus)
Tibia
A. tibialis anterior
N. peronaeus profundus

Fig. 766.—Cross Section Through the Upper Third of the Right Leg to Show the Subdivisions Formed by the Intermuscular Septa. (After Corning.)

eczema or may be markedly indurated and adherent to the deeper tissues. Under normal conditions, the great saphenous vein sometimes can be made out through the overlying skin; in a varicose state, it stands out prominently and, with its tributaries, forms dilated coils beneath the skin.

The **anterolateral region,** especially in its upper portion, is rounded into a muscle prominence by the bellies of the tibialis anterior and extensor digitorum longus muscles. The feeling of resistance in the tissues over this area is explained by the density of the overlying deep fascia investing the muscles. When the ankle is dorsiflexed actively, the fleshy part of the tibialis anterior muscle forms a prominent elevation, and the tendon can be traced distally and mesially across the dorsum of the ankle joint (p. 777). The course of the *anterior tibial artery* coincides with the lateral margin of this muscle.

The **lateral or peroneal region** is very narrow and is limited in front and behind by the anterior and posterior peroneal sulci. In eversion of the foot, the peroneal muscles applied to the lateral surface of the fibular shaft form a surface bulge, the upper part of which corresponds to the fleshy part of the peroneus longus muscle. The lower part contains the tendon of this muscle and the fleshy belly of the peroneus brevis. The *common peroneal nerve* can be rolled against the fibula behind the head and lateral to the neck of this bone. At the fibular neck, the nerve divides into its two main branches, the superficial peroneal (musculocutaneous) and deep peroneal (anterior tibial). The superficial position of the common peroneal nerve and its close relationship to the fibula render it liable to injury from minor trauma or fracture of the fibular neck. Undue pressure over the nerve must be avoided.

The **posterior region** is rendered broad and prominent in its upper half, the "calf of the leg," by the two fleshy heads of the gastrocnemius muscle and by the soleus muscle. Halfway down the leg, the fleshy part of the gastrocnemius muscle merges into its tendon, which narrows rapidly. The soleus muscle remains fleshy below the middle of the leg, and its lateral margin, in contraction, projects somewhat in front of the gastrocnemius. The median groove in the upper part of the region indicates the area between the two heads of the gastrocnemius and is the surface guide to the termination of the *small (posterior) saphenous vein.* In the foot and above the ankle, this vein lies at the lateral side, but as it ascends, it gradually approaches a posterior position and occupies the median line for some distance before terminating in the popliteal vein. Below the calf of the leg, the *tendo calcaneus* stands out in bold relief, flanked on each side by a furrow, the retromalleolar groove.

3. **Deep Fascia.**—The deep fascia of the leg closely resembles that of the thigh, with which it is continuous. It is attached above to the condyles and tuberosity of the tibia,

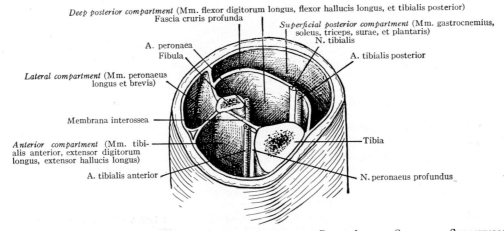

Deep posterior compartment (Mm. flexor digitorum longus, flexor hallucis longus, et tibialis posterior)
Fascia cruris profunda
Superficial posterior compartment (Mm. gastrocnemius, soleus, triceps, surae, et plantaris)
N. tibialis
A. peronaea
Fibula
A. tibialis posterior
Lateral compartment (Mm. peronaeus longus et brevis)
Membrana interossea
Anterior compartment (Mm. tibialis anterior, extensor digitorum longus, extensor hallucis longus)
Tibia
A. tibialis anterior
N. peronaeus profundus

FIG. 767.—CROSS SECTION THROUGH THE UPPER THIRD OF THE RIGHT LEG TO SHOW THE SUBDIVISIONS FORMED BY THE INTERMUSCULAR SEPTA. (After Corning.)

and to the head of the fibula. Its strength and density vary in different parts of the leg Over the subcutaneous medial surface of the tibia and the lower exposed surface of the fibula, the fascia is absent; over the lateral and anterior aspect of the leg it is developed strongly and is especially dense over the upper part of the tibialis anterior muscle. The fascia furnishes origin for the tibialis anterior and extensor digitorum communis muscles.

From its deep surface, the fascia gives off *anterior and posterior intermuscular (peroneal) septa* which attach it to the corresponding borders of the fibula. The anterior septum separates the peroneal muscles from the anterior group of leg muscles, and the posterior septum demarcates the peroneal group from the muscles of the calf. Subsidiary septa pass between the individual muscles.

At the ankle, the deep fascia is strengthened into ligamentous bands, the *transverse* and *cruciate ligaments* (p. 781) which maintain the various tendons in position.

4. **Muscles of the Anterior Compartment.**—The anterior compartment, on transverse section, is an irregular four-sided figure, bounded anteriorly by the enveloping fascia, posteriorly by the interosseous membrane and the anterior surface of the fibula, mesially by the lateral surface of the tibia, and laterally by the anterior intermuscular septum. It contains the tibialis anterior, extensor digitorum longus, extensor hallucis longus, and per-

oneus tertius muscles, the anterior tibial vessels, and the deep peroneal (anterior tibial) nerve. The anterior branch of the peroneal artery enters the compartment just above the lateral malleolus.

The *tibialis anterior muscle* arises from the mesial part of the anterior compartment. from the upper two thirds of the lateral surface of the tibia and adjoining part of the interosseous membrane, and from the deep surface of the overlying deep fascia. Its tendon

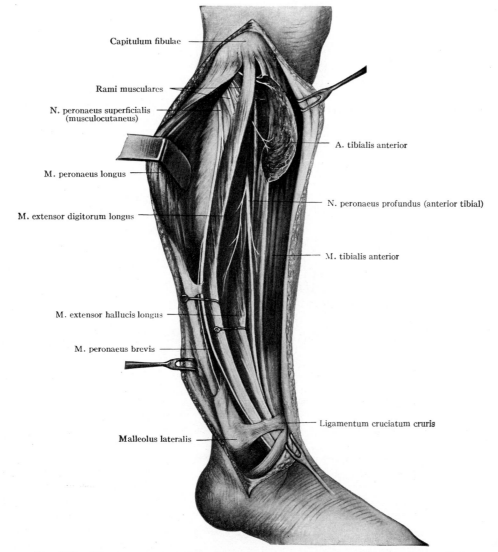

Capitulum fibulae

Rami musculares

N. peronaeus superficialis (musculocutaneus)

A. tibialis anterior

M. peronaeus longus

N. peronaeus profundus (anterior tibial)

M. extensor digitorum longus

M. tibialis anterior

M. extensor hallucis longus

M. peronaeus brevis

Ligamentum cruciatum cruris

Malleolus lateralis

FIG. 768.—STRUCTURES OF THE ANTEROLATERAL AND PROXIMAL REGIONS OF THE LEG.
Part of the anterior tibial muscle is removed to show the anterior tibial artery and deep peroneal nerve; the small hooks retract the extensor digitorum longus and the extensor hallucis longus muscles; the wide retractor is drawing aside the peroneal group of muscles.

runs downward and mesially behind the transverse and cruciate ligaments to an insertion into the adjoining medial aspect of the first metatarsal and the first cuneiform. The muscle is separated above from the extensor digitorum longus muscle and below from the extensor hallucis longus muscle by a septum of deep fascia leading to the cellular interspace which contains the neurovascular structures of the space. This muscle dorsiflexes and inverts the foot.

The *extensor digitorum longus*, *extensor hallucis longus*, and *peroneus tertius muscles* occupy the lateral part of the compartment. The extensors insert into the terminal phalanges, dorsiflex the foot at the ankle, and extend the toes. The peroneus tertius inser' into the dorsum of the base of the fifth metatarsal and dorsiflexes and everts the foot. All of the muscles of this compartment are supplied by the deep peroneal (anterior tibial) nerve (L_4, $_5$, S_1).

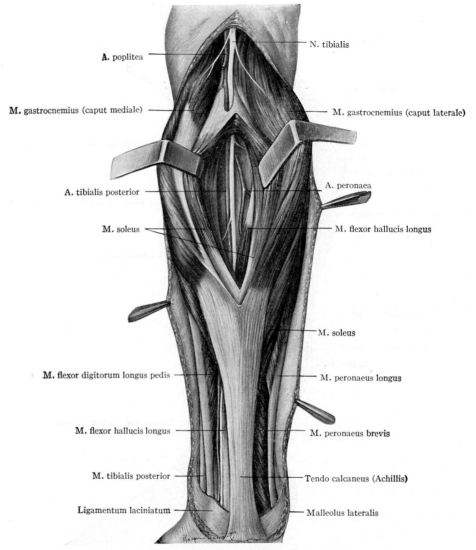

FIG. 769.—SUPERFICIAL STRUCTURES IN THE POSTERIOR REGION OF THE LEG.
The bellies of the gastrocnemius are separated and the soleus muscle is split to show the vessels and nerves in the deep muscle layers.

5. **Muscles of the Lateral Compartment.**—The lateral compartment is the smallest and is situated between the peroneal intermuscular septa. It contains the termination of the common peroneal nerve, the superficial peroneal (musculocutaneous) nerve, and the *peroneus longus and brevis muscles*. Both muscles arise from the lateral aspect of the fibula and run downward in the retromalleolar groove. In the groove, they possess a common synovial sheath, and are maintained against the fibula by the superior retinaculum (p. 782). Below the malleolus, they incline forward over the lateral surface of the cal-

caneus.   The peroneus brevis inserts into the dorsal aspect of the tuberosity of the fifth
metatarsal.   The tendon of the peroneus longus crosses the sole of the foot obliquely to an
insertion into the lateral aspect of the base of the first metatarsal and the first cuneiform
Both muscles permit plantar flexion, abduction, and eversion of the foot and are supplied
by the superficial peroneal (musculocutaneous) nerve (L_4, $_5$, S_1).

6. **Muscles of the Posterior Compartment.**—The posterior compartment is the largest,
but it diminishes very markedly as it approaches the ankle.   Its superficial boundary is the

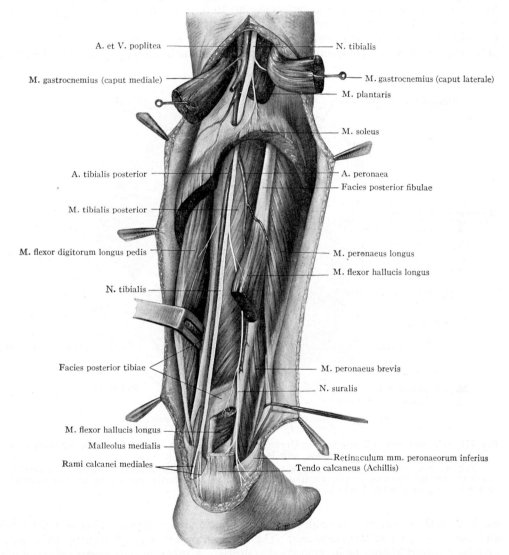

FIG. 770.—VESSELS, NERVES, AND DEEP MUSCULATURE OF THE POSTERIOR REGION OF THE LEG
Much of the gastrocnemius and soleus muscles has been removed.

deep fascia; the deep boundaries are formed by the posterior surface of the shaft of the
tibia and fibula, the interosseous membrane, and the posterior (peroneal) intermuscular
septum.

The muscles of this compartment operate as if in two groups.   The superficial group
comprises the gastrocnemius, soleus, and plantaris muscles, and the deep group consists
of the flexor digitorum longus, flexor hallucis longus, and the tibialis posterior muscles.
Between the two groups is a frontally placed sheet of deep fascia, about which there is a

quantity of areolar tissue. This tissue space communicates with the popliteal space through the fibrous ring in the soleus muscle, allowing the reciprocal spread of infection between these two regions.

Of the **superficial group of muscles,** the *gastrocnemius* arises from the distal part of the femur by two heads which unite in a common tendon halfway down the leg. The broad, flat *soleus* arises from the upper posterior surfaces of the tibia and fibula and lies under cover of the gastrocnemius. It terminates in a broad aponeurosis which is applied to, and blended with, that of the gastrocnemius to form the *triceps surae.* Their combined tendon is the *tendo calcaneus* or Achilles tendon which inserts into the distal half of the posterior surface of the calcaneus. The fusion of the soleus to the gastrocnemius is the only stay which resists contracture in the gastrocnemius in its long span from the femoral

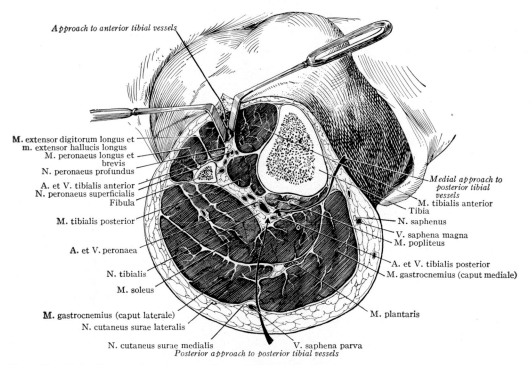

FIG. 771.—CROSS SECTION THROUGH THE UPPER PART OF THE RIGHT LEG TO SHOW THE APPROACH TO THE ANTERIOR AND POSTERIOR TIBIAL VESSELS.

The anterior arrow indicates the approach to the anterior tibial vessels; the medially placed arrow marks the medial approach to the posterior tibial vessels; the posterior arrow indicates the posterior approach to the posterior tibial vessels.

condyles to the calcaneus. A small precalcaneal bursa always is present between the tendon and the upper part of the calcaneus. This bursa may become inflamed by irritation, or may be involved in gout or in gonorrheal arthritis. A subcutaneous or *retrocalcaneal bursa* sometimes is present between the insertion of the calcaneal tendon and the skin, and is affected by the same lesions as those which affect the precalcaneal bursa. The stiff counter of a low shoe frequently irritates this bursa.

The *plantaris* is a muscle strip on the back of the leg applied to, and in line with, the medial border of the lateral head of the gastrocnemius. It ends in a long filiform tendon which is inserted into the calcaneus at the mesial margin of the tendo calcaneus. Isolated rupture of the plantaris tendon may occur. All three muscles are innervated by the tibial (internal popliteal) nerve ($L_{4, 5}$, $S_{1, 2}$). They act as plantar flexors of the foot. The gastrocnemius and plantaris also assist in flexing the leg.

The **deep group of muscles** is demarcated from the superficial muscles by a fascial septum which extends between the fibula and the mesial border of the tibia. The *tibialis posterior* arises from the interosseous membrane and adjoining part of the tibia and fibula. Its tendon passes distally and medially in a separate space behind the laciniate ligament to a principal insertion into the navicular tuberosity. The *flexor digitorum longus* arises from the fascia on the surface of the tibialis posterior muscle and the adjoining surface of the tibia. The tendon passes mesially and distally behind the medial malleolus through a space in the laciniate ligament (p. 781), lateral and posterior to the posterior tibial tendon. The *flexor hallucis longus* arises from the distal two thirds of the posterior surface of the fibula. At the ankle joint, it passes through a separate space in the laciniate ligament, separated from the flexor digitorum longus by the tibial nerve and the posterior tibial vessels. These muscles are supplied by the tibial nerve (L_5, S_2) and act as plantar flexors of the foot. The tibialis posterior is a powerful invertor as well, and the two other muscles flex the toes.

7. **Arteries.**—The leg receives a bountiful arterial supply from the popliteal artery through its anterior and posterior tibial branches. The branches are given off just after the parent trunk has penetrated the tendinous arch of the soleus muscle. They anastomose very freely, especially about the ankle and in the foot, so that circulation is adequate when one or the other main trunk is occluded. These large arteries lie close to the shafts of the bones where they are exposed to injury by sharp fragments in cases of fracture. An embolus conveyed along the popliteal artery may lodge at its point of bifurcation and block both tibial arteries. Should the succeeding thrombosis extend along the tibial arteries and occlude the recurrent branches, the remaining collateral channels may be insufficient to maintain circulation.

The **anterior tibial artery** arises from the popliteal artery at the lower border of the popliteus muscle (p. 738) and passes through the upper part of the interosseous membrane into the anterior compartment of the leg. The artery lies at first upon this membrane close to the neck of the fibula, but inclines medially and forward as it descends and rests against the anterior surface of the shaft of the tibia in the lower quarter of the leg. [Throughout its course, it is surrounded by the two interlacing venae comites, and is accompanied by the deep peroneal (anterior tibial) nerve, after that nerve has wound around the head of the fibula. Proximally, the artery lies deep between the tibialis anterior and the extensor digitorum longus muscles. In the middle of the leg, the artery is located between the tibialis anterior and the extensor hallucis longus muscles. As it approaches the ankle, it is crossed by the tendon of the latter muscle, and, just above the transverse ligament, is comparatively superficial. In front of the ankle, the anterior tibial artery is continued into the dorsal pedis.

The *course* of the anterior tibial artery corresponds to a line joining a point just mesial to the head of the fibula and a point at the ankle midway between the malleoli. The incision for ligation of the artery is made along this line. After the deep fascia has been divided, the tibialis anterior muscle is retracted medially and the other muscles are retracted laterally. In its upper third, the artery is exposed on the interosseous membrane; the deep peroneal nerve lies lateral to it. In the middle third, the deep peroneal nerve lies anterior to it. In the distal third, the artery lies on the tibia, crossed obliquely by the tendon of the extensor digitorum longus. The deep peroneal nerve is on the lateral side.

Collateral circulation is established through the anastomosis about the malleoli and the connection between the dorsalis pedis artery and the plantar arch (p. 796).

The **posterior tibial artery** is the larger of the two terminal branches of the popliteal. It originates just distal to the ring in the soleus muscle and inclines medially as it descends in the posterior compartment. At its termination, it lies midway between the medial malleolus and the medial tubercle of the calcaneus, where it divides into its terminal medial and lateral plantar arteries (p. 796). In its downward course, the artery lies on the deep group of posterior muscles, bound down by the fascial septum which separates these muscles from the gastrocnemius and soleus. In its upper two thirds, the artery is deep; in the rest

49

of its course, it is superficial. Near its termination, it lies beneath the laciniate ligament among the tendons of the deep leg muscles.

The course of the posterior tibial artery corresponds to a line extending from the center of the back of the leg, a palmbreadth below the bend of the knee, to a point at the ankle midway between the calcaneal tendon and the medial malleolus. The incision for *ligation* of the artery in its upper two thirds is not made exactly in the course of the artery, since the incision would entail an extensive division of the gastrocnemius and soleus muscles, but it is made a fingerbreadth behind the medial border of the tibia. Retraction of the skin and fascia exposes the free margin of the medial head of the gastrocnemius muscle which overlaps the origin of the soleus muscle from the medial border of the tibia. The wound is deepened through the soleus, exposing the strong fascia covering the deep muscles. This fascia is split carefully and its lateral part is raised from the underlying muscles, ex-

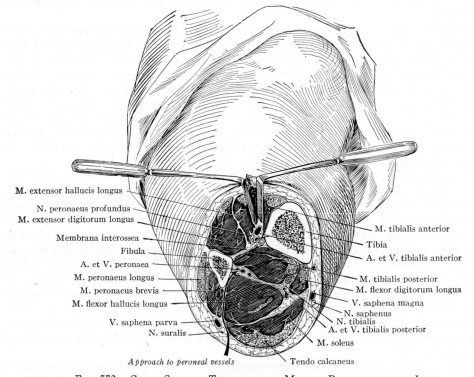

M. extensor hallucis longus
N. peronaeus profundus
M. extensor digitorum longus
Membrana interossea
Fibula
A. et V. peronaea
M. peronaeus longus
M. peronaeus brevis
M. flexor hallucis longus
V. saphena parva
N. suralis
Approach to peroneal vessels

M. tibialis anterior
Tibia
A. et V. tibialis anterior
M. tibialis posterior
M. flexor digitorum longus
V. saphena magna
N. saphenus
N. tibialis
A. et V. tibialis posterior
M. soleus
Tendo calcaneus

FIG. 772.—CROSS SECTION THROUGH THE MIDDLE PORTION OF THE LEG.
The incision is widened by retraction to indicate the approach to the anterior tibial vessels; the arrow indicates the path of approach to the peroneal vessels.

posing the posterior tibial vessels which lie on the posterior tibial muscle. In the upper third of the leg, the tibial nerve lies close to the medial side of the artery and must be avoided in applying the ligature.

For a deep wound in the upper posterior part of the leg, it may be necessary to make a long straight incision in the midline of the upper leg, beginning two or three fingerbreadths below the bend of the knee. After drawing aside the small saphenous vein, the deep fascia is incised, and the interval between the two heads of the gastrocnemius muscle is brought into view. The gastrocnemius is divided vertically as far as the wound will permit. By retracting the wound margins, the deeper structures are exposed. Within this area are found the lower part of the popliteal artery, its two branches, and the origin of the peroneal artery from the posterior tibial artery. The first part of the tibial nerve is exposed.

The **peroneal artery,** arising about 2.5 cm. below the bifurcation of the popliteal, is the largest branch of the posterior tibial artery. It follows the medial edge of the fibula within the fibers of origin of the flexor hallucis longus and remains in close relation with the posterior aspect of the bone, and with the interosseous membrane throughout the rest of its course. Just proximal to the ankle joint, it gives off a branch which pierces the interosseous membrane, and descends in front of the lateral malleolus to be distributed to the anterolateral part of the ankle and to the tarsal region. Both branches contribute to the malleolar anastomoses.

The incision for ligation is made over the posteromesial edge of the fibula. After the edge of the soleus muscle is drawn medially and the fibers of the flexor hallucis longus muscle are divided, the artery is found at the junction of the medial edge of the fibula and the interosseous membrane.

8. **Veins.**—The veins of the leg are arranged in two groups, deep and superficial. The deep veins lie beneath the deep fascia and accompany the arteries in the lower extremity. Each of the arteries below the popliteal has two accompanying veins, while the femoral and popliteal arteries have but one.

The *great (internal) saphenous vein* begins in the foot and ankle and ascends superficially on the medial aspect of the tibia. It passes along the posterior border of the medial tibial condyle and thence up the thigh to empty into the femoral vein at the saphenous opening. Under normal conditions, the vein cannot be distinguished under the skin, but, when markedly varicose, it and its tributaries stand out prominently. It communicates in the leg with the deep veins accompanying the tibial and peroneal arteries and with the small saphenous vein. From the leg down, it is associated with the saphenous nerve ($L_{3, 4}$). The *small (external) saphenous vein* begins at the ankle behind the lateral malleolus and ascends at first along the lateral aspect of the leg. It gradually approaches its posterior aspect and occupies the median line for a short distance before terminating in the popliteal vein. Through its superficial branches and by its deep connection with the venae comites, it anastomoses with the great saphenous vein. It is accompanied by the sural (short saphenous) nerve.

9. **Large Nerves.**—Each of the three muscle compartments of the leg has its own nerve as well as arterial trunk. The *tibial (internal popliteal) nerve* ($L_4, _5, S_1, _2, _3$) passes distally through the posterior compartment in close relation to the posterior tibial vessels. It lies at first on their medial side, but lower down crosses them superficially to lie on their lateral aspect at the ankle. It supplies all the muscles of the posterior compartment, and divides under the laciniate (internal annular) ligament into lateral and medial plantar branches (p. 796).

Within the lateral or peroneal compartments opposite the neck of the fibula, the common peroneal nerve divides into its two terminals, the superficial and deep peroneal nerves. The *superficial peroneal (musculocutaneous) nerve* ($L_4, _5, S_1, _2$) passes forward between the fibula and the peroneus longus muscle and descends immediately behind the anterior intermuscular (peroneal) septum where it supplies the peroneus longus and brevis muscles. At the junction of the middle and lower thirds of the septum, it pierces the deep fascia and passes downward and inward across the extensor tendons. The *deep peroneal (anterior tibial) nerve* ($L_4, _5, S_1$) is derived from the common peroneal nerve on the lateral aspect of the fibular neck, and descends through the anterior compartment in company with the anterior tibial artery. It innervates all the muscles of the anterior compartment and terminates in front of the ankle joint by dividing into medial and lateral branches.

10. **Shafts of the Fibula and Tibia.**—The fibula and tibia are united at their extremities by the proximal and distal tibiofibular joints and between them by the interosseous ligament. The *interosseous ligament* is a strong fibrous membrane formed by criss-crossing fibers which transmit indirect violence from the tibia to the fibula.

The slender *fibula* reinforces the tibia and enables it to withstand extreme bending and twisting; without fibular support, tibial fracture would occur much more frequently. The fibula is an exception to the general rule that the epiphysis toward which the nutrient artery is directed is the last to appear and the first to unite with the shaft. In the fibula, the nutrient artery is directed downward, yet growth takes place at the lower epiphysis, which is the first of the fibular epiphyses to appear and the first to unite. The upper three fourths of the fibula furnish extensive muscle attachments. The lower extremity of the fibula, the lateral malleolus, enters into the formation of the ankle joint, and, with the tibia, maintains a strong mortise for the reception of the talus. Occasionally, the fibula is congenitally absent, so that the tibia is devoid of support and the ankle joint lacks normal stability.

The *tibia* is much the stronger and more important bone, for it alone articulates with the femur and transmits the body weight through the ankle to the foot. The shaft of the tibia is composed of a strong shell of compact bone enclosing a central medullary cavity. Its sturdy anterior margin or crest is a thickened part of the compact cortex and is most dense in the middle of the shaft. Because of its strength and accessibility, grafts commonly are taken from it for bony transplants. Near each articular extremity, the outer shell diminishes considerably in thickness and encloses a quantity of cancellous tissue which extends upward and downward a considerable distance from the articular margin. The tibia is not straight but is convex medially in the upper half and laterally in the lower half. These curves are important to maintain the reduction of fractures. The mesial and lateral twisting of the tibial shaft in congenital clubfoot or in paralytic deformities so disturbs the alignment of the foot that corrective osteotomies may be required.

The nutrient foramen of the tibia is the largest in the skeleton; it lies on the posterior surface of the upper third of the bone. The nutrient canal runs a long downward course in the compact bone before opening into the medullary cavity. Fracture of the tibia through the nutrient canal predisposes to nonunion.

In addition to its susceptibility to all varieties of direct injury, the tibia is especially liable to certain forms of disease, one of the most devastating of which is *acute osteomyelitis*. The tibial shaft often is the site of a *syphilitic lesion* which manifests itself as a chronic osteitis and periostitis, and may lead to a marked thickening. The nodes of localized periosteal elevation make the smooth surface of the tibial shaft uneven. In the "sabre shin" of hereditary syphilis, the tibia is thickened, roughened, and flattened from side to side so that it presents a marked anterior convexity. The tibia, especially at its extremities, occasionally is the seat of local inflammatory disease which terminates in the formation of a central abscess (*Brodie abscess*).

Surgical Considerations

1. **Varicose Veins.**—Varicose veins are characterized by dilation and loss of the normal valvular mechanism. The consequent stagnation and back-pressure of venous blood cause fibrosis, overstretching, elongation, and sacculation of the walls.

The great frequency of varicosity in the saphenous veins may be caused by the high back-pressure within these vessels, which is attributed to long maintained erect posture and the great distance separating the veins from the heart. The great saphenous vein may be regarded as the lower part of a tube, the upper part of which coincides with the opening of the inferior vena cava into the heart. It differs from an open tube in that its interior is segmented by a series of bicuspid valves, each pair of which supports the column of blood immediately above and removes the weight from the column below. In a normal set of saphenous veins, the suction of the diaphragm and the direct pressure of muscle action are adequate to maintain the flow. Under abnormal conditions, these forces may prove inadequate, and, in consequence, the veins may become distended unduly. In some persons, the vein walls appear to be congenitally weak and they may dilate even though their interior pressure is not great. In others, the tendency of the superficial veins to dilate is augmented by the laxity of their surroundings. If the large venous trunks are subjected to pressure by tumors such as, for example, the pregnant uterus, varicosity is prone to manifest itself. When the deep veins of the leg are varicose, the distention in the superficial veins is aggravated by the current passing into them from the communicating channels from the deeper system. Superficial varices usually are noted first at the sites of entrance of these communicating veins. The upward thrust below one of these sites has to overcome not only the downward pressure of the superimposed column of blood, but also the resistance offered by the blood forcing its way outward from the deep veins. Varicosity rarely affects the deep veins, which are well adapted to emergency loads because they lie among muscles which support their walls and their valve mechanism.

As a result of varicosity, the skin over the lower and medial part of the leg may develop chronic eczema or become markedly indurated, deeply pigmented, and adherent to the deeper tissues. A chronic type of ulceration often is present over a varicose vein. Varicose ulcers are found typically in the lower half of the leg and syphilitic ulcers in the upper half of the leg. A chronic ulcer may spread over a considerable area, which is surrounded by edema and scar tissue. Although the fascia may be thickened greatly, the inflammatory process rarely extends beneath it. When ulceration overlies the tibia, its slowness to heal is explained by the tendency of the base of the ulcer to become fixed so that the amount of cicatricial contraction necessary to the healing process cannot take place. The periosteum may be thickened and new periosteal bone may be laid down.

The *treatment* of varicose veins by the injection of thrombosing chemicals is exceptionally satisfactory. The operative treatment consists in the removal of the great saphenous vein from the saphenous opening nearly to the ankle. The elimination of the varicose veins of the thigh is as important as elimination of those in the leg. The severe pain sometimes noted with varicose veins apparently is explained by the proximity of the veins to sensory nerves. A varicose ulcer is resected with a wide margin and with the deep fascia covering the muscles. The exposed heavily granulating surface is covered with skin grafts.

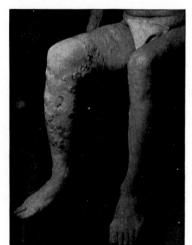

Fig. 773.—Varicosities of the Right Great Saphenous Vein. (Babcock, "Textbook of Surgery.")

2. **Surgical Approaches to the Tibia and Fibula.**—
The *approach to the tibia* for exploration or resection is along the exposed medial surface of the bone. Care is taken to avoid the saphenous nerve and the great saphenous vein lying in front of the medial malleolus. The incisions which *expose the fibula* are planned to avoid injury to the superficial (musculocutaneous) peroneal nerve. The approach to the proximal and middle thirds is made through an incision along the line of the posterior intermuscular (peroneal) septum. In the upper third of the shaft, the incision is developed between the adjoining borders of the soleus and peroneus longus muscles. Injury to the common peroneal (external popliteal) nerve, where it winds around the neck of the fibula, must be avoided. In the middle third of the shaft, a lateral incision is made through the interval between the peroneus longus and flexor hallucis longus; the latter muscle projects laterally beyond the lateral margin of the soleus. The incision for the distal third of the shaft is made just behind the anterior intermuscular septum in the interval between the peroneus brevis and tertius muscles.

3. **Amputation Through the Leg.**—Amputation through the leg may be required for a variety of conditions: irremediable tuberculosis of the ankle, gangrene of the lower part of the limb, or severe injury in which the bones and soft tissues are damaged hopelessly. The leg is divided into lower, middle, and upper thirds in the selection of standard methods of amputation through these levels. Stump length is measured from the insertion of the medial hamstring tendons into the tibia, to the end of the bone in the stump.

Pirogoff's and Syme's amputations just above the ankle joint may be classified as amputations through the *lower third* of the leg, but they are discussed topographically as amputations through the ankle (p. 791).

An amputation through the *middle third* of the leg is preferable to any other amputation between the knee and the base of the metatarsal bones. The saw-line is selected to give a 15-cm. stump length. The favorite amputation is that in which there is raised from the back of the leg a flap, sufficiently long to fold around the lower end of the stump and meet, upon the front of the limb, the tissues which have been divided transversely to form the short anterior flap. The fibula is sawed 2.5 cm. shorter than the tibia and the crest of the tibia is bevelled. This amputation has the advantage of providing an adequate musculotendinous fascial covering for the divided bones and an anterior scar line. A long anterior and a short posterior flap throw the suture line well behind the stump end. To prevent flexion contracture, a posterior leg splint is maintained in position, or traction is

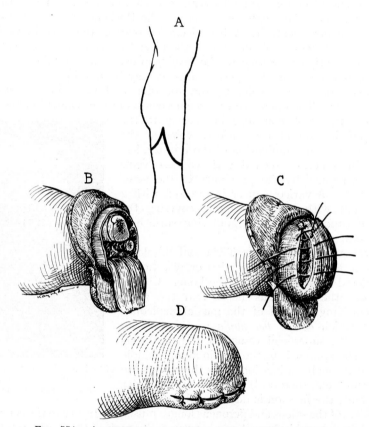

FIG. 774.—AMPUTATION OF THE LEG IN THE MIDDLE THIRD.

A, Skin incision at the optimum level. B, The skin and subcutaneous tissue flaps have been turned back; the musculotendinous flap has been taken from the gastrocnemius muscle; the deep fascia and the antero-external muscles are cut at the saw-line; the crest of the tibia is bevelled and a cuff of periosteum has been removed. C, The musculotendinous flap has been swung forward across the end of the tibia where it can be fixed by sutures to the base of the anterior skin flap. D, The appearance of the stump after closure.

applied until the wound heals; this splinting is necessary in all amputations below the knee.

All amputations through the *upper third* of the leg are above the site of election. They afford less leverage than amputations at a lower level, but provide more and better function than amputations above the knee. The "site of election," as referred to in older writings, is a line a handbreadth below the knee joint. This provided a stump well adapted to support the weight of the body in the flexed-knee pylon, and had little unsightly stump projecting behind. This stump is too short for maximum function in a modern prosthesis, for which a 10-cm. length is necessary.

The fibula often is the cause of a painful stump in amputations in the upper third because its prominent lower end tends to become more prominent and to protrude at an angle from the tibia. Removal of the fibula is advisable in all amputations in the upper third of the leg.

At the level of the upper third of the leg, there are large posterior and antero-external muscle masses mainly consisting of the gastrocnemius and soleus and the tibialis anterior and peroneus longus. With the exception of the gastrocnemius and plantaris, the muscles at this level are fixed to the bones and deep fascia, and cannot retract when divided. The operative treatment of an amputation in the upper third is the same as that in the middle, save that the fibula is removed. The tibialis anterior muscle is cut long enough to swing across the bevelled crest of the tibia. The other muscles in the anterior group are cut to retract to the saw-line, and the calf muscles are severed so that their posterior surfaces

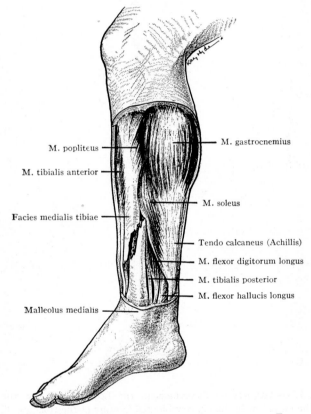

M. popliteus
M. tibialis anterior
Facies medialis tibiae
Malleolus medialis

M. gastrocnemius
M. soleus
Tendo calcaneus (Achillis)
M. flexor digitorum longus
M. tibialis posterior
M. flexor hallucis longus

FIG. 775.—OBLIQUE FRACTURE OF THE SHAFT OF THE TIBIA.

retract above the saw-line. The muscle bellies slope gradually from this level downward and forward to the saw-line.

4. Fractures of the Shafts of the Tibia and Fibula.—Fracture of the leg bones presents a problem different from that in fracture of the forearm, for the leg has no rotary motion to preserve. Any angulation of its bones may result in a change in the axis of weight-bearing, which throws an undue stress upon the ankle and knee joints. Fracture of one bone rarely results in deformity, as overriding of the fragments is opposed by the splinting effect of the intact bone. If both bones are broken, the advantages of easy palpation and access are overcome by the tendency to compounding.

Both bones of the leg may be broken by the *direct violence* of a severe blow or a crushing injury at any level between their upper and lower extremities. The site of break coincides with that of the injury and both bones are broken at the same level. Fractures caused in this fashion usually are transverse and often are comminuted. As a rule, they are not accompanied by much displacement. If displacement does take place, the upper tibial fragment usually is thrown forward, and sometimes pierces the skin. The lower fragment rides to the outer side. Overriding and displacement usually are the result of muscle action; therefore, fractures should be immobilized as quickly as possible to obviate deformity from muscle spasm. When only the tibia is broken and the line of fracture is transverse, there may be little recognizable displacement. If the finger is carried along the crest of the bone, the line of fracture may be located by a surface irregularity and by point-tenderness over the site of the lesion.

Fractures frequently are caused by the *indirect violence* of a bending strain or powerful torsion. When the leg is bent forcibly, as when the foot and ankle are fixed and the body

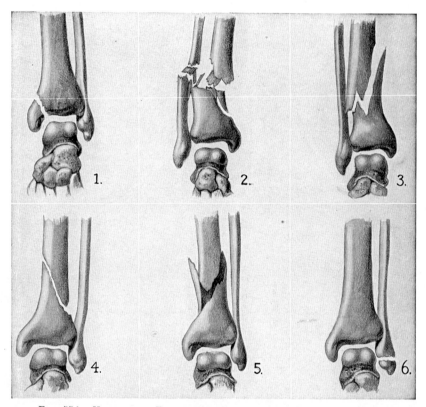

FIG. 776.—VARIETY OF FRACTURES IN THE LOWER THIRD OF THE LEG.

1, F cture of the medial malleolus; 2, comminuted fracture of the tibia and fibula at the junction of the lower and middle third; 3, oblique fracture of the tibia, with outward displacement of the upper fragments; 4, oblique fracture of the tibia without displacement; 5, spiral fracture of the lower third of the tibia; 6, fracture of the lateral malleolus. (Eisendrath in "Keen's Surgery.")

falls, the site of the tibial fracture usually is at the junction of the middle and lower thirds where the bone is most slender. When the tibia breaks, the fibula bends, and, if the force is exhausted rapidly, may not fracture. If the acting force is excessive and fracture of both bones occurs, the fibular fracture generally does not occur at the same level, but at a point higher up. Tibial fracture most often is oblique, and the pointed extremity of the upper fragment, which is superficial, may compound readily. The compounding may occur at the time of injury, but frequently a fracture, primarily simple, is made compound by the person's attempts to stand upright. In this type of fracture, displacement may be very marked. The weight of the foot causes the leg to bend and the direct traction exercised by the calf muscles draws the heel backward and angulates the leg forward at the fracture line. If the fracture is very oblique, there sometimes is much overriding. The obstacle to reduction of this and other leg fractures with displacement is the contraction of the posterior muscles of the leg. To overcome their tension, the leg is flexed to a right angle. With the leg maintained in this position by countertraction, extension can be made steadily in a downward direction until reduction is effected. The essential principle in treatment is that reduction be obtained without deviation in the normal plane of weight-bearing at the ankle joint. If the plane is altered, the weight of the body no longer falls perpendicularly upon the arch of the foot, and strain occurs, rendering the foot, ankle, and knee painful in weight-bearing. If preservation of the normal curves of the tibia (p. 772) is impossible, it is better that deformity consist of an exaggeration of the normal curves rather than that they be obliterated. If deformity in the anteroposterior plane occurs, angulation with the convexity forward always is preferable in any portion of the tibial shaft.

V. ANKLE

The ankle presents for consideration the ankle joint, composed of the tibia and fibula proximally, the talus (astragalus) distally, and the structures surrounding it. The subcutaneous tissue is scant and the skin is molded over the soft parts so closely that the contour of the bones and the direction taken by the principal tendons can be distinguished readily. Unless the swelling is too great, deviations from normal bony relationships, such as occur from fracture or dislocation, or both, are evident. The malleoli are the most obvious landmarks and serve as important guides in operations about the ankle. They subdivide the soft parts into anterior and posterior divisions.

A. STRUCTURES ABOUT THE ANKLE JOINT

1. **Structures about the Anterior Region of the Ankle.**—The landmarks of the anterior region of the ankle are of considerable surgical importance. The lateral malleolus is small and very thinly covered. It tapers into a point which lies about 0.5 cm. below and 2 cm. behind the plane of the tip of the medial malleolus. Above its tip for a distance of 7.5 cm., the shaft of the fibula is subcutaneous and is palpated readily. Anterior to the malleolus and lateral to the tendon of the peroneus tertius is a shallow depression indicating the level of the ankle joint. A similar depression lies between the medial malleolus and the tibialis anterior tendon. At these two points, the ankle joint is very superficial, and, in joint effusion or in intra-articular overgrowth of granulation tissue, these areas become filled out and form soft projections which may be elevated by the distended capsule When the foot is plantar-flexed actively, the talus (astragalus) glides forward out of its socket and forms a distinct prominence, most apparent in front of the lateral malleolus.

The medial malleolus is large, flat, and prominent. The resistant surface immediately in front of it corresponds to the medial aspect of the head and neck of the talus. On deep pressure about a fingerbreadth below the malleolus, the sustentaculum tali of the calcaneus is felt. It is obscured somewhat by the tendon of the flexor digitorum longus which crosses its medial aspect. The flexor hallucis longus tendon grooves the plantar surface of the sustentaculum. When the dorsiflexed foot is inverted actively, the tendon of the tibialis anterior stands out strongly and can be traced downward across the medial part of the ankle joint to a medial insertion into the first metatarsal and the corresponding cuneiform bone. The tendons of the extensor digitorum communis and extensor hallucis longus stand out in bold relief. The dorsalis pedis artery is very superficial and its pulsations can be felt readily. The internal saphenous vein begins in the medial part of the venous arch of the dorsum of the foot and ascends in front of the medial malleolus, where it usually can be recognized.

2. **Structures about the Posterior Region of the Ankle.**—The prominent tendo calcaneus is the structure of chief importance in the posterior region of the ankle. That part of the calcaneus intervening on each side between the calcaneal tendon and the corresponding malleolus is grooved considerably, and that on the lateral side is overlain by the tendons of the peroneus brevis and longus muscles, both of which are bound down tightly by a stout

derivation of the deep fascia, the superior retinaculum, or external annular ligament. This ligament stretches between the posterior border of the malleolus and the lateral aspect of the calcaneus, converting the groove behind the malleolus into an osteo-aponeurotic canal. The peroneus brevis tendon is the deeper and more anterior of the two and is in direct contact with the bone. Both tendons can be felt winding around the malleolus, but they diverge a little farther forward. The tendon of the peroneus brevis, which is uppermost at this level, passes anterior to the trochlear process of the calcaneus, and across the calcaneocuboid joint to an insertion into the upper aspect of the base of the prominent tuberosity of the fifth metatarsal bone. The tendon of the peroneus longus passes forward and downward beneath the trochlear process to the lateral margin of the foot, where it hooks around the lateral border of the cuboid. It crosses the sole obliquely forward and medially to the base of the first metatarsal. These tendons become prominent when the foot is everted actively.

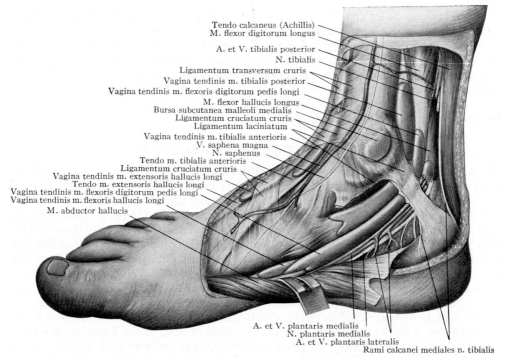

Tendo calcaneus (Achillis)
M. flexor digitorum longus
A. et V. tibialis posterior
N. tibialis
Ligamentum transversum cruris
Vagina tendinis m. tibialis posterior
Vagina tendinis m. flexoris digitorum pedis longi
M. flexor hallucis longus
Bursa subcutanea malleoli medialis
Ligamentum cruciatum cruris
Ligamentum laciniatum
Vagina tendinis m. tibialis anterioris
V. saphena magna
N. saphenus
Tendo m. tibialis anterioris
Ligamentum cruciatum cruris
Vagina tendinis m. extensoris hallucis longi
Tendo m. extensoris hallucis longi
Vagina tendinis m. flexoris digitorum pedis longi
Vagina tendinis m. flexoris hallucis longi
M. abductor hallucis
A. et V. plantaris medialis
N. plantaris medialis
A. et V. plantaris lateralis
Rami calcanei mediales n. tibialis

FIG. 777.—SUPERFICIAL STRUCTURES OF THE ANTEROMEDIAL REGION OF THE ANKLE AND FOOT.

The synovial sheaths of the peroneus muscles sometimes are involved by tuberculosis. It is important that the disease be recognized and eradicated at an early stage, lest the infection spread along the sheath of the peroneus longus into the plantar region and infect the tarsal joints. Access to the sheaths is afforded by the lateral J-shaped incision of Kocher (p. 790). To insure complete removal of the involved tissues, the retinacula must be severed and the synovia dissected away.

The interval between the medial malleolus and the calcaneus is bridged by the laciniate (internal annular) ligament which contributes to the formation of an osteo-aponeurotic canal to hold the tendons of the tibialis posterior, the flexor digitorum longus and the flexor hallucis longus muscles, and the posterior tibial vessels.

The tendon of the tibialis posterior lies immediately against the back of the malleolus and can be traced from this point to the medial margin of the foot and into the tuberosity of the navicular, its principal point of insertion. This tendon is succeeded by those of the flexor digitorum longus and the flexor hallucis longus. Between the last two tendons are the posterior tibial vessels and nerve.

The calcaneus tendon with the small plantaris tendon is brought into prominent relief by flexing the foot. It is narrowest opposite the base of the malleoli, but widens out a

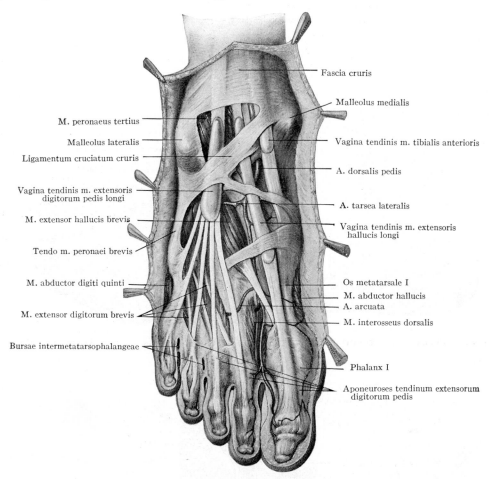

M. peronaeus tertius

Malleolus lateralis

Ligamentum cruciatum cruris

Vagina tendinis m. extensoris digitorum pedis longi

M. extensor hallucis brevis

Tendo m. peronaei brevis

M. abductor digiti quinti

M. extensor digitorum brevis

Bursae intermetatarsophalangeae

Fascia cruris

Malleolus medialis

Vagina tendinis m. tibialis anterioris

A. dorsalis pedis

A. tarsea lateralis

Vagina tendinis m. extensoris hallucis longi

Os metatarsale I

M. abductor hallucis

A. arcuata

M. interosseus dorsalis

Phalanx I

Aponeuroses tendinum extensorum digitorum pedis

FIG. 778.—SUPERFICIAL STRUCTURES ABOUT THE ANTERIOR REGION OF THE ANKLE AND THE DORSAL REGION OF THE FOOT.

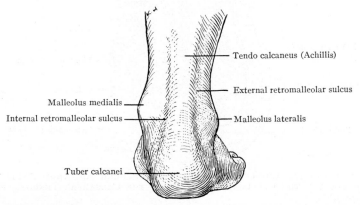

Tendo calcaneus (Achillis)

External retromalleolar sulcus

Malleolus medialis

Internal retromalleolar sulcus

Malleolus lateralis

Tuber calcanei

FIG. 779.—LANDMARKS ABOUT THE POSTERIOR REGION OF THE ANKLE AND FOOT.

little as it approaches its insertion. By splitting the deep fascia, the tendon is found in a space surrounded by a synovial sheath which greatly facilitates its movements. Synovitis

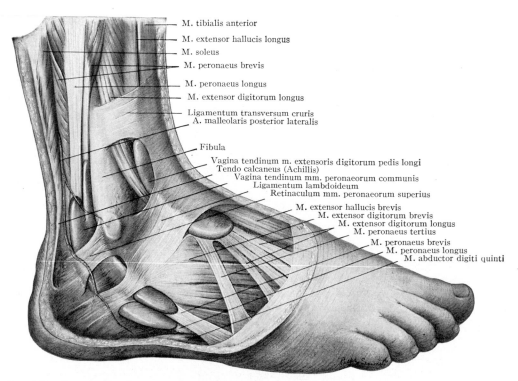

M. tibialis anterior
M. extensor hallucis longus
M. soleus
M. peronaeus brevis
M. peronaeus longus
M. extensor digitorum longus
Ligamentum transversum cruris
A. malleolaris posterior lateralis
Fibula
Vagina tendinum m. extensoris digitorum pedis longi
Tendo calcaneus (Achillis)
Vagina tendinum mm. peronaeorum communis
Ligamentum lambdoideum
Retinaculum mm. peronaeorum superius
M. extensor hallucis brevis
M. extensor digitorum brevis
M. extensor digitorum longus
M. peronaeus tertius
M. peronaeus brevis
M. peronaeus longus
M. abductor digiti quinti

FIG. 780.—SUPERFICIAL STRUCTURES OF THE ANTERO-EXTERNAL REGION OF THE ANKLE AND FOOT.

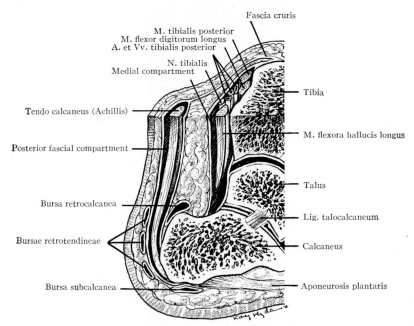

Fascia cruris
M. tibialis posterior
M. flexor digitorum longus
A. et Vv. tibialis posterior
N. tibialis
Medial compartment
Tendo calcaneus (Achillis)
Posterior fascial compartment
Bursa retrocalcanea
Bursae retrotendineae
Bursa subcalcanea
Tibia
M. flexora hallucis longus
Talus
Lig. talocalcaneum
Calcaneus
Aponeurosis plantaris

FIG. 781.—COMBINED SAGITTAL AND TRANSVERSE SECTION THROUGH THE RIGHT ANKLE TO SHOW THE SYNOVIAL BURSAE AND THE CELLULAR SPACES ABOUT THE CALCANEAL TENDON. (Modified from Testut and Jacob.)

of the sheath accounts for one variety of *achillodynia*. Whereas the other tendons lie in close relation to the ankle joint, the calcaneal tendon is separated from it by a considerable interval. A fairly wide gap filled with fatty areolar tissue, also intervenes between the tendon and the posterior tibial vessels so that there is little risk of damaging these vessels in operating upon the tendon.

3. **Deep Fascia.**—The strong deep fascia at the ankle is directly continuous with the fascia investing the leg and foot. It forms well-defined bands in front of and at each side of the ankle which maintain the ankle tendons in contact with the bones and assist in forming osteo-aponeurotic canals, through which the tendons and their synovial sheaths move with the greatest freedom.

The anterior thickening has two divisions, an upper and a lower. The upper division or *transverse ligament* stretches between the anterior borders of the tibia and fibula immediately above the ankle joint. It possesses two compartments, a medial, occupied by the tibialis anterior muscle, and a lateral, occupied by the extensor hallucis longus, extensor digitorum longus, and peroneus tertius muscles. The lower division or *cruciate ligament* is attached laterally to the prominent anterior tuberosity of the calcaneus and, at first,

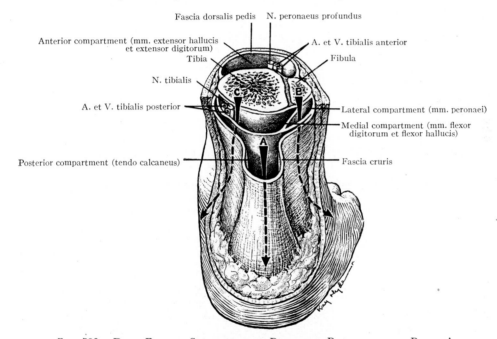

FIG. 782.—DEEP FASCIAL SPACES OF THE POSTERIOR REGION OF THE RIGHT ANKLE.

A indicates that the median space terminates below on the upper surface of the calcaneus; B marks the lateral space which passes to the plantar region; C indicates that the medial fascial compartment leads to the plantar region. (Modified from Testut and Jacob.)

consists of a single band. As it crosses in front of the joint, it divides into two limbs which diverge from each other like the limbs of a "Y." The upper limb of the ligament attaches to the medial malleolus and the lower fuses with the deep fascia along the medial margin of the foot and with the plantar fascia. The cruciate ligament forms three distinct compartments. The medial of these is occupied by the tendon of the tibialis anterior, the lateral by the tendons of the extensor hallucis longus. Each compartment is lined with a synovial sheath. Infection in the tendon sheaths about the ankle extends easily to the ankle joint. Synovial membrane involvement by tuberculosis usually is secondary to tuberculosis in the astragalus.

On the medial side of the ankle joint, the *laciniate (internal lateral) ligament* bridges the hollow between the medial malleolus and the calcaneus, to both of which it is attached. It holds in place the tendons of the tibialis posterior, flexor digitorum longus, and flexor hallucis longus. Synovial sheaths inclose these tendons where they lie under the ligament and where they extend forward into the sole of the foot.

On the lateral side of the ankle joint, two thickened bands or retinacula (external annular ligaments) bridge the groove between the lateral malleolus and the calcaneus, which holds the tendons of the peroneus longus and brevis. The *superior retinaculum* has a single compartment lined by a common synovial sheath. The *inferior retinaculum* holds the tendons to the lateral aspect of the calcaneus above and to the trochlear process (peroneal tubercle) below. The process divides the retinaculum into two compartments, each lined with synovial membrane, which are continuous with the common sheath above. Violent contraction of the peronei may rupture either or both of the retinacula and dislocate the tendons from their position.

4. **Vessels about the Ankle.**—The *anterior tibial artery* is continued into the dorsalis pedis beyond the line of the ankle joint. Just proximal to the joint line, the anterior tibial artery is crossed by the tendon of the extensor hallucis longus. At a lower level, it lies between the tendon of this muscle and that of the extensor digitorum longus. About the ankle, it gives off the malleolar branches.

The *posterior tibial artery* corresponds to the center of a line connecting the internal malleolus and the most prominent part of the heel. Opposite the lower margin of the laciniate ligament, the artery terminates in medial and lateral plantar arteries (p. 796). The calcaneal branches of the parent trunk and of its lateral plantar branch nourish the tissues at the medial side of the heel.

The anterior branch of the *peroneal artery* crosses the ankle joint in front of the interosseous ligament between the lower extremities of the tibia and fibula. The anterior and posterior tibial arteries and the peroneal artery form anastomotic networks about the ankle and heel.

5. **Injury and Repair of the Calcaneal Tendon.**—Violent muscle effort sometimes ruptures the calcaneal tendon and the plantaris tendon in the constricted portion slightly above their insertions. Occasionally, instead of rupturing, the calcaneal tendon tears off the postero-inferior part of the calcaneus (fracture by avulsion). To approximate the fragments of the tendon, it may be necessary to lengthen the tendon by a series of hemisections along each margin. After tendon suture, the knee is flexed and the foot is placed in the equinus position to relax the gastrocnemius and soleus muscles.

The retrocalcaneal bursa often becomes inflamed, tender, and painful (achillodynia) from injury to the tendon sheath. Mild forms of this condition, calcaneal bursitis or periostitis, occur from the strain of prolonged walking when the heel of the shoe is much lower than the heel usually worn. The condition is relieved by rest or by taking some of the strain off the tendon by elevating the heel or by placing a felt lift within the shoe.

B. BONES AND JOINTS

Within the ankle are the lower extremities of the tibia and fibula and that part of the talus (astragalus) with which they articulate to form the ankle joint. It is difficult to differentiate the ankle from the foot because the talus is related equally to the bones of both. Weight-bearing, proper alignment, and motion at the ankle joint depend not only upon the subtaloid and other tarsal joints, but also upon the integrity of the ankle joint mortise. The securing ligaments extend beyond the proper confines of the joint to the navicular and cuboid bones in front and to the calcaneus below.

1. **Articular Extremities.**—The medial surface of the *lower extremity of the tibia* extends into the strong, blunt, pyramidal medial malleolus. The lateral surface presents the fibular notch, a rough depression for the attachment of the inferior interosseous ligament of the distal tibiofibular joint. The posterior margin of the inferior extremity of the tibia is prominent and sometimes is known as the third or "posterior malleolus" of the ankle. This process often is fractured in eversion fracture of the ankle (p. 787). Only the inferior part of the notch has a cartilaginous covering. The inferior or articular surface is concave, and its cartilage extends mesially to merge with that covering the joint surface of the medial malleolus.

The *lower extremity of the fibula* forms the lateral malleolus, which extends to a lower level than the medial malleolus. Above the articular surface for the talus, the fibula is rough and convex for attachment to the tibia.

Ossification centers for the distal extremities of the tibia and fibula appear about the second year and the epiphyses formed are fused to the shafts between the sixteenth and nineteenth years. The tibia has an epiphysis for the medial malleolus and part of the shaft, but the fibula has one for the lateral malleolus only.

Because the fibula projects below the tibia, the epiphyseal lines are located at different levels, in consequence of which the distal extremity of the fibular diaphysis is related to the tibial epiphysis and to the cavity of the distal tibiofibular joint, when that joint is present. The fibular diaphysis sometimes is intracapsular. These considerations are important in connection with ankle joint involvement from osteomyelitis originating in the juxta-epiphyseal parts of the diaphyses. Separation of the epiphyses may result from violent

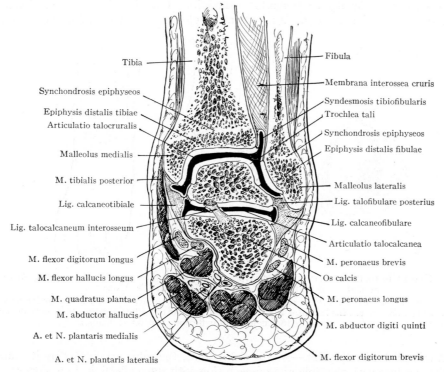

Tibia — Fibula

Synchondrosis epiphyseos — Membrana interossea cruris

Epiphysis distalis tibiae — Syndesmosis tibiofibularis

Articulatio talocruralis — Trochlea tali

Malleolus medialis — Synchondrosis epiphyseos

M. tibialis posterior — Epiphysis distalis fibulae

Lig. calcaneotibiale — Malleolus lateralis

Lig. talocalcaneum interosseum — Lig. talofibulare posterius

M. flexor digitorum longus — Lig. calcaneofibulare

M. flexor hallucis longus — Articulatio talocalcanea

M. quadratus plantae — M. peronaeus brevis

M. abductor hallucis — Os calcis

A. et N. plantaris medialis — M. peronaeus longus

A. et N. plantaris lateralis — M. abductor digiti quinti

— M. flexor digitorum brevis

Fig. 783.—Frontal Section Through the Ankle Joint.

displacements of the foot medially or laterally, but the accident is rare because of the difference in level between the two epiphyseal lines. The more usual occurrence is lateral displacement of the tibial epiphysis with transverse fracture of the fibula at a higher level.

The *talus (astragalus)* consists of a body which articulates with the tibia and fibula by its upper or trochlear surface, a forward projecting neck, and a head which articulates with the navicular (scaphoid). The inferior surface of the body of the talus rests upon the calcaneus, which is able to rotate slightly beneath it. Because of the inversion and eversion which takes place between the talus, navicular, and calcaneus, the ankle joint is spared much wear and tear. However, the movements are not sufficient to protect the ankle joint from severe and sudden strains. The superior surface of the talus, which is arched evenly anteroposteriorly, rocks in the tibiofibular notch and is broader anteriorly than posteriorly. Should ankylosis in the ankle joint occur from disease, injury, or arthrodesis, the tarsal joints replace ankle joint function to a slight degree.

The talus is covered entirely with the cartilage of its numerous articular surfaces except for a small surface of periosteum through which it receives its blood supply. Like the other bones of the tarsus, it usually develops from one center of ossification. The bone often is a site for tuberculosis.

2. **Distal Tibiofibular Joint.**—The distal tibiofibular joint usually is a simple apposition of the convex fibular surface and the concave tibial surface without the interposition of an articular cartilage. This type of joint, a syndesmosis, is very resistant and permits no movement save elasticity. This feature is important in maintaining the stability of the ankle mortise in trauma.

The tibia and fibula are connected by the strong *interosseous ligament* which is the inferior prolongation of the interosseous membrane, and by the *inferior transverse ligament* which extends from the posterior part of the medial surface of the lateral malleolus to the posterior margin of the distal extremity of the tibia. The inferior transverse ligament is a stout band which aids materially in increasing the extent of the tibiofibular arch. Anterior and posterior tibiofibular ligaments reinforce the joint. Occasionally, there is a tibiofibular joint cavity; its synovial membrane is an upward prolongation of that lining the ankle joint

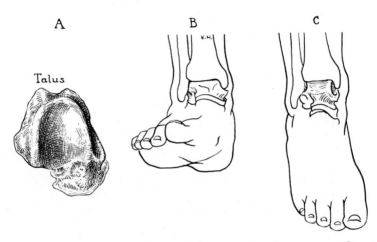

FIG. 784.—DIAGRAMS TO ILLUSTRATE THE RELATIONS BETWEEN THE SUPERIOR AND LATERAL ARTICULAR SURFACES OF THE TALUS AND THE TIBIOFIBULAR MORTISE.

A is a view of the superior surface of the talus showing that the anterior part of the articular surface is wider than the posterior. B illustrates the tightness of the mortise when the foot is in dorsiflexion. C shows that the mortise is loose when the foot is in plantar flexion. (After Homans.)

3. **Ankle (Talocrural) Joint.**—At the ankle joint, the talus articulates by its superior or trochlear surface with the tibia and on each side with the malleoli, as in a mortise. The roof or bearing surface of the joint is formed entirely of the tibia. The necessary stability of the joint is obtained by the downward projection of the malleoli which form the clasping surfaces of the mortise on each side of the talus and permit only a slight amount of lateral movement. The fibular malleolus is considerably the deeper, and the articular surface of the astragalus applied to it is correspondingly larger than that applied to the medial malleolus. This conformation doubtless is a factor in the mechanism of fracture of the lower end of the fibula resulting from forced movements of the foot.

The superior surface of the talus is wider in front than behind; hence, lateral movements at the ankle mortise occur more freely when the foot is plantar-flexed than when it is dorsiflexed. When the foot is flexed to a right angle, the broad anterior part of the trochlear surface of the talus fits tightly into the tibiofibular mortise; when the foot is extended, the narrow posterior part of the upper surface of the talus lies loosely in the mortise and admits of a small amount of play between the malleoli. Motion at the ankle is only in an anteroposterior direction. Flexion and extension takes place about a slightly oblique anteroposterior axis through the body of the talus, so that the foot points slightly mesially **in** flexion and somewhat laterally in dorsiflexion.

4. **Ligaments and Synovia of the Ankle.**—The *capsular ligament* is relatively weak, particularly anteriorly and posteriorly. It is attached proximally to the margins of the articular

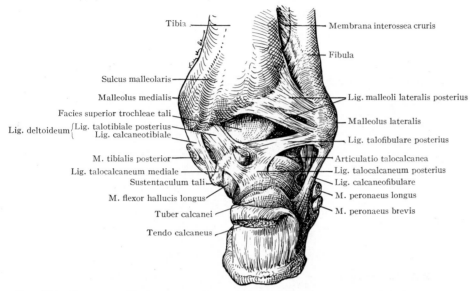

Tibia
Membrana interossea cruris
Fibula
Sulcus malleolaris
Malleolus medialis
Facies superior trochleae tali
Lig. deltoideum { Lig. talotibiale posterius
Lig. calcaneotibiale
M. tibialis posterior
Lig. talocalcaneum mediale
Sustentaculum tali
M. flexor hallucis longus
Tuber calcanei
Tendo calcaneus
Lig. malleoli lateralis posterius
Malleolus lateralis
Lig. talofibulare posterius
Articulatio talocalcanea
Lig. talocalcaneum posterius
Lig. calcaneofibulare
M. peronaeus longus
M. peronaeus brevis

FIG. 785.—Posterior View of the Ligaments and Tendons about the Right Ankle Joint.

surfaces of the tibial and fibular epiphyses and distally to the margin of the superior articular surface of the talus, except at the anterior aspect of the joint where it extends forward to the neck of the bone. The *synovial membrane* is lax in front and behind where it is covered by the anterior and posterior ligaments and where the capsule is thin and loose

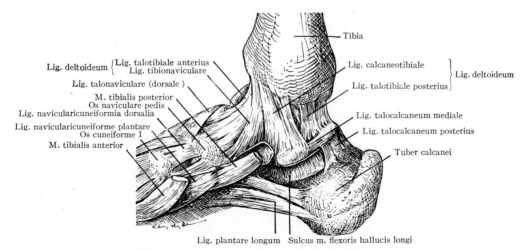

Tibia
Lig. deltoideum { Lig. talotibiale anterius
Lig. tibionaviculare
Lig. talonaviculare (dorsale)
M. tibialis posterior
Os naviculare pedis
Lig. navicularicuneiformia dorsalia
Lig. navicularicuneiforme plantare
Os cuneiforme I
M. tibialis anterior
Lig. calcaneotibiale
Lig. talotibiale posterius } Lig. deltoideum
Lig. talocalcaneum mediale
Lig. talocalcaneum posterius
Tuber calcanei
Lig. plantare longum   Sulcus m. flexoris hallucis longi

FIG. 786.—Medial Ligaments of the Right Ankle Joint.

It is directly continuous with the synovial membrane of the distal tibiofibular joint. **A** joint effusion bulges the synovial membrane and the weak capsule anteriorly and posteriorly. *Aspiration* of the ankle joint is performed between the tip of either malleolus and the corresponding articular surface of the astragalus.

50

The *anterior ligament* of the ankle is a thin membrane attached to the anterior aspect of the malleoli and the lower extremity of the tibia, and below to the rough upper surface of the neck of the talus. The *posterior ligament* is the weakest of the ankle ligaments, and is represented by a few ligamentous bands connecting the inferior surface of the tibia and the posterior tibiofibular ligament to the posterior aspect of the talus below. The tendon of the flexor hallucis longus is a strong posterior support of the joint.

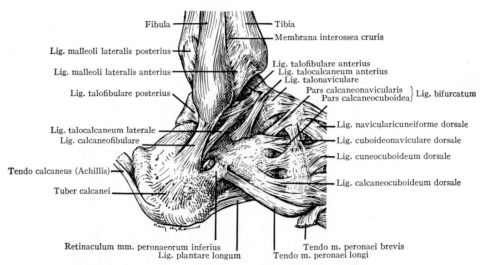

FIG. 787.—LIGAMENTS OF THE LATERAL REGION OF THE ANKLE AND FOOT.

The ligaments which reinforce the medial and lateral aspects of the joint are very strong and pass fanlike from the malleoli to the tarsal bones. The *deltoid (internal lateral) ligament* strengthens the mesial side of the joint to a great degree. It is an extensive triangular sheet of ligamentous fibers, inseparable from the joint capsule. The apical extremity of the ligament attaches to the medial malleolus. The lower or basal extremity anteroposteriorly presents an unbroken line of attachment to the navicular, talus, susten-

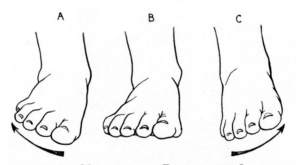

FIG. 788.—DIAGRAM OF THE MOVEMENTS OF EVERSION AND INVERSION OF THE FOOT.
A, Eversion; B, normal position; C, inversion.

taculum tali, and to the plantar calcaneonavicular ("spring") ligament. It is reinforced by the tendons of the tibialis posterior and flexor digitorum longus. Violent strains upon the deltoid ligament, when the foot is overeverted, usually pull off the medial malleolus instead of rupturing the ligament.

The *lateral ligament* is weaker and less complete; it is divided into anterior, middle, and posterior fasciculi. The anterior talofibular ligament extends from the anterior border of the lateral malleolus to the lateral surface of the neck of the talus. The calcaneofibular ligament is a band extending obliquely downward and backward from the malleolus to the lateral surface of the calcaneus. It is overlain by the peroneal tendons. The posterior talofibular ligament binds the fibula to the talus rigidly and rarely is torn. In the extremes of dorsiflexion and plantar flexion, the impingement of the edges of the tibia prevents further movement. The deltoid and lateral ligaments restrict motion.

5. **Lateral Movements at the Foot and Ankle.**—*Inversion* or tibial flexion turns the sole of the foot medially, and *eversion* or fibular flexion turns it laterally. In both of these lateral movements, the foot rotates around an anteroposterior axis in a very limited range of motion in the subastragaloid joint. Movements of this nature are checked by the lateral ligaments of the ankle. *Adduction* and *abduction* refer to those movements which turn the front of the foot medially and laterally, respectively. They are confined mainly to the joints between the anterior and posterior segments of the tarsus—the midtarsal joint (p. 799).

The combined movement of inversion and adduction is *supination;* that of eversion and abduction is *pronation.*

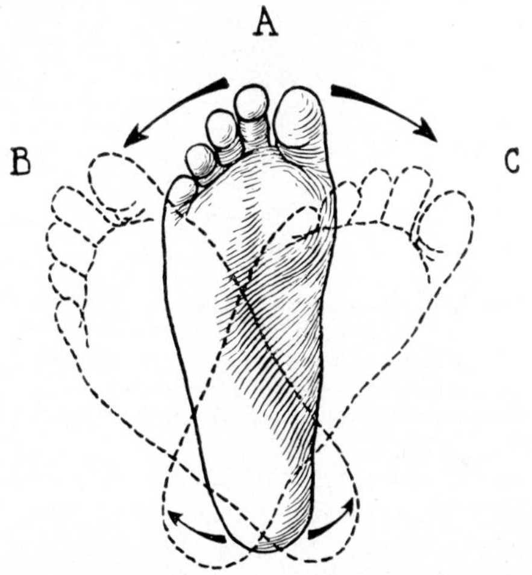

SURGICAL CONSIDERATIONS

Injuries about the ankle commonly follow twists and falls in which the body weight is transmitted in a direction out of line with the usual axis. Their nature often depends upon the position into which the foot is forced by the violence, whether it is one of overinversion and adduction or overeversion and abduction. Lesions are prevented to a large extent by the strength of the lateral ligaments of the joint, the adaptability of the talus in its mortise, and the support given by the powerful tendons surrounding the joint. In the presence of deformity, the direction toward which the foot is displaced is the clue to the nature of the fracture and governs the manipulation by which reduction is secured.

1. **Sprains.**—A sprained ankle usually is an inversion injury in which the foot is rocked

FIG. 789.—DIAGRAM TO SHOW THE MOVEMENTS OF ADDUCTION AND ABDUCTION OF THE FOOT.

A, Normal position; B, abduction; C, adduction. Since the heel is diagrammed as moving, there is in addition, rotation at the knee joint or at the hip joint.

toward the median line and some part of a ligament is torn. A violent motion of this sort puts a strain on the lateral ligament until its talofibular, and sometimes its calcaneofibular, components are ruptured. Avulsion of the lip of the lateral malleolus may be associated with the sprain and is known as a *sprain fracture.* Should the lateral ligament remain intact, the strain is transferred to the fibula and an inversion fracture occurs in which the lateral malleolus is broken off at its base. Injuries sustained by violent eversion of the foot rarely take the form of sprains since the medial or deltoid ligament is very strong. They usually result in some form of Pott's fracture.

In sprain, point-tenderness is elicited on palpation over the attachments of the torn ligament, but none is elicited over the subcutaneous surface of the fibula. Swelling and ecchymosis often are more marked than when a fracture is present.

2. **Pott's Eversion Fracture.**—A Pott's fracture is a combination of injuries to the tibia and fibula caused by forcible eversion or abduction of the foot, or a combination of these closely related movements. It may be caused by a stumble or fall in which the foot fails to receive the weight of the body squarely.

Pott's fracture varies in its clinical manifestations according to whether it is caused by eversion or abduction of the foot. In the *abduction form,* the foot is subjected to an outward rotary strain. The anterior part of the talus, maintaining its normal relations with the tarsal bones, impinges against the lateral malleolus, causing an oblique separation of the malleolus from the shaft above. The strain then falls on the medial or deltoid liga-

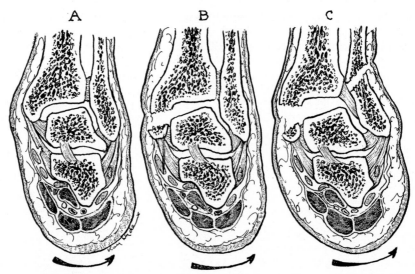

FIG 790.—SCHEMATIC FRONTAL SECTIONS THROUGH THE RIGHT ANKLE TO SHOW THE MECHANISM OF SPRAIN AND FRACTURES CAUSED BY ABDUCTION AND EVERSION OF THE FOOT.
A is an abduction sprain in which the deltoid (medial) ligament is torn. B is an abduction fracture of the tip of the medial malleolus, the ligaments remaining intact. C is a typical abduction and eversion fracture with fracture of the shaft of the fibula. (Modified from Testut and Jacob.)

ment, which tears off the medial malleolus or is ruptured. A continuation of the rotating force tears away a part of the posterior margin of the tibia along with the lower fragment of the fibula. In either instance, the talus slips backward, producing a posterior dislocation of the foot.

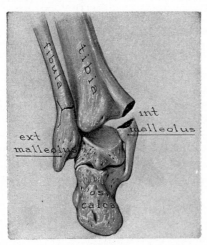

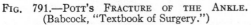

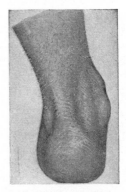

FIG. 791.—POTT'S FRACTURE OF THE ANKLE.
(Babcock, "Textbook of Surgery.")

FIG. 792.—POTT'S FRACTURE OF THE ANKLE WITH ABDUCTION AND EVERSION OF THE FOOT. (Babcock, "Textbook of Surgery.")

When *eversion* is the prevailing mechanism, great strain is thrown at once upon the deltoid ligament. This ligament rarely gives way, but the internal malleolus very frequently snaps across. Abduction without the check of the internal malleolus presses the talus (astragalus) against the tip of the lateral malleolus. The inferior tibiofibular ligament remains intact, and the lower part of the fibular shaft is bent medially toward the tibia and is broken across, allowing the foot to be deflected laterally. In an eversion fracture in which the leg is in forward motion and the foot maintains contact with the ground, the posterior edge of the tibia sometimes is broken off by the astragalus. This edge of the tibia is known as the third or posterior malleolus. A Pott's fracture with fracture of the posterior malleolus is known as a "trimalleolar" fracture (Henderson). In this fracture, there is a partial posterior dislocation of the foot.

Should the tibiofibular ligaments rupture or tear off a fragment of tibia, the tibia and fibula separate and the fibula is broken by bending in its lower third. In this case, the talus is carried to the lateral side of the tibial articular surface and upward to a varying extent. The foot also is drawn upward on the lateral side of the leg. The lower extremity of the fibula retains its connection with the talus.

Pott's fracture is recognized easily by its characteristic deformity. In the erect attitude, the medial border of the foot is directed toward the ground and its lateral edge is raised. The lower end of the tibia projects prominently on the medial side, and there is an angular depression between the foot and leg at the site of the fibular fracture.

Since all fractures of this group enter the joint, only an accurate *reduction* can restore the planes of the articulating surfaces to normal weight-bearing alignment. Accumulation of blood and exudate and fixation of the part by muscle spasm oppose reposition of the fragments unless reduction is made at the earliest possible moment. In this type of fracture, the foot usually is everted, abducted, and not infrequently is displaced backward, and the tibia and fibula tend to separate. In reduction, the knee is flexed to relax the pull of the gastrocnemius muscle; traction is made on the foot in plantar flexion, and the foot as a whole is displaced medially if lateral dislocation is present and anteriorly if posterior dislocation exists. The foot then is adducted, inverted, and dorsiflexed.

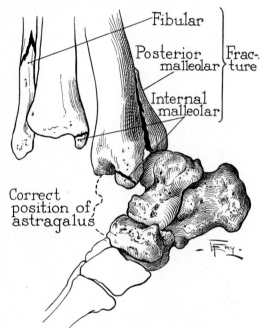

FIG. 793.—TRIMALLEOLAR FRACTURE OF THE ANKLE WITH POSTERIOR DISPLACEMENT OF THE FOOT. (Henderson, Surg., Gynec. and Obst., Feb. 15, 1935.)

In standing or walking after union of a Pott's fracture in malposition, the weight of the trunk no longer is transmitted through the tibia and the center of the ankle joint to the sole of the foot, but is supported by the lateral part of the tibiofibular mortise and is transferred to the medial border of the foot. The greater the use of the limb under these conditions, the greater becomes the deformity and disability.

3. **Reversed Pott's or Inversion Fracture.**—A reversed Pott's or inversion fracture results from turning the foot violently medially. Adduction may be a feature adding a medial rotation to the inversion of the foot. The force causing the fracture is that which causes the common sprain or sprain fracture. Traction on the lateral ligament may rupture it partially or completely without avulsion of the tip of the lateral malleolus, or a tearing off of its base below the attachment of the interosseous ligament. The force, continuing to act without opposition, presses the talus against the medial malleolus, and knocks off its tip or splits the malleolus from the tibia in a longitudinal direction. In addition, there may be fracture of the anterior articular edge of the tibia. In these injuries, there is none

of the separation of the tibia and fibula which may occur in eversion fractures, and there is little tendency to posterior displacement of the foot. *Reduction* is effected by abduction, eversion, and full dorsiflexion.

4. **Dislocations.**—Lateral and posterior displacements, with the talus maintaining its normal relations with the associated tarsal bones, have been described in connection with Pott's fracture. The extreme rarity of medial dislocation probably is accounted for by the fact that a great amount of force is required for its production. Simple dislocation unassociated with fracture sometimes occurs.

Posterior and anterior dislocations of the foot at the ankle without fracture are very unusual, contrary to what might be expected from the configuration of the joint. *Posterior dislocation* is much more frequent than anterior dislocation and results from sudden arrest or fixation of the foot while moving forward. In the simple dislocation, there is extensive tearing of ligaments until the talus is enabled to slide out behind the posterior edge of the tibia. The characteristic deformity is prominence of the heel, apparent shortening of the foot, and broadening of the ankle. From the anatomical nature of the joint, an *anterior dislocation* of the foot at the ankle could occur readily. However, as violence to the foot

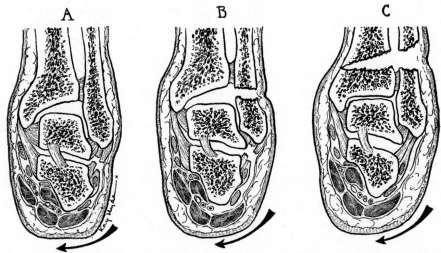

A   B   C

FIG. 794.—SCHEMATIC SAGITTAL SECTIONS THROUGH THE RIGHT ANKLE TO SHOW THE MECHANISM OF SPRAIN AND FRACTURE (REVERSED POTT'S) CAUSED BY ADDUCTION AND INVERSION OF THE FOOT.

A is a sprain from a tear of the lateral ligament. B is a lesion in which the lateral ligament is lacerated and the lateral malleolus is wrenched off. C is a transverse supramalleolar fracture. (Modified from Testut and Jacob.)

usually occurs with the patient moving forward, this type of dislocation is seen rarely. For reduction, the knee is flexed to relax the calf muscles. Extension of the foot with traction and manipulation reduces the dislocation.

Upward dislocation with the talus forced upward between the malleoli may result from falls upon the feet. The lower end of the tibia is split but the fibula usually is not broken. Unless the foot is drawn downward by skate or pin traction to narrow the mortise, the lateral malleolus impinges against the os calcis and the ankle is broadened greatly.

5. **Approach for Arthrodesis of the Ankle Joint.**—Arthrodesis of the ankle by removal of joint cartilage reduces the size of the talus and at the same time increases the size of the mortise into which it is to be received. Adequate exposure for extensive resection may be obtained through the *lateral J-shaped incision* (of Kocher). This incision begins behind the fibula and extends downward below the lateral malleolus to the trochlear process (peroneal tubercle) of the calcaneus. It then curves forward and ends behind the insertion of the peroneus tertius muscle into the tuberosity of the fifth metatarsal. The curved flap thus outlined, consisting of the skin, deep fascia, and periosteum of the lateral malleolus, is dissected forward from the peronei and lateral malleolus.

In the *lateral transfibular approach* to the ankle joint for arthrodesis, the incision is similar to the lateral J-shaped incision of Kocher. After division of the skin and subcutaneous tissue, the fibula and the peroneal tendons are exposed. The periosteum is incised longitudinally upward for a distance of 6 cm. from the tip of the lateral malleolus. In the upper third of the periosteal incision, subperiosteal dissection is carried completely around the shaft of the fibula. Osteotomy of the fibula, obliquely downward and medially, then is performed. After levering the distal fragment of the shaft of the fibula laterally, the terminal portion of the interosseous membrane and the distal tibiofibular joint are divided by sharp dissection. Continued leverage on the malleolar fragment exposes the ankle joint. The foot now is displaced medially; the taut peroneal tendons may require division. The articular surfaces of the tibia and fibula, together with the trochlear surface of the talus, are denuded of their cartilage. In order to obtain bony contact for a snug

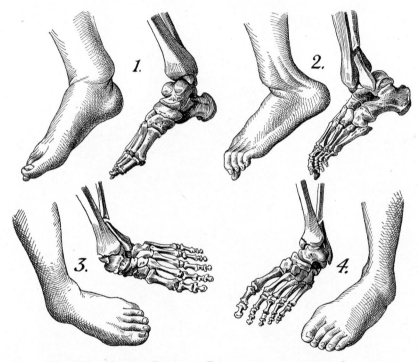

FIG. 795.—VARIOUS FORMS OF DISLOCATIONS ABOUT THE ANKLE.

1, Forward dislocation of the foot; 2, backward dislocation of the foot, associated with fracture of the fibula; 3, lateral dislocation of the foot, associated with fracture of the tibia and fibula; 4, medial dislocation of the foot, associated with fracture of the tibia and fibula. (Hoffa.)

tibiofibular mortise, the lateral surface of the distal end of the tibia is removed. The fragments of the fibula are replaced and sutured and the limb is immobilized in plaster.

In *excision of the talus*, the posterior part of the extensor digitorum brevis muscle is elevated and the talonavicular joint is opened. The head of the talus is drawn upward, so that when the talocalcaneal interosseous ligament is divided, it is held only by the attachment of the deltoid ligament to its mesial aspect. After excision of the talus, the sustentaculum tali is removed and the calcaneus is trimmed to allow it to fit the new position in the tibiofibular mortise. The lateral malleolus projects downward too far and requires shortening. The peroneal tendons are approximated and sutured and the retinacula are stitched into place over them.

6. Amputation through the Ankle Joint.—Syme's amputation through the ankle joint constitutes disarticulation of the foot at the ankle, with removal of the malleoli and the articular surface of the tibia. The flap to cover these surfaces is taken from the heel and is sutured to the divided tissues at the anterior surface of the ankle. The important point of this procedure is to insure vitality of the heel flap, which is nourished mainly by the medial calcaneal branches of the posterior tibial artery and, to some degree, by the lateral calcaneal branches of the peroneal artery.

The incision is carried across the sole of the foot from the tip of the lateral malleolus, or a point a little posterior to it, to the corresponding point at the medial malleolus. The extremities of the incision are connected by an incision directly across the front of the

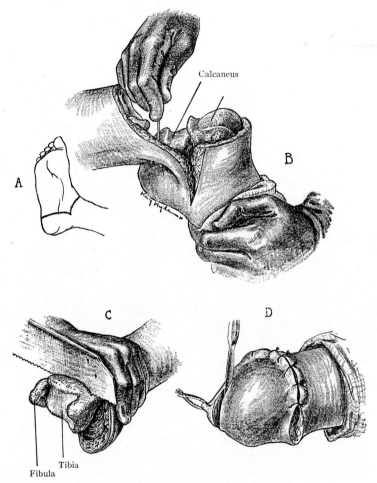

FIG. 796.—SYME'S AMPUTATION AT THE ANKLE.

A, The skin incision for flap formation. B, Disarticulation at the ankle joint and the shelling-out of the calcaneus from the heel flap. C, The skin flaps have been retracted upward to expose the inferior extremities of the tibia and fibula; these bones are sectioned 1 cm. proximal to their articular surfaces. D, The heel flap has been drawn forward over the ends of the bones and has been sutured anteriorly; the dog ears at the corners of the flap are removed. (After Wilson.)

ankle joint. The capsule is incised anteriorly, and the lateral deltoid ligament is divided from within outward. By drawing the foot forward and downward, the upper nonarticular surface of the posterior portion of the calcaneus behind the talocalcaneal joint is brought into view. The calcaneal tendon is cut close to the bone and the calcaneus is dissected out. The malleoli are cleared and sawed off along with a thin layer of the articular surface of the tibia. The incision on the sole must not be so far posterior as to injure the medial calcaneal branch of the lateral plantar artery and threaten the integrity of the flap.

The *Pirogoff amputation*, which may be regarded as a modification of Syme's, differs from it in the fact that part of the calcaneus is retained in the heel flap and subsequently is brought into contact with the divided lower extremities of the tibia and fibula. In this operation, the calcaneus is sawed through in the line of the incision in the sole. A larger piece is cut from the tibia than is taken in Syme's amputation.

VI. FOOT

The features of the foot adapting it to sustain the great weight thrown upon it in standing and locomotion are: a comparatively large size, a position at right angles to the leg, a distinctive architectural plan of construction, and a broad base of support. The foot has also a remarkable springiness because of the arrangement of the constituent bones and the ingenious interlocking of tendons, ligaments, and muscles maintaining the arches.

The movements of the foot sometimes are very rapid. Treading on an uneven or unstable surface requires almost instantaneous adjustment in balance lest sprain or even fracture result. In running, the position of its component elements must be accommodated very rapidly, and in jumping, the elements incur a special strain.

Whereas the hand is essentially an organ of touch and prehension with a remarkable freedom of movement, the foot is an organ of locomotion endowed with strength and solidity; its movements are neither intricate nor numerous. Strength in the foot is enhanced by the fact that its constituent bones are short, solid, and well integrated into a double arch, joined by strong ligaments and supported by powerful tendons. Knowledge of this structure enables one to understand the diseases, injuries, and deformities to which the foot is subject, and the means available for their prevention and cure.

A. SOFT PARTS OF THE FOOT

In general outline, the foot is triangular—narrowest at the heel and widest at the toes. The soft parts on the medial, lateral, and dorsal surfaces are so superficial as to warrant their description under the heading of regional landmarks.

1. **Landmarks on the Mesial Aspect of the Foot.**—The mesial aspect of the foot is arched anteroposteriorly and rests upon the ground only at its anterior and posterior extremities—the heel and the ball of the great toe. The skin over the mesial aspect of the foot is thin and delicate and often is marked by numerous small vessels, which give it a wavy appearance. The *sustentaculum tali* can be located by feeling 2.5 cm. below the medial malleolus. The distinct prominence of the *tuberosity of the navicular* is encountered by pressing about 2.5 cm. in front of, and slightly below the level of, the medial malleolus. This tuberosity is a useful guide in many operations on the foot, and is the principal point of insertion for the tendon of the tibialis posterior. The depression below and behind the tuberosity is an absolute guide to the *talonavicular joint*. This angular interval separates the anterior from the posterior segment of the tarsus and is the level at which Chopart's disarticulation (p. 799) is performed. Nearer the malleolus, another bony prominence, the *head and neck of the astragalus*, is palpable, particularly when the foot is extended and everted.

The first metatarsal lies distal to the *first cuneiform* which is palpated anterior to the navicular. The *tendon of the tibialis anterior* is recognized readily when the foot is inverted actively, and can be followed to its insertion into the contiguous plantar areas of the first cuneiform and the base of the first metatarsal. The head of the first metatarsal is very prominent if the great toe deviates from the midline an abnormal degree (hallux valgus) (p. 810).

2. **Landmarks on the Lateral Surface of the Foot.**—The lateral margin of the foot is thin in contrast with the medial margin, and rests in contact with the ground over its entire extent. Near the middle of the lateral border, the prominent *tuberosity of the base of the fifth metatarsal* marks the *tarsometatarsal joint* (of Lisfranc). A point on this margin of the foot just anterior to the middle of the interval between this tuberosity and the tip of the lateral malleolus defines the joint between the calcaneus and the *cuboid midtarsal*

joint (of Chopart). The *trochlear process* (peroneal tubercle) can be felt indistinctly as a small bony prominence, 2.5 cm. below and a little in front of the lateral malleolus.

3. Landmarks on the Dorsum of the Foot.—The skin on the dorsum of the foot is very thin, but is much less sensitive than that on the plantar surface. The subcutaneous tissue is remarkably loose in texture so that the edema of cardiorenal disease or that of inflammatory lesions of the foot usually is very pronounced. The veins are arranged in an arch, the outline of which often is apparent in the erect posture. The large and small saphenous veins arise from the marginal veins of this arch.

The tendons of the front of the ankle may be traced readily to their insertions. That for the tibialis anterior has been described. The tendon of the extensor hallucis longus passes forward to the dorsal aspect of the great toe, and the tendons of the extensor digitorum longus are directed to the four outer toes. On the posterolateral aspect of the dorsum of the foot, the soft inelastic mass of the fleshy belly of the extensor digitorum brevis muscle can be felt. The tendon of the peroneus brevis muscle passes forward under the lateral malleolus to an insertion into the projecting tuberosity of the fifth metatarsal.

The dorsalis pedis artery, a continuation of the anterior tibial artery into the foot, runs a course indicated on the surface by a line beginning midway between the two malleoli and ending at the posterior extremity of the first interosseous space. On the lateral side of the vessel is the anterior tibial nerve.

4. Superficial Structures of the Sole of the Foot.—The plantar surface of the foot is triangular in outline and is hollowed out considerably along its mesial border. The parts supporting the superincumbent weight are the heel, the ball of the great toe, and the lateral margin of the sole along its entire extent.

The *skin* over these supporting areas is thick and often horny in character. The rest of the plantar skin is thin, highly sensitive, and, like that of the palm of the hand, contains numerous sweat glands. The *subcutaneous tissue*, similar to that over the scalp and the palm of the hand, is dense because of the many fibrous septa traversing it. This tough and elastic tissue is reinforced by the strong central portion of the plantar aponeurosis and is thickest over the weight-bearing areas.

5. Plantar Aponeurosis.—The plantar aponeurosis (deep fascia) of the sole of the foot consists of a strong central portion and two weaker lateral divisions. It covers and protects the soft parts which play over the plantar surface of the bones and joints, and affords an origin to the intrinsic muscles of the sole. The *central portion* is attached behind to the plantar surface of the calcaneal tuberosity, and divides anteriorly into slips connected to the fibrous flexor sheaths of the five toes and to the sides of the metatarsophalangeal joints. This portion is a strong support of the longitudinal arch and is shortened considerably in the deformity known as *pes cavus* and in certain other varieties of talipes. The *medial division*, which covers the abductor hallucis, is weak. It extends from the calcaneal tubercle to the base of the proximal phalanx of the great toe. The *lateral division* is a fairly strong band extending between the calcaneus and the tuberosity of the fifth metatarsal. Because of the density of the central parts of the fascia, swelling in inflammatory conditions of the sole early becomes apparent on the dorsum of the foot.

6. Muscles of the Foot and Their Actions.—The foot is controlled by the small short muscles intrinsic to the foot and by long extrinsic muscles which arise in the leg. The *small muscles* of the dorsum and sole of the foot are less important than the corresponding muscles in the hand, since the foot is a mechanism for the stable support of the body weight, and movements of the individual toes are of secondary consequence. Most of the small muscles of the sole run longitudinally and strengthen the long arch, while a few run across the foot to support the transverse arch.

The *long muscles* bear most of the weight of the body in locomotion and direct the movement of the foot. They subserve three main functions: supporting the arch of the foot; dorsiflexing and plantar-flexing the foot; and abducting, adducting, everting, and inverting the foot. The action of the individual muscles is not simple, as they act on the ankle, the midtarsal, and the talo-calcaneo-navicular (subastragaloid) joints. If the ankle joint is stationary, the muscles abduct and evert, and adduct and invert, and if the subastragaloid joint is fixed, they dorsiflex, plantar-flex, abduct, and adduct the foot. When both joints are free, the long muscles act in combination with the small muscles.

The *muscles supporting the tarsal arch* do not belong to any single group. They include the tibialis anterior and posterior, the flexor digitorum longus, flexor hallucis longus, peroneus longus, and all the intrinsic muscles of the foot. The tibialis anterior muscle inserts almost into the summit of the arch and supports it by drawing it upward. The flexor hallucis longus and flexor digitorum longus muscles run lengthwise beneath the arch and support it from below. The tibialis posterior and peroneus longus muscles, one from the medial and one from the lateral side, cross in the sole of the foot to opposite sides. They form a cruciate sling immediately under the arch, upon which the arch rests when these muscles contract. Under the strain of locomotion, the arch is dependent upon these muscles for support. If they cannot meet the demand made upon them, the strain falls upon the ligaments. The ligaments are static, not dynamic structures like muscles, and quickly weaken, allowing the arch to flatten.

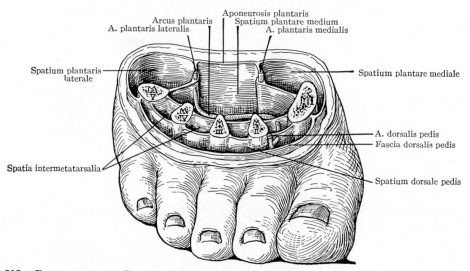

FIG. 797.—DIAGRAM OF THE FASCIAL SPACES IN THE METATARSAL REGION. (Modified from Corning.)

Each of the tarsal bones entering into the tarsal arch slightly underlags its proximal neighbor. The effect of all the supporting muscles, except the tibialis anterior, is to shorten the foot by their bowstring action beneath the arch, thus crowding together and locking the tarsal articulations against the downward thrust of the body weight, conveyed through the neck and head of the talus.

Although all the joints of the foot act to some degree in all movements of the foot, single joints permit the cardinal motions. The following table indicates the motion of the foot, the muscles producing them, and the joints in which they occur.

Action.	Joints involved.	Muscles.			
Dorsiflexion.....	talocrural (ankle joint)	Tibialis anterior	Extensor digitorum longus		
		Peroneus tertius	Extensor hallucis longus		
Plantarflexion....	talocrural (ankle joint)	Gastrocnemius	Tibialis posterior	Flexor digitorum longus	
		Soleus	Peroneus brevis	Flexor hallucis longus	
		Plantaris	Peroneus longus		
Adduction.......	midtarsal	Tibialis posterior and anterior			
Abduction.......	midtarsal	Peroneus longus, brevis, and tertius			
Inversion........	subastragaloid	Tibialis anterior and tibialis posterior			
Eversion........	subastragaloid	Peroneus tertius, brevis, and longus			

7. Plantar Vessels and Nerves.—The posterior tibial artery divides into the lateral and medial plantar arteries at the distal border of the laciniate (internal annular) ligament, midway between the medial malleolus and the most prominent part of the mesial surface of the calcaneus. From this midpoint, the *medial plantar artery*, usually a small vessel, passes forward between the abductor hallucis and the flexor digitorum brevis muscles. Its terminal branches join the digital arteries. The *lateral plantar artery* runs deep to the flexor digitorum muscle, anterior and lateral to the base of the fifth metatarsal, where it bends sharply mesially and becomes the *plantar arch*, which extends over the bases of the three middle metatarsals. It can be ligated through an incision at the mesial side of the base of the fifth metatarsal where it lies between the flexor digitorum brevis and the abductor digiti quinti muscles.

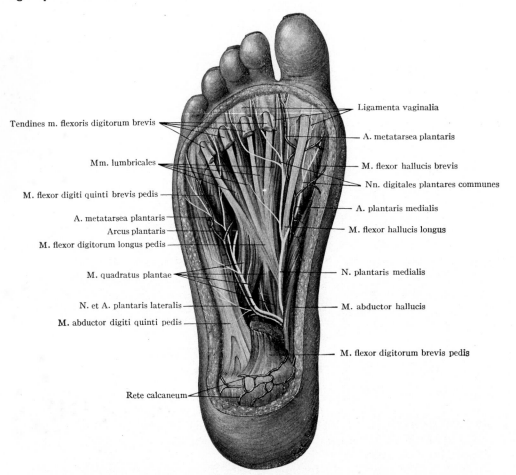

Tendines m. flexoris digitorum brevis

Mm. lumbricales

M. flexor digiti quinti brevis pedis

A. metatarsea plantaris
Arcus plantaris
M. flexor digitorum longus pedis

M. quadratus plantae

N. et A. plantaris lateralis
M. abductor digiti quinti pedis

Rete calcaneum

Ligamenta vaginalia

A. metatarsea plantaris

M. flexor hallucis brevis
Nn. digitales plantares communes
A. plantaris medialis
M. flexor hallucis longus

N. plantaris medialis

M. abductor hallucis

M. flexor digitorum brevis pedis

FIG. 798.—DEEP MUSCLES, VESSELS, AND NERVES OF THE PLANTAR REGION OF THE FOOT.
The flexor digitorum brevis has been removed to show the deeper structures.

Hemorrhage from the plantar arteries usually can be arrested by packing the wound, applying pressure, and elevating the leg. Care must be exercised in making deep incisions in the groove to the medial and lateral sides of the flexor digitorum brevis muscle, for fear of wounding these arteries. They are not endangered in subcutaneous operations on the plantar fascia, because this structure is superficial to the flexor brevis muscle and the arteries are deep to that muscle.

The *medial plantar nerve* (L_4, $_5$, S_1) arises from the tibial nerve under the laciniate (internal annular) ligament and runs forward with the medial plantar artery. The *lateral plantar nerve* supplies most of the muscles of the sole.

8. **Plantar Abscess.**—Plantar abscesses usually result from infected puncture wounds

or from upward extension from infection in the webs of the toes. The strong central portion of the plantar aponeurosis overlies and gives origin to the flexor digitorum brevis

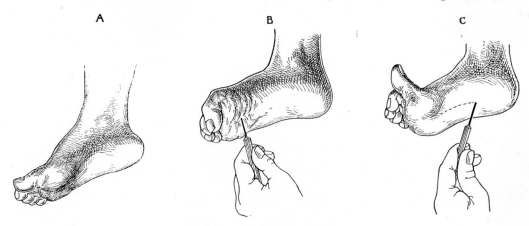

A   B   C

FIG. 799.—PLANTAR REFLEX (OF BABINSKI).
    A, The position of the toes before irritation of the plantar surface. B, The normal response to irritation is plantar flexion of the toes, particularly of the great toe. C, Pathologic response; irritation of the plantar surface causes extension of the toes.

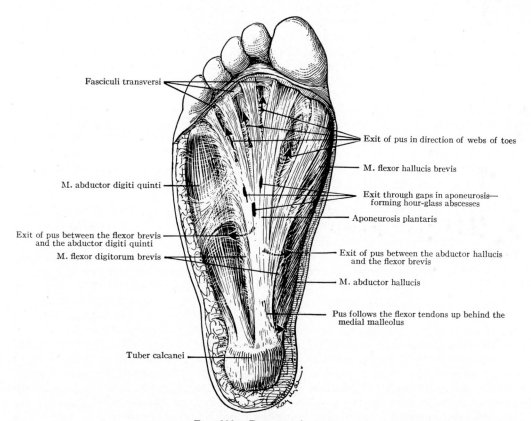

Fasciculi transversi

Exit of pus in direction of webs of toes

M. flexor hallucis brevis

M. abductor digiti quinti

Exit through gaps in aponeurosis—forming hour-glass abscesses

Aponeurosis plantaris

Exit of pus between the flexor brevis and the abductor digiti quinti

Exit of pus between the abductor hallucis and the flexor brevis

M. flexor digitorum brevis

M. abductor hallucis

Pus follows the flexor tendons up behind the medial malleolus

Tuber calcanei

FIG. 800.—PLANTAR ABSCESS.
Diagram shows the points of exit of pus beneath the plantar aponeurosis.

muscles. A puncture wound penetrating the aponeurosis may enter but not traverse the underlying short flexor. so that the tendons of the long flexors escape. Infection arising in this wound may form a *superficial plantar abscess*, from which pus points in several directions. The pus may come directly through gaps in the plantar aponeurosis and form an hour-glass or collar-button abscess, part lying deep to the aponeurosis in the substance of the flexor brevis and part in the subcutaneous tissue; it may burrow forward between the slips of the plantar fascia in the direction of the webs of the toes; it may appear in the groove on the outer part of the sole between the flexor brevis and the abductor digiti quinti muscles; or it may appear in the groove on the medial side of the foot between the abductor hallucis and the flexor brevis muscle.

The pus in a *deep plantar abscess* accumulates beneath the flexor brevis muscle and about the deep flexor tendons. It tends to pass up the leg along the flexor tendon, but may present in the webs of the toes or in the groove, to one side or the other of the flexor brevis muscle.

After *incision* of the skin and division of the plantar aponeurosis, the abscess may be located and evacuated by blunt hemostat dissection which avoids wounding arteries. Incisions should not be made over weight-bearing areas; hence, incision on the metatarsal heads and on the lateral border of the sole is avoided.

B. BONES AND JOINTS OF THE FOOT

The numerous bones and joints of the foot endow it with mobility and a capacity for lessening shock. If the bones become ankylosed, walking and balancing become difficult, and great care is required in locomotion to avoid strain and injury. The bone groups of the foot are the tarsus, metatarsus, and phalanges; the first two are the more essential. The toes are used more in balancing, running, and climbing than in walking, and, although they add to the efficiency of the intricate movements of the foot, their loss does not produce serious impairment, for the firmer more deliberate movements of walking remain almost normal.

The bones of the foot are divided longitudinally into two groups, a medial and a lateral. Most of the weight of the body is borne through the *medial group* which is in relation with the tibia. The bones of this group are the talus (astragalus), navicular (scaphoid), three cuneiforms, three medial metatarsals, and three medial phalanges. The talus and the navicular are the most likely to be injured. The *lateral group* is in relation with the fibula and is composed of the calcaneus, the cuboid, and the outer two metatarsals with their corresponding phalanges. The lateral group of bones balances the superimposed body weight. Of this group, the calcaneus is most liable to injury.

1. **Bones of the Tarsus and Metatarsus.**—The *calcaneus* (*os calcis*) is the long, arched heel-bone, the posterior extremity of which rests upon the ground. The tendo calcaneus inserts on the medial part of the tubercle of the calcaneus which is a considerable distance behind the articular surface for the talus. This arrangement is designed to give a great deal of leverage for the action of the calcaneal tendon. The calcaneus articulates anteriorly with the cuboid. On the mesial margin of the calcaneus, the shelflike sustentaculum tali juts out to support part of the neck of the talus and to serve as an attachment for the plantar calcaneonavicular (spring) ligament. This ligament is very strong and supports part of the head of the talus and that part of the body weight transmitted to it.

The *talus* (*astragalus*) is described in the ankle region (p. 783). Its body is rounded anteroposteriorly to articulate with the tibia and its sides are grasped by the malleoli. The inferior surface of its body articulates with the calcaneus. The head of the talus is thrust forward on a short neck to articulate with the navicular anteriorly and the plantar calcaneonavicular ligament inferiorly. The *navicular* (*scaphoid*) receives the forward thrust from the talus in weight-bearing and transmits it to the three cuneiforms in front. The tubercle of the navicular is a prominent landmark. The *cuboid* and *cuneiforms* rarely are involved surgically.

Of the *metatarsals*, the first is short, strong, and of greatest importance in weight-bearing. Its joints are long and solid. Between it and the ground are two sesamoid bones. The base of the fifth metatarsal is proximal to the main metatarsal joint line and is a prominent landmark on the outer margin of the foot.

The slight impairment of the function of the foot and the slight loss of firmness and stability consequent upon removal of some of its bony elements are remarkable. The talus may be removed completely without causing serious disability. The navicular, the neck of the talus, and the first and second cuneiform bones have been resected with good results. It is not desirable to interfere with the calcaneus because of its importance as a base of support and its attachments to important ligaments and muscles.

At birth, *centers of ossification* are present in the talus, calcaneus, and cuboid bones. The lateral cuneiform ossifies during the first year, the medial during the second, and the middle cuneiform and navicular ossify during the third or fourth year. A secondary center for the calcaneus appears in the eighth year in the posterior cartilaginous extremity of the bone, and forms an epiphysis which unites with the main bone between the sixteenth and twentieth years. A separate center for the posterior tubercle of the talus sometimes is present and remains separate; it is known as the os trigonum. Each of the metatarsals possesses a single epiphysis which appears during the third year and is united to the diaphysis during the eighteenth year. In the first metatarsal, the epyphysis forms the base of the bone, but in all the others, it forms the rounded head of the bone. The ossification of the phalanges is similar to that of the first metatarsal.

2. **Joints and Ligaments of the Foot.**—The extent of movement in the foot is less than would be expected, considering the number of joints. Only in the talocalcaneal and the talonavicular joints does any considerable movement take place. The little lateral motion existing occurs principally at the calcaneocuboid and talonavicular joints, which lie in the same plane and form the midtarsal joint. The many smaller joints enhance flexibility and, in the aggregate, permit a fair degree of motion.

The **talocalcaneonavicular (subastragaloid) joint** is a large region of articulation between the talus above and the calcaneus and navicular below and in front. The talus is not a keystone bone and is not wedged in between the calcaneus and navicular. It allows the foot to play freely beneath it. In the talocalcaneal segment, the under surface of the talus articulates with anterior and posterior facets of the calcaneus, which are quite distinct from each other. The anterior talocalcaneal joint is continuous with the talonavicular joint. The two parts of the joint are separated by the powerful interosseous talocalcaneal ligament, which is the main bond of union between the talus and calcaneus and partially fills the obliquely directed groove (tarsal sinus) which passes between these bones. The removal of the areolovascular tissue, which also occupies this cleft, is an important step in arthrodesis. The remaining ligaments investing the joint on its peripheral aspect are very weak. They are reinforced to some extent by the deltoid and lateral ligaments of the ankle joint (p. 786). The *talonavicular segment* of the joint is of the ball and socket variety. In it, the convex head of the talus articulates with the concave facet on the posterior aspect of the navicular, while the lower part of the head of the talus articulates with the plantar calcaneonavicular (spring) ligament, which plays a major rôle in maintaining the integrity of the arch.

The **midtarsal joint** (of Chopart) has two divisions, the *talonavicular* portion of the subtaloid joint and the *calcaneocuboid joint*. In the latter, the apposing bony surfaces present a concavoconvex outline. The midtarsal joint is supported by the long and short plantar ligaments which separate the posterior and anterior parts of the foot.

3. **Arched Structure of the Foot.**—The clearest conception of the arched structure of the foot is obtained from examining a well-shaped specimen from which the tissues have been removed and in which the connecting ligaments and tendon insertions are preserved. The plantar surface appears dome-shaped with a well-defined arch extending anteroposteriorly, and a less highly developed arch crossing the foot from side to side.

The nature and extent of the **longitudinal arch** are displayed best by resting the foot on a flat surface. Its height and length are greatest at the mesial border of the foot and diminish laterally until, at the lateral margin, the arch almost has disappeared. The arch is made up of medial and lateral columns. The *medial column* is more important and consists of the calcaneus, talus, navicular, the three cuneiforms, and the three medial meta-

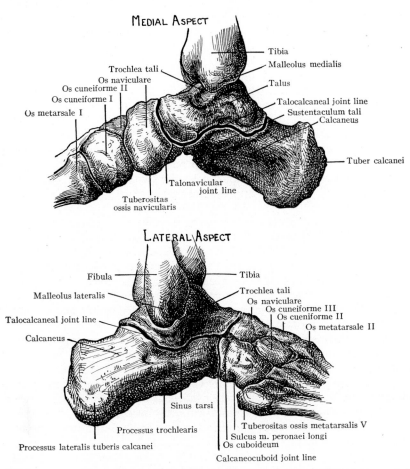

FIG. 801.—MEDIAL AND LATERAL VIEWS OF THE TALOCALCANEONAVICULAR (SUBASTRAGALOID) JOINT.

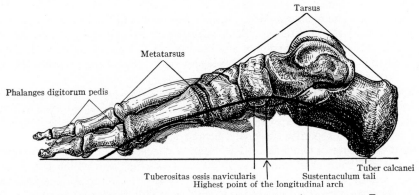

FIG. 802.—MEDIAL COLUMN OF THE LONGITUDINAL ARCH OF THE FOOT.

tarsals. The *lateral column* consists of the calcaneus, the cuboid, and the two outer metatarsals. This column is low and rests on the ground.

The body of the talus rests upon the calcaneus and its head on the inferior calcaneonavicular (spring) ligament. When the spring ligament is stretched, the head of the talus presses downward and medially, causing stretching of the mesial component of the arch with lengthening and flattening of the foot. The front of the foot turns outward into eversion (pronation) and the medial malleolus becomes prominent. In general, inverting and adducting movements of the foot raise and strengthen the arch, while everting and abducting movements lower and weaken it.

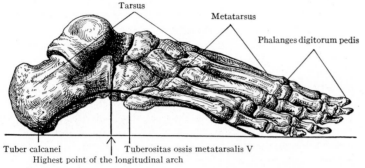

FIG. 803.—LATERAL COLUMN OF THE LONGITUDINAL ARCH OF THE FOOT.

The **transverse arch** owes its existence to the wedge-shaped formation of certain of its bones, especially the middle and lateral cuneiforms and the second, third, and fourth metatarsal bones. Their broad surfaces are directed toward the dorsum of the foot and their narrow surfaces toward the plantar aspect. This arch is relatively high and narrow in the middle of the foot, where the wedge-shaped middle and lateral cuneiforms are

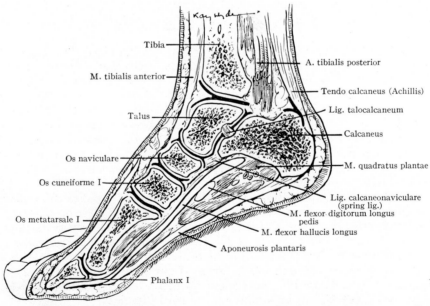

FIG. 804.—SAGITTAL SECTION THROUGH THE MEDIAL COLUMN OF THE LONGITUDINAL ARCH OF THE RIGHT FOOT TO SHOW THE PLANTAR CALCANEONAVICULAR (SPRING) LIGAMENT.

strong. The forward part of the arch is broad, flat, and weak. It often gives way, letting down one or more of the metatarsal heads, beneath which painful calluses form.

4. **Ligamentous and Muscular Support of the Arches of the Foot.**—In maintaining the arches of the foot, the **ligaments** of the tarsus and the metatarsus play an important rôle. The most essential ligaments are the plantar calcaneonavicular, the long plantar, and the plantar calcaneocuboid (short plantar). They are reinforced by the strong plantar

51

fascia which stretches like a tight cord from one extremity of the long bony arch to the other. The ligaments act only as passive agents, in contrast to the muscles which take an active part and are indispensable for the maintenance of the proper shape of the arch. Because of the elasticity of the ligamentous apparatus, the arches flatten out when the foot has to sustain a heavy weight, but they regain their original shape immediately when the weight is removed.

The *plantar calcaneonavicular* (*spring*) *ligament* stretches from the anterior border of the sustentaculum tali of the calcaneus to the plantar surface of the navicular bone. It is a very strong fibrocartilaginous band blending with the deltoid (internal lateral) ligament of the ankle joint. With the posterior articular surface of the navicular, it forms a pocket for the head of the talus.

The *long plantar ligament* is a very powerful structure attached to the under surface of the calcaneus and to the ridge on the inferior surface of the cuboid, whence it continues forward to the bases of the second, third, and fourth metatarsal bones. The *plantar calcaneocuboid* (*short plantar*) *ligament* runs obliquely forward and medially from the under surface of the calcaneus to the posterior part of the cuboid, where it is concealed by the long plantar ligament which separates the two bones. The support of the transverse arch is maintained by the plantar intertarsal and tarsometatarsal ligaments.

The **muscle support** of the longitudinal arch is derived from the strong tendons of the tibialis anterior, tibialis posterior, flexor digitorum longus and brevis, and the flexor hallucis longus. The principal muscle supporting the transverse arch is the peroneus longus, the tendon of which stretches across the arch like a bowstring and acts to approximate its extremities. Additional support comes from the tendinous sling, formed by the crossing of the flexor digitorum longus and the flexor hallucis longus tendons and from slips from the tibialis posterior which tend to contract the arch.

Surgical Considerations

The causes for alteration in the anatomical relationship of the structures of the foot are many, and require careful analysis for proper correction. Any disturbance in muscle equilibrium results in distortion and deformity because the muscles, which ordinarily are balanced in tension, are not opposed and draw structures toward the uninvolved side. Upset of the delicately balanced muscle mechanism may occur from injury, fracture, dislocation, or paralysis. In spastic birth palsies, the muscles are contracted, and in anterior horn cell degeneration, the muscles are flaccid. Deformity also results when the bones and ligaments are affected, because the arch construction of the foot gives way. This type of deformity obtains in rickets, gout, and tuberculosis. The foot sometimes is weakened without apparent cause.

1. **Flatfoot, Pronated Foot.**—The arches of the foot show considerable variability in different individuals. In some, the arches are very well developed, and, in others, so poorly developed as to be almost absent. In infants, the arches are poorly developed and the sole of the foot is almost flat. The subsequent arch development proceeds with the general growth of the foot. In some races, the negro for example, the arching never assumes striking proportions. A departure from the so-called "normal shape of foot" may appear as a deformity, but present no real pathologic change and cause no pain. Deformity is in no wise as important as functional disability.

If impressions of a foot with a well-developed arch are studied, the area of contact is found to vary much in accordance with the amount of pressure brought to bear on the foot. In withstanding heavy pressure, the arches flatten, and the foot lengthens and broadens. Foot strain causes the anterior pillar of the longitudinal arch to deviate outward. Most of the movement takes place at the midtarsal joint, and the head of the talus becomes more prominent on the medial margin of the foot.

If the foot has assumed the position of complete pronation (pes planus), the entire medial aspect of the sole from the great toe to the heel lies in contact with the ground.

The long axis of the talus is directed definitely medially, and the head and tubercle of the navicular project very prominently on the medial border. The normal slight concavity of the medial border is changed to a marked convexity. The medial malleolus is unduly prominent. The lateral border of the foot is raised slightly from the ground. The calcaneus, instead of resting squarely on the ground, is everted, bringing its lateral surface into direct contact with the extremity of the lateral malleolus, even to the degree of articulation by two lateral facets. This condition transmits a great part of the superincumbent weight to the calcaneus through the lateral malleolus.

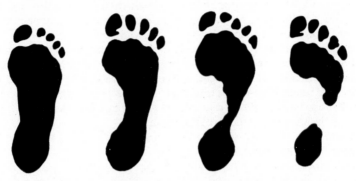

FIG. 805.—VARIETIES OF PLANTAR IMPRESSIONS.

The factors entering into the causation of acquired flatfoot are many. Debilitating illnesses, improper shoes, and improper posture, by weakening and relaxation of the ligaments and loss of tone in the muscles whose tendons maintain the arches, predispose to this condition. The tendency for its development is augmented when the foot is subjected to increased or prolonged strain, such as occurs in a rapid increase in body weight, unaccustomed standing for long periods, and carrying heavy loads.

The pain in a pronated foot is not necessarily confined to the foot, but may occur in the knee or even in the back. The pain, commonly referred to the medial side of the foot, may pass readily to the medial side of the knee, for, as the body weight falls farther to the

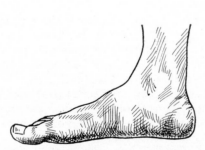

FIG. 806.—PES PLANUS (FLATFOOT).

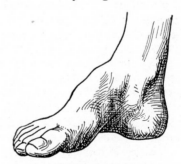

FIG. 807.—PES CAVUS.

medial side of the foot, strain is put on the tibial collateral (internal lateral) ligament of the knee joint. Painful calluses develop over pressure points on bony prominences of the foot which are not intended to touch the ground.

In the *treatment* of painfully pronated feet, the arches are supported by padding or bracing. The heels of the shoes are raised on the mesial side (Thomas heel). When pain is relieved, exercises are instituted, based on the tendency of adduction, inversion, and supination to strengthen the muscle supports of the foot. The transverse arch may be strengthened by flexion movements of the toes.

2. **Talipes in General.**—The deformities of the foot are grouped under the heading of talipes. The common foot deformities are those in which the affected parts are turned

to an abnormal degree in the direction of their normal movements. Most of these defor-mities are *congenital*, but a great many are *acquired*, and present at various periods after birth. It is not always easy to separate the two varieties. A deformity may be thought to have existed from birth and yet unquestionably have developed from infantile paralysis before the child walked.

A deformed foot usually presents two associated characteristics—paralysis or weak-ness, and contracture or strength. Paralysis can occur without contracture, but the muscle system functions on the principle of balance, and eventually the paralyzed muscle or muscle group is overpowered by the opposing muscles, which then produce contracture. Similarly, if contracture exists as the most prominent and perhaps the primary element, the opposing muscles and ligaments must, in time, be weakened and stretched.

The recognition of the shift of muscle balance furnishes the proper rationale for treatment. If weakness of the foot muscles predominates, support and even tendon trans-plantation and arthrodesis are required. If contracture exists, operation to weaken the stronger tissues and forcible manipulative measures are employed. A contracture may be overcome and the foot be brought to a normal position, but function cannot be normal until the overstretched tissues have regained their tone.

There are four simple forms of talipes—equinus, calcaneus, valgus, and varus. Com-binations of these forms are common.

3. Talipes Equinus.—In talipes equinus, the simple form of which rarely is congenital, the tendo calcaneus is contracted and nonyielding, and prevents the foot being placed squarely on the ground. The balls of the toes contact the ground, so that in walking the toes are at right angles to the foot. In advanced equinus, the foot may form an almost straight line with the leg. A contracture of the plantar aponeurosis is a frequent secondary occurrence which leads to an accentuation of the dorsal convexity of the foot with a deep hollow of the sole (talipes cavus). If adduction and inversion are superimposed on an equinus deformity, the condition is known as *talipes equinovarus*. If abduction and eversion are superimposed, the condition is *talipes equinovalgus*.

In congenital talipes equinus, the posterior muscles and the plantar aponeurosis are shortened secondarily to congenital malformation. In acquired talipes equinus, the pos-terior leg muscles enter into unopposed contracture because of paresis or paralysis of the anterior leg muscles. Treatment consists in stretching the calf muscles or performing a tenotomy upon the Achilles tendon.

4. Talipes Calcaneus.—Acute flexion of the foot on the leg constitutes the rare form of talipes calcaneus, which usually is secondary to infantile paralysis involving the calf muscles. The dorsiflexion of the foot at the ankle may be of such a degree that the foot and leg lie against each other. In the more common form of talipes calcaneus, there is partial or complete paralysis of all the muscles which act upon the foot (flatfoot). In this condition, the calcaneus and talus are in dorsiflexion. The remaining tarsal bones and the forward part of the foot are plantar-flexed by the contracture of the plantar structures. The typical gait is pounding, because the protecting spring action of the calf group of muscles and of the forefoot is absent. A large fat pad develops beneath the heel.

A varus or valgus position may be superimposed upon this deformity, with or without modification of the arches. In *talipes calcaneovarus*, the hollow of the foot generally is exaggerated because of the pull of the tibialis anterior and posterior muscles upon the long arch of the foot. The drawing of the pillars together by the flexor digitorum brevis muscle causes the arch to ascend and the plantar ligaments to contract. In *talipes calcaneovalgus*, the arch is lowered.

When the deformity is *congenital*, the tendons of the muscles of the anterior compart-ment of the leg are contracted, while those of the posterior compartment are overstretched. When the deformity is *acquired*, it results from the unopposed action of the anterior leg muscles.

Talipes calcaneus is the most disabling and resistant acquired foot deformity. Cor-rection of this condition requires operation upon the tarsal bones.

5. **Talipes Valgus.**—In talipes valgus, the lateral border of the foot is raised and the medial border is depressed into contact with the ground. When the condition is *congenital*, the peronei are shortened and the two tibialis muscles are overstretched. The *acquired* form is caused by paralysis of the tibialis anterior and posterior muscles. In the combined varieties, the muscles of more than one compartment of the leg are involved. In the *treatment* of minor deformities of the congenital type, manipulation to overcorrect the faulty position and the use of a splint to maintain the correction may suffice. In a more pro-

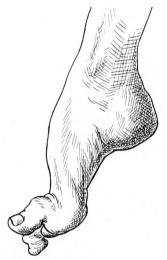

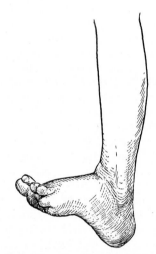

FIG. 808.—TALIPES EQUINUS.

FIG. 809.—TALIPES CALCANEUS.

nounced deformity, manipulations must be more vigorous, and plastic lengthening of the shortened structures may be necessary before the foot can be wrenched into proper position. In advanced cases, osteotomy and arthrodesis through the midtarsal and subastragaloid joints are required to align and stabilize the foot.

6. **Talipes Varus.**—The deformity of talipes varus is one of adduction and inversion. The foot is twisted upon itself at the midtarsal joint, in consequence of which the con-

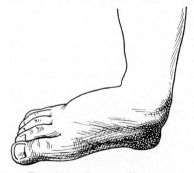

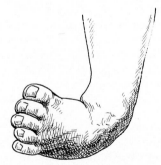

FIG. 810.—TALIPES VALGUS.

FIG. 811.—TALIPES VARUS.

cavity of the foot is increased along its upwardly directed medial border and becomes more convex along its dorsum and its lateral aspect. In walking, the dorsum of the foot is directed forward and the sole backward. Talipes varus rarely is met with alone; it is associated most often with talipes equinus. This combination constitutes by far the commonest of all clubfoot deformities.

In the *congenital* variety, the tendons of the tibialis muscles and the deltoid ligament are shortened. The distal end of the tibial shaft often is twisted medially. In the *acquired* variety, there is overcontraction of the tibialis muscles against the paralyzed peroneus longus or brevis muscles.

The tibialis tendons may require lengthening or transplantation to prevent their drawing the foot medially; division of the plantar fascia and the deltoid ligament often is necessary. To strengthen the abducting mechanism, the tendon of the tibialis anterior is detached and transplanted from the medial to the lateral side of the foot. When the abductor muscles are paralyzed completely, the tibialis anterior tendon is transplanted to the center of the dorsum of the foot, the tibialis posterior tendon is transplanted to the insertion of the Achilles tendon into the calcaneus, and arthrodesis of the subastragaloid joint frequently is required.

7. Talipes Equinovarus.—In well-marked talipes equinovarus, the heel is elevated and the foot is adducted and inverted so that its medial border looks upward, and its lateral margin downward. The whole foot is bent upon itself. There is, in addition, a more or less pronounced medial rotation of the tibia or even of the entire lower extremity. This rotation may be estimated readily by noticing the direction of the plane of the anterior aspect of the patella and comparing it with the line uniting the tips of the malleoli.

The deformity may be caused by the persistence of the attitude which the foot assumes in early uterine life, or by retarded development. If treated early, the condition usually can be corrected by manipulation and immobilization of the foot in the position of calcaneovalgus. Many elements conspire to render the foot rigid in the deformed condition. The deltoid and inferior calcaneonavicular ligaments on the medial aspect of the foot become contracted, and the tendons of the leg muscles, especially those of the tibialis anterior, the calf group, and the flexor digitorum longus, are shortened. Contracture takes place in the plantar aponeurosis and even in the skin of the sole. There often is an alteration in the shape of the bones and in the direction of their articular processes. The talus is modified strikingly and its neck deviates inward. The calcaneus becomes curved until its medial surface is concave and its lateral surface is convex. The dorsal aspect of the cuboid presses upon the ground and the overlying skin becomes hard and horny.

8. Fractures of the Talus and Navicular.—The tarsal bones, because of their cancellous structures, yield readily to direct and indirect injury. Fracture occurs commonly in falls from a height upon the feet. Compounding is a frequent complication from crushing injuries to the scantily protected dorsum of the foot.

The neck of the *talus* may be broken transversely or obliquely, with a resulting displacement of the foot laterally into a painful valgus position. Treatment of this fracture consists in remolding the foot properly and retaining it in plaster. When the body of the talus is crushed, the deformity cannot be corrected and immobilization or even excision is required. Talus fractures cause considerable limitation of motion at the ankle joint. The posterior process of the talus, the os trigonum, sometimes is an independent bone connected to the body of the main bone by fibrous tissue; in an *x*-ray film, it may be mistaken for a fracture.

Navicular fracture occurs occasionally; it results from landing on the toes in a fall from a height. The acting force is the downward thrust of the talus against the resistance of the anterior part of the foot, in which the navicular is compressed against the cuneiforms. The mushrooming results in a bony prominence on the dorsum of the foot. Treatment consists in careful manipulation, remolding, and fixation of the long arch. A more common fracture of the navicular is a sprain fracture of the dorsal surface, caused by forced plantar flexion. Fixation in dorsiflexion usually is sufficient treatment. Occasionally, a bony process at the tuberosity of the navicular (os tibiale externum) fails to unite with the main bone and may be mistaken for a fracture.

9. Fracture of the Calcaneus.—Fracture of the calcaneus is the commonest fracture in the tarsus, and frequently is bilateral. It occurs usually in falling or jumping from a height and alighting upon the heel. The fracture almost always is comminuted and involves the joints; even with extensive comminution, the degree of deformity need not be marked. In a severe fracture, the transverse diameter of the foot is increased palpably because of the lateral spread of the fragments, even to the levels of the malleoli. All motions of abduction and adduction are restricted. If there is little comminution, the fracture may be overlooked unless roentgenograms are taken in a posterior view with the patient prone, in order to reveal the exact condition of the bone. In many instances, the presence of a comminuted fracture is indicated by a lessening of the vertical and an increase in the transverse diameter of the heel. In x-ray examinations, the presence of the os trigonum and the calcaneal epiphysis must be kept in mind.

In the production of compressed and comminuted fractures, the talus, which is held tightly within the tibiofibular mortise, suddenly strikes the calcaneus. The wedge-shaped inferior surface of the talus fractures the calcaneus longitudinally and transversely. The calcaneus is widened, often to twice its normal width, and is shortened definitely.

In the normal foot, the angle subtended by the dorsal projection of the line of the posterior articular surfaces of the calcaneus and the plane of the superior surface of the body of the calcaneus measures from 27 to 33 degrees. When the calcaneus is fractured, the heel may be so crumpled that its arched shape is broken and becomes horizontal, this angle then becomes smaller or disappears. The tuberosity of the calcaneus even may be elevated above the line of the posterior projection of the posterior articular surfaces. The upward displacement of the fragment which holds the tuberosity is maintained by the trac-

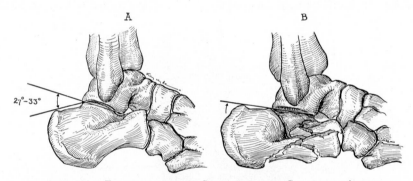

Fig. 812.—Fracture of the Calcaneus and Calcaneal Angle.

In A, the normal relations between the talus and calcaneus are indicated. Attention is directed to the posterior continuation of a line parallel with the posterior articular surface of the talocalcaneal joint. This line makes a small angle with a line parallel to the superior surface of the body of the calcaneus. In B, the calcaneus is fractured. The posterior continuation of the articular line coincides with the line along the superior surface of the calcaneus. The angle which normally exists between the two lines is obliterated.

tion of the Achilles tendon. The widening and shortening displacement is maintained by the intrinsic plantar muscles of the foot. The pull of these two muscle groups can be overcome only by traction in a direction opposite to the combined actions of the opposing muscles. By exerting traction along the axis of the normal calcaneus, both displacements can be remedied. The widening of the bone can be corrected by adequate lateral pressure on both sides.

10. Dislocation and Fracture of the Metatarsal Bones.—There is little likelihood of *dislocation* of the metatarsals because of their attachment to the tarsus at different levels and the security with which they are bound up with the transverse arch of the foot. In a severe injury, however, one or more may be fractured near the proximal end and the distal fragments be displaced laterally and forward. The fifth metatarsal may be fractured near its proximal end or its prominent tuberosity may be torn away by violent eversion of the foot. *Fractures* of the shaft sometimes occur from curiously trivial causes, such as the sudden assumption of a heavy load.

Plaster immobilization is the *treatment* for fractures without displacement. Displacements are corrected by manipulation, and the proper position is maintained by immobilization in plaster.

11. Tarsal Dislocations.—In dislocation at the talocalcaneonavicular joint, the talus maintains the normal relation to the malleoli. In the most usual form, the foot is dislocated posteriorly, and the talus overrides the navicular. If the ligaments binding the talus to the calcaneus rupture, the calcaneus is allowed to thrust backward. The foot may be dislocated to either side as well as forward, but usually only with associated fractures. Midtarsal dislocations at the talonavicular and calcaneocuboid joints are rare indeed, and are part of crushing compound injuries.

12. **Amputation Through the Midtarsal Joint (of Chopart).**—In Chopart's amputation through the interval between the anterior and posterior parts of the tarsus, the talonavicular and calcaneocuboid joints are divided. This double articular interval presents a concavo-convex outline, clearly seen when the tarsus is viewed from the dorsum. The medial landmark for the midtarsal joint line corresponds to a point just behind the tubercle of the navicular, and that for the lateral margin of the joint line is indicated by a point on the lateral border of the foot, about a fingerbreadth behind the prominent tuberosity of the fifth metatarsal. The operation consists in raising a long plantar and a short dorsal flap and in disarticulation at the joint line.

The short *dorsal flap* is defined by an incision beginning on each side at the points just indicated. The incision follows the border of the foot for a short distance forward on each side, then sweeps across the dorsum at the level of the metatarsal bases. The long *plantar flap* begins also at the level of the joint and is marked out by an incision fol-

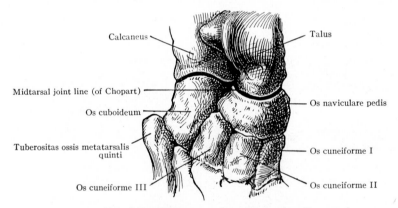

Calcaneus Talus

Midtarsal joint line (of Chopart)

Os cuboideum Os naviculare pedis

Tuberositas ossis metatarsalis quinti

Os cuneiforme I

Os cuneiforme III Os cuneiforme II

FIG. 813.—MIDTARSAL JOINT LINE (OF CHOPART)

lowing the border of the foot forward on each side and crossing the sole at the level of the middle of the metatarsus. The flap is made longer on the medial side to allow for the greater thickness of the foot on that side. By beginning the disarticulation at the medial margin of the foot, the ankle joint is protected more surely. The extensor tendons are sutured into the stump. Frequently the tendo calcaneus is cut in an attempt to prevent subsequent elevation of the heel.

The operation does not provide a satisfactory weight-bearing stump, as the talus, no longer supported, is tilted forward by the weight of the body and the calcaneus is tilted upward posteriorly, despite the division of the tendo calcaneus.

13. **Tarsometatarsal Amputation (of Lisfranc).**—In the tarsometatarsal amputation (of Lisfranc), disarticulation is effected between the tarsus and metatarsus, and flaps similar to those just described are raised. The dorsal incision extends forward about 1 cm. from a point on the medial border of the foot just behind the base of the first metatarsal. It then curves over the metatarsus to a point just behind the base of the fifth metatarsal. The plantar flap, which is much the longer, extends forward almost to the webs of the toes. In both flaps, all the tissues are divided down to the bone.

The important step of anatomical interest is that related to the disarticulation of the metatarsus. The tarsometatarsal joint line extends obliquely laterally and backward across the foot. It describes a somewhat zigzag course, an irregularity dependent mainly upon the backward extension of the base of the second metatarsal between the first and second cuneiform bones. The remaining articular interval between the tarsus and the lateral three metatarsal bones is fairly regular and can be followed readily by the knife. The joint between the first metatarsal and the first cuneiform is approximately transverse and can be delineated readily. When the metatarsal has been removed, the first cuneiform projects prominently on the medial side. The projecting portion of this bone is sawed off.

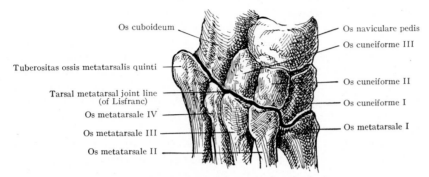

Os cuboideum
Os naviculare pedis
Os cuneiforme III
Tuberositas ossis metatarsalis quinti
Os cuneiforme II
Tarsal metatarsal joint line (of Lisfranc)
Os cuneiforme I
Os metatarsale IV
Os metatarsale III
Os metatarsale I
Os metatarsale II

FIG. 814.—TARSOMETATARSAL JOINT LINE (OF LISFRANC).

An alternative, and far more satisfactory, procedure (of Cowper) consists in sawing across the metatarsal bones distal to their bases. This operation has the great advantage of leaving the great synovial cavity of the anterior tarsus unopened and of preserving the insertions of very important muscles which actively control the foot. These insertions are those of the peroneus brevis and tertius into the tuberosity of the fifth metatarsal and those of the peroneus longus and part of the tibialis anterior into the base of the first metatarsal.

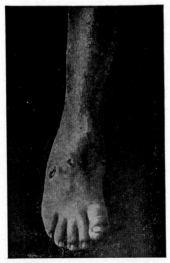

FIG. 815.—TUBERCULOSIS OF THE ANKLE WITH SINUS FORMATION. (Lovett in "Keen's Surgery.")

14. Tuberculosis of the Tarsus.—Tuberculosis of the tarsus is very common and appears usually as a rarefying osteitis (caries) in one or another of the bones. One of the determining factors may be the preponderance of poorly vascularized cancellous bone. It would appear that the bones most subject to disease are those which bear the greatest strain, the calcaneus, navicular, cuboid, the base of the first metatarsal, and, less frequently, the talus. The disease, however, may involve the tarsus en masse. Tuberculosis of the calcaneus tends to remain localized in the posterior half of the bone. The lesion sometimes is represented by several abscesses surrounded by sclerosed bone. As the process advances, it invades the neighboring talocalcaneal or the calcaneocuboid joint.

Tuberculosis beginning in the neck of the talus may spread upward and involve the synovial membrane of the ankle joint; backward and infect the body of the bone, whence it spreads through the articular cartilage upward into the ankle joint; downward to the talocalcaneal joint; or forward into the talonavicular joint. Caries of the navicular is serious, as it may involve the complex synovial membrane of the anterior part of the foot.

The signs of tarsal tuberculosis, especially when the forward part of the foot is involved, usually are most evident upon the dorsum and sides of the foot because these areas are covered thinly. The heel and toes remain essentially unchanged, but the intervening area is swollen. The skin over the dorsum has a glazed appearance and may present the openings of many sinuses.

Caries of the tarsal bones and joints may extend through the periosteum and the joint coverings and into the synovial tendon sheaths, especially those of the tibialis and the peroneus muscles, rendering treatment complicated.

15. Reconstructive Surgery.—The foot presents a variety of faulty functional positions, for which reconstructive surgical procedures must be instituted to satisfy the cardinal requirements of painless function and to give as much mobility as is compatible with stability.

In localized paralyses, *tendon lengthening, shortening,* and *transplantation* are performed. Tendons for transplantation must have normal tone and functional integrity. The normal tendon may be inserted subperiosteally to a fresh attachment on bone, or be sutured to other normal tendons, but never to paralyzed ones.

The joints, in a variety of paralytic conditions, must be obliterated to secure stability. In the foot, the outstanding *arthrodeses* immobilize the talocalcaneonavicular (subastragaloid), talonavicular, and calcaneocuboid (midtarsal) joints, where much of the normal movement of the foot occurs. If bony deformity accompanies instability, wedges of bone are removed from denuded joint surfaces in such a manner as to restore the weight-bearing lines of the foot. Finally, the whole foot is set backward through the subastragaloid joint to bring the weight more nearly over the longitudinal arch. Another recognized form of stabilization is *astragalectomy.* Arthrodesis and astragalectomy may be performed through Kocher's lateral J-shaped incision at the ankle (p. 790). In severe or neglected paralytic foot deformities of the acquired type, external tibial torsion regularly is present, and requires correction by tibial *osteotomy.*

In certain types of deformity, particularly congenital talipes equinovarus, a wedge of tarsus may be removed to restore balance to the foot (*cuneiform tarsectomy*). In equinus deformities of the drop foot or flatfoot type, a wedge of bone may be elevated from the dorsal surface of the calcaneus between the Achilles tendon and the back of the ankle so as to impinge upon the tibia and limit plantar flexion (*bone-block*).

C. TOES

The toes are prehensile structures which are of no great use to man, although they aid considerably in walking and to a greater degree in balancing, climbing, and running. They increase the efficiency of the foot, but their loss impairs it to no great degree. Intricate and delicate movements are hindered by their loss, but the firmer and more deliberate movements of walking remain nearly normal. The great toe with its two instead of three phalanges acquires strength at the expense of mobility.

1. Hallux Valgus.—In hallux valgus, the great toe deviates laterally to an abnormal extent, rendering the head of the first metatarsal prominent. This abnormal relationship produces an unsightly, angular projection which commonly is exaggerated by the development of osteophytic overgrowths upon the metatarsal head. In hallux valgus, there usually is a deformity of the head of the metatarsal in which the joint surface is inclined obliquely laterally. Congenital metatarsus varus frequently may be the etiologic factor.

In general, the condition is thought to be occasioned by ill-fitting shoes. Such shoes, in addition to being too short, have the axis of the toe of the shoe in line with the third rather than with the first toe. The shoe thus squeezes the toes against one another and displaces the great toe laterally. The distortion is increased by the action of the long flexor, extensor,

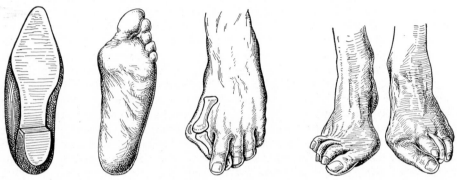

FIG. 816.—HALLUX VALGUS.

and adductor muscles. These muscles and the lateral metacarpophalangeal ligament may become shortened permanently.

An adventitious bursa known as a *bunion* is likely to develop over the projecting head of the first metatarsal, further accentuating the deformity. This bursa is irritated constantly by pressure and friction, and infection in it may involve the metatarsophalangeal joint.

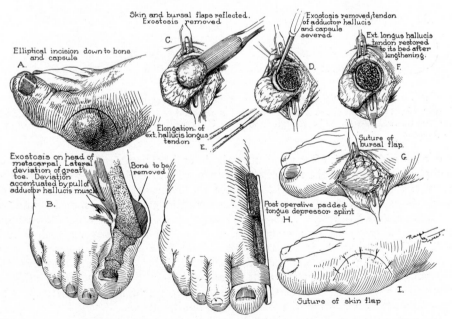

FIG. 817.—OPERATIVE CORRECTION OF HALLUX VALGUS.

Operations designed to cure hallux valgus contemplate reducing the prominence of the metatarsal head by removal of a large part of its medial surface and reconstruction of its articulating surface so that the phalanx may be brought into proper alignment. A curved incision with the concavity toward the sole is made over the prominence of the joint, and the flap of skin and fascia is retracted downward. The bursa is dissected free, save for its proximal attachment, so that it can be stitched into position between the phalanx and the remodelled metatarsal head. To keep the toe straight, the tendon of the extensor hallucis is displaced medially and maintained in position by suture, so that its contraction keeps the great toe aligned.

2. **Hammer Toe.**—A hammer toe is one contracted into sharp angulation. The contraction usually occurs in the second or third toe, and may be present alone or in combination with hallux valgus. When it affects the four lateral digits of each foot, it commonly is congenital in origin. All the toes tend toward this contracture in the presence of pes cavus or equinus. In these conditions, the common extensor muscle is stretched, elevating the proximal phalanx, but leaving the other phalanges in flexion. In the typical deformity, the metatarsophalangeal joint and the distal interphalangeal joint are hyperextended, but the proximal interphalangeal joint is flexed acutely. Over the acutely flexed joint, and occasionally upon the tip of the toe, a painful corn develops.

In the *operative treatment* of this condition, it generally is necessary to excise the prominent head of the proximal phalanx to shorten the toe and allow it to be straightened. The skin and the dorsal expansion of the extensor tendon which cover the dorsum of the joint are divided through a dorsilateral incision and are retracted medially. Thus the

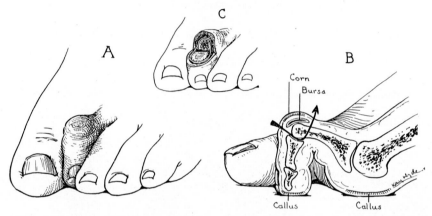

FIG. 818.—FRONT VIEW AND SCHEMATIC SAGITTAL SECTION OF A HAMMER TOE.
The arrow in B indicates the excision of the prominent head of the proximal phalanx; this is necessary to shorten the toe and allow it to be straightened out. C shows the method of removal of the head of the proximal phalanx.

joint is opened widely, and, after division of the lateral ligament and further flexion of the middle phalanx, the head of the first phalanx can be dislocated into the wound and excised. Where pes cavus and equinus are the cause of the deformity, elongation of the Achilles tendon and transplantation of the extensor digitorum longus tendons may be indicated.

3. **Metatarsalgia (Morton's Disease).**—The painful affection of the metatarsophalangeal joints, probably caused by a collapse of that part of the transverse arch formed by the heads of the metatarsals, is known as metatarsalgia or Morton's disease. Treatment is based upon the assumption that the falling of the arch brings pressure upon the plantar nerves passing forward between the metatarsal heads to the toes. Relief is afforded by supporting the arch with a pad placed beneath and just proximal to the metatarsal heads. Exercises designed to strengthen the foot muscles are instituted.

4. **Dislocation of the Toes.**—*Dislocation of the great toe dorsally* at the metatarsophalangeal joint is a common injury from direct violence, and often is compound. The same difficulty may be experienced in reducing it as is encountered in the reduction of a similar lesion in the thumb—the head of the metatarsal may be caught in the fibrous tissues of the capsule or between the two heads of the flexor hallucis brevis, each of which has a sesamoid bone. In reduction, the great toe should be hyperflexed into an exaggeration of the dislocation deformity and, at the same time, the base of the phalanx must be

pushed forward until it slips over the large metatarsal head. If one of the heads of the short flexor has slipped between the phalanx and the metatarsal head, the detachment of the muscle head from the base of the first phalanx is necessary before replacement can be effected.

Dislocation of the other toes, caused by jumping from a height, is common. The proximal phalanx usually is displaced upon the metatarsal, and the symptoms may be those of a sprain, but the head of the projecting metatarsal can be felt in the sole, and the toes are shortened. The space between them and the adjacent toes is increased. Diagnosis is not always easy, and is established best by the use of the *x*-ray. Reduction is difficult and is hard to maintain.

5. **Ingrowing Toenail.**—This condition is confined to the great toe, because it alone lies flat and parallel to the plantar surface. The other toes rest upon their extremities. In the great toe, the soft parts have a natural tendency to crowd around the borders of the

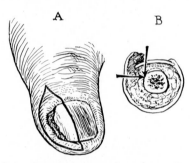

FIG. 819.—OPERATION FOR INGROWING TOENAIL.
A marks out the area to be removed. B, Cross section to show the area to be removed.

nail. Pressure from the sole upward or from above downward presses the nail margin into the flesh until ulceration and, later, infection set in. The pressure of a badly shaped shoe may be responsible. In mild cases, the cuticle encroaches upon the nail; in advanced cases, the skin of the nail bed is inflamed, thickened and overhanging, and is the seat of suppurative exuberant granulation. The pain is intense and the discharge is foul.

In the *treatment* of mild cases, a wisp of antiseptic cotton placed under the offending edge of the nail usually suffices to clear up the condition. In severer cases, longitudinal incision is made through the nail and the overlying skin, separating a marginal strip, about 0.5 cm. wide, from the main body of the nail. The incision extends through the matrix of the nail, a dense white layer easily distinguished from the subcutaneous fat. The overlying skin at this side is dissected free from the marginal strip of nail and from its matrix. After the strip of matrix and nail is excised, the skin flaps are retracted carefully and the wound is inspected for any bit of matrix that may remain. Sutures may be used, but are not necessary.

INDEX